DIAGNOSTIC ULTRASOUND

FOURTH EDITION

Carol M. Rumack, MD, FACR
Professor of Radiology and Pediatrics
University of Colorado Denver School of Medicine
Denver, Colorado

Stephanie R. Wilson, MD, FRCPC
Clinical Professor of Radiology
University of Calgary
Staff Radiologist
Foothills Medical Centre
Calgary, Alberta, Canada

J. William Charboneau, MD, FACR
Professor of Radiology
Mayo Clinic College of Medicine
Consultant in Radiology
Mayo Clinic
Rochester, Minnesota

Deborah Levine, MD, FACR
Professor of Radiology
Harvard Medical School
Associate Radiologist-in-Chief of Academic Affairs
Director of Ob/Gyn Ultrasound
Beth Israel Deaconess Medical Center
Boston, Massachusetts

ELSEVIER
MOSBY

ELSEVIER
MOSBY

1600 John F. Kennedy Blvd.
Ste 1800
Philadelphia, PA 19103-2899

DIAGNOSTIC ULTRASOUND, FOURTH EDITION   ISBN: 978-0-323-05397-6
Copyright © 2011 by Mosby, Inc., an affiliate of Elsevier Inc.

Notices

Knowledge and best practice in this field are constantly changing. As new research and experience broaden our understanding, changes in research methods, professional practices, or medical treatment may become necessary.

Practitioners and researchers must always rely on their own experience and knowledge in evaluating and using any information, methods, compounds, or experiments described herein. In using such information or methods they should be mindful of their own safety and the safety of others, including parties for whom they have a professional responsibility.

With respect to any drug or pharmaceutical products identified, readers are advised to check the most current information provided (i) on procedures featured or (ii) by the manufacturer of each product to be administered, to verify the recommended dose or formula, the method and duration of administration, and contraindications. It is the responsibility of practitioners, relying on their own experience and knowledge of their patients, to make diagnoses, to determine dosages and the best treatment for each individual patient, and to take all appropriate safety precautions. To the fullest extent of the law, neither the Publisher nor the authors, contributors, or editors, assume any liability for any injury and/or damage to persons or property as a matter of products liability, negligence or otherwise, or from any use or operation of any methods, products, instructions, or ideas contained in the material herein.

Previous editions copyrighted 2005, 1998, 1993 by Mosby, Inc.

Library of Congress Cataloging in Publication Data
Diagnostic ultrasound / [edited by] Carol M. Rumack ... [et al.].—4th ed.
    p. ; cm
    Includes bibliographical references and index.
    ISBN 978-0-323-05397-6 (hardcover : alk. paper)   1. Diagnostic ultrasonic imaging.   I. Rumack, Carol M.
    [DNLM: 1. Ultrasonography. WN 208]
    RC78.7.U4D514 2011
    616.07′543—dc22   2010034851

Acquisitions Editor: *Rebecca Gaertner*
Developmental Editor: *Lisa Barnes*
Publishing Services Manager: *Patricia Tannian*
Team Manager: *Radhika Pallamparthy*
Senior Project Manager: *John Casey*
Project Manager: *Anitha Sivaraj*
Designer: *Steven Stave*

Printed in United States of America

Last digit is the print number: 9 8 7 6 5 4 3 2 1

About the Editors

Carol M. Rumack, MD, is Professor of Radiology and Pediatrics at the University of Colorado Denver School of Medicine in Denver, Colorado. Her clinical practice is based at the University of Colorado Hospital. Her primary research has been in neonatal sonography of high-risk infants, particularly 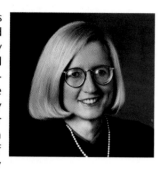 the brain. Dr. Rumack has published widely in this field and lectured frequently on pediatric ultrasound. She is a fellow and past president of the American College of Radiology, a fellow of both the American Institute of Ultrasound in Medicine and the Society of Radiologists in Ultrasound. She and her husband, Barry, have two children, Becky and Marc.

Stephanie R. Wilson, MD, is Clinical Professor of Radiology at the University of Calgary where she heads a specialty ultrasound clinic at the Foothills Medical Centre devoted primarily to the imaging of diseases of the gastrointestinal tract and gynecologic organs. With support from the 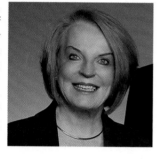 Canadian Institute of Health Research (CIHR), Dr. Wilson worked with Dr. Peter Burns in Toronto on the characterization and detection of focal liver masses with contrast-enhanced ultrasound (CEUS) and is an established authority in this field. A recognized expert on ultrasound of the gastrointestinal tract and abdominal and pelvic viscera, she is the recipient of many university teaching awards and is a frequent international speaker and author. Dr. Wilson was the first woman president of the Canadian Association of Radiologists (CAR) and is the current president-elect of the International Contrast Ultrasound Society (ICUS). She has received the gold medal from CAR in recognition of her contribution to radiology. A golf enthusiast, she and her husband Ken, have two children, Jessica and Jordan.

J. William Charboneau, MD, is Professor of Radiology at the Mayo Clinic in Rochester, Minnesota. His current research interests include image-guided tumor biopsy and ablation, as well as sonography of the liver and small parts. He is coauthor of over 200 publications, assistant editor of the 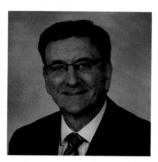 Mayo Clinic Family Health Book, and an active lecturer nationally and internationally. He is a fellow in the American College of Radiology and the Society of Radiologists in Ultrasound. He and his wife, Cathy, have three children, Nick, Ben, and Laurie.

Deborah Levine, MD, is Professor of Radiology at Beth Israel Deaconess Medical Center, Boston, and Harvard Medical School. At Beth Israel Deaconess Medical Center she is Associate Radiologist-in-Chief of Academic Affairs, Co-Chief of Ultrasound, and Director of Ob/Gyn Ultrasound. Her 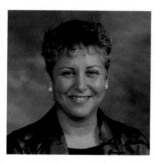 main areas of clinical interest are obstetric and gynecologic ultrasound. Her research has focused on fetal magnetic resonance imaging as an aid to improving ultrasound diagnosis. Dr. Levine is an American College of Radiology Chancellor, Chair of the American College of Radiology Commission on Ultrasound, a fellow of the American Institute of Ultrasound in Medicine and Society of Radiologists in Ultrasound. She and her husband, Alex, have two children, Becky and Julie.

Contributors

Jodi F. Abbott, MD
Associate Professor
Boston University School of Medicine
Director of Antenatal Testing
Boston Medical Center
Boston, Massachusetts

Jacques S. Abramowicz, MD, FACOG
Frances T. & Lester B. Knight Professor
Rush University
Director, Ob/Gyn Ultrasound
Rush University Medical Center
Co-Director, Rush Fetal and Neonatal Medicine Program
Rush University
Chicago, Illinois

Ronald S. Adler, PhD, MD
Professor of Radiology
Weill Medical College of Cornell University
Chief, Division of Ultrasound and Biology Imaging
Department of Radiology and Imaging
Hospital for Special Surgery
Attending Radiologist
Department of Radiology
New York Presbyterian Hospital
New York City, New York

Amit R. Ahuja, MD
Diagnostic Imaging Resident
Foothills Medical Centre
Calgary, Alberta, Canada

Jean M. Alessi-Chinetti, BS, RDMS, RVT
Technical Director
Vascular Laboratory
Tufts Medical Center
Boston, Massachusetts

Thomas Atwell, MD
Assistant Professor of Radiology
Mayo Clinic College of Medicine
Consultant in Radiology
Mayo Clinic
Rochester, Minnesota

Diane S. Babcock, MD
Professor of Radiology and Pediatrics
University of Cincinnati College of Medicine
Professor of Radiology and Pediatrics
Cincinnati Children's Hospital Medical Center
Cincinnati, Ohio

Carol E. Barnewolt, MD
Assistant Professor of Radiology
Harvard Medical School
Director, Division of Ultrasound
Children's Hospital Boston
Boston, Massachusetts

Daryl J. Barth, RVT, RDMS
Ultrasound Assistant
Department of Sonography
OSI St. Francis Medical Center
Ultrasound Assistant
Central Illinois Radiological AssociatesPeoria, Illinois

Beryl Benacerraf, MD
Clinical Professor of Obstetrics and Gynecology and
    Radiology
Brigham and Women's Hospital
Massachusetts General Hospital
Harvard Medical School
Boston, Massachusetts

Carol B. Benson, MD
Professor of Radiology
Harvard Medical School
Director of Ultrasound and Co-Director of High Risk
    Obstetrical Ultrasound
Brigham and Women's Hospital
Boston, Massachusetts

Raymond E. Bertino, MD, FACR, FSRU
Medical Director of Vascular and General Ultrasound
OSF Saint Francis Medical Center
Clinical Professor of Radiology and Surgery
University of Illinois College of Medicine
Peoria, Illinois

Edward I. Bluth, MD, FACR
Clinical Professor
Tulane University School of Medicine
Chairman Emeritus Radiology
Ochsner Health System
New Orleans, Louisiana

J. Antonio Bouffard, MD
Senior Staff Radiologist
Henry Ford Hospital
Detroit, Michigan
Consultant Radiologist
James Andrews Orthopedics and Sports Medicine Center
Pensacola, Florida

Bryann Bromley, MD
Clinical Associate Professor of Obstetrics and Gynecology
Massachusetts General Hospital
Clinical Associate Professor of Obstetrics and Gynecology
    and Radiology
Brigham and Women's Hospital
Boston, Massachusetts

Dorothy I. Bulas, MD
Professor of Radiology and Pediatrics
George Washington University Medical Center
Pediatric Radiologist
Children's National Medical Center
Washington, District of Columbia

Peter N. Burns, PhD
Professor and Chairman
Department of Medical Biophysics
University of Toronto
Senior Scientist
Department of Imaging Research
Sunnybrook Health Sciences Centre
Toronto, Ontario, Canada

Barbara A. Carroll, MD
Professor Emeritus of Radiology
Department of Radiology
Duke University Medical Center
Durham, North Carolina

J. William Charboneau, MD, FACR
Professor of Radiology
Mayo Clinic College of Medicine
Consultant in Radiology
Mayo Clinic
Rochester, Minnesota

Humaira Chaudhry, MD
Fellow in Abdominal Imaging
Duke University Medical Center
Durham, North Carolina

Tanya P. Chawla, MD, FRCPC
Assistant Professor
University of Toronto
Toronto, Ontario, Canada

David Chitayat, MD, FABMG, FACMG, FCCMG, FRCPC
Professor
University of Toronto
Prenatal Diagnosis and Medical Genetics Program
Department of Obstetrics and Gynecology
Mount Sinai Hospital
Toronto, Ontario, Canada

Peter L. Cooperberg, MD
Chief of Radiology
St. Paul's Hospital
Chief of Radiology
University of British Columbia
Vancouver, British Columbia, Canada

Peter M. Doubilet, MD, PhD
Professor of Radiology
Harvard Medical School
Senior Vice Chair
Department of Radiology
Brigham and Women's Hospital
Boston, Massachusetts

Julia A. Drose, BA, RDMS, RDCS, RVT
Associate Professor of Radiology
University of Colorado at Denver Health Sciences Center
Chief Sonographer
Divisions of Ultrasound and Prenatal Diagnosis & Genetics
University of Colorado Hospital
Aurora, Colorado

Beth S. Edeiken-Monroe, MD
Professor of Radiology
Department of Diagnostic Radiology
The University of Texas Houston Medical School
MD Anderson Cancer Center
Houston, Texas

Judy Estroff, MD
Associate Professor of Radiology
Harvard Medical School
Division Chief, Fetal Neonatal Radiology
Children's Hospital Boston
Radiologist
Department of Radiology
Beth Israel Deaconess Medical Center
Radiologist
Department of Radiology
Brigham and Women's Hospital
Boston, Massachusetts

Amy Symons Ettore, MD
Consultant
Department of Radiology
Mayo Clinic College of Medicine
Rochester, Minnesota

Katherine W. Fong, MBBS, FRCPC
Associate Professor of Medical Imaging and Obstetrics and Gynecology
University of Toronto Faculty of Medicine
Co-director, Centre of Excellence in Obstetric Ultrasound
Mount Sinai Hospital
Toronto, Ontario; Canada

Bruno D. Fornage, MD
Professor of Radiology and Surgical Oncology
M. D. Anderson Cancer Center
Houston, Texas

J. Brian Fowlkes, PhD
Associate Professor
University of Michigan
Department of Radiology
Ann Arbor, Michigan

Phyllis Glanc, MDCM
Assistant Professor
Department of Medical Imaging
University of Toronto
Assistant Professor
Department of Obstetrics & Gynecology
University of Toronto
Site Director
Body Imaging
Women's College Hospital
Toronto, Ontario, Canada

Brian Gorman, MB, BCh, FRCR, MBA
Assistant Professor of Radiology
Mayo Clinic College of Medicine
Consultant in Radiology
Mayo Clinic
Rochester, Minnesota

S. Bruce Greenberg, MD
Professor
University of Arkansas for Medical Sciences
Professor
Arkansas Children's Hospital
Little Rock, Arkansas

Leslie E. Grissom, MD
Clinical Professor of Radiology and Pediatrics
Department of Radiology
Thomas Jefferson Medical College
Thomas Jefferson University Hospital
Philadelphia, Pennsylvania;
Chair, Medical Imaging Department
Medical Imaging Department—Radiology
Alfred I. DuPont Hospital for Children
Wilmington, Delaware;
Pediatric Radiologist
Medical Imaging Department—Radiology
Christiana Care Health System
Newark, Delaware

Benjamin Hamar, MD
Instructor of Obstetrics, Gynecology, and Reproductive
   Biology
Beth Israel–Deaconess Medical Center
Boston, Massachusetts

Anthony E. Hanbidge, MB, BCh, FRCPC
Associate Professor
University of Toronto
Head, Division of Abdominal Imaging
University Health Network
Mount Sinai Hospital and Women's College Hospital
Toronto, Ontario, Canada

H. Theodore Harcke, MD, FACR, FAIUM
Professor of Radiology and Pediatrics
Jefferson Medical College
Philadelphia, Pennsylvania
Chief of Imaging Research
Department of Medical Imaging
Alfred I. DuPont Hospital for Children
Wilmington, Delaware

Ian D. Hay, MD
Professor of Medicine
Dr. R. F. Emslander Professor in Endocrinology Research
Division of Endocrinology and Internal Medicine
Mayo Clinic
Consultant in Endocrinology and Internal Medicine
Department of Medicine
Mayo ClinicRochester, Minnesota

Christy K. Holland, PhD
Professor
Departments of Biomedical Engineering and Radiology
University of Cincinnati
Cincinnati, Ohio

Caroline Hollingsworth, MD
Assistant Professor of Radiology
Duke University Medical Center
Durham, North Carolina

Bonnie J. Huppert, MD
Assistant Professor of Radiology
Mayo Clinic College of Medicine
Consultant in Radiology
Mayo Clinic
Rochester, Minnesota

E. Meridith James, MD, FACR
Professor of Radiology
Mayo Clinic College of Medicine
Consultant in Radiology
Mayo Clinic
Rochester, Minnesota

Susan D. John, MD
Professor of Radiology and Pediatrics
Chair, Department of Diagnostic and Interventional
   Imaging
University of Texas Medical School at Houston
Houston, Texas

Neil D. Johnson, MBBS, MMed, FRANZCR
Professor, Radiology and Pediatrics
Cincinnati Children's Hospital Medical Center
Cincinnati, Ohio

Korosh Khalili, MD, FRCPC
Assistant Professor
University of Toronto
Staff Radiologist
University Health Network
Toronto, Ontario, Canada

Beth M. Kline-Fath, MD
Assistant Professor of Radiology
Cincinnati Children's Hospital Medical Center
Cincinnati, Ohio

Clifford S. Levi, MD, FRCPC
Section Head
Health Sciences Centre
Professor
University of Manitoba
Winnipeg, Manitoba, Canada

Deborah Levine, MD, FACR
Professor of Radiology
Harvard Medical School
Associate Radiologist-in-Chief of Academic Affairs
Director of Ob/Gyn Ultrasound
Beth Israel Deaconess Medical Center
Boston, Massachusetts

Bradley D. Lewis, MD
Associate Professor of Radiology
Mayo Clinic College of Medicine
Consultant in Radiology
Mayo Clinic
Rochester, Minnesota

Ana Lourenco, MD
Assistant Professor of Diagnostic Imaging
Alpert Medical School of Brown University
Providence, Rhode Island

Edward A. Lyons, OC, FRCPC, FACR
Professor of Radiology
Obstetrics & Gynecology and Anatomy
University of Manitoba
Radiologist
Health Sciences Center
Winnipeg, Manitoba, Canada

Giancarlo Mari, MD
Professor and Vice-Chair, Department of Obstetrics and
    Gynecology
Director, Division of Maternal-Fetal Medicine
University of Tennessee Health Science Center
Memphis, Tennessee

John R. Mathieson, MD, FRCPC
Medical Director and Chief Radiologist
Vancouver Island Health Authority
Royal Jubilee Hospital
Victoria, British Columbia, Canada

Cynthia V. Maxwell, MD, FRCSC, RDMS, DABOG
Assistant Professor
Obstetrics and Gynecology
University of Toronto
Staff Perinatologist
Obstetrics and Gynecology
Division of Maternal Fetal Medicine
Toronto, Ontario, Canada

John McGahan, MD
Professor and Vice Chair of Radiology
University of California Davis Medical Center
Sacramento, California

Tejas S. Mehta, MD, MPH
Assistant Professor of Radiology
Beth Israel Deaconess Medical Center
Boston, Massachusetts

Christopher R. B. Merritt, BS, MS, MD
Professor
Thomas Jefferson University
Philadelphia, Pennsylvania

Norman L. Meyer, MD, PhD
Associate Professor, Division of Maternal-Fetal Medicine
Vice Chair, Department of OBGYN
University of Tennessee Health Science Center
Memphis, Tennessee

Derek Muradali, MD, FRCPC
Head, Division of Ultrasound
St. Michael's Hospital
Associate Professor
University of Toronto
Toronto, Ontario Canada

Sara M. O'Hara, MD, FAAP
Associate Professor of Radiology and Pediatrics
University of Cincinnati
Director, Ultrasound Division
Cincinnati Children's Hospital Medical Center
Cincinnati, Ohio

†Heidi B. Patriquin, MD
Department of Medical Imaging,
Sainte-Justine Hospital
Quebec, Canada

Joseph F. Polak, MD, MPH
Professor of Radiology
Tufts University School of Medicine
Chief of Radiology
Tufts Medical Center
Research Affiliation
Director, Ultrasound Reading Center
Tufts University School of Medicine
Boston, Massachusetts

Philip Ralls, MD
Radiology Professor
University of Southern California
Keck School of Medicine
Los Angeles, California

Cynthia T. Rapp, BS, RDMS, FAIUM, FSDMS
VP of Clinical Product Development
Medipattern
Toronto, Ontario, Canada

Carl C. Reading, MD, FACR
Professor of Radiology
Mayo Clinic College of Medicine
Consultant in Radiology
Mayo Clinic
Rochester, Minnesota

Maryam Rivaz, MD
Post Doctoral Fellow
Department of Obstetrics and Gynecology
University of Tennessee Health Science Center
Memphis, Tennessee

Julie E. Robertson, MD, FRCSC
Fellow
Division of Maternal Fetal Medicine
Obstetrics and Gynecology
University of Toronto
Toronto, Ontario, Canada

Henrietta Kotlus Rosenberg, MD, FACR, FAAP
Professor of Radiology and Pediatrics
The Mount Sinai School of Medicine
Director of Pediatric Radiology
The Mount Sinai Medical Center
New York, New York

Carol M. Rumack, MD, FACR
Professor of Radiology and Pediatrics
University of Colorado Denver School of Medicine
Denver, Colorado

†Deceased.

Shia Salem, MD, FRCPC
Associate Professor
University of Toronto
Radiologist
Mount Sinai Hospital
University Health Network
Women's College Hospital
Department of Medical Imaging
Mount Sinai Hospital
Toronto, Ontario, Canada

Nathan A. Saucier, MD
R4 Resident
Diagnostic Radiology
University of Illinois College of Medicine at Peoria
Peoria, Illinois

Eric E. Sauerbrei, BSc, MSc, MD, FRCPC
Professor of Radiology, Adjunct Professor of Obstetrics
    and Gynecology
Queen's University
Director of Ultrasound
Kingston General Hospital and Hotel Dieu Hospital
Director of Residents Research
Queen's University
Kingston, Ontario, Canada

Joanna J. Seibert, MD
Professor of Radiology and Pediatrics
Arkansas Children's Hospital
University of Arkansas for Medical Sciences
Little Rock, Arkansas

Chetan Chandulal Shah, MBBS, DMRD, MBA
Assistant Professor
Arkansas Children's Hospital
University of Arkansas for Medical Sciences
Little Rock, Arkansas

Rola Shaheen, MB, BS, MD
Radiology Instructor
Harvard Medical School
Chief of Radiology and
Director of Women's Imaging
Harrington Memorial Hospital
Boston, Massachusetts

William E. Shiels II, DO
Chairman, Department of Radiology
Nationwide Children's Hospital
Clinical Professor of Radiology, Pediatrics, and
    Biomedical Engineering
The Ohio State University College of Medicine
Columbus, Ohio;
Adjunct Professor of Radiology
The University of Toledo Medical Center
Toledo, Ohio

Thomas D. Shipp, MD
Associate Professor of Obstetrics, Gynecology, and
    Reproductive Biology
Harvard Medical School
Boston, Massachusetts
Associate Obstetrician and Gynecologist
Brigham & Women's Hospital
Boston, Massachusetts

Luigi Solbiati, MD
Director, Department of Diagnostic Imaging
General Hospital of Busto Arsizio
Busto Arsizio, (VA) Italy

Elizabeth R. Stamm, MD
Associate Professor of Radiology
University of Colorado at Denver Health Sciences Center
Aurora, Colorado

A. Thomas Stavros, MD, FACR
Medical Director, Ultrasound Invision
Sally Jobe Breast Center
Englewood, Colorado

George A. Taylor, MD
John A. Kirkpatrick Professor of Radiology (Pediatrics)
Harvard Medical School
Radiologist-in-Chief
Children's Hospital Boston
Boston, Massachusetts

Wendy Thurston, MD
Assistant Professor
Department of Medical Imaging
University of Toronto
Chief, Diagnostic Imaging
Department of Diagnostic Imaging
St. Joseph's Health Centre
Courtesy Staff
Department of Medical Imaging
University Health Network
Toronto, Ontario, Canada

Ants Toi, MD, FRCPC
Associate Professor of Radiology and Obstetrics and
    Gynecology
University of Toronto
Staff Radiologist
University Health Network and Mt. Sinai Hospital
Toronto, Ontario, Canada

Didier H. Touche, MD
Chief Radiologist
Centre Sein Godinot
Godinot Breast Cancer Center
Reims, France

Mitchell Tublin, MD
Professor of Radiology
Chief, Abdominal Imaging Section
Department of Radiology
University of Pittsburgh School of Medicine
Pittsburgh, Pennsylvania

Rebecca A. Uhlmann, MS
Program Administrator
Obstetrics and Gynecology
University of Tennessee Health Science Center
Memphis, Tennessee

Sheila Unger, MD
Clinical Geneticist
Institute of Human Genetics
University of Freiburg
Freiburg, Germany

Marnix T. van Holsbeeck, MD
Professor of Radiology
Wayne State University School of Medicine
Detroit, Michigan
Division Head, Musculoskeletal Radiology
Henry Ford Hospital
Detroit, Michigan

Patrick M. Vos, MD
Clinical Assistant Professor
University of British Columbia
Vancouver, British Columbia, Canada

Dzung Vu, MD, MBBS, Dip Anat
Senior Lecturer
University of New South Wales
Sydney, New South Wales, Australia

Wendy L. Whittle, MD
Maternal Fetal Medicine Specialist
Department of Obstetrics and Gynecology
Mount Sinai Hospital
University of Toronto
Toronto, Ontario, Canada

Stephanie R. Wilson, MD, FRCPC
Clinical Professor of Radiology
University of Calgary
Staff Radiologist
Foothills Medical Centre
Calgary, Alberta, Canada

Rory Windrim, MD, MSc, FRCSC
Professor
Department of Obstetrics & Gynecology
University of Toronto
Staff Perinatologist
Mount Sinai Hospital
Toronto, Ontario, Canada

Cynthia E. Withers
Staff Radiologist
Department of Radiology
Santa Barbara Cottage Hospital
Santa Barbara, California

*In memory of **my parents, Drs. Ruth and Raymond Masters,** who encouraged me to enjoy the intellectual challenge of medicine and the love of making a difference in patients' lives.*

CMR

*To a lifetime of **clinical colleagues, residents, and fellows** who have provided me with a wealth of professional joy. And **to my wonderful family,** for your love and never-ending support.*

SRW

*To **Cathy, Nicholas, Ben, and Laurie,** for all the love and joy you bring to my life. You are all I could ever hope for.*

JWC

*To **Alex, Becky, and Julie**—your love and support made this work possible.*

DL

Preface

The fourth edition of *Diagnostic Ultrasound* is a major revision. Previous editions have been very well accepted as a reference textbook and have been the most commonly used reference in ultrasound education and practices worldwide. We are pleased to provide a new update of images and text with new areas of strength. For the first time we are including video clips in the majority of chapters. The display of real-time ultrasound has helped to capture those abnormalities that require a sweep through the pathology to truly appreciate the lesion. It is similar to scrolling through images on a PACS and has added great value to clinical imaging. Daily we find that cine or video clips show important areas between still images that help to make certain a diagnosis or relationships between lesions. Now we rarely need to go back to reevaluate a lesion with another scan, making patient imaging more efficient.

We are pleased to announce that a new editor, Deborah Levine, has joined us, providing expertise in fetal imaging, in both obstetrical sonography and fetal MRI. Prenatal diagnosis is one of the frontiers of medicine that continues to grow as a field and has pushed our understanding of what happens to the fetus before we see a lesion at birth. These antecedents of disease in children and adults help us to arrange care for patients long before the mother goes into labor.

Approximately 90 outstanding new and continuing authors have contributed to this edition, and all are recognized experts in the field of ultrasound. We have replaced at least 50% of the images without increasing the size of the two volumes, so new value has been added to all of the chapters, particularly for obstetrics and gynecology. The fourth edition now includes over 5000 images, many in full color. The layout has been exhaustively revamped, and there are highly valuable multipart figures or key figure collages. These images all reflect the spectrum of sonographic changes that may occur in a given disease instead of the most common manifestation only.

The book's format has been redesigned to facilitate reading and review. There are again color-enhanced boxes to highlight the important or critical features of sonographic diagnoses. Key terms and concepts are emphasized in boldface type. To direct the readers to other research and literature of interest, comprehensive reference lists are organized by topic.

Diagnostic Ultrasound is again divided into two volumes. Volume I consists of Parts I to III. Part I contains chapters on physics and biologic effects of ultrasound, as well as more of the latest developments in ultrasound contrast agents. Part II covers abdominal, pelvic, and thoracic sonography, including interventional procedures and organ transplantation. Part III presents small parts imaging including thyroid, breast, scrotum, carotid, peripheral vessels, and particularly MSK imaging. Newly added is a chapter on musculoskeletal intervention.

Volume II begins with Part IV, where the greatest expansion of text and images has been on obstetric and fetal sonography, including video clips for the first time. Part V comprehensively covers pediatric sonography.

Diagnostic Ultrasound is for practicing physicians, residents, medical students, sonographers, and others interested in understanding the vast applications of diagnostic sonography in patient care. Our goal is for *Diagnostic Ultrasound* to continue to be the most comprehensive reference book available in the sonographic literature with a highly readable style and superb images.

Carol M. Rumack
Stephanie R. Wilson
J. William Charboneau
Deborah Levine

Acknowledgments

Our deepest appreciation and sincerest gratitude:

To all of our outstanding authors who have contributed extensive, newly updated, and authoritative text and images. We cannot thank them enough for their efforts on this project.

To Sharon Emmerling in Denver, Colorado, whose outstanding secretarial and communication skills with authors and editors have facilitated the review and final revision of the entire manuscript. Her enthusiastic attention to detail and accuracy has made this our best edition ever.

To Gordana Popovich and Dr. Hojun Yu for their artwork and schematics in Chapter 8, The Gastrointestinal Tract.

To Dr. Hojun Yu for his schematics on liver anatomy in Chapter 4, The Liver.

To Lisa Barnes, developmental editor at Elsevier, who has worked closely with us on this project from the very beginning of the fourth edition. We also thank the enthusiastic participation of many other Elsevier experts including **Rebecca Gaertner**, Elsevier's guiding hand overseeing the project. She has patiently worked with us through all the final stages of development and production. It has been an intense year for everyone, and we are very proud of this superb edition of *Diagnostic Ultrasound*.

Contents

Online Video Contents

Part I

Physics

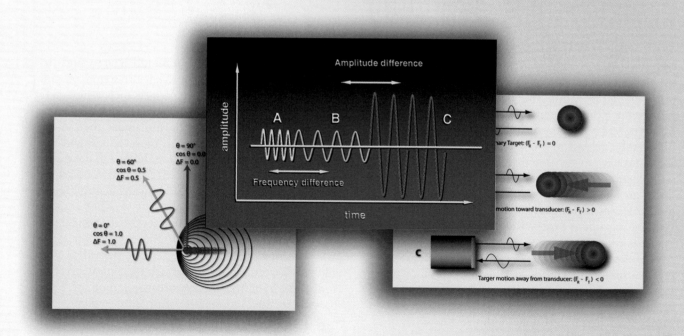

CHAPTER 1

Physics of Ultrasound

Christopher R. B. Merritt

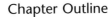

Chapter Outline

*A*ll diagnostic ultrasound applications are based on the detection and display of acoustic energy reflected from interfaces within the body. These interactions provide the information needed to generate high-resolution, gray-scale images of the body, as well as display information related to blood flow. Its unique imaging attributes have made ultrasound an important and versatile medical imaging tool. However, expensive state-of-the-art instrumentation does not guarantee the production of high-quality studies of diagnostic value. Gaining maximum benefit from this complex technology requires a combination of skills, including knowledge of the physical principles that empower ultrasound with its unique diagnostic capabilities. The user must understand the fundamentals of the interactions of acoustic energy with tissue and the methods and instruments used to produce and optimize the ultrasound display. With this knowledge the user can collect the maximum information from each examination, avoiding pitfalls and errors in diagnosis that may result from the omission of information or the misinterpretation of artifacts.

Ultrasound imaging and Doppler ultrasound are based on the scattering of sound energy by interfaces of materials with different properties through interactions governed by acoustic physics. The amplitude of reflected energy is used to generate ultrasound images, and frequency shifts in the backscattered ultrasound provide information relating to moving targets such as blood. To produce, detect, and process ultrasound data, users must manage numerous variables, many under their direct control. To do this, operators must understand the methods used to generate ultrasound data and the theory and operation of the instruments that detect, display, and store the acoustic information generated in clinical examinations.

This chapter provides an overview of the fundamentals of acoustics, the physics of ultrasound imaging and flow detection, and ultrasound instrumentation with emphasis on points most relevant to clinical practice. A discussion of the therapeutic application of high-intensity focused ultrasound concludes the chapter.

BASIC ACOUSTICS

Wavelength and Frequency

Sound is the result of mechanical energy traveling through matter as a wave producing alternating **compression** and **rarefaction.** Pressure waves are propagated by limited physical displacement of the material through

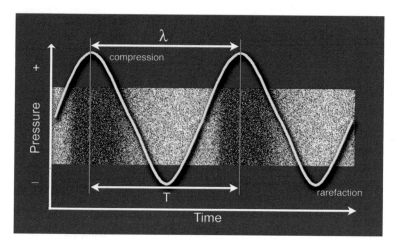

FIGURE 1-1. Sound waves. Sound is transmitted mechanically at the molecular level. In the resting state the pressure is uniform throughout the medium. Sound is propagated as a series of alternating pressure waves producing compression and rarefaction of the conducting medium. The time for a pressure wave to pass a given point is the period, *T*. The frequency of the wave is 1/T. The wavelength, λ, is the distance between corresponding points on the time-pressure curve.

which the sound is being transmitted. A plot of these changes in pressure is a sinusoidal waveform (Fig. 1-1), in which the Y axis indicates the pressure at a given point and the X axis indicates time. **Changes in pressure with time define the basic units of measurement for sound.** The distance between corresponding points on the time-pressure curve is defined as the **wavelength** (λ), and the time (T) to complete a single cycle is called the **period.** The number of complete cycles in a unit of time is the **frequency** (*f*) of the sound. Frequency and period are inversely related. If the period (T) is expressed in seconds, $f = 1/T$, or $f = T \times sec^{-1}$. The unit of **acoustic frequency** is the **hertz** (Hz); 1 Hz = 1 cycle per second. High frequencies are expressed in kilohertz (kHz; 1 kHz = 1000 Hz) or megahertz (MHz; 1 MHz = 1,000,000 Hz).

In nature, acoustic frequencies span a range from less than 1 Hz to more than 100,000 Hz (100 kHz). Human hearing is limited to the lower part of this range, extending from 20 to 20,000 Hz. Ultrasound differs from audible sound only in its frequency, and it is 500 to 1000 times higher than the sound we normally hear. Sound frequencies used for diagnostic applications typically range from 2 to 15 MHz, although frequencies as high as 50 to 60 MHz are under investigation for certain specialized imaging applications. In general, the frequencies used for ultrasound imaging are higher than those used for Doppler. Regardless of the frequency, the same basic principles of acoustics apply.

Propagation of Sound

In most clinical applications of ultrasound, brief bursts or pulses of energy are transmitted into the body and propagated through tissue. Acoustic pressure waves can travel in a direction perpendicular to the direction of the particles being displaced (**transverse** waves), but in tissue and fluids, sound propagation is along the direction of particle movement (**longitudinal** waves). The speed at which the pressure wave moves through tissue varies greatly and is affected by the physical properties of the tissue. **Propagation velocity** is largely determined by the

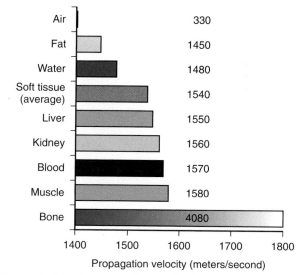

FIGURE 1-2. Propagation velocity. In the body, propagation velocity of sound is determined by the physical properties of tissue. As shown, this varies considerably. Medical ultrasound devices base their measurements on an assumed average propagation velocity of 1540 m/sec.

resistance of the medium to compression, which in turn is influenced by the density of the medium and its stiffness or elasticity. Propagation velocity is increased by increasing stiffness and reduced by decreasing density. In the body, propagation velocity may be regarded as constant for a given tissue and is not affected by the frequency or wavelength of the sound.

Figure 1-2 shows typical propagation velocities for a variety of materials. In the body the propagation velocity of sound is assumed to be 1540 meters per second (m/sec). This value is the average of measurements obtained from normal tissues.[1,2] Although this value represents most soft tissues, such tissues as aerated lung and fat have propagation velocities significantly less than 1540 m/sec, whereas tissues such as bone have greater velocities. Because a few normal tissues have propagation values significantly different from the average value assumed by the ultrasound scanner, the display of such tissues may be subject to measurement errors or **artifacts** (Fig. 1-3). The propagation velocity of sound (c) is related to frequency and wavelength by the following simple equation:

$$c = f\lambda \quad 1$$

Thus a frequency of 5 MHz can be shown to have a wavelength of 0.308 mm in tissue: $\lambda = c/f = 1540$ m/sec $\times 5,000,000$ sec$^{-1} = 0.000308$ m $= 0.308$ mm.

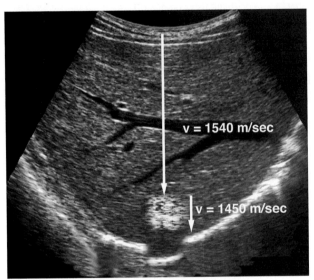

FIGURE 1-3. Propagation velocity artifact. When sound passes through a lesion containing fat, echo return is delayed because fat has a propagation velocity of 1450 m/sec, which is less than the liver. Because the ultrasound scanner assumes that sound is being propagated at the average velocity of 1540 m/sec, the delay in echo return is interpreted as indicating a deeper target. Therefore the final image shows a **misregistration artifact** in which the diaphragm and other structures deep to the fatty lesion are shown in a deeper position than expected (simulated image).

Distance Measurement

Propagation velocity is a particularly important value in clinical ultrasound and is critical in determining the distance of a reflecting interface from the transducer. Much of the information used to generate an ultrasound scan is based on the precise measurement of time and employs the principles of **echo-ranging.** If an ultrasound pulse is transmitted into the body and the time until an echo returns is measured, it is simple to calculate the depth of the interface that generated the echo, provided the propagation velocity of sound for the tissue is known. For example, if the time from the transmission of a pulse until the return of an echo is 0.145 millisecond (ms; 0.000145 sec) and the velocity of sound is 1540 m/sec, the distance that the sound has traveled must be 22.33 cm (1540 m/sec × 100 cm/m × 0.000145 sec = 22.33 cm). Because the time measured includes the time for sound to travel to the interface and then return along the same path to the transducer, the distance from the transducer to the reflecting interface is 22.33 cm/2 = 11.165 cm (Fig. 1-4). The accuracy of this measurement is therefore highly influenced by how closely the presumed velocity of sound corresponds to the true velocity in the tissue being observed (see Figs. 1-2 and 1-3), as well as by the important assumption that the sound pulse travels in a straight path to and from the reflecting interface.

Acoustic Impedance

Current diagnostic ultrasound scanners rely on the detection and display of **reflected sound or echoes.** Imaging based on transmission of ultrasound is also possible, but this is not used clinically at present. To produce an echo, a reflecting interface must be present. Sound passing through a **totally homogeneous medium**

FIGURE 1-4. Ultrasound ranging. The information used to position an echo for display is based on the precise measurement of time. Here the time for an echo to travel from the transducer to the target and return to the transducer is 0.145 ms. Multiplying the velocity of sound in tissue (1540 m/sec) by the time shows that the sound returning from the target has traveled 22.33 cm. Therefore the target lies half this distance, or 11.165 cm, from the transducer.

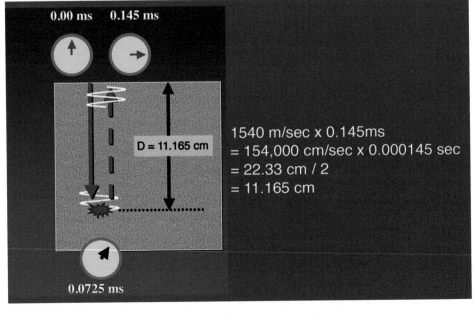

1540 m/sec x 0.145ms
= 154,000 cm/sec x 0.000145 sec
= 22.33 cm / 2
= 11.165 cm

encounters no interfaces to reflect sound, and the medium appears **anechoic** or **cystic.** At the junction of tissues or materials with different physical properties, acoustic interfaces are present. These interfaces are responsible for the reflection of variable amounts of the incident sound energy. Thus, when ultrasound passes from one tissue to another or encounters a vessel wall or circulating blood cells, some of the incident sound energy is reflected. The amount of reflection or **backscatter** is determined by the difference in the acoustic impedances of the materials forming the interface.

Acoustic impedance (Z) is determined by product of the density (ρ) of the medium propagating the sound and the propagation velocity (c) of sound in that medium (Z = ρc). Interfaces with large acoustic impedance differences, such as interfaces of tissue with air or bone, reflect almost all the incident energy. Interfaces composed of substances with smaller differences in acoustic impedance, such as a muscle and fat interface, reflect only part of the incident energy, permitting the remainder to continue onward. As with propagation velocity, acoustic impedance is determined by the properties of the tissues involved and is independent of frequency.

Reflection

The way ultrasound is reflected when it strikes an acoustic interface is determined by the size and surface features of the interface (Fig. 1-5). If large and relatively smooth, the interface reflects sound much as a mirror reflects light. Such interfaces are called **specular reflectors** because they behave as "mirrors for sound." The amount of energy reflected by an acoustic interface can be expressed as a fraction of the incident energy; this is termed the **reflection coefficient** (R). If a specular reflector is perpendicular to the incident sound beam, the amount of energy reflected is determined by the following relationship:

$$R = (Z_2 - Z_1)^2 / (Z_2 + Z_1)^2 \quad \textbf{2}$$

where Z_1 and Z_2 are the acoustic impedances of the media forming the interface.

Because ultrasound scanners only detect reflections that return to the transducer, **display of specular interfaces is highly dependent on the angle of insonation** (exposure to ultrasound waves). Specular reflectors will return echoes to the transducer only if the sound beam is perpendicular to the interface. If the interface is not at a 90-degree angle to the sound beam, it will be reflected away from the transducer, and the echo will not be detected (see Fig. 1-5, *A*).

Most echoes in the body do not arise from specular reflectors but rather from much smaller interfaces within solid organs. In this case the acoustic interfaces involve structures with individual dimensions much smaller than

---

EXAMPLES OF SPECULAR REFLECTORS

Diaphragm
Wall of urine-filled bladder
Endometrial stripe

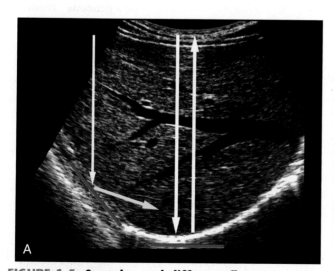

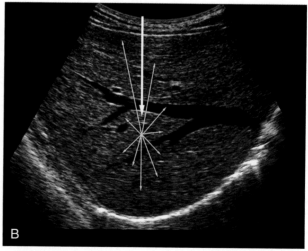

FIGURE 1-5. Specular and diffuse reflectors. A, Specular reflector. The diaphragm is a large and relatively smooth surface that reflects sound like a mirror reflects light. Thus, sound striking the diaphragm at nearly a 90-degree angle is reflected directly back to the transducer, resulting in a strong echo. Sound striking the diaphragm obliquely is reflected away from the transducer, and an echo is not displayed *(yellow arrow).* **B, Diffuse reflector.** In contrast to the diaphragm, the liver parenchyma consists of acoustic interfaces that are small compared to the wavelength of sound used for imaging. These interfaces scatter sound in all directions, and only a portion of the energy returns to the transducer to produce the image.

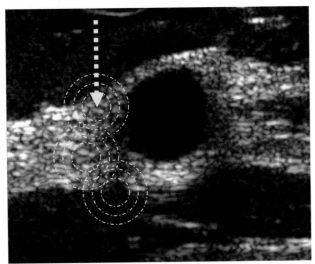

FIGURE 1-6. Ultrasound speckle. Close inspection of an ultrasound image of the breast containing a small cyst reveals it to be composed of numerous areas of varying intensity (speckle). Speckle results from the constructive *(red)* and destructive *(green)* interaction of the acoustic fields *(yellow rings)* generated by the scattering of ultrasound from small tissue reflectors. This interference pattern gives ultrasound images their characteristic grainy appearance and may reduce contrast. Ultrasound speckle is the basis of the texture displayed in ultrasound images of solid tissues.

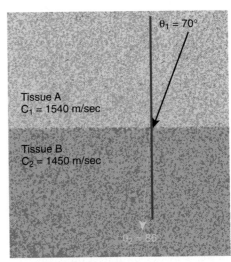

FIGURE 1-7. Refraction. When sound passes from tissue A with one acoustic propagation velocity (c_1) to tissue B with a different propagation velocity (c_2), there is a change in the direction of the sound wave because of refraction. The degree of change is related to the ratio of the propagating velocities of the media forming the interface ($\sin\theta_1/\sin\theta_2 = c_1/c_2$).

the wavelength of the incident sound. The echoes from these interfaces are scattered in all directions. Such reflectors are called **diffuse reflectors** and account for the echoes that form the characteristic echo patterns seen in solid organs and tissues (see Fig. 1-5, *B*). The constructive and destructive interference of sound scattered by diffuse reflectors results in the production of **ultrasound speckle,** a feature of tissue texture of sonograms of solid organs (Fig. 1-6). For some diagnostic applications, the nature of the reflecting structures creates important conflicts. For example, most vessel walls behave as specular reflectors that require insonation at a 90-degree angle for best imaging, whereas Doppler imaging requires an angle of less than 90 degrees between the sound beam and the vessel.

Refraction

Another event that can occur when sound passes from a tissue with one acoustic propagation velocity to a tissue with a higher or lower sound velocity is a change in the direction of the sound wave. This change in direction of propagation is called refraction and is governed by Snell's law:

$$\sin\theta_1/\sin\theta_2 = c_1/c_2 \quad 3$$

where θ_1 is the angle of incidence of the sound approaching the interface, θ_2 is the angle of refraction, and c_1 and c_2 are the propagation velocities of sound in the media

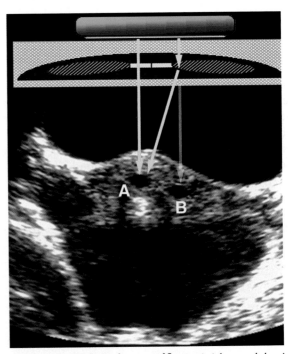

FIGURE 1-8. Refraction artifact. Axial transabdominal image of the uterus shows a small gestational sac *(A)* and what appears to be a second sac *(B)*. In this case, the artifact *B* is caused by refraction at the edge of the rectus abdominis muscle. The bending of the path of the sound results in the creation of a duplicate of the image of the sac in an unexpected and misleading location (simulated image).

forming the interface (Fig. 1-7). Refraction is important because it is one cause of **misregistration** of a structure in an ultrasound image (Fig. 1-8). When an ultrasound scanner detects an echo, it assumes that the source of the echo is along a fixed line of sight from the transducer. If the sound has been refracted, the echo detected may be coming from a different depth or location than the image shown in the display. If this is suspected, increasing the scan angle so that it is perpendicular to the interface minimizes the artifact.

Attenuation

As the acoustic energy moves through a uniform medium, work is performed and energy is ultimately transferred to the transmitting medium as heat. The capacity to perform work is determined by the quantity of acoustic energy produced. **Acoustic power**, expressed in watts (W) or milliwatts (mW), describes the amount of acoustic energy produced in a unit of time. Although measurement of power provides an indication of the energy as it relates to time, it does not take into account the spatial distribution of the energy. **Intensity** (I) is used to describe the spatial distribution of power and is calculated by dividing the power by the area over which the power is distributed, as follows:

$$I\,(W/cm^2) = Power\,(W)/Area\,(cm^2) \quad 4$$

The **attenuation** of sound energy as it passes through tissue is of great clinical importance because it influences the *depth* in tissue, from which useful information can be obtained. This in turn affects transducer selection and a number of operator-controlled instrument settings, including time (or depth) gain compensation, power output attenuation, and system gain levels. Attenuation is measured in relative rather than absolute units. The **decibel** (dB) notation is generally used to compare different levels of ultrasound power or intensity. This value is 10 times the log_{10} of the ratio of the power or intensity values being compared. For example, if the intensity measured at one point in tissues is 10 mW/cm² and at a deeper point is 0.01 mW/cm², the difference in intensity is as follows:

$$(10)(log_{10}\,0.01/10) = (10)(log_{10}\,0.001) =$$
$$(10)(-log_{10}\,1000) = (10)(-3) = -30\ dB$$

As it passes through tissue, sound loses energy, and the pressure waves decrease in amplitude as they travel farther from their source. Contributing to the attenuation of sound are the transfer of energy to tissue, resulting in heating (absorption), and the removal of energy by reflection and scattering. Attenuation is therefore the result of the combined effects of **absorption, scattering, and reflection.** Attenuation depends on the insonating frequency as well as the nature of the attenuating medium. High frequencies are attenuated more rapidly than lower frequencies, and transducer frequency is a major determinant of the useful depth from which information can be obtained with ultrasound. Attenuation determines the efficiency with which ultrasound penetrates a specific tissue and varies considerably in normal tissues (Fig. 1-9).

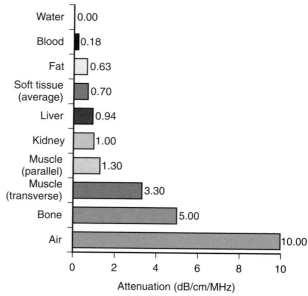

FIGURE 1-9. Attenuation. As sound passes through tissue, it loses energy through the transfer of energy to tissue by heating, reflection, and scattering. Attenuation is determined by the insonating frequency and the nature of the attenuating medium. Attenuation values for normal tissues show considerable variation. Attenuation also increases in proportion to insonating frequency, resulting in less penetration at higher frequencies.

INSTRUMENTATION

Ultrasound scanners are complex and sophisticated imaging devices, but all consist of the following basic components to perform key functions:
- Transmitter or pulser to energize the transducer
- Ultrasound transducer itself
- Receiver and processor to detect and amplify the backscattered energy and manipulate the reflected signals for display
- Display that presents the ultrasound image or data in a form suitable for analysis and interpretation
- Method to record or store the ultrasound image

Transmitter

Most clinical applications use pulsed ultrasound, in which brief bursts of acoustic energy are transmitted into the body. The source of these pulses, the ultrasound transducer, is energized by application of precisely timed, high-amplitude voltage. The maximum voltage that may be applied to the transducer is limited by federal regulations that restrict the acoustic output of diagnostic scanners. Most scanners provide a control that permits attenuation of the output voltage. Because the use of maximum output results in higher exposure of the patient to ultrasound energy, prudent use dictates use of the output attenuation controls to reduce power levels to the lowest levels consistent with the diagnostic problem.[3]

The transmitter also controls the rate of pulses emitted by the transducer, or the **pulse repetition frequency** (PRF). The PRF determines the time interval between ultrasound pulses and is important in determining the depth from which unambiguous data can be obtained both in imaging and Doppler modes. The ultrasound pulses must be spaced with enough time between the pulses to permit the sound to travel to the depth of interest and return before the next pulse is sent. For imaging, PRFs from 1 to 10 kHz are used, resulting in an interval of 0.1 to 1 ms between pulses. Thus, a PRF of 5 kHz permits an echo to travel and return from a depth of 15.4 cm before the next pulse is sent.

Transducer

A transducer is any device that converts one form of energy to another. In ultrasound the transducer converts electric energy to mechanical energy, and vice versa. In diagnostic ultrasound systems the transducer serves two functions: (1) converting the electric energy provided by the transmitter to the acoustic pulses directed into the patient and (2) serving as the receiver of reflected echoes, converting weak pressure changes into electric signals for processing.

Ultrasound transducers use **piezoelectricity,** a principle discovered by Pierre and Jacques Curie in 1880. Piezoelectric materials have the unique ability to respond to the action of an electric field by changing shape. They also have the property of generating electric potentials when compressed. Changing the polarity of a voltage applied to the transducer changes the thickness of the transducer, which expands and contracts as the polarity changes. This results in the generation of mechanical pressure waves that can be transmitted into the body. The piezoelectric effect also results in the generation of small potentials across the transducer when the transducer is struck by returning echoes. Positive pressures cause a small polarity to develop across the transducer; negative pressure during the rarefaction portion of the acoustic wave produces the opposite polarity across the transducer. These tiny polarity changes and the associated voltages are the source of all the information processed to generate an ultrasound image or Doppler display.

When stimulated by the application of a voltage difference across its thickness, the transducer vibrates. The frequency of vibration is determined by the transducer material. When the transducer is electrically stimulated, a range or **band** of frequencies results. The preferential frequency produced by a transducer is determined by the propagation speed of the transducer material and its thickness. In the **pulsed wave** operating modes used for most clinical ultrasound applications, the ultrasound pulses contain additional frequencies that are both higher and lower than the preferential frequency. The range of frequencies produced by a given transducer is termed its **bandwidth.** Generally, the shorter the pulse of ultrasound produced by the transducer, the greater is the bandwidth.

Most modern digital ultrasound systems employ broad-bandwidth technology. **Ultrasound bandwidth** refers to the range of frequencies produced and detected by the ultrasound system. This is important because each tissue in the body has a characteristic response to ultrasound of a given frequency, and different tissues respond differently to different frequencies. The range of frequencies arising from a tissue exposed to ultrasound is referred to as the **frequency spectrum bandwidth** of the tissue, or tissue signature. Broad-bandwidth technology provides a means to capture the frequency spectrum of insonated tissues, preserving acoustic information and tissue signature. Broad-bandwidth beam formers reduce speckle artifact by a process of **frequency compounding.** This is possible because speckle patterns at different frequencies are independent of one another, and combining data from multiple frequency bands (i.e., compounding) results in a reduction of speckle in the final image, leading to improved contrast resolution.

The length of an ultrasound pulse is determined by the number of alternating voltage changes applied to the transducer. For **continuous wave** (CW) ultrasound devices, a constant alternating current is applied to the transducer, and the alternating polarity produces a continuous ultrasound wave. For imaging, a single, brief voltage change is applied to the transducer, causing it to vibrate at its preferential frequency. Because the transducer continues to vibrate or "ring" for a short time after it is stimulated by the voltage change, the ultrasound pulse will be several cycles long. The number of cycles of sound in each pulse determines the **pulse length.** For imaging, short pulse lengths are desirable because longer pulses result in poorer axial resolution. To reduce the pulse length to no more than two or three cycles, **damping** materials are used in the construction of the transducer. In clinical imaging applications, very short pulses are applied to the transducer, and the transducers have highly efficient damping. This results in very short pulses of ultrasound, generally consisting of only two or three cycles of sound.

The ultrasound pulse generated by a transducer must be propagated in tissue to provide clinical information. Special transducer coatings and ultrasound coupling gels are necessary to allow efficient transfer of energy from the transducer to the body. Once in the body, the ultrasound pulses are propagated, reflected, refracted, and absorbed, in accordance with the basic acoustic principles summarized earlier.

The ultrasound pulses produced by the transducer result in a series of wavefronts that form a three-dimensional (3-D) beam of ultrasound. The features of this beam are influenced by constructive and destructive interference of the pressure waves, the curvature of the transducer, and acoustic lenses used to shape the beam.

Interference of pressure waves results in an area near the transducer where the pressure amplitude varies greatly. This region is termed the **near field,** or **Fresnel zone.** Farther from the transducer, at a distance determined by the radius of the transducer and the frequency, the sound field begins to diverge, and the pressure amplitude decreases at a steady rate with increasing distance from the transducer. This region is called the **far field,** or **Fraunhofer zone.** In modern multielement transducer arrays, precise timing of the firing of elements allows correction of this divergence of the ultrasound beam and focusing at selected depths. Only reflections of pulses that return to the transducer are capable of stimulating the transducer with small pressure changes, which are converted into the voltage changes that are detected, amplified, and processed to build an image based on the echo information.

Receiver

When returning echoes strike the transducer face, minute voltages are produced across the piezoelectric elements. The receiver detects and amplifies these weak signals. The receiver also provides a means for compensating for the differences in echo strength, which result from attenuation by different tissue thickness by control of **time gain compensation** (TGC) or **depth gain compensation** (DGC).

Sound is attenuated as it passes into the body, and additional energy is removed as echoes return through tissue to the transducer. The attenuation of sound is proportional to the frequency and is constant for specific tissues. Because echoes returning from deeper tissues are weaker than those returning from more superficial structures, they must be amplified more by the receiver to produce a uniform tissue echo appearance (Fig. 1-10). This adjustment is accomplished by TGC controls that permit the user to selectively amplify the signals from deeper structures or to suppress the signals from super-

ficial tissues, compensating for tissue attenuation. Although many newer machines provide for some means of automatic TGC, the manual adjustment of this control is one of the most important user controls and may have a profound effect on the quality of the ultrasound image provided for interpretation.

Another important function of the receiver is the compression of the wide range of amplitudes returning to the transducer into a range that can be displayed to the user. The ratio of the highest to the lowest amplitudes that can be displayed may be expressed in decibels and is referred to as the **dynamic range.** In a typical clinical application, the range of reflected signals may vary by a factor of as much as $1:10^{12}$, resulting in a dynamic range of up to 120 dB. Although the amplifiers used in ultrasound machines are capable of handling this range of voltages, gray-scale displays are limited to display a signal intensity range of only 35 to 40 dB. **Compression and remapping of the data** are required to adapt the dynamic range of the backscattered signal intensity to the dynamic range of the display (Fig. 1-11). Compression is performed in the receiver by selective amplification of weaker signals. Additional manual postprocessing controls permit the user to map selectively the returning signal to the display. These controls affect the brightness of different echo levels in the image and therefore determine the image contrast.

Image Display

Ultrasound signals may be displayed in several ways.[4] Over the years, imaging has evolved from simple A-mode and bistable display to high-resolution, real-time, grayscale imaging. The earliest A-mode devices displayed the voltage produced across the transducer by the backscattered echo as a vertical deflection on the face of an oscilloscope. The horizontal sweep of the oscilloscope was calibrated to indicate the distance from the transducer to the reflecting surface. In this form of display, the

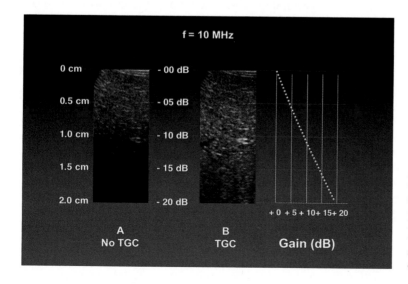

FIGURE 1-10. Time gain compensation (TGC). Without TGC, tissue attenuation causes gradual loss of display of deeper tissues *(A)*. In this example, tissue attenuation of 1 dB/cm-MHz is simulated for a transducer of 10 MHz. At a depth of 2 cm, the intensity is −20 dB (1% of initial value). By applying increasing amplification or gain to the backscattered signal to compensate for this attenuation, a uniform intensity is restored to the tissue at all depths *(B)*.

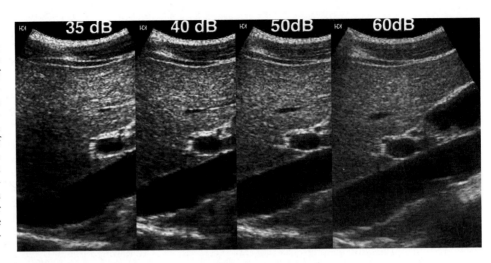

FIGURE 1-11. Dynamic range. The ultrasound receiver must compress the wide range of amplitudes returning to the transducer into a range that can be displayed to the user. Here, compression and remapping of the data to display dynamic ranges of 35, 40, 50, and 60 dB are shown. The widest dynamic range shown (60 dB) permits the best differentiation of subtle differences in echo intensity and is preferred for most imaging applications. The narrower ranges increase conspicuity of larger echo differences.

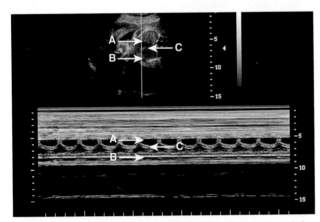

FIGURE 1-12. M-mode display. M-mode ultrasound displays changes of echo amplitude and position with time. Display of changes in echo position is useful in the evaluation of rapidly moving structures such as cardiac valves and chamber walls. Here, the three major moving structures in an M-mode image of the fetal heart correspond to the near ventricular wall *(A)*, the interventricular septum *(B)*, and the far ventricular wall *(C)*. The baseline is a time scale that permits the calculation of heart rate from the M-mode data.

strength or amplitude of the reflected sound is indicated by the height of the vertical deflection displayed on the oscilloscope. With **A-mode ultrasound,** only the position and strength of a reflecting structure are recorded.

Another simple form of imaging, **M-mode ultrasound,** displays echo amplitude and shows the position of moving reflectors (Fig. 1-12). M-mode imaging uses the brightness of the display to indicate the intensity of the reflected signal. The time base of the display can be adjusted to allow for varying degrees of temporal resolution, as dictated by clinical application. M-mode ultrasound is interpreted by assessing motion patterns of specific reflectors and determining anatomic relationships from characteristic patterns of motion. Currently, the major application of M-mode display is evaluation of the rapid motion of cardiac valves and of cardiac chamber and vessel walls. M-mode imaging may play a future role in measurement of subtle changes in vessel wall elasticity accompanying atherogenesis.

The mainstay of imaging with ultrasound is provided by **real-time, gray-scale, B-mode display,** in which variations in display intensity or brightness are used to indicate reflected signals of differing amplitude. To generate a two-dimensional (2-D) image, multiple ultrasound pulses are sent down a series of successive scan lines (Fig. 1-13), building a 2-D representation of echoes arising from the object being scanned. When an ultrasound image is displayed on a black background, signals of greatest intensity appear as white; absence of signal is shown as black; and signals of intermediate intensity appear as shades of gray. If the ultrasound beam is moved with respect to the object being examined and the position of the reflected signal is stored, the brightest portions of the resulting 2-D image indicate structures reflecting more of the transmitted sound energy back to the transducer.

In most modern instruments a digital memory of 512 × 512 or 512 × 640 pixels is used to store values that correspond to the echo intensities originating from corresponding positions in the patient. At least 2^8, or 256, shades of gray are possible for each pixel, in accord with the amplitude of the echo being represented. The image stored in memory in this manner can then be sent to a video monitor for display.

Because B-mode display relates the strength of a backscattered signal to a brightness level on the display device (usually a video display monitor), it is important that the operator understand how the amplitude information in the ultrasound signal is translated into a brightness scale in the image display. Each ultrasound manufacturer offers several options for the way the dynamic range of the target is compressed for display, as well as the transfer function that assigns a given signal amplitude to a shade of gray. Although these technical details vary among machines, the way the operator uses them may greatly affect the clinical value of the final image. In general, it

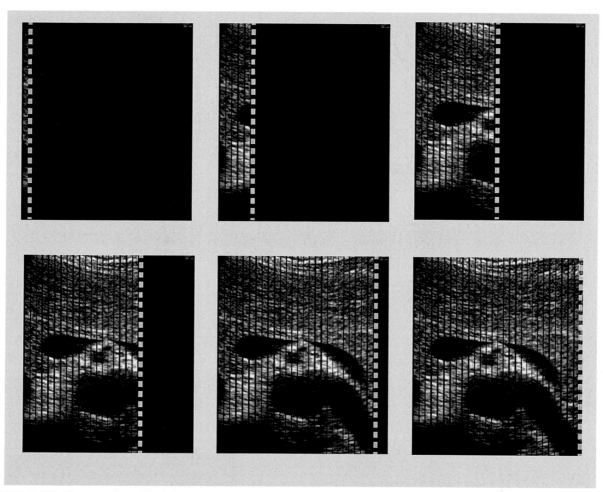

FIGURE 1-13. B-mode imaging. A 2-D, real-time image is built by ultrasound pulses sent down a series of successive scan lines. Each scan line adds to the image, building a 2-D representation of echoes from the object being scanned. In real-time imaging, an entire image is created 15 to 60 times per second.

is desirable to display as *wide* a dynamic range as possible, to identify subtle differences in tissue echogenicity (see Fig. 1-11).

Real-time ultrasound produces the impression of motion by generating a series of individual 2-D images at rates of 15 to 60 frames per second. Real-time, 2-D, B-mode ultrasound is now the major method for ultrasound imaging throughout the body and is the most common form of B-mode display. Real-time ultrasound permits assessment of both anatomy and motion. When images are acquired and displayed at rates of several times per second, the effect is dynamic, and because the image reflects the state and motion of the organ at the time it is examined, the information is regarded as being shown in real time. In cardiac applications the terms "2-D echocardiography" and "2-D echo" are used to describe real-time, B-mode imaging; in most other applications the term "real-time ultrasound" is used.

Transducers used for real-time imaging may be classified by the method used to steer the beam in rapidly generating each individual image, keeping in mind that as many as 30 to 60 complete images must be generated

per second for real-time applications. **Beam steering** may be done through mechanical rotation or oscillation of the transducer or by electronic means (Fig. 1-14). **Electronic beam steering** is used in linear array and phased array transducers and permits a variety of image display formats. Most electronically steered transducers currently in use also provide electronic focusing that is adjustable for depth. **Mechanical beam steering** may use single-element transducers with a fixed focus or may use annular arrays of elements with electronically controlled focusing. For real-time imaging, transducers using mechanical or electronic beam steering generate displays in a rectangular or pie-shaped format. For obstetric, small parts, and peripheral vascular examinations, linear array transducers with a rectangular image format are often used. The rectangular image display has the advantage of a larger field of view near the surface but requires a large surface area for transducer contact. Sector scanners with either mechanical or electronic steering require only a small surface area for contact and are better suited for examinations in which access is limited.

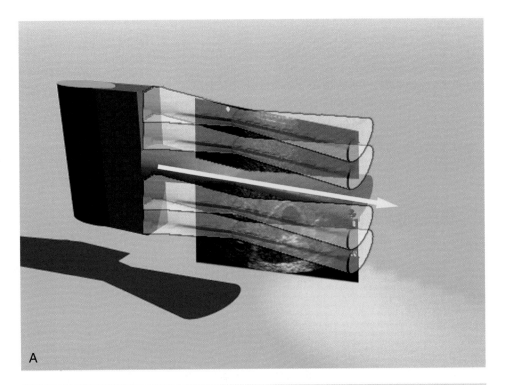

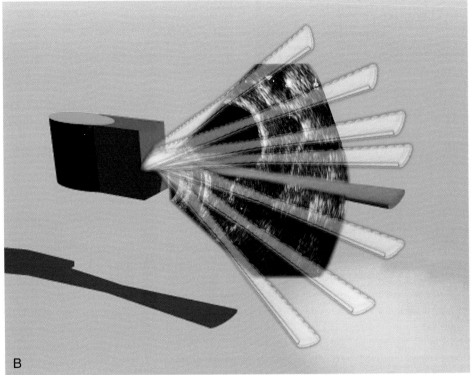

FIGURE 1-14. Beam steering. A, Linear array. In a linear array transducer, individual elements or groups of elements are fired in sequence. This generates a series of parallel ultrasound beams, each perpendicular to the transducer face. As these beams move across the transducer face, they generate the lines of sight that combine to form the final image. Depending on the number of transducer elements and the sequence in which they are fired, focusing at selected depths from the surface can be achieved. **B, Phased array.** A phased array transducer produces a sector field of view by firing multiple transducer elements in precise sequence to generate interference of acoustic wavefronts. The ultrasound beam that results generates a series of lines of sight at varying angles from one side of the transducer to the other, producing a sector image format.

Mechanical Sector Scanners

Early ultrasound scanners used transducers consisting of a single piezoelectric element. To generate real-time images with these transducers, mechanical devices were required to move the transducer in a linear or circular motion. Mechanical sector scanners using one or more single-element transducers do not allow variable focusing. This problem is overcome by using annular array transducers. Although important in the early days of real-time imaging, mechanical sector scanners with fixed-focus, single-element transducers are not presently in common use.

Arrays

Current technology uses a transducer composed of multiple elements, usually produced by precise slicing of a piece of piezoelectric material into numerous small units, each with its own electrodes. Such transducer arrays may be formed in a variety of configurations. Typically, these are linear, curved, phased, or annular arrays. High-density 2-D arrays have also been developed. By precise timing of the firing of combinations of elements in these arrays, interference of the wavefronts generated by the individual elements can be exploited to change the direction of the ultrasound beam, and this can be used to provide a steerable beam for the generation of real-time images in a linear or sector format.

Linear Arrays

Linear array transducers are used for small parts, vascular, and obstetric applications because the rectangular image format produced by these transducers is well suited for these applications. In these transducers, individual elements are arranged in a linear fashion. By firing the transducer elements in sequence, either individually or in groups, a series of parallel pulses is generated, each forming a line of sight perpendicular to the transducer face. These individual lines of sight combine to form the image field of view (see Fig. 1-14, *A*). Depending on the number of transducer elements and the sequence in which they are fired, focusing at selected depths from the surface can be achieved.

Curved Arrays

Linear arrays that have been shaped into convex curves produce an image that combines a relatively large surface field of view with a sector display format. Curved array transducers are used for a variety of applications, the larger versions serving for general abdominal, obstetric, and transabdominal pelvic scanning. Small, high-frequency, curved array scanners are often used in transvaginal and transrectal probes and for pediatric imaging.

Phased Arrays

In contrast to mechanical sector scanners, phased array scanners have no moving parts. A sector field of view is produced by multiple transducer elements fired in precise sequence under electronic control. By controlling the time and sequence at which the individual transducer elements are fired, the resulting ultrasound wave can be steered in different directions as well as focused at different depths (see Fig. 1-14, *B*). By rapidly steering the beam to generate a series of lines of sight at varying angles from one side of the transducer to the other, a sector image format is produced. This allows the fabrication of transducers of relatively small size but with large fields of view at depth. These transducers are particularly useful for intercostal scanning, to evaluate the heart, liver, or spleen, and for examinations in other areas where access is limited.

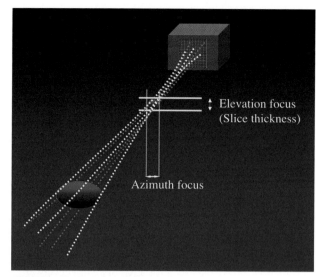

FIGURE 1-15. Two-dimensional array. High-density 2-D arrays consist of a 2-D matrix of transducer elements, permitting acquisition of data from a volume rather than a single plane of tissue. Precise electronic control of individual elements permits adjustable focusing on both azimuth and elevation planes.

Two-Dimensional Arrays

Transducer arrays can be formed (1) by slicing a rectangular piece of transducer material perpendicular to its long axis to produce a number of small rectangular elements or (2) by creating a series of concentric elements nested within one another in a circular piece of piezoelectric material to produce an annular array. The use of multiple elements permits precise focusing. A particular advantage of 2-D array construction is that the beam can be focused in both the elevation plane and the lateral plane, and a uniform and highly focused beam can be produced (Fig. 1-15). These arrays improve spatial resolution and contrast, reduce clutter, and are well suited for the collection of data from volumes of tissue for use in 3-D processing and display. Unlike linear 2-D arrays, in which delays in the firing of the individual elements may be used to steer the beam, annular arrays do not permit beam steering and, to be used for real-time imaging, must be steered mechanically.

Transducer Selection

Practical considerations in the selection of the optimal transducer for a given application include not only the requirements for spatial resolution, but also the distance of the target object from the transducer because penetration of ultrasound diminishes as frequency increases. In general, the **highest ultrasound frequency permitting penetration to the depth of interest should be selected.** For superficial vessels and organs, such as the thyroid, breast, or testicle, lying within 1 to 3 cm of the surface, imaging frequencies of 7.5 to 15 MHz are typically used. These high frequencies are also ideal for intraoperative applications. For evaluation of deeper structures in the abdomen or pelvis more than 12 to 15 cm from the surface, frequencies as low as 2.25 to 3.5 MHz may be required. When maximal resolution is needed, a high-frequency transducer with excellent lateral and elevation resolution at the depth of interest is required.

IMAGE DISPLAY AND STORAGE

With real-time ultrasound, user feedback is immediate and is provided by video display. The brightness and contrast of the image on this display are determined by the ambient lighting in the examination room, the brightness and contrast settings of the video monitor, the system gain setting, and the TGC adjustment. The factor most affecting image quality in many ultrasound departments is probably improper adjustment of the video display, with a lack of appreciation of the relationship between the video display settings and the appearance of hard copy or images viewed on a workstation. Because of the importance of the real-time video display in providing feedback to the user, it is essential that the display and the lighting conditions under which it is viewed are standardized and matched to the display used for interpretation. Interpretation of images and archival storage of images may be in the form of transparencies printed on film by optical or laser cameras and printers, videotape, or digital **picture archiving and communications system** (PACS). Increasingly, digital storage is being used for archiving of ultrasound images.

SPECIAL IMAGING MODES

Tissue Harmonic Imaging

Variation of the propagation velocity of sound in fat and other tissues near the transducer results in a **phase aberration** that distorts the ultrasound field, producing noise and clutter in the ultrasound image. Tissue harmonic imaging provides an approach for reducing the effects of phase aberrations.[5] Nonlinear propagation of ultrasound through tissue is associated with the more rapid propagation of the high-pressure component of the ultrasound pressure wave than its negative (rarefactional) component. This results in increasing distortion of the acoustic pulse as it travels within the tissue and causes the generation of multiples, or **harmonics,** of the transmitted frequency (Fig. 1-16).

Tissue harmonic imaging takes advantage of the generation, at depth, of these harmonics. Because the generation of harmonics requires interaction of the transmitted field with the propagating tissue, harmonic generation is not present near the transducer/skin interface, and it only becomes important some distance from the transducer. In most cases the near and far fields of

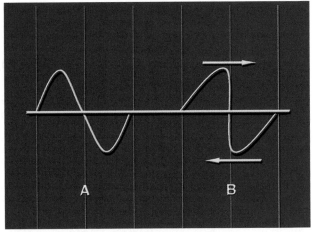

FIGURE 1-16. Harmonic generation. The transmitted waveform is shown in *A*. As the sound is propagated through tissue, the high-pressure component of the wave travels more rapidly than the rarefactional component, producing distortion *(B)* of the wave and generating higher-frequency components (harmonics). *(From Merritt CR: Technology update. Radiol Clin North Am 2001;39:385-397.)*

the image are affected less by harmonics than by intermediate locations. Using broad-bandwidth transducers and signal filtration or coded pulses, the harmonic signals reflected from tissue interfaces can be selectively displayed. Because most imaging artifacts are caused by the interaction of the ultrasound beam with superficial structures or by aberrations at the edges of the beam profile, these artifacts are eliminated using harmonic imaging because the artifact-producing signals do not consist of sufficient energy to generate harmonic frequencies and therefore are filtered out during image formation. Images generated using tissue harmonics often exhibit reduced noise and clutter (Fig. 1-17). Because harmonic beams are narrower than the originally transmitted beams, spatial resolution is improved and side lobes are reduced.

Spatial Compounding

An important source of image degradation and loss of contrast is **ultrasound speckle.** Speckle results from the constructive and destructive interaction of the acoustic fields generated by the scattering of ultrasound from small tissue reflectors. This interference pattern gives ultrasound images their characteristic grainy appearance (see Fig. 1-6), reducing contrast (Fig. 1-18) and making the identification of subtle features more difficult. By summing images from different scanning angles through **compound scanning** (Fig. 1-19), significant improvement in the **contrast-to-noise (speckle) ratio** can be achieved (Fig. 1-20). This is because speckle is random, and the generation of an image by compounding will reduce speckle noise because only the signal is reinforced. In addition, spatial compounding may reduce artifacts that result when an ultrasound beam strikes a specular

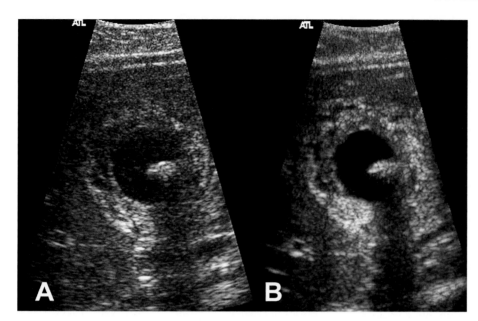

FIGURE 1-17. Tissue harmonic imaging. A, Conventional image, and **B, tissue harmonic image,** of gallbladder of patient with acute cholecystitis. Note the reduction of noise and clutter in the tissue harmonic image. Because harmonic beams do not interact with superficial structures and are narrower than the originally transmitted beam, spatial resolution is improved and clutter and side lobes are reduced. *(From Merritt CR: Technology update. Radiol Clin North Am 2001;39:385-397.)*

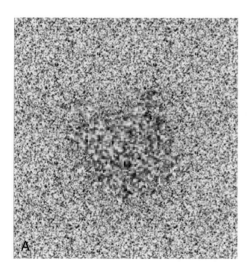

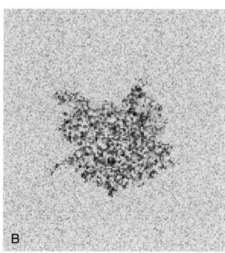

FIGURE 1-18. Effect of speckle on contrast. A, Speckle noise partially obscures the simulated lesion. **B,** The speckle has been reduced, increasing contrast resolution between the lesion and the background. *(From Merritt CR: Technology update. Radiol Clin North Am 2001;39:385-397.)*

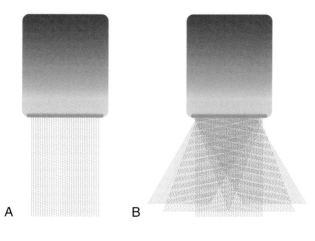

FIGURE 1-19. Spatial compounding. A, Conventional **imaging** is limited to a fixed angle of incidence of ultrasound scan lines to tissue interfaces, resulting in poor definition of specular reflectors that are not perpendicular to the beam. **B, Spatial compounding** combines images obtained by insonating the target from multiple angles. In addition to improving detection interfaces, compounding reduces speckle noise because only the signal is reinforced; speckle is random and not reinforced. This improves contrast.

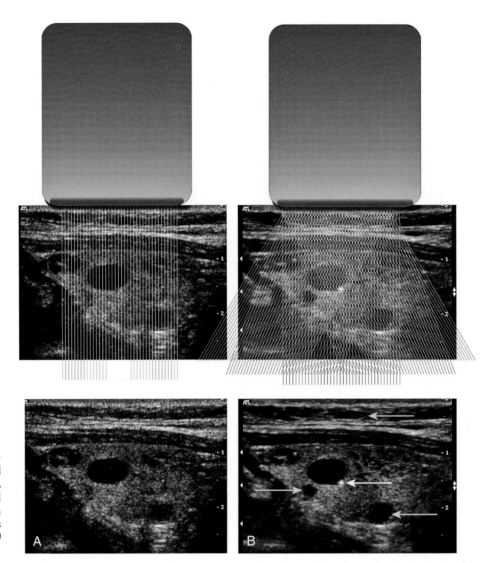

FIGURE 1-20. Spatial compounding. A, **Conventional image,** and B, **compound image,** of the thyroid. Note the reduced speckle as well as better definition of superficial tissue *(blue arrow)* as well as small cysts *(yellow arrows)* and calcifications *(white arrow).*

reflector at an angle greater or less than 90 degrees. In conventional real-time imaging, each scan line used to generate the image strikes the target at a constant, fixed angle. As a result, strong reflectors that are not perpendicular to the ultrasound beam scatter sound in directions that prevent their clear detection and display. This in turn results in poor margin definition and less distinct boundaries for cysts and other masses. Compounding has been found to reduce these artifacts. Limitations of compounding are diminished visibility of shadowing and enhancement; however, these are offset by the ability to evaluate lesions, both with and without compounding, preserving shadowing and enhancement when these features are important to diagnosis.[6]

Three-Dimensional Ultrasound

Dedicated 3-D scanners used for fetal, gynecologic, and cardiac scanning may employ hardware-based image registration, high-density 2-D arrays, or software registration of scan planes as a tissue volume is acquired. 3-D

imaging permits volume data to be viewed in multiple imaging planes and allows accurate measurement of lesion volume (Fig. 1-21).

IMAGE QUALITY

The key determinants of the quality of an ultrasound image are its spatial, contrast, and temporal resolution, as well as freedom from certain artifacts.

Spatial Resolution

The ability to differentiate two closely situated objects as distinct structures is determined by the spatial resolution of the ultrasound device. Spatial resolution must be considered in three planes, with different determinants of resolution for each. Simplest is the resolution along the axis of the ultrasound beam, or **axial resolution.** With pulsed wave ultrasound, the transducer introduces a series of brief bursts of sound into the body. Each

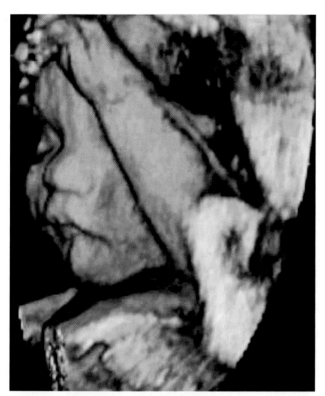

FIGURE 1-21. 3-D ultrasound image, 24-week fetus. Three-dimensional ultrasound permits collection and review of data obtained from a volume of tissue in multiple imaging planes, as well as a rendering of surface features.

ultrasound pulse typically consists of two or three cycles of sound. The pulse length is the product of the wavelength and the number of cycles in the pulse. Axial resolution, the maximum resolution along the beam axis, is determined by the pulse length (Fig. 1-22). Because ultrasound frequency and wavelength are inversely related, the pulse length decreases as the imaging frequency increases. Because the pulse length determines the maximum resolution along the axis of the ultrasound beam, **higher transducer frequencies provide higher image resolution**. For example, a transducer operating at 5 MHz produces sound with a wavelength of 0.308 mm. If each pulse consists of three cycles of sound, the pulse length is slightly less than 1 mm, and this becomes the maximum resolution along the beam axis. If the transducer frequency is increased to 15 MHz, the pulse length is less than 0.4 mm, permitting resolution of smaller details.

In addition to axial resolution, resolution in the planes perpendicular to the beam axis must also be considered. **Lateral resolution** refers to resolution in the plane perpendicular to the beam and parallel to the transducer and is determined by the **width** of the ultrasound beam. Azimuth resolution, or **elevation resolution**, refers to the slice **thickness** in the plane perpendicular to the beam and to the transducer (Fig. 1-23). Ultrasound is a tomographic method of imaging that produces thin slices of information from the body, and the width and thickness of the ultrasound beam are important determinants of image quality. Excessive beam width and thickness limit the ability to delineate small features and may obscure shadowing and enhancement from small structures, such as breast microcalcifications and small thyroid cysts. The width and thickness of the ultrasound beam determine lateral resolution and elevation resolution, respectively. Lateral and elevation resolutions are significantly poorer than the axial resolution of the beam. Lateral resolution is controlled by focusing the beam, usually by electronic phasing, to alter the beam width at a selected depth of interest. Elevation resolution is determined by the construction of the transducer and generally cannot be controlled by the user.

IMAGING PITFALLS

In ultrasound, perhaps more than in any other imaging method, the quality of the information obtained is determined by the user's ability to recognize and avoid artifacts and pitfalls.[7] Many imaging artifacts are induced by errors in scanning technique or improper use of the instrument and are preventable. Artifacts may cause misdiagnosis or may obscure important findings. Understanding artifacts is essential for correct interpretation of ultrasound examinations.

Many artifacts suggest the presence of structures not actually present. These include reverberation, refraction, and side lobes. **Reverberation artifacts** arise when the ultrasound signal reflects repeatedly between highly reflective interfaces that are usually, but not always, near the transducer (Fig. 1-24). Reverberations may also give the false impression of solid structures in areas where only fluid is present. Certain types of reverberation may be helpful because they allow the identification of a specific type of reflector, such as a surgical clip. Reverberation artifacts can usually be reduced or eliminated by changing the scanning angle or transducer placement to avoid the parallel interfaces that contribute to the artifact.

Refraction causes bending of the sound beam so that targets not along the axis of the transducer are insonated. Their reflections are then detected and displayed in the image. This may cause structures to appear in the image that actually lie outside the volume the investigator assumes is being examined (see Fig. 1-7). Similarly, side lobes may produce confusing echoes that arise from sound beams that lie outside the main ultrasound beam (Fig. 1-25). These **side lobe artifacts** are of clinical importance because they may create the impression of structures or debris in fluid-filled structures (Fig. 1-26). Side lobes may also result in errors of measurement by reducing lateral resolution. As with most other artifacts, repositioning the transducer and its focal zone or using a different transducer will usually allow the differentiation of artifactual from true echoes.

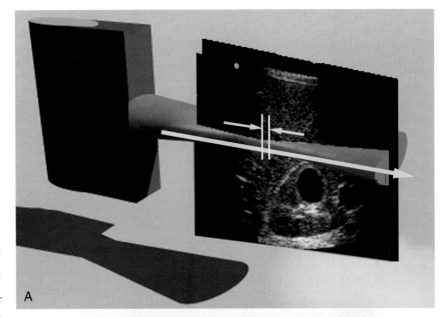

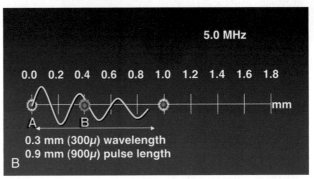

FIGURE 1-22. Axial resolution. Axial resolution is the resolution along the beam axis (**A**) and is determined by the pulse length (**B**). The pulse length is the product of the wavelength (which decreases with increasing frequency) and the number of waves (usually two to three). Because the pulse length determines axial resolution, higher transducer frequencies provide higher image resolution. In **B,** for example, a transducer operating at 5 MHz produces sound with a wavelength of 0.31 mm. If each pulse consists of three cycles of sound, the pulse length is slightly less than 1 mm, and objects *A* and *B*, which are 0.5 mm apart, cannot be resolved as separate structures. If the transducer frequency is increased to 15 MHz, the pulse length is less than 0.3 mm, permitting *A* and *B* to be identified as separate structures.

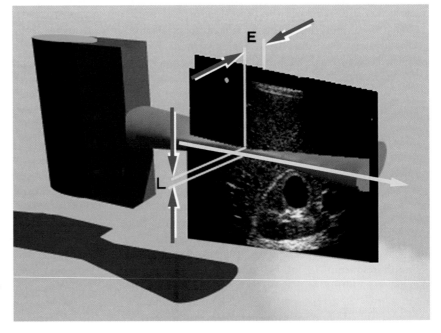

FIGURE 1-23. Lateral and elevation resolution. Resolution in the planes perpendicular to the beam axis is an important determinant of image quality. **Lateral resolution** *(L)* is resolution in the plane perpendicular to the beam and parallel to the transducer and is determined by the width of the ultrasound beam. Lateral resolution is controlled by focusing the beam, usually by electronic phasing to alter the beam width at a selected depth of interest. Azimuth or **elevation resolution** *(E)* is determined by the slice thickness in the plane perpendicular to the beam and the transducer. Elevation resolution is controlled by the construction of the transducer. Both lateral and elevation resolution are less than the axial resolution.

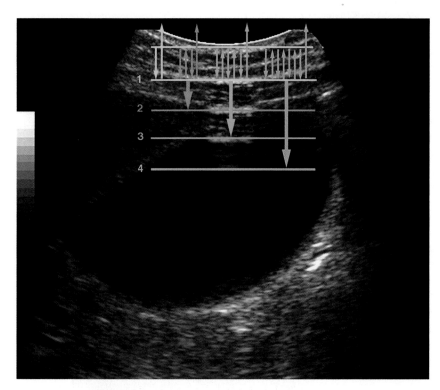

FIGURE 1-24. Reverberation artifact. Reverberation artifacts arise when the ultrasound signal reflects repeatedly between highly reflective interfaces near the transducer, resulting in delayed echo return to the transducer. This appears in the image as a series of regularly spaced echoes at increasing depth. The echo at depth *1* is produced by simple reflection from a strong interface. Echoes at levels *2, 3,* and *4* are produced by multiple reflections between this interface and the surface (simulated image).

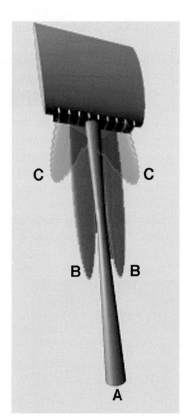

FIGURE 1-25. Side lobes. Although most of the energy generated by a transducer is emitted in a beam along the central axis of the transducer *(A),* some energy is also emitted at the periphery of the primary beam *(B* and *C).* These are called side lobes and are lower in intensity than the primary beam. Side lobes may interact with strong reflectors that lie outside of the scan plane and produce artifacts that are displayed in the ultrasound image (see also Fig. 1-26).

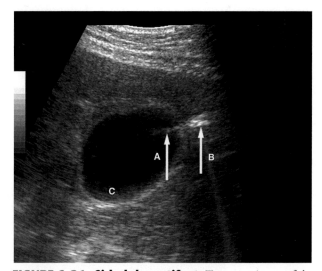

FIGURE 1-26. Side lobe artifact. Transverse image of the gallbladder reveals a **bright internal echo** *(A)* that suggests a band or septum within the gallbladder. This is a side lobe artifact related to the presence of a **strong out-of-plane reflector** *(B)* medial to the gallbladder. The low-level echoes in the dependent portion of the gallbladder *(C)* are also artifactual and are caused by the same phenomenon. Side lobe and slice thickness artifacts are of clinical importance because they may create the impression of debris in fluid-filled structures. As with most other artifacts, repositioning the transducer and its focal zone or using a different transducer will usually allow the differentiation of artifactual from true echoes.

Artifacts may also remove real echoes from the display or obscure information, and important pathology may be missed. **Shadowing** results when there is a marked reduction in the intensity of ultrasound deep to a strong reflector or attenuator. Shadowing causes partial or complete loss of information due to attenuation of the sound by superficial structures. Another common cause of loss of image information is **improper adjustment of system gain and TGC settings**. Many low-level echoes are near the noise levels of the equipment, and considerable skill and experience are needed to adjust instrument settings to display the maximum information with the minimum noise. **Poor scanning angles, inadequate penetration,** and **poor resolution** may also result in loss of significant information. **Careless selection of transducer frequency** and **lack of attention to the focal characteristics of the beam** will cause loss of clinically important information from deep, low-amplitude reflectors and small targets. Ultrasound artifacts may alter the size, shape, and position of structures. For example, a **multipath artifact** is created when the path of the returning echo is not the one expected, resulting in display of the echo at an improper location in the image (Fig. 1-27).

Shadowing and Enhancement

Although most artifacts degrade the ultrasound image and impede interpretation, two artifacts of clinical value are shadowing and enhancement. Again, shadowing results when an object (e.g., calculus) attenuates sound more rapidly than surrounding tissues. **Enhancement** occurs when an object (e.g., cyst) attenuates less than surrounding tissues. Failure of TGC applied to normal tissue to compensate properly for the attenuation of more highly attenuating (shadowing) or poorly attenuating (enhancing) structures produces the artifact (Fig. 1-28). Because attenuation increases with frequency, the effects of shadowing and enhancement are greater at higher than at lower frequencies. The conspicuity of

shadowing and enhancement is reduced by excessive beam width, improper focal zone placement, and use of spatial compounding.

DOPPLER SONOGRAPHY

Conventional B-mode ultrasound imaging uses pulse-echo transmission, detection, and display techniques. Brief pulses of ultrasound energy emitted by the transducer are reflected from acoustic interfaces within the body. Precise timing allows determination of the depth from which the echo originates. When pulsed wave ultrasound is reflected from an interface, the backscattered (reflected) signal contains amplitude, phase, and frequency information (Fig. 1-29). This information permits inference of the position, nature, and motion of the interface reflecting the pulse. B-mode ultrasound imaging uses only the amplitude information in the backscattered signal to generate the image, with differences in the strength of reflectors displayed in the image in varying shades of gray. Rapidly moving targets, such as red cells in the bloodstream, produce echoes of low amplitude that are not usually displayed, resulting in a relatively anechoic pattern within the lumens of large vessels.

Although gray-scale display relies on the amplitude of the backscattered ultrasound signal, additional information is present in the returning echoes that can be used to evaluate the motion of moving targets. When high-frequency sound impinges on a stationary interface, the reflected ultrasound has essentially the same frequency or wavelength as the transmitted sound (Fig. 1-30, *A*). If the reflecting interface is moving with respect to the sound beam emitted from the transducer, however, there is a change in the frequency of the sound scattered by the moving object (Fig. 1-30, *B* and *C*). This change in frequency is directly proportional to the velocity of the reflecting interface relative to the transducer and is a

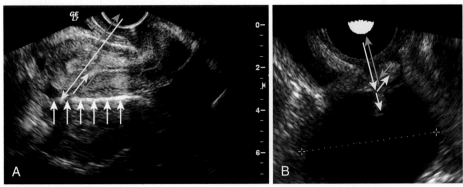

FIGURE 1-27. Multipath artifact. A, Mirror image of the uterus is created by reflection of sound from an interface produced by gas in the rectum. **B,** Echoes reflected from the wall of an ovarian cyst create complex echo paths that delay return of echoes to the transducer. In both examples, the longer path of the reflected sound results in the display of echoes at a greater depth than they should normally appear. In **A** this results in an artifactual image of the uterus appearing in the location of the rectum. In **B** the effect is more subtle and more likely to cause misdiagnosis because the artifact suggests a mural nodule in what is actually a simple ovarian cyst.

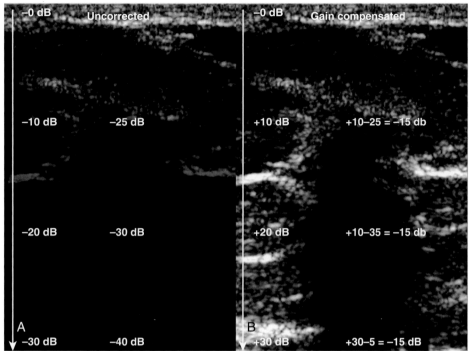

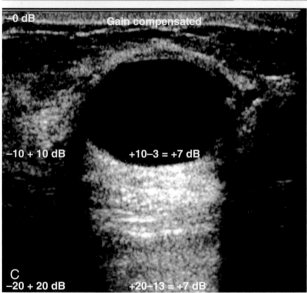

FIGURE 1-28. Shadowing and enhancement. A, Uncorrected image of a shadowing breast mass shows that the mass attenuates 15 dB more than the surrounding normal tissue. **B,** Application of appropriate TGC results in proper display of the normal breast tissue. However, because of the increased attenuation of the mass, a shadow results. **C,** Similarly, the cyst attenuates 7 dB less than the normal tissue, and TGC correction for normal tissue results in overamplification of the signals deep to the cyst, producing enhancement of these tissues.

result of the **Doppler effect.** The relationship of the returning ultrasound frequency to the velocity of the reflector is described by the Doppler equation, as follows:

$$\Delta F = (F_R - F_T) = 2 \cdot F_T \cdot v/c \quad 5$$

The **Doppler frequency shift** is ΔF; F_R is the frequency of sound reflected from the moving target; F_T is the frequency of sound emitted from the transducer; v is the velocity of the target toward the transducer; and c is the velocity of sound in the medium. The Doppler frequency shift (ΔF), as just described, applies only if the target is moving directly toward or away from the transducer (Fig. 1-31, *A*). In most clinical settings the direction of the ultrasound beam is seldom directly toward or

away from the direction of flow, and the ultrasound beam usually approaches the moving target at an angle designated as the **Doppler angle** (Fig. 1-31, *B*). In this case, ΔF is reduced in proportion to the cosine of this angle, as follows:

$$\Delta F = (F_R - F_T) = 2 \cdot F_T \cdot v \cdot \cos\theta/c \quad 6$$

where θ is the angle between the axis of flow and the incident ultrasound beam. If the Doppler angle can be measured, estimation of flow velocity is possible. Accurate estimation of target velocity requires precise measurement of both the Doppler frequency shift and the angle of insonation to the direction of target movement. As the Doppler angle (θ) approaches 90 degrees, the

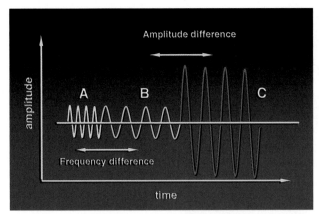

FIGURE 1-29. Backscattered information. The back-scattered ultrasound signal contains amplitude, phase, and frequency information. Signals *B* and *C* differ in amplitude but have the same frequency. Amplitude differences are used to generate B-mode images. Signals *A* and *B* differ in frequency but have similar amplitudes. Such frequency differences are the basis of Doppler ultrasound.

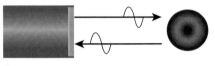

A   Stationary target: $(F_R - F_T) = 0$

B   Target motion toward transducer: $(F_R - F_T) > 0$

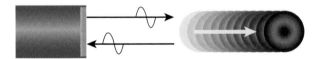

C   Target motion away from transducer: $(F_R - F_T) < 0$

FIGURE 1-30. Doppler effect. A, Stationary target. If the reflecting interface is stationary, the backscattered ultrasound has the same frequency or wavelength as the transmitted sound, and there is no difference in the transmitted (F_T) and reflected (F_R) frequencies. **B and C, Moving targets.** If the reflecting interface is moving with respect to the sound beam emitted from the transducer, there is a change in the frequency of the sound scattered by the moving object. When the interface moves toward the transducer **(B),** the difference in reflected and transmitted frequencies is greater than zero. When the target is moving away from the transducer **(C),** this difference is less than zero. The Doppler equation is used to relate this change in frequency to the velocity of the moving object.

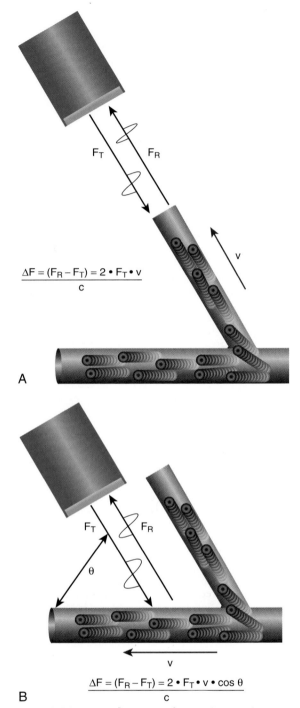

$$\Delta F = (F_R - F_T) = \frac{2 \cdot F_T \cdot v}{c}$$

A

$$\Delta F = (F_R - F_T) = \frac{2 \cdot F_T \cdot v \cdot \cos \theta}{c}$$

B

FIGURE 1-31. Doppler equations. The Doppler equation describes the relationship of the Doppler frequency shift to target velocity. **A,** In its simplest form, it is assumed that the direction of the ultrasound beam is parallel to the direction of movement of the target. This situation is unusual in clinical practice. More often, the ultrasound impinges on the vessel at angle θ. **B,** In this case the Doppler frequency shift detected is reduced in proportion to the cosine of θ.

cosine of θ approaches 0. At an **angle of 90 degrees,** there is no relative movement of the target toward or away from the transducer, and **no Doppler frequency shift** is detected (Fig. 1-32). Because the cosine of the Doppler angle changes rapidly for angles more than 60

degrees, accurate angle correction requires that Doppler measurements be made at angles of less than 60 degrees. Above 60 degrees, relatively small changes in the Doppler angle are associated with large changes in cosθ, and therefore a small error in estimation of the Doppler angle

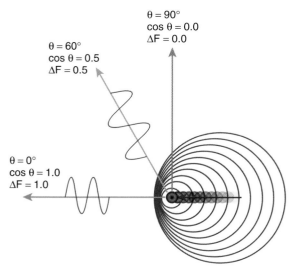

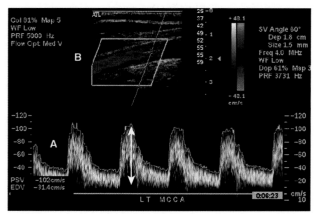

FIGURE 1-32. Effect of Doppler angle on frequency shift. At an angle of 60 degrees, the detected frequency shift detected by the transducer is only 50% of the shift detected at an angle of 0 degrees. At 90 degrees, there is no relative movement of the target toward or away from the transducer, and no frequency shift is detected. The detected Doppler frequency shift is reduced in proportion to the cosine of the Doppler angle. Because the cosine of the angle changes rapidly at angles above 60 degrees, the use of Doppler angles of less than 60 degrees is recommended in making velocity estimates.

FIGURE 1-33. Doppler display. A, Doppler frequency **spectrum waveform** shows changes in flow velocity and direction by vertical deflections of the waveform above and below the baseline. The width of the spectral waveform (spectral broadening) is determined by the range of frequencies present at any instant in time *(arrow)*. A brightness (gray) scale is used to indicate the amplitude of each frequency component. **B,** Color Doppler **imaging.** Amplitude data from stationary targets provide the basis for the B-mode image. Signal phase provides information about the presence and direction of motion, and changes in frequency relate to the velocity of the target. Backscattered signals from red blood cells are displayed in color as a function of their motion toward or away from the transducer, and the degree of the saturation of the color is used to indicate the frequency shift from moving red cells.

may result in a large error in the estimation of velocity. These considerations are important in using both duplex and color Doppler instruments. Optimal imaging of the vessel wall is obtained when the axis of the transducer is perpendicular to the wall, whereas maximal Doppler frequency differences are obtained when the transducer axis and the direction of flow are at a relatively small angle.

In peripheral vascular applications, it is highly desirable that measured **Doppler frequencies be corrected for the Doppler angle to provide velocity measurement.** This allows comparison of data from systems using different Doppler frequencies and eliminates error in interpretation of frequency data obtained at different Doppler angles. For abdominal applications, angle-corrected velocity measurements are encouraged, although qualitative assessments of flow are often made using only the Doppler frequency shift data. The interrelation of transducer frequency (FT) and the Doppler angle (θ) to the Doppler frequency shift (ΔF) and target velocity described by the Doppler equation are important in proper clinical use of Doppler equipment.

Doppler Signal Processing and Display

Several options exist for the processing of ΔF, the Doppler frequency shift, to provide useful information regarding the direction and velocity of blood. Doppler frequency shifts encountered clinically are in the audible

range. This audible signal may be analyzed by ear and, with training, the operator can identify many flow characteristics. More often, the Doppler shift data are displayed in graphic form as a time-varying plot of the frequency spectrum of the returning signal. A fast Fourier transformation is used to perform the frequency analysis. The resulting Doppler frequency spectrum displays the following (Fig. 1-33, *A*):

- Variation with time of the Doppler frequencies present in the volume sampled.
- The **envelope of the spectrum,** representing the maximum frequencies present at any given point in time.
- The **width of the spectrum** at any point, indicating the range of frequencies present.

The amplitude of the Doppler signal is related to the number of targets moving at a given velocity. In many instruments the amplitude of each frequency component is displayed in gray scale as part of the spectrum. The presence of a large number of different frequencies at a given point in the cardiac cycle results in **spectral broadening**.

In color Doppler imaging systems, a representation of the Doppler frequency shift is displayed as a feature of the image itself (Fig. 1-33, *B*). In addition to the detection of Doppler frequency shift data from each pixel in the image, these systems may also provide range-gated pulsed wave Doppler with spectral analysis for display of Doppler data.

Doppler Instrumentation

In contrast to A-mode, M-mode, and B-mode gray-scale ultrasonography, which display the information from tissue interfaces, Doppler ultrasound instruments are optimized to display **flow** information. The simplest Doppler devices use continuous wave rather than pulsed wave ultrasound, using two transducers that transmit and receive ultrasound continuously (**continuous wave or CW Doppler**). The transmit and receive beams overlap in a sensitive volume at some distance from the transducer face (Fig. 1-34, *A*). Although direction of flow can be determined with CW Doppler, these devices do not allow discrimination of motion coming from various depths, and the source of the signal being detected is difficult, if not impossible, to ascertain with certainty. Inexpensive and portable, CW Doppler instruments are used primarily at the bedside or intraoperatively to confirm the presence of flow in superficial vessels.

Because of the limitations of CW systems, most applications use range-gated, pulsed wave Doppler. Rather than a continuous wave of ultrasound emission, pulsed wave Doppler devices emit brief pulses of ultrasound energy (Fig. 1-34, *B*). Using pulses of sound permits use of the time interval between the transmission of a pulse and the return of the echo as a means of determining the depth from which the Doppler shift arises. The principles are similar to the echo-ranging principles used for imaging (see Fig. 1-4). In a pulsed wave Doppler system the sensitive volume from which flow data are sampled can be controlled in terms of shape, depth, and position. When pulsed wave Doppler is combined with a 2-D,

real-time, B-mode imager in the form of a **duplex scanner**, the position of the Doppler sample can be precisely controlled and monitored.

The most common form of Doppler ultrasound to be used for radiology applications is **color Doppler imaging**[8] (Fig. 1-35, *A*). In color Doppler imaging systems, frequency shift information determined from Doppler measurements is displayed as a feature of the image itself. Stationary or slowly moving targets provide the basis for the B-mode image. **Signal phase** provides information about the presence and direction of motion, and changes in echo signal frequency relate to the velocity of the target. Backscattered signals from red blood cells are displayed in color as a function of their motion toward or away from the transducer, and the degree of the saturation of the color is used to indicate the relative frequency shift produced by the moving red cells.

Color Doppler flow imaging (CDFI) expands conventional duplex sonography by providing additional capabilities. The use of color saturation to display variations in Doppler shift frequency allows an estimation of relative velocity from the image alone, provided that variations in the Doppler angle are noted. The display of flow throughout the image field allows the position and orientation of the vessel of interest to be observed at all times. The display of spatial information with respect to velocity is ideal for display of small, localized areas of turbulence within a vessel, which provide clues to stenosis or irregularity of the vessel wall caused by atheroma, trauma, or other disease. Flow within the vessel is observed at all points, and stenotic jets and focal areas of turbulence are displayed that might be overlooked with duplex instrumentation. The contrast of

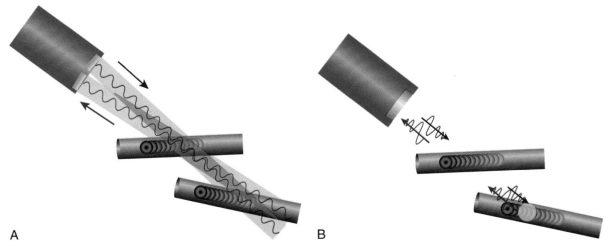

A   B

FIGURE 1-34. Continuous wave and pulsed wave Doppler. A, Continuous wave (CW) Doppler uses separate transmit and receive crystals that continuously transmit and receive ultrasound. Although able to detect the presence and direction of flow, CW devices are unable to distinguish signals arising from vessels at different depths *(green-shaded area).* **B,** Using the principle of ultrasound ranging (see Fig. 1-4), **pulsed wave Doppler** permits the sampling of flow data from selected depths by processing only the signals that return to the transducer after precisely timed intervals. The operator is able to control the position of the sample volume and, in duplex systems, to view the location from which the Doppler data are obtained.

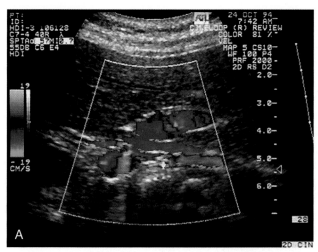
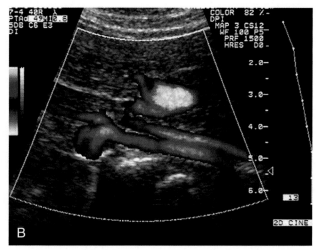

FIGURE 1-35. Color flow and power mode Doppler. A, Color flow Doppler imaging uses a color map to display information based on the detection of frequency shifts from moving targets. Noise in this form of display appears across the entire frequency spectrum and limits sensitivity. **B, Power mode Doppler** uses a color map to show the distribution of the power or amplitude of the Doppler signal. Flow direction and velocity information are not provided in power mode Doppler display, but noise is reduced, allowing higher gain settings and improved sensitivity for flow detection.

LIMITATIONS OF COLOR DOPPLER FLOW IMAGING

Angle dependence
Aliasing
Inability to display entire Doppler spectrum in the image
Artifacts caused by noise

ADVANTAGES OF POWER MODE DOPPLER

No aliasing
Much less angle dependence
Noise: a homogeneous background color
Increased sensitivity for flow detection

---

flow within the vessel lumen (1) permits visualization of small vessels that are invisible when using conventional imagers and (2) enhances the visibility of wall irregularity. CDFI aids in determination of the direction of flow and measurement of the Doppler angle.

Power Mode Doppler

An alternative to the display of frequency information with color Doppler imaging is to use a color map that displays the **integrated power** of the Doppler signal instead of its mean frequency shift[9] (Fig. 1-35, *B*). Because frequency shift data are not displayed, there is no aliasing. The image does not provide information related to flow direction or velocity, and power mode Doppler imaging is much less angle dependent than frequency-based color Doppler display. In contrast to color Doppler, where noise may appear in the image as any color, power mode Doppler permits noise to be assigned to a homogeneous background color that does not greatly interfere with the image. This results in a significant increase in the usable dynamic range of the scanner, permitting higher effective gain settings and increased sensitivity for flow detection (Fig. 1-36).

Interpretation of the Doppler Spectrum

Doppler data components that must be evaluated both in spectral display and in color Doppler imaging include the Doppler shift frequency and amplitude, the Doppler angle, the spatial distribution of frequencies across the vessel, and the temporal variation of the signal. Because the Doppler signal itself has no anatomic significance, the examiner must interpret the Doppler signal and then determine its relevance in the context of the image.

The detection of a Doppler frequency shift indicates movement of the target, which in most applications is related to the presence of flow. The sign of the frequency shift (positive or negative) indicates the direction of flow relative to the transducer. **Vessel stenosis** is typically associated with large Doppler frequency shifts in both systole and diastole at the site of greatest narrowing, with turbulent flow in poststenotic regions. In peripheral vessels, analysis of the Doppler changes allows accurate prediction of the degree of vessel narrowing. Information related to the resistance to flow in the distal vascular tree can be obtained by analysis of changes of blood velocity with time, as shown in the **Doppler spectral display.**

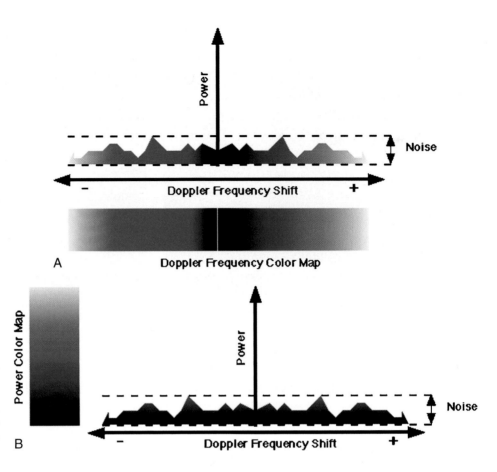

FIGURE 1-36. Frequency and power mode color mapping. A, Conventional color Doppler uses the color map to show differences in flow direction and Doppler frequency shift. Because noise appears over the entire frequency spectrum, gain levels are limited to those that do not introduce excessive noise. **B, Power mode Doppler** color map, in contrast, indicates the amplitude of the Doppler signal. Because most noise is of low amplitude, it is possible to map this to colors near the background. This permits the use of high gain settings that offer significant improvements over conventional color Doppler in flow detection.

Figure 1-37 provides a graphic example of the changes in the Doppler spectral waveform resulting from physiologic changes in the resistance of the vascular bed supplied by a normal brachial artery. A blood pressure cuff has been inflated to above systolic pressure to occlude the distal branches supplied by the brachial artery. This **occlusion** causes reduced systolic amplitude and cessation of diastolic flow, resulting in a waveform different than that found in the normal resting state. During the period of ischemia induced by pressure cuff occlusion of the forearm vessels, **vasodilation** has occurred. The Doppler waveform now reflects a low-resistance peripheral vascular bed with increased systolic amplitude and rapid flow throughout diastole, typical for vasodilation.

Doppler indices include the systolic/diastolic ratio, resistive index, and pulsatility index (Fig. 1-38). These compare blood flow in systole and diastole, show resistance to flow in the peripheral vascular bed, and help evaluate the perfusion of tumors, renal transplants, the placenta, and other organs. With Doppler ultrasound, it is therefore possible to identify vessels, determine the direction of blood flow, evaluate narrowing or occlusion, and characterize blood flow to organs and tumors. Analysis of the Doppler shift frequency with time can be used to infer both proximal stenosis and changes in distal vascular impedance. Most work using pulsed wave Doppler imaging has emphasized the detection of stenosis, thrombosis, and flow disturbances in major peripheral arteries and veins. In these applications, measurement of peak systolic and end diastolic frequency or velocity, analysis of the Doppler spectrum, and calculation of certain frequency or velocity ratios have been the basis of analysis. Changes in the spectral waveform measured by indices comparing flow in systole and diastole indicate the resistance of the vascular bed supplied by the vessel and the changes resulting from a variety of pathologies.

Changes in Doppler indices from normal may help in the early identification of rejection of transplanted organs, parenchymal dysfunction, and malignancy. Although useful, these measurements are influenced not only by the resistance to flow in peripheral vessels, but also by heart rate, blood pressure, vessel wall length and elasticity, extrinsic organ compression, and other factors. Therefore, interpretation must always take into account these variables.

Interpretation of Color Doppler

Although the graphic presentation of color Doppler imaging suggests that interpretation is made easier, the complexity of the color Doppler image actually makes this a more demanding image to evaluate than the simple Doppler spectrum. Nevertheless, color Doppler imaging has important advantages over pulsed wave duplex Doppler imaging, in which flow data are obtained only from a small portion of the area being imaged. To be

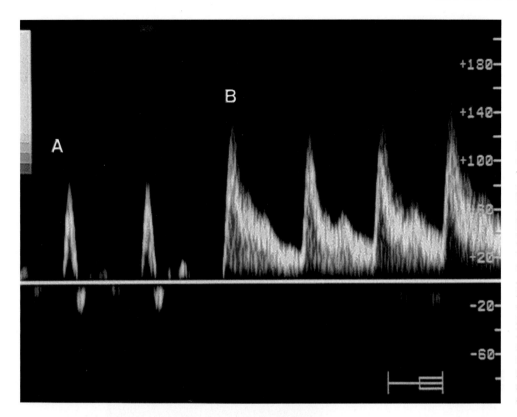

FIGURE 1-37. Impedance. *A,* **High-resistance waveform in brachial artery** produced by inflating forearm blood pressure cuff to a pressure above the systolic blood pressure. As a result of high peripheral resistance, there is low systolic amplitude and reversed diastolic flow. *B,* **Low-resistance waveform in peripheral vascular bed** caused by vasodilation stimulated by the prior ischemia. Immediately after release of 3 minutes of occluding pressure, the Doppler waveform showed increased amplitude and rapid antegrade flow throughout diastole.

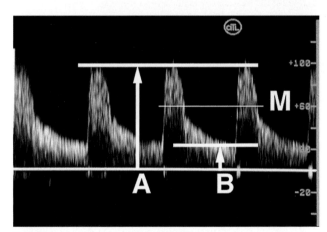

FIGURE 1-38. Doppler indices. Doppler imaging can provide information about blood flow in both large and small vessels. Small vessel impedance is reflected in the Doppler spectral waveform of afferent vessels. Doppler flow indices used to characterize peripheral resistance are based on the **peak systolic frequency** or **velocity** *(A),* the **minimum** or **end diastolic frequency** or **velocity** *(B),* and the **mean frequency** or **velocity** *(M).* The most frequently used indices are the **systolic/diastolic ratio** (A/B); **resistive index** [(A-B)/A]; and **pulsatility index** [(A-B)/M]. In calculation of the pulsatility index, the minimum diastolic velocity or frequency is used; calculation of the systolic/diastolic ratio and resistive index use the end diastolic value.

confident that a conventional Doppler study has achieved reasonable sensitivity and specificity in detection of flow disturbances, a methodical search and sampling of multiple sites within the field of interest must be performed. In contrast, CDFI devices permit simultaneous sampling of multiple sites and are less susceptible to this error.

Although color Doppler can indicate the presence of blood flow, misinterpretation of color Doppler images may result in significant errors. Each color pixel displays a representation of the Doppler frequency shift detected at that point. The frequency shift displayed is not the peak frequency present at sampling but rather a **weighted mean frequency** that attempts to account for the range of frequencies and their relative amplitudes at sampling. Manufacturers use different methods to derive the weighted mean frequency displayed in their systems. In addition, the pulse repetition frequency (PRF) and the color map selected to display the detected range of frequencies affect the color displayed. The color assigned to each Doppler pixel is determined by the Doppler frequency shift (which in turn is determined by target velocity and Doppler angle), the PRF, and the color map selected for display; therefore the interpretation of a color Doppler image must consider each of these variables. Although most manufacturers provide on-screen indications suggesting a relationship between the color displayed and flow velocity, this is misleading because color Doppler does not show velocity and only indicates the weighted mean frequency shift measured in the vessel; without correction for the effect of the Doppler angle, velocity cannot be estimated (Fig. 1-39). Since the frequency shift at a given point is a function of velocity and the Doppler angle, depending on the frequency shift present in a given pixel and the PRF, *any* velocity may be represented by *any* color, and under certain circumstances, low-velocity flow may not be shown at all. As with spectral Doppler, **aliasing** is determined by PRF.

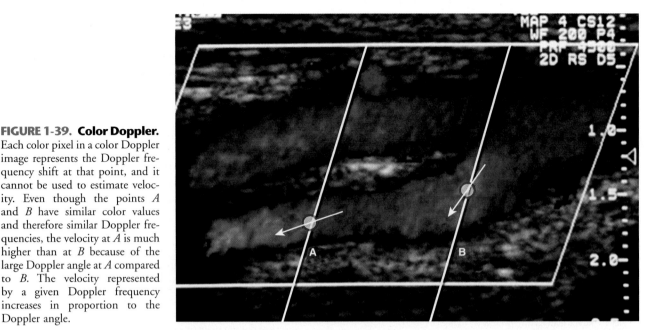

FIGURE 1-39. Color Doppler. Each color pixel in a color Doppler image represents the Doppler frequency shift at that point, and it cannot be used to estimate velocity. Even though the points *A* and *B* have similar color values and therefore similar Doppler frequencies, the velocity at *A* is much higher than at *B* because of the large Doppler angle at *A* compared to *B*. The velocity represented by a given Doppler frequency increases in proportion to the Doppler angle.

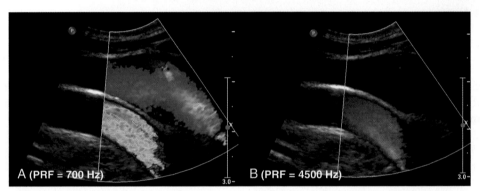

FIGURE 1-40. Pulse repetition frequency (PRF). Depending on the color map selected, velocity of the target, Doppler angle, and PRF, a given velocity may appear as any color with color Doppler. **A** and **B** are sonograms of identical vessels. **A,** PRF is 700 Hz, which results in aliasing of the higher Doppler frequency shifts in the carotid artery, but permits the identification of relatively slow flow in the jugular vein. **B,** PRF is 4500 Hz, eliminating aliasing in the artery but also suppressing the display of the low Doppler frequencies in the internal jugular vein.

With color Doppler, aliasing causes frequencies greater than twice the PRF to "wrap around" and to be displayed in the opposite colors of the color map. Inexperienced users tend to associate color Doppler aliasing with elevated velocity, but even low velocities may show marked aliasing if PRF is sufficiently low. As PRF is increased, aliasing of high Doppler frequency shifts is reduced; however, low frequency shifts may be eliminated from the display, resulting in diagnostic error (Fig. 1-40).

Other Technical Considerations

Although many problems and artifacts associated with B-mode imaging (e.g., shadowing) are encountered with Doppler sonography, the detection and display of frequency information related to moving targets present additional technical considerations. It is important to

understand the source of these artifacts and their influence on the interpretation of the flow measurements obtained in clinical practice.

Doppler Frequency

A primary objective of the Doppler examination is the accurate measurement of characteristics of flow within a vascular structure. The moving red blood cells that serve as the primary source of the Doppler signal act as **point scatterers** of ultrasound rather than specular reflectors. This interaction results in the intensity of the scattered sound varying in proportion to the fourth power of the frequency, which is important in selecting the Doppler frequency for a given examination. As the transducer frequency increases, Doppler **sensitivity** improves, but attenuation by tissue also increases, resulting in dimin-

MAJOR SOURCES OF DOPPLER IMAGING ARTIFACTS

DOPPLER FREQUENCY
Higher frequencies lead to more tissue attenuation.
Wall filters remove signals from low-velocity blood flow.

INCREASE IN SPECTRAL BROADENING
Excessive system gain or changes in dynamic range of the gray-scale display.
Excessively large sample volume.
Sample volume too near the vessel wall.

INCREASE IN ALIASING
Decrease in pulse repetition frequency PRF.
Decrease in Doppler angle.
Higher Doppler frequency transducer.

DOPPLER ANGLE
Relatively inaccurate above 60 degrees.

SAMPLE VOLUME SIZE
Large sample volumes increase vessel wall noise.

ished **penetration.** Careful balancing of the requirements for sensitivity and penetration is an important responsibility of the operator during a Doppler examination. Because many abdominal vessels lie several centimeters beneath the surface, Doppler frequencies in the range of 3 to 3.5 MHz are usually required to permit adequate penetration.

Wall Filters

Doppler instruments detect motion not only from blood flow but also from adjacent structures. To eliminate these low-frequency signals from the display, most instruments use **high pass filters,** or "wall" filters, which remove signals that fall below a given frequency limit. Although effective in eliminating low-frequency noise, these filters may also remove signals from low-velocity blood flow (Fig. 1-41). In certain clinical situations the measurement of these slower flow velocities is of clinical importance, and the improper selection of the wall filter may result in serious errors of interpretation. For example, low-velocity venous flow may not be detected if an improper filter is used, and low-velocity diastolic flow in certain arteries may also be eliminated from the display, resulting in errors in the calculation of Doppler indices, such as the systolic/diastolic ratio or resistive index. In general, the filter should be kept at the lowest practical level, usually 50 to 100 Hz.

Spectral Broadening

Spectral broadening refers to the presence of a large range of flow velocities at a given point in the pulse cycle and, by indicating turbulence, is an important criterion of high-grade vessel narrowing. Excessive system gain or changes in the dynamic range of the gray-scale display of the Doppler spectrum may suggest spectral broadening; opposite settings may mask broadening of the Doppler spectrum, causing diagnostic inaccuracy. Spectral broadening may also be produced by the selection

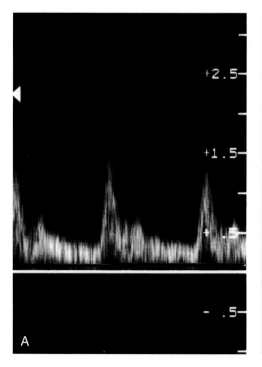
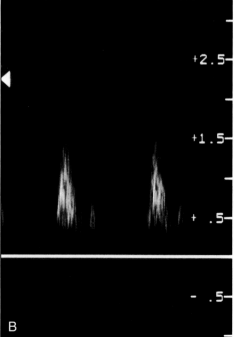

FIGURE 1-41. Wall filters. Wall filters are used to eliminate low-frequency noise from the Doppler display. Here the effect on the display of low-velocity flow is shown with wall filter settings of **A,** 100 Hz, and **B,** 400 Hz. High wall filter settings remove signal from low-velocity blood flow and may result in interpretation errors. In general, wall filters should be kept at the lowest practical level, usually in the range of 50 to 100 Hz.

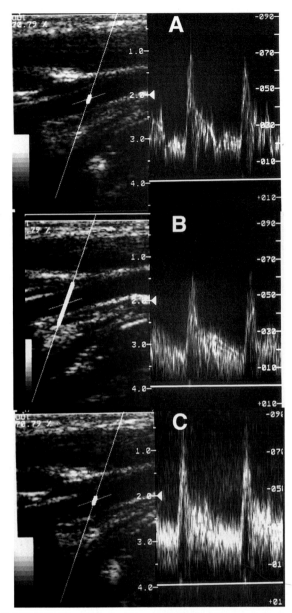

FIGURE 1-42. Spectral broadening. The range of velocities detected at a given time in the pulse cycle is reflected in the Doppler spectrum as spectral broadening. **A, Normal spectrum.** Spectral broadening may arise from turbulent flow in association with vessel stenosis. **B and C, Artifactual spectral broadening** may be produced by improper positioning of the sample volume near the vessel wall, use of an excessively large sample volume (**B**), or excessive system gain (**C**).

of an excessively large sample volume or by the placement of the sample volume too near the vessel wall, where slower velocities are present (Fig. 1-42).

Aliasing

Aliasing is an artifact arising from ambiguity in the measurement of high Doppler frequency shifts. To ensure that samples originate from only a selected depth when using a pulsed wave Doppler system, it is necessary to wait for the echo from the area of interest before trans-

mitting the next pulse. This limits the rate with which pulses can be generated, a lower PRF being required for greater depth. The PRF also determines the maximum depth from which unambiguous data can be obtained. If PRF is less than twice the maximum frequency shift produced by movement of the target (Nyquist limit), aliasing results (Fig. 1-43, A and B). When PRF is less than twice the frequency shift being detected, lower frequency shifts than are actually present are displayed. Because of the need for lower PRFs to reach deep vessels, signals from deep abdominal arteries are prone to aliasing if high velocities are present. In practice, aliasing is usually readily recognized (Fig. 1-43, C and D). Aliasing can be reduced by increasing the PRF, by increasing the Doppler angle—thereby decreasing the frequency shift—or by using a lower-frequency Doppler transducer.

Doppler Angle

When making Doppler measurement of velocity, it is necessary to correct for the Doppler angle. The accuracy of a velocity estimate obtained with Doppler is only as great as the accuracy of the measurement of the Doppler angle. This is particularly true as the Doppler angle exceeds 60 degrees. In general, the **Doppler angle is best kept at 60 degrees or less** because small changes in the Doppler angle above 60 degrees result in significant changes in the calculated velocity. Therefore, measurement inaccuracies result in much greater errors in velocity estimates than do similar errors at lower Doppler angles. Angle correction is not required for the measurement of Doppler indices such as the resistive index, because these measurements are based only on the relationship of the systolic and diastolic amplitudes.

Sample Volume Size

With pulsed wave Doppler systems, the length of the Doppler sample volume can be controlled by the operator, and the width is determined by the beam profile. Analysis of Doppler signals requires that the sample volume be adjusted to exclude as much of the unwanted clutter as possible from near the vessel walls.

Doppler Gain

As with imaging, proper gain settings are essential to accurate and reproducible Doppler measurements. *Excessive* Doppler gain results in noise appearing at all frequencies and may result in overestimation of velocity. Conversely, *insufficient* gain may result in underestimation of peak velocity (Fig. 1-44). A consistent approach to setting Doppler gain should be used. After placing the sample volume in the vessel, the Doppler gain should be increased to a level where noise is visible in the image, then gradually reduced to the point at which the noise first disappears completely.

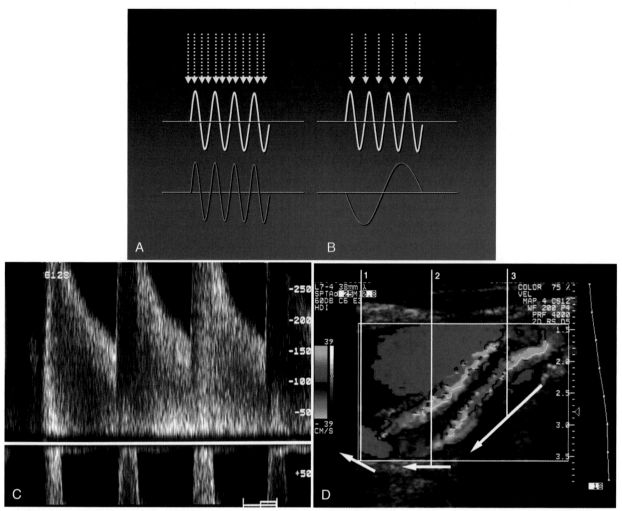

FIGURE 1-43. Aliasing. Pulse repetition frequency (PRF) determines the sampling rate of a given Doppler frequency. **A,** If PRF *(arrows)* is sufficient, the sampled waveform *(orange curve)* will accurately estimate the frequency being sampled *(yellow curve)*. **B,** If PRF is less than half the frequency being measured, **undersampling** will result in a lower frequency shift being displayed *(orange curve)*. **C,** In a clinical setting, **aliasing** appears in the spectral display as a "wraparound" of the higher frequencies to display below the baseline. **D,** In color Doppler display, aliasing results in a wraparound of the frequency color map from one flow direction to the opposite direction, passing through a transition of unsaturated color. The velocity throughout the vessel is constant, but aliasing appears only in portions of the vessel because of the effect of the Doppler angle on the Doppler frequency shift. As the angle increases, the Doppler frequency shift decreases, and aliasing is no longer seen.

OPERATING MODES: CLINICAL IMPLICATIONS

Ultrasound devices may operate in several modes, including real-time, color Doppler, spectral Doppler, and M-mode imaging. Imaging is produced in a *scanned* mode of operation. In scanned modes, pulses of ultrasound from the transducer are directed down lines of sight that are moved or steered in sequence to generate the image. This means that the number of ultrasound pulses arriving at a given point in the patient over a given interval is relatively small, and relatively little energy is deposited at any given location. In contrast, spectral Doppler imaging is an *unscanned* mode of operation in which multiple ultrasound pulses are sent in repetition

along a line to collect the Doppler data. In this mode the beam is stationary, resulting in considerably greater potential for heating than in imaging modes. For imaging, PRFs are usually a few thousand hertz with very short pulses. Longer pulse durations are used with Doppler than with other imaging modes. In addition, to avoid aliasing and other artifacts with Doppler imaging, it is often necessary to use higher PRFs than with other imaging applications. **Longer pulse duration and higher PRF** result in higher duty factors for Doppler modes of operation and increase the amount of energy introduced in scanning. Color Doppler, although a scanned mode, produces exposure conditions between those of real-time and Doppler imaging because color Doppler devices tend to send more pulses down each scan line and may use longer pulse durations than

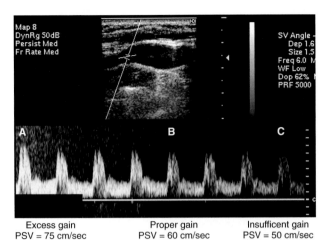

Excess gain
PSV = 75 cm/sec

Proper gain
PSV = 60 cm/sec

Insufficient gain
PSV = 50 cm/sec

FIGURE 1-44. Doppler gain. Accurate estimation of velocity requires proper Doppler gain adjustment. **Excessive gain** will cause an overestimation of peak velocity *(A)*, and **insufficient gain** will result in underestimation of velocity *(C)*. To adjust gain properly, the sample volume and Doppler angle are first set at the sample site. The gain is turned up until noise appears in the background *(A)*, then is gradually reduced just to the point where the background noise disappears from the image *(B)*.

imaging devices. Clearly, every user needs to be aware that switching from an imaging to a Doppler mode changes the exposure conditions and the potential for biologic effects (bioeffects).

With current devices operating in imaging modes, concerns about bioeffects are minimal because intensities sufficient to produce measurable heating are seldom used. **With Doppler ultrasound, the potential for thermal effects is greater.** Preliminary measurements on commercially available instruments suggest that at least some of these instruments are capable of producing temperature rises of greater than 1° C at soft tissue/bone interfaces, if the focal zone of the transducer is held stationary. Care is therefore warranted when Doppler measurements are obtained at or near soft tissue/bone interfaces, as in the second and third trimester of pregnancy. These applications require thoughtful application of the principle of ALARA (as low as reasonably achievable). Under ALARA the user should use the lowest possible acoustic exposure to obtain the necessary diagnostic information.

Bioeffects and User Concerns

Although users of ultrasound need to be aware of bioeffects concerns, another key factor to consider in the safe use of ultrasound is the user. The knowledge and skill of the user are major determinants of the risk-to-benefit implications of the use of ultrasound in a specific clinical situation. For example, an unrealistic emphasis on risks may discourage an appropriate use of ultrasound, resulting in harm to the patient by preventing the acquisition of useful information or by subjecting the patient to

another, more hazardous examination. The skill and experience of the individual performing and interpreting the examination are likely to have a major impact on the overall benefit of the examination. In view of the rapid growth of ultrasound and its proliferation into the hands of minimally trained clinicians, many more patients are likely to be harmed by misdiagnosis resulting from improper indications, poor examination technique, and errors in interpretation than from bioeffects. Failure to diagnose a significant anomaly or misdiagnosis (e.g., of ectopic pregnancy) are real dangers, and poorly trained users may be the greatest current hazard of diagnostic ultrasound.

Understanding bioeffects is essential for the prudent use of diagnostic ultrasound and is important in ensuring that the excellent risk-to-benefit performance of diagnostic ultrasound is preserved. All users of ultrasound should be prudent, understanding as fully as possible the potential risks and obvious benefits of ultrasound examinations, as well as those of alternate diagnostic methods. With this information, operators can monitor exposure conditions and implement the principle of ALARA to keep patient and fetal exposure as low as possible while fulfilling diagnostic objectives.

THERAPEUTIC APPLICATIONS: HIGH-INTENSITY FOCUSED ULTRASOUND

Although the primary medical application of ultrasound has been for diagnosis, therapeutic applications are developing rapidly, particularly the use of high-intensity focused ultrasound (HIFU). HIFU is based on three important capabilities of ultrasound: (1) focusing the ultrasound beam to produce highly localized energy deposition, (2) controlling the location and size of the focal zone, and (3) using intensities sufficient to destroy tissue at the focal zone. This has led to an interest in HIFU as a means of destroying noninvasive tumor and controlling bleeding and cardiac conduction anomalies.

High-intensity focused ultrasound exploits **thermal** (heating of tissues) and **mechanical** (cavitation) bioeffect mechanisms. As ultrasound passes through tissue, attenuation occurs through scattering and absorption. Scattering of ultrasound results in the return of some of the transmitted energy to the transducer, where it is detected and used to produce an image, or Doppler display. The remaining energy is transmitted to the molecules in the acoustic field and produces heating. At the **spatial peak temporal average** (SPTA), intensities of 50 to 500 mW/cm^2 used for imaging and Doppler, heating is minimal, and no observable bioeffects related to tissue heating in humans have yet been documented with clinical devices. With higher intensities, however, tissue heating sufficient to destroy tissue may be achieved. Using HIFU at 1 to 3 mHz, focal peak intensities of 5000 to 20,000 W/

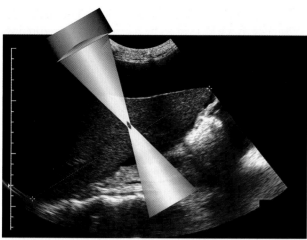

FIGURE 1-45. High-intensity focused ultrasound (HIFU). Local tissue destruction by heating may be achieved using HIFU delivered with focal peak intensities of several thousand W/cm². Tissue destruction can be confined to a small area a few millimeters in size without injury to adjacent tissues. HIFU is a promising tool for minimally invasive treatment of bleeding sites, uterine fibroids, and tumors in the prostate, liver, and breast.

cm² may be achieved. This energy can be delivered to a small point several millimeters in size, producing rapid temperature elevation and resulting in tissue coagulation, with little damage to adjacent tissues (Fig. 1-45). The destruction of tissue is a function of the temperature reached and the duration of the temperature elevation. In general, elevation of tissue to a temperature of 60° C for 1 second is sufficient to produce **coagulation necrosis.** These conditions are readily achieved with HIFU.

Because of its ability to produce highly localized tissue destruction, HIFU has been investigated as a tool for noninvasive or minimally invasive treatment of bleeding sites, uterine fibroids, and tumors in the prostate, liver, and breast.[10,11] As with diagnostic ultrasound, HIFU is limited by the presence of gas or bone interposed between the transducer and the target tissue. The reflection of high-energy ultrasound from strong interfaces produced

by bowel gas, aerated lung, or bone may result in tissue heating along the reflected path of the sound, producing unintended tissue damage.

Major challenges with HIFU include image guidance and accurate monitoring of therapy as it is being delivered. Magnetic resonance imaging (MRI) provides a means of monitoring temperature elevation during treatment, which is not possible with ultrasound. Guidance of therapy may be done with ultrasound or MRI, with ultrasound guidance having the advantage of verification of the acoustic window and sound path for the delivery of HIFU.

References

Basic Acoustics

1. Chivers RC, Parry RJ. Ultrasonic velocity and attenuation in mammalian tissues. J Acoust Soc Am 1978;63:940-953.
2. Goss SA, Johnston RL, Dunn F. Comprehensive compilation of empirical ultrasonic properties of mammalian tissues. J Acoust Soc Am 1978;64:423-457.
3. Merritt CR, Kremkau FW, Hobbins JC. Diagnostic ultrasound: bioeffects and safety. Ultrasound Obstet Gynecol 1992;2:366-374.
4. Medical diagnostic ultrasound instrumentation and clinical interpretation. Report of the Ultrasonography Task Force, Council on Scientific Affairs. JAMA 1991;265:1155-1159.

Instrumentation

5. Krishan S, Li PC, O'Donnell M. Adaptive compensation of phase and magnitude aberrations. IEEE Trans Ultrasonics Fer Freq Control 1996;43:44.
6. Merritt CR. Technology update. Radiol Clin North Am 2001;39:385-397.
7. Merritt CR. Doppler US: the basics. Radiographics 1991;11:109-119.
8. Merritt CR. Doppler color flow imaging. J Clin Ultrasound 1987;15:591-597.
9. Rubin JM, Bude RO, Carson PL, et al. Power Doppler US: a potentially useful alternative to mean frequency-based color Doppler US. Radiology 1994;190:853-856.

Therapeutic Applications: High-Intensity Focused Ultrasound

10. Dubinsky TJ, Cuevas C, Dighe MK, et al. High-intensity focused ultrasound: current potential and oncologic applications. AJR Am J Roentgenol 2008;190:191-199.
11. Kennedy JE, Ter Haar GR, Cranston D. High-intensity focused ultrasound: surgery of the future? Br J Radiol 2003;76:590-599.

CHAPTER 2

Biologic Effects and Safety

J. Brian Fowlkes and Christy K. Holland

Chapter Outline

*U*ltrasound has provided a wealth of knowledge in diagnostic medicine and has greatly impacted medical practice, particularly obstetrics. Millions of sonographic examinations are performed each year, and ultrasound remains one of the fastest-growing imaging modalities because of its low cost, real-time interactions, portability, and apparent lack of biologic effects (bioeffects). No casual relationship has been established between clinical applications of diagnostic ultrasound and bioeffects on the patient or operator.

REGULATION OF ULTRASOUND OUTPUT

At present, the U.S. Food and Drug Administration (FDA) regulates the maximum output of ultrasound devices to an established level. The marketing approval process requires devices to be equivalent in efficacy and output to those produced before 1976. This historic regulation of sonography has provided a safety margin for ultrasound while allowing clinically useful performance. The mechanism has restricted ultrasound exposure to levels that apparently produce few, if any, obvious bioeffects based on the epidemiologic evidence, although animal studies have shown some evidence for biologic effects.

In an effort to increase the efficacy of diagnostic ultrasound, the maximum acoustic output for some applications has increased through an additional FDA market approval process termed "510K Track 3." The vast majority of ultrasound systems currently in use were approved through this process. The Track 3 process provides the potential for better imaging performance and, as discussed later, requires that additional information be reported to the operator regarding the relative potential for bioeffects. Therefore, informed decision making is important concerning the possible adverse effects of ultrasound in relation to the desired diagnostic information. Current FDA regulations that limit the maximum output are still in place, but in the future, systems might allow sonographers and physicians the discretion to increase acoustic output beyond a level that might induce a biologic response.

Although the choices made during sonographic examinations may not be equivalent to the risk-versus-benefit decisions associated with imaging modalities using ionizing radiation, the operator will be increasingly responsible for determining the diagnostically required amount of ultrasound exposure. Thus the operator should know the potential bioeffects associated with ultrasound exposure. Patients also need to be reassured about the safety of a diagnostic ultrasound scan. The scientific community has identified some potential bioeffects from sonography, and although no causal relation has been established, it does not mean that no effects exist. Therefore it is important to understand the interaction of ultrasound with biologic systems.

PHYSICAL EFFECTS OF SOUND

The physical effects of sound can be divided into two principal groups: **thermal** and **nonthermal.** Most medical professionals recognize the thermal effects of elevated temperature on tissue, and the effects caused by ultrasound are similar to those of any localized heat source. With ultrasound the heating mainly results from the absorption of the sound field as it propagates through tissue. However, "nonthermal" sources can generate heat as well.

Many nonthermal mechanisms for bioeffects exist. Acoustic fields can apply **radiation forces** (not ionizing radiation) on the structures within the body both at the macroscopic and the microscopic level, resulting in exerted pressure and torque. The temporal average pressure in an acoustic field is different than the hydrostatic pressure of the fluid, and any object in the field is subject to this change in pressure. The effect is typically considered smaller than other effects because it relies on less significant factors in the formulation of the acoustic field. Acoustic fields can also cause motion of fluids. Such acoustically induced flow is called **streaming.**

Acoustic cavitation is the action of acoustic fields within a fluid to generate bubbles and cause volume pulsation or even collapse in response to the acoustic field. The result can be heat generation and associated free radical generation, microstreaming of fluid around the bubble, radiation forces generated by the scattered acoustic field from the bubble, and mechanical actions from bubble collapse. The interaction of acoustic fields with bubbles or "gas bodies" (as they are generally called) has been a significant area of bioeffects research in recent years.

THERMAL EFFECTS

Ultrasound Produces Heat

As ultrasound propagates through the body, energy is lost through **attenuation.** Attenuation causes loss of penetration and the inability to image deeper tissues. Attenuation is the result of two processes, scattering and absorption. **Scattering** of the ultrasound results from the redirection of the acoustic energy by tissue encountered during propagation. With diagnostic ultrasound, some of the acoustic energy transmitted into the tissue is scattered back in the direction of the transducer, termed **backscatter,** which allows a signal to be detected and images made. Energy also is lost along the propagation

path of the ultrasound by **absorption.** Absorption loss occurs substantially through the conversion of the ultrasound energy into heat. This heating provides a mechanism for ultrasound-induced bioeffects.

Factors Controlling Tissue Heating

The rate of temperature increase in tissues exposed to ultrasound depends on a several factors, including spatial focusing, ultrasound frequency, exposure duration, and tissue type.

Spatial Focusing

Ultrasound systems use multiple techniques to concentrate or focus ultrasound energy and improve the quality of measured signals. The analogy for light is that of a magnifying glass. The glass collects all the light striking its surface and concentrates it into a small region. In sonography and acoustics in general, the term **intensity** is used to describe the spatial distribution of ultrasonic **power** (energy per unit time), where **intensity = power/area** and the **area** refers to the cross-sectional area of the ultrasound beam. Another common beam dimension is the **beam width** at a specified location of the field. If the same ultrasonic power is concentrated into a smaller area, the intensity will increase.

Focusing in an ultrasound system can be used to improve the spatial resolution of the images. The side effect is an increased potential for bioeffects caused by heating and cavitation. In general, the greatest heating potential is between the scanhead and the focus, but the exact position depends on the focal distance, tissue properties, and heat generated within the scanhead itself.

Returning to the magnifying glass analogy, most children learn that the secret to incineration is a steady hand. Movement distributes the power of the light beam over a larger area, thereby reducing its intensity. The same is true in ultrasound imaging. Thus, imaging systems that scan a beam through tissue reduce the spatial average intensity. **Spectral Doppler** and **M-mode** ultrasound imaging maintain the ultrasound beam in a stationary position (both considered **unscanned modes**) and therefore provide no opportunity to distribute the ultrasonic power spatially, whereas **color flow Doppler, power mode Doppler,** and **B-mode** (often called **gray-scale**) ultrasound imaging require that the beam be moved to new locations (**scanned modes**) at a rate sufficient to produce the real-time nature of these imaging modes.

Temporal Considerations

The ultrasound power is the temporal rate at which ultrasound energy is produced. Therefore, controlling how ultrasound is produced in time seems a reasonable method for limiting its effects.

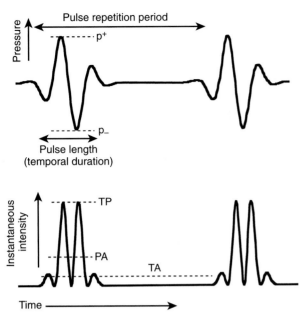

FIGURE 2-1. Pressure and intensity parameters measured in medical ultrasound. The variables are defined as follows: *p+*, peak positive pressure in waveform; *p–*, peak negative pressure in waveform; *TP*, temporal peak; *PA*, pulse average; and *TA*, temporal average.

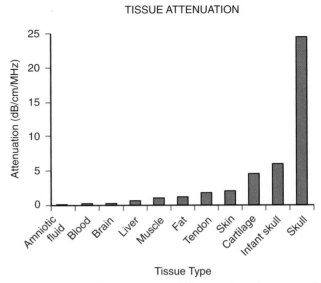

TISSUE ATTENUATION

FIGURE 2-2. Tissue attenuation. Values for types of human tissue at body temperature. *(Data from Duck FA, Starritt HC, Anderson SP. A survey of the acoustic output of ultrasonic Doppler equipment. Clin Phys Physiol Meas 1987;8:39-49.)*

Ultrasound can be produced in bursts rather than continuously. Ultrasound imaging systems operate on the principle of **pulse-echo,** in which a burst of ultrasound is emitted, followed by a quiescent period listening for echoes to return. This **pulsed wave** ultrasound is swept through the image plane numerous times during an imaging sequence. On the other hand, ultrasound may be transmitted in a **continuous wave** (CW) mode, in which the ultrasound transmission is not interrupted. The **temporal peak intensity** refers to the largest intensity at any time during ultrasound exposure (Fig. 2-1). The **pulse average intensity** is the average value over the ultrasound pulse. The **temporal average** is the average over the entire pulse repetition period (elapsed time between onset of ultrasound bursts). The **duty factor** is defined as the fraction of time the ultrasound field is "on." With significant time "off" between pulses (small duty factor), the temporal average value will be significantly smaller. For example, a duty factor of 10% will reduce the temporal average intensity by a factor of 10 compared to the pulse average. The time-averaged quantities are the variables most related to the potential for thermal bioeffects. Combining temporal and spatial information results in common terms such as the **spatial peak, temporal average intensity** (I_{SPTA}) and **spatial average, temporal average intensity** (I_{SATA}).

The overall duration, or **dwell time,** of the ultrasound exposure to a particular tissue is important because longer exposure of the tissue may increase the risk of bioeffects. The motion of the scanhead during an examination reduces the dwell time within a particular region of the body and can minimize the potential for bioeffects

of ultrasound. Therefore, performing an efficient scan, spending only the time required for diagnosis, is a simple way to reduce exposure.

Tissue Type

Numerous physical and biologic parameters control heating of tissues. Absorption is normally the dominant contributor to attenuation in soft tissue. The **attenuation coefficient** is the attenuation per unit length of sound travel and is usually given in decibels per centimeters-megahertz (dB/cm-MHz). The attenuation typically increases with increasing ultrasound frequency. The attenuation ranges from a negligible amount for fluids (e.g., amniotic fluid, blood, urine) to the highest value for bone, with some variation among different soft tissue types (Fig. 2-2).

Another important factor is the body's ability to cool tissue through blood perfusion. Well-perfused tissue will more effectively regulate its temperature by carrying away the excess heat produced by ultrasound. The exception is when heat is deposited too rapidly, as in therapeutic thermal ablation.[1]

Bone and soft tissue are two specific areas of interest based on the differences in heating phenomena. **Bone** has high attenuation of incident acoustic energy. In examinations during pregnancy, calcified bone is typically subjected to ultrasound, as in measurement of the biparietal diameter (BPD) of the skull. Fetal bone contains increasing degrees of mineralization as gestation progresses, thereby increasing risk of localized heating. Special heating situations relevant to obstetric ultrasound examinations may also occur in **soft tissue,** where overlying structures provide little attenuation of the field, such as the fluid-filled amniotic sac.

Bone Heating

The absorption of ultrasound at bone allows for rapid deposition of energy from the field into a limited volume of tissue. The result can be a significant temperature rise. For example, Carstensen et al.[2] combined an analytic approach and experimental measurements of the temperature rise in mouse skull exposed to CW ultrasound to estimate the temperature increments in bone exposures. Because bone has a large absorption coefficient, the incident ultrasonic energy is assumed to be absorbed in a thin planar sheet at the bone surface. The temperature rise of mouse skull has been studied in a 3.6-MHz focused beam with a beam width of 2.75 mm (Fig. 2-3). The temporal average intensity in the focal region was 1.5 W/cm^2. One of two models (upper curve in Fig. 2-3) in common use[3] predicts values for the temperature rise about 20% greater than that actually measured in this experiment.[1] Thus the theoretical model is conservative in nature.

Similarly for the fetal femur, Drewniak et al.[4] indicated that the size and calcification state of the bone contributed to the ex vivo heating of bone (Table 2-1). To put this in perspective and to illustrate the operator's role in controlling potential heating, consider the following scenario. By reducing the output power of an ultrasound scanner by 10 dB, the predicted temperature rise would be reduced by a factor of 10, making the increase of 3° C seen by these researchers (Table 2-1) virtually nonexistent. **This strongly suggests the use of maximum gain and reduction in output power during ultrasound examinations** (see later section on controlling ultrasound output). In fetal examinations an attempt should be made to maximize amplifier gain because this comes at no cost to the patient in terms of exposure. Distinctions are often made between bone positioned deep to the skin at the focal plane of the transducer and bone near the skin surface, as when considering transcranial applications. This distinction is discussed later with regard to the thermal index.

Soft Tissue Heating

Two clinical situations for ultrasound exposure in soft tissue are particularly relevant to obstetric/gynecologic applications. First, a common scenario involves **scanning through a full bladder.** The urine is a fluid with a relatively low ultrasound attenuation coefficient. The reduced attenuation allows larger acoustic amplitudes to be applied deeper within the body. Second, the propagating wave may experience **finite amplitude distortion,** resulting in energy being shifted by a nonlinear process from lower to higher frequencies. The result is a **shockwave** where a gradual wave steepening results in a waveform composed of higher-frequency components (Fig. 2-4). Attenuation increases with increasing frequency; therefore the absorption of a large portion of the energy in such a wave occurs over a much shorter distance, concentrating the energy deposition in the first tissue encountered, which may include the fetus.

Ultrasound imaging systems now include specific modalities that rely on nonlinear effects. In **tissue harmonic imaging,** or native harmonic imaging, the image is created using the backscatter of harmonic components induced by nonlinear propagation of the ultrasound field. This has distinct advantages in terms of reducing image artifacts and improving lateral resolution in particular. In these nonlinear imaging modes the acoustic

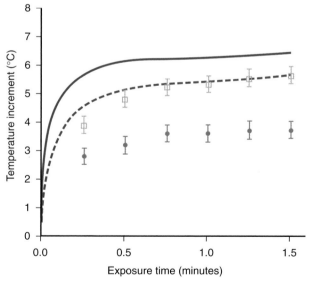

FIGURE 2-3. Heating of mouse skull in a focused sound field. For these experiments, frequency was 3.6 MHz, and temporal average focal intensity was 1.5 W/cm^2. *Solid circles:* Young (<17 wks) mice (N = 7); *open squares:* old (>6 mo) mice (N = 4); *vertical bars:* two standard errors in height; *top curves:* theoretical estimation of the temperature increases by Nyborg.[3] *(From Carstensen EL, Child SZ, Norton S, et al. Ultrasonic heating of the skull. J Acoust Soc Am 1990;87:1310-1317.)*

TABLE 2-1. FETAL FEMUR TEMPERATURE INCREMENTS* AT 1 W/cm^2

Gestational Age (days)	Diameter (mm)	Temperature Increments (° C)
59	0.5	0.10
78	1.2	0.69
108	3.3	2.92

From Drewniak JL, Carnes KI, Dunn F. In vitro ultrasonic heating of fetal bone. J Acoust Soc Am 1989;86:1254-1258.

*Temperature increments in human fetal femur exposed for 20 seconds were found to be approximately proportional to incident intensity.

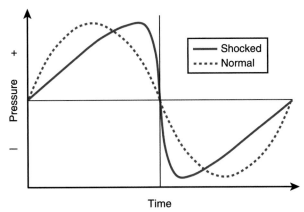

FIGURE 2-4. Effect of finite amplitude distortion on a propagating ultrasound pulse. Note the increasing steepness in the pulse, which contains higher-frequency components.

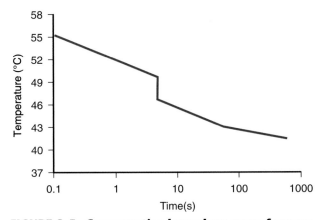

FIGURE 2-5. Conservative boundary curve for nonfetal bioeffects caused by a thermal mechanism. Note the increase in temperature tolerance associated with shorter durations of exposures, a modification to the earlier AIUM Conclusions Regarding Heat statement (March 26, 1997). AIUM approved a revised thermal statement on April 6, 2009. For a complete description of the origins of this curve, see O'Brien et al.[10] *(From O'Brien WD Jr, Deng CX, Harris GR, et al. The risk of exposure to diagnostic ultrasound in postnatal subjects: thermal effects. J Ultrasound Med 2008;27:517-535.)*

output must be sufficiently high to produce the effect. The acoustic power currently used is still within the FDA limits, but improvements in image quality using such modes may create the need to modify or relax the regulatory restrictions.

Transvaginal ultrasound is important to note because of the proximity of the transducer to sensitive tissues such as the ovaries. As discussed later, temperature increases near the transducer may provide a heat source at sites other than the focus of the transducer. In addition, the transducer face itself may be a significant heat source because of inefficiencies in its conversion of electric to acoustic energy. Therefore, such factors must be considered in the estimation of potential thermal effects in transvaginal ultrasound and other endocavitary applications.

Hyperthermia and Ultrasound Safety

Knowledge of the bioeffects for ultrasound heating is based on the experience available from other, more common forms of hyperthermia, which serve as a basis for safety criteria. Extensive data exist on the effects of short-term and extended temperature increases, or hyperthermia. Teratogenic effects from hyperthermia have been demonstrated in birds, all the common laboratory animals, farm animals, and nonhuman primates.[5] The wide range of observed bioeffects, from subcellular chemical alterations to gross congenital abnormalities and fetal death, is an indication of the effectiveness or universality of hyperthermic conditions for perturbing living systems.[6]

The National Council on Radiation Protection and Measurements (NCRP) Scientific Committee on Biological Effects of Ultrasound compiled a comprehensive list of the lowest reported thermal exposures producing teratogenic effects.[7,8] Examination of these data indicated a lower boundary for observed thermally

induced bioeffects. Questions remain, however, about the relevance of this analysis of hyperthermia to the application of diagnostic ultrasound.[9] More recently, after a careful literature review, O'Brien et al.[10] suggested a more detailed consideration of thermal effects with regard to short-duration exposures. Figure 2-5 shows the recommended approach to addressing the combination of temperature and duration of exposure. Note that the tolerance of shorter durations and higher temperatures suggests a substantial safety margin for diagnostic ultrasound. Regardless, it is beneficial to provide feedback to the ultrasound operator as to the relative potential for a temperature rise in a given acoustic field under conditions associated with a particular examination. This will allow an informed decision as to the exposure needed to obtain diagnostically relevant information.

Thermal Index

Based on analysis of hyperthermia data, NCRP proposed a general statement concerning the safety of ultrasound examinations in which no temperature rise greater than 1° C is expected. In an afebrile patient within this limit, NCRP concluded that there was no basis for expecting an adverse effect. In cases where the temperature rise might be greater, the operator should weigh the benefit against the potential risk. To assist in this decision, given the range of different imaging conditions seen in practice, a **thermal index** (TI) was approved as part of the Standard for Real-Time Display of Thermal and Mechanical Acoustical Output Indices on Diagnostic Ultrasound Equipment of the American Institute of Ultrasound in Medicine (AIUM).[11] This standard provides the operator with an indication of the relative potential risk of heating tissue, with calculations based on the imaging conditions and an on-screen display showing the TI.

THE THERMAL INDEX

To more easily inform the physician of the operating conditions that could, in some cases, lead to a temperature elevation of 1°C, a thermal index is defined as

$$TI = \frac{W_0}{W_{deg}}$$

where W_{deg} is the ultrasonic source power (in watts) calculated as capable of producing a 1°C temperature elevation under specific conditions. W_0 is the ultrasonic source power (in watts) being used during the current exam.

Reproduced with permission of American Institute of Ultrasound in Medicine (AIUM).

The NCRP ultrasound committee introduced the TI concept.[7] The purpose of the TI is to provide an indication of the *relative* potential for increasing tissue temperature, but it is not meant to provide the *actual* temperature rise. The NCRP recommended two tissue models to aid in the calculation of the ultrasound power that could raise the temperature in tissue by 1° C: (1) a homogeneous model in which the attenuation coefficient is uniform throughout the region of interest, and (2) a fixed-attenuation model in which the minimum attenuation along the path from transducer to a distant anatomic structure is independent of the distance because of a low-attenuation fluid path (e.g., amniotic fluid).[7,12,13] Because of concern for the patient, it was recommended that "reasonable worst case" assumptions be made with respect to estimation of temperature elevations in vivo. The FDA, AIUM, and National Electrical Manufacturers Association (NEMA) adopted the TI as part of the output display standard. They advocate estimating the effect of attenuation in the body by reducing the acoustic power/output of the scanner (W_0) by a derating factor equal to 0.3 dB/cm-MHz for the soft tissue model.[11]

The AIUM Thermal Index Working Group considered three tissue models: (1) the homogeneous tissue or soft tissue model, (2) a tissue model with bone at the focus, and (3) a tissue model with bone at the surface, or transcranial model.[11] The TI takes on three different forms for these tissue models.

Homogeneous Tissue Model (Soft Tissue)

The assumption of homogeneity helps simplify the determination of the effects of acoustic propagation and attenuation, as well as the heat transfer characteristics of the tissue. Providing one of the most common applications for ultrasound imaging, this model applies to situations where bone is not present and can generally be used for fetal examinations during the first trimester (low calcification in bone). In the estimation of potential heating, many assumptions and compromises had to be made to calculate a single quantity that would guide the operator. Calculations of the temperature rise along the axis of a focused beam for a simple, spherically curved, single-element transducer result in two thermal peaks. The first is in the near field (between the transducer and the focus), and the second appears close to the focal region.[14,15] The **first thermal peak** occurs in a region with low ultrasound intensity and wide beam width. When the beam width is large, cooling will occur mainly because of perfusion. In the near field the magnitude of the local intensity is the chief determinant of the degree of heating. The **second thermal peak** occurs at the location of high intensity and narrow beam width at or near the focal plane. Here the cooling is dominated by conduction, and the total acoustic power is the chief determinant of the degree of heating.

Given the thermal "twin peaks" dilemma, the AIUM Thermal Index Working Group compromised in creating a TI that included contributions from both heating domains.[11] Their rationale was based on the need to minimize the acoustic measurement load for manufacturers of ultrasound systems. In addition, adjustments had to be made to compensate for effects of the large range of potential apertures. The result is a complicated series of calculations and measurements that must be performed, and to the credit of the many manufacturers, there has been considerable effort in implementing a display standard to provide user feedback. Different approaches to these calculations are being considered,[10] but changes will require that the currently accepted implementation be reexamined and approved for use by the FDA and considered by the International Electrotechnical Commission (IEC), a standards organization.

Tissue Model with Bone at the Focus (Fetal Applications)

Applications of ultrasound in which the acoustic beam travels through soft tissue for a fixed distance and impinges on bone occur most often in obstetric scanning during the second and third trimesters. Carson et al.[13] recorded sonographic measurements of the maternal abdominal wall thickness in various stages of pregnancy. Based on their results, the NCRP recommended that the attenuation coefficients for the first, second, and third trimesters be 1.0, 0.75, and 0.5 dB/MHz, respectively.[7] These values represent "worst case" estimates. In addition, Siddiqi et al.[16] determined the average tissue attenuation coefficient for transabdominal insonification (exposure to ultrasound waves) in a patient population of nonpregnant, healthy volunteers was 2.98 dB/MHz. This value represents an average measured value and is much different than the worst-case estimates previously listed. This leads to considerable debate on how such parameters should be included in an index.

In addition, bone is a complex, hard connective tissue with a calcified collagenous intercellular substance. Its absorption coefficient for longitudinal waves is a factor of 10 greater than that for most soft tissues (see Fig. 2-2). **Shear waves** are also created in bone as sound waves strike bone at oblique incidence. The absorption coefficients for shear waves are even greater than those for longitudinal waves.[17-19]

Based on the data of Carstensen et al.[2] described earlier, the NCRP proposed a thermal model for bone heating. Using this model, the **thermal index for bone (TIB)** is estimated for conditions in which the focus of the beam is at or near bone. Again, assumptions and compromises had to be made to develop a functional TI for the case of bone exposure, as follows:

- For **unscanned mode** transducers (operating in a fixed position) with bone in the focal region, the location of the maximum temperature increase is at the surface of the bone. Therefore the TIB is calculated at an axial distance where it is maximized, a worst-case assumption.
- For **scanned modes**, the **thermal index for soft tissue (TIS)** is used because the temperature increase at the surface is either greater than or approximately equal to the temperature increase with bone in the focus.

Tissue Model with Bone at the Surface (Transcranial Applications)

For adult cranial applications, the same model as that with bone at the focus is used to estimate the temperature distribution in situ. However, because the bone is located at the surface, immediately after the acoustic beam enters the body, attenuation of the acoustic power output is not included.[11] In this situation the equivalent beam diameter at the surface is used to calculate the acoustic power.

Estimate of Thermal Effects

Ultrasound users should keep in mind several points when referring to the thermal index as a means of estimating the potential for thermal effects. First, the TI is not synonymous with temperature rise. A TI equal to 1 does not mean the temperature will rise 1° C. An increased potential for thermal effects can be expected as TI increases. Second, a high TI does not mean that bioeffects are occurring, but only that the potential exists. Factors that may reduce the actual temperature rise may not be considered by the thermal models employed for TI calculation. However, TI should be

monitored during examinations and minimized when possible. Finally, there is no consideration in the TI for the duration of the scan, so minimizing the overall examination time will reduce the potential for effects.

Summary Statement on Thermal Effects

The AIUM statement concerning thermal effects of ultrasound includes several conclusions that can be summarized as follows[20]:

- Adult examinations resulting in a temperature rise of up to 2° C are not expected to cause bioeffects. (Many ultrasound examinations fall within these parameters.)
- A significant number of factors control heat production by diagnostic ultrasound.
- Ossified bone is a particularly important concern for ultrasound exposure.
- A labeling standard now provides information concerning potential heating in soft tissue and bone.
- Even though an FDA limit exists for fetal exposures, predicted temperature rises can exceed 2° C.
- Thermal indices are expected to track temperature increases better than any single ultrasonic field parameter.

EFFECTS OF ACOUSTIC CAVITATION

Potential Sources for Bioeffects

Knowledge concerning the interaction of ultrasound with **gas bodies** (which many term "cavitation") has significantly increased recently, although it is not as extensive as that for ultrasound thermal effects and other sources of hyperthermia. **Acoustic cavitation inception** is demarcated by a specific threshold value: the minimum acoustic pressure necessary to initiate the growth of a cavity in a fluid during the rarefaction phase of the cycle. Several parameters affect this threshold, including **initial bubble** or **cavitation nucleus size**, acoustic pulse characteristics (e.g., center frequency, pulse repetition frequency, pulse duration), ambient hydrostatic pressure, and host fluid parameters (e.g., density, viscosity, compressibility, heat conductivity, surface tension). **Inertial cavitation** refers to bubbles that undergo large variations from their equilibrium sizes in a few acoustic cycles. Specifically during contraction, the surrounding fluid inertia controls the bubble motion.[21] Large acoustic pressures are necessary to generate inertial cavitation, and the collapse of these cavities is often violent.

The effect of **preexisting cavitation nuclei** may be one of the principal controlling factors in mechanical effects that result in biologic effects. The body is such an excellent filter that these nucleation sites may be found

AIUM STATEMENT ON HEAT—THERMAL BIOEFFECTS

Approved April 6, 2009

1. Excessive temperature increase can result in toxic effects in mammalian systems. The biological effects observed depend on many factors, such as the exposure duration, the type of tissue exposed, its cellular proliferation rate, and its potential for regeneration. Age and stage of development are important factors when considering fetal and neonatal safety. Temperature increases of several degrees Celsius above the normal core range can occur naturally. The probability of an adverse biological effect increases with the duration of the temperature rise.

2. In general, adult tissues are more tolerant of temperature increases than fetal and neonatal tissues. Therefore, higher temperatures and/or longer exposure durations would be required for thermal damage. The considerable data available on the thermal sensitivity of adult tissues support the following inferences:

   For exposure durations up to 50 hours, there have been no significant, adverse biological effects observed due to temperature increases less than or equal to 2°C above normal.

   For temperature increases between 2°C and 6°C above normal, there have been no significant, adverse biological effects observed due to temperature increases less than or equal to $6 - \log_{10}(t/60)/0.6$ where t is the exposure duration in seconds. For example, for temperature increases of 4°C and 6°C, the corresponding limits for the exposure durations t are 16 min and 1 min, respectively.

   For temperature increases greater than 6°C above normal, there have been no significant, adverse biological effects observed due to temperature increases less than or equal to $6 - \log_{10}(t/60)/0.3$ where t is the exposure duration in seconds. For example, for temperature increases of 9.6°C and 6.0°C, the corresponding limits for the exposure durations t are 5 and 60 seconds, respectively.

   For exposure durations less than 5 seconds, there have been no significant, adverse biological effects observed due to temperature increases less than or equal to $9 - \log_{10}(t/60)/0.3$ where t is the exposure duration in seconds. For example, for temperature increases of 18.3°C, 14.9°C, and 12.6°C, the corresponding limits for the exposure durations t are 0.1, 1, and 5 seconds, respectively.

3. Acoustic output from diagnostic ultrasound devices is sufficient to cause temperature elevations in fetal tissue. Although fewer data are available for fetal tissues, the following conclusions are justified:

   In general, temperature elevations become progressively greater from B-mode to color Doppler to spectral Doppler applications.

   For identical exposure conditions, the potential for thermal bioeffects increases with the dwell time during examination.

   For identical exposure conditions, the temperature rise near bone is significantly greater than in soft tissues, and it increases with ossification development throughout gestation. For this reason, conditions where an acoustic beam impinges on ossifying fetal bone deserve special attention due to its close proximity to other developing tissues.

   The current FDA regulatory limit for $I_{SPTA.3}$ is 720 mW/cm^2. For this, and lesser intensities, the theoretical estimate of the maximum temperature increase in the conceptus can exceed 2°C.

   Although, in general, an adverse fetal outcome is possible at any time during gestation, most severe and detectable effects of thermal exposure in animals have been observed during the period of organogenesis. For this reason, exposures during the first trimester should be restricted to the lowest outputs consistent with obtaining the necessary diagnostic information.

   Ultrasound exposures that elevate fetal temperature by 4°C above normal for 5 minutes or more have the potential to induce severe developmental defects. Thermally induced congenital anomalies have been observed in a large variety of animal species. In current clinical practice, using commercially available equipment, it is unlikely that such thermal exposure would occur at a specific fetal anatomic site.

   Transducer self-heating is a significant component of the temperature rise of tissues close to the transducer. This may be of significance in transvaginal scanning, but no data for the fetal temperature rise are available.

4. The temperature increase during exposure of tissues to diagnostic ultrasound fields is dependent upon (a) output characteristics of the acoustic source such as frequency, source dimensions, scan rate, power, pulse repetition frequency, pulse duration, transducer self-heating, exposure time, and wave shape and (b) tissue properties such as attenuation, absorption, speed of sound, acoustic impedance, perfusion, thermal conductivity, thermal diffusivity, anatomical structure, and nonlinearity parameter.

5. Calculations of the maximum temperature increase resulting from ultrasound exposure *in vivo* are not exact because of the uncertainties and approximations associated with the thermal, acoustic, and structural characteristics of the tissues involved. However, experimental evidence shows that calculations are generally capable of predicting measured values within a factor of two. Thus, such calculations are used to obtain safety guidelines for clinical exposures where direct temperature measurements are not feasible. These guidelines, called *thermal indices,** provide a real-time display of the relative probability that a diagnostic system could induce thermal injury in the exposed subject. Under most clinically relevant conditions, the soft tissue thermal index, TIS, and the bone thermal index, TIB, either overestimate or closely approximate the best available estimate of the maximum temperature increase (ΔT_{max}). For example, if TIS = 2, then $\Delta T_{max} \leq 2°C$.

Reprinted with permission of AIUM.

*Thermal indices are the nondimensional ratios of the estimated temperature increases to 1°C for specific tissue models. See American Institute of Ultrasound in Medicine. Standard for real-time display of thermal and mechanical acoustic output indices on diagnostic ultrasound equipment, Revision 2, Rockville, Md, 2001, AIUM and National Electrical Manufacturers Association.

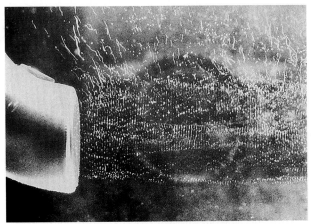

FIGURE 2-6. Acoustic cavitation bubbles. This cavitation activity is being generated in water using a common therapeutic ultrasound device. *(Courtesy National Center for Physical Acoustics, University of Mississippi.)*

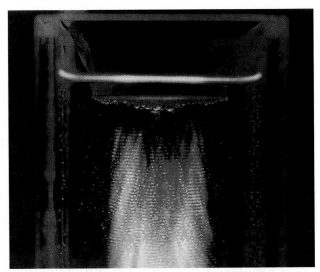

FIGURE 2-7. Chemical reaction induced by cavitation producing visible light. The reaction is the result of free radical production. *(Courtesy National Center for Physical Acoustics, University of Mississippi.)*

only in small numbers and at selected sites. For example, if water is filtered down to 2 μm, the cavitation threshold doubles.[22] Theoretically, the tensile strength of water that is devoid of cavitation nuclei is about 100 megapascals (MPa).[23] Various models have been suggested to explain bubble formation in animals,[24,25] and these models have been used extensively in cavitation threshold determination. One model is used in the prediction of SCUBA diving tables and may also have applicability to patients.[26] It remains to be seen how well such models will predict the nucleation of bubbles from diagnostic ultrasound in the body.

Figure 2-6 shows a 1-MHz therapeutic ultrasound unit generating bubbles in gas-saturated water. The particular medium and ultrasound parameters were chosen to optimize the conditions for cavitation. Using continuous wave ultrasound and many preexisting gas pockets in the water set the stage for the production of cavitation. Even though these acoustic pulses are longer than those typically used in diagnostic ultrasound, cavitation effects have also been observed with diagnostic pulses in fluids.[27] **Ultrasound contrast agents** composed of stabilized gas bubbles should provide a source of cavitation nuclei, as discussed later.

Sonochemistry

Free radical generation and detection provide a means to observe cavitation and to gauge its strength and potential for damage. The sonochemistry of free radicals is the result of very high temperatures and pressures within the rapidly collapsing bubble. These conditions can even generate light, or **sonoluminescence.**[28] With the addition of the correct compounds, chemical luminescence can also be used for free radical detection and can be generated with short pulses similar to that used in diagnostic ultrasound.[29] Figure 2-7 shows **chemiluminescence** generated by a therapeutic ultrasound device; the

setup is backlighted (in red) to show the bubbles and experimental apparatus. The chemiluminescence emissions are the blue bands seen through the middle of the liquid sample holder. The light emitted is sufficient to be seen by simply adapting one's eyes to darkness. Electron spin resonance can also be used with molecules that trap free radicals to detect cavitation activity capable of free radical production.[30] A number of other chemical detection schemes are presently employed to detect cavitation from diagnostic devices in vitro.

Evidence of Cavitation from Lithotripters

It is possible to generate bubbles in vivo using short pulses with high amplitudes of an extracorporeal shockwave lithotripter (ESWL). The peak positive pressure for lithotripsy pulses can be as high as 50 MPa, with the negative pressure about 20 MPa. **Finite amplitude distortion** causes high frequencies to appear in high-amplitude ultrasound fields. Although ESWL pulses have significant energy at high frequencies because of finite amplitude distortion, a large portion of the energy is actually in the 100-kHz range, much lower than frequencies in diagnostic scanners. The lower frequency makes cavitation more likely. Aymé and Carstensen[31] showed that the higher-frequency components in nonlinearly distorted pulses contribute little to the killing of *Drosophila* larvae.

Interestingly, increasing evidence indicates that collapsing bubbles play a role in stone disruption.[32-34] A bubble collapsing near a surface may form a liquid jet through its center, which strikes the surface (Fig. 2-8). Placing a sheet of aluminum foil at the focus of a lithotripter generates small pinholes.[32] The impact is even sufficient to pit solid brass and aluminum plates.

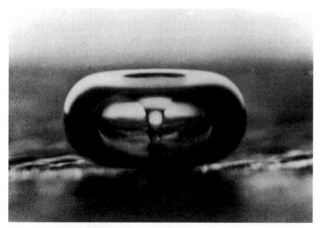

FIGURE 2-8. Collapsing bubble near a boundary. When cavitation is produced near boundaries, a liquid jet may form through the center of a bubble and strike the boundary surface. *(Courtesy Lawrence A. Crum.)*

Clearly, lithotripsy and diagnostic ultrasound differ in the acoustic power generated and are not comparable in the bioeffects produced. However, some diagnostic devices produce peak rarefactional pressures greater than 3 MPa, which is in the lower range of lithotripter outputs.[35-37] Lung damage and surface petechiae have been noted as side effects of ESWL in clinical cases.[38] Inertial cavitation was suspected as the cause, prompting several researchers to study the effects of diagnostic ultrasound exposure on the lung parenchyma.[39,40]

Bioeffects in Lung and Intestine

Lung tissue and intestinal tissue are key locations for examining for bioeffects of diagnostic ultrasound.[39] The presence of air in the alveolar spaces constitutes a significant source of gas bodies. Child et al.[40] measured threshold pressures for hemorrhage in mouse lung exposed to 1- to 4-MHz short-pulse diagnostic ultrasound (i.e., 10- and 1-μm pulse durations). The threshold of damage in murine lung at these frequencies was 1.4 MPa. Pathologic features of this damage included extravasation of blood cells into the alveolar spaces.[41] The authors hypothesized that cavitation, originating from gas-filled alveoli, was responsible for the damage. Their data provided the first direct evidence that clinically relevant, pulsed ultrasound exposures produce deleterious effects in mammalian tissue in the absence of significant heating. Hemorrhagic foci induced by 4-MHz pulsed Doppler ultrasound have also been reported in the monkey.[42] Damage in the monkey lung was of a significantly lesser degree than that in the mouse. In these studies it was impossible to show categorically that bubbles induced these effects because the cavitation-induced bubbles were not observed. Thresholds for petechial hemorrhage in the lung caused by ultrasound have been measured in mouse, rat, rabbit and pig.[43-45] Direct mechanical stresses associated with

propagation of ultrasound in the lung were believed to contribute to the damage observed.[39,46] Thresholds for hemorrhage in the murine intestine exposed to pulsed ultrasound have also been determined.[47]

Kramer et al.[48] assessed cardiopulmonary function in rats exposed to pulsed ultrasound well above the acoustic output threshold of damage, at a mechanical index (MI) of 9.7 (see later discussion). Measurements of cardiopulmonary function included arterial blood pressure, heart rate, respiratory rate, and arterial blood gases (P_{CO_2} and P_{O_2}). If only one side of the rat lung was exposed, the cardiopulmonary measurements did not change significantly between baseline and postexposure values because of the functional respiratory reserve in the unexposed lobes. However, when both sides of the lung had significant ultrasound-induced lesions, the rats were unable to maintain systemic arterial pressure or resting levels of arterial P_{O_2}.

Further studies are required to determine the relevance of these findings to humans. In general, tissues containing air (or stabilized gas) are more susceptible to damage than those tissues without gas. Also, no confirmed reports of petechial hemorrhage have been noted in animal studies below an MI of 0.4.

Ultrasound Contrast Agents

The apparent absence of cavitation in many locations in the body can result from the lack of available cavitation nuclei. Based on evidence in the lung and intestine in mammalian models described earlier, the presence of gas bodies clearly reduces the requisite acoustic field for producing bioeffects. Many ultrasound contrast agents are composed of stabilized gas bubbles, so they could provide readily available nuclei for potential cavitation activity. This makes the investigation of bioeffects in the presence of ultrasound contrast agents an important area of research.[49-51] Studies have also shown that ultrasound exposure in the presence of contrast agents produces small vascular petechiae and endothelial damage in mammalian systems.[52-57] Acoustic emissions from activated microbubbles correlate with the degree of vascular damage.[54,55]

As a result, the AIUM has updated a safety statement on the bioeffects of diagnostic ultrasound with gas body contrast agents. This bioeffect may occur, but the issue remains whether it constitutes a significant physiologic risk. The safety statement is designed to make sonographers and physicians aware of the potential for bioeffects in the presence of gas contrast agents and allow them to make an informed decision based on a risk/benefit assessment.

Some research also indicates the production of premature ventricular contractions (PVCs) during cardiac scanning in the presence of ultrasound contrast agents. At least one human study indicated an increase in PVCs only when ultrasound imaging was performed with a

AIUM STATEMENT ON BIOEFFECTS OF DIAGNOSTIC ULTRASOUND WITH GAS BODY CONTRAST AGENTS

Approved November 8, 2008

Presently available ultrasound contrast agents consist of suspensions of gas bodies (stabilized gaseous microbubbles). The gas bodies have the correct size for strong echogenicity with diagnostic ultrasound and also for passage through the microcirculation. Commercial agents undergo rigorous clinical testing for safety and efficacy before Food and Drug Administration approval is granted, and they have been in clinical use in the United States since 1994. Detailed information on the composition and use of these agents is included in the package inserts. To date, diagnostic benefit has been proven in patients with suboptimal echocardiograms to opacify the left ventricular chamber and to improve the delineation of the left ventricular endocardial border. Many other diagnostic applications are under development or clinical testing.

Contrast agents carry some potential for nonthermal bioeffects when ultrasound interacts with the gas bodies. The mechanism for such effects is related to the physical phenomenon of acoustic cavitation. Several published reports describe adverse bioeffects in mammalian tissue *in vivo* resulting from exposure to diagnostic ultrasound with gas body contrast agents in the circulation. Induction of premature ventricular contractions by triggered contrast echocardiography in humans has been reported for a noncommercial agent and in laboratory animals for commercial agents. Microvascular leakage, killing of cardiomyocytes, and glomerular capillary hemorrhage, among other bioeffects, have been reported in animal studies. Two medical ultrasound societies have examined this

potential risk of bioeffects in diagnostic ultrasound with contrast agents and provide extensive reviews of the topic: the World Federation for Ultrasound in Medicine and Biology (WFUMB) Contrast Agent Safety Symposium* and the American Institute of Ultrasound in Medicine 2005 Bioeffects Consensus Conference.[49] Based on review of these reports and of recent literature, the Bioeffects Committee issues the following statement:

Induction of premature ventricular contractions, microvascular leakage with petechiae, glomerular capillary hemorrhage, and local cell killing in mammalian tissue *in vivo* have been reported and independently confirmed for diagnostic ultrasound exposure with a mechanical index (MI) above about 0.4 and a gas body contrast agent present in the circulation.

Although the medical significance of such microscale bioeffects is uncertain, minimizing the potential for such effects represents prudent use of diagnostic ultrasound. In general, for imaging with contrast agents at an MI above 0.4, practitioners should use the minimal agent dose, MI, and examination time consistent with efficacious acquisition of diagnostic information. In addition, the echocardiogram should be monitored during high-MI contrast cardiac-gated perfusion echocardiography, particularly in patients with a history of myocardial infarction or unstable cardiovascular disease. Furthermore, physicians and sonographers should follow all guidance provided in the package inserts of these drugs, including precautions, warnings, and contraindications.

Reprinted with permission of AIUM.

*Barnett SB. Safe use of ultrasound contrast agents. WFUMB Symposium on Safety of Ultrasound in Medicine: Ultrasound Contrast Agents. Ultrasound Med Biol 2007;33:171-172.

contrast agent, and not with ultrasound imaging alone or during injection of the agent without imaging.[58] Another study[59] revealed that oscillating microbubbles affect stretch activation channels[60,61] in cardiac cells, which generates membrane depolarization and triggers action potentials and thus PVCs. The importance of this bioeffect is also being debated because there is a naturally occurring rate of PVCs, and a small increase may not be considered significant, particularly if the patient benefits from using the agent. Additional consideration might be given to patients with specific conditions in whom additional PVCs should be avoided.

The consequences of the ultrasound contrast agent bioeffects reported thus far require more study. Although the potential exists for a bioeffect, its scale and influence on human physiology remain unclear. Contrast agents have demonstrated efficacy for specific indications, facilitating patient management.[62] In addition, clinical trials

and marketing follow-up of many patients receiving ultrasound and contrast agents have reported few effects. In fact, recent evidence confirms the safety of ultrasound contrast agent use.[63-66]

Mechanical Index

Calculations for cavitation prediction have yielded a trade-off between peak rarefactional pressure and frequency.[67] This predicted trade-off assumes short-pulse (a few acoustic cycles) and low-duty cycle ultrasound (<1%). This relatively simple result can be used to gauge the potential for the onset of cavitation from diagnostic ultrasound. The mechanical index was adopted by the FDA, AIUM, and NEMA as a real-time output display to estimate the potential for bubble formation in vivo, in analogy to the thermal index. As previously stated, the collapse temperature for inertial cavitation is very high.

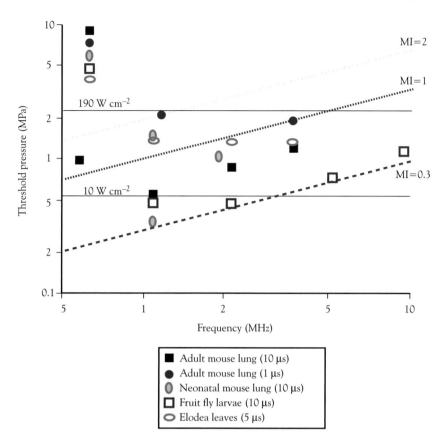

FIGURE 2-9. Threshold for bioeffects from pulsed ultrasound scan using low temporal average intensity. Data shown are the threshold for effects measured in peak rarefactional pressures (*p*– in Fig. 2-1) as a function of ultrasound frequency used in the exposure. Pulse durations are shown in parentheses in the key below the graph. Also shown for reference purposes are the values for the mechanical index *(MI)* and the local spatial peak, pulse average intensity (I$_{SPPA}$). *(From American Institute of Ultrasound in Medicine. Bioeffects and safety of diagnostic ultrasound. Rockville, Md, 1993, AIUM.)*

For MI, a collapse temperature of 5000 kelvins (K) was chosen based on the potential for free radical generation, and the frequency dependence of the pressure required to generate this thermal threshold takes a relatively simple form. The MI is a type of "mechanical energy index" because the square of the MI is about proportional to mechanical work that can be performed on a bubble in the acoustic rarefaction phase.

Results from several investigators have specified the MI value above which bioeffects associated with cavitation are observed in animals and insects.[66] In Figure 2-9 the dotted lines are calculations for several MI values, where all the effects appear to occur at an MI value of 0.3 or greater. In many of these cases, however, stable pockets of gas (gas bodies) are known to exist in the exposed tissues. Also, other body areas containing gas bodies might also be particularly susceptible to ultrasound damage, including the intestinal lining.[68]

In response to this potential, the AIUM issued a safety statement related to the potential for bioeffects related to the interaction of ultrasound with naturally occurring nuclei. Experimentation continues, and it remains to be seen if such damage occurs in human tissue.

Inherent in the formulation of the MI are the conditions only for the onset of inertial cavitation. The degree to which the threshold is exceeded, however, relates to the degree of potential bubble activity, which may correlate with the probability of a bioeffect. Note that, given present knowledge, exceeding the cavitation threshold

does not mean there will be a bioeffect. Below an MI of about 0.4, the physical conditions do not favor bubble growth, even in the presence of a broad bubble nuclei distribution in the body, which is in reasonable agreement with the results of Figure 2-9. Moreover, whereas the TI is a time-averaged measure of the interaction of ultrasound with tissue, the MI is a peak measure of this interaction. Thus, there is a desirable parallel between these two measures, one thermal and one mechanical, for informing the user of the extent to which the diagnostic tool can produce undesirable changes in the body.

Summary Statement on Gas Body Bioeffects

The AIUM statements concerning bioeffects in body areas with gas bodies include several conclusions,[20] summarized as follows:

1. Current ultrasound systems can produce cavitation in vitro and in vivo and can cause blood extravasation in animal tissues.
2. A mechanical index can gauge the likelihood for cavitation and apparently works better than other field parameters in predicting cavitation.
3. Several interesting results have been observed concerning animal models for lung damage, which indicate a very low threshold for damage, but the implications for human exposure are not yet determined.

AIUM STATEMENT ON NATURALLY OCCURRING GAS BODIES

Approved November 8, 2008

Biologically significant, adverse, nonthermal effects have only been identified with certainty for diagnostically relevant exposures in tissues that have well-defined populations of stabilized gas bodies. Such gas bodies either may occur naturally or may be injected from an exogenous source such as an ultrasound contrast agent. This statement concerns the former, while a separate statement deals with contrast agents [Ed. note: *see the box on p. 44*].

1. The outputs of some currently available diagnostic ultrasound devices can generate levels that produce hemorrhage in the lungs and intestines of laboratory animals.
2. A mechanical index (MI)* has been formulated to assist users in evaluating the likelihood of cavitation-related adverse biological effects for diagnostically relevant exposures. The MI is a better indicator than single-parameter measures of exposure, e.g., derated spatial-peak pulse-average intensity ($I_{SPPA.3}$) or derated peak rarefactional pressure ($p_{r.3}$), for known adverse nonthermal biological effects of ultrasound.
3. The threshold value of the current MI for lung hemorrhage in the mouse is approximately 0.4. The corresponding threshold for the intestine is MI = 1.4. The implications of these observations for human exposure are yet to be determined.
4. Thresholds for adverse nonthermal effects depend upon tissue characteristics, exposure duration (ED),

and ultrasound parameters such as frequency (f_c), pulse duration (PD), and pulse repetition frequency (PRF). For lung hemorrhage in postnatal laboratory animals, an empirical relation for the threshold value of *in situ* acoustic pressure is

$$P^\wedge_r = (2.4\ f_c^{0.28}PRF^{0.04})/(PD^{0.27}ED^{0.23})\text{MPa},$$

where the ranges and units of the variables investigated are f_c = 1 to 5.6 MHz, PRF = 0.017 to 1.0 kHz, PD = 1.0 to 11.7 μs, and ED = 2.4 to 180 s. The above relationship differs significantly from the corresponding form used for the MI, and a lung-specific MI is in development.

5. The worst-case theoretical threshold for bubble nucleation and subsequent inertial cavitation in soft tissue is MI = 3.9 at 1 MHz. The threshold decreases to MI approximately 1.9 at 5 MHz and above, a level equal to the maximum output permitted by the U.S. Food and Drug Administration for diagnostic ultrasound devices. Experimental values for the cavitation threshold correspond to MI > 4 for extravasation of blood cells in mouse kidneys, and MI > 5.1 for hind limb paralysis in the mouse neonate.
6. For diagnostically relevant exposures (MI ≤ 1.9), no independently confirmed, biologically significant adverse nonthermal effects have been reported in mammalian tissues that do not contain well-defined gas bodies.

Reprinted with permission of AIUM.

*The MI is equal to the derated peak rarefactional pressure (in MPa) at the point of the maximum derated pulse intensity integral divided by the square root of the ultrasonic center frequency (in MHz). See American Institute of Ultrasound in Medicine. Standard for real-time display of thermal and mechanical acoustic output indices on diagnostic ultrasound equipment, Revision 2. Rockville, Md, 2004, AIUM and National Electrical Manufacturers Association.

4. In the absence of gas bodies, the threshold for damage is much higher. (This is significant because ultrasound examinations may be performed predominantly in tissues with no identifiable gas bodies.)

OUTPUT DISPLAY STANDARD

Several groups, including the FDA, AIUM, and NEMA, have developed the Standard for Real-Time Display of Thermal and Mechanical Acoustical Output Indices on Diagnostic Ultrasound Equipment, which introduces a method to provide the user with information concerning the thermal and mechanical indices. Real-time display of the MI and TI will allow a more informed decision on the potential for bioeffects during ultrasound examinations (Fig. 2-10). The standard requires dynamic updates

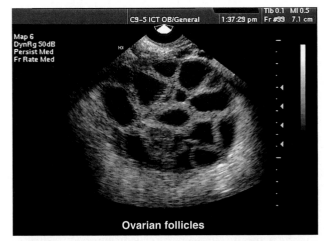

FIGURE 2-10. Display of bioeffects indices. Typical appearance of an ultrasound scanner display showing *(right upper corner)* the thermal index in bone *(TIb)* and mechanical index *(MI)* for an endocavitary transducer.

of the indices as instrument output is modified and allows the operator to learn how controls will affect these indices. Important points to remember about this display standard include the following:

- The mechanical index should be clearly visible on the screen (or alert the operator by some other means) and should begin to appear when the instrument exceeds a value of 0.4. An exception is made for instruments incapable of exceeding index values of 1; these are not required to display the bioeffects indices such as MI.
- Sometimes only one index (MI or TI) will be displayed at a time. The choice is often based on whether a given output condition is more likely to produce an effect by either mechanism.
- The standard also requires that appropriate default output settings be in effect at power-up, new patient entry, or when changing to a fetal examination. After that time the operator can adjust the instrument output as necessary to acquire clinically useful information while attempting to minimize the index values.
- As indicated previously, the bioeffects indices do not include any factors associated with the time taken to perform the scan. Efficient scanning is still an important component in limiting potential bioeffects.

In the document Medical Ultrasound Safety, AIUM suggests that the operator ask the following four questions to use the output display effectively[69]:

1. Which index should be used for the examination being performed?
2. Are there factors present that might cause the reading to be too high or low?
3. Can the index value be reduced further even when it is already low?
4. How can the ultrasound exposure be minimized without compromising the scan's diagnostic quality?

Sonographers and physicians are being presented with real-time data on acoustic output of diagnostic scanners and are being asked not only to understand the manner in which ultrasound propagates through and interacts with tissue, but also to gauge the potential for adverse bioeffects. The output display is a tool that can be used to guide an ultrasound examination and control for potential adverse effects. The thermal and mechanical indices provide the user with more information and more responsibility in limiting output.

GENERAL AIUM SAFETY STATEMENTS

It is important to consider some official positions concerning the status of bioeffects resulting from ultrasound. Most important is the high level of confidence in the safety of ultrasound in official statements. For example,

---

AIUM SAFETY STATEMENTS ON DIAGNOSTIC ULTRASOUND

AIUM STATEMENT ON PRUDENT USE AND CLINICAL SAFETY
Approved October 1982; Revised and approved March 2007

Diagnostic ultrasound has been in use since the late 1950s. Given its known benefits and recognized efficacy for medical diagnosis, including use during human pregnancy, the American Institute of Ultrasound in Medicine herein addresses the clinical safety of such use: No independently confirmed adverse effects caused by exposure from present diagnostic ultrasound instruments have been reported in human patients in the absence of contrast agents. Biological effects (such as localized pulmonary bleeding) have been reported in mammalian systems at diagnostically relevant exposures, but the clinical significance of such effects is not yet known. Ultrasound should be used by qualified health professionals to provide medical benefit to the patient.

AIUM STATEMENT ON SAFETY IN TRAINING AND RESEARCH
Approved March 1983; Revised and approved March, 2007

Diagnostic ultrasound has been in use since the late 1950s. There are no confirmed adverse biological effects on patients resulting from this usage. Although no hazard has been identified that would preclude the prudent and conservative use of diagnostic ultrasound in education and research, experience from normal diagnostic practice may or may not be relevant to extended exposure times and altered exposure conditions. It is therefore considered appropriate to make the following recommendation:

> When examinations are carried out for purposes of training or research, the subject should be informed of the anticipated exposure conditions and how these compare with normal diagnostic practice.

Reprinted with permission of AIUM.

---

in 2007 the AIUM reiterated its earlier statement concerning the clinical use of diagnostic ultrasound by stating that no known bioeffects have been confirmed with the use of present diagnostic equipment, and the patient benefits resulting from prudent use outweigh the risks, if any. Similarly, in commenting on the use of diagnostic ultrasound in research, by AIUM recommends that in the case of ultrasound exposure for other than direct medical benefit, the person should be informed concerning the exposure conditions and how these relate to normal exposures. For the most part, even examinations for research purposes are comparable to normal diagnostic exams and pose no additional risk. In fact, many research exams can be performed in conjunction with routine exams.

The effects based on in vivo animal models can be summarized by the AIUM Statements on Heat—Thermal Bioeffects, Bioeffects of Diagnostic Ultrasound with Gas Body Contrast Agents, and Naturally Occurring Gas Bodies.[20] No independently confirmed experimental evidence indicates damage in animal models below certain prescribed levels (temperature rises <2° C; MI <0.4). The value for the MI is strict because tissues containing gas bodies exhibit damage at much lower levels than tissues devoid of gas bodies. Biologic effects have not been detected even at an MI of 4.0 in the absence of gas bodies.

EPIDEMIOLOGY

With all the potential causes for bioeffects, we must now examine the epidemiologic evidence that has been used in part to justify the apparent safety of ultrasound. In 1988, Ziskin and Petitti[70] reviewed the epidemiologic studies conducted until then and concluded, "Epidemiologic studies and surveys in widespread clinical usage over 25 years have yielded no evidence of any adverse effect from diagnostic ultrasound." A 2008 review[71] of the epidemiology literature conducted by an AIUM subcommittee reiterated the AIUM statement regarding the epidemiology of diagnostic ultrasound safety in obstetrics.[72] This statement is similar to that approved in 1995 and differs slightly from that approved in 1987, which stated that no confirmed effects associated with ultrasound exposure existed at that time. The distinction being made is that although some effects may have been detected now, one cannot justify a conclusion of a causal relationship based on this evidence.

Epidemiologic studies are difficult to conduct, and data analysis and interpretation of results can be even more difficult. Several epidemiologic studies of fetal exposure to ultrasound have claimed to detect certain bioeffects and have also been criticized. Only one indication of an unspecified effect was reported in a general survey involving an estimated 1.2 million examinations in Canada.[73] However, this is an extremely low incidence, with no follow-up to determine the nature of the effect. In addition, an earlier study that included 121,000 fetal exams reported no effect.[74] Moore et al.[75] reported an increased incidence of low birth weight, whereas Stark et al.[76] examined the same data using a different statistical treatment and found no significant increase. Scheidt et al.[77] noted abnormal grasp and tonic neck reflexes. These results are difficult to interpret, however, given the statistical treatment of the data. Stark et al.[76] detected an increased incidence of dyslexia, but the same children exhibited below-average birth weights. General problems also plague the epidemiologic studies, including the lack of clearly stated exposure conditions and gestational age, problems in statistical sampling (with both positive and negative results), and use of older scanning systems, particularly with fetal Doppler ultrasound. Dyslexia was examined as part of two randomized trials, including specific long-term follow-up that showed no statistical difference between ultrasound-exposed and control subjects.[78,79]

Ziskin and Petitti[70] also summarized the factors in evaluating epidemiologic evidence. It is important to recognize that epidemiologic evidence can be used to identify an association between exposures and biologic effects, but that this does not prove the exposure caused the bioeffect. The strength of the association is established by the statistical significance of the relationship. Hill[80] and Abramowicz et al.[71] have developed the following seven criteria for judging **causality:**
1. Strength of the association.
2. Consistency in reproducibility and with previous, related research.
3. Specificity to a particular bioeffect or exposure site.
4. Classic time relationship of cause followed by effect.
5. Existence of a dose response.
6. Plausibility of the effect.
7. Supporting evidence from laboratory studies.
When considering these factors, no clear causal relationship seems to exist between an adverse biologic response and ultrasound exposure of a diagnostic nature.

Newnham et al.[81] reported higher intrauterine growth restriction during a study designed to determine the efficacy of ultrasound in reducing the number of neonatal days and prematurity rate. Therefore the study was not designed to detect an adverse bioeffect, but a statistically significant effect was observed as a result of subsequent data analysis. Several other deficiencies in methodology are evident in the selection and exposure of the experimental groups, but in general, some association might be inferred from the results of this well-conducted, randomized clinical trial. In a case-control study, Campbell et al.[82] reported a statistically significant higher rate of delayed speech in children who were insonified in utero. Evidence of association is not as strong in case-control studies as in prospective studies, and measures of delayed speech are difficult. Subsequently, Salvesen et al.[83] found no significant differences in delayed speech, limited vocabulary, or stuttering in a study of 1107 children exposed in utero (1033 controls).

CONTROLLING ULTRASOUND OUTPUT

The most important issue regarding potential bioeffects involves actions the physician or sonographer can take to minimize these effects. It is essential that operators understand the risks involved in the process, but without some ability to control the output of the ultrasound system, this knowledge has limited use. Some specific methods can be used to limit ultrasound exposure while maintaining diagnostically relevant images.

Controls for the ultrasound system can be divided into direct controls and indirect controls. The **direct controls** are the application types and output intensity. **Application types** are those broad system controls that allow convenient selection of a particular examination type. These often come in the form of icons that are selected by the user. These default settings help minimize the time required to optimize the imaging parameters for the myriad of applications for diagnostic ultrasound. These settings should be used only as indicated (e.g., do not use the cardiac settings for a fetal exam). **Output intensity** (also called "power," "output," or "transmit") controls the overall ultrasonic power emitted by the transducer. This control will generally affect the intensity at all points in the image to varying degrees, depending on the focusing. The lowest output intensity that produces a good image should be used, to minimize the exposure intensity. Focusing of the system is controlled by the operator and can be used to improve image quality while limiting required acoustic intensity. Focusing at the correct depth can improve the image without requiring increased intensity.

OPTIMUM ULTRASOUND OUTPUT: LOWEST POWER OUTPUT THAT CREATES GOOD IMAGES

DIRECT CONTROLS
Application type: fetal, cardiac, etc.
Output intensity: power, output, transmit
Focusing: allows increasing output intensity only at the focal zone

INDIRECT CONTROLS
Ultrasound mode
Unscanned modes (deposits heat in one area)
  Continuous wave Doppler
  Spectral or pulsed Doppler
  M-mode
Scanned modes
  B-mode or gray-scale
  Color flow Doppler
  Power mode Doppler
Pulse repetition frequency
Increases bursts of energy per time
Pulse length
Increasing sample volume in Doppler studies
Appropriate transducer
High frequency: requires more output for depth
Lower frequency: less output needed at depth
Gain controls
Time gain compensation (TGC) can improve image without more output.
Receiver gain increases echo amplitudes without more output.

The many **indirect controls** greatly affect the ultrasound exposure by dictating how the ultrasonic energy is distributed temporally and spatially. By choosing the mode of ultrasound used (e.g., B-mode, pulsed Doppler, color Doppler), the operator controls whether the beam is scanned. Unscanned modes deposit energy along a single path and increase the potential for heating. The **pulse repetition frequency** (PRF) indicates how often the transducer is excited. Increasing the number of ultrasound bursts per second will increase the temporal average intensity. PRF is usually controlled by changing the maximum image depth in B-mode or the velocity range in Doppler modes. **Burst length** (also called "pulse length" or "pulse duration") controls the duration of on-time for each ultrasonic burst transmitted. Increasing the burst length while maintaining the same PRF will increase the temporal average intensity. The control of burst length may not be obvious. For example, in pulsed Doppler ultrasound, increasing the Doppler sample volume length will increase the burst length.

The selection of the **appropriate transducer** will also limit the need for high acoustic power. Even though higher frequencies provide better spatial resolution, the attenuation of tissue increases with increasing ultrasound frequency, so penetration may be lost. Perhaps most important are the **receiver gain controls.** The receiver gain control has no effect on the amplitude of the acoustic output. Therefore, before turning up the acoustic output intensity, try increasing receiver gain first. It should be noted that some system controls actually interact with the acoustic output intensity without direct control. Check to see whether the manufacturer provides separate controls for receiver gain, **time gain compensation** (TGC), and acoustic output intensity. The TGC can improve image quality without increasing the output.

There is really no substitute for a well-instructed operator. The indices and requirements of output display standards will help only those willing to use and understand them. Real-time display of the mechanical and thermal indices on diagnostic scanners will help clinicians evaluate and minimize potential risks in the use of such instrumentation. Physicians and sonographers are encouraged to learn more about how to minimize potential bioeffects.

ULTRASOUND ENTERTAINMENT VIDEOS

Of concern is the growing use of diagnostic ultrasound for the nonmedical scanning of pregnant women to provide a fetal "keepsake" video. Unfortunately, entertainment ultrasound is promoted most vigorously in the second and third trimesters, when bone calcification can increase thermal effects. Also, women with the economic means to schedule multiple ultrasound imaging sessions may be exposing both themselves and their fetus to even

AIUM STATEMENT ON KEEPSAKE FETAL IMAGING

Approved June 22, 2005

The AIUM advocates the responsible use of diagnostic ultrasound for all fetal imaging. The AIUM understands the growing pressures from patients for the performance of ultrasound examinations for bonding and reassurance purposes, largely driven by the improving image quality of 3D sonography and by more widely available information about these advances. Although there is only preliminary scientific evidence that 3D sonography has a positive impact on parental-fetal bonding, the AIUM recognizes that many parents may pursue scanning for this purpose.

Such "keepsake imaging" currently occurs in a variety of settings, including the following:

1. Images or video clips given to parents during the course of a medically indicated ultrasound examination;
2. Freestanding commercial fetal imaging sites, usually without any physician review of acquired images and with no regulation of the training of the individuals obtaining the images; these images are sometimes called "entertainment videos"; and
3. As added cost visits to a medical facility (office or hospital) outside the coverage of contractual arrangements between the provider and the patient's insurance carrier.

The AIUM recommends that appropriately trained and credentialed medical professionals (either licensed physicians, registered sonographers, or sonography registry candidates) who have received specialized training in fetal imaging perform all fetal ultrasound scans. These individuals have been trained to recognize medically important conditions, such as congenital anomalies, artifacts associated with ultrasound scanning that may mimic pathology, and techniques to avoid ultrasound exposure beyond what is considered safe for the fetus. Any other use of "limited medical ultrasound" may constitute practice of medicine without a license. The AIUM reemphasizes that all imaging requires proper documentation and a final report for the patient medical record signed by a physician.

Although the general use of ultrasound for medical diagnosis is considered safe, ultrasound energy has the potential to produce biological effects. Ultrasound bioeffects may result from scanning for a prolonged period, inappropriate use of color or pulsed Doppler ultrasound without a medical indication, or excessive thermal or mechanical index settings. The AIUM encourages patients to make sure that practitioners using ultrasound have received specific training in fetal imaging to ensure the best possible results.

The AIUM also believes that added cost arrangements other than those of providing patients images or copies of their medical records at cost may violate the principles of medical ethics of the American Medical Association[85,86] (E-8.062 and E-8.063) and the American College of Obstetricians and Gynecologists.[87] The AIUM[88] therefore reaffirms the *Prudent Use* statement and recommends that only scenario 1 above is consistent with the ethical principles of our professional organizations.

The market for keepsake images is driven in part by past medical approaches that have used medicolegal concerns as a reason not to provide images to patients. Sharing images with patients is unlikely to have a detrimental medicolegal impact. Although these concerns need further analysis and evaluation, we encourage sharing images with patients as appropriate when indicated obstetric ultrasound examinations are performed.[89]

Reprinted with permission of AIUM.

---

greater risk if ultrasound bioeffects are shown to be additive, or just by increasing the chances for a bioeffect. If there is no clinical benefit in such entertainment ultrasound, the benefit/risk ratio is clearly zero. In addition, because often the ultrasound equipment used is identical to diagnostic equipment used by clinicians, the consumer may be unaware that no medical information is being generated, interpreted, or referred to her obstetrician. (It is recognized that release forms are signed to the contrary.) The FDA[84] views this as an unapproved use of a medical device and refers users to the AIUM statement regarding keepsake videos.

References

Thermal Effects

1. Hynynen K. Ultrasound therapy. In: Goldman LE, Fowlkes JB, editors: Medical CT and ultrasound: current technology and applications. Madison, Wis: Advanced Medical Publishing; 1995. p. 249-265.
2. Carstensen EL, Child SZ, Norton S, Nyborg W. Ultrasonic heating of the skull. J Acoust Soc Am 1990;87:1310-1317.
3. Nyborg WL. Solutions of the bio-heat transfer equation. Phys Med Biol 1988;33:785-792.
4. Drewniak JL, Carnes KI, Dunn F. In vitro ultrasonic heating of fetal bone. J Acoust Soc Am 1989;86:1254-1258.
5. Edwards MJ. Hyperthermia as a teratogen: a review of experimental studies and their clinical significance. Teratog Carcinog Mutagen 1986;6:563-582.
6. Miller MW, Ziskin MC. Biological consequences of hyperthermia. Ultrasound Med Biol 1989;15:707-722.
7. National Council on Radiation Protection and Measurements, Scientific Committee on Biological Effects of Ultrasound. Exposure criteria for medical diagnostic ultrasound. I. Criteria based on thermal mechanisms. Report No 113. Bethesda, Md: NCRP; 1992.
8. National Council on Radiation Protection and Measurements, Scientific Committee on Biological Effects of Ultrasound. Exposure criteria for medical diagnostic ultrasound. II. Criteria based on all known mechanisms. Report No 140. Bethesda, Md: NCRP; 2002.
9. Miller MW, Nyborg WL, Dewey WC, et al. Hyperthermic teratogenicity, thermal dose and diagnostic ultrasound during pregnancy: implications of new standards on tissue heating. Int J Hyperthermia 2002;18:361-384.
10. O'Brien Jr WD, Deng CX, Harris GR, et al. The risk of exposure to diagnostic ultrasound in postnatal subjects: thermal effects. J Ultrasound Med 2008;27:517-535.

11. American Institute of Ultrasound in Medicine. Standard for real-time display of thermal and mechanical acoustical output indices on diagnostic ultrasound equipment. Rockville, Md: AIUM and National Electrical Manufacturers Association; 1992.

12. Carson PL. Medical ultrasound fields and exposure measurements. In: Nonionizing electromagnetic radiations and ultrasound. Bethesda, Md, 1988, National Council on Radiation Protection and Measurements, NCRP Proc 8:287-307.

13. Carson PL, Rubin JM, Chiang EH. Fetal depth and ultrasound path lengths through overlying tissues. Ultrasound Med Biol 1989;15:629-639.

14. Thomenius KE. Scientific rationale for the TIS index model. Presented at the National Electrical Manufacturers Association Output Display Standard Seminar. Rockville, Md, 1993.

15. Thomenius KE. Estimation of the potential for bioeffects. In: Ziskin MC, Lewin PA, editors. Ultrasonic exposimetry. Ann Arbor, Mich: CRC Press; 1993.

16. Siddiqi TA, O'Brien Jr WD, Meyer RA, et al. In situ exposimetry: the ovarian ultrasound examination. Ultrasound Med Biol 1991;17:257-263.

17. Chan AK, Sigelmann RA, Guy AW, Lehmann JF. Calculation by the method of finite differences of the temperature distribution in layered tissues. IEEE Trans Biomed Eng 1973;20:86-90.

18. Chan AK, Sigelmann RA, Guy AW. Calculations of therapeutic heat generated by ultrasound in fat-muscle-bone layers. IEEE Trans Biomed Eng 1974;21:280-284.

19. Frizzell LA. Ultrasonic heating of tissues (dissertation). Rochester, NY: University of Rochester; 1975.

20. American Institute of Ultrasound in Medicine. Bioeffects and safety of diagnostic ultrasound. Rockville, Md, 2008. Current versions are available to the public on request or at http://www.aium.org.

Effects of Acoustic Cavitation

21. Flynn HG. Cavitation dynamics. I. A mathematical formulation. J Acoust Soc Am 1975;57:1379-1396.

22. Roy RA, Atchley AA, Crum LA, et al. A precise technique for the measurement of acoustic cavitation thresholds and some preliminary results. J Acoust Soc Am 1985;78:1799-1805.

23. Kwak HY, Panton RL. Tensile strength of simple liquids predicted by a model of molecular interactions. J Phys D 1985;18:647.

24. Harvey EN, Barnes DK, McElroy WD, et al. Bubble formation in animals. I. Physical factors. J Cell Compar Phys 1944;24:1-22.

25. Harvey EN, Barnes DK, McElroy WD, et al. Bubble formation in animals. II. Gas nuclei and their distribution in blood and tissues. J Cell Compar Phys 1944;24:23-34.

26. Yount DE. Skins of varying permeability: a stabilization mechanism for gas cavitation nuclei. J Acoust Soc Am 1978;65:1429-1439.

27. Holland CK, Roy RA, Apfel RE, Crum LA. In vitro detection of cavitation induced by a diagnostic ultrasound system. IEEE Trans Ultrason Ferroelectr Freq Control 1992;39:95-101.

28. Walton AJ, Reynolds GT. Sonoluminescence. Adv Physics 1984;33:595-660.

29. Crum LA, Fowlkes JB. Acoustic cavitation generated by microsecond pulses of ultrasound. Nature 1986;319:52-54.

30. Carmichael AJ, Mossoba MM, Riesz P, Christman CL. Free radical production in aqueous solutions exposed to simulated ultrasonic diagnostic conditions. IEEE Trans Ultrason Ferroelectr Freq Control 1986;33:148-155.

31. Aymé EJ, Carstensen EL. Occurrence of transient cavitation in pulsed sawtooth ultrasonic fields. J Acoust Soc Am 1988;84:1598-1605.

32. Coleman AJ, Saunders JE, Crum LA, et al. Acoustic cavitation generated by an extracorporeal shockwave lithotripter. Ultrasound Med Biol 1987;13(2):69-76.

33. Delius M, Brendel W, Heine G. A mechanism of gallstone destruction by extracorporeal shock waves. Naturwissenschaften 1988;75:200-201.

34. Williams AR, Delius M, Miller DL, Schwarze W. Investigation of cavitation in flowing media by lithotripter shock waves both in vitro and in vivo. Ultrasound Med Biol 1989;15:53-60.

35. Duck FA, Starritt HC, Aindow JD, et al. The output of pulse-echo ultrasound equipment: a survey of powers, pressures and intensities. Br J Radiol 1985;58:989-1001.

36. Duck FA, Starritt HC, Anderson SP. A survey of the acoustic output of ultrasonic Doppler equipment. Clin Phys Physiol Meas 1987;8:39-49.

37. Patton CA, Harris GR, Phillips RA. Output levels and bioeffects indices from diagnostic ultrasound exposure data reported to the FDA. IEEE Trans Ultrason Ferroelectr Freq Control 1994;41:353-359.

38. Chaussy C, Schmiedt E, Jocham D, et al. Extracorporeal shock wave lithotripsy. Basel: Karger; 1986.

39. Church CC, Carstensen EL, Nyborg WL, et al. The risk of exposure to diagnostic ultrasound in postnatal subjects: nonthermal mechanisms. J Ultrasound Med 2008;27:565-592.

40. Child SZ, Hartman CL, Schery LA, Carstensen EL. Lung damage from exposure to pulsed ultrasound. Ultrasound Med Biol 1990;16:817-825.

41. Penney DP, Schenk EA, Maltby K, et al. Morphological effects of pulsed ultrasound in the lung. Ultrasound Med Biol 1993;19:127-135.

42. Tarantal AF, Canfield DR. Ultrasound-induced lung hemorrhage in the monkey. Ultrasound Med Biol 1994;20:65-72.

43. O'Brien Jr WD, Yang Y, Simpson DG, et al. Threshold estimation of ultrasound-induced lung hemorrhage in adult rabbits and comparison of thresholds in mice, rats, rabbits and pigs. Ultrasound Med Biol 2006;32:1793-1804.

44. Baggs R, Penney DP, Cox C, et al. Thresholds for ultrasonically induced lung hemorrhage in neonatal swine. Ultrasound Med Biol 1996;22:119-128.

45. Dalecki D, Child SZ, Raeman CH, et al. Ultrasonically induced lung hemorrhage in young swine. Ultrasound Med Biol 1997;23:777-781.

46. O'Brien Jr WD, Frizzell LA, Weigel RM, Zachary JF. Ultrasound-induced lung hemorrhage is not caused by inertial cavitation. J Acoust Soc Am 2000;108:1290-1297.

47. Dalecki D, Raeman CH, Child SZ, Carstensen EL. Intestinal hemorrhage from exposure to pulsed ultrasound. Ultrasound Med Biol 1995;21:1067-1072.

48. Kramer JM, Waldrop TG, Frizzell LA, et al. Cardiopulmonary function in rats with lung hemorrhage induced by pulsed ultrasound exposure. J Ultrasound Med 2001;20:1197-1206.

49. Miller DL, Averkiou MA, Brayman AA, et al. Bioeffects considerations for diagnostic ultrasound contrast agents. J Ultrasound Med 2008;27:611-632; quiz 633-636.

50. Ter Haar G. Safety and bio-effects of ultrasound contrast agents. Med Biol Eng Comput 2009;47:893-900.

51. Dalecki D: Bioeffects of ultrasound contrast agents in vivo. WFUMB Safety Symposium on Echo-Contrast Agents. Ultrasound Med Biol 2007;33:205-213.

52. Skyba DM, Price RJ, Linka AZ, et al. Direct in vivo visualization of intravascular destruction of microbubbles by ultrasound and its local effects on tissue. Circulation 1998;98:290-293.

53. Miller DL, Quddus J. Diagnostic ultrasound activation of contrast agent gas bodies induces capillary rupture in mice. Proc Natl Acad Sci USA 2000;97:10179-10184.

54. Hwang JH, Brayman AA, Reidy MA, et al. Vascular effects induced by combined 1-MHz ultrasound and microbubble contrast agent treatments in vivo. Ultrasound Med Biol 2005;31:553-564.

55. Samuel S, Cooper MA, Bull JL, et al. An ex vivo study of the correlation between acoustic emission and microvascular damage. Ultrasound Med Biol 2009;35:1574-1586.

56. Miller DL, Dou C, Wiggins RC, et al. An in vivo rat model simulating imaging of human kidney by diagnostic ultrasound with gas-body contrast agent. Ultrasound Med Biol 2007;33:129-135.

57. Hwang JH, Tu J, Brayman AA, et al. Correlation between inertial cavitation dose and endothelial cell damage in vivo. Ultrasound Med Biol 2006;32:1611-1619.

58. Van der Wouw PA, Brauns AC, Bailey SE, et al. Premature ventricular contractions during triggered imaging with ultrasound contrast. J Am Soc Echocardiogr 2000;13:288-294.

59. Tran TA, Le Guennec JY, Babuty D, et al. On the mechanisms of ultrasound contrast agents–induced arrhythmias. Ultrasound Med Biol 2009;35:1050-1056.

60. Tran TA, Le Guennec JY, Bougnoux P, et al. Characterization of cell membrane response to ultrasound-activated microbubbles. IEEE Trans Ultrason Ferroelectr Freq Control 2008;55:43-49.

61. Tran TA, Roger S, Le Guennec JY, et al. Effect of ultrasound-activated microbubbles on the cell electrophysiological properties. Ultrasound Med Biol 2007;33:158-163.

62. Kurt M, Shaikh KA, Peterson L, et al. Impact of contrast echocardiography on evaluation of ventricular function and clinical

management in a large prospective cohort. J Am Coll Cardiol 2009; 53:802-810.

63. Abdelmoneim SS, Bernier M, Scott CG, et al. Safety of contrast agent use during stress echocardiography: a 4-year experience from a single-center cohort study of 26,774 patients. JACC Cardiovasc Imaging 2009;2:1048-1056.

64. Grayburn PA. Product safety compromises patient safety (an unjustified black box warning on ultrasound contrast agents by the Food and Drug Administration). Am J Cardiol 2008;101:892-893.

65. Kusnetzky LL, Khalid A, Khumri TM, et al. Acute mortality in hospitalized patients undergoing echocardiography with and without an ultrasound contrast agent: results in 18,671 consecutive studies. J Am Coll Cardiol 2008;51:1704-1706.

66. Main ML, Ryan AC, Davis TE, et al. Acute mortality in hospitalized patients undergoing echocardiography with and without an ultrasound contrast agent (multicenter registry results in 4,300,966 consecutive patients). Am J Cardiol 2008;102:1742-1746.

67. Apfel RE, Holland CK. Gauging the likelihood of cavitation from short-pulse, low-duty cycle diagnostic ultrasound. Ultrasound Med Biol 1991;17:179-185.

68. Dalecki D, Raeman CH, Child SZ, Carstensen EL. A test for cavitation as a mechanism for intestinal hemorrhage in mice exposed to a piezoelectric lithotripter. Ultrasound Med Biol 1996;22:493-496.

Output Display Standard

69. American Institute of Ultrasound in Medicine. Medical ultrasound safety. 2nd ed. Rockville, Md: AIUM; 2009.

Epidemiology

70. Ziskin MC, Petitti DB. Epidemiology of human exposure to ultrasound: a critical review. Ultrasound Med Biol 1988;14:91-96.

71. Abramowicz JS, Fowlkes JB, Skelly AC, et al. Conclusions regarding epidemiology for obstetric ultrasound. J Ultrasound Med 2008;27: 637-644.

72. American Institute of Ultrasound in Medicine. Conclusions regarding epidemiology for obstetric ultrasound. Approved June 2005. Current versions are available to the public on request or at http://www.aium.org.

73. EDH Environment Health Directorate. Canada-wide survey of non-ionizing radiation emitting medical devices. II. Ultrasound devices. Report No 80-EDH-53, 1980, EDH.

74. Ziskin MC. Survey of patient exposure to diagnostic ultrasound. In: Reid JM, Sikov MR, editors. Interaction of ultrasound and biological tissues. Pub No FDA 78-8008. Washington, DC: US Department of Health, Education and Welfare; 1972. p. 203.

75. Moore Jr R, Barrick M, Hamilton P. Effects of sonic radiation on growth and development. Am J Epidemiol 1982;116:571 (abstract).

76. Stark CR, Orleans M, Haverkamp AD, Murphy J. Short- and long-term risks after exposure to diagnostic ultrasound in utero. Obstet Gynecol 1984;63:194-200.

77. Scheidt PC, Stanley F, Bryla DA. One-year follow-up of infants exposed to ultrasound in utero. Am J Obstet Gynecol 1978;131: 743-748.

78. Bakketeig LS, Eik-Nes SH, Jacobsen G, et al. Randomised controlled trial of ultrasonographic screening in pregnancy. Lancet 1984;2: 207-211.

79. Eik-Nes SH, Okland O, Aure JC, Ulstein M. Ultrasound screening in pregnancy: a randomised controlled trial. Lancet 1984;1:1347.

80. Hill AB: The environment and disease: association or causation? Proc R Soc Med 1965;58:295-300.

81. Newnham JP, Evans SF, Michael CA, et al. Effects of frequent ultrasound during pregnancy: a randomised controlled trial. Lancet 1993; 342:887-891.

82. Campbell JD, Elford RW, Brant RF. Case-control study of prenatal ultrasonography exposure in children with delayed speech. CMAJ 1993;149:1435-1440.

83. Salvesen KA, Vatten LJ, Bakketeig LS, Eik-Nes SH. Routine ultrasonography in utero and speech development. Ultrasound Obstet Gynecol 1994;4:101-103.

Ultrasound Entertainment Videos

84. FDA Statement on Fetal Keepsake Videos. http://www.fda.gov/MedicalDevices/Safety/AlertsandNotices/PatientAlerts/ucm064756.htm.

85. American Medical Association. E-8.062: Sale of non-health-related goods from physician's offices. Chicago: AMA; 1998.

86. American Medical Association. E-8.063: Sale of health-related products from physician's offices. Chicago: AMA; 1999.

87. American College of Obstetricians and Gynecologists. Commercial enterprises in medical practice. In: Ethics in obstetrics and gynecology. Washington, DC: ACOG; 2004.

88. American Institute of Ultrasound in Medicine. Prudent use. Laurel, Md: AIUM; 1999.

89. American Institute of Ultrasound in Medicine. Providing images to patients. Laurel, Md: AUIM; 1998.

CHAPTER 3

Contrast Agents for Ultrasound

Peter N. Burns

Chapter Outline

*T*he injection of a contrast agent forms a routine part of clinical x-ray, CT, MR, and radionuclide imaging in radiology. Despite the obvious significance of the vascular component of many ultrasound examinations in radiology, however, and despite the widespread availability of contrast agents for echocardiography, noncardiac ultrasound imaging has only begun to exploit the potential benefit of contrast enhancement. The reason is that ultrasound, unlike x-ray imaging, benefits from an intrinsically high contrast between blood and solid tissue, and therefore large vessels can be visualized without a contrast agent and associated subtraction imaging method. Furthermore, color Doppler sonographic imaging offers a powerful and effective tool, with the additional ability to quantify hemodynamic parameters such as the direction and velocity of blood flow.

It is precisely these capabilities that the new generation of ultrasound contrast agents has extended into the microcirculation, redefining the role of ultrasound in resolving vascular questions until now left to contrast-enhanced computed tomography (CT) and magnetic resonance imaging (MRI). Contrast agents can help delineate vascular structures and enhance Doppler signals from small volumes of blood. More importantly, for the first time, these agents allow ultrasound imaging of organ and lesion perfusion in real time. This chapter provides both a tutorial and a reference for the practical use of contrast agents for these new indications.

REQUIREMENTS AND TYPES

The principal requirements for an ultrasound contrast agent are (1) being easily introducible into the vascular system, (2) being stable for the duration of the diagnostic examination, (3) having low toxicity, and (4) modifying one or more acoustic properties of tissues that can be detected by ultrasound imaging. Although applications might be found for ultrasound contrast agents to justify their injection into arteries, the clinical context for contrast ultrasonography requires that agents be capable of **intravenous** administration and intact passage through the heart and lungs. These constitute a demanding specification that has been met only in the past decade. Currently, more than 60 countries have approved the use of at least one contrast agent for abdominal ultrasound diagnosis. The technology universally adopted is that of encapsulated bubbles of gas that are smaller than red blood cells and therefore capable of circulating freely in the systemic vasculature.

Contrast agents act by their presence in the vascular system, from where they are ultimately metabolized (**blood pool** agents) or by their **selective uptake** in tissue after a vascular phase. The most important properties of tissue that influence the ultrasound image are **linear and nonlinear backscatter coefficient, attenuation,** and **acoustic propagation velocity.**[1,2] Most agents work to enhance the echo from blood by increasing the backscatter of the tissue as much as possible while increasing the attenuation in the tissue as little as possible.

Blood Pool Contrast Agents

Free Gas Bubbles

Gramiak and Shah[3] first used bubbles to enhance the echo from blood in 1968. They injected agitated saline into the left ventricle during an echocardiographic examination and saw strong echoes within the lumen of the aorta. It was subsequently shown that these echoes originated from free bubbles of air arising from solution either during agitation or at the catheter tip during injection.[4] Agitated solutions of compounds such as indocyanine green and diatrizoate sodium/meglumine (Renografin)—already approved for intra-arterial injection—were also used. The application of free gas as a contrast agent was confined to the heart, including evaluation of valvular insufficiency,[5] intracardiac shunts,[6] and cavity dimensions.[7] The fundamental limitations of bubbles produced in this way are that they are *large,* and thus effectively filtered by the lungs, and *unstable,* and thus go back into solution in about 1 second. Apart from occasional use to identify shunts, free bubbles are rarely used at present as a contrast agent.

Encapsulated Air Bubbles

To overcome the natural instability of free gas bubbles, various shell coatings were investigated to create a more stable particle. In 1980, Carroll et al.[8] encapsulated nitrogen bubbles in gelatin and injected them into the femoral artery of rabbits with VX2 tumors in the thigh. Although echo enhancement of the tumor rim was identified, the large diameter of the coated bubbles (80 μm) precluded intravenous administration. In 1984, Feinstein et al.[9] first produced a stable encapsulated microbubble that was comparable in size to a red blood cell (RBC) and that could survive passage through the heart and pulmonary capillary network. They produced microbubbles by sonication of a solution of human serum albumin and showed that it could be detected in the left side of the heart after peripheral venous injection. This agent was subsequently developed commercially as **Albunex** (Mallinckrodt Medical, St. Louis) (Table 3-1).

Another approach to stabilizing an air bubble is to add a **lipid shell** on dissolution of a dry powder. **Levovist** (Schering AG, Berlin), is a dry mixture comprising 99.9% microcrystalline galactose microparticles and 0.1% palmitic acid. On dissolving in sterile water, the galactose disaggregates into microparticles, which provide an irregular surface for the adherence of microbubbles 3 to 4 μm in size. Stabilization of the microbubbles takes place as they become coated with palmitic acid, which separates the gas-liquid interface and slows their dissolution.[10] The resulting microbubbles have a median bubble diameter of about 3 μm, with the 97th centile at approximately 6 μm, and are sufficiently stable for transit through the pulmonary circuit. The agent is chemically related to its predecessor **Echovist** (SHU454, Schering AG), a galactose agent that forms larger bubbles and is used principally for visualization of nonvascular ductal structures such as the fallopian tubes.[11,12] Numerous early studies with Levovist demonstrated its capacity to traverse the pulmonary bed in sufficient concentrations

TABLE 3-1. REGULATORY AND MARKETING STATUS OF ULTRASOUND CONTRAST AGENTS, 2009

NAME	COMPANY	LIPID SHELL/GAS	STATUS
Albunex	Mallinckrodt	Sonicated albumin/air	Approved in EU, USA, Canada *Not marketed*
Echovist	Schering	Galactose matrix/air	Approved in EU, Canada
Levovist	Schering	Lipid/air	Approved in EU, Canada, Japan *Not marketed*
Definity	Lantheus Medical Imaging	Liposome/perfluoropropane	Approved in US for cardiology; in Canada, Australasia, Americas for radiology/cardiology
SonoVue	Bracco	Phospholipid/sulfur hexafluoride	Approved in EU for radiology/cardiology; in US for clinical development in USA
Optison	GE Healthcare	Sonicated albumin/octafluoropropane	Approved in EU, USA, Canada for cardiology
Imagent	Schering	Surfactant/perfluorohexane-air	Approved in USA for cardiology *Not marketed*
Sonavist	Schering	Polymer/air	Suspended development suspended
Sonazoid	GE Healthcare/ Daiichi-Sankyo	Lipid/perflubutane	Approved in Japan for radiology
Bisphere	Point Biomedical	Polymer bilayer/air	Clinical development[100]
Imagify	Acusphere	Polymer/perflubutane	Clinical development[101]
PESDA	[Porter et al[102]]	Sonicated albumin/perfluorocarbon	Not commercially developed

EU, European Union; *USA,* United States.

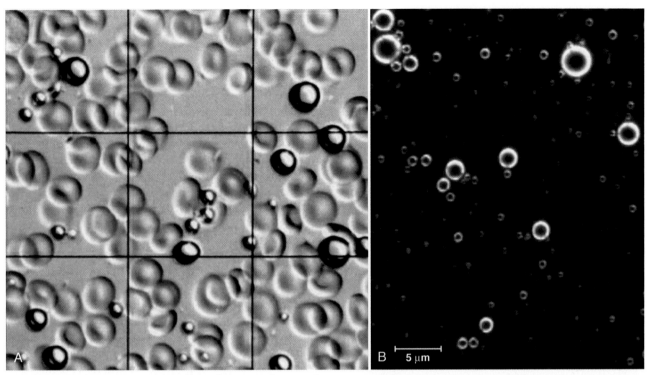

FIGURE 3-1. Contrast agents for ultrasound. A, Perfluoropropane bubbles with a protein shell (Optison), seen here against a background of red blood cells. **B,** Lipid-coated microbubbles of perfluoropropane gas (Definity) are seen under darkfield microscope.

to enhance both color and spectral Doppler signals, as well as gray-scale examinations using nonlinear imaging modes such as pulse inversion.[13,14] Levovist remains approved for use in the European Union (EU), Canada, Japan, and numerous other countries, although not in the United States. Many clinical applications of intravenous contrast were pioneered using Levovist, which has now given way to the so-called second-generation agents and is no longer marketed.

Low-Solubility Gas Bubbles

The shells that stabilize microbubbles are extremely thin and allow a gas such as air to diffuse through and fall back into solution in the blood. How fast this happens depends on a number of factors, including the nature of the fluid medium and the bubble under insonation. After venous injection, the typical duration in the systemic circulation of Levovist and Echovist is only a few minutes. Because these agents are introduced as a **bolus** and the maximum effect of the agent is in the first pass, the useful imaging time is usually considerably less than this duration. Second-generation agents were designed both to increase backscatter enhancement and to last longer in the bloodstream by taking advantage of low-solubility gases such as the **perfluorocarbons.** These heavier gases diffuse more slowly through the bubble shell and have much lower solubility in blood. **Optison** (GE Healthcare, Milwaukee) is a perfluoropropane-filled albumin shell with a size distribution similar to that of

its predecessor, Albunex, and is currently approved for "cardiology" indications in the EU, United States, and Canada (Fig. 3-1, *A*). **SonoVue** (Bracco Imaging SpA, Milan) uses sulfur hexafluorane in a phospholipid shell and is available for "cardiology and radiology" indications in the EU, China, and a number of other countries. **Definity** (Lantheus Medical Imaging, Billerica, Mass) comprises a perfluoropropane microbubble coated with a flexible bilipid shell, which also showed improved stability and high enhancement at low doses[15] (Fig. 3-1, *B*). Definity is currently approved for "cardiology and radiology" indications in Canada, Australasia, and a number of Central and South American countries, and for cardiology in the United States. **Sonazoid** (Daiichi Sankyo, Tokyo) consists of a perfluorobutane bubble in a lipid shell[16] and is currently approved for radiology in Japan.

Although tiny, these bubbles are large compared with the molecules and particles used as contrast agents for CT and MRI. The contrast agents for these modalities are sufficiently small to be able to diffuse through the fenestrated endothelium of blood vessels into the interstitium. Thus, x-ray and MR contrast-enhanced images frequently show a **parenchymal** phase of enhancement, which is used to identify hyperpermeable vascular structures, such as those involved with tumor angiogenesis.[17] **Microbubbles,** on the other hand, are of a size comparable to that of an RBC, so they go where an RBC goes (Fig. 3-2) and, more significantly, do *not* go where an RBC does not go. Microbubbles are clinical radiology's first pure "blood pool" contrast agent.

Selective Uptake Contrast Agents

An ideal blood pool agent displays the same flow dynamics as blood itself, and ultimately it is metabolized from the blood pool. Agents such as Definity, SonoVue, and Optison are generally not detected outside the vascular system and therefore come close to this ideal. However, contrast preparations can be made that are capable of providing ultrasound enhancement during their metabo-

lism as well as while in the blood pool. Colloidal suspensions of liquid droplets such as perfluoroctylbromide[18] and microbubble agents with certain shell properties[16,19,20] are taken up by the reticuloendothelial system (RES), from where they ultimately are excreted. In the RES they may provide contrast from within the liver parenchyma, demarcating the distribution of Kupffer cells.[21] Agents such as Levovist and Sonazoid provide "late phase" enhancement in the parenchyma of the liver and spleen after having cleared from the vascular system,[22] allowing detection of Kupffer cell–poor lesions such as cancers.[23,24] Other strategies for more specific uptake and targeted imaging are discussed later.

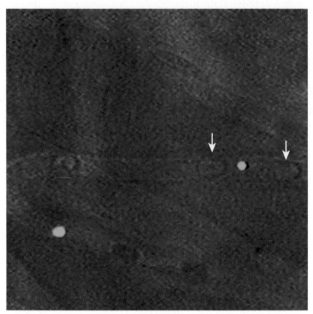

FIGURE 3-2. Bubbles are relatively large as contrast agents and remain within the blood pool. Intravital microscopy of fluorescent-labeled perfluoropropane bubbles (Definity) shows them in capillaries, being transported much as red blood cells nearby *(arrows). (Courtesy J Lindner, Oregon Health Sciences.)*

NEED FOR BUBBLE-SPECIFIC IMAGING

A typical dose of an ultrasound contrast agent is of the order of tens of microliters (μL) of bubble suspension per kilogram (kg) body weight, so that a whole-body dose might be of the order of 0.1 to 1.0 milliliter (mL). Figure 3-3 shows the enhancement of the echo from systemic arterial blood after a peripheral venous injection of a second-generation agent. A first-pass peak is seen, followed by recirculation and washout as the agent is eliminated over the next few minutes. By infusing the bubbles through a saline drip or pump, a steady enhancement lasting up to 20 minutes can also be obtained.[25] The small amount of perfluorocarbon gas goes into solution in the blood and is ultimately excreted by the lungs and liver. The trace amount of shell material is reduced to biocompatible elements that, in the case of the common agents, are already present in the blood.[26]

FIGURE 3-3. Contrast-enhanced arterial flow. Arterial blood echo enhancement after intravenous bolus of Optison at increasing doses. The peak enhancement is 30 dB, corresponding to a 1000-fold increase of echo power. Note that increasing the dose by a factor of 10 does not have the same effect on the peak enhancement. Instead, it is the washout time that is increased.

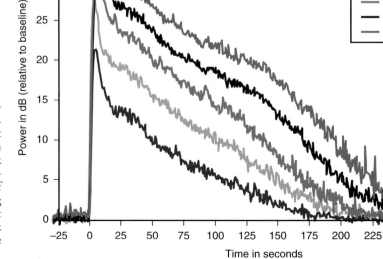

One of the major diagnostic objectives in using an ultrasound contrast agent in a solid organ is to detect flow at the **perfusion**—that is, the arteriolar and capillary—level. The peak enhancement in Figure 3-3 is about 30 dB, corresponding to a 1000-fold increase in the power of the ultrasound echo from blood. Although this may seem impressive, it does not necessarily help ultrasound to image perfusion. The echoes from blood associated with such flow, such as in the hepatic sinusoids, exist in the midst of echoes from the surrounding solid structures of the liver parenchyma, echoes that are almost always stronger than even the contrast-enhanced blood echo. When they can be seen, blood vessels in a nonenhanced image have a low echo level; thus an **echo-enhancing agent** actually **lowers** the contrast between blood and the surrounding tissue, making the lumen of the blood vessel less visible. Therefore, to image flow in small vessels of the liver, a contrast agent is required that either (1) enhances the blood echo to a level that is substantially higher than that of the surrounding tissue or (2) can be used with a method for suppressing the echo from non-contrast-bearing structures.

Doppler offers a method that successfully separates the echoes from blood from those of tissue. It was originally thought that microbubbles would be used as an "echo-enhancing" agent, enabling perfusion to be revealed.[27] However, Doppler relies on the relatively high velocity of moving blood compared to that of the surrounding tissue. This distinction allows use of a high pass (or wall) filter to separate the Doppler signals caused by blood flow from those caused by tissue motion and is valid for flow in large vessels, but it does not work for flow at the parenchymal level, where the tissue is moving at the same speed or faster than the blood that perfuses it. In this case the Doppler shift frequency from the moving solid tissue is comparable to or higher than that of the moving blood itself. Because the wall filter cannot be used without eliminating both the flow and the tissue echoes, the use of Doppler in such circumstances is defeated by the overwhelming signal from tissue movement: the **flash artifact** in color or the **thump artifact** in spectral Doppler.[28] Despite some hopeful claims to the contrary, these fundamental limitations mean that true parenchymal flow cannot be imaged using Doppler at clinical frequencies, with or without intravenous contrast agents[29] (see Fig. 3-1).

How then might contrast agents be used to improve the visibility of perfused small structures within tissue? Clearly, a method that could identify the echo from the contrast agent and suppress that from solid tissue would provide both a real-time "subtraction" mode for contrast-enhanced B-mode imaging and a means of suppressing Doppler **clutter,** without the use of a velocity-dependent filter in spectral and color modes. **Contrast-specific imaging,** often referred to as **nonlinear imaging,** has provided such a method and thus the means for detecting flow in smaller vessels.

Bubble Behavior and Incident Pressure

The key to understanding contrast-specific imaging modes and their successful clinical use lies in the unique interaction between a microbubble contrast agent and the imaging process. Controlling and exploiting this interaction are central to all contrast-specific methods. Unlike tissue, microbubbles scatter ultrasound in a manner dependent on the amplitude of the sound to which they are exposed by the imaging process. The result is three broad regimens of bubble behavior, resulting in three types of echoes (Table 3-2).

The regimens depend primarily on the intensity, or more precisely, the **peak negative pressure,** of the incident sound field produced by the scanner. At low incident pressures (corresponding to low transmit power of the scanner) the agents produce **linear backscatter enhancement,** which augments the echo from blood. This is the behavior originally envisioned by contrast agent manufacturers. As the transmit intensity control of the scanner is increased and the negative pressure incident on a bubble goes beyond 50 to 100 kilopascals (kPa), which is still below the level used in most diagnostic scans, the contrast agent backscatter begins to show nonlinear characteristics, such as the **emission of harmonics.** The detection of these forms the basis of contrast-specific imaging modes, such as harmonic and

TABLE 3-2. THREE REGIMENS OF ACOUSTIC BEHAVIOR OF TYPICAL PERFLUOROCARBON GAS/LIPID-SHELLED AGENT IN ULTRASOUND FIELD

PEAK PRESSURE (APPROX)	MECHANICAL INDEX (MI) (AT 2 MHz)	BUBBLE BEHAVIOR	ACOUSTIC BEHAVIOR	APPLICATION
<100 kPa	<0.07	Linear oscillation	Linear backscatter enhancement	Doppler signal enhancement
0.1-0.4 MPa	0.07-0.3	Nonlinear oscillation	Nonlinear backscatter	Real-time (low MI) perfusion imaging
>0.5 MPa	>0.4	Disruption	Transient nonlinear echoes	Triggered perfusion/disruption-replenishment flow measurement

pulse inversion and Doppler. As the peak pressure reaches and passes about 300 kPa, or 0.3 megapascal (MPa), and approaches the level emitted by a typical ultrasound imaging system in conventional B-mode imaging, bubbles will produce a strong but brief echo as they are disrupted by the ultrasound beam. This behavior forms the basis of the most common way of quantifying perfusion.

In practice, because of the different sizes present in a realistic population of bubbles,[30] as well as the additional effect of frequency, the borders between these acoustic behaviors are not sharp and vary among different bubble types, whose behavior strongly depends on the gas and shell properties.[31]

Mechanical Index

For reasons unrelated to contrast imaging, ultrasound scanners marketed in the United States are required by the Food and Drug Administration (FDA) to carry an on-screen label of the estimated normalized peak negative pressure to which tissue is exposed. This pressure changes according to the tissue through which the sound travels as well as the amplitude and geometry of the ultrasound beam: the higher the attenuation, the less the peak pressure in tissue. A scanner cannot "know" the tissue being imaged, so an index has been defined that reflects the approximate exposure to ultrasound pressure at the focus of the beam in average tissue.

The **mechanical index** (MI) is defined as the peak rarefactional (i.e., negative) pressure, divided by the square root of the ultrasound frequency. This quantity is related to the amount of mechanical work that can be performed on a bubble during a negative half-cycle of sound.[32] MI is thought to indicate the propensity of the sound to cause cavitation in the medium. In clinical ultrasound systems, MI is usually 0.05 to 2.0. Although a single value is displayed for each image, in practice the actual MI varies throughout the image. In the absence of attenuation, the MI is maximal at the focus of the beam. Attenuation shifts this maximum toward the transducer. Furthermore, because of the complex procedure to calculate MI, which is itself only an estimate of the actual quantity within the body, the indices displayed by different machines are not precisely comparable. Thus, for example, more bubble disruption might be observed at a displayed MI of 0.5 using one machine but at 0.6 with the same patient using another machine. For this reason, recommendations of machine settings for a specific examination are not transferable between manufacturers' instruments. Nonetheless, the MI is the operator's most important indication of the expected behavior of the contrast agent bubbles. Therefore, it is usually incorporated into the preset initial settings for a contrast imaging mode on the scanner and the "output power" adjustment at the operator's front line of controls.

MECHANICAL INDEX (MI) IN ULTRASOUND IMAGING

- Defined as follows:

$$MI = \frac{P_{neg}}{\sqrt{f}}$$

where P_{neg} is the peak negative ultrasound pressure in MPa, and f is the ultrasound frequency in MHz.
- Reflects the normalized negative pressure to which a target, such as a bubble, is exposed in an ultrasound field.
- Is defined for the focus of the ultrasound beam.
- Varies with depth in the image (lessens with increasing depth).
- Varies with lateral location in the image (lessens at the sector edges).
- Is estimated differently in systems from different manufacturers.

NONLINEAR BACKSCATTER: HARMONIC IMAGING

The behavior of bubbles in an acoustic field offers two important pieces of evidence. First, as shown in Figure 3-4, the size of the echo enhancement is much larger than would be expected from such sparse scatterers of this size in blood. Second, investigations of the acoustic characteristics of early agents[33] demonstrated peaks in the spectra of attenuation and scattering that depend on both ultrasound frequency and size of the microbubbles. This evidence suggests that the bubbles **resonate** in an ultrasound field. As the ultrasound wave (comprising alternate compressions and rarefactions) propagates over the bubbles, the bubbles experience a periodic change in their radius in sympathy with the oscillations of the incident sound. Like vibrations of the string of a musical instrument, these oscillations have a natural or **resonant** frequency of oscillation at which they will both absorb and scatter ultrasound with a peculiarly high efficiency. Considering the linear oscillation of a free bubble of air in water, a simple theory[1,2] can predict the resonant frequency of radial oscillation of a bubble of 3-μm diameter (median diameter of typical transpulmonary microbubble agent): about 3 MHz, approximately the center frequency of ultrasound used in a typical abdominal scan (Fig. 3-5). This coincidence explains why ultrasound contrast agents are so efficient and can be administered in such small quantities. It also predicts that bubbles undergoing resonant oscillation in an ultrasound field can be induced to nonlinear motion, the basis of harmonic imaging.

It has long been recognized[34] that if bubbles are "driven" by an ultrasound field at sufficiently high acoustic pressures, the oscillatory excursions of the bubble

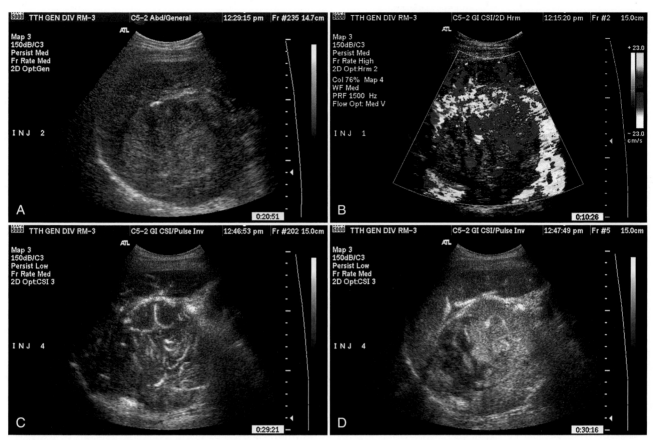

FIGURE 3-4. Need for contrast-specific imaging. A, Conventional image of liver shows a large, solid mass. **B,** Administration of contrast increases the echogenicity of blood but creates Doppler artifacts due to blooming and tissue motion. **C,** Contrast-specific imaging shows blood vessels not seen by Doppler. **D,** Initiating high-MI imaging after a pause reveals perfusion of the mass and a necrotic area. The lesion is a hepatocellular carcinoma. *(Modified from Burns PN, Wilson SR, Simpson DH. Pulse inversion imaging of liver blood flow: improved method for characterizing focal masses with microbubble contrast. Invest Radiol 2000;35:58-71.)*

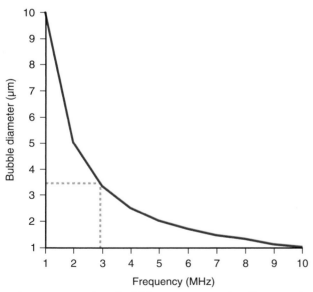

FIGURE 3-5. Microbubbles resonate in diagnostic ultrasound field. This graph shows that the resonant (or natural) frequency of oscillation of a bubble of air in an ultrasound field depends on its size. For a 3.5-μm diameter, the size needed for an intravenously injectable contrast agent, the resonant frequency is about 3 MHz.

reach a point at which the alternate expansions and contractions in bubble size are not equal. Lord Rayleigh, whose original theoretical understanding of sound is the basis for ultrasound imaging, first investigated this in 1917, curious about the creaking noises in a tea kettle as water boils.[35] The consequence of such **nonlinear motion** is that the sound emitted by the bubble, and detected by the transducer, contains **harmonics,** just as the resonant strings of a musical instrument, depending on how they are bowed or plucked, will produce a timbre comprising overtones (the musical term for harmonics), exact octaves above the pitch of the fundamental note. The origin of this phenomenon is the asymmetry that begins to affect bubble oscillation as the amplitude becomes large. As a bubble is compressed by the ultrasound pressure wave, it becomes stiffer and thus resists further reduction in its radius. Conversely, in the rarefaction phase of the ultrasound pulse, the bubble becomes less stiff and therefore enlarges much more (Fig. 3-6).

Figure 3-7 shows the frequency spectrum of an echo produced by a microbubble contrast agent after exposure to a 3-MHz burst of sound. The particular agent is Optison, although most microbubble agents behave

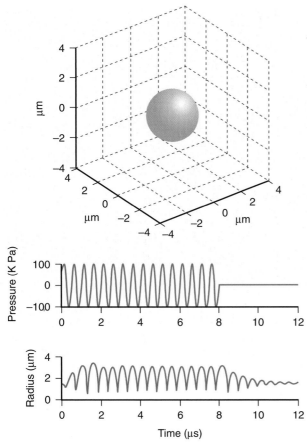

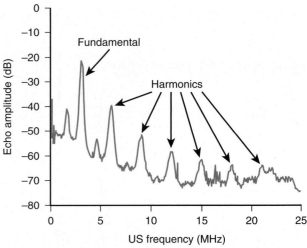

FIGURE 3-7. Harmonic emission from Optison. Sample of contrast agent is insonated at 3 MHz and the echo analyzed for its frequency content. It is seen that the largest peak of the energy in the echo is at the 3-MHz fundamental, but that there are clear secondary peaks in the spectrum at 6, 9, 12, 15, and 18 MHz, as well as peaks between these harmonics (known as "ultraharmonics") and below the fundamental (the "subharmonic"). The second harmonic echo is about 18 dB less than that of the main, or fundamental, echo. Harmonic imaging and Doppler aim to separate and process this signal alone. *(From Becher H, Burns PN. Handbook of contrast echocardiography. Berlin, 2000, Springer.)*

FIGURE 3-6. Microbubble in acoustic field. Bubbles respond asymmetrically to diagnostic sound waves *(top graph)*, stiffening when compressed by sound and yielding only small changes in radius *(bottom graph)*. During the low-pressure portion of the sound wave, the bubble stiffness decreases and changes in radius can be large. This asymmetric response leads to the production of harmonics in the scattered wave.

similarly. Ultrasound frequency is on the horizontal axis, with the relative amplitude on the vertical axis. In addition to the **fundamental echo** at 3 MHz, a series of echoes are seen at whole multiples of the transmitted frequency, known as **higher harmonics**.

Therefore, one simple method to distinguish bubbles from tissue is to excite the bubbles so as to produce harmonics and then detect these in preference over the fundamental echo from tissue. Key factors in the harmonic response of an agent are the incident pressure of the ultrasound field, the frequency, the size distribution of the bubbles, and the mechanical properties of the bubble capsule (e.g., a stiff capsule will dampen oscillations and attenuate its nonlinear response).

Harmonic B-Mode Imaging

An imaging and Doppler method based on this phenomenon, called **harmonic imaging**,[36] is widely available on modern ultrasound scanners. In harmonic mode the system transmits normally at one frequency but is tuned to receive echoes preferentially at double that frequency,

where the echoes from the bubbles lie. Typically, the transmit frequency lies between 1.5 and 3.0 MHz, and the receive frequency is selected by means of a detection strategy (originally, simple radiofrequency bandpass filter with center frequency at second harmonic), between 3 and 6 MHz. Harmonic imaging uses the same array transducers as conventional imaging and, for most current ultrasound systems, involves only software changes. Echoes from solid tissue, as well as red blood cells themselves, are suppressed. **Real-time harmonic spectral Doppler and color Doppler modes** have also been implemented on a number of commercially available systems. Clearly, an exceptional transducer bandwidth is needed to operate over such a large range of frequencies. Fortunately, recent efforts have increased the bandwidth of transducer arrays because of its significant bearing on conventional imaging performance, so harmonic imaging modes do not require the additional expense of dedicated transducers.

Harmonic Spectral and Power Doppler Imaging

In harmonic images the echo from tissue mimicking material is reduced, but not eliminated, reversing the contrast between the agent and its surroundings (Fig. 3-8). The value of this effect is to increase the conspicuity of the agent when it is in blood vessels normally hidden by the strong echoes from tissue. In spectral

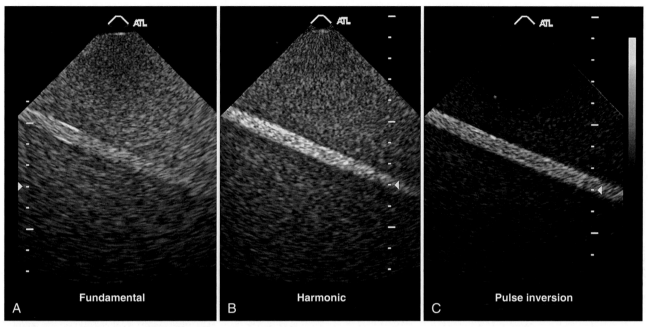

FIGURE 3-8. Pulse inversion imaging. In vitro images of a vessel phantom containing stationary perfluorocarbon contrast agent surrounded by tissue equivalent material (biogel and graphite). **A,** Conventional image, mechanical index (MI) = 0.2. **B,** Harmonic imaging, MI = 0.2, provides improved contrast between agent and tissue. **C,** Pulse inversion imaging, MI = 0.2. By suppressing linear echoes from stationary tissue, pulse inversion imaging provides better contrast between agent and tissue than both conventional and harmonic imaging. *(From Becher H, Burns PN.* Handbook of contrast echocardiography. *Berlin, 2000, Springer.)*

Doppler, one would expect the suppression of the tissue echo to reduce the tissue motion or "thump" artifact familiar to all Doppler sonographers that limits the detection of flow in moving vessels. In vivo spectral Doppler measurements show that the signal-to-clutter ratio is improved by a combination of harmonic imaging and the contrast agent by as much as 35 dB.[37] Applications of this method include detection of blood flow in small vessels surrounded by tissue that is moving, such as the branches of the coronary arteries.[38] It remains a somewhat specialized technique.

In conventional color Doppler studies using a contrast agent, the increased echo signal does nothing to suppress the clutter "flash" from moving tissue, but instead adds to it a "blooming" artifact of flow signals as the receiver is overloaded with the enhanced echo from blood (see Fig. 3-4, *C*). Harmonic power Doppler mode effectively overcomes this clutter problem by suppressing the signal from tissue, revealing better detail of small vessels. Combining the harmonic method with power Doppler produces an especially effective tool for the detection of flow in the small vessels of the abdominal organs, which may be moving with cardiac pulsation or respiration (Fig. 3-9). A study comparing flow on contrast-enhanced power harmonic images with histologically sized arterioles in the corresponding regions of the renal cortex concluded that the method is capable of demonstrating flow in vessels less than 40 μm in diameter; about 10 times smaller than the corresponding imaging resolution limit, even as the organ was moving with normal respira-tion.[39] Using this power mode method in the heart allows flow imaging in the myocardium.[40,41]

Tissue Harmonic Imaging

In **second harmonic imaging** an ultrasound scanner transmits at one frequency and receives at double this frequency. The improved detection of the microbubble echo results from the peculiar behavior of a gas bubble in an ultrasound field. However, any source of a received signal at the harmonic frequency that does not come from the bubble will clearly reduce the efficacy of this method. Such unwanted signals can come from nonlinearities in the transducer or its associated electronics, and these must be tackled effectively in a good harmonic imaging system. However, **tissue itself can produce harmonics** that will be received by the transducer and that develop as a wave **propagates** through tissue. Again, this is caused by asymmetry; in this case, sound travels slightly faster through tissue during the compressional (where it is denser and thus stiffer) than during the rarefactional half-cycle. Although very small, the effect is sufficient to produce substantial harmonic components in the transmitted wave by the time it reaches deep tissue. Therefore, when the sound wave is scattered by a linear target such as the myocardium, there is a harmonic component in the echo, which is detected by the scanner along with the harmonic echo from the bubble.[42] This is the reason that solid tissue is not completely dark in a typical harmonic image. The effect is to reduce the

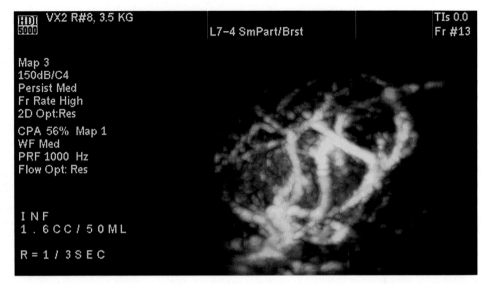

FIGURE 3-9. Harmonic power Doppler. Doppler image of experimental tumor (VX2 carcinoma) 1 cm in diameter shows clear separation of the enhanced blood signal by contrast-specific harmonic imaging.

contrast between the bubble and tissue, complicating the problem of detecting perfusion in tissue.

Tissue harmonics, although a hindrance to contrast imaging, are not necessarily a drawback. In fact, an image formed from tissue harmonics without the presence of contrast agents has many advantages over conventional imaging. These arise from the tissue harmonics that develop as the beam penetrates tissue, in contrast to the conventional beam, which is generated at the transducer surface.[43,44] Artifacts that accrue from the first few centimeters of tissue, such as reverberations, are reduced by using tissue harmonic imaging. Side lobe and other low-level interference is also suppressed, making tissue harmonic imaging the modality of choice in many situations, especially when visualizing fluid-filled structures.[45]

For contrast studies, however, the tissue harmonic limits the visibility of bubbles within tissue and therefore can be considered an **artifact.** In considering how to reduce it, the operator must keep in mind the differences between harmonics produced by tissue propagation and those created by bubble echoes. First, tissue harmonics require a high peak pressure and thus are only evident at high MI. Using low-MI contrast imaging, as is usually the case, leaves only the bubble harmonics. Second, harmonics from tissue at high MI are continuous and sustained, whereas those from bubbles at high MI are transient as the bubble disrupts.

Pulse Inversion Imaging

The most obvious, and historically the first, way to make an imaging method that preferentially displays harmonic echoes is simply to filter the transmitted sound so that it is centered around one frequency. The received sound is then filtered so that only components of about double that frequency will be detected (higher harmonics, although present in the echo, are too high in frequency

to be detected by the transducer). This is second harmonic imaging.

However, this imaging mode has problems. First, a pulse-echo system cannot transmit one frequency and must transmit a pulse containing a band of frequencies (Fig. 3-10, *A*). Similarly, the received band of frequencies must be restricted to those lying around the second harmonic. If these two regions overlap (Fig. 3-10, *B*), the **harmonic filter** will receive echoes from ordinary tissue, thus reducing the contrast between the agent and the tissue. If the two regions do not overlap, the range of frequencies (or bandwidth) of the echoes displayed will be so narrow as to compromise the resolution of the image. A further drawback of the filtering approach is that if the received echo is weak, the overlapping region between the transmit and receive frequencies becomes a larger portion of the entire received signal (Fig. 3-10, *C*).

Thus, contrast in the harmonic image depends on how strong the echo is from the bubbles, which is determined by the concentration of bubbles and the intensity of the incident ultrasound pulse. In practice, this forces use of a **high MI in harmonic mode,** resulting in transient, irreversible disruption of the bubbles.[46] As the bubbles enter the scan plane of a real-time ultrasound image, they provide an echo but then disappear. Thus, in such a harmonic image, vessels that lie within the scan plane are not visualized as continuous tubular structures, but instead have a punctate appearance (Fig. 3-11).

Pulse inversion imaging overcomes the conflict between the requirements of contrast and resolution in harmonic imaging and provides greater sensitivity, thus allowing low–incident power, nondestructive, continuous imaging of microbubbles in an organ such as the liver. The method also relies on the asymmetric oscillation of an ultrasound bubble in an acoustic field, although it detects "even" nonlinear components of the echo over the entire bandwidth of the transducer.

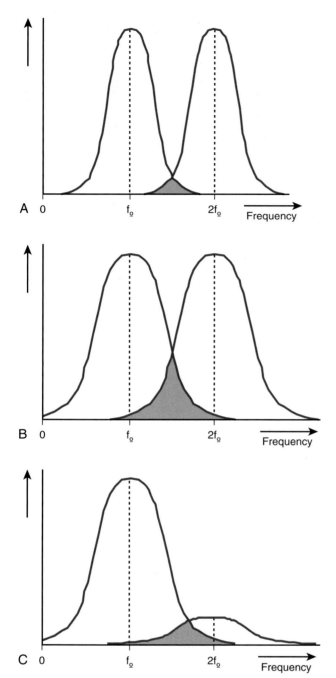

FIGURE 3-10. Compromises forced by harmonic imaging. A, In harmonic imaging the transmitted frequencies must be restricted to a band around the fundamental echo, and the received frequencies must be limited to a band around the second harmonic. This limits resolution. **B,** If the transmit and receive bandwidths are increased to improve resolution, some fundamental echoes from tissue will overlap the receive bandwidth and will be detected, reducing contrast between agent and tissue. **C,** When the harmonic echoes are weak because of low agent concentration or low incident pulse intensity, this overlap will be especially large, and the harmonic signal may be composed mainly of tissue echoes.

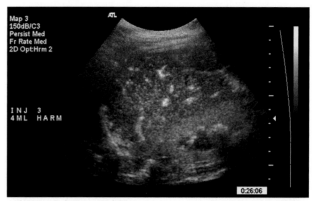

FIGURE 3-11. Appearance of blood vessels using harmonic B-mode imaging in patient with incidental hemangioma. Note that large vessels have a punctate appearance as the high-MI ultrasound disrupts the bubbles as they enter the scan plane. *(From Becher H, Burns PN. Handbook of contrast echocardiography. Berlin, 2000, Springer.)*

In pulse inversion (also known as **phase inversion**) imaging, two pulses are sent in rapid succession into the tissue. The second pulse is a mirror image of the first (Fig. 3-11); that is, it has undergone a 180-degree phase change. The scanner detects the echo from these two successive pulses and forms their sum. For ordinary tissue, which behaves in a linear manner, the sum of two inverted pulses is simply zero. For an echo with nonlinear components, such as from a bubble, the echoes produced from these two pulses will not be simple mirror images of each other, because of the asymmetric behavior of the bubble radius with time. The result is that the sum of these two echoes is not zero. Thus, a signal is detected from a bubble but not from tissue. It can be shown mathematically that this summed echo contains the nonlinear "even" harmonic components of the signal, including the second harmonic.[47] One advantage of pulse inversion over the filter approach to detect harmonics from bubbles is eliminating the restriction of bandwidth. The full frequency range of sound emitted from the transducer can be detected in this way, providing a full-bandwidth, high-resolution image of the echoes from bubbles.[48]

Pulse inversion imaging provides better suppression of linear echoes than harmonic imaging and is effective over the full bandwidth of the transducer, showing improvement of image resolution over harmonic mode (Fig. 3-12). Because this detection method is a more efficient means of isolating the bubble echo, weaker echoes from bubbles insonated at low, nondestructive intensities can be detected. As the MI increases, however, tissue harmonic renders the tissue brighter. Indeed, pulse inversion is now the preferred method in many systems for tissue harmonic imaging. Optimal **pulse inversion contrast imaging** thus is often performed at low MI. The principle of pulse inversion is the basis of many imaging modes, including **coherent contrast imaging** and **ensemble harmonic imaging**.

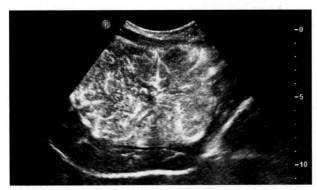

FIGURE 3-12. Pulse inversion image of a hypervascular liver mass in the arterial phase, made in real time at low MI. Note that the spatial resolution of this image is comparable to that of conventional imaging, reflecting the advantage of a broad-bandwidth, contrast-specific image.

Pulse Inversion Doppler Imaging

Despite the improvements offered by pulse inversion over harmonic imaging for suppressing stationary tissue, the method is somewhat sensitive to echoes from moving tissue. Tissue motion causes linear echoes to change slightly between pulses, so they do not cancel perfectly. Furthermore, at high MI, nonlinear propagation also causes harmonic echoes to appear in pulse inversion images, even from linear-scattering structures such as the liver parenchyma. Although tissue motion artifacts can be minimized by using a short pulse repetition interval, nonlinear tissue echoes can mask the echoes from bubbles, reducing the efficacy of microbubble contrast, especially when a high MI is used.

A recent development to address these problems involves a generalization of the pulse inversion method, called pulse inversion Doppler.[47] This technique, also known as **power pulse inversion imaging,** combines the nonlinear detection performance of pulse inversion imaging with the motion discrimination capabilities of power Doppler. Multiple transmit pulses of alternating polarity are used, and Doppler signal-processing techniques are applied to distinguish between bubble echoes and echoes from moving tissue or tissue harmonics, as determined by the operator. This method offers potential improvements in the contrast agent–to-tissue contrast and signal-to-noise performance, although at the cost of a somewhat reduced frame rate. The most dramatic manifestation of this method's ability to detect very weak harmonic echoes has been its first demonstration of real-time perfusion imaging of the myocardium.[49] By lowering the MI to 0.1 or less, bubbles undergo stable, nonlinear oscillation, emitting continuous harmonic signals. Because of the low MI, very few bubbles are disrupted, so imaging can take place at real-time rates. Because sustained, stable, nonlinear oscillation is required for this method, perfluorocarbon gas bubbles work best.

Amplitude and Phase Modulation Imaging

On receiving the echoes from a pulse inversion sequence, the receiver combines them in a way that ensures that the mirrorlike echoes from tissues sum to zero. What remains is some combination of the nonlinear components of the bubble echo. Changing (or modulating) the pulse from one transmission to the next by flipping its phase is only one of many available strategies. For example, by changing the amplitude of the pulse in consecutive transmissions and amplifying the echoes to compensate for this, linear echoes can also be canceled out. What is left now, however, is not just the even but *all* components of the nonlinear echoes from bubbles.[50] Precisely what nonlinear components are produced by a particular sequence of pulses can be determined mathematically, and the contrast-specific imaging mode can be optimized for specific applications.[51]

Almost all diagnostic systems now use some form of multipulse modulation processing in their contrast-specific imaging modes, known as **power modulation pulse inversion** (PMPI) and **contrast pulse sequence** (CPS). As long as the peak negative pressure is kept low (<100 kPa) so that the bubble is not disrupted by the pulses, real-time imaging of perfusion can be achieved in many organ beds, including the myocardium, liver, kidney, skin, prostate, and breast, even in the presence of tissue motion. Because one performance criterion that improves detection of perfusion is complete suppression of background tissue, many contrast-specific images are quite black before the contrast agent is injected, making it difficult to scan the patient. Thus, **side-by-side imaging,** in which a simultaneous, low-MI, fundamental image is seen alongside (or superimposed on) the contrast image (Fig. 3-13), has become a preferred method for detecting small lesions or guiding interventional devices such as needles or ablation probes, whose echoes are visible in the fundamental image but suppressed in the contrast image.

The technology for low-MI, real-time, bubble-specific imaging in commercial ultrasound systems has stabilized over recent years, but clinical applications are still expanding, especially in tumor imaging, which in turn presents new challenges for this imaging methodology.

Temporal Maximum-Intensity Projection Imaging

One clinically striking elaboration of contrast-specific imaging exploits the sufficient sensitivity of detecting and displaying echoes from individual bubbles in real time. By creating the equivalent of an "open shutter" photograph, where bright objects create tracks of their own motion, the bubbles can be made to trace the morphology of the microvessels that contain them. The result, known as temporal maximum-intensity

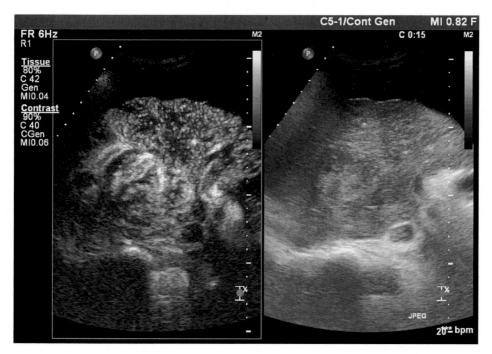

FIGURE 3-13. Side-by-side imaging shows a low-MI real-time conventional image *(right)* at the same time as low-MI contrast-specific image *(left)*. This is particularly useful for characterizing small lesions and for guiding interventional devices. The contrast mode here combines phase and amplitude modulation.

projection (**temporal MIP**) imaging, can produce a detailed picture of vascular morphology lasting a few seconds or the duration of a breath hold (Fig. 3-14). Usually, the MIP process is initiated after a "flash," which disrupts the bubbles within the scan plane. As new bubbles wash into the plane, their tracks are traced in an image that is integrated over a selected period of 100 milliseconds to a few seconds.[52] These images can also provide dynamic information; for example, revealing whether the pattern of arterial enhancement of a liver lesion is centripetal or centrifugal, the implications of which are under clinical investigation.[53]

TRANSIENT DISRUPTION: INTERMITTENT IMAGING

As the incident pressure to which a resonating bubble is exposed increases, its oscillation becomes wilder, with the radius increasing in some bubbles by a factor of five or more during the rarefaction phase of the incident sound. Just as a good soprano can shatter a wine glass by singing at its resonant frequency, so a microbubble, if driven by higher-amplitude ultrasound, will sustain irreversible disruption of its shell. A physical picture of precisely what happens to a disrupted bubble has emerged from video studies using cameras with frame rates up to 25 million pictures per second[54,55] (Fig. 3-15). It seems certain, however, that the bubble shell disappears (not instantly, but over a period determined by bubble composition) and releases free gas, which forms a highly effective acoustic scatterer, giving strong, nonlinear

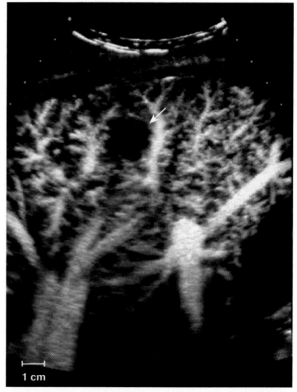

FIGURE 3-14. Temporal maximum-intensity projection (MIP). Temporal MIP image of normal liver vasculature shows accumulated enhancement in 11 seconds after contrast material arrives in liver. Unprecedented depiction of vessel structure to fifth-order branching is evident. Focal unenhanced region *(arrow)* is a slowly perfusing hemangioma. *(From Wilson SR, Jang HJ, Kim TK, et al. Real-time temporal maximum-intensity-projection imaging of hepatic lesions with contrast-enhanced sonography. AJR Am J Roentgenol 2008;190:691-695.)*

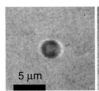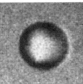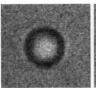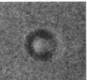

5 µm

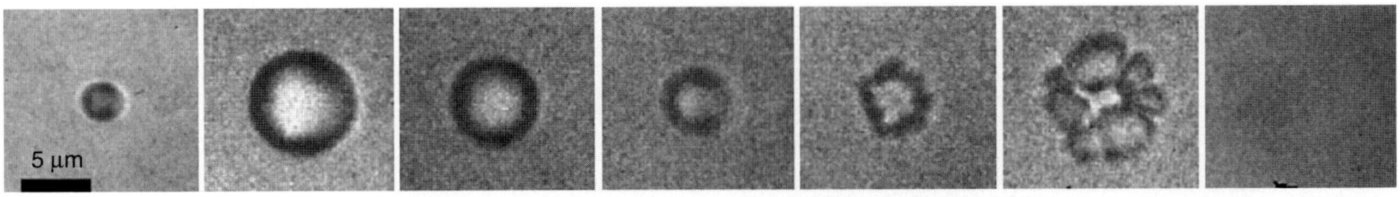

FIGURE 3-15. Fragmentation of contrast agent. These frame images were captured over 50 nanoseconds with a high-speed camera by researchers at the University of California, Davis. The bubble is insonated with 2.4-MHz ultrasound with a peak negative pressure of 1.1 MPa (MI ~0.7). The bubble is initially 3 µm in diameter and fragments during compression after the first expansion. Resulting bubble fragments are not seen after insonation, because they are either fully dissolved or below the optical resolution. *(From Becher H, Burns PN. Handbook of contrast echocardiography. Berlin, 2000, Springer.)*

echoes for a brief time. This process was once incorrectly thought to constitute a release of energy, like a balloon bursting, and was wrongly termed "stimulated acoustic emission."

Intermittent imaging has a twofold use. First, it represents a very sensitive way to detect a bubble,[56] but because it results in the bubble's disruption, it cannot be performed continuously. Replenishment of bubbles in a typical microvascular bed takes 5 to 10 seconds. The technique of imaging with high MI every few seconds to display perfusion is called triggered or "interval delay" imaging.[57] Second, the degree to which a region is replenished by bubbles between insonations separated by a fixed interval reflects the flow rate of blood into the scan plane and provides a unique method to measure tissue perfusion.

Triggered Imaging

Early studies of harmonic imaging found that pressing the **freeze** button on a scanner for a few moments, thus interrupting the acquisition of ultrasound images during a contrast study, could increase the effectiveness of a contrast agent. So dramatic is this effect that it was responsible for the first ultrasound images of myocardial perfusion using harmonic imaging.[58] This results from the ability of the ultrasound field, if its peak pressure is sufficiently high, to disrupt a bubble's shell and destroy it.[46] As the bubble is disrupted, it releases energy, creating a strong, transient echo rich in harmonics. This process is also incorrectly referred to as "stimulated acoustic emission." The transient nature of this echo can be exploited for its detection. One simple method is to subtract from a disruption image a baseline image obtained either before or (more usefully) immediately after insonation. Such a method requires offline processing of stored ultrasound images, together with software that can align the ultrasound images before subtraction, and is useful only in rare circumstances.[57]

Intermittent Harmonic Power Doppler for Bubble Detection

Power Doppler imaging was developed as a way to detect the movement of targets such as red blood cells in a vessel. It works by a simple, pulse-to-pulse subtraction method,[59] in which two or more pulses are sent successively along each scan line of the image. Pairs of received echo trains are compared for each line. If they are identical, nothing is displayed, but if there is a change (from tissue motion between pulses), a color is displayed whose saturation is related to the amplitude of the echo that has changed. This method, although not designed for the detection of bubble disruption, is ideally suited for high-MI "disruption" imaging. The first pulse receives an echo from the bubble, and the second receives none, so the comparison yields a strong signal. Power Doppler may be seen as a line-by-line subtraction procedure on the radiofrequency echo detected by the transducer. Interestingly, pulse inversion imaging, the most common method at low MI, becomes equivalent to power Doppler if the MI is high and the bubble disrupted. Figure 3-16 clearly shows that if the echo from the second pulse is absent (because the bubble is gone), the sum of the two bubble echoes is the same as their difference, which is what is measured by power Doppler. The fact that the second transmitted pulse is inverted is immaterial for the bubble that has disappeared! Thus, at high MI, power or pulse inversion Doppler becomes a sensitive way to detect bubbles, whether they are moving or not.

This method has been incorporated into modes specifically adapted to detect the distribution of bubbles taken up in the Kupffer cells in the postvascular phase of such agents as Levovist and Sonazoid. The transducer is slowly swept through the liver minutes after the agent has left the vascular system; as it does so, the high-MI pulses disrupt the in situ bubbles and are detected in the image. Figure 3-17 shows such an image, in which the defect in liver uptake represents the Kupffer cell–poor region of a cholangiocarcinoma. The preferred modes for this method are pulse inversion, which has the advantage of high-resolution imaging but the disadvantage of a strong tissue harmonic background, or power Doppler modes, such as **Harmonic Power Angio** or **Agent Detection Imaging** (ADI). Many systems offer a low-MI "monitor" mode that can be used to provide a contrast-specific or fundamental image of the liver during the scan sweep that, when blended with the high-MI contrast mode, can be helpful to keep the scan plane aligned in the region of interest.

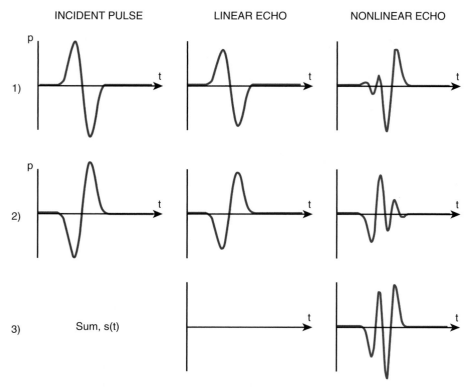

FIGURE 3-16. Basic principle of pulse inversion imaging. A pulse of sound is transmitted into the body, and echoes are received from agent and tissue. A second pulse, which is an inverted copy of the first, is then transmitted in the same direction, and the two resulting echoes are summed. Linear echoes from tissue are inverted copies of each other and cancel to zero. The microbubble echoes are distorted copies of each other, so that the even nonlinear components of these echoes will reinforce each other when summed, producing a strong harmonic signal.

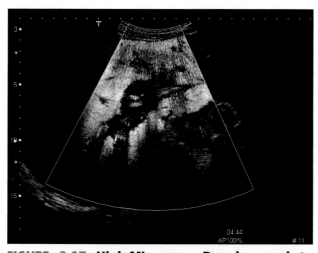

FIGURE 3-17. High-MI power Doppler used to detect Levovist bubbles by disruption during their postvascular phase in the liver. The bubbles are detected within the Kupffer cells. The signal defect around the porta hepatis is a cholangiocarcinoma that was not detected in the precontrast image.

Disruption-Replenishment Imaging: Measuring Perfusion

By disrupting bubbles and monitoring replenishment to a region of tissue, contrast ultrasound offers a unique, noninvasive, and validated[60] method for the measurement of microvascular perfusion. In the disruption-replenishment method,[61] microbubbles are infused at a steady rate until a steady enhancement is achieved

throughout the vascular system. The bubbles are then disrupted by a high-MI "flash," which clears them from the scan plane (Fig. 3-18). Immediately, new bubbles begin to wash in, at a rate related to the local flow velocity and flow rate, which can be extracted from a physical model of the process.[62]

An important application for such measurement is in assessing the response of tumors and other organs to therapies that target the vasculature. In cancer therapy, many new treatment strategies have been proposed that target the proliferating vasculature of a developing tumor, including drugs specifically designed to inhibit the angiogenic transformation itself.[63] Such antiangiogenic or vascular-disrupting drugs have the effect of shutting down the tumor circulation and inhibiting further growth. They do not in themselves kill cancer cells, so the tumor often responds without shrinking in size; thus the need for a functional test to determine drug response. Experience to date suggests that dynamic contrast-enhanced ultrasound, with its advantage of high sensitivity, portability, and a pure intravascular tracer, is a strong candidate for this role.[64-68]

SUMMARY OF BUBBLE-SPECIFIC IMAGING

Three regimens of behavior of bubbles in an acoustic field have been defined, which depend on the amplitude and frequency of the transmitted ultrasound beam (see Table 3-2). In practice, this exposure is best monitored

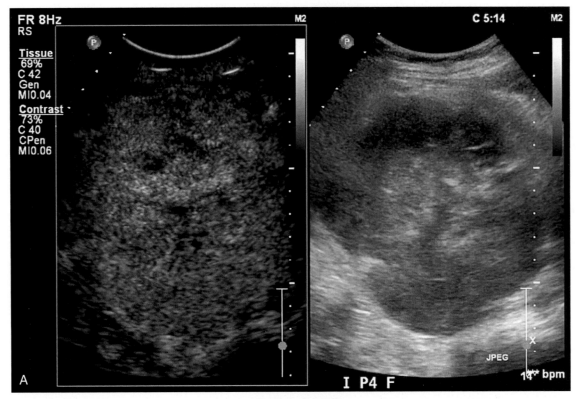

t = −1 sec (enhanced)

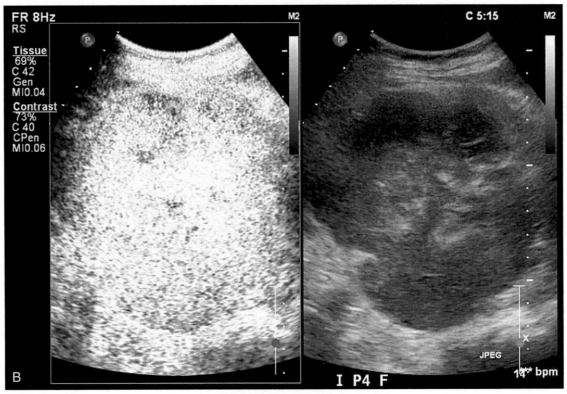

t = 0 sec (flash)

FIGURE 3-18. Disruption-replenishment imaging to quantify blood flow. Patient with renal cell carcinoma is undergoing antiangiogenic treatment. Sequence of side-by-side contrast images (*right,* conventional image; *left,* simultaneous contrast enhanced sonogram) of a large renal cell carcinoma is made during a steady intravenous infusion of the agent Definity. **A,** Time *(t)* = −1 second; the tumor is enhanced. **B,** Time = 0 second; a brief, high-MI "flash" disrupts bubbles within the scan plane.

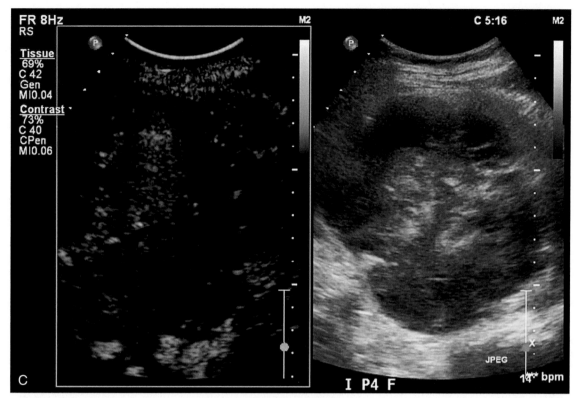

t = 1 sec after flash

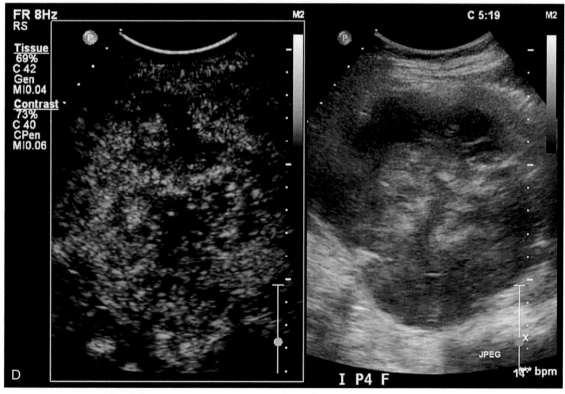

t = 4 sec after flash

FIGURE 3-18, cont'd. C, Time = 1 second; new bubbles begin to wash into the scan plane. **D, E,** and **F,** Time = 4, 8, and 18 seconds, respectively, after flash; the scan plane is fully replenished.

Continued

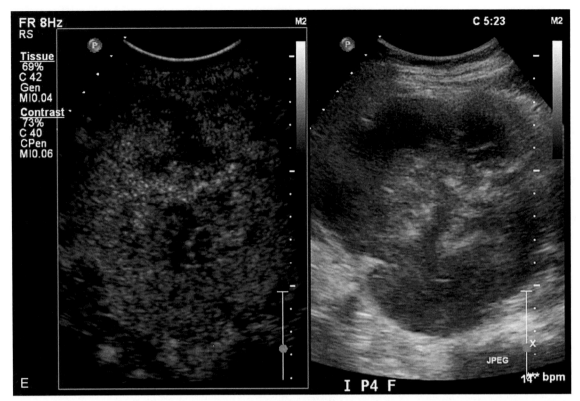

t = 8 sec after flash

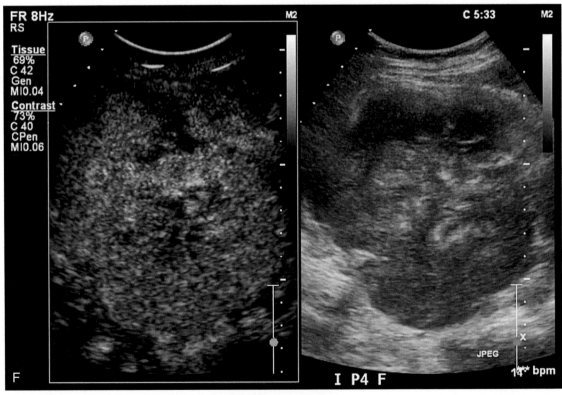

t = 18 sec after flash

FIGURE 3-18, cont'd.

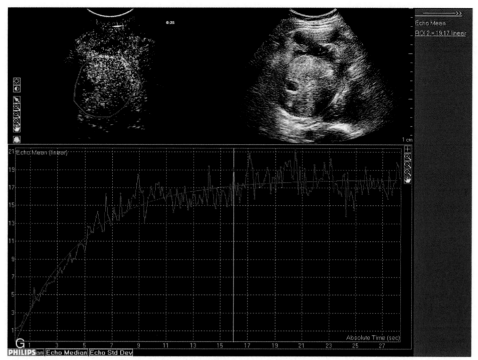

FIGURE 3-18, cont'd. G, Analysis software (Q-Lab, Philips Ultrasound, Bothell, Wash) measures wash-in of a region of interest from the cineloop record in a similar case. The steeper the slope, the greater the flow rate; the higher the asymptote, the greater the vascular volume. Disruption-replenishment imaging thus allows quantitation of changes in tumor flow and total vascular volume.

by means of the mechanical index displayed by the scanner. At very low MI, the bubbles act as simple but powerful echo enhancers. This regimen is most useful for spectral Doppler enhancement but is rarely used in the abdominal organs. At slightly higher intensities (bottom of range of those used diagnostically), the bubbles emit harmonics as they undergo nonlinear oscillation. These nonlinear echoes can be detected by contrast-specific imaging modes, which generally rely on trains of low-MI pulses modulated in phase and/or amplitude. Pulse inversion imaging is an example of such a method. Finally, at the higher-intensity settings, comparable to those used in conventional scanning, the bubbles can be disrupted deliberately, creating a strong, transient echo. Detecting this echo with harmonic power Doppler is one of the most sensitive means available to image bubbles in very low concentration, but it comes at the price of destroying the bubble. Because of the long replenishment periods of tissue flow, intermittent imaging using an interval delay (in which the high-MI imaging is arrested) becomes necessary.

SAFETY CONSIDERATIONS AND REGULATORY STATUS

Contrast ultrasound examinations expose patients to ultrasound in a way that is identical to that of a normal ultrasound examination. However, the use of ultrasound pulses to disrupt bubbles that sit in microscopic vessels raises new questions about the hazard potential. When a bubble produces the brief echo associated with its disruption, it releases energy that it has stored during its exposure to the ultrasound field. Can this energy damage the surrounding tissue? At higher exposure levels, ultrasound is known to produce biologic effects (bioeffects) in tissue, the thresholds for which have been studied extensively.[69] Do these thresholds change when bubbles are present in the vasculature? Whereas the safety of ultrasound contrast agents as drugs has been established to the satisfaction of the most stringent requirements of the regulating authorities in a number of countries, much remains to be learned about the interaction between ultrasound and tissue when bubbles are present.

The most extreme of these interactions is known as **inertial cavitation,** which refers to the rapid formation, growth, and collapse of a gas cavity in fluid as a result of ultrasound exposure. It was studied extensively before the development of microbubble contrast agents.[70] In fact, most of the mathematical models used to describe contrast microbubbles were originally developed to describe cavitation.[71] When sound waves of sufficient intensity travel through a fluid, the rarefactional half-cycle of the sound wave can actually tear the fluid apart, creating spherical cavities within the fluid. The subsequent rapid collapse of these cavities during the compressional half-cycle of the sound wave can focus large amounts of energy into a very small volume, raising the temperature at the center of the collapse to thousands of kelvins, forming free radicals, and even emitting electromagnetic radiation.[72]

The concern over potential cavitation-induced bioeffects in diagnostic ultrasound has led to many experimental studies assessing whether the presence of contrast microbubbles can act as cavitation seeds, potentiating bioeffects.[73-78] This work has been reviewed by ter Haar[79] and twice by the World Federation for Ultrasound in Medicine and Biology.[80,81] Although it has been shown that adding contrast agents to blood decreases the threshold for cavitation and related bioeffects (e.g., hemolysis, platelet lysis), no significant effects have been reported in conditions that are comparable to the bubble concentrations and ultrasound exposure of a low-MI diagnostic clinical examination. It nonetheless remains prudent to practice an extension of the **ALARA (as low as reasonably achievable)** exposure principle to contrast ultrasound. The contrast ultrasound examination should expose the patient to the **lowest MI**, the **shortest total acoustic exposure time**, the **lowest contrast agent dose,** and the **highest ultrasound frequency**, consistent with obtaining adequate diagnostic information.

In the meantime, at least 3 million injections of microbubble contrast for clinical diagnosis have been performed worldwide. These injections are very well tolerated and have an excellent safety record, with postmarket surveillance suggesting that the predominant cause of severe adverse events is anaphylactoid reaction, with an estimated rate of 1 in 7000 for both the perflutren microspheres approved for cardiac indications in the United States[82] and the sulfur hexafluoride microspheres approved in Europe.[83] This rate is comparable to that of most analgesics and antibiotics and lower than that for other imaging contrast agents, such as those used in CT imaging.[84] A 2006 study of more than 23,000 injections of a microbubble contrast agent for abdominal diagnosis in Europe showed no deaths and two serious adverse events, giving a measured serious adverse event rate of less than 1:10,000.[83]

Although there is currently no FDA-approved radiologic indication in the United States, there is extensive experience with ultrasound contrast in the echocardiology laboratory. In 2008, Kusnetsky et al.[85] reviewed more than 18,671 hospitalized patients undergoing echocardiography in an acute setting in a single U.S. center and reported no effect on mortality from using contrast in this group.[85] In 2008, Main et al.[86] analyzed registry data from 4,300,966 consecutive patients who underwent transthoracic echocardiography at rest during hospitalization; 58,254 of these patients were given the contrast agent Definity. Acute crude mortality was no different between groups, but multivariate analysis revealed that in patients undergoing echocardiography, those receiving the contrast agent were 24% less likely to die within 1 day than patients not receiving contrast. Nonetheless, after four deaths of acutely ill cardiac patients, North American labeling currently advises caution when using microbubble agents in patients with severe cardiopulmonary compromise.[87-89]

At least one contrast agent is under current clinical development in the United States, seeking the first FDA approval for a "radiology" indication.

FUTURE OF MICROBUBBLE TECHNOLOGY

Development of microbubble technology is likely to focus on at least two main areas. First, the potential for functional information yielded by the bubbles is increased by active targeting to a specific cellular or molecular process. Thus a bubble attaches itself to the cells lining blood vessels (endothelial cells) that are involved in a disease process such as inflammation (in atherosclerosis)[90] or proliferation (in cancer).[91] This is achieved by attaching ligands to the surface of the lipid shell, such as a peptide and an antibody.[92] Antibodies to factors such as VCAM, a marker of inflammation, and VEGF receptor 2, a marker of vascular proliferation, have already been shown to effectively make bubbles "stick" selectively to the endothelial surface[93] (Fig. 3-19). This form of molecular imaging has potential applications in identifying the target and assessing the effectiveness of new therapies.[94]

In the second application, the bubbles are used as a potentiator of the therapy itself. Bubbles can concentrate and lower the threshold for thermal tissue damage in high-intensity focused ultrasound (HIFU) treatments. They can also have the effect of opening or making the endothelial layer permeable, even the blood-brain barrier.[95] This allows drugs to pass through into a region of tissue selected by the ultrasound beam. The drugs may be circulating in the bloodstream or incorporated into the bubbles themselves. In the latter case, plasmid DNA, which cannot survive in the blood, can be carried in the bubble shell and released by acoustic disruption.[96] Oscillation of the free gas near the cell membrane makes it permeable and allows the DNA to enter the cell. Both endothelial cells and myocytes have been successfully transfected in this potentially new form of gene therapy.[97] Finally, the barrier of the endothelium itself can be overcome by injecting liquid **nanodroplets,** precursors of the gas contrast agents, allowing them to diffuse into the interstitium and then using external acoustic energy to activate them into gas bodies, which are both targeted and detectable[98] and can be used to enhance therapy.[99]

The use of bubbles as molecular and cellular probes, their targeting as a means of detection as well as drug and gene delivery, and their use as focal potentiators for minimally invasive therapies are all applications in their infancy. The coming years are likely to see an unprecedented union of ultrasound imaging with a unique series of injectable constructs that will transport an already-

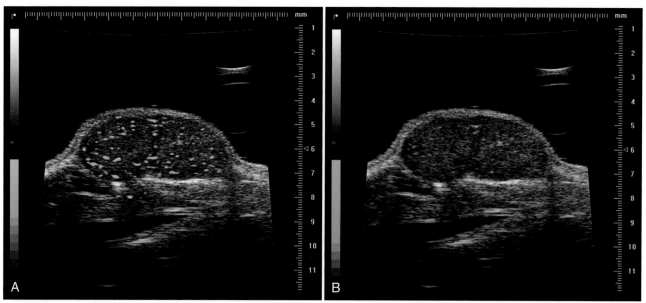

FIGURE 3-19. Molecular ultrasound imaging of receptor with targeted microbubbles. Images (40 MHz) of MeWo subdermal tumor derived from human melanoma cells in mouse after injection of vascular endothelial growth factor receptor 2 (VEGF-R2)–targeted microbubbles. **A,** Circulating bubbles have left the vascular system; those imaged are adhering to the receptor target. Microbubble-specific signal is shown as a green overlay. **B,** After disruption "flash," the bubble echoes disappear. The difference in bubble signal between these two images quantifies adhesion of the tracer to the target receptor. Scale units are millimeters. *(From Rychak JJ, Graba J, Cheung AM, et al. Microultrasound molecular imaging of vascular endothelial growth factor receptor 2 in a mouse model of tumor angiogenesis. Mol Imaging 2007;6:289-296.)*

versatile imaging modality to the forefront of the interface between diagnosis and therapy.

CONCLUSION

Contrast agents for ultrasound are safe, effective, and well tolerated by patients. Unlike contrast agents for other imaging modalities, microbubbles are modified by the process used to image them. Understanding the behavior of bubbles while exposed to an ultrasound imaging beam is the key to performing an effective contrast ultrasound examination. The appropriate choice of a contrast-specific imaging method is based on the behavior of the agent and the requirements of the examination. The mechanical index (MI) is the major determinant of the response of contrast bubbles to ultrasound. Low-MI harmonic and multipulse imaging offer real-time, contrast-specific B-mode methods for perfusion imaging using perfluorocarbon agents approved for clinical use in many countries. Future developments offer the intriguing prospect of molecular and cellular imaging, potentiated therapy, and drug and gene delivery, all with ultrasound and microbubbles.

References

Requirements and Types
1. Ophir J, Parker KJ. Contrast agents in diagnostic ultrasound. Ultrasound Med Biol 1989;15:319-333.
2. Ophir J, Parker KJ. Contrast agents in diagnostic ultrasound. Ultrasound Med Biol 1990;16:209 (erratum).
3. Gramiak R, Shah PM. Echocardiography of the aortic root. Invest Radiol 1968;3:356-366.
4. Kremkau FW, Carstensen EL. Ultrasonic detection of cavitation at catheter tips. Am J Roentgenol 1968;3:159-167.
5. Kerber RE, Kioschos JM, Lauer RM. Use of an ultrasonic contrast method in the diagnosis of valvular regurgitation and intracardiac shunts. Am J Cardiol 1974;34:722-727.
6. Valdes-Cruz LM, Sahn DJ. Ultrasonic contrast studies for the detection of cardiac shunts. J Am Coll Cardiol 1984;3:978-985.
7. Roelandt J. Contrast echocardiography. Ultrasound Med Biol 1982;8:471-492.
8. Carroll BA, Turner RJ, Tickner EG, et al. Gelatin encapsulated nitrogen microbubbles as ultrasonic contrast agents. Invest Radiol 1980;15:260-266.
9. Feinstein SB, Shah PM, Bing RJ, et al. Microbubble dynamics visualized in the intact capillary circulation. J Am Coll Cardiol 1984;4:595-600.
10. Schurmann R, Schlief R. Saccharide-based contrast agents: characteristics and diagnostic potential. Radiol Med 1994;87:15-23.
11. Fritzsch T, Schartl M, Siegert J. Preclinical and clinical results with an ultrasonic contrast agent. Invest Radiol 1988;23(Suppl 1):302-305.
12. Deichert U, Schleif R, van de Sandt M, Juhnke I. Transvaginal hysterosalpingo-contrast-sonography (Hy-Co-Sy) compared with conventional tubal diagnostics. Hum Reprod 1989;4:418-424.
13. Goldberg BB, Liu JB, Burns PN, et al. Galactose-based intravenous sonographic contrast agent: experimental studies. J Ultrasound Med 1993;12:463-470.
14. Fobbe F, Ohnesorge O, Reichel M, et al. Transpulmonary contrast agent and color-coded duplex sonography: first clinical experience. Radiology 1992;185:142.
15. Unger E, Shen D, Fritz T, et al. Gas-filled lipid bilayers as ultrasound contrast agents. Invest Radiol 1994;29:134-136.
16. Sontum PC. Physicochemical characteristics of Sonazoid, a new contrast agent for ultrasound imaging. Ultrasound Med Biol 2008;34:824-833.
17. Folkman J, Beckner K. Angiogenesis imaging. Acad Radiol 2000;7:783-785.

18. Mattrey RF, Scheible FW, Gosink BB, et al. Perfluoroctylbromide: a liver/spleen-specific and tumor-imaging ultrasound contrast material. Radiology 1982;145:759-762.
19. Fritsch T, Hauff P, Heldmann F, et al. Preliminary results with a new liver specific ultrasound contrast agent. Ultrasound Med Biol 1994;20:137.
20. Yanagisawa K, Moriyasu F, Miyahara T, et al: Phagocytosis of ultrasound contrast agent microbubbles by Kupffer cells. Ultrasound Med Biol 2007;33:318-325.
21. Leen ELS, Albrecht T, Harvey CJ, et al. Multi-center study of Sonazoid-enhanced pulse inversion harmonic imaging in the characterisation of focal hepatic lesions: preliminary results. Radiology 2000;217:458.
22. Iijima H, Moriyasu F, Miyahara T, Yanagisawa K. Ultrasound contrast agent Levovist microbubbles are phagocytosed by Kupffer cells: in vitro and in vivo studies. Hepatol Res 2006;35:235-237.
23. Albrecht T, Blomley MJ, Burns PN, et al. Improved detection of hepatic metastases with pulse-inversion US during the liver-specific phase of SHU 508A: multicenter study. Radiology 2003;227: 361-370.
24. Moriyasu F, Itoh K. Efficacy of perflubutane microbubble-enhanced ultrasound in the characterization and detection of focal liver lesions: Phase 3 multicenter clinical trial. AJR Am J Roentgenol 2009;193: 86-95.

Need for Bubble-Specific Imaging
25. Correas JM, Burns PN, Lai X, Qi X. Infusion versus bolus of an ultrasound contrast agent: in vivo dose-response measurements of BR1. Invest Radiol 2000;35:72-79.
26. Schlief R. Ultrasound contrast agents. Curr Opin Radiol 1991;3: 198-207.
27. Schlief R. Echo enhancement: agents and techniques: basic principles. Adv Echo-Contrast 1994;4:5-19.
28. Becher H, Burns PN. Contrast agents for echocardiography: principles and instrumentation. In: Handbook of contrast echocardiography. Berlin: Springer; 2000. p. 1-47. http://www.sunnybrook.utoronto.ca/EchoHandbook/.
29. Cosgrove DO, Bamber JC, Davey JB, et al. Color Doppler signals from breast tumors: work in progress. Radiology 1990;176: 175-180.
30. Chin CT, Burns PN. Predicting the acoustic response of a microbubble population for contrast imaging. Proc IEEE Ultrasonics Symposium, 1997.
31. De Jong N. Physics of microbubble scattering. In: Nanda NC, Schlief R, Goldberg BB, editors. Advances in echo imaging using contrast enhancement. 2nd ed. Dubai: Kluwer Academic Publishers; 1997. p. 39-64.
32. Apfel RE, Holland CK. Gauging the likelihood of cavitation from short-pulse, low-duty cycle diagnostic ultrasound. Ultrasound Med Biol 1991;17:179-185.

Nonlinear Backscatter: Harmonic Imaging
33. Bleeker HJ, Schung KK, Barnhart JL. Ultrasonic characterization of Albunex, a new contrast agent. J Acoust Soc Am 1990;87:1792-1797.
34. Neppiras EA, Nyborg WL, Miller PL. Nonlinear behavior and stability of trapped micron-sized cylindrical gas bubbles in an ultrasound field. Ultrasonics 1983;21:109-115.
35. Rayleigh L. On the pressure developed in a liquid during the collapse of a spherical cavity. Philosophy Magazine, 1917;Series 6:94-98.
36. Burns PN, Powers JE, Fritzsch T. Harmonic imaging: a new imaging and Doppler method for contrast-enhanced ultrasound. Radiology 1992;185:142 (abstract).
37. Burns PN, Powers JE, Hope Simpson D, et al. Harmonic contrast-enhanced Doppler as a method for the elimination of clutter: in vivo duplex and color studies. Radiology 1993;189:285.
38. Mulvagh SL, Foley DA, Aeschbacher BC, et al. Second harmonic imaging of an intravenously administered echocardiographic contrast agent: visualization of coronary arteries and measurement of coronary blood flow. J Am Coll Cardiol 1996;27:1519-1525.
39. Burns PN, Powers JE, Hope Simpson D, et al. Harmonic power mode Doppler using microbubble contrast agents: an improved method for small vessel flow imaging. Proc IEEE UFFC 1994: 1547-1550.

40. Burns PN, Wilson SR, Muradali D, et al. Intermittent US harmonic contrast-enhanced imaging and Doppler improves sensitivity and longevity of small vessel detection. Radiology 1996;201: 159.
41. Becher H, editor. Second harmonic imaging with Levovist: initial clinical experience. Second European Symposium on Ultrasound Contrast Imaging. Book of abstracts. Rotterdam: Erasmus University; 1997.
42. Hamilton MF, Blackstock DT, editors. Nonlinear acoustics. San Diego: Academic Press; 1998.
43. A new imaging technique based on the nonlinear properties of tissues. Proc IEEE Ultrasonics Symposium, 1997.
44. Burns PN, Hope Simpson D, Averkiou MA. Nonlinear imaging. Ultrasound Med Biol 2000;26(Suppl 1):19-22.
45. Ortega D, Burns PN, Hope Simpson D, Wilson SR. Tissue harmonic imaging: is it a benefit for bile duct sonography? AJR Am J Roentgenol 2001;176:653-659.
46. Burns PN, Wilson SR, Muradali D, et al. Microbubble destruction is the origin of harmonic signals from FS069. Radiology 1996;201:158.
47. Simpson DH, Chin CT, Burns PN. Pulse inversion Doppler: a new method for detecting nonlinear echoes from microbubble contrast agents. IEEE Trans Ultrason Ferroelectr Freq Control 1999;46: 372-382.
48. Burns PN, Wilson SR, Simpson DH. Pulse inversion imaging of liver blood flow: improved method for characterizing focal masses with microbubble contrast. Invest Radiol 2000;35:58-71.
49. Tiemann K, Lohmeier S, Kuntz S, et al. Real-time contrast echo assessment of myocardial perfusion at low emission power: first experimental and clinical results using power pulse inversion imaging. Echocardiography 1999;16:799-809.
50. Thomas DH, Butler MB, Anderson T, et al. Single microbubble response using pulse sequences: initial results. Ultrasound Med Biol 2009;35:112-119.
51. Eckersley RJ, Chin CT, Burns PN. Optimising phase and amplitude modulation schemes for imaging microbubble contrast agents at low acoustic power. Ultrasound Med Biol 2005;31:213-219.
52. Wilson SR, Jang HJ, Kim TK, et al. Real-time temporal maximum-intensity-projection imaging of hepatic lesions with contrast-enhanced sonography. AJR Am J Roentgenol 2008;190:691-695.
53. Kim TK, Jang HJ, Burns PN, et al. Focal nodular hyperplasia and hepatic adenoma: differentiation with low-mechanical-index contrast-enhanced sonography. AJR Am J Roentgenol 2008;190: 58-66.

Transient Disruption: Intermittent Imaging
54. Dayton PA, Morgan KE, Klibanov AL, et al. Optical and acoustical observations of the effects of ultrasound on contrast agents. IEEE Trans Ultrason Ferroelectr Freq Control 1999;46:220-232.
55. De Jong N, Frinking PJ, Bouakaz A, et al. Optical imaging of contrast agent microbubbles in an ultrasound field with a 100-MHz camera. Ultrasound Med Biol 2000;26:487-492.
56. Uhlendorf V, Scholle FD. Imaging of spatial distribution and flow of microbubbles using nonlinear acoustic properties. Acoustical Imaging 1996;22:233-238.
57. Becher H, Burns PN. Handbook of contrast echocardiography. Berlin: Springer; 2000. http://www.sunnybrook.utoronto.ca/EchoHandbook/.
58. Porter TR, Xie F. Transient myocardial contrast after initial exposure to diagnostic ultrasound pressures with minute doses of intravenously injected microbubbles: demonstration and potential mechanisms. Circulation 1995;92:2391-2395.
59. Burns PN. Interpretation of Doppler ultrasound signals. In: Burns PN, Taylor KJ, Wells PNT, editors. Clinical applications of Doppler ultrasound. 2nd ed. New York: Raven Press; 1996.
60. Masugata H, Peters B, Lafitte S, et al. Quantitative assessment of myocardial perfusion during graded coronary stenosis by real-time myocardial contrast echo refilling curves. J Am Coll Cardiol 2001;37:262-269.
61. Wei K, Jayaweera AR, Firoozan S, et al. Quantification of myocardial blood flow with ultrasound-induced destruction of microbubbles administered as a constant venous infusion. Circulation 1998; 97:473-483.
62. Hudson JM, Karshafian R, Burns PN. Quantification of flow using ultrasound and microbubbles: a disruption-replenishment model

based on physical principles. Ultrasound Med Biol 2009;35(12): 2007-2020.

63. Kerbel R, Folkman J. Clinical translation of angiogenesis inhibitors. Nat Rev Cancer 2002;2:727-739.

64. Goertz DE, Yu JL, Kerbel RS, et al. High-frequency Doppler ultrasound monitors the effects of antivascular therapy on tumor blood flow. Cancer Res 2002;62:6371-6375.

65. Lassau N, Lamuraglia M, Vanel D, et al. Doppler US with perfusion software and contrast medium injection in the early evaluation of isolated limb perfusion of limb sarcomas: prospective study of 49 cases. Ann Oncol 2005;16:1054-1060.

66. Lassau N, Lamuraglia M, Chami L, et al. Gastrointestinal stromal tumors treated with imatinib: monitoring response with contrast-enhanced sonography. AJR Am J Roentgenol 2006;187:1267-1273.

67. Eggermont AM. Evolving imaging technology: contrast-enhanced Doppler ultrasound is early and rapid predictor of tumour response. Ann Oncol 2005;16:995-996.

68. Weskott HP. Emerging roles for contrast-enhanced ultrasound. Clin Hemorheol Microcirc 2008;40:51-71.

Safety Considerations and Regulatory Status

69. Section 6. Mechanical bioeffects in the presence of gas-carrier ultrasound contrast agents. American Institute of Ultrasound in Medicine. J Ultrasound Med 2000;19:120-142, 154-168.

70. Brennan CE. Cavitation and bubble dynamics. New York: Oxford University Press; 1995.

71. Plesset MS. The dynamics of cavitation bubbles. J Appl Mech 1949;16:272-282.

72. Poritsky H, editor. The collapse or growth of a spherical bubble or cavity in a viscous fluid. First US National Congress on Applied Mechanics, 1951.

73. Williams AR, Kubowicz G, Cramer E, Schlief R. The effects of the microbubble suspension SH U 454 (Echovist) on ultrasound-induced cell lysis in a rotating tube exposure system. Echocardiography 1991;8:423-433.

74. Miller DL, Thomas RM. Ultrasound contrast agents nucleate inertial cavitation in vitro. Ultrasound Med Biol 1995;21:1059-1065.

75. Miller MW, Miller DL, Brayman AA. A review of in vitro bioeffects of inertial ultrasonic cavitation from a mechanistic perspective. Ultrasound Med Biol 1996;22:1131-1154.

76. Miller DL, Gies RA, Chrisler WB. Ultrasonically induced hemolysis at high cell and gas body concentrations in a thin-disc exposure chamber. Ultrasound Med Biol 1997;23:625-633.

77. Holland CK, Roy RA, Apfel RE, Crum LA. In vitro detection of cavitation induced by a diagnostic ultrasound system. IEEE Trans Ultrason Ferroelectr Freq Control 1992;29:95-101.

78. Everbach EC, Makin IR, Francis CW, Meltzer RS. Effect of acoustic cavitation on platelets in the presence of an echo-contrast agent. Ultrasound Med Biol 1998;24:129-136.

79. Ter Haar GR. Ultrasonic contrast agents: safety considerations reviewed. Eur J Radiol 2002;41:217-221.

80. Barnett SB, Ter Haar GR, Ziskin MC, et al. International recommendations and guidelines for the safe use of diagnostic ultrasound in medicine. Ultrasound Med Biol 2000;26:355-366.

81. Bouakaz A, de Jong N. WFUMB Safety Symposium on Echo-Contrast Agents: nature and types of ultrasound contrast agents. Ultrasound Med Biol 2007;33:187-196.

82. Kitzman DW, Goldman ME, Gillam LD, et al. Efficacy and safety of the novel ultrasound contrast agent perflutren (Definity) in patients with suboptimal baseline left ventricular echocardiographic images. Am J Cardiol 2000;86:669-674.

83. Piscaglia F, Bolondi L. The safety of SonoVue in abdominal applications: retrospective analysis of 23,188 investigations. Ultrasound Med Biol 2006;32:1369-1375.

84. Risk of anaphylaxis in a hospital population in relation to the use of various drugs: an international study. Pharmacoepidemiol Drug Saf 2003;12:195-202.

85. Kusnetzky LL, Khalid A, Khumri TM, et al. Acute mortality in hospitalized patients undergoing echocardiography with and without an ultrasound contrast agent: results in 18,671 consecutive studies. J Am Coll Cardiol 2008;51:1704-1706.

86. Main ML, Ryan AC, Davis TE, et al. Acute mortality in hospitalized patients undergoing echocardiography with and without an ultrasound contrast agent: multicenter registry results in 4,300,966 consecutive patients. Am J Cardiol 2008;102:1742-1746.

87. Main ML. Ultrasound contrast agent safety: from anecdote to evidence. JACC Cardiovasc Imaging 2009;2:1057-1059.

88. Health Canada. Updated safety information on Definity (Perflutren Injectable Suspension). Accessed November 2009. http://www.hc-sc.gc.ca/dhp-mps/medeff/advisories-avis/prof/_2008/definity_hpc-cps_2-eng.php. 2008.

89. US Food and Drug Administration. Microbubble contrast agents marketed as Definity (Perflutren Lipid Microsphere) Injectable Suspension and Optison (Perflutren Protein-Type Microspheres for Injection). Accessed November 2009. http://www.fda.gov/Safety/MedWatch/SafetyInformation/SafetyAlertsforHumanMedicalProducts/ucm092270.htm. 2008.

Future of Microbubble Technology

90. Rychak JJ, Lindner JR, Ley K, Klibanov AL. Deformable gas-filled microbubbles targeted to P-selectin. J Control Release 2006;114:288-299.

91. Christiansen JP, Lindner JR. Molecular and cellular imaging with targeted contrast ultrasound. Proc IEEE UFFC 2005;9.

92. Klibanov AL, Rychak JJ, Yang WC, et al. Targeted ultrasound contrast agent for molecular imaging of inflammation in high-shear flow. Contrast Media Mol Imaging 2006;1:259-266.

93. Rychak JJ, Graba J, Cheung AM, et al. Microultrasound molecular imaging of vascular endothelial growth factor receptor 2 in a mouse model of tumor angiogenesis. Mol Imaging 2007;6:289-296.

94. Behm CZ, Lindner JR. Cellular and molecular imaging with targeted contrast ultrasound. Ultrasound Q 2006;22:67-72.

95. Hynynen K, McDannold N, Vykhodtseva N, et al. Focal disruption of the blood-brain barrier due to 260-kHz ultrasound bursts: a method for molecular imaging and targeted drug delivery. J Neurosurg 2006;105:445-454.

96. Liu Y, Miyoshi H, Nakamura M. Encapsulated ultrasound microbubbles: therapeutic application in drug/gene delivery. J Control Release 2006;114:89-99.

97. Leong-Poi H, Kuliszewski MA, Lekas M, et al. Therapeutic arteriogenesis by ultrasound-mediated VEGF165 plasmid gene delivery to chronically ischemic skeletal muscle. Circ Res 2007;101:295-303.

98. Kawabata K-I, Asami R, Azuma T, et al. Site-specific contrast imaging with phase change nano particle. Proc IEEE Ultrasonics Symposium 2006:517-520.

99. Giesecke T, Hynynen K. Ultrasound-mediated cavitation thresholds of liquid perfluorocarbon droplets in vitro. Ultrasound Med Biol 2003;29:1359-1365.

100. Wei K, Crouse L, Weiss J, et al. Comparison of usefulness of dipyridamole stress myocardial contrast echocardiography to technetium-99m sestamibi single-photon emission computed tomography for detection of coronary artery disease (PB127 Multicenter Phase 2 Trial results). Am J Cardiol 2003;91:1293-1298.

101. Senior R, Monaghan M, Main ML, et al. Detection of coronary artery disease with perfusion stress echocardiography using a novel ultrasound imaging agent: two Phase 3 international trials in comparison with radionuclide perfusion imaging. Eur J Echocardiogr 2009;10:26-35.

102. Porter TR, Xie F, Kricsfeld A, Kilzer K. Noninvasive identification of acute myocardial ischemia and reperfusion with contrast ultrasound using intravenous perfluoropropane-exposed sonicated dextrose albumin. J Am Coll Cardiol 1995;26:33-40.

Part II

Abdominal, Pelvic, and Thoracic Sonography

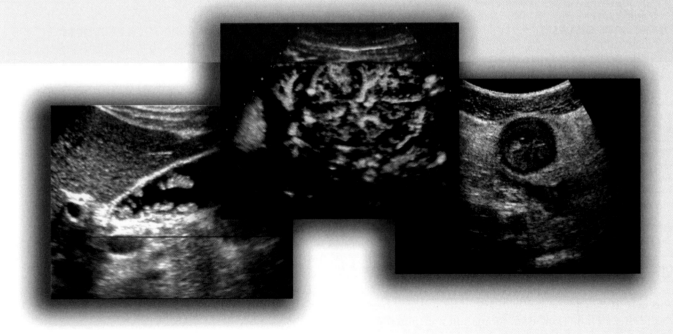

CHAPTER 4

The Liver

Stephanie R. Wilson and Cynthia E. Withers

Chapter Outline

$\mathcal{T}$he liver is the largest organ in the human body, weighing approximately 1500 g in the adult. Because it is frequently involved in systemic and local disease, sonographic examination is often requested to assess hepatic abnormality.

SONOGRAPHIC TECHNIQUE

The liver is best examined with real-time sonography, ideally after a 6-hour fast. Both supine and right anterior oblique views should be obtained. Sagittal, transverse, coronal, and subcostal oblique views are suggested using both a standard abdominal transducer and a higher-frequency transducer. Many patients' liver is tucked beneath the lower right ribs, so a transducer with a small scanning face, allowing an intercostal approach, is invaluable. Further, the recent introduction of **volumetric imaging** to ultrasound contributes greatly to the evalu-

ation of the liver as a single, appropriately selected acquisition and may show virtually the entire liver, allowing for a rapid portrayal of liver anatomy, size, texture, and surface characteristics.[1] Therefore, differentiation of the diffuse changes of cirrhosis and fatty liver from normal are enhanced by review of the videos (**Videos 4-1 and 4-2**) of the acquisitions as well as the multiplanar reconstructions (Fig. 4-1). Ultrasound also best demonstrates the relationship of focal liver masses to the vital vascular structures if surgical resection is contemplated.

NORMAL ANATOMY

The liver lies in the right upper quadrant of the abdomen, suspended from the right hemidiaphragm. Functionally, it can be divided into three lobes: right, left, and caudate. The **right lobe** of the liver is separated from the left by the **main lobar fissure**, which passes through the gall-

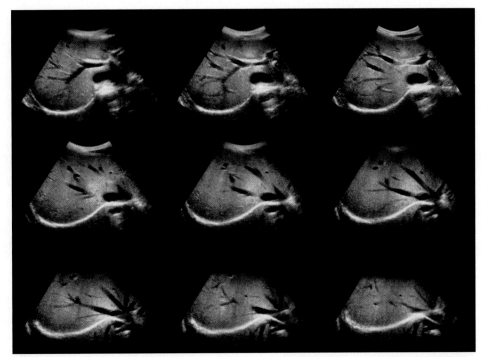

FIGURE 4-1. Normal liver. Liver shown in a nine-on-one format from a volumetric acquisition acquired in the axial plane, with the center point on the long axis of the portal veins at the porta hepatis.

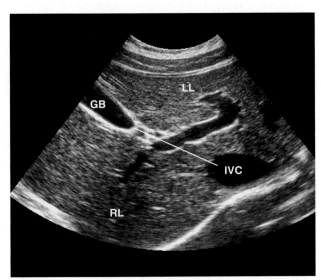

FIGURE 4-2. Normal lobar anatomy. Right lobe of the liver *(RL)* can be separated from left lobe of the liver *(LL)* by the main lobar fissure that passes through the gallbladder fossa *(GB)* and inferior vena cava *(IVC)*.

bladder fossa to the **inferior vena cava** (IVC) (Fig. 4-2). The right lobe of the liver can be further divided into anterior and posterior segments by the **right intersegmental fissure**. The **left intersegmental fissure** divides the **left lobe** into medial and lateral segments. The **caudate lobe** is situated on the posterior aspect of the liver, with the IVC as its posterior border and the fissure for the ligamentum venosum as its anterior border (Fig.

4-3). The **papillary process** is the anteromedial extension of the caudate lobe, which may appear separate from the liver and mimic lymphadenopathy.

Understanding the vascular anatomy of the liver is essential to an appreciation of the relative positions of the hepatic segments. The major **hepatic veins** course between the lobes and segments (interlobar and intersegmental). They are ideal segmental boundaries but are visualized only when scanning the superior liver (Fig. 4-4). The **middle hepatic vein** courses within the main lobar fissure and separates the anterior segment of the right lobe from the medial segment of the left. The **right hepatic vein** runs within the right intersegmental fissure and divides the right lobe into anterior and posterior segments. In more caudal sections of the liver, the right hepatic vein is no longer identified; therefore the segmental boundary becomes a poorly defined division between the anterior and posterior branches of the right portal vein. The major branches of the right and left **portal veins** run centrally within the segments (**intrasegmental**), with the exception of the ascending portion of the left portal vein, which runs in the left intersegmental fissure. The left intersegmental fissure, which separates the medial segment of the left lobe from the lateral segment, can be divided into cranial, middle, and caudal sections. The **left hepatic vein** forms the boundary of the cranial third, the ascending branch of the left portal vein represents the middle third, and the fissure for the ligamentum teres acts as the most caudal division of the left lobe[2] (Table 4-1).

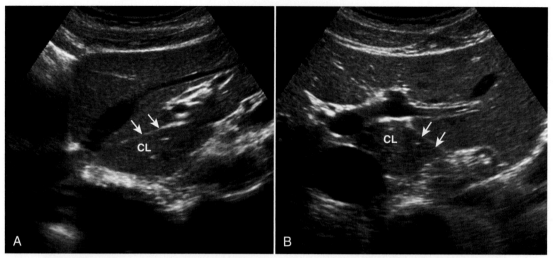

FIGURE 4-3. Caudate lobe. A, Sagittal view, and **B,** transverse view, show the caudate lobe *(CL)* separated from the left lobe by the fissure for the ligamentum venosum *(arrows)* anteriorly. Posterior is the inferior vena cava.

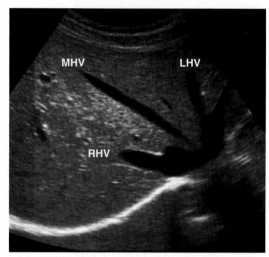

FIGURE 4-4. Hepatic venous anatomy. The three hepatic veins—right *(RHV)*, middle *(MHV)*, and left *(LHV)*—are interlobar and intersegmental, separating the lobes and segments. At the level of the hepatic venous confluence with the inferior vena cava, the right hepatic vein separates the right posterior segment (segment 7) from the right anterior segment (segment 8). The left hepatic vein separates the left medial segment from the left lateral segment. The middle hepatic vein separates the right and left lobes. As shown here, the hepatic veins are best seen on a subcostal oblique view.

Couinaud's Anatomy

Because sonography allows evaluation of liver anatomy in multiple planes, the radiologist can precisely localize a lesion to a given segment for the surgeon. **Couinaud's anatomy** is now the universal nomenclature for hepatic lesion localization[3] (Table 4-2). This description is based on **portal segments** and is of both **functional** and **pathologic** importance. Each segment has its own blood supply (arterial, portal venous, and hepatic venous), lym-

phatics, and biliary drainage. Thus the surgeon may resect a segment of a hepatic lobe, providing the vascular supply to the remaining lobe is left intact. Each segment has a branch or branches of the portal vein at its center, bounded by a hepatic vein. There are **eight segments**. The right, middle, and left hepatic veins divide the liver longitudinally into four sections. Each of these sections is further divided transversely by an imaginary plane through the right main and left main portal pedicles. **Segment I** is the caudate lobe, **segments II and III** are the left superior and inferior lateral segments, respectively, and **segment IV**, which is further divided into IVa and IVb, is the medial segment of the left lobe. The right lobe consists of **segments V and VI**, located caudal to the transverse plane, and **segments VII and VIII**, which are cephalad[4-6] (Fig. 4-5). The caudate lobe (segment I) may receive branches of both the right and the left portal vein. In contrast to the other segments, segment I has one or several hepatic veins that drain directly into the IVC.

The portal venous supply for the left lobe can be visualized using an oblique, cranially angled subxiphoid view (recurrent subcostal oblique projection). A "recumbent H" is formed by the main left portal vein, the ascending branch of the left portal vein, and the branches to segments, II, III, and IV[7] (Fig. 4-6). Segments II and III are separated from segment IV by the left hepatic vein, as well as by the ascending branch of the left portal vein and the falciform ligament. Segment IV is separated from segments V and VIII by the middle hepatic vein and the main hepatic fissure.

The portal venous supply to the right lobe of the liver can also be seen as a recumbent H. The main right portal vein gives rise to branches that supply segments V and VI (inferiorly) and VII and VIII (superiorly). They are seen best in a sagittal or oblique sagittal plane[7] (Fig. 4-6).

TABLE 4-1. NORMAL HEPATIC ANATOMY: STRUCTURES USEFUL FOR IDENTIFYING HEPATIC SEGMENTS

Structure	Location	Usefulness
RHV	Right intersegmental fissure	Divides cephalic aspect of anterior and posterior segments of right lobe
MHV	Main lobar fissure	Separates right and left lobes
LHV	Left intersegmental fissure	Divides cephalic aspect of medial and lateral segments of left lobe
RPV (anterior branch)	Intrasegmental in anterior segment of right lobe	Courses centrally in anterior segment of right lobe
RPV (posterior branch)	Intrasegmental in posterior segment of right lobe	Courses centrally in posterior segment of right lobe
LPV (horizontal segment)	Anterior to caudate lobe	Separates caudate lobe posteriorly from medial segment of left lobe anteriorly
LPV (ascending segment)	Left intersegmental fissure	Divides medial from lateral segment of left lobe
GB fossa	Main lobar fissure	Separates right and left lobes
Fissure for ligamentum teres	Left intersegmental fissure	Divides caudal aspect of left lobe into medial and lateral segments
Fissure for ligamentum venosum	Left anterior margin of caudate lobe	Separates caudate lobe posteriorly from left lobe anteriorly

Modified from Marks WM, Filly RA, Callen PW. Ultrasonic anatomy of the liver: a review with new applications. J Clin Ultrasound 1979;7:137-146.
RHV, Right hepatic vein; *MHV,* middle hepatic vein; *LHV,* left hepatic vein; *RPV,* right portal vein; *LPV,* left portal vein; *GB,* gallbladder.

TABLE 4-2. HEPATIC ANATOMY

Couinaud	Traditional
Segment I	Caudate lobe
Segment II	Lateral segment left lobe (superior)
Segment III	Lateral segment left lobe (inferior)
Segment IV	Medial segment left lobe
Segment V	Anterior segment right lobe (inferior)
Segment VI	Posterior segment right lobe (inferior)
Segment VII	Posterior segment right lobe (superior)
Segment VIII	Anterior segment right lobe (superior)

The oblique subxiphoid view shows the right portal vein in cross section and enables identification of the more superiorly located segment VIII (closer to confluence of hepatic veins) from segment V. Segments V and VIII are separated from segments VI and VII by the right hepatic vein.[7]

Ligaments

The liver is covered by a thin connective tissue layer called **Glisson's capsule**. The capsule surrounds the entire liver and is thickest around the IVC and the porta hepatis. At the porta hepatis, the main portal vein, the proper hepatic artery, and the common bile duct are contained within investing peritoneal folds known as the **hepatoduodenal ligament** (Fig. 4-7). The **falciform ligament** conducts the umbilical vein to the liver during fetal development (Fig. 4-8). After birth, the umbilical vein atrophies, forming the **ligamentum teres** (Fig 4-9). As it reaches the liver, the leaves of the falciform ligament separate. The right layer forms the upper layer of the coronary ligament; the left layer forms the upper layer

of the left triangular ligament. The most lateral portion of the coronary ligament is known as the right triangular ligament (Fig. 4-10). The peritoneal layers that form the coronary ligament are widely separated, leaving an area of the liver not covered by peritoneum. This posterosuperior region is known as the **bare area** of the liver. The **ligamentum venosum** carries the obliterated ductus venosus, which until birth shunts blood from the umbilical vein to the IVC.

Hepatic Circulation

Portal Veins

The liver receives a **dual blood supply** from both the portal vein and the hepatic artery. Although the portal vein carries incompletely oxygenated (80%) venous blood from the intestines and spleen, it supplies up to half the oxygen requirements of the hepatocytes because of its greater flow. This dual blood supply explains the low incidence of hepatic infarction.

The **portal triad** contains a branch of the portal vein, hepatic artery, and bile duct. These are contained within a connective tissue sheath that gives the portal vein an echogenic wall on sonography and that distinguishes it from the hepatic veins, which have an almost imperceptible wall. The **main portal vein** divides into right and left branches. The **right portal vein** has an anterior branch that lies centrally within the anterior segment of the right lobe and a posterior branch that lies centrally within the posterior segment of the right lobe. The **left portal vein** initially courses anterior to the caudate lobe. The ascending branch of the left portal vein then travels anteriorly in the left intersegmental fissure to divide the medial and lateral segments of the left lobe.

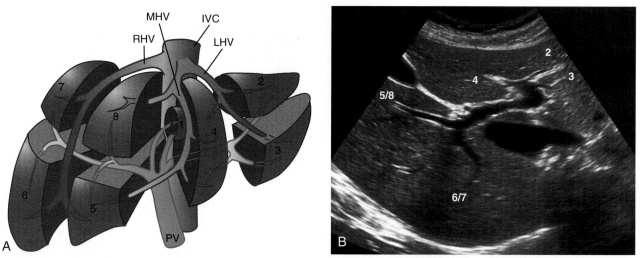

FIGURE 4-5. Couinaud's functional segmental anatomy. A, The liver is divided into nine segments. Blue longitudinal boundaries (right, middle, and left scissurae) are three hepatic veins. Transverse plane is defined by right main and left main portal pedicles. Segment I, caudate lobe, is situated posteriorly. *RHV,* Right hepatic vein; *MHV,* middle hepatic vein; *LHV,* left hepatic vein; *RPV,* right portal vein; *LPV,* left portal vein; *GB,* gallbladder. **B,** Corresponding sonogram shows the main portal vein with its right and left branches. The plane through the right and left branches is the transverse separation of the liver segments. Cephalad to this level lie segments II, IVa, VII, and VIII. Caudally located are segments III, IVb, V, and VI. *(From Sugarbaker PH: Toward a standard of nomenclature for surgical anatomy of the liver. Neth J Surg 1988;PO:100.)*

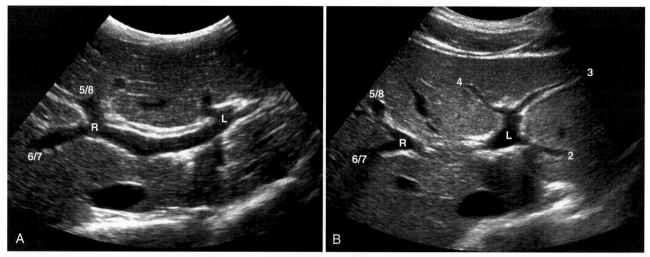

FIGURE 4-6. Portal venous anatomy in two patients. A, Best seen with a subcostal oblique view, the main portal vein is formed by the union of the right and left portal venous branches at the porta hepatis. **B,** Segmental branches of the right and left portal veins are marked. Well seen is the recumbent-H shape of the left portal venous bifurcation, made from the ascending and horizontal left portal vein and the segmental branches to 2, 3, and 4.

Arterial Circulation

The branches of the **hepatic artery** accompany the portal veins. The terminal branches of the portal vein and their accompanying hepatic arterioles and bile ducts are known as the **acinus.**

Hepatic Venous System

Blood perfuses the liver parenchyma through the sinusoids and then enters the terminal hepatic venules. These terminal branches unite to form sequentially larger veins.

The hepatic veins vary in number and position. However, in the general population, there are three major veins: the right, middle, and left hepatic veins (see Fig. 4-4). All drain into the IVC and, as with the portal veins, are without valves. As discussed earlier, the right hepatic vein is usually single and runs in the right intersegmental fissure, separating the anterior and posterior segments of the right lobe. The middle hepatic vein, which courses in the main lobar fissure, forms a common trunk with the left hepatic vein in most cases. The left hepatic vein forms the most cephalad boundary between the medial and lateral segments of the left lobe.

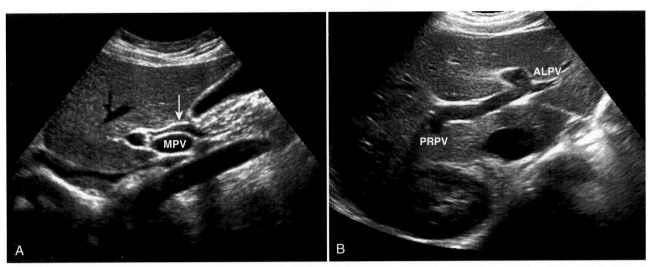

FIGURE 4-7. Porta hepatis. A, Sagittal image of the porta hepatis shows the common bile duct *(arrow)* and main portal vein *(MPV)*, which are enclosed within the hepatoduodenal ligament. **B,** Transverse image of the porta hepatis shows the right and left portal vein branches. *PRPV,* Posterior right portal vein; *ALPV,* ascending left portal vein.

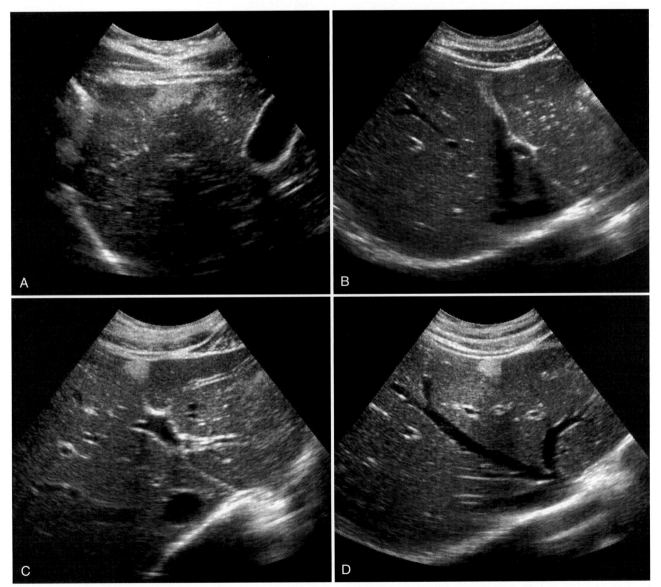

FIGURE 4-8. Falciform ligament. Contained fat helps in its localization. **A,** Sagittal image through falciform ligament. **B,** Subcostal oblique view of falciform ligament. **C,** Location of the fat just anterior to the ascending branch of the left ascending portal vein branch. **D,** Cephalad extent of the fat in the location of the ligament between the middle and the left hepatic veins.

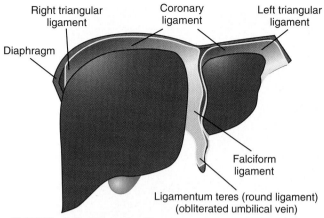

FIGURE 4-9. **Hepatic ligaments.** Diagram of anterior surface of the liver.

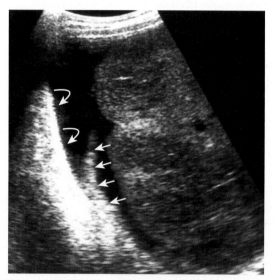

FIGURE 4-10. **Right triangular ligament.** Subcostal oblique scan near dome of right hemidiaphragm *(curved arrows)*. Note lobulated contour and inhomogeneity of liver in this patient with cirrhosis. Right triangular ligament *(straight arrows)* is visualized because of ascites.

Normal Liver Size and Echogenicity

The upper border of the liver lies approximately at the level of the fifth intercostal space at the midclavicular line. The lower border extends to or slightly below the costal margin. An accurate assessment of **liver size** is difficult with real-time ultrasound equipment because of the limited field of view. Gosink and Leymaster[8] proposed measuring the liver length in the midhepatic line. In 75% of patients with a liver length of greater than 15.5 cm, hepatomegaly is present. Niederau et al.[9] measured the liver in a longitudinal and anteroposterior diameter in both the midclavicular line and the midline and correlated these findings with gender, age, height, weight, and body surface area. They found that organ size increases with height and body surface area and decreases with age. The **mean longitudinal diameter** of the liver in the midclavicular line in this study was

10.5 cm, with standard deviation (SD) of 1.5 cm, and the mean midclavicular anteroposterior diameter was 8.1 cm (SD 1.9 cm). In most patients, measurement of the liver length suffices to measure liver size. **Reidel's lobe** is a tonguelike extension of the inferior tip of the right lobe of the liver, frequently found in asthenic women.

The normal liver is homogeneous, contains fine-level echoes, and is either minimally hyperechoic or isoechoic compared to the normal renal cortex (Fig. 4-11, *A*). The liver is hypoechoic compared to the spleen. This relationship is evident when the lateral segment of the left lobe is elongated and wraps around the spleen (Fig. 4-11, *B*).

DEVELOPMENTAL ANOMALIES

Agenesis

Agenesis of the liver is incompatible with life. Agenesis of both right and left lobes has been reported.[10,11] In three of five reported cases of agenesis of the right lobe, the caudate lobe was also absent.[11] Compensatory hypertrophy of the remaining lobes normally occurs, and liver function tests are normal.

Anomalies of Position

In **situs inversus totalis (viscerum),** the liver is found in the left hypochondrium. In congenital **diaphragmatic hernia** or **omphalocele,** varying amounts of liver may herniate into the thorax or outside the abdominal cavity.

Accessory Fissures

Although invaginations of the dome of the diaphragm have been called "accessory fissures," these are not true fissures but rather **diaphragmatic slips.** They are a cause of pseudomasses on sonography if the liver is not carefully examined in both sagittal and transverse planes (Fig. 4-12). *True* accessory fissures are uncommon and are caused by an infolding of peritoneum. The inferior accessory hepatic fissure is a true accessory fissure that stretches inferiorly from the right portal vein to the inferior surface of the right lobe of the liver.[12]

Vascular Anomalies

The **common hepatic artery** arises from the celiac axis and divides into right and left branches at the porta hepatis. This classic textbook description of the hepatic arterial anatomy occurs in only 55% of the population. The remaining 45% have some variation of this anatomy, the main patterns of which are (1) replaced left hepatic artery originating from the left gastric artery (10%); (2)

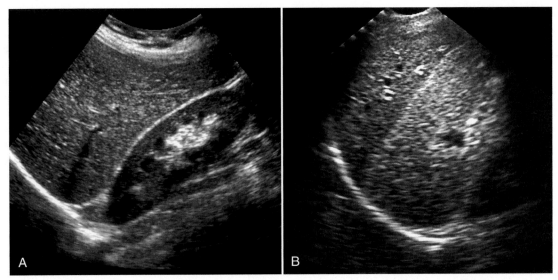

FIGURE 4-11. Normal liver echogenicity. A, The liver is more echogenic than the renal cortex. **B,** The liver is less echogenic than the spleen, as seen in many thin women, whose left lobe of the liver wraps around the spleen.

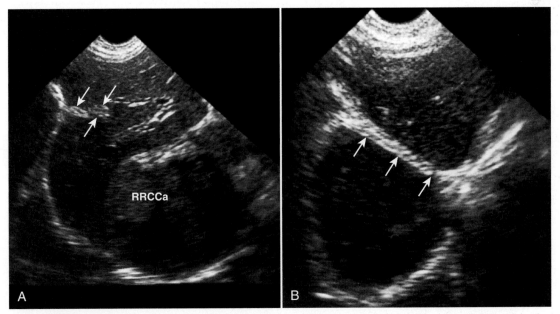

FIGURE 4-12. Diaphragmatic slip. A, Sagittal sonogram shows echogenic mass *(arrows)* adjacent to right hemidiaphragm in this patient with right renal cell carcinoma *(RRCCa)*. **B,** Subcostal oblique image reveals mass is diaphragmatic slip *(arrows)*.

replaced right hepatic artery originating from the superior mesenteric artery (11%); and (3) replaced common hepatic artery originating from the superior mesenteric artery (2.5%).

Congenital portal vein anomalies include atresias, strictures, and obstructing valves, all of which are uncommon. Sonographic variations include absence of the right portal vein, with anomalies of branching from the main and left portal veins, and absence of the horizontal segment of the left portal vein.[13]

In contrast, variations in the branching of the hepatic veins and accessory hepatic veins are relatively common. The most common accessory vein drains the superoante-

rior segment of the right lobe (segment VIII) and is seen in approximately one third of the population. It usually empties into the middle hepatic vein, although occasionally it joins the right hepatic vein.[14] An inferior right hepatic vein, which drains the inferoposterior portion of the liver (segment VI), is observed in 10% of individuals. This inferior right hepatic vein drains directly into the IVC and may be as large as the right hepatic vein or larger.[15] Left and right marginal veins, which drain into the left and right hepatic veins, occur in about 12% and 3% of individuals, respectively. Absence of the main hepatic veins is relatively less common, occurring in about 8% of people.[15] Awareness of the normal variations of the hepatic venous system is helpful in accurately defining the location of focal liver lesions and aids the surgeon in segmental liver resection.

CONGENITAL ABNORMALITIES

Liver Cyst

A liver cyst is defined as a fluid-filled space with an epithelial lining. Abscesses, parasitic cysts, and posttraumatic cysts therefore are not *true* cysts. The frequent presence of columnar epithelium within simple hepatic cysts suggests they have a ductal origin, although their precise cause is unclear. Their presentation at middle age is also unclear. Although once thought to be relatively uncommon, ultrasound examination has shown that liver cysts occur in 2.5% of the general population, increasing to 7% in the population older than 80 years.[16]

On sonographic examination, **benign hepatic cysts** are anechoic with a thin, well-demarcated wall and posterior acoustic enhancement. Occasionally, the patient may develop pain and fever secondary to cyst hemorrhage or infection. In these patients the cyst may contain internal echoes (Fig. 4-13, *A*) and septations, may have

a thickened wall, or may appear solid (Fig. 4-13, *B*). Active intervention is recommended only in symptomatic patients. Although aspiration will yield fluid for evaluation, the cyst with an epithelial lining will recur. Cyst ablation with alcohol can be performed using ultrasound guidance.[17] Alternatively, surgical excision is indicated. If thick septae or nodules are seen within liver cysts, computed tomography (CT) or contrast-enhanced ultrasound is recommended because **biliary cystadenomas** and **cystic metastases** must be considered in the differential diagnosis of complex-appearing liver cysts (Fig. 4-14).

Peribiliary Cysts

Peribiliary cysts have been described in patients with severe liver disease.[18] These cysts are small, 0.2 to 2.5 cm, and are usually located centrally within the porta hepatis or at the junction of the main right and left hepatic ducts. They generally are asymptomatic but may rarely cause biliary obstruction.[18] Pathologically, peribiliary cysts are believed to represent small, obstructed periductal glands. Sonographically, they may be seen as discrete, clustered cysts or as tubular-appearing structures with thin septae, paralleling the bile ducts and portal veins.

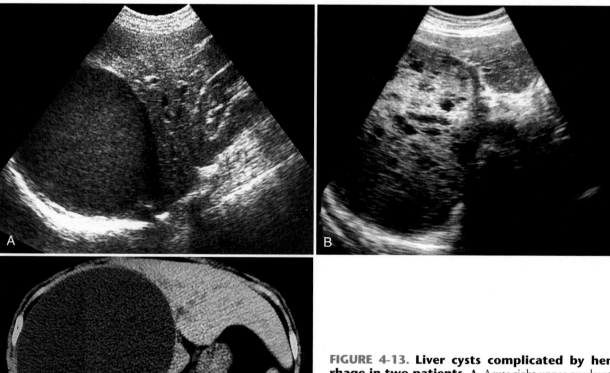

FIGURE 4-13. Liver cysts complicated by hemorrhage in two patients. A, Acute right upper quadrant pain in 46-year-old woman. Sagittal right lobe sonogram shows a well-defined, subdiaphragmatic mass with uniform low-level internal echoes. This appearance could be misinterpreted as a solid mass. **B,** Transverse sonogram shows a large, well-defined mass with a complex but predominantly solid internal character. **C,** Enhanced computed tomography (CT) scan of the same patient in **B** shows a nonenhancing low-density mass consistent with a cyst. Ultrasound is superior to CT scan at characterization of a cystic mass.

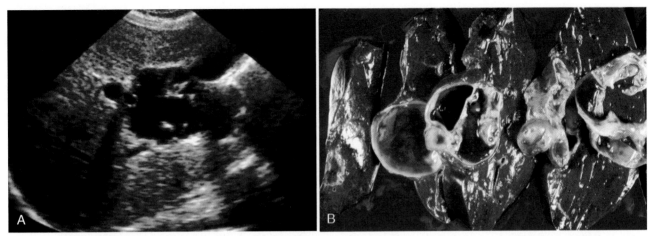

FIGURE 4-14. Biliary cystadenoma. A, Sagittal sonogram shows irregular liver cyst with thick septa and mural nodules. **B,** Surgical specimen.

Adult Polycystic Disease

The adult form of polycystic kidney disease is inherited in an autosomal dominant pattern. Liver cysts are associated with this condition in 57% to 74% of patients.[19] No correlation exists between the severity of the renal disease and the extent of liver involvement. Liver function tests (LFTs) are usually normal and, unlike the infantile autosomal recessive form of polycystic kidney disease, there is no association with hepatic fibrosis and portal hypertension. Indeed, if LFTs are abnormal, complications of polycystic liver disease, such as tumor, cyst infection, and biliary obstruction, should be excluded.[19]

Biliary Hamartomas (von Meyenburg Complexes)

Bile duct hamartomas, first described by von Meyenburg in 1918,[20] are small, focal developmental lesions of the liver composed of groups of dilated intrahepatic bile ducts set within a dense collagenous stroma.[21] These benign liver malformations are detected incidentally in 0.6% to 5.6% of reported autopsy series.[22]

Imaging features of von Meyenburg complexes (VMCs) are described in the literature in isolated case reports and a few small series, including sonographic, CT, and magnetic resonance imaging (MRI) appearances.[23] VMCs are often confused with metastatic cancer, and reports describe single, multiple, or most often innumerable well-defined solid nodules usually less than 1 cm in diameter (Fig. 4-15). Nodules are usually uniformly hypoechoic[23] and less frequently hyperechoic on sonography[24,25] and hypodense on contrast-enhanced CT scan. Bright echogenic foci in the liver with distal "ringdown" artifact without obvious mass effect are also documented on sonograms on patients with VMCs (Fig. 4-16). We believe that these echogenic foci could be related to the presence of tiny cysts beyond the resolution of the ultrasound equipment. VMCs are usually isolated,

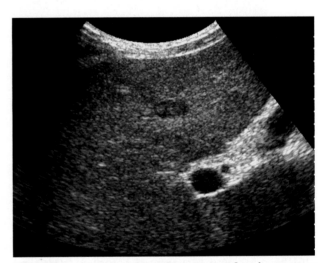

FIGURE 4-15. Von Meyenburg complex in cancer patient. Sonogram shows a single, small, hypoechoic liver mass. With no other evidence of metastatic disease, a biopsy was performed and proved the benign, insignificant nature of this lesion.

insignificant observations and may occur with other congenital disorders, such as congenital hepatic fibrosis and polycystic kidney or liver disease.[22] Association of VMCs with cholangiocarcinoma has been suggested.[26]

INFECTIOUS DISEASES

Viral Hepatitis

Viral hepatitis is a common disease that occurs worldwide. It is responsible for millions of deaths secondary to acute hepatic necrosis or chronic hepatitis, which in turn may lead to portal hypertension, cirrhosis, and hepatocellular carcinoma (HCC). Recent medical advances have identified at least six distinct hepatitis viruses: hepatitis A through E and G.[27]

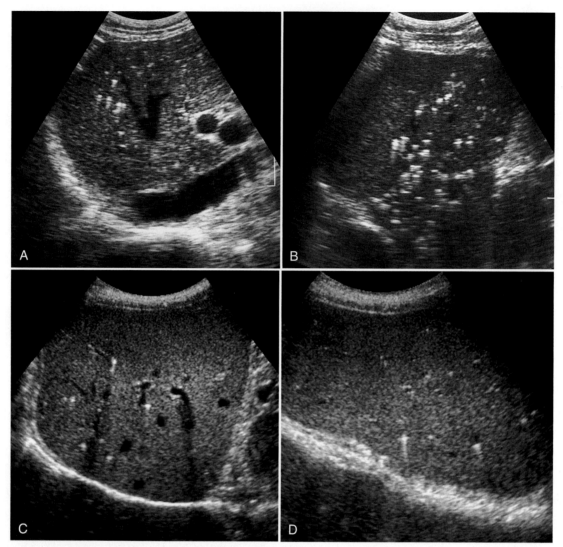

FIGURE 4-16. Von Meyenburg complex (VMC) artifacts in two patients. A, Sagittal, and **B,** transverse, images of the left lobe of the liver show multiple bright echogenic foci with "ringdown" artifact. Biopsy showed VMC. **C,** Sagittal, and **D,** transverse, images of the right lobe in an asymptomatic patient show echogenic foci with distal ringdown artifact.

Hepatitis A occurs throughout the world and can be diagnosed using serosurveys with the antibody to hepatitis A virus (anti-HAV) as the marker. The primary mode of spread is the fecal-oral route. In developing countries the disease is endemic and infection occurs early in life. Hepatitis A is an acute infection leading to complete recovery or death from acute liver failure.

Hepatitis B is transmitted parenterally (e.g., blood transfusions, needle punctures) as well as by nonpercutaneous exposure through sexual contact and at birth. Hepatitis B virus (HBV), unlike HAV, has a carrier state, which is estimated worldwide at 300 million. The regions of highest carrier rates (5%-20%) are Southeast Asia, China, sub-Saharan Africa, and Greenland. The two most useful markers for acute infection are hepatitis B surface antigen (HBsAg) and antibody to hepatitis B core antigen (anti-HBc).

Hepatitis C (predominantly) and **hepatitis E** were formerly called non-A, non-B (NANB) hepatitis, first recognized in 1974. U.S. investigators were sur-prised to learn that the majority of cases of post-transfusion hepatitis were not secondary to hepatitis B but to an unknown virus or viruses. It is now known that many cases do not result from percutaneous transmission, and that no source could be identified in almost 50% of patients with posttransfusion hepatitis. Acutely infected patients have a much greater risk of chronic infection, with up to 85% progressing to chronic liver disease. Chronic hepatitis C virus (HCV) infection is diagnosed by the presence of antibody to HCV (anti-HCV) in the blood. Hepatitis C is a major health problem in Italy and other Mediterranean countries.

Hepatitis D, or delta hepatitis, is entirely dependent on HBV for its infectivity, requiring the HBsAg to provide an envelope coat for the hepatitis D virus (HDV). Its geographic distribution is therefore similar to that of hepatitis B. HDV is an uncommon infection in North America, occurring primarily in intravenous (IV) drug users.

Clinical Manifestations

Uncomplicated **acute hepatitis** implies clinical recovery within 4 months. It is the outcome of 99% of cases of hepatitis A.

Subfulminant and fulminant **hepatic failure** follows the onset of jaundice and includes worsening jaundice, coagulopathy, and hepatic encephalopathy. Most cases of hepatic failure are caused by hepatitis B or drug toxicity and are characterized by hepatic necrosis. Death occurs if the loss of hepatic parenchyma is greater than 40%.[28]

Chronic hepatitis is defined as the persistence of biochemical abnormalities beyond 6 months. It has many etiologies other than viral, including metabolic (e.g., Wilson's disease, alpha-1 antitrypsin deficiency, hemochromatosis), autoimmune, and drug induced. The prognosis and treatment of chronic hepatitis depend on the specific etiology.[29]

In acute hepatitis, there is diffuse swelling of the hepatocytes, proliferation of Kupffer cells lining the sinusoids, and infiltration of the portal areas by lymphocytes and monocytes. The sonographic features parallel the histologic findings. The liver parenchyma may have a diffusely decreased echogenicity, with accentuated brightness of the portal triads or **periportal cuffing** (Figs. 4-17 and 4-18, A and B). Hepatomegaly and thickening of the gallbladder wall are associated findings[30] (Figs. 4-17 and 4-18, C and D). In most patients the liver appears normal.[31] Most cases of chronic hepatitis are also sonographically normal. When cirrhosis develops, sonography may demonstrate a coarsened echotexture and other morphologic changes of cirrhosis.

Bacterial Diseases

Pyogenic bacteria reach the liver by several routes, the most common being direct extension from the biliary tract in patients with suppurative cholangitis and cholecystitis. Other routes are through the portal venous system in patients with diverticulitis or appendicitis and

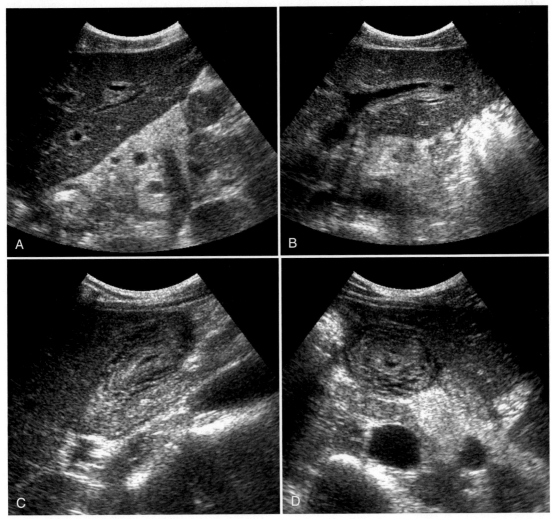

FIGURE 4-17. Acute hepatitis. A, Sagittal, and **B,** transverse, images of the left lobe of the liver show marked increased thickness and echogenicity of the soft tissue surrounding the portal vein branch, called periportal cuffing. **C,** Sagittal, and **D,** transverse, views of the gallbladder with marked mural thickening, such that the lumen is virtually obliterated. The gallbladder wall shows a multilayered appearance with extensive hypoechoic pockets of edema fluid. (*From Wilson SR. The liver. Gastrointestinal disease. 6th series. Test and syllabus. Reston, Va, 2004, American College of Radiology.*)

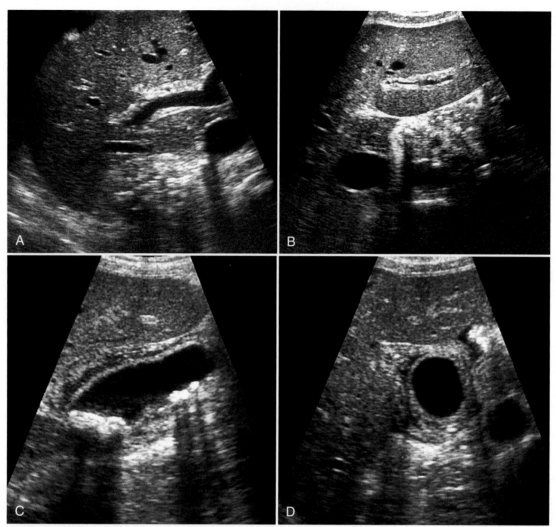

FIGURE 4-18. Acute hepatitis. Acute hepatitis in patient with fever, abnormal liver function tests, and incidental gallstones. **A,** Transverse view of porta hepatis, and **B,** transverse view of left lobe of liver, show thick, prominent echogenic bands surrounding the portal veins in the portal triads, called periportal cuffing. **C,** Sagittal, and **D,** transverse, views of the gallbladder show moderate edema and thickening of the gallbladder wall. The gallbladder is not large or tense, and the patient does not have acute cholecystitis. As this case illustrates, incidental cholelithiasis may be confusing.

through the hepatic artery in patients with osteomyelitis and subacute bacterial endocarditis. Pyogenic bacteria may also be present in the liver as a result of blunt or penetrating trauma. No cause can be found in approximately 50% of **hepatic abscesses;** the rest are mainly caused by anaerobic infection. Diagnosis of bacterial liver infection is often delayed. The most common presenting features of pyogenic liver abscess are fever, malaise, anorexia, and right upper quadrant pain. Jaundice may be present in approximately 25% of these patients.

Sonography has proved to be extremely helpful in the detection of liver abscesses. The ultrasound features of pyogenic abscesses are varied (Fig. 4-19, A-F). Frankly purulent abscesses appear cystic, with the fluid ranging from echo free to highly echogenic. Regions of early suppuration may appear solid with altered echogenicity, usually hypoechoic, related to the presence of necrotic hepatocytes.[32] Occasionally, gas-producing organisms

give rise to echogenic foci with a **posterior reverberation artifact** (Fig. 4-19, G-I). Fluid-fluid interfaces, internal septations, and debris have all been observed. The abscess wall can vary from well defined to irregular and thick.

The differential diagnosis of pyogenic liver abscess includes amebic or echinococcal infection, simple cyst with hemorrhage, hematoma, and necrotic or cystic neoplasm. Ultrasound-guided liver aspiration is an expeditious means to confirm the diagnosis. Specimens should be sent for both aerobic and anaerobic culture. In the past, 50% of abscesses were considered sterile, probably caused by failure to transport the specimen in an oxygen-free container; thus, anaerobic organisms were not identified.[33] Once the diagnosis of liver abscess is made by the identification of pus or a positive Gram stain and culture, the collection can be drained percutaneously using ultrasound or CT guidance.

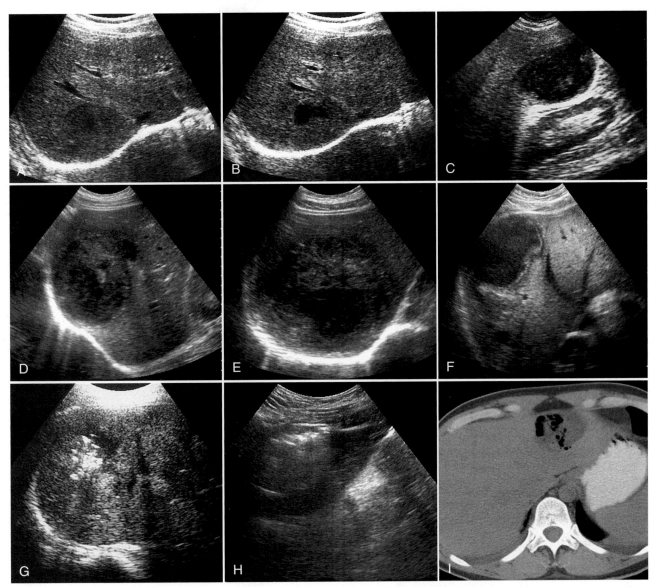

FIGURE 4-19. Pyogenic abscesses: spectrum of appearances. *Top row,* **Early lesions. A** and **B,** Rapid evolution from phlegmon to liquefaction. **A,** Poorly defined mass effect or phlegmon in segment 7 of the liver. **B,** At 24 hours later, there is a central area of liquefaction. **C,** Early abscess is poorly marginated and bulges the liver capsule. It is difficult to characterize this mass as solid or cystic. There was no vascularity within this or other masses. *Middle row,* **Mature abscess cavities in three patients. D** to **F,** Classic mature abscess as a well-defined mass with liquefaction and internal debris. *Bottom row,* **Abscesses related to gas-forming organisms. G,** Multiple gas bubbles seen as innumerable bright echogenic foci within a poorly defined hypoechoic liver mass. **H,** Sagittal image of the left lobe of the liver, and **I,** confirmatory CT scan, show a liver mass with extensive gas content.

Fungal Diseases: Candidiasis

The liver is frequently involved secondary to hematogenous spread of mycotic infections in other organs, most often the lungs. Patients are generally **immunocompromised,** although systemic candidiasis may occur in pregnancy or after hyperalimentation. The clinical characteristics include persistent fever in a neutropenic patient whose leukocyte count is returning to normal.[34]

The ultrasound features of **hepatic candidiasis** include the following[35]:

• "Wheel within a wheel": peripheral hypoechoic zone with inner echogenic wheel and central hypoechoic nidus. The central nidus represents focal necrosis in which fungal elements are found. This is seen early in the disease.

• Bull's-eye: 1 to 4 cm lesion with hyperechoic center and hypoechoic rim. It is present when neutrophil counts return to normal. The echogenic center contains inflammatory cells (Fig. 4-20).

• Uniformly hypoechoic: most common, corresponding to progressive fibrosis (Fig. 4-21, *A*).

• Echogenic: variable calcification, representing scar formation (Fig. 4-21, *B*).

Although percutaneous liver aspiration is helpful in obtaining the organism in pyogenic liver abscesses, it

HEPATIC CANDIDIASIS: SONOGRAPHIC FEATURES

"WHEEL WITHIN A WHEEL"
Peripheral hypoechoic zone
Inner echogenic wheel
Central hypoechoic nidus

BULL'S-EYE
Hyperechoic center
Hypoechoic rim

UNIFORMLY HYPOECHOIC
Progressive fibrosis

ECHOGENIC
Calcification representing scar formation

frequently yields false-negative results for the presence of *Candida* organisms.[35] This may be caused by failure to sample the central necrotic portion of the lesion, where the pseudohyphae are found.[34]

Parasitic Diseases

Amebiasis

Hepatic infection by the parasite *Entamoeba histolytica* is the most common extraintestinal manifestation of amebiasis. Transmission is by the fecal-oral route. The protozoan reaches the liver by penetrating through the colon, invading the mesenteric venules, and entering the portal vein. However, in more than one half of patients with amebic abscesses of the liver, the colon appears normal and stool culture results are negative, thus

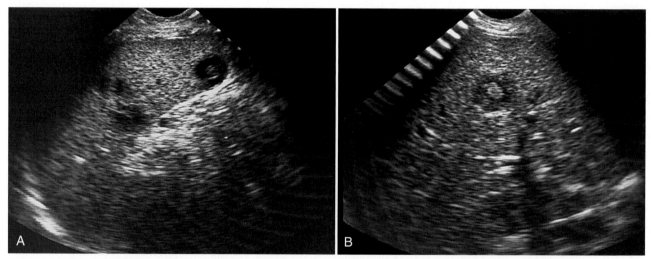

FIGURE 4-20. Fungal infection. "Bull's-eye" fungal morphology in 24-year-old man with acute lymphoblastic leukemia and fever. **A,** Sagittal sonogram through the spleen shows focal hypoechoic target lesions. **B,** The liver showed multiple masses. This magnified view shows a thick, echogenic rim and a thin, hypoechoic inner rim with a dense echogenic nidus. Biopsy revealed pseudohyphae.

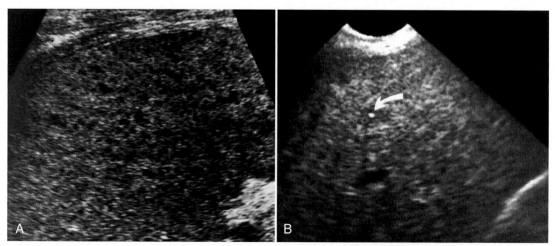

FIGURE 4-21. Candidiasis. A, Uniformly hypoechoic pattern. Multiple hypoechoic hepatic lesions are present in this young patient with acute myelogenous leukemia. **B,** Echogenic pattern after medical therapy. Small calcified lesion *(arrow)* is visualized in another immunocompromised patient.

delaying diagnosis. The most common presenting symptom, **pain** occurs in 99% of patients with amebic abscess. Approximately 15% of patients have diarrhea at diagnosis.

Sonographic features include a round or oval-shaped lesion, absence of a prominent abscess wall, hypoechogenicity compared to normal liver, fine low-level internal echoes, distal sonic enhancement, and contiguity with the diaphragm[36,37] (Fig. 4-22). These features, however, can all be found in pyogenic abscess.

In a review of 112 amebic lesions, Ralls et al.[38] reported that two sonographic patterns were significantly more prevalent in amebic abscesses: (1) round or oval shapes in 82%, versus 60% of pyogenic abscesses, and (2) hypoechoic appearance with fine internal echoes at high gain in 58%, versus 36% of pyogenic abscesses. Most amebic abscesses occur in the right lobe of the liver. Diagnosis is made using a combination of the clinical features, ultrasound findings, and serologic results. The indirect hemagglutination test is positive in 94% to 100% of patients.

Amebicidal drugs are effective therapy. Symptoms improve in 24 to 48 hours, and most patients are afebrile in 4 days. Those who exhibit clinical deterioration may also benefit from catheter drainage, although this is unusual. The majority of hepatic amebic abscesses disappear with adequate medical therapy.[39] The time from termination of therapy to resolution varies from 1.5 to 23 months (median, 7 months).[40] A minority of patients have residual hepatic cysts and focal regions of increased or decreased echogenicity.

Hydatid Disease

The most common cause of hydatid disease in humans is infestation by the parasite *Echinococcus granulosus*, which has a worldwide distribution. It is most prevalent in sheep- and cattle-raising countries, notably in the Middle East, Australia, and the Mediterranean. Endemic regions in the United States include the central valley in California, the lower Mississippi River Valley, Utah, and Arizona. Northern Canada is also endemic. *E. granulosus* is a tapeworm 3 to 6 mm in length that lives in the intestine of the definitive host, usually the dog. Its eggs are excreted in the dog's feces and swallowed by the intermediate hosts—sheep, cattle, goats, or humans. The embryos are freed in the duodenum and pass through the mucosa to reach the liver through the portal venous system. Most of the embryos remain trapped in the liver, although the lungs, kidneys, spleen, central nervous system, and bone may become secondarily involved. In the liver the right lobe is more frequently involved. The surviving embryos form slow-growing cysts. The cyst wall consists of an external membrane that is approximately 1 mm thick, which may calcify (ectocyst). The host forms a dense connective tissue capsule around the cyst (pericyst). The inner germinal layer (endocyst) gives rise to brood capsules that enlarge to form protoscolices. The brood capsules may separate from the wall and form a fine sediment called **hydatid sand.** When hydatid cysts within the organs of a herbivore are eaten, the scolices attach to the intestine and grow to adult tapeworms, thus completing the life cycle.

Several reports describe the sonographic features of hepatic hydatid disease[41-43] (Figs. 4-23 and 4-24). Lewall[42] proposed the following four groups for hydatid cysts:

- Simple cysts containing no internal architecture except sand
- Cysts with detached endocyst secondary to rupture (Fig. 4-23, *B*)
- Cysts with daughter cyst matrix (echogenic material between daughter cysts)
- Densely calcified masses

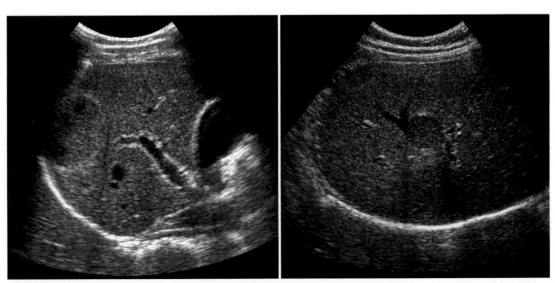

FIGURE 4-22. Amebic liver abscess: classic morphology. Transverse sonograms show a well-defined oval subdiaphragmatic mass with increased through transmission. There are uniform low-level internal echoes and absence of a well-defined abscess wall.

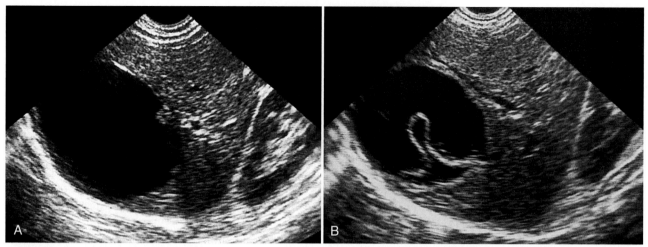

FIGURE 4-23. Hydatid cyst. A, Baseline sonogram shows a fairly simple cyst in the right lobe with a small mural nodule and a fleck of peripheral calcium anteriorly. **B,** Three weeks later the patient presented with right upper quadrant pain and eosinophilia. The detached endocyst is floating within the lesion.

SONOGRAPHIC MORPHOLOGY OF HYDATID CYSTS

1. Simple cysts
2. Cysts with detached endocyst secondary to rupture
3. Cysts with daughter cysts
4. Densely calcified masses

Surgery is the conventional treatment in echinococcal disease, although recent reports describe success with percutaneous drainage.[44-46] Although reported, anaphylaxis from hydatid cyst rupture is rare. Ultrasound has been used to monitor the course of medical therapy in patients with abdominal hydatid disease.[47] A reappearance or persistence of fluid within the cavity may signify inadequate therapy and viability of the parasites.[48]

Hepatic alveolar echinococcus is a rare parasitic infestation by the larvae of *E. multilocularis.* The fox is the main host. The sonographic features include echogenic lesions, which may be single or multiple; necrotic, irregular lesions without a well-defined wall; clusters of calcification within lesions; and dilated bile ducts.[49]

Schistosomiasis

Schistosomiasis is one of the most common parasitic infections in humans, estimated to affect 200 million people worldwide.[50] Hepatic schistosomiasis is caused by *Schistosoma mansoni, S. japonicum, S. mekongi,* and *S. intercalatum.* Hepatic involvement by *S. mansoni* is particularly severe. *S. mansoni* is prevalent in Africa, including Egypt, and South America, particularly in Venezuela and Brazil. The ova reach the liver through the portal vein and incite a chronic granulomatous reaction, first described by Symmers in 1904 as "clay-pipestem fibrosis."[51] The terminal portal vein branches become occluded, leading to presinusoidal portal hypertension, splenomegaly, varices, and ascites.

The sonographic features of schistosomiasis are widened echogenic portal tracts, sometimes reaching a thickness of 2 cm.[52,53] The porta hepatis is the region most often affected. Initially the liver size is enlarged. As the periportal fibrosis progresses, however, the liver becomes contracted, and the features of portal hypertension prevail.

Pneumocystis carinii

Pneumocystis carinii is the most common organism causing **opportunistic infection** in patients with acquired immunodeficiency syndrome (AIDS). *Pneumocystis* pneumonia is the most common cause of life-threatening infection in patients with human immunodeficiency virus (HIV). *P. carinii* also affects patients undergoing bone marrow and organ transplantation, as well as those receiving corticosteroids or chemotherapy.[54] Extrapulmonary *P. carinii* infection was being reported with frequency about 1990.[55-58] It was postulated that the use of maintenance aerosolized pentamidine achieved lower systemic levels than the intravenous form, allowing subclinical pulmonary infections and systemic dissemination of the protozoa. This treatment is now infrequently used by AIDS patients, so disseminated infection is rarely seen. Extrapulmonary *P. carinii* infection has been documented in the liver, spleen, renal cortex, thyroid gland, pancreas, and lymph nodes.

The sonographic findings of *P. carinii* involvement of the liver range from tiny, diffuse, nonshadowing echogenic foci to extensive replacement of the normal hepatic parenchyma by echogenic clumps representing dense calcification (Fig. 4-25). A similar sonographic pattern

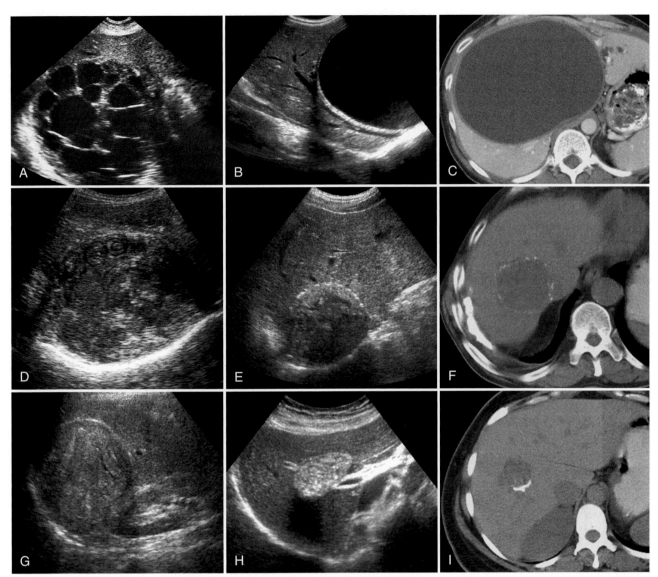

FIGURE 4-24. Hydatid liver disease: spectrum of appearances. A, Classic appearance showing a cyst containing multiple daughter cysts. **B,** Sonogram, and **C,** confirmatory CT scan, show a unilocular and simple cyst, a fairly uncommon morphology for hydatid disease. **D,** Sonogram shows a complex mass. Anteriorly, multiple ringlike structures suggest hydatid disease. At surgery, cystic mass showed thick debris and innumerable scolices. **E,** Sonogram, and **F,** confirmatory CT scan, show an indeterminate mass with a thin rim of calcification. **G,** Complex mass similar to that seen in **D.** There are fingerlike projections within, again suggestive of hydatid disease. **H,** Sonogram, and **I,** confirmatory CT scan, show a central liver mass with rim and internal punctate calcification.

has been identified with hepatic infection by *Mycobacterium avium-intracellulare* and cytomegalovirus.[59]

DISORDERS OF METABOLISM

Fatty Liver

Fatty liver is an acquired, reversible disorder of metabolism, resulting in an accumulation of triglycerides within the hepatocytes. The most common cause likely is **obesity**. Fatty liver is recognized as a significant component of the **metabolic syndrome,** which has recently increased in significance. Excessive alcohol intake produces a fatty liver by stimulating lipolysis, as

does starvation. Other causes of fatty infiltration include poorly controlled hyperlipidemia, diabetes, excess exogenous or endogenous corticosteroids, pregnancy, total parenteral hyperalimentation, severe hepatitis, glycogen storage disease, jejunoileal bypass procedures for obesity, cystic fibrosis, congenital generalized lipodystrophy, several chemotherapeutic agents, including methotrexate, and toxins such as carbon tetrachloride and yellow phosphorus.[60] Correction of the primary abnormality will usually reverse the process, although it is now recognized that fatty infiltration of the liver is the precursor for significant chronic disease and hepatocellular carcinoma in some patients.

Sonography of fatty infiltration varies depending on the amount of fat and whether deposits are diffuse or

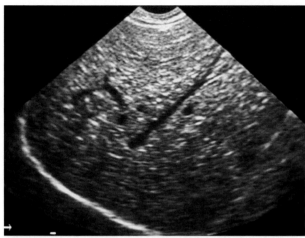

FIGURE 4-25. *Pneumocystis carinii.* Disseminated *P. carinii* infection in AIDS patient who previously used pentamidine inhaler. Sonogram shows innumerable tiny, bright echogenic foci without shadowing throughout the liver parenchyma.

focal[61] (Fig. 4-26). **Diffuse steatosis** may appear as follows:

DIFFUSE STEATOSIS

MILD
Minimal diffuse increase in hepatic echogenicity

MODERATE
Moderate diffuse increase in hepatic echogenicity
Slightly impaired visualization of intrahepatic vessels and diaphragm

SEVERE
Marked increase in echogenicity
Poor penetration of posterior liver
Poor or no visualization of hepatic vessels and diaphragm

- **Mild**—Minimal diffuse increase in hepatic echogenicity with normal visualization of diaphragm and intrahepatic vessel borders.
- **Moderate**—Moderate diffuse increase in hepatic echogenicity with slightly impaired visualization of intrahepatic vessels and diaphragm.
- **Severe**—Marked increase in echogenicity with poor penetration of posterior segment of right lobe of liver and poor or no visualization of hepatic vessels and diaphragm.

Focal fatty infiltration and focal fatty sparing may mimic neoplastic involvement.[62] In **focal fatty infiltration,** regions of increased echogenicity are present within a background of normal liver parenchyma. Conversely, islands of normal liver parenchyma may appear as hypoechoic masses within a dense, fatty infiltrated liver (**Videos 4-3** and **4-4**). Features of **focal fatty change** include the following (Fig. 4-27):

FOCAL FATTY CHANGE: SONOGRAPHIC FEATURES

Rapid change with time, both in appearance and resolution
No alteration of course or caliber of regional vessels
No contour abnormality

PREFERRED SITE FOR FOCAL FATTY SPARING
Anterior to portal vein at porta hepatis
Gallbladder fossa
Liver margins

PREFERRED SITE FOR FOCAL FAT
Anterior to portal vein at porta hepatis

GEOGRAPHIC FAT: MAPLIKE BOUNDARIES

- Focal fatty sparing and focal fatty liver most often involve the periportal region of the medial segment of the left lobe (segment IV).[63,64]
- Sparing also frequently occurs by the gallbladder fossa and along the liver margins.
- Focal subcapsular fat may occur in diabetic patients receiving insulin in peritoneal dialysate[65] (Fig. 4-27, *H* and *I*).
- Lack of mass effect; hepatic vessels generally are not displaced, although traversing vessels in metastases have been reported.[66]
- Geometric margins are present, although focal fat may appear round, nodular, or interdigitated with normal tissue.[67]
- Rapid change with time; fatty infiltration may resolve as early as 6 days.
- Liver CT scans demonstrate corresponding regions of low attenuation.

Contrast-enhanced ultrasound (CEUS) is valuable in the differentiation of fatty change from neoplasia, because the fatty or spared regions will all appear isovascular in both the arterial and the portal venous phase of enhancement. Chemical shift MRI techniques are useful in distinguishing diffuse from focal fatty infiltration. Radionuclide liver and spleen scintigraphic examination will yield normal results, indicating adequate numbers of Kupffer cells within the fatty regions.[61] Some postulate that these focal spared areas are caused by a regional decrease in portal blood flow, as demonstrated by CT scans during arterial portographic examinations.[68] Knowledge of typical patterns and use of CT, CEUS, MRI, or nuclear medicine scintigraphy will avoid the necessity for biopsy in most patients with focal fatty alteration.

Glycogen Storage Disease (Glycogenosis)

Von Gierke first recognized glycogen storage disease (GSD) affecting the kidneys and liver in 1929. Type 1

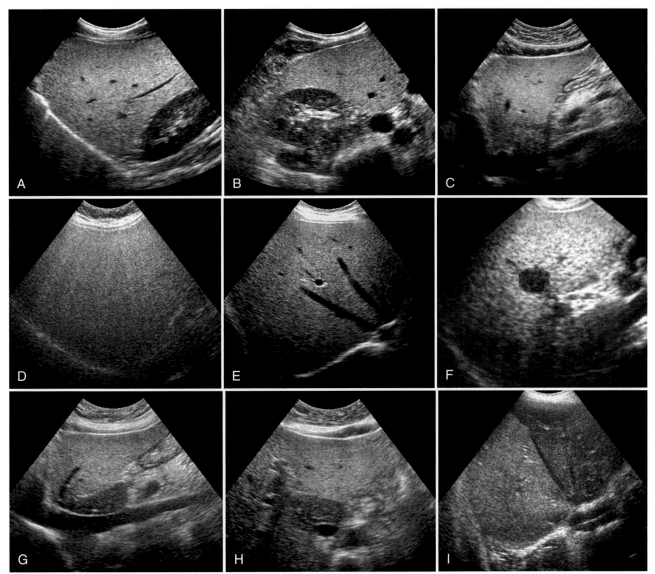

FIGURE 4-26. Diffuse fat: spectrum of appearances. **Mild fatty infiltration: A,** sagittal right lobe; **B,** transverse right lobe; **C,** sagittal left lobe. The liver is diffusely bright and echogenic; sound penetration remains good. **Marked fatty infiltration: D,** sagittal right lobe; **E,** subcostal oblique view. The liver is enlarged and attenuating; sound penetration is poor; and the walls of the hepatic veins are not defined. **Focal fatty sparing: F,** mimicking a hypoechoic mass; normal liver on biopsy and follow-up. **G,** Sagittal, and **H,** transverse, images show focal fatty sparing of the caudate lobe. **I,** Geographic fatty sparing of the entire left lobe marginated by the middle hepatic vein.

GSD (von Gierke's disease, glucose 6-phosphatase deficiency) is manifested in the neonatal period by hepatomegaly, nephromegaly, and hypoglycemic convulsions. Because of the enzyme deficiency, large quantities of glycogen are deposited in the hepatocytes and proximal convoluted tubules of the kidney.[69] With dietary management and supportive therapy, more patients currently survive to childhood and young adulthood. As a result, several patients have developed benign adenomas or less often HCC.[70]

Sonographically, type 1 GSD appears indistinguishable from other causes of diffuse fatty infiltration. Secondary hepatic adenomas are well-demarcated, solid masses of variable echogenicity. Malignant transforma-

tion can be recognized by rapid growth of the lesions, which may become more poorly defined.[70]

Cirrhosis

The World Health Organization (WHO) defines cirrhosis as a diffuse process characterized by fibrosis and the conversion of normal liver architecture into structurally abnormal nodules.[71] Three major pathologic mechanisms combine to create cirrhosis: **cell death, fibrosis,** and **regeneration.** Cirrhosis has been classified as **micronodular,** in which nodules are 0.1 to 1 cm in diameter, and **macronodular,** characterized by nodules of varying size, up to 5 cm in diameter. Alcohol

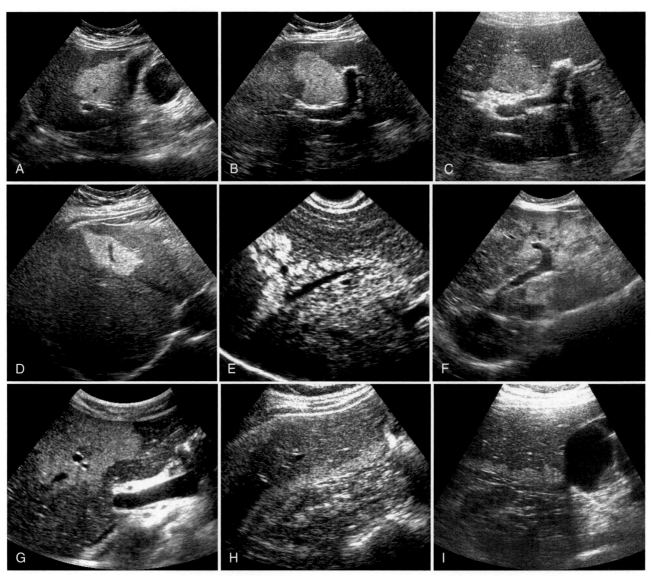

FIGURE 4-27. Focal fat: spectrum of appearances. A, Sagittal, and **B,** subcostal oblique, images show the most common location for **classic focal fat,** in segment 4, anterior to the portal venous bifurcation at the porta hepatis, where it is large and masslike. **C,** Another patient showing a more common, milder form of the same fat deposition. **D** to **G, Tumoral fat.** Fat deposits in all images suggest a focal liver mass. The liver vasculature is unaltered in its course at the location of the fatty masses. **E,** Focal fat of pregnancy. **H** and **I, Hepatic steatonecrosis** shown in views of the right lobe of the liver is a rare observation in diabetic patients who receive insulin in their peritoneal dialysate.

consumption is the most common cause of micronodular cirrhosis, and chronic viral hepatitis is the most frequent cause of the macronodular form.[72] Patients who continue to drink may go on to end-stage liver disease, which is indistinguishable from cirrhosis of other causes. Other etiologies are **biliary cirrhosis** (primary and secondary), Wilson's disease, primary sclerosing cholangitis, and hemochromatosis. The classic clinical presentation of cirrhosis is hepatomegaly, jaundice, and ascites. However, serious liver injury may be present without any clinical clues. In fact, only 60% of patients with cirrhosis have signs and symptoms of liver disease.

Because liver biopsy is invasive, the ability to detect cirrhosis by noninvasive means, such as sonography, holds great clinical interest. The sonographic patterns

associated with cirrhosis include the following (Fig. 4-28):
• **Volume redistribution.** In the early stages of cirrhosis the liver may be enlarged, whereas in advanced stages the liver is often small, with relative enlargement of the caudate lobe, left lobe, or both, compared with the right lobe. Several studies have evaluated the ratio of the caudate lobe width to the right lobe width (C/RL) as an indicator of cirrhosis.[73] A C/RL value of 0.65 is considered indicative of cirrhosis. The specificity is high (100%), but the sensitivity is low (43%-84%), indicating that the C/RL ratio is a useful measurement if it is abnormal.[73] However, no patients in these studies had Budd-Chiari syndrome, which may also cause caudate lobe enlargement.

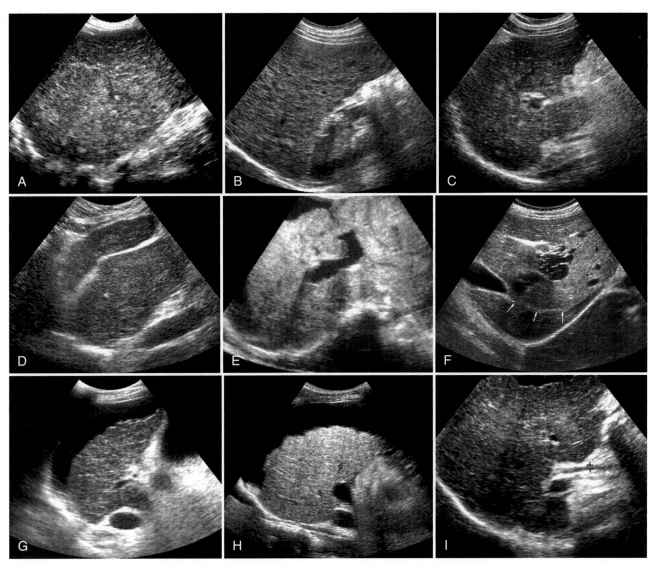

FIGURE 4-28. Cirrhosis: spectrum of appearances. *Top row,* **Parenchymal changes. A,** Coarse parenchyma and innumerable tiny, hyperechoic nodules. **B,** Coarse parenchyma and innumerable tiny, hypoechoic nodules. **C,** Coarse parenchyma and surface nodularity. *Middle row,* **Lobar redistribution. D,** Sagittal image showing an enormous caudate lobe. **E,** Transverse sonogram shows the right lobe is small, with enlargement of the left lateral segment. **F,** Subcostal oblique view showing a tiny right lobe of the liver, which is separated from the large left lobe by the main lobar fissure *(arrows). Bottom row,* **Contour abnormality. G** and **H,** Small, end-stage livers with surface nodularity, best appreciated in patients with ascites, as shown here. **I,** Liver contour varies greatly, as shown here, where a large nodule protrudes from the deep liver border.

- **Coarse echotexture.** Increased echogenicity and coarse echotexture are frequent observations in diffuse liver disease. These are subjective findings, however, and may be confounded by inappropriate time gain compensation (TGC) settings and overall gain. Liver attenuation is correlated with the presence of fat, not fibrosis.[74] Cirrhotic livers without fatty infiltration had attenuation values similar to those of controls. This accounts for the relatively low accuracy in distinguishing diffuse liver disease[75] and the conflicting reports regarding attenuation values in cirrhosis.
- **Nodular surface.** Irregularity of the liver surface during routine scanning has been appreciated as a sign of cirrhosis when the appearance is gross or when ascites is present.[76] The nodularity

CIRRHOSIS: SONOGRAPHIC FEATURES

Volume redistribution
Coarse echotexture
Nodular surface
Nodules: regenerative and dysplastic
Portal hypertension: ascites, splenomegaly, and varices

corresponds to the presence of regenerating nodules and fibrosis.
- **Regenerating nodules** (RNs). These regenerating hepatocytes are surrounded by fibrotic septae. Because RNs have a similar architecture to the normal liver, ultrasound and CT have limited ability

in their detection. RNs tend to be isoechoic or hypoechoic with a thin, echogenic border that corresponds to fibrofatty connective tissue.[76] MRI has a greater sensitivity than both CT and ultrasound in RN detection. Because some RNs contain iron, gradient echo sequences demonstrate these nodules as hypointense.[77]

• **Dysplastic nodules.** Dysplastic nodules or adenomatous hyperplastic nodules are larger than RNs (diameter of 10 mm) and are considered premalignant.[78] They contain well-differentiated hepatocytes, a portal venous blood supply, and atypical or frankly malignant cells. The portal venous blood supply can be detected with color Doppler flow imaging and distinguished from the hepatic artery–supplied HCC.[79] In a patient with cirrhosis and a liver mass, percutaneous biopsy is often performed to exclude or diagnose HCC.

Doppler Ultrasound Characteristics

The normal Doppler waveform of the hepatic veins reflects the hemodynamics of the right atrium. The waveform is triphasic: two large antegrade diastolic and systolic waves and a small retrograde wave corresponding to the atrial "kick." Because the walls of the hepatic veins are thin, disease of the hepatic parenchyma may alter their compliance. In many patients with compensated cirrhosis (no portal hypertension), the Doppler waveform is abnormal. **Two abnormal patterns** have been described: decreased amplitude of phasic oscillations with loss of reversed flow and a flattened waveform.[80,81] These abnormal patterns have also been found in patients with fatty infiltration of the liver.[81]

As cirrhosis progresses, luminal narrowing of the hepatic veins may be associated with flow alterations visible on color and spectral Doppler ultrasound. High-velocity signals through an area of narrowing produce color aliasing and turbulence (Fig. 4-29).

The hepatic artery waveform also shows altered flow dynamics in cirrhosis and chronic liver disease. Lafortune et al.[82] found an increase in the resistive index of the hepatic artery after a meal in patients with a normal liver. The vasoconstriction of the hepatic artery occurs as a normal response to the increased portal venous flow stimulated by eating (20% change). In patients with cirrhosis and chronic liver disease, the normal increase in postprandial resistive index is blunted.[83]

VASCULAR ABNORMALITIES

Portal Hypertension

Normal portal vein pressure is 5 to 10 mm Hg (14 cm H_2O). Portal hypertension is defined by (1) wedge hepatic vein pressure or direct portal vein pressure more than 5 mm Hg greater than IVC pressure, (2) splenic vein pressure greater than 15 mm Hg, or (3) portal vein pressure (measured surgically) greater than 30 cm H_2O. Pathophysiologically, portal hypertension can be divided into presinusoidal and intrahepatic groups, depending on whether the hepatic vein wedge pressure is normal (presinusoidal) or elevated (intrahepatic).

Presinusoidal portal hypertension can be subdivided into extrahepatic and intrahepatic forms. The causes of extrahepatic presinusoidal portal hypertension include thrombosis of the portal or splenic veins. This

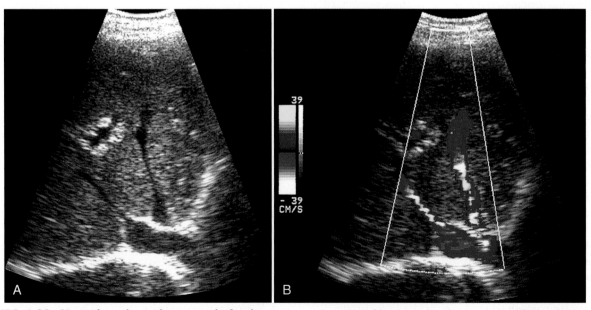

FIGURE 4-29. Hepatic vein strictures: cirrhosis. A, Gray-scale image of hepatic veins shows a tapered luminal narrowing. **B,** Color Doppler image shows appropriately directed blood flow toward the inferior vena cava in blue. There is color aliasing from the rapid-velocity flow through the points of narrowing.

should be suspected in any patient who presents with clinical signs of portal hypertension—ascites, splenomegaly, and varices—and a normal liver biopsy. Thrombosis of the portal venous system occurs in children secondary to umbilical vein catheterization, omphalitis, and neonatal sepsis. In adults the causes of portal vein thrombosis include trauma, sepsis, HCC, pancreatic carcinoma, pancreatitis, portacaval shunts, splenectomy, and hypercoagulable states. The **intrahepatic presinusoidal** causes of portal hypertension are the result of diseases affecting the portal zones of the liver, notably schistosomiasis, primary biliary cirrhosis, congenital hepatic fibrosis, and toxic substances, such as polyvinyl chloride and methotrexate.[84]

Cirrhosis is the most common cause of **intrahepatic portal hypertension** and accounts for greater than 90% of all cases of portal hypertension in the West. In cirrhosis the distorted vascular channels increase resistance to portal venous blood flow and obstruct hepatic venous outflow. Diffuse metastatic liver disease also produces portal hypertension by the same mechanism. Over time, thrombotic diseases of the IVC and hepatic veins, as well as constrictive pericarditis and other causes of severe right-sided heart failure, will lead to centrilobular fibrosis, hepatic regeneration, cirrhosis, and finally portal hypertension.

Sonographic findings of portal hypertension include the **secondary signs** of splenomegaly, ascites, and portosystemic venous collaterals (Figs. 4-30 and 4-31). When the resistance to blood flow in the portal vessels exceeds the resistance to flow in the small communicating channels between the portal and systemic circulations, portosystemic collaterals form. Thus, although the caliber of the portal vein initially may be increased (>1.3 cm) in portal hypertension,[85] with the development of portosystemic shunts, the portal vein caliber will decrease.[86] Five **major sites of portosystemic venous collaterals** are visualized by ultrasound[87-89] (see Fig. 4-30).

- **Gastroesophageal junction:** Between the coronary and short gastric veins and the systemic esophageal veins. These varices are of particular importance because they may lead to life-threatening or fatal hemorrhage. Dilation of the coronary vein (>0.7 cm) is associated with severe portal hypertension (portohepatic gradient >10 mm Hg)[86] (Fig. 4-31, *C* and *D*).
- **Paraumbilical vein:** Runs in the falciform ligament and connects the left portal vein to the systemic epigastric veins near the umbilicus (Cruveilhier-Baumgarten syndrome)[90] (Fig. 4-31, *A*). Some suggest that, if the hepatofugal flow in the patent paraumbilical vein exceeds the hepatopetal flow in the portal vein, patients may be protected from developing esophageal varices.[91,92]
- **Splenorenal and gastrorenal:** Tortuous veins may be seen in the region of the splenic and left renal

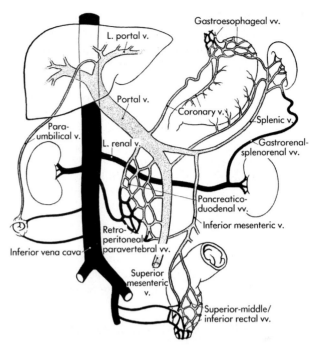

FIGURE 4-30. Portal hypertension. Major sites of portosystemic venous collaterals. *(From Subramanyam BR, Balthazar EJ, Madamba MR, et al: Sonography of portosystemic venous collaterals in portal hypertension. Radiology 1983;146:161-166.)*

PORTOSYSTEMIC VENOUS COLLATERALS: MAJOR SITES IDENTIFIED ON ULTRASOUND

1. Gastroesophageal junction
2. Paraumbilical vein in falciform ligament
3. Splenorenal and gastrorenal veins
4. Intestinal-retroperitoneal anastomoses
5. Hemorrhoidal veins

hilus (Fig. 4-31, *E* and *F*), which represent collaterals between the splenic, coronary, and short gastric veins and the left adrenal or renal veins.
- **Intestinal:** Regions in which the gastrointestinal tract becomes retroperitoneal so that the veins of the ascending and descending colon, duodenum, pancreas, and liver may anastomose with the renal, phrenic, and lumbar veins (systemic tributaries).
- **Hemorrhoidal:** The perianal region where the superior rectal veins, which extend from the inferior mesenteric vein, anastomose with the systemic middle and inferior rectal veins.

Duplex Doppler sonography provides additional information regarding direction of portal flow. False results may occur, however, when sampling is obtained from periportal collaterals in patients with portal vein thrombosis or hepatofugal portal flow.[93] Normal portal venous flow rates will vary in the same individual, increasing postprandially and during inspiration[83,94] and decreasing after exercise or in the upright position.[95] An increase of less than 20% in the diameter of the portal

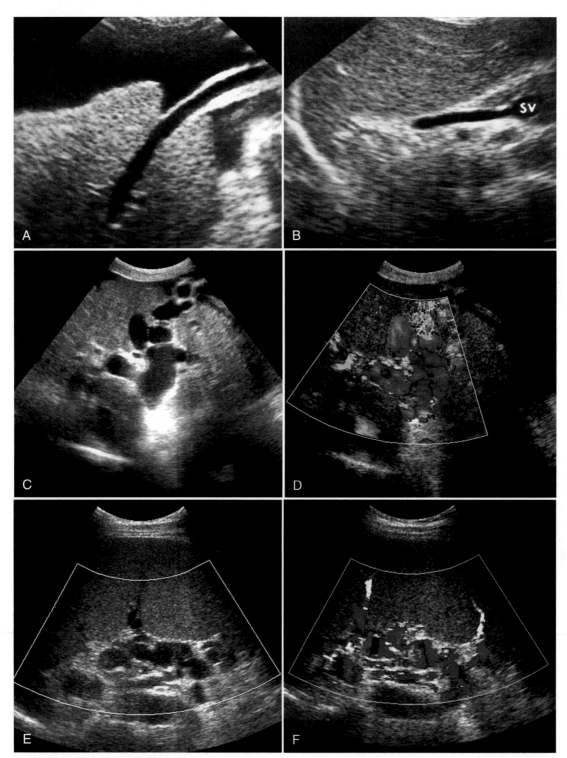

FIGURE 4-31. Portal hypertension. A, Sagittal image of recanalized paraumbilical vein in patient with gross ascites. **B,** Sagittal image shows enlarged coronary vein running cephalad from the splenic vein *(SV)*. **C,** Gray-scale image, and **D,** color Doppler image, show extensive varices in the distribution of the coronary vein. **E,** Gray-scale image, and **F,** color Doppler image, show splenic hilar varices.

vein with deep inspiration indicates portal hypertension with 81% sensitivity and 100% specificity.[96]

The **normal portal vein** demonstrates an undulating **hepatopetal** (toward the liver) flow. Mean portal venous flow velocity is approximately 15 to 18 cm/sec and varies with respiration and cardiac pulsation. As portal hyper-

tension develops, the flow in the portal vein loses its undulatory pattern and becomes monophasic. As the severity of portal hypertension increases, flow becomes biphasic and finally **hepatofugal** (away from the liver). Intrahepatic arterial-portal venous shunting may also be seen.

Chronic liver disease is also associated with increased splanchnic blood flow. Recent evidence suggests that portal hypertension is partly caused by the hyperdynamic flow state of cirrhosis. Zweibel et al.[97] found that blood flow was increased in the superior mesenteric arteries and splenic arteries of patients with cirrhosis and splenomegaly, compared with normal controls. Of interest, in patients with cirrhosis and normal-sized livers, splanchnic blood flow was not increased. Patients with isolated splenomegaly and normal livers were not included in this study.

The limitations of Doppler sonography in the evaluation of portal hypertension include the inability to determine vascular pressures and flow rates accurately. Patients with portal hypertension are often ill, with contracted livers, abundant ascites, and floating bowel, all of which create a technical challenge. In a comparison of duplex Doppler sonography with MR angiography, MR imaging was superior in the assessment of patency of the portal vein and surgical shunts, as well as in detection of varices.[98] However, when technically adequate, the Doppler study was accurate in the assessment of normal portal anatomy and flow direction. Duplex Doppler sonography has the added advantages of decreased cost and portability of the equipment and therefore should be used as the initial screening method for portal hypertension.

Portal Vein Thrombosis

Portal vein thrombosis has been associated with malignancy, including HCC, metastatic liver disease, carcinoma of the pancreas, and primary leiomyosarcoma of the portal vein,[99] as well as with chronic pancreatitis, hepatitis, septicemia, trauma, splenectomy, portacaval shunts, hypercoagulable states such as pregnancy and in neonates, omphalitis, umbilical vein catheterization, and acute dehydration.[100]

Sonographic findings of portal vein thrombosis include echogenic thrombus within the lumen of the vein, portal vein collaterals, expansion of the caliber of the vein, and cavernous transformations[100] (Figs. 4-32 and 4-33). **Cavernous transformation of the portal vein** refers to numerous wormlike vessels at the porta

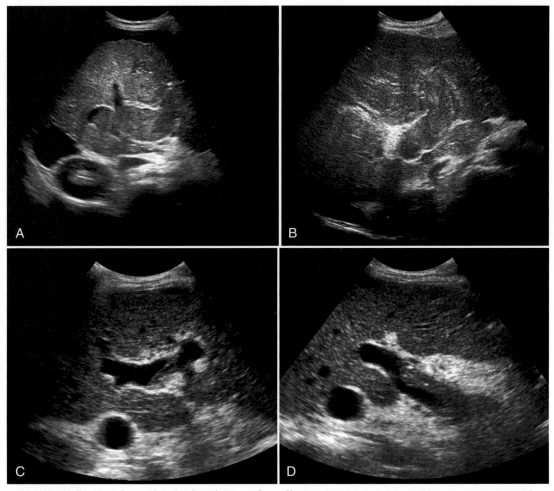

FIGURE 4-32. Portal vein thrombosis: benign and malignant. Malignant thrombus: transverse views of **A,** the vein at the porta hepatis, and **B,** left ascending left portal vein. Both are distended with occlusive thrombus. **Benign thrombus: C,** transverse, and **D,** sagittal, images of simple, bland nonocclusive thrombus in the left portal vein at the porta hepatis.

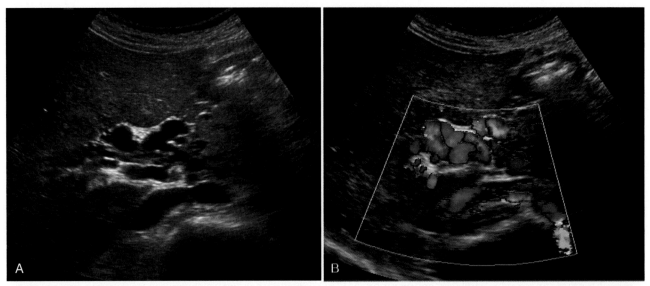

FIGURE 4-33. Cavernous transformation of portal vein. A, Gray-scale image, and **B,** Color Doppler image. Numerous periportal collateral vessels are present.

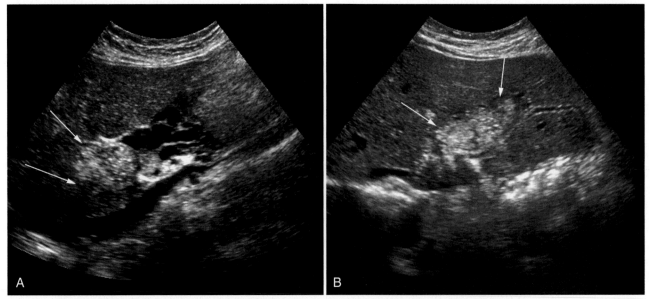

FIGURE 4-34. Metastasis to the portal vein from colon cancer. A, Sagittal view of the main portal vein at the porta hepatis, and **B,** subcostal oblique sonogram of the left ascending branch of the portal vein, show the portal vein is distended and highly echogenic *(arrows).* There is also evidence of cavernous transformation, an uncommon accompaniment of malignant portal vein occlusion.

hepatis, which represent periportal collateral circulation.[101] This pattern is observed in long-standing thrombosis, requiring up to 12 months to occur, and thus is more likely to develop with benign disease.[102] **Acute thrombus** may appear relatively anechoic and thus may be overlooked unless Doppler ultrasound interrogation is performed. **Malignant thrombosis** of the portal vein has a high association with HCC and is often expansive, as is malignant occlusion from other primary or secondary disease (Fig. 4-34).

Doppler sonography is useful in distinguishing between benign and malignant portal vein thrombi in patients with cirrhosis. Both bland and malignant thrombi may demonstrate continuous blood flow. Pulsatile flow, however, has been found to be 95% specific for the diagnosis of malignant portal vein thrombosis (see Fig. 4-32). The sensitivity was only 62% because many malignant thrombi are hypovascular.[103]

Budd-Chiari Syndrome

The Budd-Chiari syndrome is a relatively rare disorder characterized by occlusion of the lumens of the hepatic veins with or without occlusion of the IVC lumen. The degree of occlusion and presence of collateral circulation predict the clinical course. Some patients die in the acute phase of liver failure. Causes of Budd-Chiari syndrome include coagulation abnormalities such as polycythemia rubra vera, chronic leukemia, and paroxysmal nocturnal hemoglobinuria; trauma; tumor extension from primary HCC, renal carcinoma, and adrenocortical carcinoma; pregnancy; congenital abnormalities; and obstructing membranes. The classic patient in North America is a young adult woman taking oral contraceptives who presents with an acute onset of ascites, right upper quadrant pain, hepatomegaly, and to a lesser extent, splenomegaly. In some cases, no etiologic factor is found. The syndrome is more common in other geographic areas, including India, South Africa, and Asia.

Sonographic evaluation of the patient with Budd-Chiari syndrome includes gray-scale and Doppler features.[104-115] Ascites is invariably seen. The liver is typically large and bulbous in the acute phase (Fig. 4-35, A). Hemorrhagic infarction may produce significant altered regional echogenicity. As infarcted areas become more fibrotic, echogenicity increases.[105] The caudate lobe is often spared in Budd-Chiari syndrome because the emissary veins drain directly into the IVC at a lower level than the involved main hepatic veins. Increased blood flow through the caudate lobe leads to relative caudate enlargement.

Real-time scanning allows the radiologist to evaluate the IVC and hepatic veins noninvasively. Sonographic features include evidence of the **hepatic vein occlusion** (Fig. 4-35, B, and Fig. 4-36) and the development of **abnormal intrahepatic collaterals** (Fig. 4-37). The extent of hepatic venous involvement in Budd-Chiari syndrome includes partial or complete inability to see the hepatic veins, stenosis with proximal dilation, intraluminal echogenicity, thickened walls, thrombosis (Figs. 4-38 and 4-39), and extensive intrahepatic collaterals[107, 108] (see Fig. 4-37). Membranous "webs" may be identified as echogenic or focal obliterations of the lumen.[108] Real-time ultrasonography, however, underestimates the presence of thrombosis and webs and may be inconclusive in a cirrhotic patient with hepatic veins that are difficult to image.[107] Intrahepatic collaterals, on gray-scale images, show as tubular vascular structures in an abnormal location and typically are seen extending from a hepatic vein to the liver surface, where they anastomose with systemic capsular vessels.

Duplex Doppler ultrasound and **color Doppler flow imaging** (CDFI) can help determine both the presence and the direction of hepatic venous flow in the evaluation of patients with suspected Budd-Chiari syndrome. The middle and left hepatic veins are best scanned in the transverse plane at the level of the xiphoid process. From this angle, the veins are almost parallel to the Doppler beam, allowing optimal reception of their Doppler signals. The right hepatic vein is best evaluated from a right intercostal approach.[110] The intricate pathways of blood flow out of the liver in the patient with Budd-Chiari syndrome can be mapped with documentation of hepatic venous occlusions, hepatic-systemic collaterals, hepatic venous–portal venous collaterals, and increased caliber of anomalous or accessory hepatic veins.

The normal blood flow in the IVC and hepatic veins is **phasic** in response to both the cardiac and respiratory cycles.[116] In Budd-Chiari syndrome, flow in the IVC, hepatic veins, or both, changes from phasic to **absent, reversed, turbulent,** or **continuous.**[112,115] Continuous flow has been called the **pseudoportal Doppler signal** and appears to reflect either partial IVC obstruction or

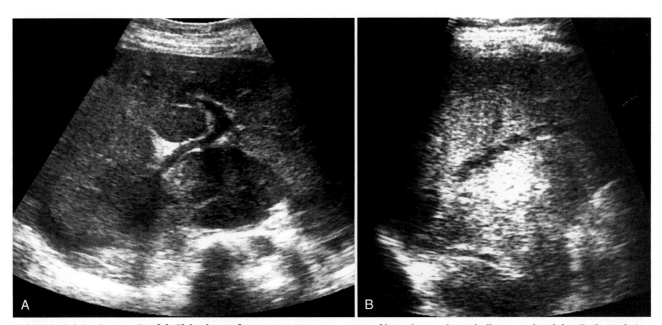

FIGURE 4-35. Acute Budd-Chiari syndrome. A, Transverse view of liver shows a large, bulbous caudate lobe. **B,** Sagittal view of right hepatic vein shows echoes within the vein lumen consistent with thrombosis, with absence of the vessel toward the inferior vena cava. Doppler ultrasound showed no flow in this vessel.

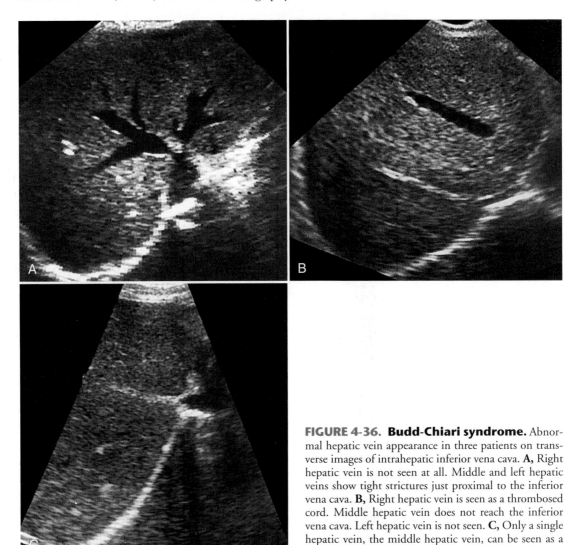

FIGURE 4-36. Budd-Chiari syndrome. Abnormal hepatic vein appearance in three patients on transverse images of intrahepatic inferior vena cava. **A,** Right hepatic vein is not seen at all. Middle and left hepatic veins show tight strictures just proximal to the inferior vena cava. **B,** Right hepatic vein is seen as a thrombosed cord. Middle hepatic vein does not reach the inferior vena cava. Left hepatic vein is not seen. **C,** Only a single hepatic vein, the middle hepatic vein, can be seen as a thrombosed cord.

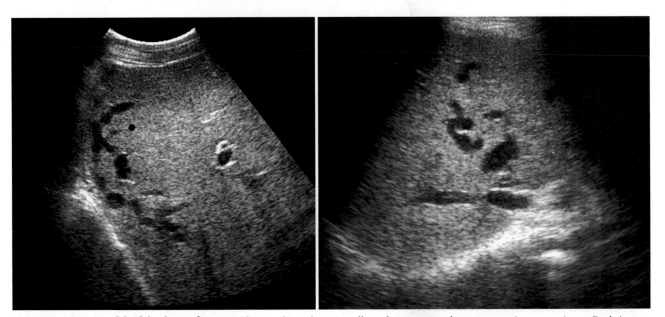

FIGURE 4-37. Budd-Chiari syndrome. Abnormal intrahepatic collaterals on gray-scale sonograms in two patients. Both images show vessels with abnormal locations and increased tortuosity compared with the normal intrahepatic vasculature.

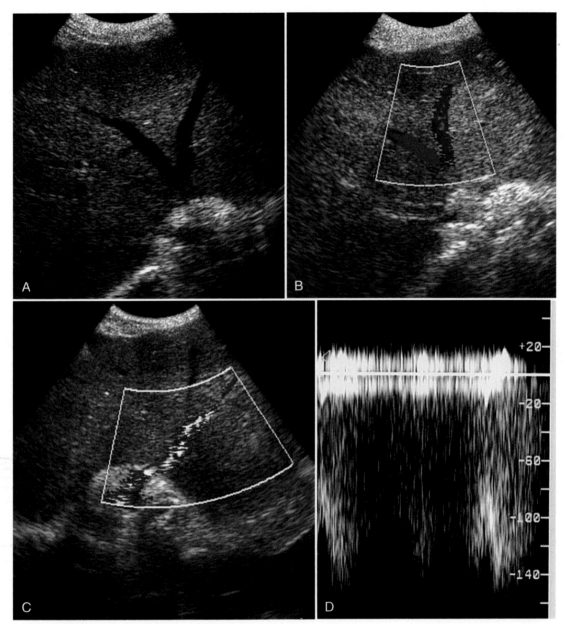

FIGURE 4-38. Budd-Chiari syndrome. A, Gray-scale transverse image of hepatic venous confluence shows complete absence of the right hepatic vein with obliteration of the lumen of a common trunk for the middle and left hepatic veins. **B,** Color Doppler image shows that blood flow in the middle hepatic vein *(blue)* is normally directed toward the inferior vena cava. As the trunk is obliterated, all the blood is flowing out of the left hepatic vein *(red),* which is abnormal. Other images showed anastomoses of the left hepatic vein with surface collaterals. **C,** Color Doppler image shows an anomalous left hepatic vein with flow to the inferior vena cava (normal direction) and aliasing from a long stricture. **D,** Spectral Doppler waveform of the anomalous left hepatic vein shows a very high abnormal velocity of approximately 140 cm/sec, confirming the tight stricture.

extrinsic IVC compression.[111] The portal blood flow also may be affected and is characteristically either slowed or reversed.[112]

The addition of Doppler to gray-scale sonography in the patient with suspected Budd-Chiari syndrome lends strong supportive evidence to the gray-scale impression of missing, compressed, or otherwise abnormal hepatic veins and IVC.[114,115] Associated reversal of flow in the portal vein and epigastric collaterals is also optimally assessed with this technique.[115]

Hepatic veno-occlusive disease causes progressive occlusion of the small hepatic venules. The disease is endemic in Jamaica, secondary to alkaloid toxicity from bush tea. In North America, most cases are iatrogenic, secondary to hepatic irradiation and chemotherapy used in bone marrow transplantation.[113] Patients with hepatic veno-occlusive disease are clinically indistinguishable from those with Budd-Chiari syndrome. Duplex Doppler sonography demonstrates normal caliber, patency, and phasic **forward** (toward the heart)

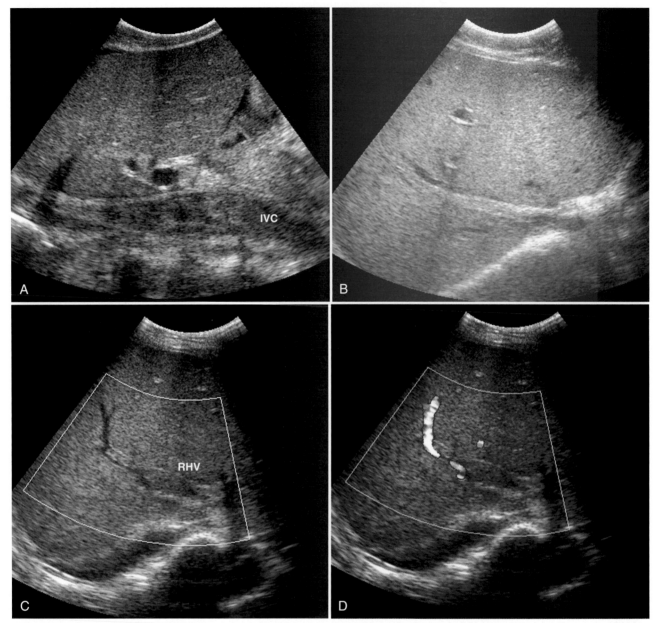

FIGURE 4-39. Budd-Chiari syndrome with extensive inferior vena cava thrombosis. A, Sagittal image of the inferior vena cava *(IVC)* shows that it is distended with echogenic thrombus. **B,** Middle hepatic vein as a thrombosed cord. **C,** Gray-scale image of right hepatic vein *(RHV),* and **D,** color Doppler image, show that anomalous right hepatic vein is distended with thrombus. There is flow in the vein proximal to the thrombus *(blue).*

flow of the main hepatic veins and IVC.[113] Flow in the portal vein, however, may be abnormal, showing either reversed or "to and fro" flow.[113,117] In addition, the diagnosis of hepatic veno-occlusive disease may be suggested in a patient with decreased portal blood flow (compared with baseline measurement before ablative therapy).[113]

Portal Vein Aneurysm

Aneurysms of the portal vein are rare. Their origin is either congenital or acquired secondary to portal hypertension.[118] Portal vein aneurysms have been described

proximally at the junction of the superior mesenteric and splenic veins and distally involving the portal venous radicles. The sonographic appearance is that of an anechoic cystic mass, which connects with the portal venous system. Pulsed Doppler sonographic examination demonstrates turbulent venous flow.[118]

Intrahepatic Portosystemic Venous Shunts

Intrahepatic arterial-portal fistulas are well-recognized complications of large-gauge percutaneous liver biopsy and trauma. Conversely, intrahepatic portohepatic venous shunts are rare. Their cause is controversial and believed to be either congenital or related to portal hypertension.[119,120] Patients typically are middle aged and present with hepatic encephalopathy. Anatomically, portohepatic venous shunts are more common in the right lobe. Sonography demonstrates a tortuous tubular vessel or complex vascular channels, which connect a branch of the portal vein to a hepatic vein or the IVC.[118-121] The diagnosis is confirmed angiographically.

Hepatic Artery Aneurysm and Pseudoaneurysm

The hepatic artery is the fourth most common site of an intra-abdominal aneurysm, following the infrarenal aorta, iliac, and splenic arteries. Eighty percent of patients with a hepatic artery aneurysm experience **catastrophic rupture** into the peritoneum, biliary tree, gastrointestinal tract, or portal vein.[122] Hepatic artery pseudoaneurysm secondary to chronic pancreatitis has been described. The duplex Doppler sonographic examination revealed turbulent arterial flow within a sonolucent mass.[122] Primary dissection of the hepatic artery is rare and in most cases leads to death before diagnosis.[123] Sonography may show the intimal flap with the true and false channels.

Hereditary Hemorrhagic Telangiectasia

Hereditary hemorrhagic telangiectasia, or **Osler-Weber-Rendu disease,** is an autosomal dominant disorder that causes arteriovenous (AV) malformations in the liver, hepatic fibrosis, and cirrhosis. Patients present with multiple telangiectasias and recurrent episodes of bleeding. Sonographic findings include a large feeding common hepatic artery up to 10 mm, multiple dilated tubular structures representing AV malformations, and large draining hepatic veins secondary to AV shunting.[124]

Peliosis Hepatis

Peliosis hepatis is a rare liver disorder characterized by blood-filled cavities ranging from less than a millimeter to many centimeters in diameter. It can be distinguished from hemangioma by the presence of portal tracts within the fibrous stroma of the blood spaces. The pathogenesis of peliosis hepatis involves rupture of the reticulin fibers that support the sinusoidal walls, secondary to cell injury or nonspecific hepatocellular necrosis.[125] The diagnosis of peliosis can be made with certainty only by histologic examination. Most cases of peliosis affect the liver, although other solid internal organs and lymph nodes may be involved in the process as well.

Although early reports described incidental detection of peliosis hepatis at autopsy in patients with chronic wasting disorders, it has now been seen following renal and liver transplantation, in association with a multitude of drugs, especially anabolic steroids, and with an increased incidence in HIV patients.[126] The HIV association may occur alone or as part of bacillary angiomatosis in the spectrum of opportunistic infections of AIDS.[127] Peliosis hepatis has the potential to be aggressive and lethal.

The imaging features of peliosis hepatis have been described in single case reports,[128-130] although often without adequate histologic confirmation. Angiographically, the peliotic lesions have been described as accumulations of contrast detected late in the arterial phase and becoming more distinct in the parenchymal phase.[131] On sonography, described lesions are nonspecific and have shown single or multiple masses of heterogeneous echogenicity.[128,129,132] Calcifications have been reported[132] (Fig. 4-40). CT scans show low-attenuation nodular

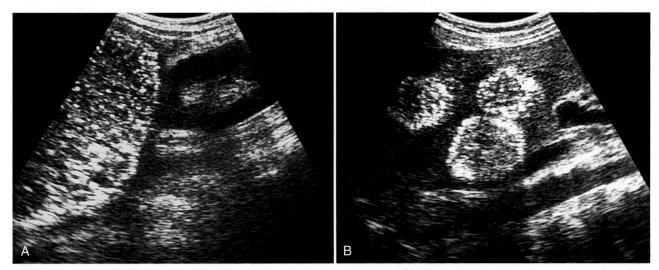

FIGURE 4-40. Peliosis hepatis. Peliosis hepatis in 34-year-old woman with deteriorating liver function necessitating transplantation. **A,** Sagittal right lobe, and **B,** sagittal left lobe, scans show multiple large liver masses with innumerable tiny punctate calcifications. *(From Muradali D, Wilson SR, Wanless IR, et al. Peliosis hepatis with intrahepatic calcifications. J Ultrasound Med 1996;15:257-260.)*

lesions that may or may not enhance with contrast injection.[128,131] Peliosis hepatis is difficult to diagnose both clinically and radiologically and must be suspected in a susceptible individual with a liver mass.

HEPATIC MASSES

Focal liver masses include a variety of malignant and benign neoplasms, as well as masses with developmental, inflammatory, and traumatic causes. In cross-sectional imaging, two basic issues relate to a focal liver lesion: **characterization** of a known liver lesion (what is it?) and **detection** (is it there?). The answer to either question requires a focused examination, often adjusted according to the clinical situation.

Liver Mass Characterization

Characterization of a liver mass on conventional sonography is based on the **appearance** of the mass on gray-scale imaging and **vascular information** derived from spectral, color, and power Doppler sonography. With excellent spatial and contrast resolution, the gray-scale morphology of a mass allows for the differentiation of cystic and solid masses, and characteristic appearances may suggest the correct diagnosis without further evaluation. More often, however, definitive diagnosis is not based on gray-scale information alone, but on vascular information obtained on conventional Doppler ultrasound examination. However, conventional Doppler often fails in the evaluation of a focal liver mass, particularly in a large patient or on a small or deep liver lesion, or on a mass with inherent weak Doppler signals. Motion artifact is also highly problematic for abdominal Doppler ultrasound studies, and a left lobe liver mass close to the pulsation of the cardiac apex, for example, is virtually always a failure for conventional Doppler. For these reasons, conventional ultrasound is not regarded highly for characterization of focal liver masses, and a mass detected on ultrasound is generally evaluated further with contrast-enhanced CT (CECT) or MRI for definitive characterization.

Role of Microbubble Contrast Agents

Worldwide, noninvasive diagnosis of focal liver masses is achieved with CECT and MRI based on recognized enhancement patterns in the arterial and portal venous phases. These noninvasive methods of characterization have become so accurate that excisional and percutaneous biopsy for diagnosis of liver masses is now rarely performed. Over the last decade, however, contrast-enhanced ultrasound has joined the ranks of CT and MRI in providing similar diagnostic information as well as information unique to CEUS.[133]

To address a failed Doppler ultrasound examination of a focal liver lesion, the two basic remedies are (1) inject a microbubble contrast agent to enhance the Doppler signal from blood and (2) use a specialized imaging technique such as pulse inversion sonography, which allows preferential detection of the signal from the contrast agent with suppression of the signal from background tissue.

Ultrasound contrast agents currently in use are second-generation agents comprising tiny bubbles of a perfluorocarbon gas contained within a stabilizing shell. Microbubble contrast agents are blood pool agents that do not diffuse through the vascular endothelium. This is of potential importance when imaging the liver because comparable contrast agents for CT and MRI may diffuse into the interstitium of a tumor. Our personal experience with perfluorocarbon microbubble agents is largely based on the use of Definity (Lantheus Medical Imaging, Billerica, Mass) and brief exposure to Optison (GE Healthcare, Milwaukee).[134,135]

Microbubble contrast agents are approved for use in liver imaging in more than 70 countries. In our clinical practice, we routinely perform CEUS for characterization of incidentally detected liver masses, those found on surveillance scans of patients at risk for HCC, and any focal mass referred by our clinicians found on outside imaging or indeterminate on CT and MRI. In the United States, however, microbubble use in abdominal imaging has not yet been approved.[136]

Microbubble contrast agents for ultrasound are unique in that they interact with the imaging process.[135] The major determinant of this interaction is the peak negative pressure of the transmitted ultrasound pulse, reflected by the **mechanical index** (MI), a number displayed on the ultrasound machine. The bubbles show stable, nonlinear oscillation when exposed to an ultrasound field with a low MI, with the production of harmonics of the transmitted frequency, including the frequency double that of the sound emitted by the transducer, the **second harmonic.** When the MI is raised sufficiently, the bubbles undergo irreversible disruption, with the production of a brief but bright, high-intensity ultrasound signal (see Chapter 3).

Liver lesion characterization with microbubble contrast agents is based on lesional vascularity and lesional enhancement in the arterial and portal venous phase. **Lesional vascularity** assessment depends on continuous imaging of the agents while they are within the vascular pool. We document the presence, number, distribution, and morphology of any lesional vessels (Figs. 4-41 and 4-42). A low MI is essential because it will preserve the contrast agent population without destruction of the bubbles in the imaging field, allowing for prolonged periods of real-time observation. The morphology of the lesional vessels is discriminatory and facilitates the diagnosis of liver lesions.

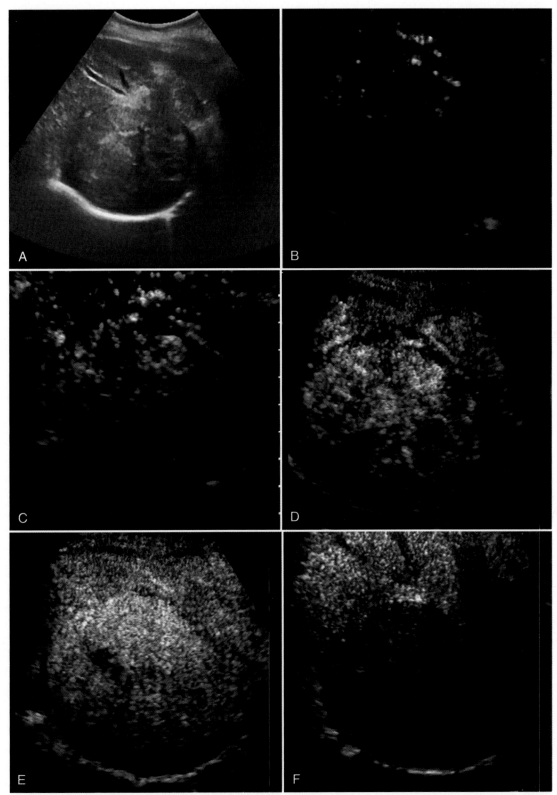

FIGURE 4-41. Hepatocellular carcinoma. Characterization of a focal liver mass with microbubble contrast agents. **A,** Baseline gray-scale image shows a posterior focal mass that is hypoechoic. **B,** Taken at the same location with low mechanical index (MI), before arrival of microbubbles, the entire image now appears black. The lesion is not visible. **C** and **D,** Real-time images obtained with low MI. **C,** As the bubbles appear in the field of view, disorganized echogenic vessels are seen in the liver and in the lesion. **D,** Later in the arterial phase, more vessels are seen in the lesion than in the liver. **E,** Arterial phase image, at the peak of enhancement, shows the mass is hypervascular. **F,** Portal venous phase image shows that the liver is enhanced. The lesion is less echogenic than the liver or has "washed out."

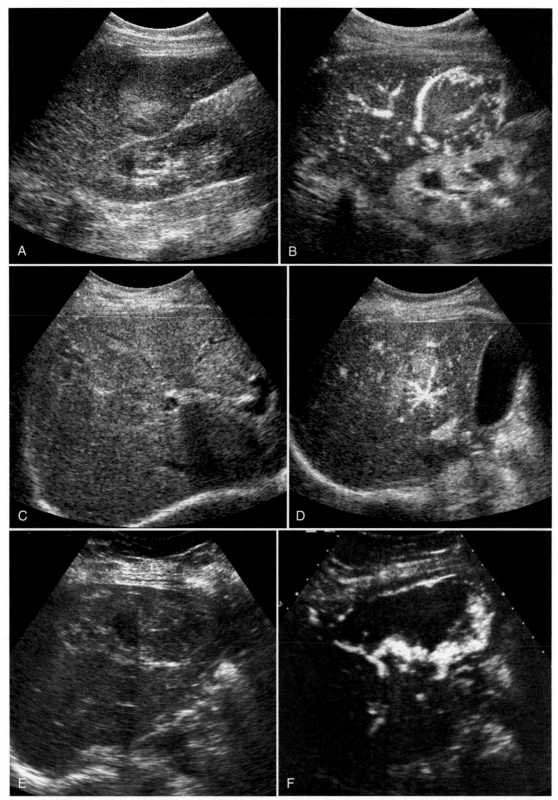

FIGURE 4-42. Discriminatory features of vascular imaging with microbubble contrast agents. *Left side,* Baseline images; *right side,* vascular images. *Top row,* **Hepatocellular carcinoma**. **A,** Baseline shows an exoplytic mass in segment 6. **B,** Vessels in the anterior part of the lesion are tortuous and dysmorphic. *Middle row,* **Focal nodular hyperplasia**. **C,** Lesion is barely visible. **D,** Stellate vessels are classic for this diagnosis. *Bottom row,* **Hemangioma**. **E,** Baseline image shows the lesion is heterogeneous with a thin, echogenic border. **F,** Low-MI vascular image shows brightly enhanced peripheral nodules and pools. There are no visible linear vessels. *(From Brannigan M, Burns PNB, Wilson SR. Blood flow patterns in focal liver lesions at microbubble enhanced ultrasound. Radiographics 2004; 24:921-935.)*

Lesional enhancement is best determined by comparing the echogenicity of the lesion to the echogenicity of the liver at a similar depth on the same frame and requires knowledge of liver blood flow. The liver has a dual blood supply from the hepatic artery and portal vein. The liver derives a larger proportion of its blood from the portal vein, whereas most liver tumors derive their blood supply from the hepatic artery. At the initiation of the injection, the low-MI technique will cause the entire field of view (FOV) to appear virtually black, regardless of the baseline appearance of the liver and the lesion in question. In fact, a known mass may be invisible at this point (see Fig. 4-41, *B*). As the microbubbles arrive in the FOV, the discrete vessels in the liver (Fig. 4-43) and then those within a liver lesion will be visualized, followed by increasing generalized enhancement as the microvascular volume of liver and lesion fills with the contrast agent. The liver parenchyma will appear more echogenic in the arterial phase than at baseline, and even more enhanced in the portal venous phase, as a reflection of its blood flow. Vascularity and enhancement patterns of a liver lesion, by comparison, will therefore reflect the actual blood flow and hemodynamics of the lesion in question, such that a hyperarterialized mass will appear more enhanced against a less enhanced liver

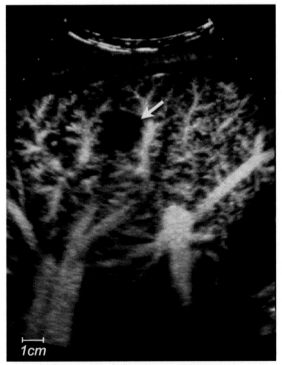

FIGURE 4-43. Normal liver vasculature. Temporal maximum-intensity projection image shows accumulated enhancement in 11 seconds after contrast material arrives in liver. Unprecedented depiction of vessel structure to fifth-order branching is evident. Focal unenhanced region *(arrow)* is slowly perfusing hemangioma. *(From Wilson SR, Jang HJ, Kim TK, et al. Real-time temporal maximum-intensity-projection imaging of hepatic lesions with contrast-enhanced sonography. AJR Am J Roentgenol 2008;190:691-695.)*

on an arterial phase sequence (see Fig. 4-41, *E*). Conversely, a hypoperfused lesion will appear as a dark or hypoechoic region within the enhanced liver on an arterial phase sequence.

Currently, evaluation of lesional enhancement is usually performed with the low-MI technique just described. However, details of vessel morphology and lesional enhancement are even more sensitively assessed using a bubble-tracking technique called **maximum-intensity projection** (MIP) imaging.[137] In this technique, performed either at wash-in of contrast or at the peak of arterial phase enhancement, a **brief high-MI exposure will destroy all the bubbles** within the FOV. Sequential frames, as the lesion and liver are reperfused, track the bubble course by adding information between sequential frames.

There are established algorithms for the diagnosis of focal liver masses with CEUS, with similarities to CT and MR algorithms but also important differences[138-140] (Table 4-3). Diagnosis of benign liver masses, hemangioma, and **focal nodular hyperplasia** (FNH) is close to 100%, showing characteristic features of enhancement in the arterial phase and sustained enhancement in the portal venous phase, such that their enhancement equals or exceeds the enhancement of the adjacent liver. Malignant tumors, by comparison, tend to show washout, such that the tumor appears unenhanced in the portal venous phase of enhancement (see Fig. 4-41, *F*). Exceptions to this general rule include frequent washout of benign hepatic adenoma and delayed or no washout of HCC. Discrimination of benign and malignant liver masses has similarly high accuracy.[141]

Liver Mass Detection

Contrary to popular belief, excellent spatial resolution allows small lesions to be well seen on sonography. Therefore it is not size but **echogenicity** that determines lesion conspicuity on a sonogram. That is, a tiny mass of only a few millimeters will be easily seen if it is increased or decreased in echogenicity compared with the adjacent liver parenchyma. Because many metastases are either hypoechoic or hyperechoic relative to the liver, a careful examination should allow for their detection. Nonetheless, many metastatic lesions are of similar echogenicity to the background liver, making their detection difficult or impossible, even if they are of a substantial size. This occurs when the backscatter from the lesion is virtually identical to the backscatter from the liver parenchyma.

To combat this inherent problem of lack of contrast between many metastatic liver lesions and the background liver on conventional sonography, the most effective method to date to improve lesion visibility is to perform contrast-enhanced liver ultrasound (Fig. 4-44). The two methods available both produce enhancement of the background liver without enhancement of the

TABLE 4-3. SCHEMATIC OF ALGORITHM FOR LIVER MASS DIAGNOSIS ON CEUS

Hemangioma

AP
Peripheral nodular enhancement
Centripetal progression of enhancement

PVP
Complete or partial fill-in

FNH

AP
Centrifugal hypervascular enhancement
Stellate arteries

PVP
Sustained enhancement
Hypoechoic central scar

Adenoma

AP
Diffuse or centripetal hypervascular enhancement
Dysmorphic arteries

PVP
Sustained enhancement
Soft wash out

Metastases

AP
Rim enhancement
Diffuse hypervascular
Hypovascular

PVP
Fast washout

Arterial phase (AP)   Portal venous phase (PVP)

(+) Enhancement   Soft wash out   (−) enhancement (wash out)

From Wilson SR, Burns PN. Microbubble contrast enhanced ultrasound in body imaging: what role? Radiology 2010.
FNH, Focal nodular hyperplasia.

metastatic lesions, thereby improving their conspicuity. Although their mechanism of action is different, in both there is microbubble enhancement of the normal liver with no enhancement of the liver metastases. This increases the backscatter from the liver compared with the liver lesions, thereby improving their detection.

The first method used the first-generation contrast agent Levovist (Schering AG, Berlin). After clearance of the contrast agent from the vascular pool, the microbubble persisted in the liver, probably within the Kupffer cells on the basis of phagocytosis. A high-MI sweep through the liver produced bright enhancement in the distribution of the bubbles. Therefore, all normal liver enhances. Liver metastases, lacking Kupffer cells, do not enhance and therefore show as black or hypoechoic holes within the enhanced parenchyma.[142] In a multicenter study conducted in Europe and Canada in which we participated, more and smaller lesions were seen than on baseline scan.[143] Overall, lesion detection was equivalent

to CT and MRI. The decibel difference between the lesions and the liver parenchyma is increased many fold because of increased backscatter from contrast agent within the normal liver tissue. Although many results were compelling, these first-generation contrast agents are no longer marketed.

Therefore, current requirements for improved lesion detection use a second technique of CEUS with a **perfluorocarbon contrast agent** and low-MI scanning in both the arterial and the portal venous phase. The use of a low-MI imaging technique for lesion detection has advantages in terms of scanning because the microbubble population is preserved and timing is not so critical. Virtually all metastases and HCCs will be unenhanced relative to the liver in the portal phase because the liver parenchyma is optimally enhanced in this phase. Therefore, all malignant lesions tend to appear hypoechoic in the portal phase, allowing for improved lesion detection (see Figs. 4-41, F, and 4-44, C and D). This observation,

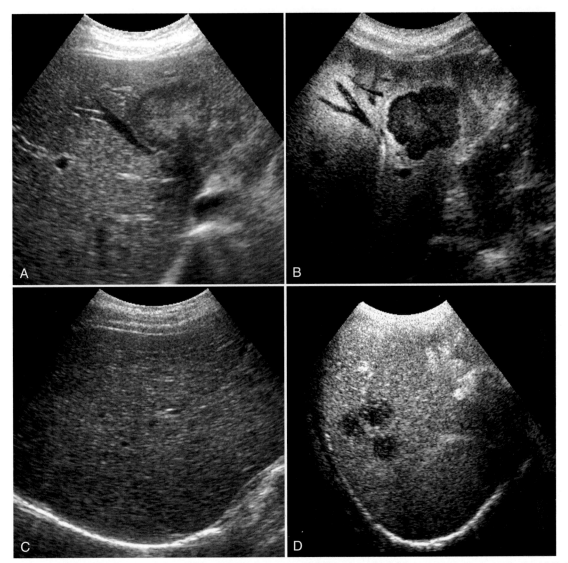

FIGURE 4-44. Improved detection of focal liver masses with microbubble contrast agents. A and **B,** Levovist (Schering, Berlin). **A,** Baseline sonogram shows a subtle isoechoic mass with a hypoechoic halo. **B,** Postvascular image shows increased echogenicity in the liver. The lesion is strikingly hypoechoic and has increased conspicuity. **C** and **D,** Definity (Lantheus Medical Imaging, Billerica, Mass). **C,** Baseline sonogram does not show any metastatic lesions in this patient with lung carcinoma. **D,** Portal venous phase image shows multiple focal unenhanced metastases.

that malignant lesions tend to be hypoechoic in the portal venous phase of perfluorocarbon liver enhancement, is helpful for both lesion detection and lesion characterization. Enhancement of benign lesions, FNH, and hemangioma generally equals or exceeds liver enhancement in the portal venous phase.

Detection of hypervascular liver masses (e.g., HCC, metastases) is also improved by scanning with perfluorocarbon agents in the arterial phase. These agents will show as hyperechoic masses relative to the liver parenchyma in the arterial phase because they are predominantly supplied by hepatic arterial flow.

HEPATIC NEOPLASMS

Sonographic visualization of a focal liver mass may occur in a variety of clinical scenarios, ranging from incidental detection to identification in a symptomatic patient or as part of a focused search in a patient at risk for hepatic neoplasm. Hemangiomas, FNH, and adenomas are the benign neoplasms typically encountered in the liver, whereas HCC and metastases account for the majority of malignant tumors.

The role of medical imaging in the evaluation of an identified focal liver mass is to determine which masses are significant, requiring confirmations of their diagnoses, and which masses are likely to be insignificant and benign, not requiring further evaluation to confirm their nature. On a sonographic study, there is considerable overlap in the appearances of focal liver masses. Once a liver mass is seen, however, the excellent contrast and spatial resolution of state-of-the-art ultrasound equipment have provided guidelines for the initial management of patients,[144] which include recognition of the following features:

- A **hypoechoic halo** identified around an echogenic or isoechoic liver mass is an ominous sonographic sign necessitating definitive diagnosis.
- A **hypoechoic and solid liver mass** is highly likely to be significant and also requires definitive diagnosis.
- **Multiple solid liver masses** may be significant and suggest metastatic or multifocal malignant liver disease. However, hemangiomas are also frequently multiple.
- **Clinical history** of malignancy, chronic liver disease or hepatitis, and symptoms referable to the liver are requisite information for interpretation of a focal liver lesion.

Benign Hepatic Neoplasms

Cavernous Hemangioma

Cavernous hemangiomas are the **most common benign tumors** of the liver, occurring in approximately 4% of the population. They occur in all age groups but are more common in adults, particularly women, with a female/male ratio of approximately 5:1.[145] The vast majority of hemangiomas are small, asymptomatic, and discovered incidentally. Large lesions may rarely produce symptoms of acute abdominal pain, caused by hemorrhage or thrombosis within the tumor. Thrombocytopenia, caused by sequestration and destruction of platelets within a large cavernous hemangioma (Kasabach-Merritt syndrome), occasionally occurs in infants and is rare in adults.

Traditional teaching suggests that once identified in the adult, hemangiomas usually have reached a stable size, rarely changing in appearance or size.[146,147] In our practice, however, we have documented substantial growth of some lesions over many years of follow-up. Hemangiomas may enlarge during pregnancy or with the administration of estrogens, suggesting the tumor is hormone dependent.

Histologically, hemangiomas consist of multiple vascular channels that are lined by a single layer of endothelium and separated and supported by fibrous septa. The vascular spaces may contain thrombi.

The **sonographic appearance** of cavernous hemangioma varies. Typically the lesion is small (<3 cm in diameter), well defined, homogeneous, and hyperechoic[148] (Fig. 4-45, A). The increased echogenicity has been related to the numerous interfaces between the walls of the cavernous sinuses and the blood within.[149] Inconsistently seen and nonspecific, posterior acoustic enhancement has been correlated with hypervascularity on angiography[150] (Fig. 4-45, H). Approximately 67% to 79% of hemangiomas are hyperechoic,[151,152] of which 58% to 73% are homogeneous.[147,150] Other now-familiar features include a nonhomogeneous central area containing hypoechoic portions, which may appear uniformly granular (Fig. 4-45, D-F) or lacelike in character (D); an echogenic border, either a thin rim or a thick rind (E-G); and a tendency to scalloping of the margin (B).[153] Larger lesions tend to be heterogeneous, with central hypoechoic foci corresponding to fibrous collagen scars (Fig. 4-45, C), large vascular spaces, or both. A hemangioma may appear hypoechoic within the background of a fatty infiltrated liver.[154] Calcification is rare (Fig. 4-45, I).

Hemangiomas are characterized by extremely slow blood flow that will not routinely be detected by either color or duplex Doppler sonography. Occasional lesions may show a low to midrange kilohertz shift from both peripheral and central blood vessels. The ability of power Doppler ultrasound, which is more sensitive to slow flow, to detect signals within a hemangioma is controversial.[155]

Cavernous hemangiomas are often observed on abdominal sonograms performed for any reason, and confirmation of all visualized lesions has proved to be costly and unnecessary. Therefore it is considered acceptable practice to manage some patients conservatively without confirmation of the diagnosis. When a hyperechoic lesion typical of a cavernous hemangioma is incidentally discovered, no further examination is usually necessary, or at most, a repeat ultrasound is performed in 3 to 6 months to document lack of change.

Conversely, potentially significant lesions may mimic the morphology of a hemangioma on ultrasound and produce a single mass or multiple masses of uniform increased echogenicity. These include metastases from a colon primary or a vascular primary tumor, such as a neuroendocrine tumor and small HCCs in particular. In a prospective evaluation of 1982 patients with newly diagnosed cirrhosis, Caturelli et al.[156] found that 50% of echogenic liver lesions with morphology suggestive of hemangioma had that diagnosis, although 50% of these proved to be HCC. The authors also showed that in 1648 patients with known cirrhosis and new appearance of an echogenic hemangioma-like mass, all were HCC. These results emphasize the extreme necessity to prove the diagnosis of all masses with this morphology in high-risk patients. Therefore, in a patient with a known malignancy, an increased risk for hepatoma, abnormal results of LFTs, clinical symptoms referable to the liver, or an atypical sonographic pattern, one of the following additional imaging techniques is generally recommended to confirm the suspicion of hemangioma: microbubble-enhanced sonography, CT, red blood cell (RBC) scintigraphy, or MRI.

In the arterial phase on **CEUS,** hemangiomas show peripheral puddles and pools that are brighter than the adjacent enhanced liver parenchyma. There are no linear vessels. Over time, centripetal progression of the enhancement leads to complete globular fill-in, with sustained enhancement equal to or better than the liver in the portal venous phase, which may last for several minutes[157] (Fig. 4-46). This enhancement may occur rapidly or

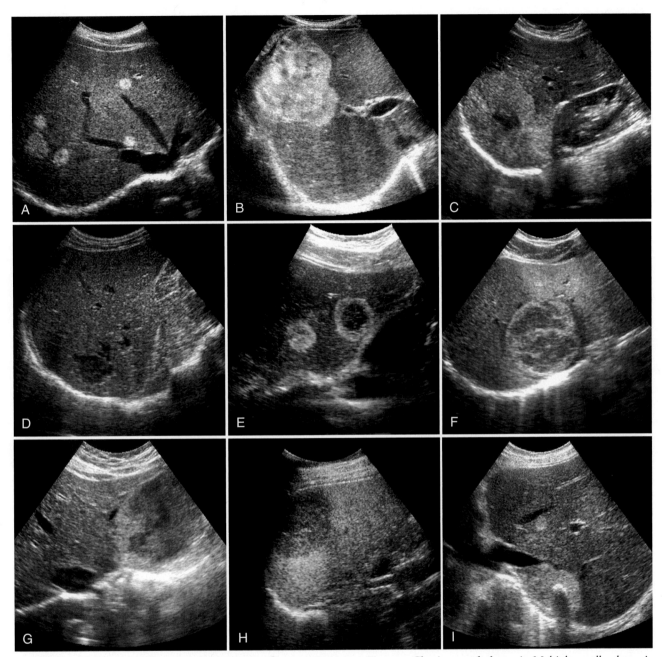

FIGURE 4-45. Hemangiomas: spectrum of appearances. *Top row,* **Classic morphology. A,** Multiple small echogenic masses. **B,** Single large, lobulated echogenic mass. **C,** Echogenic lobulated mass with a hypoechoic area centrally, probably related to central thrombosis or scarring. *Middle row,* **Atypical morphology. D,** Atypical hemangioma. It is hypoechoic and has a thin echogenic border. **E, Classic and atypical morphologies.** The atypical hemangioma has a thick, uniform echogenic border. **F,** Atypical hemangioma is partially hypoechoic centrally with an irregular echogenic rim. *Bottom row,* **Infrequent observations. G,** Exophytic hemangioma bulging from the left lateral lobe of the liver. **H,** Hypoechoic mass with increased through transmission, a suggestive but infrequently encountered sign of hemangioma. **I,** Central calcification in a hemangioma with distal acoustic shadowing. This is a rare ending in hemangiomas.

slowly and may be incomplete, even in the delayed portal venous phase **(Video 4-5).** We have diagnosed almost 100% of hemangiomas with CEUS, including those of small size, removing the necessity for CT, MRI, or labeled-RBC scintigraphy for confirmation of diagnosis, particularly in incidentally detected lesions. We hope that in the future, most hemangiomas seen on ultrasound will be confirmed with CEUS.

In a small minority of patients, imaging will not allow definitive diagnosis of hemangioma. Percutaneous biopsy of hepatic hemangiomas has been safely performed.[158,159] Cronan et al.[159] performed biopsies on 15 patients (12 of whom were outpatients) using a 20-gauge Franseen needle. In all patients the histologic sample was diagnostic and was characterized by large spaces with an endothelial lining. It is recommended that normal liver be

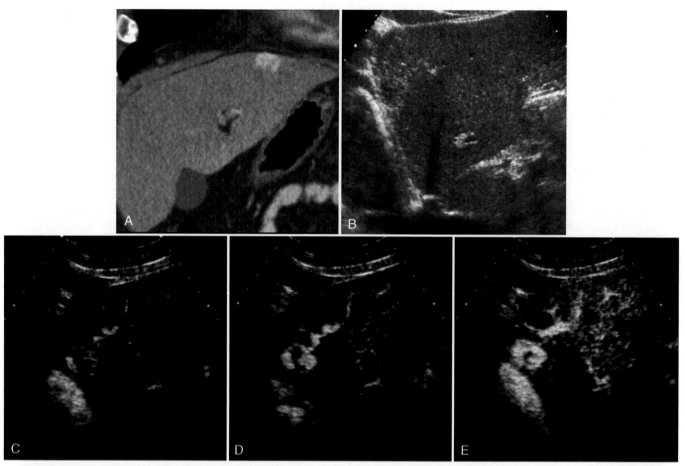

FIGURE 4-46. Characterization of hemangioma with Definity enhancement. Resolution of an indeterminate mass on CT scan is shown in a 65-year-old man with carcinoma of the esophagus. **A,** CT scan of the thorax shows an indeterminate incidental enhanced mass in the left lobe of the liver. **B,** Sagittal sonogram shows the mass is hypoechoic. **C, D,** and **E,** are frames taken between 10 and 14 seconds after the injection of contrast agent. They show peripheral nodular enhancement and centripetal progression of enhancement in spite of the rapidity of lesion filling. This is a classic flash-filling hemangioma. The lesion remained enhanced to 5 minutes *(not shown).* See also Video 4-5. *(From Wilson SR, Burns PN. Microbubble enhanced ultrasound imaging: what role? Radiology 2010 [in press].)*

interposed between the abdominal wall and the hemangioma to allow hepatic tamponade of any potential bleeding.

Focal Nodular Hyperplasia

Focal nodular hyperplasia is the **second most common benign liver mass** after hemangioma.[160] These masses are believed to be developmental hyperplastic lesions related to an area of congenital vascular malformation, probably a preexisting arterial spiderlike malformation.[161] Hormonal influences may be a factor because FNH is much more common in women than men, particularly in the childbearing years.[162-164] As with hemangioma, FNH is invariably an incidentally detected liver mass in an asymptomatic patient.[162]

Focal nodular hyperplasia is typically a solitary well-circumscribed mass with a central scar.[162] Most lesions are less than 5 cm in diameter. Although usually single,

multiple FNH masses have been reported. Microscopically, lesions include normal hepatocytes, Kupffer cells, biliary ducts, and the components of portal triads, although no normal portal venous structures are found. As a hyperplastic lesion, there is proliferation of normal, nonneoplastic hepatocytes that are abnormally arranged. Bile ducts and thick-walled arterial vessels are prominent, particularly in the central fibrous scar. The excellent blood supply makes hemorrhage, necrosis, and calcification rare.[162] These lesions often produce a contour abnormality to the surface of the liver or may displace the normal blood vessels within the parenchyma.

On **sonography,** FNH is often a subtle liver mass that is difficult to differentiate in echogenicity from the adjacent liver parenchyma. Considering the histologic similarities to normal liver, this is not a surprising fact and has led to descriptions of FNH on all imaging as a "stealth lesion" that may be extremely subtle or completely hidden.[165] Subtle contour abnormalities (Figs. 4-47 and 4-48, *E* and *F*) and displacement of vascular structures should immediately raise the possibility of FNH. The central scar may be seen on gray-scale sonograms as a hypoechoic, linear or stellate area within the central portion of the mass[166] (Fig. 4-48, *A*). On occasion, the scar may appear hyperechoic. FNH may also display a range of gray-scale appearances, from hypoechoic to rarely hyperechoic.

Doppler ultrasound features of FNH are highly suggestive, in that well-developed peripheral and central blood vessels are seen. Pathologic studies in FNH describe an anomalous arterial blood vessel larger than expected for the location in the liver.[161] Our experience suggests that this feeding vessel is usually quite obvious on color Doppler imaging, although other vascular masses may appear to have unusually large feeding vessels as well.[167] The blood vessels can be seen to course within the central scar with either a linear or a stellate configuration. Spectral interrogation usually shows predominantly arterial signals centrally, with a midrange (2-4 kHz) shift.

Similar to hemangioma, FNH is consistently diagnosed with **CEUS**.[168-171] In the arterial phase, lesions are hypervascular, and highly suggestive morphologies include the presence of stellate lesional vessels, a tortuous feeding artery, and a centrifugal filling direction (Fig. 4-49). Arterial phase enhancement is homogeneous and in excess of the adjacent liver. Portal venous enhancement is sustained such that lesion enhancement equals or exceeds that of adjacent liver with a nonenhancing scar **(Video 4-6).** Infrequently, FNH may show washout, which is often weak and delayed. An unenhanced scar may be seen in both arterial and portal phases. Ultrasound alone should be able to suggest the presence of

these insignificant lesions without referral for further imaging.

Sulfur colloid scanning is invaluable in patients with suspect FNH because 50% of lesions will take up sulfur colloid similar to the adjacent normal liver, and another 10% will be "hot." Therefore, only 40% of patients with FNH will lack confirmation of their diagnosis after performing a sulfur colloid scan.[171,172] In these patients, CECT or MRI may be performed for diagnosis. Primovist-enhanced MRI shows improved specificity for the diagnosis of FNH.[173]

Biopsy may be required in a minority of patients with FNH who do not have a hot or a warm lesion on sulfur colloid scanning, especially if CT or MRI features are not specific. Cytologic biopsy is not confirmatory because normal hepatocytes may be found in normal liver, adenoma, and FNH. Core liver biopsy is required to show the disorganized pattern characteristic of this pathology. Because FNH rarely leads to clinical problems and does not undergo malignant transformation, conservative management is recommended.[174]

Hepatic Adenoma

Hepatic adenomas are **much less common** than FNH. However, a dramatic rise in their incidence since the 1970s clearly established a link to oral contraceptive (OC) use. As expected, therefore, hepatic adenomas, similar to FNH, are more common in women. The tumor may be asymptomatic, but often the patient or the physician feels a mass in the right upper quadrant. Pain may occur as a result of bleeding or infarction within the lesion. The most alarming manifestation is shock caused by tumor rupture and hemoperitoneum. Hepatic adenomas have also been reported in association

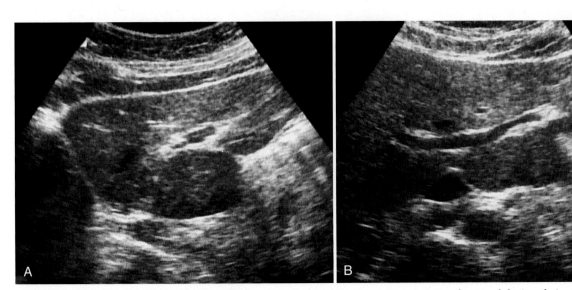

FIGURE 4-47. Focal nodular hyperplasia. A, Sagittal, and **B,** transverse, sonograms show a subtle, isoechoic caudate lobe mass. The contour variation is the key to appreciating the presence of this mass.

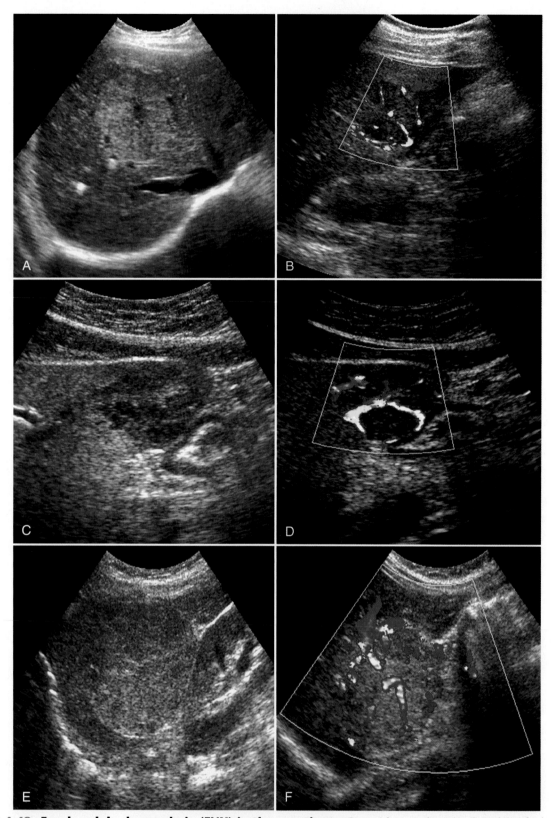

FIGURE 4-48. Focal nodular hyperplasia (FNH) in three patients. Gray-scale equivalents (**A, C,** and **E**) of color Doppler images (**B, D,** and **F**). **A,** Virtually normal image only suggests an isoechoic and subtle mass. **B,** Doppler image shows a stellate arterial pattern and confirms the authenticity of the observation. **C,** Fatty liver and focal hypoechoic region in the tip of segment 3. Fatty sparing was considered. **D,** Doppler features show a hypervascular mass with a stellate appearance, the classic finding in FNH. **E,** Contour-altering mass in the right lobe of the liver. **F,** Doppler image again shows the central stellate vascularity suggesting FNH. This hypervascularity with stellate vasculature is usually readily observed with conventional sonography in FNH.

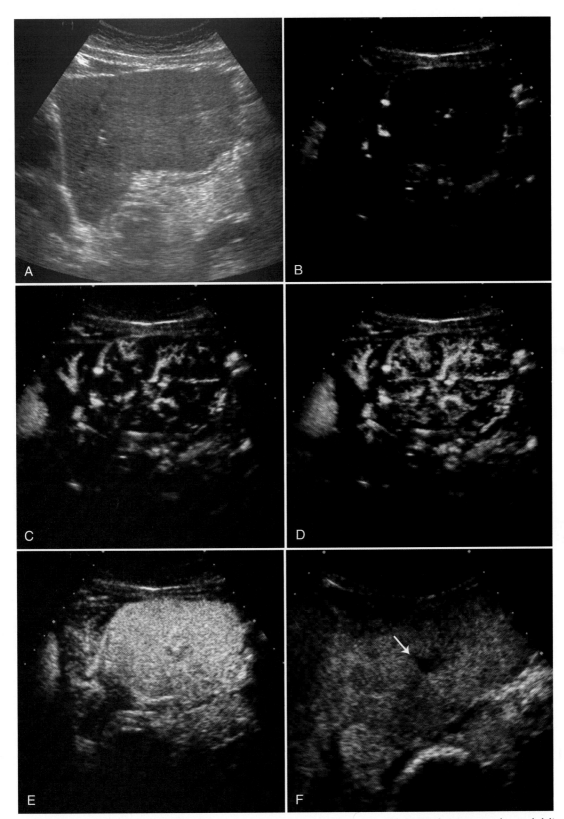

FIGURE 4-49. Focal nodular hyperplasia. Asymptomatic 22-year-old woman with FNH showing superb vessel delineation on arterial phase contrast-enhanced ultrasound (CEUS) images taken with temporal maximum-intensity projection (MIP) technique. **A,** Baseline sagittal image shows bulbous expansion of tip of left lobe of liver. **B** to **E,** Sequential images taken in the arterial phase of CEUS showing stellate vascularity and centrifugal filling. **F,** Image in portal venous phase at 3 minutes shows sustained enhancement and central unenhancing scar *(arrow).* See also Video 4-6. *(From Wilson SR, Greenbaum LD, Goldberg BB. Contrast-enhanced ultrasound: what is the evidence and what are the obstacles? AJR Am J Roentgenol 2009;193:55-60.)*

with glycogen storage disease. In particular, the frequency of adenoma for type 1 GSD (von Gierke's disease) is 40%.[175] Because of its propensity to hemorrhage and risk of malignant degeneration,[174] surgical resection is recommended.

Pathologically, a hepatic adenoma is usually solitary, 8 to 15 cm, and well encapsulated. Microscopically, the tumor consists of normal or slightly atypical hepatocytes. Bile ducts and Kupffer cells are few or absent.[176] Hepatic adenomas may show either calcification or fat (Fig. 4-50), both of which appear echogenic on sonography, making their gray-scale appearance suggestive in some cases.

The **sonographic appearance** of hepatic adenoma is nonspecific. The echogenicity may be hyperechoic (Figs. 4-50 and 4-51), hypoechoic, isoechoic, or mixed.[172]

With hemorrhage, a fluid component may be evident within or around the mass (Fig. 4-52), and free intraperitoneal blood may be seen. The sonographic changes with bleeding are variable, depending on the duration and amount of hemorrhage.

Differentiation of hepatic adenomas from FNH is often not possible by their gray-scale or Doppler characteristics. Further, both have a similar demographic, occurring in young women in their childbearing years, often with a history of OC use. Both demonstrate well-defined perilesional and intralesional blood vessels with shifts in the midrange (2-4 kHz). Golli et al.[167] described increased venous structures within the center of hepatic adenomas and a paucity of arterial vessels. In our experience, this has not been a constant finding; although we believe hepatic adenomas are substantially less vascular

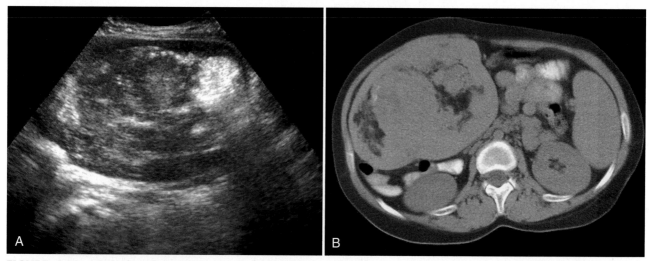

FIGURE 4-50. Hepatic adenoma. A, Sonogram, and **B,** confirmatory CT scan, show a large exophytic liver mass in an asymptomatic young woman. The mass shows highly echogenic foci, which correspond to areas of fat and calcification on the CT scan.

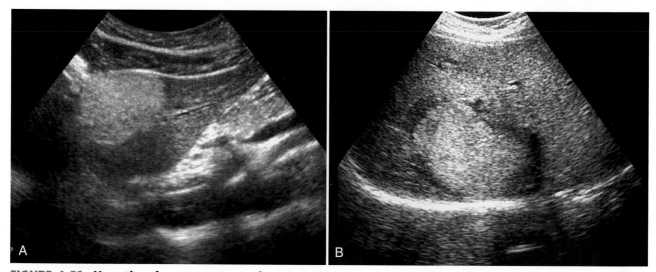

FIGURE 4-51. Hepatic adenoma: gray-scale appearances. A, Sagittal sonogram of the left lobe of the liver of an asymptomatic 35-year-old man shows a highly echogenic mass. It is unusual to see an adenoma in an otherwise normal man. **B,** Oblique sonogram of a 26-year-old Chinese woman shows a highly echogenic mass with a hypoechoic halo. The hypoechoic halo was related to a surrounding zone of liver atrophy on biopsy.

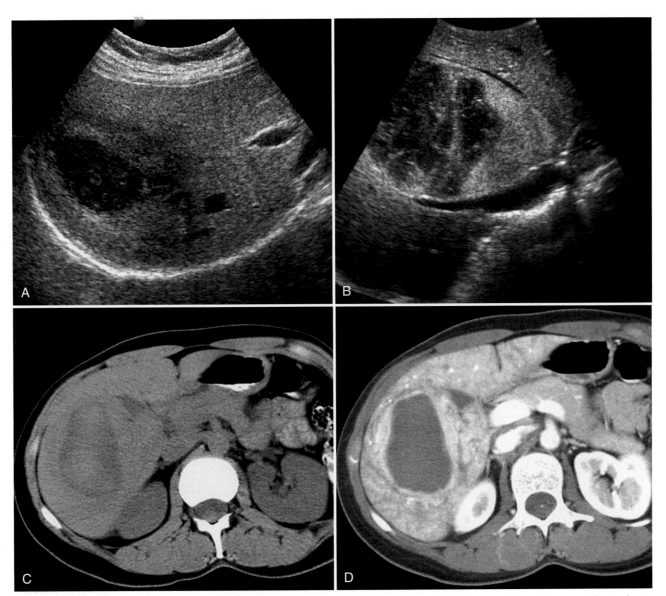

FIGURE 4-52. Bleeding hepatic adenomas. A and **B,** Sonograms of two young women presenting with acute abdominal pain from hemorrhage into hepatic adenomas. The masses are highly complex, and their appearance in a patient with pain suggests hemorrhage into a preexisting lesion. **C,** Unenhanced, and **D,** enhanced, CT scans of the patient in **B** show the value of the unenhanced scan, which confirms the high-attenuation blood within the adenoma.

than most FNH masses and certainly do not show either the intralesional or perilesional vascular tortuosity associated with FNH. Most adenomas are cold on technetium-99m sulfur colloid imaging as a result of absent or greatly decreased numbers of Kupffer cells. Isolated cases of radiocolloid uptake by the adenoma have been reported.[177] Hepatobiliary scans may be helpful in the diagnosis of hepatic adenomas. Because these lesions do not contain bile ducts, the tracer is not excreted, and the mass persists as a photon-active region.

In the typical clinical scenario, differentiation of FNH from adenoma poses a regular problem. Both masses are frequently incidentally detected in asymptomatic women, and both produce a hypervascular mass in the arterial phase. Their significance and management are totally different, and therefore more subtle features are

required to distinguish them. Differentiation is generally possible with **CEUS;** although it shows a hypervascular mass in the arterial phase similar to FNH,[178] hepatic adenoma is characterized by centripetal filling and nonhomogeneity. Also, multiple reports document possible portal venous phase washout, although with differing likelihood **(Video 4-7).** Our impression also is that hepatic adenoma, although hypervascular, does not show the profuse vascularity typical of FNH (Fig. 4-53).

In a patient with right upper quadrant (RUQ) pain and possible hemorrhage, it is important to perform an unenhanced CT scan of the liver before contrast injection. The hemorrhage will appear as high-density regions within the mass (see Fig. 4-52, *C*). The lesion often demonstrates rapid, transient enhancement during the arterial phase.[179] Hepatic adenomas have a variable

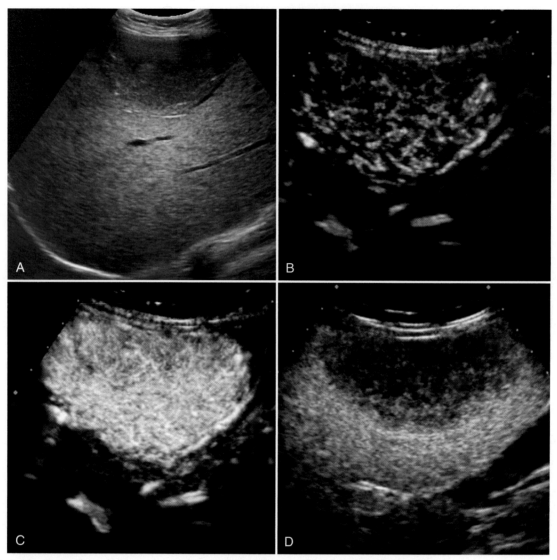

FIGURE 4-53. Hepatic adenoma: maximum-intensity projection (MIP) imaging. A, Baseline scan on an asymptomatic 29-year-old woman with abnormal liver function tests shows a fatty liver and superficial hypoechoic focal mass. **B,** Early arterial phase MIP image shows diffuse vascularity. **C,** At the peak of arterial phase enhancement, the mass is hypervascular and homogeneous. **D,** In the portal venous phase the mass shows washout, necessitating confirmation of diagnosis with biopsy. See also Video 4-7. *(From Wilson SR, Burns PN. Microbubble enhanced ultrasound imaging: what role? Radiology 2010 [in press].)*

appearance on MRI and cannot always be distinguished from HCC.

Fatty Tumors: Hepatic Lipomas and Angiomyolipomas

Hepatic lipomas are extremely rare, and only isolated cases have been reported in the radiologic literature.[180-182] There is an association between hepatic lipomas and renal angiomyolipomas and tuberous sclerosis. The lesions are asymptomatic. Ultrasound demonstrates a well-defined echogenic mass indistinguishable from a hemangioma, echogenic metastasis, or focal fat, unless the mass is large and near the diaphragm, in which case differential sound transmission through the fatty mass will produce a **discontinuous or broken diaphragm**

echo[181] (Fig. 4-54, *A*). CT confirms the diagnosis and reveals the fatty nature of the mass by the negative Hounsfield units (−30 HU)[180,183] (Fig. 4-54, *B*). Angiomyolipomas, by comparison, may also appear echogenic on sonography (Fig. 4-54, *C*), although they may have insufficient fat to appear consistently with fatty attenuation on CT, making diagnostic confirmation more difficult without biopsy.

Malignant Hepatic Neoplasms

Hepatocellular Carcinoma

Hepatocellular carcinoma is one of the most common malignant tumors, particularly in Southeast Asia, sub-Saharan Africa, Japan, Greece, and Italy. HCC occurs

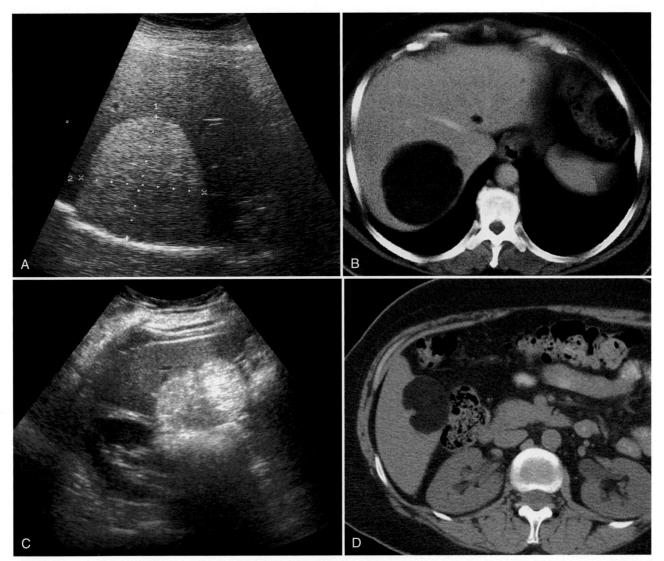

FIGURE 4-54. Fatty tumors of liver: lipoma and angiomyolipoma. A, Sonogram shows a highly echogenic, solid focal liver mass, which initially suggests a hemangioma. The **discontinuity of the diaphragm echo** caused by the altered rate of sound transmission is a clue to the correct diagnosis. **B,** Confirmatory CT scan shows the fat density of the mass, a confirmed hepatic lipoma. **C** and **D,** Another highly echogenic and slightly exophytic mass in the liver, initially suggesting a hemangioma. *(A and B from Reinhold C, Garant M. Hepatic lipoma. Can Assoc Radiol J 1996;47:140-142; C and D from Wilson SR. The liver. Gastrointestinal disease. 6th series. Test and syllabus. Reston, Va, 2004, American College of Radiology.)*

predominantly in men, with a male/female ratio of approximately 5:1.[176] Etiologic factors depend on the geographic distribution. Although alcoholic cirrhosis remains a common predisposing cause for hepatoma in the West, both hepatitis C and hepatitis B are now of worldwide significance. These viral infections also account for the high incidence of HCC in sub-Saharan Africa, Southeast Asia, China, Japan, and in the Mediterranean. Of growing importance in the Western world, fatty liver with the development of steatohepatitis is increasing in significance as an antecedent to the development of cirrhosis and HCC. Aflatoxins, toxic metabolites produced by fungi in certain foods, have also been implicated in the pathogenesis of hepatomas in developing countries.[176]

The **clinical presentation** of HCC is often delayed until the tumor reaches an advanced stage. Symptoms include RUQ pain, weight loss, and abdominal swelling when ascites is present.

Pathologically, HCC occurs in the following three forms:

Solitary tumor
Multiple nodules
Diffuse infiltration

There is a propensity toward venous invasion. The portal vein is involved in 30% to 60% of cases and more often than the hepatic venous system.[184-186]

The **sonographic appearance of** HCC is variable. The masses may be hypoechoic, complex, or echogenic. Most small (<5 cm) HCCs are hypoechoic (Fig. 4-55,

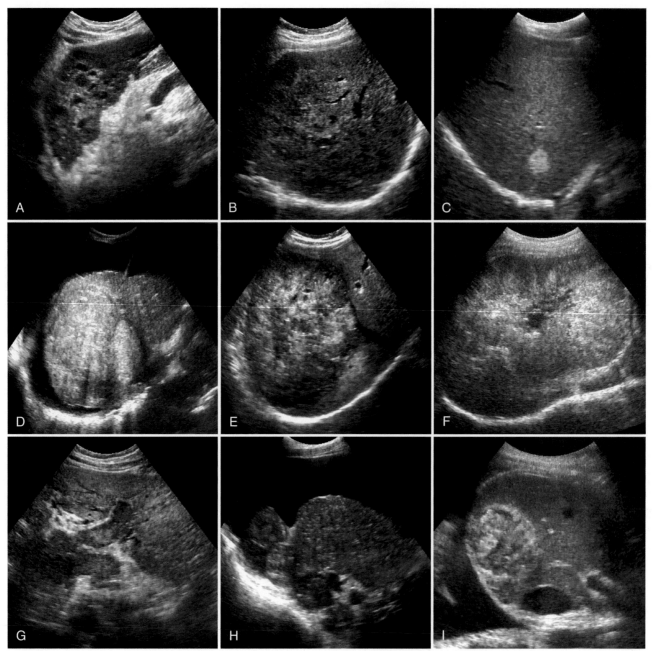

FIGURE 4-55. Hepatocellular carcinoma: spectrum of appearances. A, Small, focal hypoechoic nodules. **B,** Multifocal hypoechoic nodules, which may be difficult to differentiate from the background cirrhotic nodules. **C,** Focal echogenic nodule mimicking hemangioma, **D,** Large echogenic nodule in a cirrhotic liver. **E,** Large mixed-echogenic mass. Hypoechoic regions corresponded at pathology to areas of necrosis. **F,** Large lobulated mass with central hypoechoic region suggesting a scar. **G,** Expansive tumor filling the portal vein is the only observation on the sonogram. **H,** Small cirrhotic liver showing exophytic tumors. **I,** Superficial mass of mixed echogenicity in a young hepatitis B patient presenting with spontaneous liver rupture.

A), corresponding histologically to a solid tumor without necrosis.[187,188] A thin, peripheral hypoechoic halo, which corresponds to a fibrous capsule, is seen most often in small HCCs.[189] With time and increasing size, the masses tend to become more complex and inhomogeneous as a result of necrosis and fibrosis (Fig. 4-55, *E*). Calcification is uncommon but has been reported.[190] Small tumors may appear diffusely hyperechoic, secondary to fatty metamorphosis or sinusoidal dilation (Fig. 4-55, *C*), making them indistinguishable from focal fatty infiltra-

tion, cavernous hemangiomas, and lipomas.[187,188,191] Intratumoral fat also occurs in larger masses; because it tends to be focal, it is unlikely to cause confusion in diagnosis. Patients with rare surface lesions may present with spontaneous rupture and hemoperitoneum (Fig. 4-55, *I*).

Studies evaluating focal liver lesions with duplex Doppler and CDFI suggest HCC has characteristic high-velocity signals.[192-194] Doppler sonography is excellent for detecting neovascularity within tumor thrombi

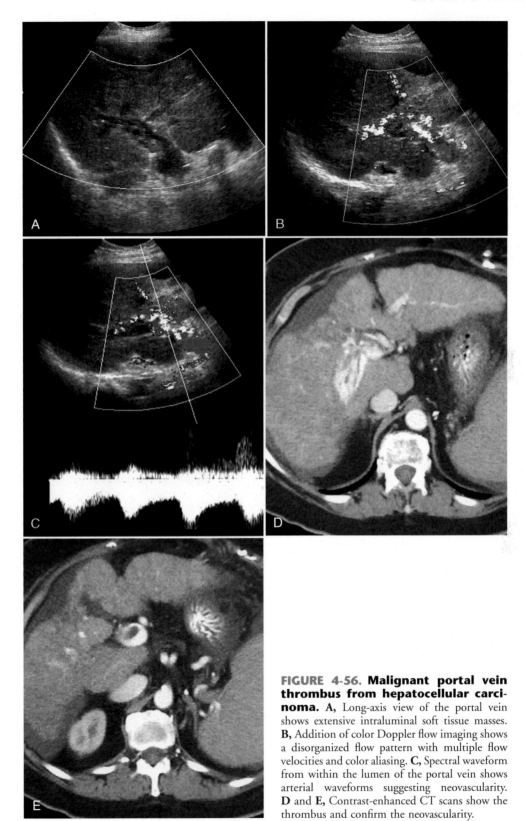

FIGURE 4-56. Malignant portal vein thrombus from hepatocellular carcinoma. A, Long-axis view of the portal vein shows extensive intraluminal soft tissue masses. **B,** Addition of color Doppler flow imaging shows a disorganized flow pattern with multiple flow velocities and color aliasing. **C,** Spectral waveform from within the lumen of the portal vein shows arterial waveforms suggesting neovascularity. **D** and **E,** Contrast-enhanced CT scans show the thrombus and confirm the neovascularity.

within the portal veins, diagnostic of HCC even without demonstration of the parenchymal lesion (Fig. 4-56).

Highly superior to conventional Doppler sonography for characterization of **HCC in the cirrhotic liver, microbubble CEUS** is much more sensitive for the detection of lesional vascularity (Table 4-4). Lesions are hypervascular, often showing dysmorphic vessels (see Fig. 4-42, *B*) and frequently showing unenhanced regions representing either necrosis or scarring[195,196] (Fig. 4-57). In the portal venous phase, lesions show washout,

TABLE 4-4. SCHEMATIC OF ALGORITHM FOR DIAGNOSIS OF NODULES IN CIRRHOTIC LIVER ON CEUS

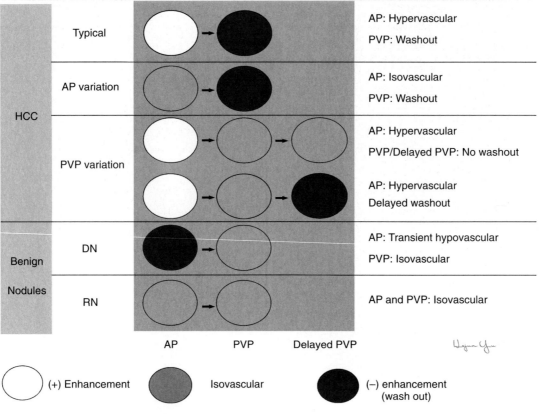

Overlap between DN and WDHCC
(Any arterial enhancing foci or dysmorphic vessels within a nodule or obvious washout during portal phase should raise a suspicion of HCC.)

From Wilson SR, Burns PN. Microbubble contrast enhanced ultrasound in body imaging: what role? Radiology 2010 (in press).
HCC, Hepatocellular carcinoma; *AP,* arterial phase; *PVP,* portal venous phase; *DN,* dysplastic nodules; *RN,* regenerative nodules; *WDHCC,* well-differentiated hepatocellular carcinoma.

such that they are less enhanced than the adjacent liver (**Video 4-8;** see Fig. 4-41, *F*). Variations to this classic pattern are now well described[195] and include arterial phase hypovascularity and delayed or no washout in the portal venous phase (Fig. 4-58). Regenerative **nodules,** by comparison, show similar arterial phase and portal venous phase vascularity and enhancement to the remainder of the cirrhotic liver. **Dysplastic nodules** may show transient arterial phase hypovascularity followed by isovascularity. Identification of this feature prompts biopsy in our institution.

Microbubble-enhanced sonography may contribute also to the detection of HCC. Sweeps of the liver in the arterial phase may detect hypervascular foci potentially representing HCC. Sweeps in the portal venous phase, by comparison, show HCC as hypoechoic or washout regions, again allowing for the detection of

unsuspected lesions. The arterialized liver of cirrhosis, however, is problematic for several reasons. First, it shows dysmorphology of all liver vessels, in general, and the appreciation of focal increased vascularity in a small nodule is more difficult. Portal venous phase imaging is also weakened when the liver receives a greater proportion of its blood supply from the hepatic artery. Therefore, washout of a specific nodule may not be as evident as in a normal liver. This area remains of high interest to us, and ongoing investigations are evaluating chronically diseased livers. CT[197] and MRI[198] are frequently performed to screen for and evaluate HCC. The importance of CEUS is recognized by the American Association for the Study of Liver Diseases (AASLD) and has been included in the practice guideline for the management of small nodules detected in the surveillance for HCC.[199]

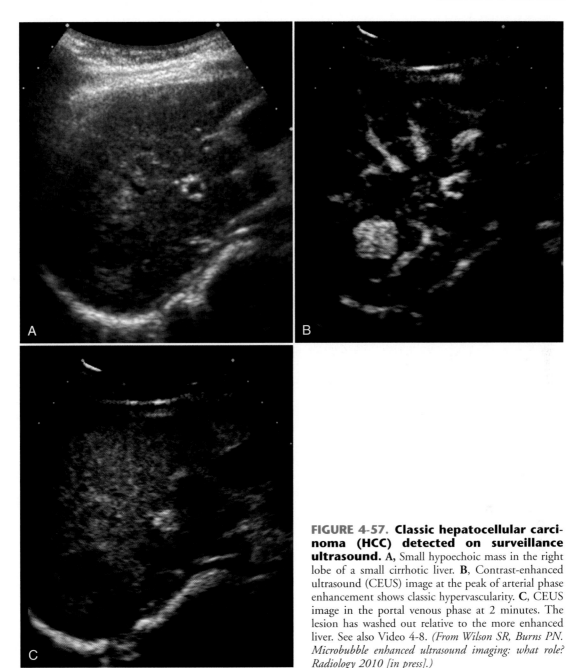

FIGURE 4-57. Classic hepatocellular carcinoma (HCC) detected on surveillance ultrasound. A, Small hypoechoic mass in the right lobe of a small cirrhotic liver. **B,** Contrast-enhanced ultrasound (CEUS) image at the peak of arterial phase enhancement shows classic hypervascularity. **C,** CEUS image in the portal venous phase at 2 minutes. The lesion has washed out relative to the more enhanced liver. See also Video 4-8. *(From Wilson SR, Burns PN. Microbubble enhanced ultrasound imaging: what role? Radiology 2010 [in press].)*

Fibrolamellar carcinoma is a histologic subtype of HCC found in younger patients (adolescents and young adults) without coexisting liver disease. The serum alpha-fetoprotein levels are usually normal. The tumors are usually solitary, 6 to 22 cm, well differentiated, and often encapsulated by fibrous tissue.[200-202] With 5-year survival rates of approximately 25% to 30%, the prognosis is generally better for fibrolamellar carcinoma than HCC.[203,204] Most patients, however, demonstrate advanced disease at diagnosis. Aggressive surgical resection of tumor is recommended at presentation as well as for recurrent disease.[202] The echogenicity of fibrolamellar carcinoma is variable. Punctate calcification and a central echogenic scar—features that are distinctly unusual in

hepatomas—are more common in the fibrolamellar subtype.

Hemangiosarcoma (Angiosarcoma)

Hepatic hemangiosarcoma is an extremely rare malignant tumor. It occurs almost exclusively in adults, reaching its peak incidence in the sixth and seventh decades of life. Hemangiosarcoma is of particular interest because of its association with specific carcinogens: **Thorotrast, arsenic,** and **polyvinyl chloride.**[176] Only a few cases of hepatic hemangiosarcoma have been reported in the radiologic literature. The sonographic appearance is a large mass of mixed echogenicity.[205,206]

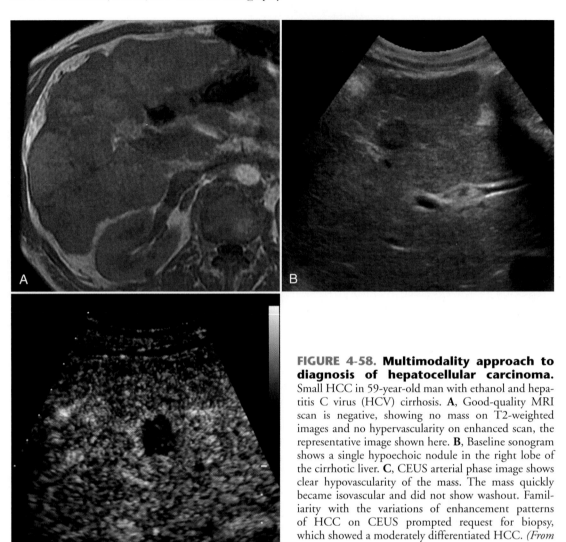

FIGURE 4-58. Multimodality approach to diagnosis of hepatocellular carcinoma. Small HCC in 59-year-old man with ethanol and hepatitis C virus (HCV) cirrhosis. **A,** Good-quality MRI scan is negative, showing no mass on T2-weighted images and no hypervascularity on enhanced scan, the representative image shown here. **B,** Baseline sonogram shows a single hypoechoic nodule in the right lobe of the cirrhotic liver. **C,** CEUS arterial phase image shows clear hypovascularity of the mass. The mass quickly became isovascular and did not show washout. Familiarity with the variations of enhancement patterns of HCC on CEUS prompted request for biopsy, which showed a moderately differentiated HCC. *(From Wilson SR, Burns PN. Microbubble enhanced ultrasound imaging: what role? Radiology 2010 [in press].)*

Hepatic Epithelioid Hemangioendothelioma

Epithelioid hemangioendothelioma (EHE) is a rare malignant tumor of vascular origin that occurs in adults. Soft tissues, lung, and liver are affected. The prognosis is variable; many patients survive longer than 5 years with or without treatment.[207] Hepatic EHE begins as multiple hypoechoic nodules, which grow and coalesce over time, forming larger, confluent masses that tend to involve the periphery of the liver. Foci of calcification may be present.[207,208] The hepatic capsule overlying the lesions of EHE may be retracted inward, secondary to fibrosis incited by the tumor; this unusual feature is highly suggestive of the diagnosis. Importantly, peripheral postchemotherapy metastases and tumors causing biliary obstruction and segmental atrophy may have a similar appearance.[209] The diagnosis of hepatic EHE is made by percutaneous liver biopsy and immunohistochemical staining.

Metastatic Liver Disease

In the United States, metastatic liver disease is 18 to 20 times more common than HCC. Detection of metastasis greatly alters the patient's prognosis and often the management. The incidence of hepatic metastases depends on the type of primary tumor and its stage at initial detection. At autopsy, 25% to 50% of patients dying from cancer have liver metastases. Patients with short-term survival (<1 year) after initial detection of liver metastases are those with HCC and carcinomas of the pancreas, stomach, and esophagus. Patients with longer-term survival are those with head and neck carcinomas and carcinoma of the colon. Most patients with melanoma have an extremely low incidence of hepatic metastases at diagnosis. Liver involvement at autopsy, however, may be as high as 70%.

The most common **primary tumors** resulting in liver metastases, in decreasing order of frequency, are gallbladder, colon, stomach, pancreas, breast, and lung. Most metastases to the liver are blood-borne through the hepatic artery or portal vein, but lymphatic spread of tumors from stomach, pancreas, ovary, or uterus may also occur. The portal vein provides direct access to the liver for tumor cells originating from the gastrointestinal tract and probably accounts for the high frequency of liver metastases from organs that drain into the portal circulation.

Advantages of ultrasound as a screening test for metastatic liver disease include its relative accuracy, speed, lack of ionizing radiation, and availability. Further, the multiplanar capability of ultrasound allows for excellent segmental localization of masses, with the ability to detect proximity to or involvement of the vital vascular structures. Although isolated reports describe detection of metastases on sonography in skilled hands as competitive with CT and MRI,[210] sonography is not uniformly used as the first-line investigative technique to search for metastatic disease worldwide; CT has filled that role. Experience suggests that ultrasound without microbubble contrast agents does not compete with triphasic CT for metastasis detection.[143] Although greatly improved with the addition of contrast agents, as described earlier, we doubt CEUS will ever be widely used in routine clinical practice for the large numbers of patients who have scans for metastatic disease. Nonetheless, on a case-by-case basis, and as a problem-solving modality, CEUS may play a contributory role in the evaluation of the patient with metastatic liver disease.

On **conventional gray-scale sonography,** patients with metastatic liver disease may present with a single liver lesion (Fig. 4-59, *A*), although more often they present with multiple focal liver masses. All metastatic lesions in a given liver may have identical sonographic morphology; however, biopsy-confirmed lesions of differing appearances may have the same underlying histology. Of importance, metastases may also be present in a liver that already has an underlying diffuse or focal abnormality, most often hemangioma. Metastatic involvement of the liver may take on different forms, showing diffuse liver involvement and rarely geographic infiltration (Fig. 4-59, *C-F*).

Knowledge of a prior or concomitant malignancy and features of disseminated malignancy at sonography are helpful in correct interpretation of a sonographically detected liver masses. Although no confirmatory features of metastatic disease are seen on sonography, suggestive features include **multiple solid lesions** of varying size and a **hypoechoic halo** surrounding a liver mass. A halo around the periphery of a liver mass on sonography is an ominous sign strongly associated with malignancy, particularly metastatic disease but also HCC.

In our investigation of 214 consecutive patients with focal liver lesions, 66 had lesions that showed a hypoechoic halo; 13 had HCCs (Fig. 4-60, *A* and *B*); 43 had metastases (Fig. 4-60, *C-F*); four had focal nodular hyperplasia; and two had adenomas (see Fig. 4-51). Four lesions were unconfirmed. In 1992, Wernecke et al.[211] described the importance of the hypoechoic halo in the differentiation of malignant from benign focal hepatic lesions. Its identification has a positive and negative predictive value of 86% and 88%, respectively. Therefore, we conclude that although not absolutely indicative of malignancy, a halo is seen with lesions that require further investigation and confirmation of their nature, regardless of the patient's presentation or status. Radiologic-histologic correlation of a hypoechoic halo surrounding a liver mass has revealed that, in the majority of cases, the hypoechoic rim corresponds to normal liver parenchyma, which is compressed by the rapidly expanding tumor. Less frequently, the hypoechoic rim represents proliferating malignant cells, tumor fibrosis or vascularization, or a fibrotic rim.[212-214]

The *sonographic appearance* of metastatic liver disease has been described as echogenic, hypoechoic, target, calcified, cystic, and diffuse. Although the ultrasound appearance is not specific for determining the origin of the metastasis, certain generalities apply (Fig. 4-61).

METASTATIC LIVER DISEASE: COMMON PATTERNS

ECHOGENIC METASTASES
Gastrointestinal tract
Hepatocellular carcinoma
Vascular primaries
Islet cell carcinoma
Carcinoid
Choriocarcinoma
Renal cell carcinoma

HYPOECHOIC METASTASES
Breast cancer
Lung cancer
Lymphoma
Esophagus, stomach, and pancreas

BULL'S-EYE OR TARGET PATTERN
Lung cancer

CALCIFIED METASTASES
Frequently: mucinous adenocarcinoma
Less frequently: osteogenic sarcoma
Chondrosarcoma
Teratocarcinoma
Neuroblastoma

CYSTIC METASTASES
Necrosis: sarcomas
Cystic growth patterns: cystadenocarcinoma of
    ovary and pancreas
Mucinous carcinoma of colon

INFILTRATIVE PATTERNS
Breast cancer
Lung cancer
Malignant melanoma

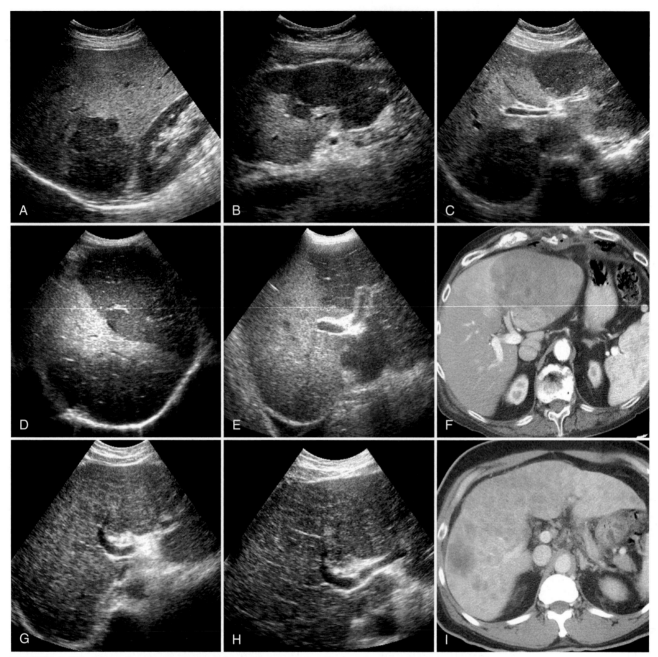

FIGURE 4-59. Liver involvement with metastases in three patients. *Top row,* **Focal liver masses:** most common variety and easiest to appreciate. **A,** Sagittal image of the right lobe shows a well-defined and lobulated hypoechoic mass. **B,** Sagittal image of the left lobe shows confluent masses in segment 3. **C,** Transverse image shows the two focal hypoechoic masses separated by normal liver. *Middle row,* **Rare geographic pattern of metastases. D** and **E,** Subcostal views show the right and left lobes of the liver. A sharp geographic or maplike border separates the normal echogenic liver from the hypoechoic tumor. The distribution and echogenicity variation both suggest possible fatty change or perfusion abnormality. **F,** Confirmatory CT scan. *Bottom row,* **Diffuse tumor involvement:** often the most difficult to appreciate on ultrasound, as shown here. **G,** Transverse sonogram; **H,** similar view with greater magnification. Both images show a coarse liver parenchyma. It is more suggestive of cirrhosis than the extensive tumor shown on **I,** CT scan.

Echogenic metastases tend to arise from a gastrointestinal origin or from HCC (Fig. 4-61, *I*). The more vascular the tumor, the more likely it is that the lesion is echogenic.[193,215] Therefore, metastases from renal cell carcinoma, neuroendocrine tumors, carcinoid, choriocarcinoma, and islet cell carcinoma also tend to be hyperechoic. It is this particular group of tumors that may mimic a hemangioma on sonography.

Hypoechoic metastases are generally hypovascular and may be monocellular or hypercellular without interstitial stroma. Hypoechoic lesions represent the typical pattern seen in untreated metastatic breast or lung cancer (see Figs. 4-60 and 4-61), as well as gastric, pancreatic, and esophageal tumors. Lymphomatous involvement of the liver may also manifest as hypoechoic masses (Fig. 4-62). The uniform cellularity of **lymphoma** without

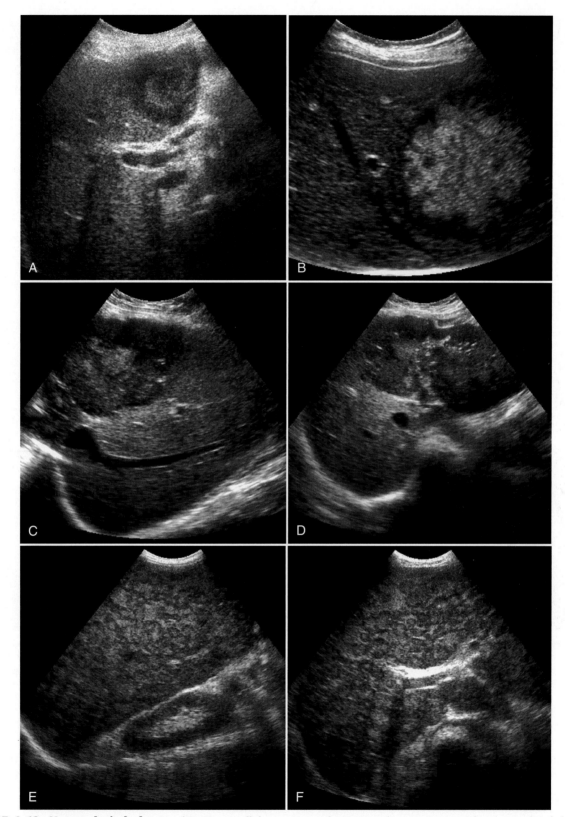

FIGURE 4-60. Hypoechoic halo. A and **B,** Hepatocellular carcinoma showing as echogenic masses with a surrounding halo. **C** and **D,** Sagittal and transverse images of a large solitary breast metastasis. **E** and **F,** Large liver full of small masses with hypoechoic halos from small cell carcinoma of the lung.

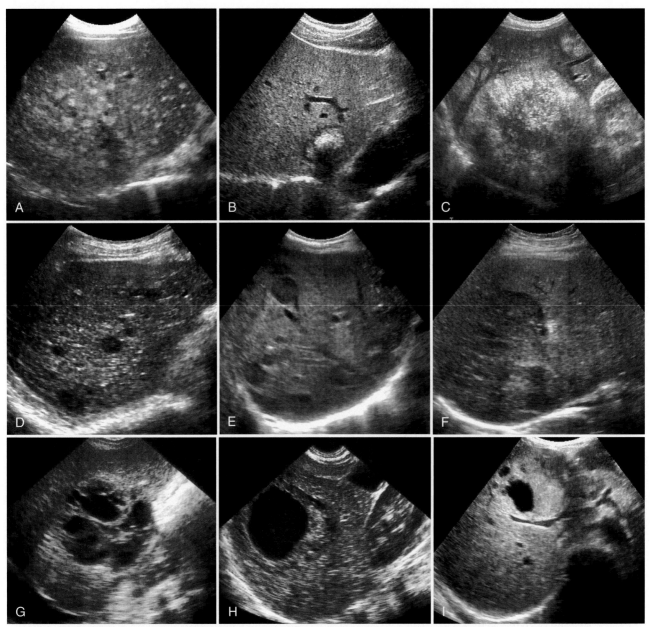

FIGURE 4-61. Patterns of metastatic liver disease. *Top row,* **Echogenic lesions. A,** Multiple tiny echogenic metastases from choriocarcinoma. **B,** Colon metastasis with clump of calcium and distal acoustic shadowing. **C,** Large, poorly differentiated metastatic adenocarcinoma, with tiny punctate echogenicities suggesting microcalcification. *Middle row,* **Hypoechoic lesions of increasing size** from **D,** pancreas; **E,** lung; and **F,** adenocarcinoma, from unknown primaries. *Bottom row,* **Cystic metastases. G,** Rare metastatic liposarcoma from the thigh. Metastasis has a cystic growth pattern. **H,** Metastatic sarcoma from the small bowel with necrosis, and **I,** highly echogenic metastasis with a well-defined cystic component, highly suggestive of metastatic carcinoid or neuroendocrine tumor.

significant background stroma is thought to be related to its hypoechoic appearance on sonography. Although at autopsy the liver is often a secondary site of involvement by Hodgkin's and non-Hodgkin's lymphoma, the disease tends to be diffusely infiltrative and undetected by sonography and CT.[216] The pattern of multiple hypoechoic hepatic masses is more typical of primary non-Hodgkin's lymphoma of the liver or lymphoma associated with AIDS.[216,217] The lymphomatous masses may appear anechoic and septated, mimicking hepatic abscesses.

The **bull's-eye or target pattern** is characterized by a peripheral hypoechoic zone (see Fig. 4-60). The appearance is nonspecific and common, although it is frequently identified in metastases from bronchogenic carcinoma.[218]

Calcified metastases are distinctive by virtue of their marked echogenicity and distal acoustic shadowing (see Fig. 4-61, *B*). Mucinous adenocarcinoma of the colon is most frequently associated with calcified metastases. Calcium may appear as large, echogenic, and shadowing foci or, more often, shows innumerable tiny punctate

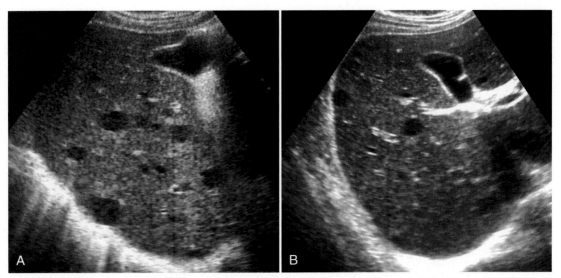

FIGURE 4-62. Lymphoma of the liver. A, Sagittal, and **B,** transverse, sonograms show small, focal hypoechoic nodules throughout the liver. Lymphoma may also involve the liver diffusely without producing a focal sonographic abnormality.

echogenicities without clear shadowing. Other primary malignancies that give rise to calcified metastases are endocrine pancreatic tumors, leiomyosarcoma, adenocarcinoma of the stomach, neuroblastoma, osteogenic sarcoma, chondrosarcoma, and ovarian cystadenocarcinoma and teratocarcinoma.[219]

Cystic metastases are uncommon and generally exhibit features that distinguish them from the ubiquitous benign hepatic cyst, including mural nodules, thick walls, fluid-fluid levels, and internal septations.[220,221] Primary neoplasms with a cystic component, such as cystadenocarcinoma of the ovary and pancreas and mucinous carcinoma of the colon, may produce cystic secondary lesions, although infrequently. More often, cystic neoplasms result from extensive necrosis, seen most often in metastatic sarcomas, which typically have low-level echoes and a thickened, shaggy wall (see Fig. 4-61, *H*). Metastatic neuroendocrine and carcinoid tumors are typically highly echogenic and often show secondary cystic change (see Fig. 4-61, *I*). Large colorectal metastases may also rarely be necrotic, producing a predominantly cystic liver mass.

Diffuse disorganization of the hepatic parenchyma reflects **infiltrative metastatic disease** and is the most difficult to appreciate on sonography, probably because of the loss of the reference normal liver for comparison (see Fig. 4-59, *G-I*). In our experience, breast and lung carcinomas, as well as malignant melanomas, are the most common primary tumors to present this pattern. The diagnosis can be even more difficult if the patient has a fatty liver from chemotherapy. In these patients, CEUS, CT, or MRI may be helpful. Segmental and lobar tumor infiltration by secondary tumor may also be difficult to detect because it may mimic other benign conditions, such as fatty infiltration (see Fig. 4-59, *D-F*) or cirrhosis (Fig. 4-63).

Contrast-enhanced ultrasound plays a major role in the diagnosis and detection of metastases.[143,222] In the portal venous phase, metastases all show washout, which tends to be complete and also rapid, beginning within the time frame typically designated as the arterial phase (Fig. 4-64 and **Video 4-9**). Therefore, metastases will appear as black punched areas within the enhanced parenchyma. Arterial phase enhancement is variable, although most metastases, regardless of their expected enhancement, show transient hypervascularity in the arterial phase, followed by rapid washout. Hypovascularity and rim enhancement can also be shown.

Peripheral cholangiocarcinoma is an infrequent tumor presenting with a solitary liver mass similar to a metastasis, both on gray scale and CEUS. Capsular retraction may be appreciated.

Hepatic involvement by **Kaposi's sarcoma,** although frequent in patients with AIDS at autopsy, is rarely diagnosed by imaging studies.[223] Sonography has demonstrated periportal infiltration and multiple small, peripheral hyperechoic nodules.[224,225]

Because of the nonspecific appearance of metastatic liver disease, **ultrasound-guided biopsy** is widely used to establish a primary tissue diagnosis. In addition, ultrasound is an excellent means to monitor the response to chemotherapy in oncology patients.

HEPATIC TRAUMA

The approach to the management of blunt hepatic injury is becoming increasingly more conservative. Surgical exploration is indicated for patients who are in shock or hemodynamically unstable.[226] In the hemodynamically stable patient, many institutions initially perform abdominal CT to assess the extent of liver

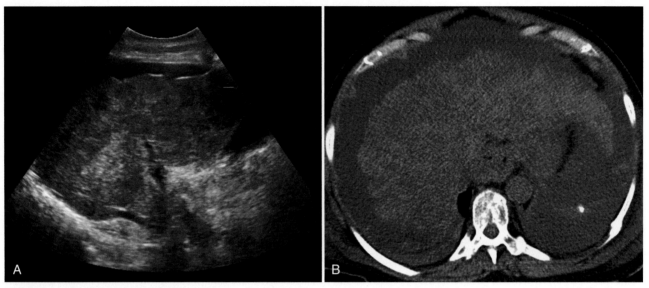

FIGURE 4-63. Pseudocirrhosis. Elderly woman presented to emergency department with increased abdominal girth. **A,** Intercostal sonogram of the liver shows heterogeneous nodular parenchyma, surface nodularity, and ascites; all suggest cirrhosis. **B,** Unenhanced CT image of the liver confirms the findings, including ascites, surface nodularity, and heterogeneous parenchyma. Contrast enhancement did not suggest focal metastatic disease. At autopsy, diffuse breast metastases were found.

trauma. Ultrasound may be used for serial monitoring of the healing pattern.

The predominant site of hepatic injury in blunt trauma is the right lobe, in particular the posterior segment.[227] Foley et al.[228] found that the most common type of injury was a perivascular laceration paralleling branches of the right and middle hepatic veins and the anterior and posterior branches of the right portal vein. Other findings were subcapsular, pericapsular, and isolated hematomas; liver fracture, defined as a laceration extending between two visceral surfaces; lacerations involving the left lobe; and hemoperitoneum[228] (Fig. 4-65). Hepatic infarcts are rarely identified after blunt abdominal trauma because of the dual blood supply of the liver.

Van Sonnenberg et al.[229] evaluated the sonographic findings of acute trauma to the liver (<24 hours after injury or transhepatic cholangiogram) and determined that fresh hemorrhage was echogenic. Within the first week, the hepatic laceration becomes more hypoechoic and distinct as a result of resorption of devitalized tissue and ingress of interstitial fluid. After 2 to 3 weeks, the laceration becomes increasingly indistinct because of fluid resorption and filling of the spaces with granulation tissue.

Portosystemic Shunts

Surgical portosystemic shunts are performed to decompress the portal system in patients with portal hypertension. The most common surgical shunts include mesocaval, distal splenorenal (Warren shunts), mesoatrial, and portacaval. Duplex Doppler sonography and

CDFI appear to be reliable noninvasive methods of assessing shunt patency or thrombosis.[230-233] Both modalities are effective in assessing portacaval, mesoatrial, and mesocaval shunts.[230] Shunt patency is confirmed by demonstrating flow at the anastomotic site. If the anastomosis cannot be visualized, hepatofugal portal flow is an indirect sign of patency.[231,232]

Distal splenorenal communications are particularly difficult to examine with duplex Doppler sonography because overlying bowel gas and fat hinder accurate placement of the Doppler cursor.[230,234] CDFI more readily locates the splenic and renal limbs of Warren shunts. The splenic limb is best imaged from a left subcostal approach, whereas the left renal vein is optimally scanned through the left flank. Grant et al.[230] reported that color Doppler sonography correctly inferred patency or thrombosis in all 14 splenorenal communications by evaluating the flow in both limbs of the shunt.

Transjugular Intrahepatic Portosystemic Shunts

Transjugular intrahepatic portosystemic shunts (**TIPS**) are the most recently developed and now the most popular technique for relief of symptomatic portal hypertension, specifically varices with gastrointestinal bleeding, and less often, refractory ascites. Performed percutaneously with insertion of an expandable metal stent, TIPS have less morbidity and mortality than surgical shunt procedures.[235]

The technique of performing TIPS requires transjugular access to the infrahepatic IVC, with selection of the

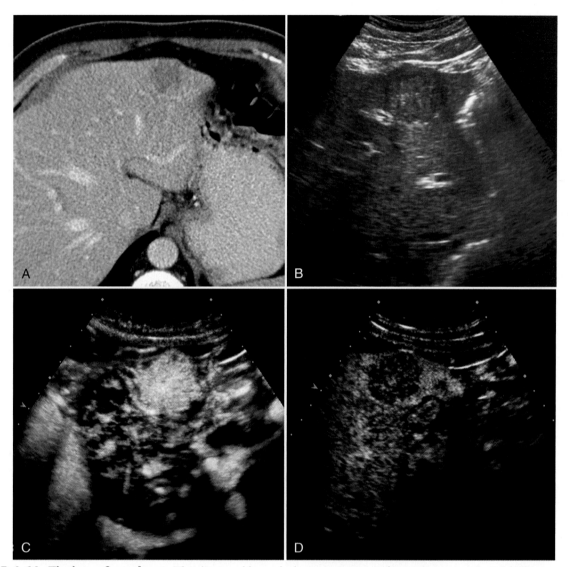

FIGURE 4-64. Timing of washout. This 49-year-old man had proven metastasis from colon cancer. **A,** Axial CT image shows a low-attenuation mass in the lateral segment of the left lobe. **B,** Baseline sonogram shows that the mass is slightly exophytic and of mixed echogenicity. **C,** CEUS arterial phase image at the peak of enhancement shows hypervascularity. **D,** Image at 45 seconds shows clear washout of the lesion, which had begun at 28 seconds. See also Video 4-9. *(From Wilson SR, Burns PN. Microbubble enhanced ultrasound imaging: what role? Radiology 2010 [in press].)*

optimal hepatic vein on the basis of its angle and diameter, most often the right hepatic vein. After targeting the portal vein with either fluoroscopy or Doppler sonography, a transjugular puncture needle is passed from the hepatic vein to the intrahepatic portal vein and a shunt created. The tract is dilated to an approximate diameter of 10 mm, with monitoring of the portal pressure gradient and filling of varices on portal venography. A bridging stent is left in place.[236]

In addition to acute problems directly attributed to the procedure itself, TIPS may be complicated by stenosis or occlusion of the stent caused by hyperplasia of the pseudointimal lining. At 1 year, primary patency rates vary from 25% to 66%, with a primary assisted patency of about 83%.[237,238] Doppler sonography provides a non-

invasive method for monitoring of TIPS patients because malfunction of the graft may be silent in its early phase. Scans should be performed immediately after the procedure, at three monthly intervals, and as indicated clinically.

Normal postprocedural Doppler findings include high-velocity, turbulent blood flow (mean peak systolic velocity, 135-200 cm/sec)[239] throughout the stent and hepatofugal flow in the intrahepatic portal venous branches, as the liver parenchyma drains through the shunt into the systemic circulation. Increased hepatic artery peak systolic velocity is also a normal observation, as is increased velocity in the main portal vein, because the stent serves as a low-resistance conduit, bypassing the high-resistance hepatic circulation. The reported mean

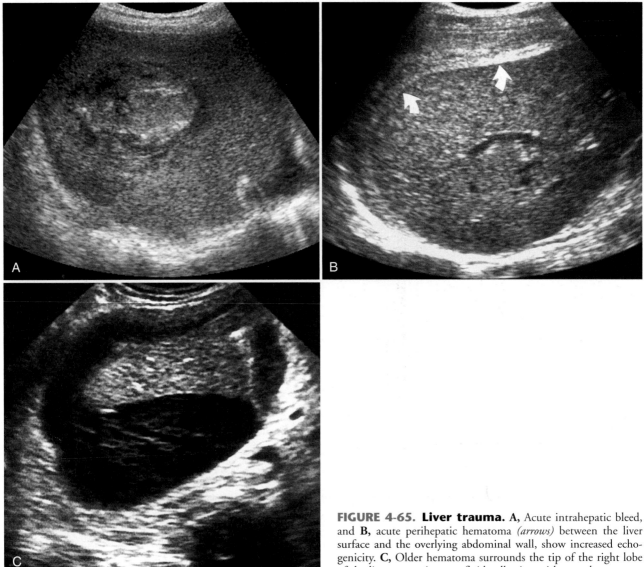

FIGURE 4-65. Liver trauma. A, Acute intrahepatic bleed, and **B,** acute perihepatic hematoma *(arrows)* between the liver surface and the overlying abdominal wall, show increased echogenicity. **C,** Older hematoma surrounds the tip of the right lobe of the liver, appearing as a fluid collection with strands.

main portal vein velocity in patients with patent shunts ranges from 37 to 47 cm/second.[240-242] Hepatic artery velocities increase from 79 cm/sec preshunt to 131 cm/ sec after the procedure.[239]

Sonographic evaluation should include measurement of angle-corrected stent velocities at three points along the stent and in the main portal vein, as well as evaluation of the direction of flow in the intrahepatic portal vein and in the involved hepatic vein (Figs. 4-66 and 4-67).

Sonographically detected complications include the following:
Stent occlusion
Stent stenosis
Hepatic venous stenosis
Detection of these complications is related to identification of both direct abnormalities and secondary signs.[243-246] **Direct signs** include no flow, abnormal

peak shunt velocity, a change in the peak shunt velocity, a low velocity in the main portal vein, reversal of hepatic vein flow, and hepatopedal intrahepatic portal venous flow. **Secondary signs** include reaccumulation of ascites and reappearance of varices and of recanalized paraumbilical vein.

PERCUTANEOUS LIVER BIOPSY

Percutaneous biopsy of malignant disease involving the liver has a sensitivity greater than 90% in most study series.[247,248] Relative contraindications to percutaneous biopsy are an uncorrectable bleeding diathesis, an unsafe access route, and an uncooperative patient. Ultrasound guidance allows real-time observation of the needle tip as it is advanced into the lesion. Several biopsy attachments allow continuous observation of the needle as it follows

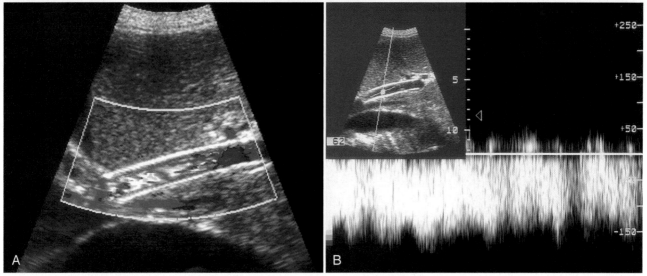

FIGURE 4-66. Transjugular intrahepatic portosystemic shunt (TIPS). A, Color Doppler image of TIPS shows flow throughout the shunt appropriately directed toward the heart, with a turbulent pattern. **B,** Angle-corrected midshunt velocity is normal at 150 cm/sec.

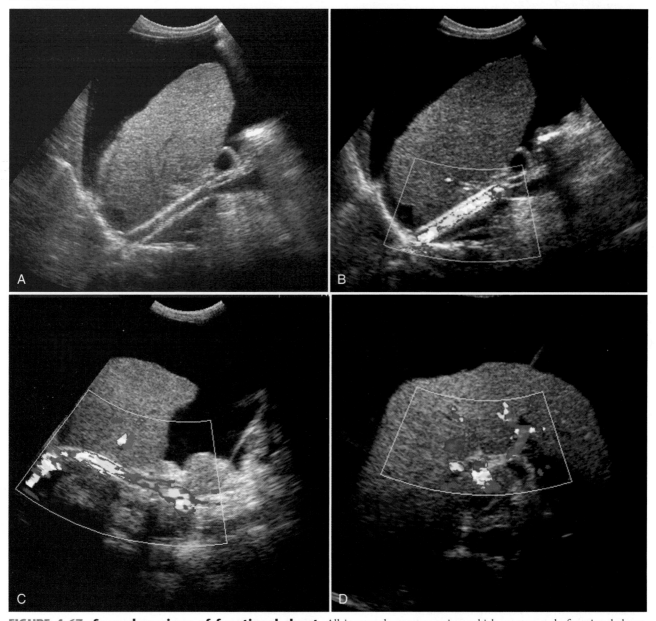

FIGURE 4-67. Secondary signs of functional shunt. All images show gross ascites, which suggests a dysfunctional shunt. **A,** Gray-scale, and **B,** color Doppler, images show a patent TIPS. Velocities throughout the shunt were about 130 cm/sec, which is normal. **C,** Sagittal image shows that flow in the main portal vein is appropriately directed toward the shunt, appearing red. **D,** Transverse image of the porta hepatis shows the ascending left portal venous branch is blue, flowing toward the shunt; this is also the correct direction. Therefore, despite the ascites, the ultrasound evaluation does not show a dysfunctional shunt.

MALFUNCTION OF TRANSJUGULAR INTRAHEPATIC PORTOSYSTEMIC SHUNTS: SONOGRAPHIC SIGNS

DIRECT SIGNS
No flow, consistent with shunt thrombosis or occlusion

Peak shunt velocity: <90 or >190 cm/sec

Change in peak shunt velocity: decrease of >40 cm/sec or increase of >60 cm/sec

Main portal vein velocity <30 cm/sec

Reversal of flow in hepatic vein away from inferior vena cava, suggesting hepatic vein stenosis

Hepatopedal intrahepatic portal venous flow

SECONDARY SIGNS
Reaccumulation of ascites

Reappearance of varices

Reappearance of recanalized paraumbilical vein

a predetermined path. Alternatively, many experienced radiologists prefer a "freehand" technique. Even small masses (2.5 cm) can undergo successful biopsy using sonographic guidance.[249] Ultrasound guidance may also be used in percutaneous aspiration and drainage of complicated fluid collections in the liver. Ultrasound-guided percutaneous ethanol injection has been used in the treatment of HCC and hepatic metastases.[250]

INTRAOPERATIVE ULTRASOUND

Intraoperative ultrasound is now an established application of ultrasound technology. The exposed liver is scanned with a sterile, 7.5-MHz transducer or one covered by a sterile sheath. Intraoperative ultrasound has been found to change the operative strategy in 31% to 49% of patients undergoing hepatic resection, either by allowing more precise resection or by indicating inoperability because of unsuspected masses or venous invasion.[251,252] Studies emphasize further improvement of surgical outcome with the addition of CEUS to intraoperative procedures.[253] Improved detection of metastases on CEUS undoubtedly accounts for this improvement.

Acknowledgment

Dr. Hojun Yu for his wonderful schematics and artwork.

References

Sonographic Technique
1. Wilson SR, Gupta C, Eliasziw M, Andrew A. Volume imaging in the abdomen with ultrasound: how we do it. AJR Am J Roentgenol 2009;193:79-85.

Normal Anatomy
2. Marks WM, Filly RA, Callen PW. Ultrasonic anatomy of the liver: a review with new applications. J Clin Ultrasound 1979;7:137-146.
3. Couinaud C. Le Foie. Paris: Masson et Cie; 1957.
4. Sugarbaker PH. Toward a standard of nomenclature for surgical anatomy of the liver. Neth J Surg 1988;PO:100.
5. Nelson RC, Chezmar JL, Sugarbaker PH, et al. Preoperative localization of focal liver lesions to specific liver segments: utility of CT during arterial portography. Radiology 1990;176:89-94.
6. Soyer P, Bluemke DA, Bliss DF, et al. Surgical segmental anatomy of the liver: demonstration with spiral CT during arterial portography and multiplanar reconstruction. AJR Am J Roentgenol 1994; 163:99-103.
7. Lafortune M, Madore F, Patriquin H, Breton G. Segmental anatomy of the liver: a sonographic approach to the Couinaud nomenclature. Radiology 1991;181:443-448.
8. Gosink BB, Leymaster CE. Ultrasonic determination of hepatomegaly. J Clin Ultrasound 1981;9:37-44.
9. Niederau C, Sonnenberg A, Muller JE, et al. Sonographic measurements of the normal liver, spleen, pancreas, and portal vein. Radiology 1983;149:537-540.

Developmental Anomalies
10. Belton RL, Van Zandt TF. Congenital absence of the left lobe of the liver: a radiologic diagnosis. Radiology 1983;147:184.
11. Radin DR, Colletti PM, Ralls PW, et al. Agenesis of the right lobe of the liver. Radiology 1987;164:639-642.
12. Lim JH, Ko YT, Han MC, et al. The inferior accessory hepatic fissure: sonographic appearance. AJR Am J Roentgenol 1987;149: 495-497.
13. Fraser-Hill MA, Atri M, Bret PM, et al. Intrahepatic portal venous system: variations demonstrated with duplex and color Doppler ultrasound. Radiology 1990;177:523-526.
14. Cosgrove DO, Arger PH, Coleman BG. Ultrasonic anatomy of hepatic veins. J Clin Ultrasound 1987;15:231-235.
15. Makuuchi M, Hasegawa H, Yamazaki S, et al. The inferior right hepatic vein: ultrasonic demonstration. Radiology 1983;148:213-217.

Congenital Abnormalities
16. Gaines PA, Sampson MA. The prevalence and characterization of simple hepatic cysts by ultrasound examination. Br J Radiol 1989;62:335-337.
17. Bean WJ, Rodan BA. Hepatic cysts: treatment with alcohol. AJR Am J Roentgenol 1985;144:237-241.
18. Baron RL, Campbell WL, Dodd 3rd GD. Peribiliary cysts associated with severe liver disease: imaging-pathologic correlation. AJR Am J Roentgenol 1994;162:631-636.
19. Levine E, Cook LT, Grantham JJ. Liver cysts in autosomal dominant polycystic kidney disease: clinical and computed tomographic study. AJR Am J Roentgenol 1985;145:229-233.
20. Von Meyenburg H. Uber die Cystenliber. Beitr Pathol Anat 1918;64:477-532.
21. Chung EB. Multiple bile-duct hamartomas. Cancer 1970;26: 287-296.
22. Redston MS, Wanless IR. The hepatic von Meyenburg complex: prevalence and association with hepatic and renal cysts among 2843 autopsies [corrected]. Mod Pathol 1996;9:233-237.
23. Lev-Toaff AS, Bach AM, Wechsler RJ, et al. The radiologic and pathologic spectrum of biliary hamartomas. AJR Am J Roentgenol 1995;165:309-313.
24. Salo J, Bru C, Vilella A, et al. Bile-duct hamartomas presenting as multiple focal lesions on hepatic ultrasonography. Am J Gastroenterol 1992;87:221-223.
25. Tan A, Shen JF, Hecht AH. Sonogram of multiple bile duct hamartomas. J Clin Ultrasound 1989;17:667-669.

Infectious Diseases
26. Burns CD, Kuhns JG, Wieman TJ. Cholangiocarcinoma in association with multiple biliary microhamartomas. Arch Pathol Lab Med 1990;114:1287-1289.
27. Seeft LB. Acute viral hepatitis. In: Kaplowitz N, editor. Liver and biliary disease. 2nd ed. Baltimore: Williams & Wilkins; 1996. p. 289-316.

28. Douglas DD. Fulminant hepatitis. In: Kaplowitz N, editor. Liver and biliary disease. 2nd ed. Baltimore: Williams & Wilkins; 1996. p. 317-326.

29. Davis GL. Chronic hepatitis. In: Kaplowitz N, editor. Liver and biliary disease. 2nd ed. Baltimore: Williams & Wilkins; 1996. p. 327-337.

30. Wilson SR. The gallbladder. In: Gastrointestinal disease. 6th series. Test and syllabus. Reston, Va: American College of Radiology; 2004.

31. Zwiebel WJ. Sonographic diagnosis of diffuse liver disease. Semin Ultrasound CT MR 1995;16:8-15.

32. Wilson SR, Arenson AM. Sonographic evaluation of hepatic abscesses. J Can Assoc Radiol 1984;35:174-177.

33. Sabbaj J, Sutter VL, Finegold SM. Anaerobic pyogenic liver abscess. Ann Intern Med 1972;77:627-638.

34. Lawrence PH, Holt SC, Levi CS, Gough JC. Ultrasound case of the day: hepatosplenic candidiasis. Radiographics 1994;14:1147-1149.

35. Pastakia B, Shawker TH, Thaler M, et al. Hepatosplenic candidiasis: wheels within wheels. Radiology 1988;166:417-421.

36. Ralls PW, Colletti PM, Quinn MF, Halls J. Sonographic findings in hepatic amebic abscess. Radiology 1982;145:123-126.

37. Berry M, Bazaz R, Bhargava S. Amebic liver abscess: sonographic diagnosis and management. J Clin Ultrasound 1986;14:239-242.

38. Ralls PW, Barnes PF, Radin DR, et al. Sonographic features of amebic and pyogenic liver abscesses: a blinded comparison. AJR Am J Roentgenol 1987;149:499-501.

39. Ralls PW, Barnes PF, Johnson MB, et al. Medical treatment of hepatic amebic abscess: rare need for percutaneous drainage. Radiology 1987;165:805-807.

40. Ralls PW, Quinn MF, Boswell Jr WD, et al. Patterns of resolution in successfully treated hepatic amebic abscess: sonographic evaluation. Radiology 1983;149:541-543.

41. Gharbi HA, Hassine W, Brauner MW, Dupuch K. Ultrasound examination of the hydatic liver. Radiology 1981;139:459-463.

42. Lewall DB, McCorkell SJ. Hepatic echinococcal cysts: sonographic appearance and classification. Radiology 1985;155:773-775.

43. Beggs I. The radiology of hydatid disease. AJR Am J Roentgenol 1985;145:639-648.

44. Mueller PR, Dawson SL, Ferrucci Jr JT, Nardi GL. Hepatic echinococcal cyst: successful percutaneous drainage. Radiology 1985;155:627-628.

45. Bret PM, Fond A, Bretagnolle M, et al. Percutaneous aspiration and drainage of hydatid cysts in the liver. Radiology 1988;168:617-620.

46. Akhan O, Ozmen MN, Dincer A, et al. Liver hydatid disease: long-term results of percutaneous treatment. Radiology 1996;198:259-264.

47. Bezzi M, Teggi A, De Rosa F, et al. Abdominal hydatid disease: ultrasound findings during medical treatment. Radiology 1987;162:91-95.

48. Jha R, Lyons EA, Levi CS. Ultrasound case of the day: hydatid cyst (*Echinococcus granulosus*) in the right lobe of the liver. Radiographics 1994;14:455-458.

49. Didier D, Weiler S, Rohmer P, et al. Hepatic alveolar echinococcosis: correlative ultrasound and CT study. Radiology 1985;154:179-186.

50. McCully RM, Barron CM, Cheever AW. Schistosomiasis. In: Binford CH, Connor DH, editors. Pathology of tropical and extraordinary disease. Washington, DC: Armed Forces Institute of Pathology; 1976. p. 482-508.

51. Symmers WSC. Note on a new form of liver cirrhosis due to the presence of the ova of *Bilharzia hematobilia*. J Pathol 1904;9:237-239.

52. Cerri GG, Alves VA, Magalhaes A. Hepatosplenic schistosomiasis mansoni: ultrasound manifestations. Radiology 1984;153:777-780.

53. Fataar S, Bassiony H, Satyanath S, Vassileva J, Hanna RM. Characteristic sonographic features of schistosomal periportal fibrosis. AJR Am J Roentgenol 1984;143:69-71.

54. Kuhlman JE. Pneumocystic infections: the radiologist's perspective. Radiology 1996;198:623-635.

55. Radin DR, Baker EL, Klatt EC, et al. Visceral and nodal calcification in patients with AIDS-related *Pneumocystis carinii* infection. AJR Am J Roentgenol 1990;154:27-31.

56. Spouge AR, Wilson SR, Gopinath N, Sherman M, Blendis LM. Extrapulmonary Pneumocystis carinii in a patient with AIDS: sonographic findings. AJR Am J Roentgenol 1990;155:76-78.

57. Telzak EE, Cote RJ, Gold JW, Campbell SW, Armstrong D. Extrapulmonary *Pneumocystis carinii* infections. Rev Infect Dis 1990;12:380-386.

58. Lubat E, Megibow AJ, Balthazar EJ, Goldenberg AS, Birnbaum BA, Bosniak MA. Extrapulmonary *Pneumocystis carinii* infection in AIDS: CT findings. Radiology 1990;174:157-160.

59. Towers MJ, Withers CE, Hamilton PA, Kolin A, Walmsley S. Visceral calcification in patients with AIDS may not always be due to *Pneumocystis carinii*. AJR Am J Roentgenol 1991;156:745-747.

Disorders of Metabolism

60. Zakim D. Metabolism of glucose and fatty acids by the liver. In: Zakim D, Boyer TD, editors. Hepatology: a textbook of liver disease. Philadelphia: Saunders; 1982. p. 76-109.

61. Wilson SR, Rosen IE, Chin-Sang HB, Arenson AM. Fatty infiltration of the liver–an imaging challenge. J Can Assoc Radiol 1982;33:227-232.

62. Yates CK, Streight RA. Focal fatty infiltration of the liver simulating metastatic disease. Radiology 1986;159:83-84.

63. Sauerbrei EE, Lopez M. Pseudotumor of the quadrate lobe in hepatic sonography: a sign of generalized fatty infiltration. AJR Am J Roentgenol 1986;147:923-927.

64. White EM, Simeone JF, Mueller PR, et al. Focal periportal sparing in hepatic fatty infiltration: a cause of hepatic pseudomass on ultrasound. Radiology 1987;162:57-59.

65. Wanless IR, Bargman JM, Oreopoulos DG, Vas SI. Subcapsular steatonecrosis in response to peritoneal insulin delivery: a clue to the pathogenesis of steatonecrosis in obesity. Mod Pathol 1989;2:69-74.

66. Apicella PL, Mirowitz SA, Weinreb JC. Extension of vessels through hepatic neoplasms: MR and CT findings. Radiology 1994;191:135-136.

67. Quinn SF, Gosink BB. Characteristic sonographic signs of hepatic fatty infiltration. AJR Am J Roentgenol 1985;145:753-755.

68. Arai K, Matsui O, Takashima T, Ida M, Nishida Y. Focal spared areas in fatty liver caused by regional decreased portal flow. AJR Am J Roentgenol 1988;151:300-302.

69. Ishak KG, Sharp HL. Metabolic errors and liver disease. In: MacSween RNM, Anthony PP, Scheuer PJ, editors. Pathology of the liver. 2nd ed. New York: Churchill Livingstone; 1987. p. 99-180.

70. Grossman H, Ram PC, Coleman RA, et al. Hepatic ultrasonography in type I glycogen storage disease (von Gierke disease): detection of hepatic adenoma and carcinoma. Radiology 1981;141:753-756.

71. Anthony PP, Ishak KG, Nayak NC, et al. The morphology of cirrhosis: definition, nomenclature, and classification. Bull WHO 1977;55:521-540.

72. Millward-Sadler GH. Cirrhosis. In: MacSween RNM, Anthony PP, Scheuer PJ, editors. Pathology of the liver. 2nd ed. New York: Churchill Livingstone; 1987. p. 342-363.

73. Giorgio A, Amoroso P, Lettieri G, et al. Cirrhosis: value of caudate to right lobe ratio in diagnosis with ultrasound. Radiology 1986;161:443-445.

74. Taylor KJ, Riely CA, Hammers L, et al. Quantitative ultrasound attenuation in normal liver and in patients with diffuse liver disease: importance of fat. Radiology 1986;160:65-71.

75. Sanford NL, Walsh P, Matis C, Baddeley H, Powell LW. Is ultrasonography useful in the assessment of diffuse parenchymal liver disease? Gastroenterology 1985;89:186-191.

76. Freeman MP, Vick CW, Taylor KJ, Carithers RL, Brewer WH. Regenerating nodules in cirrhosis: sonographic appearance with anatomic correlation. AJR Am J Roentgenol 1986;146:533-536.

77. Murakami T, Kuroda C, Marukawa T, et al. Regenerating nodules in hepatic cirrhosis: MR findings with pathologic correlation. AJR Am J Roentgenol 1990;155:1227-1231.

78. Theise ND. Macroregenerative (dysplastic) nodules and hepatocarcinogenesis: theoretical and clinical considerations. Semin Liver Dis 1995;15:360-371.

79. Tanaka S, Kitamra T, Fujita M, et al. Small hepatocellular carcinoma: differentiation from adenomatous hyperplastic nodule with color Doppler flow imaging. Radiology 1992;182:161-165.

80. Bolondi L, Li Bassi S, Gaiani S, et al. Liver cirrhosis: changes of Doppler waveform of hepatic veins. Radiology 1991;178:513-516.

81. Colli A, Cocciolo M, Riva C, et al. Abnormalities of Doppler waveform of the hepatic veins in patients with chronic liver disease:

correlation with histologic findings. AJR Am J Roentgenol 1994;162: 833-837.

82. Lafortune M, Dauzat M, Pomier-Layrargues G, et al. Hepatic artery: effect of a meal in healthy persons and transplant recipients. Radiology 1993;187:391-394.

83. Joynt LK, Platt JF, Rubin JM, et al. Hepatic artery resistance before and after standard meal in subjects with diseased and healthy livers. Radiology 1995;196:489-492.

Vascular Abnormalities

84. Boyer TD. Portal hypertension and its complications. In: Zakim D, Boyer TD, editors. Hepatology: a textbook of liver disease. Philadelphia: Saunders; 1982. p. 464-499.

85. Bolondi L, Gandolfi L, Arienti V, et al. Ultrasonography in the diagnosis of portal hypertension: diminished response of portal vessels to respiration. Radiology 1982;142:167-172.

86. Lafortune M, Marleau D, Breton G, et al. Portal venous system measurements in portal hypertension. Radiology 1984;151: 27-30.

87. Juttner HU, Jenney JM, Ralls PW, et al. Ultrasound demonstration of portosystemic collaterals in cirrhosis and portal hypertension. Radiology 1982;142:459-463.

88. Subramanyam BR, Balthazar EJ, Madamba MR, et al. Sonography of portosystemic venous collaterals in portal hypertension. Radiology 1983;146:161-166.

89. Patriquin H, Lafortune M, Burns PN, Dauzat M. Duplex Doppler examination in portal hypertension: technique and anatomy. AJR Am J Roentgenol 1987;149:71-76.

90. Lafortune M, Constantin A, Breton G, et al. The recanalized umbilical vein in portal hypertension: a myth. AJR Am J Roentgenol 1985;144:549-553.

91. DiCandio G, Campatelli A, Mosca F. Ultrasound detection of unusual spontaneous portosystemic shunts associated with uncomplicated portal hypertension. J Ultrasound Med 1985;4:297-305.

92. Mostbeck GH, Wittich GR, Herold C, et al. Hemodynamic significance of the paraumbilical vein in portal hypertension: assessment with duplex ultrasound. Radiology 1989;170:339-342.

93. Nelson RC, Lovett KE, Chezmar JL, et al. Comparison of pulsed Doppler sonography and angiography in patients with portal hypertension. AJR Am J Roentgenol 1987;149:77-81.

94. Bellamy EA, Bossi MC, Cosgrove DO. Ultrasound demonstration of changes in the normal portal venous system following a meal. Br J Radiol 1984;57:147-149.

95. Ohnishi K, Saito M, Nakayama T, et al. Portal venous hemodynamics in chronic liver disease: effects of posture change and exercise. Radiology 1985;155:757-761.

96. Bolondi L, Mazziotti A, Arienti V, et al. Ultrasonographic study of portal venous system in portal hypertension and after portosystemic shunt operations. Surgery 1984;95:261-269.

97. Zweibel WJ, Mountford RA, Halliwell MJ, Wells PN. Splanchnic blood flow in patients with cirrhosis and portal hypertension: investigation with duplex Doppler ultrasound. Radiology 1995;194:807-812.

98. Finn JP, Kane RA, Edelman RR, et al. Imaging of the portal venous system in patients with cirrhosis: MR angiography vs duplex Doppler sonography. AJR Am J Roentgenol 1993;161:989-994.

99. Wilson SR, Hine AL. Leiomyosarcoma of the portal vein. AJR Am J Roentgenol 1987;149:183-184.

100. Van Gansbeke D, Avni EF, Delcour C, et al. Sonographic features of portal vein thrombosis. AJR Am J Roentgenol 1985;144:749-752.

101. Kauzlaric D, Petrovic M, Barmeir E. Sonography of cavernous transformation of the portal vein. AJR Am J Roentgenol 1984;142:383-384.

102. Aldrete JS, Slaughter RL, Han SY. Portal vein thrombosis resulting in portal hypertension in adults. Am J Gastroenterol 1976;65:236-243.

103. Dodd 3rd GD, Memel DS, Baron RL, et al. Portal vein thrombosis in patients with cirrhosis: does sonographic detection of intrathrombus flow allow differentiation of benign and malignant thrombus? AJR Am J Roentgenol 1995;165:573-577.

104. Stanley P. Budd-Chiari syndrome. Radiology 1989;170:625-627.

105. Becker CD, Scheidegger J, Marincek B. Hepatic vein occlusion: morphologic features on computed tomography and ultrasonography. Gastrointest Radiol 1986;11:305-311.

106. Makuuchi M, Hasegawa H, Yamazaki S, et al. Primary Budd-Chiari syndrome: ultrasonic demonstration. Radiology 1984;152:775-779.

107. Menu Y, Alison D, Lorphelin JM, et al. Budd-Chiari syndrome: ultrasound evaluation. Radiology 1985;157:761-764.

108. Park JH, Lee JB, Han MC, et al. Sonographic evaluation of inferior vena caval obstruction: correlative study with vena cavography. AJR Am J Roentgenol 1985;145:757-762.

109. Murphy FB, Steinberg HV, Shires 3rd GT, et al. The Budd-Chiari syndrome: a review. AJR Am J Roentgenol 1986;147:9-15.

110. Grant EG, Perrella R, Tessler FN, et al. Budd-Chiari syndrome: the results of duplex and color Doppler imaging. AJR Am J Roentgenol 1989;152:377-381.

111. Keller MS, Taylor KJ, Riely CA. Pseudoportal Doppler signal in the partially obstructed inferior vena cava. Radiology 1989;170:475-477.

112. Hosoki T, Kuroda C, Tokunaga K, et al. Hepatic venous outflow obstruction: evaluation with pulsed duplex sonography. Radiology 1989;170:733-737.

113. Brown BP, Abu-Yousef M, Farner R, et al. Doppler sonography: a noninvasive method for evaluation of hepatic venocclusive disease. AJR Am J Roentgenol 1990;154:721-724.

114. Ralls PW, Johnson MB, Radin DR, et al. Budd-Chiari syndrome: detection with color Doppler sonography. AJR Am J Roentgenol 1992;159:113-116.

115. Millener P, Grant EG, Rose S, et al. Color Doppler imaging findings in patients with Budd-Chiari syndrome: correlation with venographic findings. AJR Am J Roentgenol 1993;161:307-312.

116. Taylor KJ, Burns PN, Woodcock JP, Wells PN. Blood flow in deep abdominal and pelvic vessels: ultrasonic pulsed-Doppler analysis. Radiology 1985;154:487-493.

117. Kriegshauser JS, Charboneau JW, Letendre L. Hepatic venocclusive disease after bone-marrow transplantation: diagnosis with duplex sonography. AJR Am J Roentgenol 1988;150:289-290.

118. Vine HS, Sequeira JC, Widrich WC, Sacks BA. Portal vein aneurysm. AJR Am J Roentgenol 1979;132:557-560.

119. Chagnon SF, Vallee CA, Barge J, et al. Aneurysmal portahepatic venous fistula: report of two cases. Radiology 1986;159:693-695.

120. Mori H, Hayashi K, Fukuda T, et al. Intrahepatic portosystemic venous shunt: occurrence in patients with and without liver cirrhosis. AJR Am J Roentgenol 1987;149:711-714.

121. Park JH, Cha SH, Han JK, Han MC. Intrahepatic portosystemic venous shunt. AJR Am J Roentgenol 1990;155:527-528.

122. Falkoff GE, Taylor KJ, Morse S. Hepatic artery pseudoaneurysm: diagnosis with real-time and pulsed Doppler ultrasound. Radiology 1986;158:55-56.

123. Garcia P, Garcia-Giannoli H, Meyran S, et al. Primary dissecting aneurysm of the hepatic artery: sonographic, CT, and angiographic findings. AJR Am J Roentgenol 1996;166:1316-1318.

124. Cloogman HM, DiCapo RD. Hereditary hemorrhagic telangiectasia: sonographic findings in the liver. Radiology 1984;150:521-522.

125. Wanless IR. Vascular disorders. In: MacSween RNM, Anthony PP, Scheuer PJ, editors. Pathology of the liver. 3rd ed. Edinburgh: Churchill Livingstone; 1994. p. 535.

126. Czapar CA, Weldon-Linne CM, Moore DM, Rhone DP. Peliosis hepatis in the acquired immunodeficiency syndrome. Arch Pathol Lab Med 1986;110:611-613.

127. Leong SS, Cazen RA, Yu GS, et al. Abdominal visceral peliosis associated with bacillary angiomatosis: ultrastructural evidence of endothelial destruction by bacilli. Arch Pathol Lab Med 1992;116:866-871.

128. Jamadar DA, D'Souza SP, Thomas EA, Giles TE. Case report: radiological appearances in peliosis hepatis. Br J Radiol 1994;67:102-104.

129. Toyoda S, Takeda K, Nakagawa T, Matsuda A. Magnetic resonance imaging of peliosis hepatis: a case report. Eur J Radiol 1993;16:207-208.

130. Lloyd RL, Lyons EA, Levi CS, et al. The sonographic appearance of peliosis hepatis. J Ultrasound Med 1982;1:293-294.

131. Tsukamoto Y, Nakata H, Kimoto T, et al. CT and angiography of peliosis hepatis. AJR Am J Roentgenol 1984;142:539-540.

132. Muradali D, Wilson SR, Wanless IR, et al. Peliosis hepatis with intrahepatic calcifications. J Ultrasound Med 1996;15:257-260.

Hepatic Masses

133. Burns PN, Wilson SR. Focal liver masses: enhancement patterns on contrast-enhanced images: concordance of ultrasound scans with CT scans and MR images. Radiology 2007;242:162-174.
134. Wilson SR, Burns PN, Muradali D, et al. Harmonic hepatic ultrasound with microbubble contrast agent: initial experience showing improved characterization of hemangioma, hepatocellular carcinoma, and metastasis. Radiology 2000;215:153-161.
135. Burns PN, Wilson SR, Simpson DH. Pulse inversion imaging of liver blood flow: improved method for characterizing focal masses with microbubble contrast. Invest Radiol 2000;35:58-71.
136. Wilson SR, Greenbaum LD, Goldberg BB. Contrast-enhanced ultrasound: what is the evidence and what are the obstacles? AJR Am J Roentgenol 2009;193:55-60.
137. Wilson SR, Jang HJ, Kim TK, et al. Real-time temporal maximum-intensity-projection imaging of hepatic lesions with contrast-enhanced sonography. AJR Am J Roentgenol 2008;190:691-695.
138. Brannigan M, Burns PN, Wilson SR. Blood flow patterns in focal liver lesions at microbubble-enhanced ultrasound. Radiographics 2004;24:921-935.
139. Wilson SR, Burns PN. An algorithm for the diagnosis of focal liver masses using microbubble contrast-enhanced pulse-inversion sonography. AJR Am J Roentgenol 2006;186:1401-1412.
140. Quaia E, Degobbis F, Tona G, et al. [Differential patterns of contrast enhancement in different focal liver lesions after injection of the microbubble ultrasound contrast agent SonoVue]. Radiol Med 2004;107:155-165.
141. Von Herbay A, Vogt C, Willers R, Haussinger D. Real-time imaging with the sonographic contrast agent SonoVue: differentiation between benign and malignant hepatic lesions. J Ultrasound Med 2004;23:1557-1568.
142. Blomley MJ, Albrecht T, Cosgrove DO, et al. Improved imaging of liver metastases with stimulated acoustic emission in the late phase of enhancement with the ultrasound contrast agent SHU 508A: early experience. Radiology 1999;210:409-416.
143. Albrecht T, Blomley MJ, Burns PN, et al. Improved detection of hepatic metastases with pulse-inversion ultrasound during the liver-specific phase of SHU 508A: multicenter study. Radiology 2003;227:361-370.

Hepatic Neoplasms

144. Charboneau JW. There is a hyperechoic mass in the liver: what does that mean? 2002 Categorical Course in Diagnostic Radiology. In: Cooperberg PL, editor. Findings at ultrasound: what do they mean? Radiological Society of North America, p. 73-78.
145. Edmondson HA. Tumours of the liver and intrahepatic bile ducts. In Atlas of tumor pathology. Washington, DC: Armed Forces Institute of Pathology; 1958.
146. Gibney RG, Hendin AP, Cooperberg PL. Sonographically detected hepatic hemangiomas: absence of change over time. AJR Am J Roentgenol 1987;149:953-957.
147. Mungovan JA, Cronan JJ, Vacarro J. Hepatic cavernous hemangiomas: lack of enlargement over time. Radiology 1994;191:111-113.
148. Bree RL, Schwab RE, Neiman HL. Solitary echogenic spot in the liver: is it diagnostic of a hemangioma? AJR Am J Roentgenol 1983;140:41-45.
149. McArdle CR. Ultrasonic appearances of a hepatic hemangioma. J Clin Ultrasound 1978;6:124.
150. Taboury J, Porcel A, Tubiana JM, Monnier JP. Cavernous hemangiomas of the liver studied by ultrasound: enhancement posterior to a hyperechoic mass as a sign of hypervascularity. Radiology 1983;149:781-785.
151. Itai Y, Ohnishi S, Ohtomo K, et al. Hepatic cavernous hemangioma in patients at high risk for liver cancer. Acta Radiol 1987;28:697-701.
152. Itai Y, Furui S, Araki T, et al. Computed tomography of cavernous hemangioma of the liver. Radiology 1980;137:149-155.
153. Moody AR, Wilson SR. Atypical hepatic hemangioma: a suggestive sonographic morphology. Radiology 1993;188:413-417.
154. Marsh JI, Gibney RG, Li DK. Hepatic hemangioma in the presence of fatty infiltration: an atypical sonographic appearance. Gastrointest Radiol 1989;14:262-264.
155. Choi BI, Kim TK, Han JK, et al. Power versus conventional color Doppler sonography: comparison in the depiction of vasculature in liver tumors. Radiology 1996;200:55-58.
156. Caturelli E, Pompili M, Bartolucci F, et al. Hemangioma-like lesions in chronic liver disease: diagnostic evaluation in patients. Radiology 2001;220:337-342.
157. Wilson SR, Burns PN. Microbubble enhanced ultrasound imaging: what role? Radiology 2010 (in press).
158. Solbiati L, Livraghi T, De Pra L, et al. Fine-needle biopsy of hepatic hemangioma with sonographic guidance. AJR Am J Roentgenol 1985;144:471-474.
159. Cronan JJ, Esparza AR, Dorfman GS, et al. Cavernous hemangioma of the liver: role of percutaneous biopsy. Radiology 1988;166:135-138.
160. Craig JR, Peters RL, Edmondson HA. Tumors of the liver and intrahepatic bile ducts. Fasc 26, 2nd series. Washington, DC: Armed Forces Institute of Pathology; 1989.
161. Wanless IR, Mawdsley C, Adams R. On the pathogenesis of focal nodular hyperplasia of the liver. Hepatology 1985;5:1194-1200.
162. Saul SH. Masses of the liver. In: Sternberg SS, editor. Diagnostic surgical pathology. 2nd ed. New York: Raven Press; 1994. p. 1517-1580.
163. Knowles 2nd DM, Casarella WJ, Johnson PM, Wolff M. The clinical, radiologic, and pathologic characterization of benign hepatic neoplasms: alleged association with oral contraceptives. Medicine (Baltimore) 1978;57:223-237.
164. Ross D, Pina J, Mirza M, et al. Regression of focal nodular hyperplasia after discontinuation of oral contraceptives (letter). Ann Intern Med 1976;85:203-204.
165. Buetow PC, Pantongrag-Brown L, Buck JL, et al. Focal nodular hyperplasia of the liver: radiologic-pathologic correlation. Radiographics 1996;16:369-388.
166. Scatarige JC, Fishman EK, Sanders RC. The sonographic "scar sign" in focal nodular hyperplasia of the liver. J Ultrasound Med 1982;1:275-278.
167. Golli M, Van Nhieu JT, Mathieu D, et al. Hepatocellular adenoma: color Doppler ultrasound and pathologic correlations. Radiology 1994;190:741-744.
168. Dietrich CF, Schuessler G, Trojan J, et al. Differentiation of focal nodular hyperplasia and hepatocellular adenoma by contrast-enhanced ultrasound. Br J Radiol 2005;78:704-707.
169. Ungermann L, Elias P, Zizka J, et al. Focal nodular hyperplasia: spoke-wheel arterial pattern and other signs on dynamic contrast-enhanced ultrasonography. Eur J Radiol 2007;63:290-294.
170. Yen YH, Wang JH, Lu SN, et al. Contrast-enhanced ultrasonographic spoke-wheel sign in hepatic focal nodular hyperplasia. Eur J Radiol 2006;60:439-444.
171. Drane WE, Krasicky GA, Johnson DA. Radionuclide imaging of primary tumors and tumor-like conditions of the liver. Clin Nucl Med 1987;12:569-582.
172. Welch TJ, Sheedy 2nd PF, Johnson CM, et al. Focal nodular hyperplasia and hepatic adenoma: comparison of angiography, CT, ultrasound, and scintigraphy. Radiology 1985;156:593-595.
173. Zech CJ, Grazioli L, Breuer J, et al. Diagnostic performance and description of morphological features of focal nodular hyperplasia in Gd-EOB-DTPA-enhanced liver magnetic resonance imaging: results of a multicenter trial. Invest Radiol 2008;43:504-511.
174. Kerlin P, Davis GL, McGill DB, et al. Hepatic adenoma and focal nodular hyperplasia: clinical, pathologic, and radiologic features. Gastroenterology 1983;84:994-1002.
175. Brunelle F, Tammam S, Odievre M, Chaumont P. Liver adenomas in glycogen storage disease in children: ultrasound and angiographic study. Pediatr Radiol 1984;14:94-101.
176. Kew MC. Tumors of the liver. In: Zakim D, Boyer TD, editors. Hepatology: a textbook of liver disease. Philadelphia: Saunders; 1982. p. 1048-1084.
177. Lubbers PR, Ros PR, Goodman ZD, Ishak KG. Accumulation of technetium-99m sulfur colloid by hepatocellular adenoma: scintigraphic-pathologic correlation. AJR Am J Roentgenol 1987;148:1105-1108.
178. Kim TK, Jang HJ, Burns PN, et al. Focal nodular hyperplasia and hepatic adenoma: differentiation with low-mechanical-index contrast-enhanced sonography. AJR Am J Roentgenol 2008;190:58-66.
179. Ito K, Honjo K, Fujita T, et al. Liver neoplasms: diagnostic pitfalls in cross-sectional imaging. Radiographics 1996;16:273-293.
180. Roberts JL, Fishman EK, Hartman DS, et al. Lipomatoultrasound tumors of the liver: evaluation with CT and ultrasound. Radiology 1986;158:613-617.

181. Marti-Bonmati L, Menor F, Vizcaino I, Vilar J. Lipoma of the liver: ultrasound, CT, and MRI appearance. Gastrointest Radiol 1989; 14:155-157.
182. Garant M, Reinhold C. Residents' corner. Answer to case of the month #36: hepatic lipoma. Can Assoc Radiol J 1996;47:140-142.
183. Wilson SR. The liver. Reston, Va: American College of Radiology; 2004.
184. Jackson VP, Martin-Simmerman P, Becker GJ, Holden RW. Real-time ultrasonographic demonstration of vascular invasion by hepatocellular carcinoma. J Ultrasound Med 1983;2:277-280.
185. Subramanyam BR, Balthazar EJ, Hilton S, et al. Hepatocellular carcinoma with venous invasion: sonographic-angiographic correlation. Radiology 1984;150:793-796.
186. LaBerge JM, Laing FC, Federle MP, et al. Hepatocellular carcinoma: assessment of resectability by computed tomography and ultrasound. Radiology 1984;152:485-490.
187. Sheu JC, Chen DS, Sung JL, et al. Hepatocellular carcinoma: ultrasound evolution in the early stage. Radiology 1985;155:463-467.
188. Tanaka S, Kitamura T, Imaoka S, et al. Hepatocellular carcinoma: sonographic and histologic correlation. AJR Am J Roentgenol 1983;140:701-707.
189. Choi BI, Takayasu K, Han MC. Small hepatocellular carcinomas and associated nodular lesions of the liver: pathology, pathogenesis, and imaging findings. AJR Am J Roentgenol 1993;160:1177-1187.
190. Teefey SA, Stephens DH, Weiland LH. Calcification in hepatocellular carcinoma: not always an indication of fibrolamellar histology. AJR Am J Roentgenol 1987;149:1173-1174.
191. Yoshikawa J, Matsui O, Takashima T, et al. Fatty metamorphosis in hepatocellular carcinoma: radiologic features in 10 cases. AJR Am J Roentgenol 1988;151:717-720.
192. Taylor KJ, Ramos I, Morse SS, et al. Focal liver masses: differential diagnosis with pulsed Doppler ultrasound. Radiology 1987;164:643-647.
193. Tanaka S, Kitamura T, Fujita M, et al. Color Doppler flow imaging of liver tumors. AJR Am J Roentgenol 1990;154:509-514.
194. Reinhold C, Hammers L, Taylor CR, et al. Characterization of focal hepatic lesions with duplex sonography: findings in 198 patients. AJR Am J Roentgenol 1995;164:1131-1135.
195. Jang HJ, Kim TK, Burns PN, Wilson SR. Enhancement patterns of hepatocellular carcinoma at contrast-enhanced US: comparison with histologic differentiation. Radiology 2007;244:898-906.
196. Nicolau C, Catala V, Vilana R, et al. Evaluation of hepatocellular carcinoma using SonoVue, a second generation ultrasound contrast agent: correlation with cellular differentiation. Eur Radiol 2004; 14:1092-1099.
197. Baron RL, Oliver 3rd JH, Dodd 3rd GD, et al. Hepatocellular carcinoma: evaluation with biphasic, contrast-enhanced, helical CT. Radiology 1996;199:505-511.
198. Johnson CD. Imaging of hepatocellular carcinoma. San Diego: American Roentgen Ray Society 96th Annual Meeting; 1996.
199. Bruix J, Sherman M. Management of hepatocellular carcinoma. Hepatology 2005;42:1208-1236.
200. Friedman AC, Lichtenstein JE, Goodman Z, et al. Fibrolamellar hepatocellular carcinoma. Radiology 1985;157:583-587.
201. Brandt DJ, Johnson CD, Stephens DH, Weiland LH. Imaging of fibrolamellar hepatocellular carcinoma. AJR Am J Roentgenol 1988;151:295-299.
202. Stevens WR, Johnson CD, Stephens DH, Nagorney DM. Fibrolamellar hepatocellular carcinoma: stage at presentation and results of aggressive surgical management. AJR Am J Roentgenol 1995;164:1153-1158.
203. Kanai T, Hirohashi S, Upton MP, et al. Pathology of small hepatocellular carcinoma: a proposal for a new gross classification. Cancer 1987;60:810-819.
204. Okuda K, Musha H, Nakajima Y, et al. Clinicopathologic features of encapsulated hepatocellular carcinoma: a study of 26 cases. Cancer 1977;40:1240-1245.
205. Mahony B, Jeffrey RB, Federle MP. Spontaneous rupture of hepatic and splenic angiosarcoma demonstrated by CT. AJR Am J Roentgenol 1982;138:965-966.
206. Fitzgerald EJ, Griffiths TM. Computed tomography of vinyl-chloride-induced angiosarcoma of liver. Br J Radiol 1987;60:593-595.
207. Furui S, Itai Y, Ohtomo K, et al. Hepatic epithelioid hemangioendothelioma: report of five cases. Radiology 1989;171:63-68.
208. Radin DR, Craig JR, Colletti PM, et al. Hepatic epithelioid hemangioendothelioma. Radiology 1988;169:145-148.
209. Oliver JH. Malignant hepatic neoplasms, excluding hepatocellular carcinoma and cholangiocarcinoma. San Diego: American Roentgen Ray Society 96th Annual Meeting; 1996.
210. Kane RA, Longmaid HE, Costello P, et al. Noninvasive imaging in patients with hepatic masses: a prospective comparison on ultrasound, CT and MR imaging (abstract). Radiological Society of North America Scientific Program, 1993.
211. Wernecke K, Vassallo P, Bick U, et al. The distinction between benign and malignant liver tumors on sonography: value of a hypoechoic halo. AJR Am J Roentgenol 1992;159:1005-1009.
212. Marchal GJ, Pylyser K, Tshibwabwa-Tumba EA, et al. Anechoic halo in solid liver tumors: sonographic, microangiographic, and histologic correlation. Radiology 1985;156:479-483.
213. Wernecke K, Henke L, Vassallo P, et al. Pathologic explanation for hypoechoic halo seen on sonograms of malignant liver tumors: an in vitro correlative study. AJR Am J Roentgenol 1992;159:1011-1016.
214. Kruskal JB, Thomas P, Nasser I, et al. Hepatic colon cancer metastases in mice: dynamic in vivo correlation with hypoechoic rims visible at ultrasound. Radiology 2000;215:852-857.
215. Rubaltelli L, Del Maschio A, Candiani F, Miotto D. The role of vascularization in the formation of echographic patterns of hepatic metastases: microangiographic and echographic study. Br J Radiol 1980;53:1166-1168.
216. Sanders LM, Botet JF, Straus DJ, et al. CT of primary lymphoma of the liver. AJR Am J Roentgenol 1989;152:973-976.
217. Townsend RR, Laing FC, Jeffrey Jr RB, Bottles K. Abdominal lymphoma in AIDS: evaluation with ultrasound. Radiology 1989;171:719-724.
218. Yoshida T, Matsue H, Okazaki N, Yoshino M. Ultrasonographic differentiation of hepatocellular carcinoma from metastatic liver cancer. J Clin Ultrasound 1987;15:431-437.
219. Bruneton JN, Ladree D, Caramella E, et al. Ultrasonographic study of calcified hepatic metastases: a report of 13 cases. Gastrointest Radiol 1982;7:61-63.
220. Wooten WB, Green B, Goldstein HM. Ultrasonography of necrotic hepatic metastases. Radiology 1978;128:1447-1450.
221. Federle MP, Filly RA, Moss AA. Cystic hepatic neoplasms: complementary roles of CT and sonography. AJR Am J Roentgenol 1981;136:345-348.
222. Murphy-Lavallee J, Jang HJ, Kim TK, et al. Are metastases really hypovascular in the arterial phase? The perspective based on contrast-enhanced ultrasonography. J Ultrasound Med 2007;26:1545-1556.
223. Nyberg DA, Federle MP. AIDS-related Kaposi sarcoma and lymphomas. Semin Roentgenol 1987;22:54-65.
224. Luburich P, Bru C, Ayuso MC, et al. Hepatic Kaposi sarcoma in AIDS: ultrasound and CT findings. Radiology 1990;175:172-174.
225. Towers MJ, Withers CE, Rachlis AR, et al. Ultrasound diagnosis of hepatic Kaposi sarcoma. J Ultrasound Med 1991;10:701-703.

Hepatic Trauma
226. Anderson CB, Ballinger WF. Abdominal injuries. In: Zuidema GD, Rutherford RB, Ballinger WF, editors. The management of trauma. 4th ed. Philadelphia: Saunders; 1985. p. 449-504.
227. Moon Jr KL, Federle MP. Computed tomography in hepatic trauma. AJR Am J Roentgenol 1983;141:309-314.
228. Foley WD, Cates JD, Kellman GM, et al. Treatment of blunt hepatic injuries: role of CT. Radiology 1987;164:635-638.
229. Van Sonnenberg E, Simeone JF, Mueller PR, et al. Sonographic appearance of hematoma in liver, spleen, and kidney: a clinical, pathologic, and animal study. Radiology 1983;147:507-510.
230. Grant EG, Tessler FN, Gomes AS, et al. Color Doppler imaging of portosystemic shunts. AJR Am J Roentgenol 1990;154:393-397.
231. Lafortune M, Patriquin H, Pomier G, et al. Hemodynamic changes in portal circulation after portosystemic shunts: use of duplex sonography in 43 patients. AJR Am J Roentgenol 1987;149:701-706.
232. Chezmar JL, Bernardino ME. Mesoatrial shunt for the treatment of Budd-Chiari syndrome: radiologic evaluation in eight patients. AJR Am J Roentgenol 1987;149:707-710.
233. Ralls PW, Lee KP, Mayekawa DS, et al. Color Doppler sonography of portocaval shunts. J Clin Ultrasound 1990;18:379-381.

234. Foley WD, Gleysteen JJ, Lawson TL, et al. Dynamic computed tomography and pulsed Doppler ultrasonography in the evaluation of splenorenal shunt patency. J Comput Assist Tomogr 1983;7:106-112.

235. Freedman AM, Sanyal AJ, Tisnado J, et al. Complications of transjugular intrahepatic portosystemic shunt: a comprehensive review. Radiographics 1993;13:1185-1210.

236. Kerlan Jr RK, LaBerge JM, Gordon RL, Ring EJ. Transjugular intrahepatic portosystemic shunts: current status. AJR Am J Roentgenol 1995;164:1059-1066.

237. LaBerge JM, Ring EJ, Gordon RL, et al. Creation of transjugular intrahepatic portosystemic shunts with the Wallstent endoprosthesis: results in 100 patients. Radiology 1993;187:413-420.

238. Haskal ZJ, Pentecost MJ, Soulen MC, et al. Transjugular intrahepatic portosystemic shunt stenosis and revision: early and midterm results. AJR Am J Roentgenol 1994;163:439-444.

239. Foshager MC, Ferral H, Nazarian GK, et al. Duplex sonography after transjugular intrahepatic portosystemic shunts (TIPS): normal hemodynamic findings and efficacy in predicting shunt patency and stenosis. AJR Am J Roentgenol 1995;165:1-7.

240. Haskal ZJ, Carroll JW, Jacobs JE, et al. Sonography of transjugular intrahepatic portosystemic shunts: detection of elevated portosystemic gradients and loss of shunt function. J Vasc Interv Radiol 1997;8:549-556.

241. Murphy TP, Beecham RP, Kim HM, et al. Long-term follow-up after TIPS: use of Doppler velocity criteria for detecting elevation of the portosystemic gradient. J Vasc Interv Radiol 1998;9:275-281.

242. Surratt RS, Middleton WD, Darcy MD, et al. Morphologic and hemodynamic findings at sonography before and after creation of a transjugular intrahepatic portosystemic shunt. AJR Am J Roentgenol 1993;160:627-630.

243. Chong WK, Malisch TA, Mazar MJ. Transjugular intrahepatic portosystemic shunts: ultrasound assessment with maximum flow velocity. Radiology 1993;189:789-793.

244. Dodd 3rd GD, Zajko AB, Orons PD, et al. Detection of transjugular intrahepatic portosystemic shunt dysfunction: value of duplex Doppler sonography. AJR Am J Roentgenol 1995;164:1119-1124.

245. Feldstein VA, LaBerge JM. Hepatic vein flow reversal at duplex sonography: a sign of transjugular intrahepatic portosystemic shunt dysfunction. AJR Am J Roentgenol 1994;162:839-841.

246. Kanterman RY, Darcy MD, Middleton WD, et al. Doppler sonography findings associated with transjugular intrahepatic portosystemic shunt malfunction. AJR Am J Roentgenol 1997;168:467-472.

Percutaneous Liver Biopsy

247. Charboneau JW, Reading CC, Welch TJ. CT and sonographically guided needle biopsy: current techniques and new innovations. AJR Am J Roentgenol 1990;154:1-10.

248. Downey DB, Wilson SR. Ultrasonographically guided biopsy of small intra-abdominal masses. Can Assoc Radiol J 1993;44:350-353.

249. Livraghi T, Festi D, Monti F, et al. Ultrasound-guided percutaneous alcohol injection of small hepatic and abdominal tumors. Radiology 1986;161:309-312.

250. Shiina S, Yasuda H, Muto H, et al. Percutaneous ethanol injection in the treatment of liver neoplasms. AJR Am J Roentgenol 1987;149:949-952.

Intraoperative Ultrasound

251. Rifkin MD, Rosato FE, Branch HM, et al. Intraoperative ultrasound of the liver: an important adjunctive tool for decision making in the operating room. Ann Surg 1987;205:466-472.

252. Parker GA, Lawrence Jr W, Horsley 3rd JS, et al. Intraoperative ultrasound of the liver affects operative decision making. Ann Surg 1989;209:569-576; discussion 576-577.

253. Leen E, Ceccotti P, Moug SJ, et al. Potential value of contrast-enhanced intraoperative ultrasonography during partial hepatectomy for metastases: an essential investigation before resection? Ann Surg 2006;243:236-240.

CHAPTER 5

The Spleen

Patrick M. Vos, John R. Mathieson, and Peter L. Cooperberg

Chapter Outline

*U*ltrasound is a very useful imaging modality to diagnose or exclude splenic abnormalities and is also extremely helpful in the follow-up of patients with known splenic abnormalities. Splenic lesions may be encountered in a variety of clinical settings, and the radiologist should be aware of the spectrum of processes that may involve the spleen as well as the clinical context in which they occur.[1]

The spleen and left upper quadrant (LUQ) should be routinely evaluated on all abdominal investigations, especially in patients with suspected splenomegaly, LUQ pain, or trauma. In general, the spleen can be examined by ultrasound without difficulty. Because the normal spleen is uniform in echogenicity, focal abnormalities stand out clearly. Similarly, perisplenic abnormalities and fluid collections are usually easily identified. Inadequate assessment of the spleen and surrounding structures is therefore relatively rare. Occasionally, because the spleen is located high in the LUQ, difficulties can be encountered. Shadowing from ribs, overlying bowel gas, and overlying lung can obscure visualization of the deeper structures. Expertise and persistence may be required to overcome these obstacles.

EMBRYOLOGY AND ANATOMY

The spleen arises from a mass of mesenchymal cells located between the layers of the **dorsal mesentery,** which connects the stomach to the posterior peritoneal surface over the aorta (Fig. 5-1, A). These mesenchymal cells differentiate to form the **splenic pulp,** the supporting connective tissue structures, and the **splenic capsule.** The **splenic artery** penetrates the primitive spleen, and arterioles branch through the connective tissue into the splenic sinusoids.

As the embryonic stomach rotates 90 degrees on its longitudinal axis, the spleen and dorsal mesentery are carried to the left along with the greater curvature of the stomach (Fig. 5-1, B). The base of the dorsal mesentery fuses with the posterior peritoneum over the left kidney, giving rise to the **splenorenal ligament.** This explains why, although the spleen is intraperitoneal, the splenic artery enters from the retroperitoneum through the splenorenal ligament (Fig. 5-1, C). In most adults, a portion of the splenic capsule is firmly attached to the fused dorsal mesentery anterior to the upper left kidney, giving rise to the **bare area** of the spleen.[2] The size of the splenic bare area varies but usually involves less than half the posterior splenic surface (Fig. 5-2). This anatomic feature is analogous to the bare area of the liver and can be helpful in distinguishing intraperitoneal from pleural fluid collections.

The normal adult spleen is convex superolaterally, is concave inferomedially, and has a homogeneous echo pattern. The spleen lies between the **fundus of the stomach** and the **diaphragm,** with its long axis in the line of the left 10th rib. The diaphragmatic surface is convex and is usually situated between the ninth and 11th ribs. The visceral or inferomedial surface has gentle indentations where it comes into contact with the stomach, left kidney, pancreas, and splenic flexure. The spleen is suspended by the splenorenal ligament, which is in contact with the **posterior peritoneal wall,** the **phrenicocolic ligament,** and the **gastrosplenic ligament.** The gastrosplenic ligament is composed of the two layers of the dorsal mesentery that separate the lesser sac posteriorly from the greater sac anteriorly.

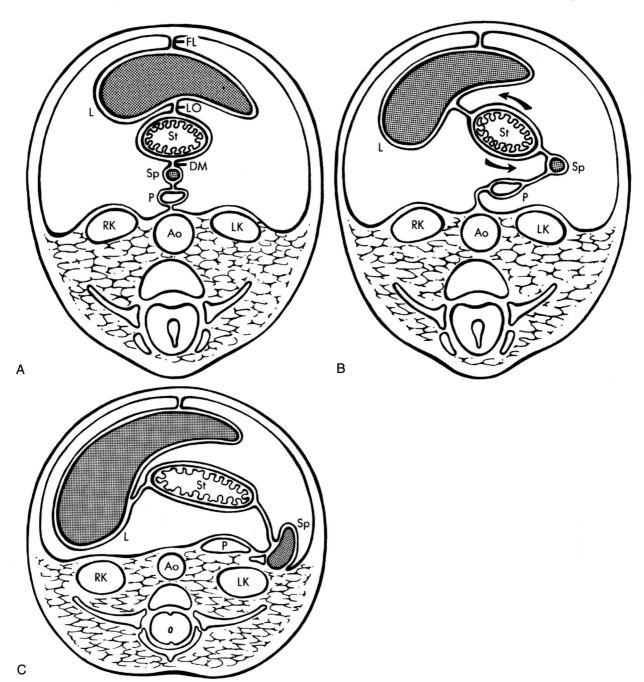

FIGURE 5-1. Embryologic development of the spleen. Schematic axial drawings of the upper abdomen. **A, Embryo: 4 to 5 weeks.** The mesentery anterior to the stomach *(St)* is the ventral mesentery. The ventral mesentery is divided into two portions by the liver *(L)* into the **falciform ligament** *(FL)* anteriorly and the **gastrohepatic ligament** or **lesser omentum** *(LO)* posteriorly. Posterior to the stomach is the **dorsal mesentery** *(DM)*, which contains the developing spleen *(Sp)* and pancreas *(P)*. The dorsal mesentery is divided into two portions by the spleen: the **splenogastric ligament** anteriorly and the **splenorenal ligament** posteriorly. The pancreas *(P)* has not yet become retroperitoneal and remains within the dorsal mesentery. *Ao,* Aorta; *RK,* right kidney; *LK,* left kidney. **B, Embryo: 8 weeks.** The stomach rotates counterclockwise, displacing the liver to the right and the spleen to the left. The portion of the dorsal mesentery containing the pancreas, splenic vessels, and spleen begins to fuse to the anterior retroperitoneal surface, giving rise to the splenogastric ligament and the "bare area" of the spleen. If fusion is incomplete, the spleen will be attached to the retroperitoneum only by a long mesentery, giving rise to a mobile or "wandering" spleen. **C, Newborn.** Fusion of the dorsal mesentery is now complete. The pancreas is now completely retroperitoneal, and a portion of the spleen has fused with the retroperitoneum. Note the close relation of the pancreatic tail to the splenic hilum.

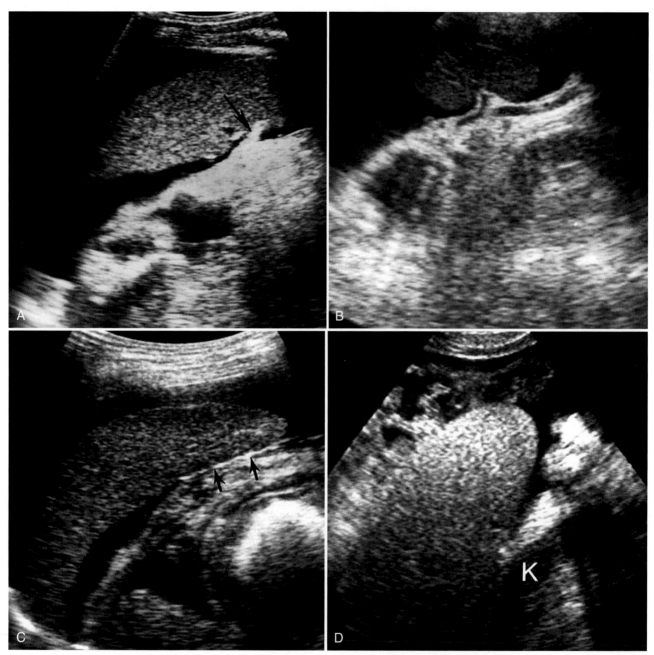

FIGURE 5-2. Bare area of the spleen. Variability in the relationship of the spleen to the anterior retroperitoneal surface is demonstrated in patients with ascites. **A,** This spleen has **no bare area**. The splenorenal ligament *(arrow)* is outlined on both sides by ascitic fluid. **B,** Part of the lower pole of the spleen is fused posteriorly. **C,** Lower pole is fused to the retroperitoneum *(arrows)*. **D,** Large proportion of this patient's spleen is fused posteriorly. Note the close relation of the spleen to the left kidney *(K)*.

Its weight is related to the patient's age and gender; the spleen usually weighs less than 150 g on autopsy (range, 80-300 g).[3] The spleen decreases in size and weight with advancing age and is smaller in women. It also increases slightly during digestion and can vary in size according to the nutritional status of the body.

Splenic functions include phagocytosis, fetal hematopoiesis, adult lymphopoiesis, immune response, and erythrocyte storage.

The spleen may be congenitally absent. Under a variety of conditions, including surgical misadventure, the spleen also may be removed. Currently, the surgical trend is toward preservation of the spleen whenever possible.[4] A person can live fully without a spleen. However, particularly in childhood, the immune response may be impaired, especially to encapsulated bacteria. Overwhelming postsplenectomy **sepsis** is a long-term risk in asplenic patients, and appropriate preventive measures should be taken to minimize this risk.[5,6]

SONOGRAPHIC TECHNIQUE

All routine abdominal sonographic examinations, regardless of the indications, should include at least one **coronal view** of the spleen and the upper pole of the left kidney. The most common and easy approach to visualize the spleen is to maintain the patient in the supine position and place the transducer in the coronal plane of section posteriorly in one of the lower left intercostal spaces. The patient can then be examined in various degrees of inspiration to maximize the window to the spleen. Deep inspiration introduces air into the lung in the lateral costophrenic angle and may obscure visualization. A modest inspiration depresses the central portion of the left hemidiaphragm and spleen inferiorly so that they can be visualized. The plane of section should then be swept posteriorly and anteriorly to view the entire volume of the spleen. We generally find that a thorough examination in the **coronal plane** of section is highly accurate for excluding any lesion within or around the spleen and for documenting the spleen's approximate size.

If an abnormality is discovered within or around the spleen, other planes of section should be used. An **oblique plane** of section along the intercostal space can avoid rib shadowing (Fig. 5-3). In some patients with narrow intercostal spaces, however, intercostal scanning can be difficult. A **transverse plane** from a lateral, usually intercostal, approach may help to localize a lesion within the spleen anteriorly or posteriorly. In this regard, especially for beginners, it must be emphasized that the *apex of the sector image is always placed at the top of the screen.* However, on a left lateral intercostal transverse image, the top of the screen—the apex of the sector—is actually to the patient's left; the right side of the sector image is posterior, and the left side of the image is anterior. To look at the image appropriately, the clinician would have to rotate it 90 degrees clockwise.

If the spleen is not enlarged and is not surrounded by a large mass, scanning from an anterior position—as one would for imaging the liver—is not helpful because of the interposition of gas within the stomach and the splenic flexure of the colon. However, if the patient has a relatively large liver, or spleen, the spleen may be visualized from an anterior approach (Fig. 5-4). If there is free intraperitoneal fluid around the spleen or a left pleural effusion, the spleen may be better visualized from an anterolateral approach. Often, it is beneficial to have the patient roll onto the right side as much as 45 degrees, or even 90 degrees, so that a more posterior approach can be used to visualize the spleen.

Generally, the same curvilinear transducers and technical settings are used for examination of the spleen as for the other abdominal organs. A high-frequency linear array transducer can be used for more detail. Advanced ultrasound imaging modalities such as harmonic and compound imaging are used to improve image quality and detect subtle lesions.

The use of contrast-enhanced ultrasound (CEUS) is increasing both in research and clinical settings. Multiple reports have recently described CEUS of the spleen and its characterization of splenic lesions.[7,8] However, its role in general practice is yet to be determined.

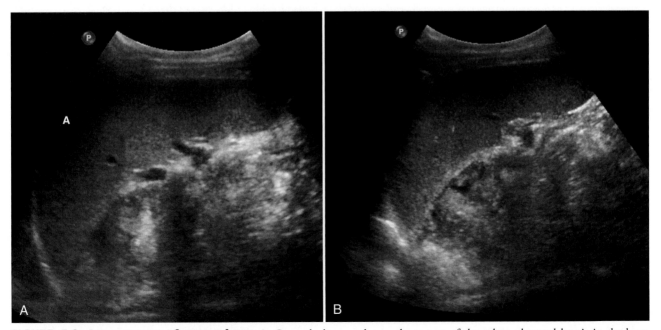

FIGURE 5-3. Importance of scan plane. A, Coronal ultrasound scan shows part of the spleen obscured by air in the lung. **B,** Improved visualization of the spleen on coronal oblique scan aligned with the 10th interspace between the ribs.

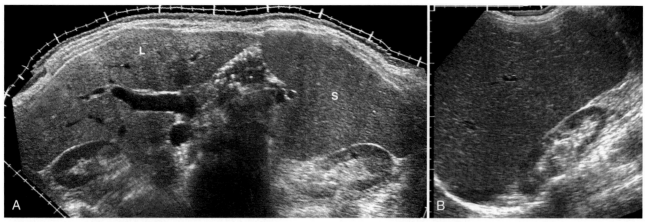

FIGURE 5-4. Splenomegaly. A, Transverse, and **B,** coronal extended–field of view (FOV) (Siescape), images demonstrate marked splenic *(S)* enlargement; *L,* liver.

SONOGRAPHIC APPEARANCE

The shape of the normal spleen is variable. The spleen consists of **two components** joined at the hilum: a **superomedial** component and an **inferolateral** component. More superiorly, on transverse scanning, the spleen has a typical fat, "inverted comma" shape, with a thin component extending anteriorly and another component extending medially, either superior to or adjacent to the upper pole of the kidney. This second component (superomedial) can be seen to indent the gastric fundus on plain films of the abdomen or in barium studies. As the scan plane moves inferiorly, only the inferior component of the spleen is seen. This component (inferolateral) can be outlined by a thin rim of fat above the splenic flexure, as seen on a plain abdominal film. It may extend inferiorly to the costal margin and present clinically as a palpable spleen. However, either the superomedial or the inferolateral component can enlarge independently, without enlargement of the other component.

It is important to recognize the **normal structures** that are related to the spleen. The diaphragm cradles the spleen posteriorly, superiorly, and laterally. The left liver lobe may extend into the left upper quadrant superior and lateral to the spleen (Fig. 5-5). The fundus of the stomach and lesser sac are medial and anterior to the splenic hilum. The gastric fundus may contain gas or fluid, which should not be confused with a fluid collection. The tail of the pancreas lies posterior to the stomach and lesser sac. It approaches the hilum of the spleen, closely related to the splenic artery and vein. Consequently, the spleen can be used as a "window" to evaluate the pancreatic tail area. The left kidney generally lies inferior and medial to the spleen. A useful landmark in identifying the spleen and splenic hilum is the **splenic vein,** which generally can be demonstrated without difficulty.

The normal splenic **parenchyma** is homogeneous. The liver is generally considered to be more echogenic than the spleen, but in fact the echogenicity of the parenchyma is higher in the spleen than in the liver. Using a dual-image setting, the operator may compare the echogenicity of these two organs. The impression that the liver has greater echogenicity results from its large number of reflective vessels.

As in measuring other body structures, it is helpful to have measurements that establish the **upper limits of normal.** The size of a normal spleen depends on gender, age, and body-height. The range of the "normal sized" adult spleen, combined with its complex three-dimensional shape, makes it difficult to establish a normal range of sonographic measurements. Ideally, the clinician would assess splenic **volume** or **weight.** Techniques have been developed to measure serial sections of the spleen by planimetry and then compute the volume of the spleen by adding the values for each section.[9] However, these techniques are cumbersome and not popular. The most frequently used method is "eyeballing" the size (Fig. 5-6; see also Fig. 5-4). Unfortunately, this method of assessment requires considerably more experience than is necessary for other imaging techniques and is relatively inaccurate. Various authors have used different methods to measure splenic size. The length of the spleen measured on a coronal or coronal oblique view that includes the hilum is the most common technique[10,11] (Fig. 5-7). This view can be obtained during deep inspiration or quiet breathing. Importantly, this method correlates well with the splenic volume, particularly when performed with the patient in the **right lateral decubitus** (RLD) position.[11]

Multiple studies have tried to establish nomograms of spleen size. In a study of 703 normal adults, the **length** of the spleen was less than 11 cm, the **width** (breadth) less than 7 cm, and the **thickness** less than 5 cm in 95% of patients.[12] Rosenberg et al.[10] established an upper limit of normal splenic length of 12 cm for girls and 13 cm for boys (≥15 years). Hosey et al.[13] demonstrated

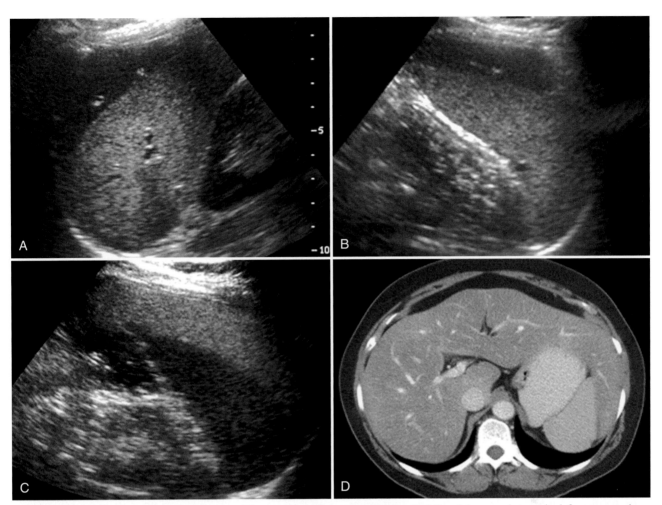

FIGURE 5-5. Relationship of spleen with surrounding structures. Left liver lobe extends into the left upper quadrant superior to the spleen. **A,** Coronal and **B,** transverse, sonograms demonstrate the left liver lobe superior to the spleen. The liver is hypoechoic compared with the spleen. **C** and **D,** Liver extends over spleen in a different patient with a fatty liver. **C,** Transverse sonogram shows an echogenic liver and a relatively hypoechoic spleen. **D,** Axial CT image shows the left liver lobe draping around the spleen.

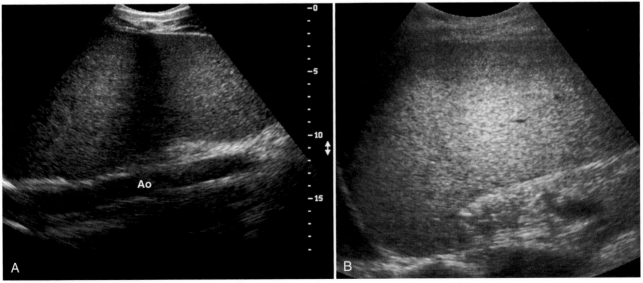

FIGURE 5-6. Splenomegaly in two patients. A, Coronal ultrasound scan shows an enlarged spleen with margins beyond the sector format. Midportion is partially obscured by a rib shadow. *Ao,* Aorta. **B,** Increased echogenicity of a large spleen.

Longitudinal section

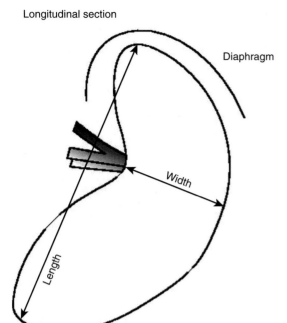

FIGURE 5-7. Splenic measurement. Diagram shows sonographic approach to measuring splenic length and width. Splenic size is best measured by obtaining a coronal view that includes the hilum. (From Lamb PM, Lund A, Kanagasabay RR, et al. Spleen size: how well do linear ultrasound measurements correlate with three-dimensional CT volume assessments? Br J Radiol 2002;75:573-577.)

TABLE 5-1. CAUSES OF SPLENOMEGALY

Splenomegaly (<18 cm)	Massive Splenomegaly (>18 cm)
HEMATOLOGIC	
Red blood cell membrane defects	Thalassemia major
Hemoglobinopathies	
Autoimmune hemolytic anemias	
RHEUMATOLOGIC	
Rheumatoid arthritis	
Systemic lupus erythematosus	
Sarcoidosis	
INFECTIOUS	
Viruses	Visceral leishmaniasis
Bacteria	Hyperreactive malarial
Mycobacteria	splenomegaly syndrome
Fungi	*Mycobacterium avium-*
Parasites	*intracellulare* complex
CONGESTIVE	
Hepatic cirrhosis	
Venous thromboses (hepatic, portal, splenic)	
Congestive heart failure	
INFILTRATIVE	
Lymphomas	Lymphomas
Myeloproliferative neoplasms	Myeloproliferative neoplasms
Metastatic cancer	Gaucher's disease
Amyloidosis	
Gaucher's disease	
Niemann-Pick disease	
Glycogen storage disease	
Hemophagocytic syndrome	
Langerhans cell histiocytosis	

Data from Pozo AL, Godfrey EM, Bowles KM. Splenomegaly: investigation, diagnosis and management. Blood Rev 2009;23:105-111; and from Abramson JS, Chatterji M, Rahemtullah A. Case records of the Massachusetts General Hospital. Case 39-2008. A 51-year-old woman with splenomegaly and anemia. N Engl J Med. 2008 Dec 18;359:2707-2718.

a mean splenic length of 10.65 cm. In this study, men also had larger spleens than women. Spielmann et al.[14] showed that the length of the spleen correlates with height and established nomograms for tall, healthy athletes. In women taller than 5 feet, 6 inches (168 cm), the mean splenic length of 10 cm increased by 0.1 cm for each 1-inch incremental increase in height. In men taller than 6 ft (180 cm), the mean splenic length of 11 cm increased by 0.2 cm for each 1-inch incremental increase in height. Upper limits of normal in splenic length were 14 cm in women 6 ft, 6 inches (198 cm) tall and 16.3 cm in men 7 ft (213 cm) tall. Finally, unlike patient height, Kaneko et al.[15] did not show correlation of splenic volume with patient weight or body surface area in adults.

PATHOLOGIC CONDITIONS

Splenomegaly

The differential diagnosis of splenomegaly is exceedingly long. It includes **infection** (e.g., mononucleosis, tuberculosis, malaria), **hematologic disorders** (myelofibrosis, lymphoma, leukemia), **congestion** (portal hypertension, portal/splenic vein thrombosis, congestive heart failure), **inflammation** (sarcoidosis), **neoplasia** (hemangioma, metastases), and **infiltration** (e.g., Gaucher's disease)[16] (Table 5-1).

Frequency and etiology of splenomegaly vary between developing and developed countries and even between hospitals in the same region.[17] Sonography is very helpful in determining the degree of enlargement. In "borderline" splenomegaly, however, diagnosis can be difficult. Useful dimensions are provided in the previous section (see Figs. 5-6 and 5-7).

The spleen is capable of growing to an enormous size. It can extend inferiorly into the left iliac fossa, and it can cross the midline and appear as a mass inferior to the left lobe of the liver on longitudinal section. The degree of splenomegaly is generally not a reliable tool in providing a more concise differential diagnosis. The differential diagnosis of **massive splenomegaly,** defined as a spleen size greater than 18 cm, is less extensive and includes hematologic disorders and infections[18] (Table 5-1). Sonographic assessment of the splenic architecture is used to differentiate between **focal** lesions (single or multiple) causing splenomegaly and **diffuse** splenomegaly.

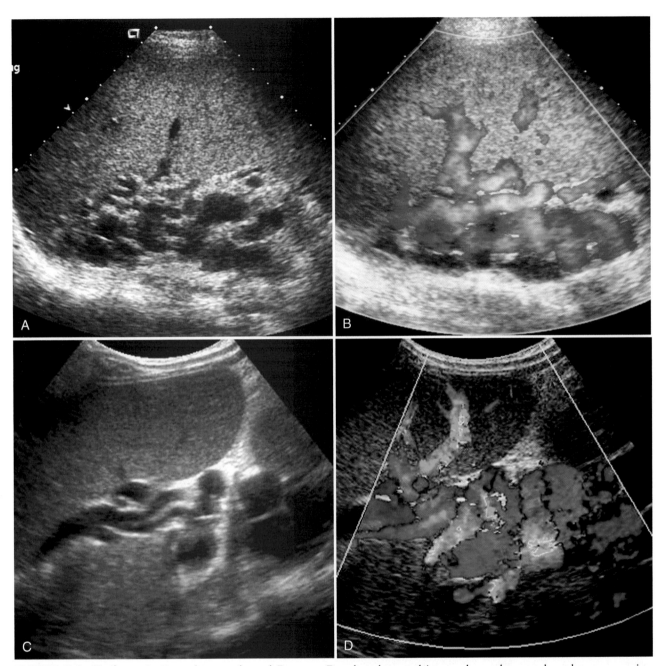

FIGURE 5-8. Varices. A, Coronal gray-scale, and **B,** power Doppler, ultrasound images show splenomegaly and tortuous varices medial to the spleen. **C** and **D,** Varices medial and inferior to the spleen representing a splenorenal shunt.

The most common finding is diffuse enlargement; in these patients, imaging is typically not helpful in providing a specific diagnosis. When the spleen enlarges, it can become more echogenic, but the clinician cannot differentiate between the different types of splenomegaly on the basis of its echogenicity (see Fig. 5-6, *B*). Experimental studies have tried to quantify the degree of fibrosis in liver and spleen using the echotexture characteristics, but no clinical applications have been established to date.[19]

Associated clinical and radiologic features can be helpful in establishing a differential diagnosis. Liver disease and evidence of portal venous collaterals can establish **portal hypertension** as the cause of spleno-megaly (Fig. 5-8). Focal lesions, multiorgan involvement, and lymphadenopathy may indicate **lymphoma.**

However, in many patients, extensive radiologic and laboratory investigations will fail to yield a diagnosis. In these cases of "isolated" splenomegaly, the risks of serious underlying disease must be balanced against the risks of further invasive investigations, such as diagnostic splenic biopsy or splenectomy.[16] In selected cases, ultrasound-guided splenic biopsy of focal abnormalities can be helpful in establishing a diagnosis, with an acceptable complication rate and high accuracy.[20]

Complications of splenomegaly include **hypersplen-ism** and **spontaneous splenic rupture.** Spontaneous splenic rupture typically occurs in patients with an enlarged spleen after minimal trauma or insignificant events such as coughing.[21]

Focal Abnormalities

Ultrasound is extremely helpful in finding and characterizing focal splenic lesions. However, because of the overlap in the appearance of splenic lesions, it is often not possible to make a specific diagnosis based on the sonographic findings alone. Splenic lesions can be solitary or multiple, diffuse, and infiltrative. Focal lesions can be cystic, complex cystic, or solid. Further, lesions can be categorized according to size as **micronodular** (<1 cm), **nodular** (1-3 cm), or **focal** (>3 cm) masses.[22] Knowledge of past medical history, clinical presentation, and sonographic findings is required to provide an appropriate

differential diagnosis and guide further management.[23] Ultimately, percutaneous biopsy or splenectomy may be required to obtain a definitive diagnosis.

Splenic Cysts

Splenic cysts, as with cysts elsewhere in the body, appear as anechoic lesions with posterior acoustic enhancement. Simple cysts are round to ovoid in shape and have a thin, sharply defined wall. **Complex cysts** do not meet these criteria and may demonstrate septations, thick walls, calcifications, solid components, or internal echoes.

Occasionally, cysts can grow to a very large size, becoming predominantly **exophytic.** It may then be difficult to appreciate their splenic origin (Fig. 5-9).

The most common splenic cystic lesions are primary congenital cysts, pseudocysts, and hydatid cysts. Uncom-

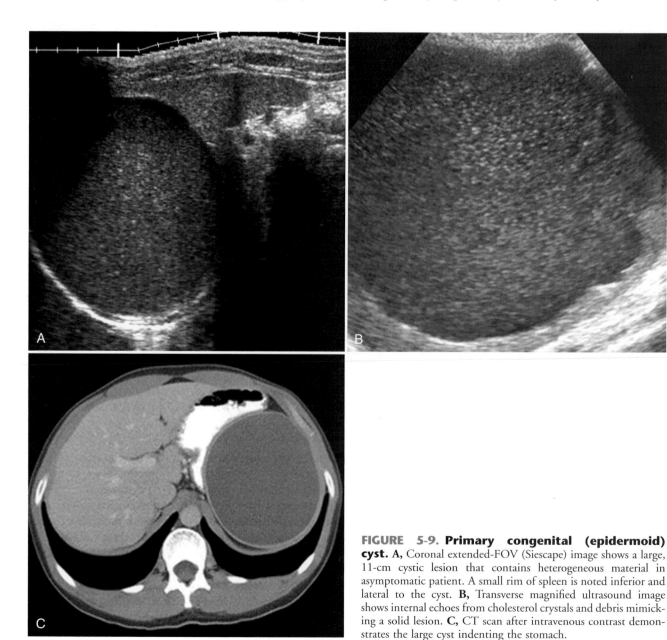

FIGURE 5-9. Primary congenital (epidermoid) cyst. A, Coronal extended-FOV (Siescape) image shows a large, 11-cm cystic lesion that contains heterogeneous material in asymptomatic patient. A small rim of spleen is noted inferior and lateral to the cyst. **B,** Transverse magnified ultrasound image shows internal echoes from cholesterol crystals and debris mimicking a solid lesion. **C,** CT scan after intravenous contrast demonstrates the large cyst indenting the stomach.

mon splenic cystic lesions include pancreatic pseudocysts, lymphangiomas, hemangiomas, peliosis, hamartomas, angiosarcomas, and cystic metastases.[24] Other lesions that can mimic cysts on ultrasound are abscesses, lymphoma, necrotic metastases and hematomas.[25]

TYPES OF SPLENIC CYSTS

Congenital cysts
Pseudocysts
Hydatid (echinococcal) cysts
Pancreatic pseudocysts
Endothelial-lined cysts
   Lymphangiomas
   Cystic hemangiomas
Peliosis
Cystic metastasis*
Abscess*
Hematoma*

*Not true cysts.

In the developed world, most splenic cysts are asymptomatic incidental findings discovered during routine imaging and generally represent congenital cysts or pseudocysts. These cysts may cause symptoms when large or when present with complications such as internal hemorrhage, infection, or rupture.

Primary congenital cysts, also called **epidermoid cysts** or **true cysts,** are characterized by the presence of an epithelial lining on pathologic examination.[26] Thought to arise from embryonic rests of primitive mesothelial cells within the spleen, typical epidermoid cysts present as well-defined, thin-walled anechoic lesions that do not change over time (Fig. 5-10, *A*). **Pseudocysts,** also known as **false cysts,** have no cellular lining and are presumably secondary to trauma, infarct, or infection.[27] These cysts are more often complex, with wall calcifications and internal echoes (Fig. 5-10, *B*). However, *differentiation between both types of cysts is usually not possible* because there is considerable overlap both on imaging and on pathologic examination[28] (Fig. 5-10, *C*). Furthermore, a history of significant trauma or

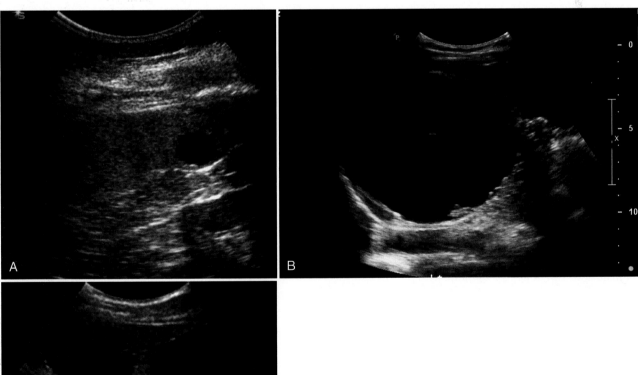

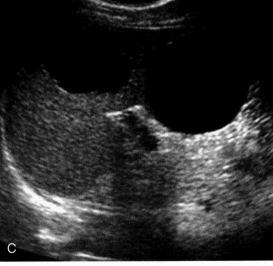

FIGURE 5-10. Splenic cysts in three patients. A, Primary congenital cyst. Coronal scan showing a small, simple 1.5-cm cyst. **B, Pseudocyst.** Large, 12-cm complex cyst after previous trauma to the left upper quadrant. **C, Two incidental cysts** in asymptomatic female. Central 5-cm cyst with irregular borders and a simple 6-cm cyst at the inferior portion of the spleen. Both congenital cysts and pseudocysts may have this appearance.

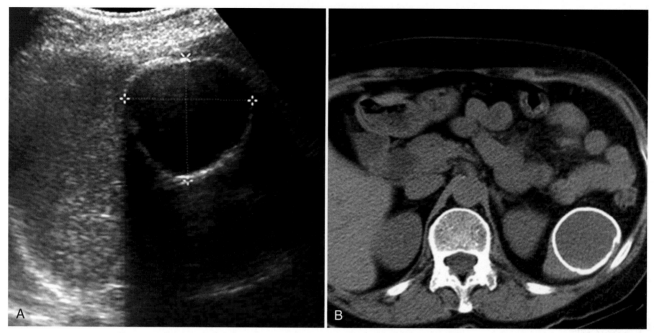

FIGURE 5-11. Calcified splenic cyst. A, Coronal ultrasound scan. Note the shadowing from the near wall. **B,** Non-contrast-enhanced CT scan demonstrates the wall calcification. Congenital cysts, pseudocysts, and "burned out" hydatid cysts may have similar appearance.

infection is rarely established in patients with a pseudocyst. Both types of cysts can be complex, with wall calcifications or increased echogenicity of the fluid caused by cholesterol crystals, inflammatory debris, or hemorrhage[29] (Fig. 5-11; see also Fig. 5-9).

Hydatid (or **echinococcal**) **disease** is the most common cause of splenic cysts in endemic areas. Isolated splenic involvement without liver and peritoneal disease is rare.[30] The appearance of a hydatid cyst depends on the stage of the disease and varies from simple to complex, with or without daughter cysts (Fig. 5-12). The diagnosis is made by combining the appropriate history, geographic background, serologic testing, and imaging appearances.[31,32] Percutaneous fine-needle aspiration can be diagnostic, provided the pathologist has been alerted to search for the scolices.

Pseudocysts related to **pancreatitis** in or adjacent to the spleen are usually diagnosed by the associated features of pancreatitis.[33] Splenic **peliosis** is very rare and characterized by multiple blood-filled cystic spaces, sometimes involving the entire spleen.[34] On ultrasound, these lesions appear as multiple indistinct hypoechoic lesions. The lesions may be hyperechoic if thrombosis is present.

Endothelial-lined cysts include lymphangiomas and cystic hemangiomas.[35,36] **Lymphangiomas** have been described as multiple cysts of varying size, ranging from a few millimeters to several centimeters, divided by thin septa.[37] **Hemangiomas** with cystic spaces of variable size have been reported.

Cystic metastases to the spleen are typically seen in patients with widespread metastatic disease, such as

ovarian or colon carcinoma. Occasionally, necrotic metastases mimic a cystic lesion.

The most common causes of **splenic abscess** are endocarditis, septicemia, and trauma.[38] Splenic pyogenic abscesses may have an appearance similar to that of simple cysts, but the diagnosis is typically made in conjunction with the clinical findings. The presence of gas indicates an infectious cause. Gas may cause a confusing picture if only a small, curvilinear or punctate hyperechoic focus is seen. The presence of a reverberation artifact (dirty shadowing) indicates the presence of gas (Fig. 5-13). However, the sonographic findings of a pyogenic abscess are variable, and in indeterminate cases, aspiration is useful for diagnosis.[39] Percutaneous catheter drainage can be used as a safe and successful treatment option.[40]

Nodular Splenic Lesions

Nodular lesions are often multiple and can be subdivided into micronodular (<1 cm) and nodular (1-3 cm). If splenic nodules are present in a patient with a known diagnosis such as lymphoma, tuberculosis, or sarcoidosis, these nodules likely represent the same disease. However, if no diagnosis has been established and the splenic nodules are an isolated finding, the diagnosis is rarely made on the imaging features alone. Most common etiologies of splenic nodules include infection (e.g., mycobacteria, histoplasmosis), sarcoidosis, and malignancy (e.g., lymphoma, metastases). Other, less common causes of splenic nodular lesions with similar imaging findings include Gamna-Gandy bodies, *Pneumocystis jir-*

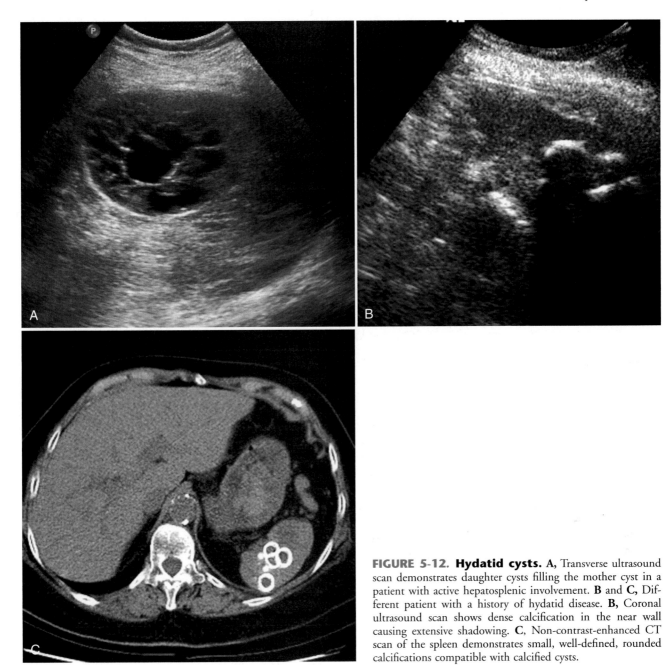

FIGURE 5-12. Hydatid cysts. A, Transverse ultrasound scan demonstrates daughter cysts filling the mother cyst in a patient with active hepatosplenic involvement. **B** and **C,** Different patient with a history of hydatid disease. **B,** Coronal ultrasound scan shows dense calcification in the near wall causing extensive shadowing. **C,** Non-contrast-enhanced CT scan of the spleen demonstrates small, well-defined, rounded calcifications compatible with calcified cysts.

oveci (formerly known as *P. carinii* pneumonia) and cat-scratch disease.[41-43]

Active **tuberculosis** involving the spleen is typically seen in miliary dissemination and can occur with both tuberculosis and atypical mycobacterial infections. The typical sonographic findings are multiple hypoechoic nodules 0.2 to 1 cm in size (Fig. 5-14). Sometimes the nodules are hyperechoic or present as larger, echo-poor or cystic lesions representing tuberculous abscesses (Figs. 5-15 and 5-16).

When the nodules or granulomas heal, they can be become calcified and appear as small, scattered, discrete, bright echogenic lesions with posterior shadowing in an otherwise normal spleen (Fig. 5-17). These probably are the most frequently encountered nodular splenic lesions. Splenic artery calcifications are also common and should not be confused with a granuloma (Fig. 5-18).

Microabscesses are typically seen in immunocompromised patients with generalized infections. They often coexist in the liver and spleen and are similar in appearance. Microabscesses usually present as multiple hypoechoic nodules (Fig. 5-19, *A*). In **hepatosplenic candidiasis** the two most common sonographic patterns are hypoechoic nodules and hyperechoic foci 2 to 5 mm in size, occasionally containing central calcification. Two other sonographic patterns have also been described. In the **wheels-within-wheels** appearance the outer hypoechoic "wheel" is thought to represent a ring of

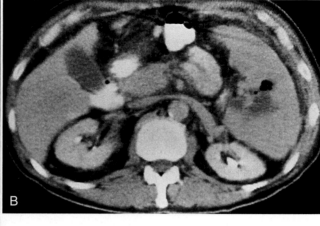

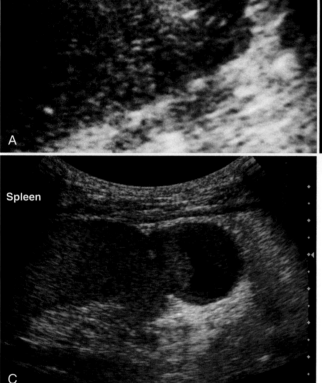

FIGURE 5-13. **Splenic abscess. A,** Coronal sonogram shows a gas collection with "dirty shadowing" *(arrowhead).* **B,** Confirmatory CT scan confirms the presence of gas and fluid within the spleen. **C,** Methicillin-resistant *Staphylococcus aureus* (MRSA) abscess in a different patient with endocarditis and septic emboli shows a complex cystic structure.

CAUSES OF SPLENIC NODULES

INFECTIOUS
Tuberculosis/*Mycobacterium avium-intracellulare*
  complex
Pyogenic abscesses
Histoplasmosis
Candida abscesses
Cat-scratch disease
Pneumocystis jiroveci (formerly *P. carinii* pneumonia)

INFLAMMATORY
Sarcoidosis

MALIGNANT
Lymphoma
Metastases

OTHER
Gamna-Gandy bodies
Gaucher's disease

fibrosis surrounding the inner echogenic "wheel" of inflammatory cells and a central hypoechoic, necrotic area.[44] The **bull's-eye** appearance consists of echogenic inflammatory cells in the center surrounded by a hypoechoic fibrotic outer rim[45] (Fig. 5-19, *B*).

Lymphoma and **metastatic disease** can also present with a small, diffuse nodular pattern, especially Hodgkin's disease and low-grade non-Hodgkin's lymphoma[46] (see Fig. 5-20, *A*).

Focal Solid Splenic Lesions

Malignancies. The spleen is frequently involved in patients with **lymphoma.** Patients with lymphomatous involvement of the spleen often present with associated abdominal lymphadenopathy and constitutional symptoms. In **Hodgkin's disease,** splenic enlargement occurs in 30% to 40% of patients, but in one third of these patients there is no lymphomatous involvement of the spleen at histopathology. Conversely, one third of patients with Hodgkin's disease and splenic involvement have a normal-sized spleen. In **non-Hodgkin's lymphoma** the spleen is involved in 40% of patients during the course of their disease. **Four sonographic patterns** of lymphomatous involvement of the spleen have been described,[47] corresponding with the pathologic findings: (1) diffuse involvement, typically an enlarged spleen with a normal echotexture or patchy inhomogeneity; (2) focal small (<3 cm) hypoechoic nodular lesions; (3) focal large (>3 cm) nodular lesions; and (4) bulky solid mass lesions (Fig. 5-20). Focal lesions in lymphoma are typically hypoechoic and hypovascular.[25] Occasionally, after

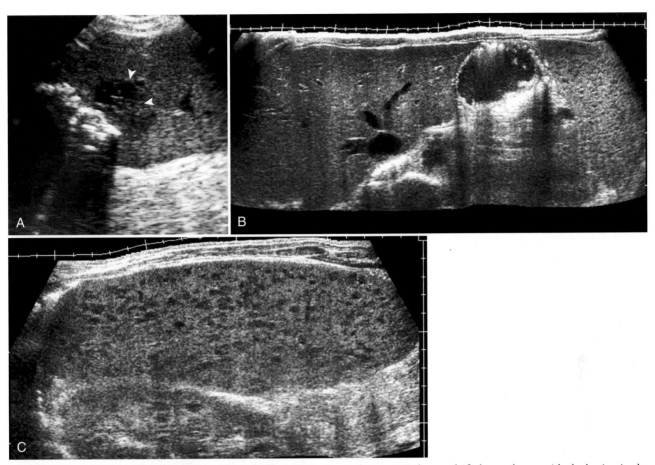

FIGURE 5-14. Tuberculosis (TB) in two patients. A, Coronal sonogram shows calcified granulomas with shadowing in the superior aspect of the spleen, and echo-poor lesions *(arrowheads)* in the midportion resulting from reactivated TB. **B,** Transverse, and **C,** coronal extended-FOV (Siescape), images in a young AIDS patient with active miliary TB. Numerous tiny hypoechoic nodules are present throughout the enlarged spleen.

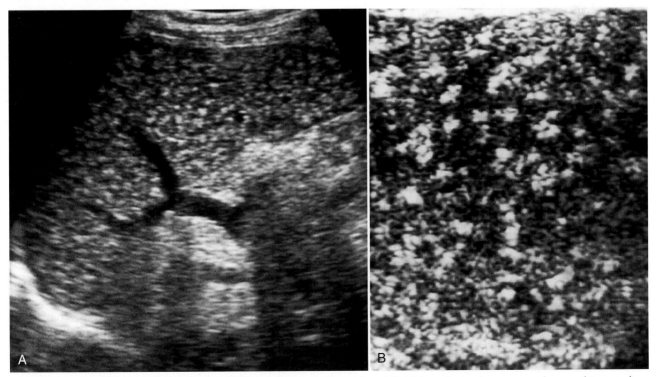

FIGURE 5-15. Miliary tuberculosis of the spleen. A, Coronal, and **B,** high-resolution linear array, ultrasound images show multiple tiny echogenic foci of tuberculous granulomata. This was active TB.

central necrosis with subsequent liquefaction, lesions may present as anechoic cysts or mimic an abscess.[48] Hyperechoic lesions are uncommon.

Primary splenic malignancies include primary lymphoma, angiosarcoma, and hemangiopericytoma. **Isolated (primary) lymphoma** of the spleen is rare and is encountered in less than 1% of all patients with lymphoma. It typically represents Hodgkin's disease.[46] **Angiosarcoma** is a rare primary malignant vascular neo-plasm of the spleen with a very poor prognosis. Sonographic findings include a heterogeneous echotexture, complex mass or masses, and splenomegaly (Fig. 5-21). Increased Doppler flow may be seen in the solid components of the tumor.[49,50] **Hemangiopericytoma** is a very rare tumor that may arise in the spleen with variable malignant potential. On ultrasound, it may appear as a hypoechoic vascular mass distinct from the surrounding splenic parenchyma.[34]

Metastases to the spleen are relatively rare and generally occur as a late phenomenon. They are typically seen

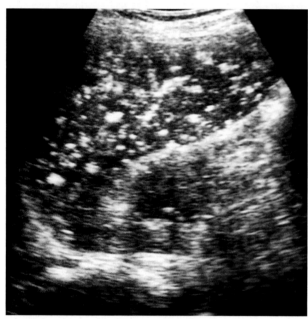

FIGURE 5-16. Atypical tuberculosis of the spleen in AIDS patient. Tiny echogenic foci throughout the spleen. Isolated foci were also identified in the liver and kidneys. Several core biopsies through the liver confirmed these to be *Mycobacterium avium-intracellulare* granulomas. Disseminated *Pneumocystis jiroveci*, formerly *P. carinii* pneumonia (PCP), can also appear in this way.

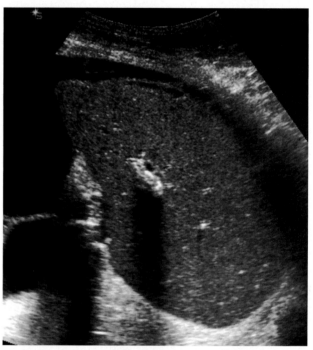

FIGURE 5-18. Calcifications. Central splenic artery calcifications in a patient on peritoneal dialysis.

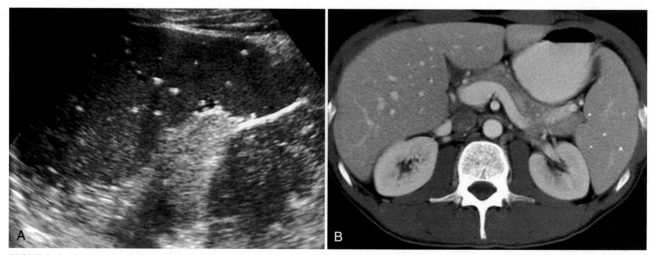

FIGURE 5-17. Calcified granulomas in a patient with sarcoidosis. A, Multiple tiny bright foci throughout the spleen, some demonstrating posterior shadowing. **B,** CT scan after IV contrast shows multiple small parenchymal calcifications throughout the spleen.

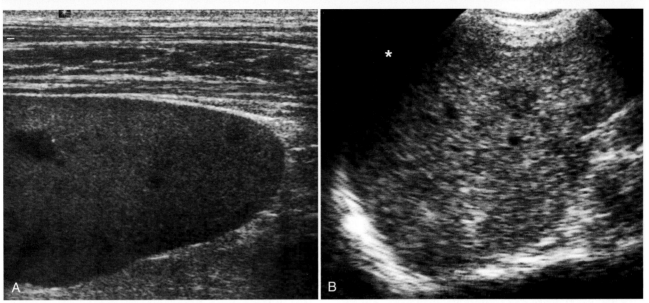

FIGURE 5-19. Microabscesses in two patients. A, High-frequency linear array ultrasound image shows multiple poorly defined microabscesses in a patient with *Klebsiella* septicemia. **B,** *Candida* abscesses of the spleen in an AIDS patient. Note that lesion in the middle has an echogenic center, characteristic of *Candida*.

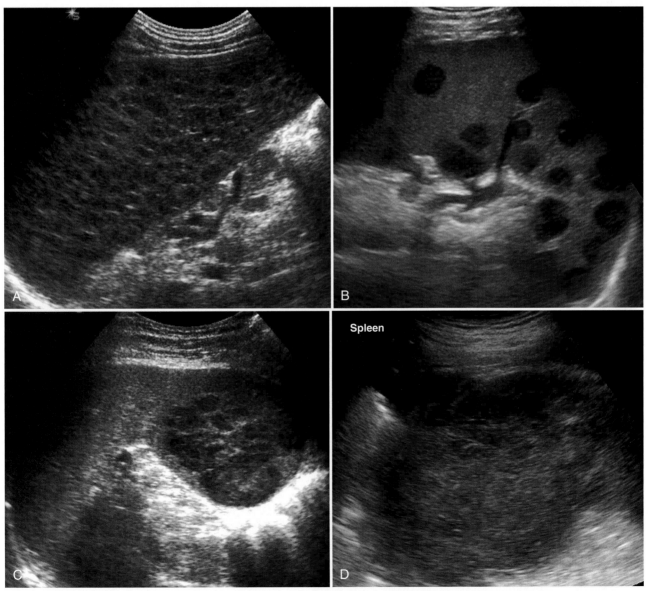

FIGURE 5-20. Patterns of lymphoma in different patients. A, Numerous small nodules resulting from T-cell lymphoma in an enlarged spleen. **B,** Multiple solid nodules in a patient with follicular lymphoma. **C,** Bulky solid mass in a patient with non-Hodgkin's lymphoma. **D,** Large, poorly defined mass caused by B-cell lymphoma replacing the spleen and extending beyond the normal contour. Lymphoma may also involve the spleen diffusely without focal abnormalities.

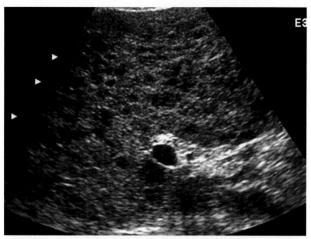

FIGURE 5-21. Primary splenic malignancy: angio-sarcoma. Transverse scan shows multiple poorly defined hypoechoic lesions. Other sonographic findings include a heterogeneous echotexture, complex masses, and splenomegaly.

in patients with widespread metastatic disease rather than as a presenting feature.[51] Isolated metastases to the spleen are very uncommon. Splenic metastases are relatively frequent in **malignant melanoma** but can be encountered in any metastatic disease, including carcinoma of the lung, breast, ovary, stomach, colon and in Kaposi's sarcoma.[52] Metastases are usually hypoechoic but may be echogenic, heterogeneous, or even cystic[1] (Fig. 5-22).

Benign Lesions. Hemangioma is the most common primary benign neoplasm of the spleen, incidence ranges from 0.3% to 14% in autopsy series.[53] Hemangiomas are usually isolated phenomena but can be part of a generalized condition, such as hemangiomatosis or Klippel-Trenaunay-Weber syndrome.[54,55] The lesions often have a well-defined echogenic appearance similar to the typical appearance of hemangiomas in the liver, but this appearance is seen much less frequently in the spleen than in

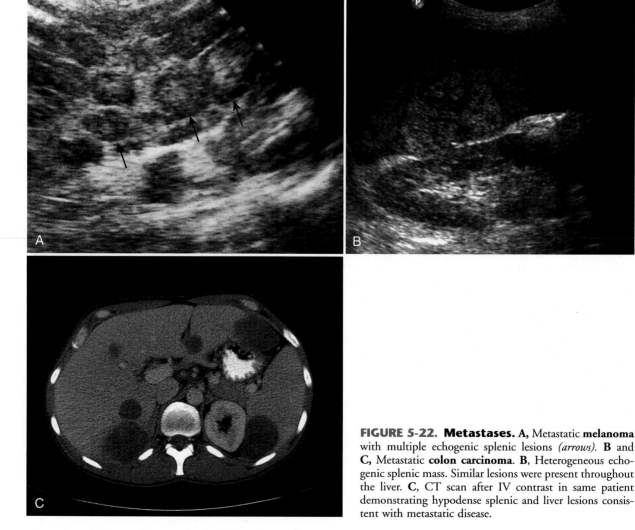

FIGURE 5-22. Metastases. A, Metastatic **melanoma** with multiple echogenic splenic lesions *(arrows).* **B** and **C,** Metastatic **colon carcinoma. B,** Heterogeneous echogenic splenic mass. Similar lesions were present throughout the liver. **C,** CT scan after IV contrast in same patient demonstrating hypodense splenic and liver lesions consistent with metastatic disease.

FOCAL SOLID SPLENIC MASSES

BENIGN
Hemangioma
Hamartoma
Littoral cell angioma
Lymphangioma
Sclerosing angiomatoid nodular transformation
  (SANT)
Inflammatory pseudotumor

MALIGNANT
Lymphoma
Metastases
Angiosarcoma
Hemangiopericytoma

OTHER
Infarct

---

the liver (Fig. 5-23). Lesions of mixed echogenicity, with cystic spaces of variable sizes and foci of calcification, have also been reported.[35,53]

Other benign tumors of the spleen are rare and include hamartomas, littoral cell angioma, sclerosing angiomatoid nodular transformation (SANT), and inflammatory pseudotumor. **Hamartomas** are typically well-defined, homogeneous, isoechoic to mildly hypoechoic or hyperechoic lesions[56] (Fig. 5-24). Hamartomas may contain cystic areas or coarse calcifications, and some demonstrate increased vascularity on color Doppler imaging.[57] The sonographic appearance of **littoral cell angioma** is

variable and includes reports of hypoechoic and hyperechoic focal lesions as well as a diffuse mottled pattern without discrete lesions[34,58] (Fig. 5-25). Sclerosing angiomatoid nodular transformation (SANT) is a recently recognized benign vascular lesion of the spleen. Information regarding the sonographic imaging findings of this condition is very limited. **Inflammatory pseudotumors** usually present as a well-defined hypoechoic mass.[59]

Splenic infarction is one of the more common causes of focal splenic lesions and may mimic a mass on ultrasound. If a typical peripheral, wedge-shaped, hypoechoic lesion is noted, splenic infarction should be the first diagnostic consideration[60,61] (Figs. 5-26 and 5-27). However, the sonographic appearance of splenic infarcts varies and includes multinodular or masslike changes with irregular margins.[62] The temporal evolution of the ultrasound appearance of splenic infarctions has shown that the echogenicity of the lesion is related to the age of the infarction. Infarctions are hypoechoic, or echo free, in early stages and progress to hyperechoic lesions when fibrosis develops over time.[63,64]

Other Abnormalities

Sickle Cell Disease

Sickle cell disease almost always affects the spleen. The most common splenic complications are autosplenectomy, acute sequestration, hypersplenism, massive infarction, and abscess. In **homozygous** sickle cell disease, multiple infarcts generally result in a small, fibrotic spleen and complete loss of function (**autosplenectomy**). Although promising new therapies are being

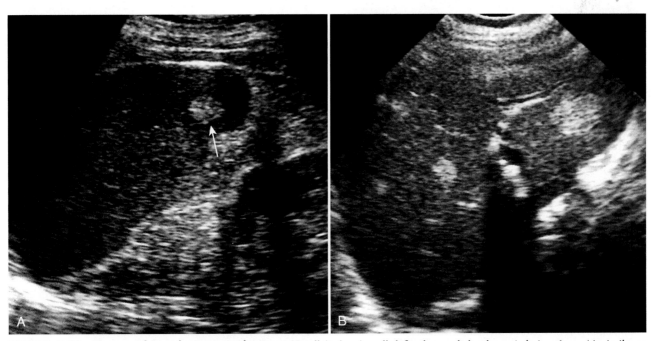

FIGURE 5-23. Hemangioma in two patients. A, Small (1.4 cm), well-defined, rounded, echogenic lesion *(arrow)* is similar to the typical liver hemangiomas. **B,** Coronal ultrasound scan shows multiple echogenic splenic hemangiomas of different sizes in the spleen. Note the calcified splenic artery adjacent to the vein.

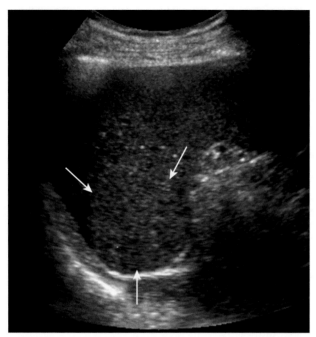

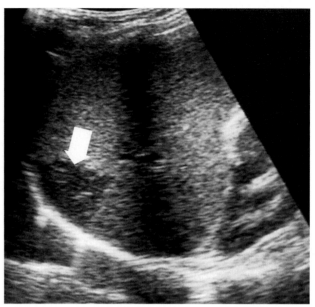

FIGURE 5-24. Hamartoma. Round, 5-cm, slightly hyper-echoic lesion *(arrows)* arising from the medial margins of the spleen.

FIGURE 5-26. Splenic infarct. Triangular hypoechoic infarct *(arrow)* in the superior aspect of the spleen extends to the splenic capsule, analogous to the pleural wedge-shaped density seen in pulmonary infarction.

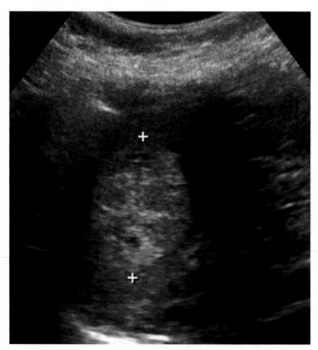

FIGURE 5-25. Littoral cell angioma. Oval, well-defined, 5-cm echogenic lesion. Splenectomy was performed when this lesion demonstrated growth during follow-up.

developed, many homozygous sickle cell patients become **asplenic** in late childhood or early adulthood. This results in a small spleen, often difficult to visualize, with a diffuse echogenic appearance. Patients with **heterozygous** sickle cell disease often present with **splenomegaly** and may demonstrate the sequelae of **infarction.**[65,66] In some patients, areas of preserved splenic tissue are present

in an otherwise small and fibrotic spleen, and these should not be mistaken for an abscess or mass.

Acute splenic sequestration is a life-threatening complication of sickle cell disease and typically occurs in infants and children with homozygous sickle cell disease. It represents sudden trapping of blood in the spleen, resulting in splenic enlargement. On ultrasound, the spleen is larger than expected and heterogeneous with multiple hypoechoic areas.[65] It is important to recognize that in homozygous sickle cell patients, an apparently normal-sized spleen may actually indicate splenomegaly.

Gaucher's Disease

In Gaucher's disease, splenomegaly occurs almost universally, and approximately one third of patients have multiple splenic nodules. These nodules frequently are well-defined hypoechoic lesions, but they may also be irregular, hyperechoic, or of mixed echogenicity[67,68] (Fig. 5-28). Pathologically, these nodules represent focal areas of Gaucher cells associated with fibrosis and infarction. Rarely, the entire spleen may be involved, with ultrasound showing a diffuse heterogeneous spleen.

Gamna-Gandy Bodies

Gamna-Gandy bodies (Gamna nodules) are siderotic nodules that result from organized focal hemorrhagic infarcts, typically seen in congestive splenomegaly and sickle cell disease. Gamna-Gandy bodies appear as multiple punctate hyperechoic foci on ultrasound but are usually better seen on magnetic resonance imaging (MRI).[69]

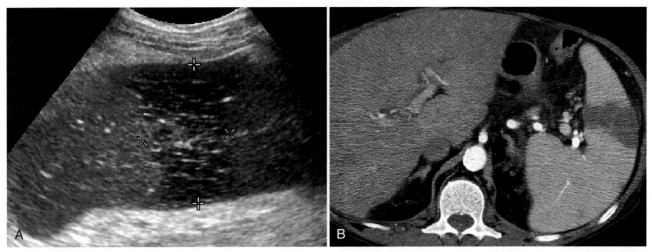

FIGURE 5-27. **Splenic infarct. A,** Coronal longitudinal scan shows a well-defined hypoechoic central area reaching the splenic capsule medial and lateral in a patient with splenomegaly receiving peritoneal dialysis. **B,** Corresponding CT scan after IV contrast demonstrates the wedge-shaped nonenhancing area in keeping with an infarct.

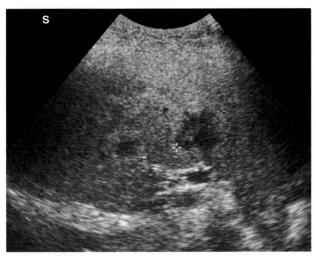

FIGURE 5-28. **Gaucher's disease.** Enlarged spleen containing a 2-cm heterogeneous nodule. *(Courtesy M. Maas, MD, Amsterdam.)*

Splenic Trauma

The spleen is the most frequently injured visceral organ in patients with blunt abdominal trauma. The spectrum of splenic injuries ranges from contusion to a completely shattered spleen. The severity of the splenic injury can be scored using the American Association for the Surgery of Trauma (AAST) **Organ Injury Scoring Scale** (OIS).[70] Treatment options depend on hemodynamic and clinical criteria and include conservative management with or without embolization and surgery.[4]

Ultrasound can be very helpful and highly accurate in the diagnosis of splenic injury. However, computed tomography (CT) has proved particularly useful in this area because the severity of splenic injury is better assessed and other abdominal injuries can be identified in one examination.[71] In addition, traumatic splenic vascular injuries (e.g., active bleeding, pseudoaneurysms, arteriovenous fistulas) are difficult to detect with ultrasound.[72] However, splenic injury is not always clinically apparent and **spontaneous splenic rupture** or **pathologic splenic rupture** can occur after negligible trauma or insignificant events such as coughing.[21] This is typically seen in patients with a pathologically enlarged spleen caused by the altered consistency and splenic extension below the rib cage.

Advantages of ultrasound are that it is fast, portable, and easily integrated into the resuscitation of patients with trauma without delaying therapeutic measures.[73] In addition, if the patient is hemodynamically unstable, obtaining a CT scan may not be feasible.[74] Therefore, ultrasound examinations performed in the emergency department after blunt abdominal trauma should not only focus on free intra-abdominal fluid, but also evaluate the solid organs. Further, now that nonsurgical management is preferred, ultrasound is helpful for numerous follow-up examinations.

When the spleen is involved in blunt abdominal trauma, two outcomes are possible. If the capsule remains intact, the result may be an **intraparenchymal or subcapsular hematoma** (Fig. 5-29). If the capsule ruptures, a **focal or free intraperitoneal hematoma** may result. With capsular rupture, it might be possible to demonstrate fluid surrounding the spleen in the left upper quadrant. Although blood often spreads within the peritoneal cavity and can be found in the pelvis or in Morison's pouch, on some occasions it becomes walled off in the left upper quadrant (Fig. 5-30).

It is important to consider the timing of the sonographic examination relative to the trauma. Immediately after the traumatic incident, the hematoma is liquid and can easily be differentiated from splenic parenchyma.

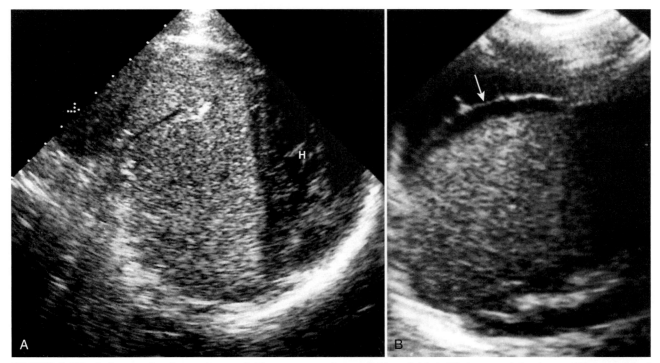

FIGURE 5-29. Subcapsular hematoma. A, Transverse scan shows a fluid- and debris-filled crescentic hematoma *(H)* in the lateral aspect of the spleen. **B,** Thin, brightly echogenic crescentic line *(arrow)* represents the splenic capsule.

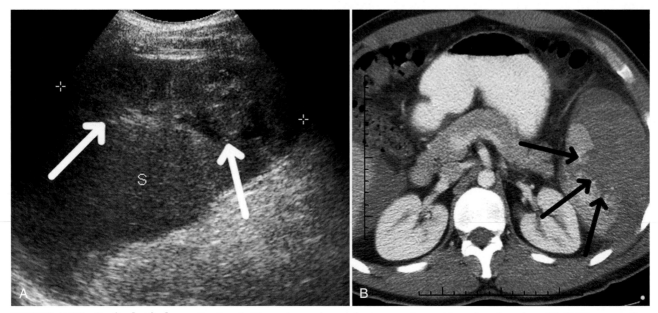

FIGURE 5-30. Perisplenic hematoma. A, Coronal scan shows a hematoma *(arrows)* lateral to the spleen *(S)*. **B,** Corresponding CT scan after IV contrast shows the splenic laceration *(arrows)* and large, perisplenic hematoma. Free fluid is also seen in the right upper abdomen.

After the blood clots, and for the subsequent 24 to 48 hours, the echogenicity of the perisplenic hematoma may closely resemble the echogenicity of normal splenic parenchyma and may mimic splenomegaly. Subsequently, the blood re-liquefies and the diagnosis becomes easy again. In splenic injuries, there are often focal areas of inhomogeneity within the spleen, but these can be subtle (Fig. 5-31).

There is no clear consensus in the literature as to whether imaging follow-up is helpful or necessary.[75] If follow-up is performed, the clinician may see the subcapsular hematoma differentiated from the pericapsular,

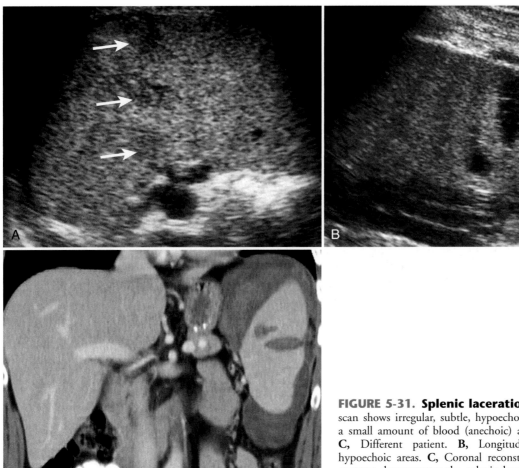

FIGURE 5-31. Splenic laceration. A, Coronal ultrasound scan shows irregular, subtle, hypoechoic areas *(arrows)*. There is a small amount of blood (anechoic) around the spleen. **B** and **C,** Different patient. **B,** Longitudinal scan shows ovoid hypoechoic areas. **C,** Coronal reconstructed CT scan after IV contrast demonstrates the splenic lacerations and a large, perisplenic hematoma.

organized hematoma by the capsule itself (see Fig. 5-29, *B*). The splenic capsule is very thin and frequently not visualized separately from adjacent fluid. In these cases the shape of the fluid collection can provide an important clue to the location of the hematoma. If the collection is crescentic and conforms to the contour of the spleen, the hematoma is likely subcapsular. Irregularly shaped collections are seen more with perisplenic hematomas.

Perisplenic fluid may persist for weeks or even months after splenic injury. Although there may actually be a condition of delayed rupture of the spleen, it is possible that all ruptures of the spleen occurred at the time of injury and were walled off initially.[76] Delayed rupture may be only the extension of blood into the peritoneal cavity after liquefaction of a perisplenic hematoma.

Aside from splenic capsule rupture, there may be internal damage to the spleen with an intact splenic capsule. This can result in intraparenchymal or subcapsular hematoma of the spleen, which initially appears only as an inhomogeneous area in the otherwise uniform splenic parenchyma. Subsequently, the hematoma may resolve, and repeat scans may show cystic change at the site of the original injury.

Sonographically, a perisplenic hematoma can closely mimic a perisplenic abscess. A hematoma can also become infected and transform into a left subphrenic abscess.[38] If the distinction cannot be made clinically, fine-needle aspiration can differentiate between a hematoma and an abscess.

CONGENITAL ANOMALIES

Accessory spleens, also known as **splenunculi,** are common normal variants found in up to 30% of autopsies. They are typically located near the splenic hilum and have similar echogenicity as the normal spleen. Splenunculi may be confused with enlarged lymph nodes around the spleen or with masses in the tail of the pancreas. When the spleen enlarges, the accessory spleens may also enlarge. **Ectopic accessory spleens** described in various locations, including the pancreas and scrotum, are typically confused with abnormal masses or may rarely undergo torsion and cause acute abdominal pain.[77,78] The vast majority of accessory spleens, however, are easy to recognize sonographically as small, rounded masses, usually less than 5 cm in diameter, with the same

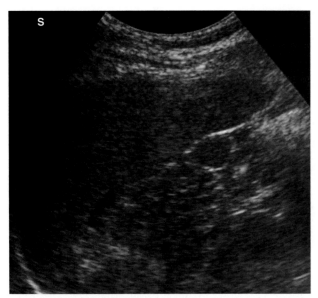

FIGURE 5-32. Accessory spleen. Coronal sonogram shows an accessory spleen (splenunculus) adjacent to the inferior medial portion of the spleen.

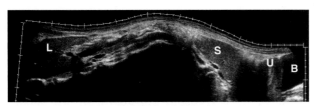

FIGURE 5-33. Wandering spleen. Sagittal extended-FOV image of midline abdomen in asymptomatic young woman; L, liver, S, spleen; U, uterus; B, bladder.

echogenicity as the spleen (Fig. 5-32). CT, MRI or in challenging cases, scintigraphy with ^{99m}Tc-labeled heat-damaged red blood cells, can confirm the diagnosis.[79]

A "wandering spleen" (or **mobile** spleen) can be found in unusual locations and may be mistaken for a mass (Fig. 5-33). It is caused by absence or extreme laxity of the supporting ligaments and a long, mobile mesentery (see Fig. 5-1, B). The mobile spleen may undergo torsion, resulting in acute or chronic abdominal pain.[80,81] If the diagnosis of a wandering spleen is made in a patient with acute abdominal pain, the diagnosis of torsion may be supported by color flow Doppler imaging showing absence of blood flow.[82]

The other two major congenital splenic anomalies are the asplenia and polysplenia syndromes. These conditions are best understood if viewed as part of the spectrum of anomalies known as **visceral heterotaxy.** A normal arrangement of asymmetrical body parts is known as situs solitus. The mirror image condition is called situs inversus. Between these two extremes is a wide spectrum of abnormalities called situs ambiguus. Splenic abnormalities in patients with visceral heterotaxy consist of polysplenia and asplenia. Interestingly, patients with **polysplenia** have **bilateral left-sidedness,** or a domi-

nance of left-sided over right-sided body structures. They may have two morphologically left lungs, left-sided azygous continuation of an interrupted inferior vena cava, biliary atresia, absence of the gallbladder, gastrointestinal malrotation, and frequently cardiovascular abnormalities. Conversely, patients with **asplenia** may have **bilateral right-sidedness.** They may have two morphologically right lungs, midline location of the liver, reversed position of the abdominal aorta and inferior vena cava, anomalous pulmonary venous return, and horseshoe kidneys. The wide range of possible anomalies accounts for the variety of presenting symptoms, but absence of the spleen itself causes impairment of the immune response, and such patients can present with serious infections, such as sepsis and bacterial meningitis.[6]

Polysplenia must be differentiated from **posttraumatic splenosis.**[83] Splenosis is an acquired condition defined as autotransplantation of viable splenic tissue throughout different anatomic compartments of the body. It occurs after traumatic or iatrogenic rupture of the spleen.[84] Nuclear medicine imaging, with technetium-labeled heat-damaged red blood cells, is the most sensitive study for both posttraumatic splenosis and congenital polysplenia. Accessory spleens as small as 1 cm can be demonstrated by this method.[79]

INTERVENTIONAL PROCEDURES

Multiple reports and case series have described percutaneous splenic interventions.[85,86] Although typically described in smaller series, safety and success rates are similar to those performed elsewhere in the abdomen.[87]

Ultrasound-guided splenic biopsy can help establish a diagnosis with a low rate of complication rates and a high diagnostic yield.[20] Fine-needle and core-needle biopsies have been performed successfully to diagnose focal abnormalities, including abscesses, sarcoidosis, primary splenic malignancies, metastases, and lymphoma.[88,89]

In patients with abscesses, cysts, hematomas, and infected necrotic tumors, percutaneous catheter drainage is often successful.[40] Even radiofrequency ablation (RFA) procedures involving the spleen have been reported recently.[90]

Despite these reports, however, many interventional radiologists remain reluctant to perform splenic interventions. The main concern has been fear of **bleeding** caused by the highly vascular nature of the organ. However, clinicians should take into consideration that a successful image-guided percutaneous procedure could prevent the need for splenectomy.[87]

PITFALLS IN INTERPRETATION

Sonographers must be wary of several ultrasound pitfalls them when scanning the left upper quadrant and spleen.

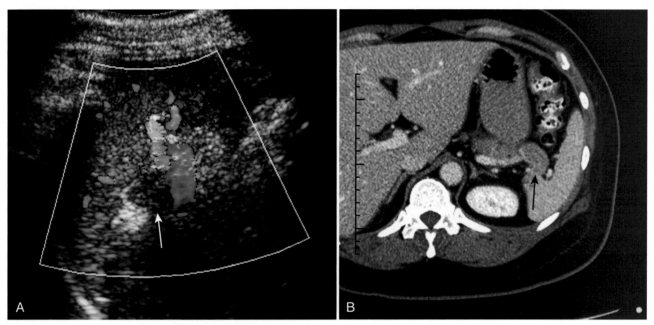

FIGURE 5-34. Pancreatic tail simulating mass. A, Sonogram shows 2-cm lesion adjacent to the splenic hilum *(arrow).* **B,** CT scan shows that "lesion" is the normal pancreatic tail *(arrow).*

The first is the crescentic, echo-poor area superior to the spleen, which can be caused by the left lobe of the liver in thin individuals[91-94] (see Fig. 5-5). The left liver lobe can mimic the appearance of a subcapsular hematoma or a subphrenic abscess. Observing the liver sliding over the more echogenic spleen during quiet respiration can make the correct diagnosis. Hepatic and portal veins may help to identify this structure as the liver.

The tail of the pancreas may simulate a mass adjacent to the hilum of the spleen (Fig. 5-34). This is particularly true if the plane of section is aimed along the long axis of the pancreatic tail. Identifying the splenic artery and vein may be helpful in confirming the normal tail of the pancreas.

Similarly, the fundus of the stomach may nestle in the hilum of the spleen. An oblique plane during scanning may pass through the spleen and include the hilum, with an echogenic portion of the stomach simulating an intrasplenic lesion. In some patients, this is just the fat around the stomach. Occasionally, fluid in the fundus of the stomach can simulate a perisplenic fluid collection. This can usually be resolved by scanning transversely or by letting the patient drink some water during the scan.

An occasional anatomic variant can occur if the inferior portion of the spleen is located posterolateral to the upper pole of the left kidney. This variant has been called the **retrorenal spleen.** Awareness of its existence can prevent the misdiagnosis of an abnormal mass. If visualized sonographically, it should be avoided in any interventional procedure performed on the left kidney.[95]

It can be very difficult to determine the site of origin of large, LUQ masses arising from the spleen, left adrenal gland, left kidney, tail of the pancreas, stomach, or ret-roperitoneum. Differential motion observed during shallow respiration may be helpful. Additionally, the identification of the splenic vein entering the splenic hilum can be definitive. CT or MRI should be used to clarify challenging cases.

References

1. Kamaya A, Weinstein S, Desser TS. Multiple lesions of the spleen: differential diagnosis of cystic and solid lesions. Semin Ultrasound CT MR 2006;27:389-403.

Embryology and Anatomy
2. Zhao Z, Liu S, Li Z, et al. Sectional anatomy of the peritoneal reflections of the upper abdomen in the coronal plane. J Comput Assist Tomogr 2005;29:430-437.
3. DeLand FH. Normal spleen size. Radiology 1970;97:589-592.
4. Gauer JM, Gerber-Paulet S, Seiler C, Schweizer WP. Twenty years of splenic preservation in trauma: lower early infection rate than in splenectomy. World J Surg 2008;32:2730-2735.
5. Cadili A, de Gara C. Complications of splenectomy. Am J Med 2008;121:371-375.
6. Spelman D, Buttery J, Daley A, et al. Guidelines for the prevention of sepsis in asplenic and hyposplenic patients. Intern Med J 2008;38:349-356.

Sonographic Technique
7. Catalano O, Sandomenico F, Vallone P, et al. Contrast-enhanced sonography of the spleen. Semin Ultrasound CT MR 2006;27:426-433.
8. Gorg C. The forgotten organ: contrast-enhanced sonography of the spleen. Eur J Radiol 2007;64:189-201.

Sonographic Appearance
9. Yetter EM, Acosta KB, Olson MC, Blundell K. Estimating splenic volume: sonographic measurements correlated with helical CT determination. AJR Am J Roentgenol 2003;181:1615-1620.
10. Rosenberg HK, Markowitz RI, Kolberg H, et al. Normal splenic size in infants and children: sonographic measurements. AJR Am J Roentgenol 1991;157:119-121.

11. Lamb PM, Lund A, Kanagasabay RR, et al. Spleen size: how well do linear ultrasound measurements correlate with three-dimensional CT volume assessments? Br J Radiol 2002;75:573-537.
12. Frank K, Linhart P, Kortsik C, Wohlenberg H. [Sonographic determination of spleen size: normal dimensions in adults with a healthy spleen]. Ultraschall Med 1986;7:134-137.
13. Hosey RG, Mattacola CG, Kriss V, et al. Ultrasound assessment of spleen size in collegiate athletes. Br J Sports Med 2006;40:251-254; discussion 254.
14. Spielmann AL, DeLong DM, Kliewer MA. Sonographic evaluation of spleen size in tall healthy athletes. AJR Am J Roentgenol 2005;184:45-49.
15. Kaneko J, Sugawara Y, Matsui Y, et al. Normal splenic volume in adults by computed tomography. Hepatogastroenterology 2002;49:1726-1727.

Pathologic Conditions
16. Pozo AL, Godfrey EM, Bowles KM. Splenomegaly: investigation, diagnosis and management. Blood Rev 2009;23:105-111.
17. Swaroop J, O'Reilly RA. Splenomegaly at a university hospital compared to a nearby county hospital in 317 patients. Acta Haematol 1999;102:83-88.
18. Abramson JS, Chatterji M, Rahemtullah A. Case records of the Massachusetts General Hospital. Case 39-2008. A 51-year-old woman with splenomegaly and anemia. N Engl J Med 2008;359:2707-2718.
19. Jeong JW, Lee S, Lee JW, et al. The echotextural characteristics for the diagnosis of the liver cirrhosis using the sonographic images. Conf Proc IEEE Eng Med Biol Soc 2007;1343-1345.
20. Tam A, Krishnamurthy S, Pillsbury EP, et al. Percutaneous image-guided splenic biopsy in the oncology patient: an audit of 156 consecutive cases. J Vasc Interv Radiol 2008;19:80-87.
21. Wehbe E, Raffi S, Osborne D. Spontaneous splenic rupture precipitated by cough: a case report and a review of the literature. Scand J Gastroenterol 2008;43:634-637.
22. Paterson A, Frush DP, Donnelly LF, et al. A pattern-oriented approach to splenic imaging in infants and children. Radiographics 1999;19:1465-1485.
23. Warshauer DM, Hall HL. Solitary splenic lesions. Semin Ultrasound CT MR 2006;27:370-388.
24. Lashbrook DJ, James RW, Phillips AJ, et al. Splenic peliosis with spontaneous splenic rupture: report of two cases. BMC Surg 2006;6:9.
25. Ishida H, Konno K, Ishida J, et al. Splenic lymphoma: differentiation from splenic cyst with ultrasonography. Abdom Imaging 2001;26:529-532.
26. Urrutia M, Mergo PJ, Ros LH, et al. Cystic masses of the spleen: radiologic-pathologic correlation. Radiographics 1996;16:107-129.
27. Williams RJ, Glazer G. Splenic cysts: changes in diagnosis, treatment and aetiological concepts. Ann R Coll Surg Engl 1993;75:87-89.
28. Morgenstern L. Nonparasitic splenic cysts: pathogenesis, classification, and treatment. J Am Coll Surg 2002;194:306-314.
29. Dachman AH, Ros PR, Murari PJ, et al. Nonparasitic splenic cysts: a report of 52 cases with radiologic-pathologic correlation. AJR Am J Roentgenol 1986;147:537-542.
30. Durgun V, Kapan S, Kapan M, et al. Primary splenic hydatidosis. Dig Surg 2003;20:38-41.
31. Akhan O, Koroglu M. Hydatid disease of the spleen. Semin Ultrasound CT MR 2007;28:28-34.
32. Celebi S, Basaranoglu M, Karaaslan H, Demir A. A splenic hydatid cyst case presented with lumbar pain. Intern Med 2006;45:1023-1024.
33. Heider R, Behrns KE. Pancreatic pseudocysts complicated by splenic parenchymal involvement: results of operative and percutaneous management. Pancreas 2001;23:20-25.
34. Abbott RM, Levy AD, Aguilera NS, et al. From the archives of the AFIP: primary vascular neoplasms of the spleen: radiologic-pathologic correlation. Radiographics 2004;24:1137-1163.
35. Willcox TM, Speer RW, Schlinkert RT, Sarr MG. Hemangioma of the spleen: presentation, diagnosis, and management. J Gastrointest Surg 2000;4:611-613.
36. Wunderbaldinger P, Paya K, Partik B, et al. CT and MR imaging of generalized cystic lymphangiomatosis in pediatric patients. AJR Am J Roentgenol 2000;174:827-832.
37. Bezzi M, Spinelli A, Pierleoni M, Andreoli G. Cystic lymphangioma of the spleen: US-CT-MRI correlation. Eur Radiol 2001;11:1187-1190.
38. Fotiadis C, Lavranos G, Patapis P, Karatzas G. Abscesses of the spleen: report of three cases. World J Gastroenterol 2008;14:3088-3091.
39. Changchien CS, Tsai TL, Hu TH, et al. Sonographic patterns of splenic abscess: an analysis of 34 proven cases. Abdom Imaging 2002;27:739-745.
40. Ferraioli G, Brunetti E, Gulizia R, et al. Management of splenic abscess: report on 16 cases from a single center. Int J Infect Dis 2009;13:524-530.
41. Koh DM, Burn PR, Mathews G, et al. Abdominal computed tomographic findings of Mycobacterium tuberculosis and Mycobacterium avium intracellulare infection in HIV seropositive patients. Can Assoc Radiol J 2003;54:45-50.
42. Thanos L, Zormpala A, Brountzos E, et al. Nodular hepatic and splenic sarcoidosis in a patient with normal chest radiograph. Eur J Radiol 2002;41:10-11.
43. O'Neal CB, Ball SC. Splenic pneumocystosis: an atypical presentation of extrapulmonary Pneumocystis infection. AIDS Read 2008;18:503-508.
44. Pastakia B, Shawker TH, Thaler M, et al. Hepatosplenic candidiasis: wheels within wheels. Radiology 1988;166:417-421.
45. Rudolph J, Rodenwaldt J, Ruhnke M, et al. Unusual enhancement pattern of liver lesions in hepatosplenic candidiasis. Acta Radiol 2004;45:499-503.
46. Matone J, Lopes Filho GD, Scalabrin M, et al. Primary splenic lymphoma in patient with hepatitis C virus infection: case report and review of the literature. Int Surg 2000;85:248-251.
47. Gorg C, Weide R, Schwerk WB. Malignant splenic lymphoma: sonographic patterns, diagnosis and follow-up. Clin Radiol 1997;52:535-540.
48. Takabe K, Al-Refaie W, Chin B, et al. Can large B-cell lymphoma mimic cystic lesions of the spleen? Int J Gastrointest Cancer 2005;35:83-88.
49. Neuhauser TS, Derringer GA, Thompson LD, et al. Splenic angiosarcoma: a clinicopathologic and immunophenotypic study of 28 cases. Mod Pathol 2000;13:978-987.
50. Thompson WM, Levy AD, Aguilera NS, et al. Angiosarcoma of the spleen: imaging characteristics in 12 patients. Radiology 2005;235:106-115.
51. Berge T. Splenic metastases: frequencies and patterns. Acta Pathol Microbiol Scand A 1974;82:499-506.
52. Lam KY, Tang V. Metastatic tumors to the spleen: a 25-year clinicopathologic study. Arch Pathol Lab Med 2000;124:526-530.
53. Ros PR, Moser Jr RP, Dachman AH, et al. Hemangioma of the spleen: radiologic-pathologic correlation in ten cases. Radiology 1987;162:73-77.
54. Jindal R, Sullivan R, Rodda B, et al. Splenic malformation in a patient with Klippel-Trenaunay syndrome: a case report. J Vasc Surg 2006;43:848-850.
55. Dufau JP, le Tourneau A, Audouin J, et al. Isolated diffuse hemangiomatosis of the spleen with Kasabach-Merritt-like syndrome. Histopathology 1999;35:337-344.
56. Tang S, Shimizu T, Kikuchi Y, et al. Color Doppler sonographic findings in splenic hamartoma. J Clin Ultrasound 2000;28:249-253.
57. Yu RS, Zhang SZ, Hua JM. Imaging findings of splenic hamartoma. World J Gastroenterol 2004;10:2613-2615.
58. Tee M, Vos P, Zetler P, Wiseman SM. Incidental littoral cell angioma of the spleen. World J Surg Oncol 2008;6:87.
59. Yan J, Peng C, Yang W, et al. Inflammatory pseudotumour of the spleen: report of 2 cases and literature review. Can J Surg 2008;51:75-76.
60. Romano S, Scaglione M, Gatta G, et al. Association of splenic and renal infarctions in acute abdominal emergencies. Eur J Radiol 2004;50:48-58.
61. Miller LA, Mirvis SE, Shanmuganathan K, Ohson AS. CT diagnosis of splenic infarction in blunt trauma: imaging features, clinical significance and complications. Clin Radiol 2004;59:342-348.
62. Gorg C, Zugmaier G. Chronic recurring infarction of the spleen: sonographic patterns and complications. Ultraschall Med 2003;24:245-249.
63. Balcar I, Seltzer SE, Davis S, Geller S. CT patterns of splenic infarction: a clinical and experimental study. Radiology 1984;151:723-729.
64. Goerg C, Schwerk WB. Splenic infarction: sonographic patterns, diagnosis, follow-up, and complications. Radiology 1990;174:803-807.

65. Lonergan GJ, Cline DB, Abbondanzo SL. Sickle cell anemia. Radiographics 2001;21:971-994.
66. Madani G, Papadopoulou AM, Holloway B, et al. The radiological manifestations of sickle cell disease. Clin Radiol 2007;62:528-538.
67. Chippington S, McHugh K, Vellodi A. Splenic nodules in paediatric Gaucher disease treated by enzyme replacement therapy. Pediatr Radiol 2008;38:657-660.
68. Patlas M, Hadas-Halpern I, Abrahamov A, et al. Spectrum of abdominal sonographic findings in 103 pediatric patients with Gaucher disease. Eur Radiol 2002;12:397-400.
69. Chan YL, Yang WT, Sung JJ, et al. Diagnostic accuracy of abdominal ultrasonography compared to magnetic resonance imaging in siderosis of the spleen. J Ultrasound Med 2000;19:543-547.
70. American Association for the Surgery of Trauma (AAST) Organ Injury Scoring Scale. http://www.trauma.org/archive/scores/ois-spleen.html. Accessed March 2010.
71. Weninger P, Mauritz W, Fridrich P, et al. Emergency room management of patients with blunt major trauma: evaluation of the multislice computed tomography protocol exemplified by an urban trauma center. J Trauma 2007;62:584-591.
72. Hamilton JD, Kumaravel M, Censullo ML, et al. Multidetector CT evaluation of active extravasation in blunt abdominal and pelvic trauma patients. Radiographics 2008;28:1603-1616.
73. Brown MA, Casola G, Sirlin CB, et al. Blunt abdominal trauma: screening us in 2,693 patients. Radiology 2001;218:352-358.
74. Farahmand N, Sirlin CB, Brown MA, et al. Hypotensive patients with blunt abdominal trauma: performance of screening ultrasound. Radiology 2005;235:436-443.
75. McCray VW, Davis JW, Lemaster D, Parks SN. Observation for nonoperative management of the spleen: how long is long enough? J Trauma 2008;65:1354-1358.
76. Gamblin TC, Wall Jr CE, Royer GM, et al. Delayed splenic rupture: case reports and review of the literature. J Trauma 2005;59:1231-1234.

Congenital Anomalies

77. Meyer-Rochow GY, Gifford AJ, Samra JS, Sywak MS. Intrapancreatic splenunculus. Am J Surg 2007;194:75-76.
78. Netto JM, Perez LM, Kelly DR, et al. Splenogonadal fusion diagnosed by Doppler ultrasonography. ScientificWorldJournal 2004;4(Suppl 1):253-257.
79. MacDonald A, Burrell S. Infrequently performed studies in nuclear medicine. Part 1. J Nucl Med Technol 2008;36:132-143; quiz 145.
80. Soleimani M, Mehrabi A, Kashfi A, et al. Surgical treatment of patients with wandering spleen: report of six cases with a review of the literature. Surg Today 2007;37:261-269.
81. Misawa T, Yoshida K, Shiba H, et al. Wandering spleen with chronic torsion. Am J Surg 2008;195:504-505.
82. Danaci M, Belet U, Yalin T, et al. Power Doppler sonographic diagnosis of torsion in a wandering spleen. J Clin Ultrasound 2000;28:246-248.
83. Gayer G, Hertz M, Strauss S, Zissin R. Congenital anomalies of the spleen. Semin Ultrasound CT MR 2006;27:358-369.
84. Fremont RD, Rice TW. Splenosis: a review. South Med J 2007;100:589-593.

Interventional Procedures

85. Lucey BC, Boland GW, Maher MM, et al. Percutaneous nonvascular splenic intervention: a 10-year review. AJR Am J Roentgenol 2002;179:1591-1596.
86. Kang M, Kalra N, Gulati M, et al. Image-guided percutaneous splenic interventions. Eur J Radiol 2007;64:140-146.
87. Lieberman S, Libson E, Sella T, et al. Percutaneous image-guided splenic procedures: update on indications, technique, complications, and outcomes. Semin Ultrasound CT MR 2007;28:57-63.
88. Lopez JI, Del Cura JL, De Larrinoa AF, et al. Role of ultrasound-guided core biopsy in the evaluation of spleen pathology. APMIS 2006;114:492-499.
89. Liang P, Gao Y, Wang Y, et al. Ultrasound-guided percutaneous needle biopsy of the spleen using 18-gauge versus 21-gauge needles. J Clin Ultrasound 2007;35:477-482.
90. Liu Q, Ma K, Song Y, et al. Two-year follow-up of splenic radiofrequency ablation in patients with cirrhotic hypersplenism: does increased hepatic arterial flow induce liver regeneration? Surgery 2008;143:509-518.

Pitfalls in Interpretation

91. Rao MG. Enlarged left lobe of the liver mistaken for a mass in the splenic region. Clin Nucl Med 1989;14:134.
92. Li DK, Cooperberg PL, Graham MF, Callen P. Pseudo perisplenic "fluid collections": a clue to normal liver and spleen echogenic texture. J Ultrasound Med 1986;5:397-400.
93. Crivello MS, Peterson IM, Austin RM. Left lobe of the liver mimicking perisplenic collections. J Clin Ultrasound 1986;14:697-701.
94. Arenson AM, McKee JD. Left upper quadrant pseudolesion secondary to normal variants in liver and spleen. J Clin Ultrasound 1986;14:558-561.
95. Dodds WJ, Darweesh RM, Lawson TL, et al. The retroperitoneal spaces revisited. AJR Am J Roentgenol 1986;147:1155-1161.

CHAPTER 6

The Biliary Tree and Gallbladder

Korosh Khalili and Stephanie R. Wilson

Chapter Outline

$\mathcal{S}$onographic evaluation of the biliary tract is one of the most appropriate and efficacious uses of the ultrasound examination. The cystic nature of both the gallbladder and the bile ducts, particularly when dilated, provides an inherently high contrast resolution in comparison to the adjacent tissues. This factor, the excellent spatial resolution of sonography, and the acoustic window provided by the liver allow for a high-quality examination in the majority of patients. Currently, sonography remains the modality of choice for the detection of gallstones, assessment of acute right upper quadrant pain, and for the initial evaluation of the patient with jaundice or elevated liver function tests. In conjunction with MRI/MRCP and contrast-enhanced CT scan, sonography also plays a key role in the multimodality evaluation of more complex biliary problems, such as the diagnosis and staging of hilar cholangiocarcinoma. The recent development of contrast-enhanced sonography for detection of hepatic masses further broadens this role. From the smallest of ultrasound departments operating in remote geographic areas to the largest of tertiary institutions, there is no other anatomic location in the body that is better studied with sonography than the biliary tract.

THE BILIARY TREE

Anatomy and Normal Variants

An understanding of the normal location of the bile ducts and common anatomic variations is important in staging of malignancies and directing intervention. In biliary terminology, **proximal** denotes the portion of the biliary tree that is in relative proximity to the liver and hepatocytes, whereas **distal** refers to the caudal end closer to the bowel. The term **branching order** applies to the level of division of the bile ducts starting from the **common hepatic duct** (CHD); first-order branches are the right and left hepatic ducts, second-order branches are their respective divisions (also known as secondary biliary **radicles**), and so on. **Central** specifies proximity to the porta hepatis, whereas **peripheral** refers to the higher-order branches of the intrahepatic biliary tree extending well into the hepatic parenchyma. Knowledge of **Couinaud's functional anatomy** of the liver is also vital in description of the intrahepatic biliary abnormalities (see Chapter 4).

The **intrahepatic ducts** are not in a fixed relation to the portal veins within the portal triads and can be anterior or posterior to the vein or even tortuous about the vein.[1] The right and left hepatic ducts, that is, the first-order branches of the CHD, are routinely seen on sonography, and normal second-order branches may be visualized[2] (Fig. 6-1). The use of spectral and color Doppler ultrasound is often needed to distinguish hepatic arteries from ducts. In our experience, visualization of third-order or higher-order branches is often an abnormal finding and requires a search for the cause of dilation. Most of the right and left hepatic ducts are extrahepatic and, along with the CHD, form the hilar or central portion of the biliary tree at the porta hepatis. This is the most common location for cholangiocarcinoma. The normal diameter of the first-order and higher-order branches of the CHD has been suggested to be 2 mm or less, and no more than 40% of the diameter of the adjacent portal vein.[2]

The most common branching pattern of the biliary tree occurs in 56% to 58% of the population[3,4] (Figs. 6-2 and 6-3). On the right side, the right hepatic duct forms from the right anterior and right posterior branches, draining the anterior (segments 5 and 8) and posterior (segments 6 and 7) segments of the right lobe, respectively. On the left side, segment 2 and 3 branches join to the left of the falciform ligament to form the left hepatic duct. This duct becomes extrahepatic in location as it extends to the right of the falciform ligament, where it is joined by ducts of segments 4 and 1.

The key to understanding the common normal variants of biliary branching lies in the variability of the site of insertion of the **right posterior duct** (RPD) (segments 6 and 7). The RPD often extends centrally toward the porta hepatis in a cranial direction. It passes superior and posterior to the **right anterior duct** (RAD) and then turns caudally, joining the RAD to form the short right hepatic duct (see Fig. 6-2). Three other common sites of insertion of the RPD account for the majority of the anatomic variations. If the RPD extends more to the left than usual, it can join the junction of the right and left hepatic ducts ("trifurcation pattern"; ~8% of normal

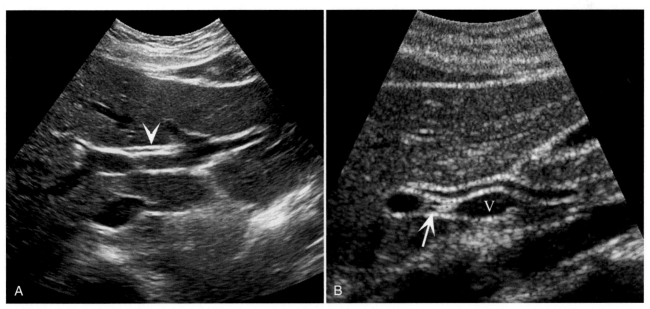

FIGURE 6-1. Normal bile ducts. A, Right and left hepatic ducts *(arrowhead)* are normally seen lying anterior to the portal veins. **B,** Common hepatic/common bile ducts of normal caliber in sagittal view lying in the typical position anterior to the portal vein *(V)* and hepatic artery *(arrow).*

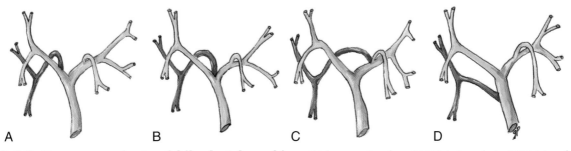

FIGURE 6-2. Common variants of bile duct branching. Right posterior duct (RPD) is in red. **A,** RPD joins the right anterior duct in 56% to 58% of population. **B,** Trifurcation pattern, 8%. **C,** RPD joins the left hepatic duct, 13%. **D,** RPD joins the common hepatic or common bile duct directly, 5%.

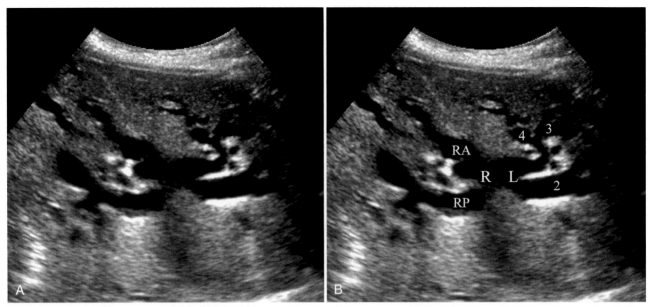

FIGURE 6-3. Typical ductal branching order. Intrahepatic biliary tree is dilated because of an obstructed common bile duct (not shown). **A** and **B,** Subcostal oblique views foreshorten the right *(R)* and left *(L)* hepatic ducts. *RA,* Right anterior duct; *RP,* right posterior duct; *2,* segment 2 duct; *3,* segment 3 duct; *4,* segment 4 duct.

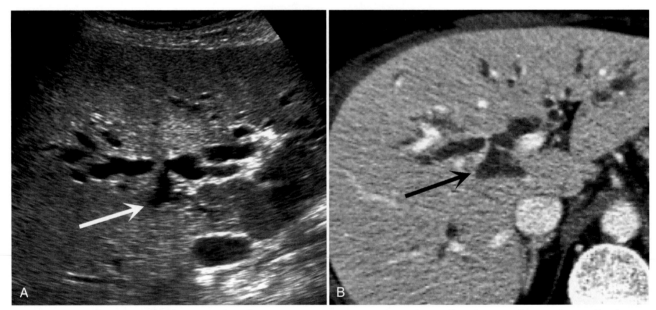

FIGURE 6-4. Aberrant right posterior duct. A, Transverse image obtained cranial to the porta hepatis depicts the aberrant right posterior duct *(arrow)* inserting into the left hepatic duct. This is the most common anomaly of the biliary tree. **B,** Corresponding enhanced CT image shows the same anomaly.

variants) or the left hepatic duct (~13%) (Fig 6-4). If the RPD extends in a caudal-medial direction instead, it can join the CHD or common bile duct (CBD) directly (~5%). Anomalous drainage of various segmental hepatic ducts directly into the common hepatic ducts is less common.

The **normal caliber** of the CHD/CBD in patients without history of biliary disease is up to 6 mm in most studies[5] (see Fig. 6-1). Controversy surrounds whether there is a normal widening of the duct with increasing age.[6] Similarly, studies on an association between cholecystectomy and a large-caliber CBD are inconclusive. Although diameters of up to 10 mm have been recorded in an asymptomatic normal population, the great majority of the diameters are under 7 mm. Therefore, a ductal diameter of 7 mm or greater should prompt further investigations, such as correlation with serum levels of cholestatic liver enzymes.

The site of insertion of the **cystic duct** into the bile duct is quite variable. The cystic duct may join the bile duct along its lateral, posterior, or medial border. It may also run a parallel course to the duct and insert into the lower one third of the duct, close to the ampulla of Vater.[7] The **common bile duct** extends caudally within the hepatoduodenal ligament, lying anterior to the portal vein and to the right of the hepatic artery. It then passes posterior to the first portion of the duodenum and the head of the pancreas, sometimes embedded in the latter. It ends in the ampulla of Vater, which is rarely identified on transabdominal ultrasound.

Sonographic Technique

Our technique for assessment of the intrahepatic ducts includes a **routine scan,** as would be performed for liver evaluation, including both sagittal and transverse scans. In addition, we perform a **focused scan** to assess the porta hepatis, recognizing that its orientation requires an oblique plane to show the length of the right and left hepatic ducts in a single image. For this we utilize a **subcostal oblique view** with the left edge of the transducer more cephalad than the right edge. The face of the transducer is directed toward the right shoulder. With a full suspended inspiration, a sweep of the transducer from the shoulder to the umbilical region will show the middle hepatic vein, then the long axis of the right and left hepatic ducts at the porta hepatis, followed by the common duct in cross section. By rotating the transducer 90 degrees to this plane, a second suspended inspi-

ration will allow for a long axis view of the CHD and CBD at the porta hepatis.

Harmonic imaging allows for improved contrast between the ducts and adjacent tissues, leading to improved visualization of the duct, its luminal contents, and wall (Fig. 6-5). We advocate routine use of harmonic imaging in the assessment of the biliary tree. Specific scanning techniques for assessment of choledocholithiasis and cholangiocarcinoma are discussed in the appropriate sections.

Choledochal Cysts

Choledochal cysts represent a heterogeneous group of congenital diseases that may manifest as **focal or diffuse cystic dilation** of the biliary tree. These cysts occur most often in East Asian populations; the incidence in Japan is 1 in 13,000 versus 1 in 100,000 in Western populations.[8,9] The female/male ratio is 3:1 to 4:1.

Although most patients present early in life, about 20% of choledochal cysts are encountered in adulthood, when sonography is performed for symptoms of gallstone disease.[10] The most widely used classification system divides choledochal cysts into **five types**[11] (Fig. 6-6). **Type I** choledochal cysts, a fusiform dilation of the CBD, are the most common (80%) and, along with type IVa, are associated with an abnormally long common channel (>20 mm) between the distal bile duct and the pancreatic duct. This long common channel could allow for reflux of pancreatic juices into the CBD, causing dilation, but this remains controversial.[8,12] **Type II** cysts

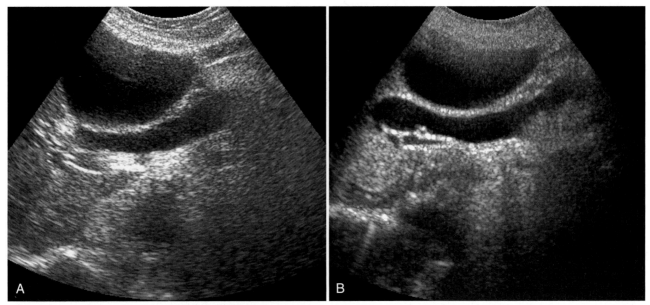

FIGURE 6-5. Harmonic imaging of biliary tree. A, Longitudinal view of the common bile duct with fundamental frequencies and **B,** with harmonic imaging. There is increased contrast to noise with harmonic imaging, effectively clearing the artifactual, low-level echoes over the fluid-filled duct. *(From Ortega D, Burns PN, Hope Simpson D, Wilson SR. Tissue harmonic imaging: is it a benefit for bile duct sonography? AJR Am J Roentgenol 2001;176:653-659.)*

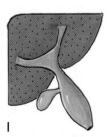 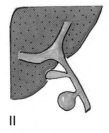 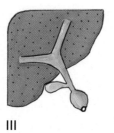 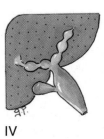

I   II   III   IV

FIGURE 6-6. Todani classification system for choledochal cysts. Type I cyst: diffuse dilation of the extrahepatic bile duct; this is the most common type (80%). **Type II cyst:** true diverticulum of the bile duct; very rare. **Type III cyst:** also called chole-dochocele; diffuse dilation of the very distal (intraduodenal) common bile duct. **Type IV cyst:** multifocal dilations of the intrahepatic and extrahepatic bile ducts. **Type V cyst,** Caroli's disease, is omitted because it is not a true choledochal cyst. *(From Todani T, Watanabe Y, Narusue M, et al. Congenital bile duct cysts, classification, operative procedures, and review of thirty-seven cases including cancer arising from choledochal cyst. Am J Surg 1977;134:263-269.)*

are true diverticula of the bile ducts and are very rare. **Type III** cysts, the "choledochoceles," are confined to the intraduodenal portion of the CBD. **Type IVa** cysts are multiple intrahepatic and extrahepatic biliary dilations, whereas **type IVb** cysts are confined to the extrahepatic biliary tree. Caroli's disease has been classified as a **type V** cyst, but it has a different embryonic origin and is not a true choledochal cyst.[9]

On sonography, a cystic structure is identified that may contain internal sludge, stones, or even solid neoplasm. In some cases the cyst is large enough that its connection to the bile duct is not immediately recognized. Use of various scanning windows and angles allows for demonstration of the relationship of the lesion to the biliary tract, differentiating it from pancreatic pseudocysts or enteric duplication cysts. Biliary scintigraphy, magnetic resonance cholangiopancreatography (MRCP), and endoscopic retrograde cholangiopancreatography (ERCP) have been used to delineate further the structure of choledochal cysts. ERCP is necessary to ensure that the dilation is not a result of distal neoplasm, especially in the case of type I choledochal cysts (Fig. 6-7). Because there is a proven risk of cholangiocarcinoma with all choledochal cysts, surgical resection is advocated.

Caroli's Disease

Caroli's disease is a rare congenital disease of the intrahepatic biliary tree that results from malformation of the ductal plates, the primordial cells that give rise to the intrahepatic bile ducts. There are two types of Caroli's disease: the simple, classic form and the second, more common form, which occurs with **periportal hepatic fibrosis.**[13] The second form has also been called **Caroli's syndrome.** Caroli's disease has been associated with cystic renal disease, most often renal tubular ectasia (medullary sponge kidneys). However, both forms may also be seen in patients with autosomal recessive polycystic kidney disease. Caroli's disease affects men and women equally, and more than 80% of patients present before the age of 30 years.[14]

Caroli's disease leads to **saccular dilation** or less often **fusiform dilation** of the intrahepatic biliary tree, resulting in biliary stasis, stone formation, and bouts of cholangitis and sepsis (Fig. 6-8). The disease most often affects the intrahepatic biliary tree diffusely, but it may be focal. The dilated ducts contain stones and sludge. Unlike recurrent pyogenic cholangitis, the ductal contents do not form a cast of the dilated system and thus are more easily identified as ductal contents.[15] Also, small portal vein branches surrounded by dilated bile ducts and bridging echogenic septa traversing the dilated ducts have been described on ultrasound. These correspond to persistent embryonic ductal structures.[16] If associated with congenital hepatic fibrosis, findings of altered hepatic architecture and portal hypertension are also present. Cholangiocarcinoma develops in 7% of patients with Caroli's disease.[14]

Overview of Biliary Tree Obstruction

Elevation of cholestatic liver parameters, which may appear clinically as jaundice, is a frequent indication for sonographic examination of the abdomen. The major objective in performing these scans is to determine if the patient has obstruction of the bile ducts, as opposed to a hepatocellular or biliary ductular disease. Sonography is highly sensitive in the detection of dilation of the biliary tree and is therefore an excellent modality for initiation of the imaging investigation (Fig. 6-9). These scans should be performed with knowledge of the patient's clinical condition, especially whether the patient has painless jaundice or has painful jaundice, as seen with acute obstruction or infection affecting the biliary tree.

The ultrasound examination should focus on answering the following three questions:
1. Are the bile ducts or gallbladder dilated?
2. If dilated, to what level?
3. What is the cause of the obstruction?

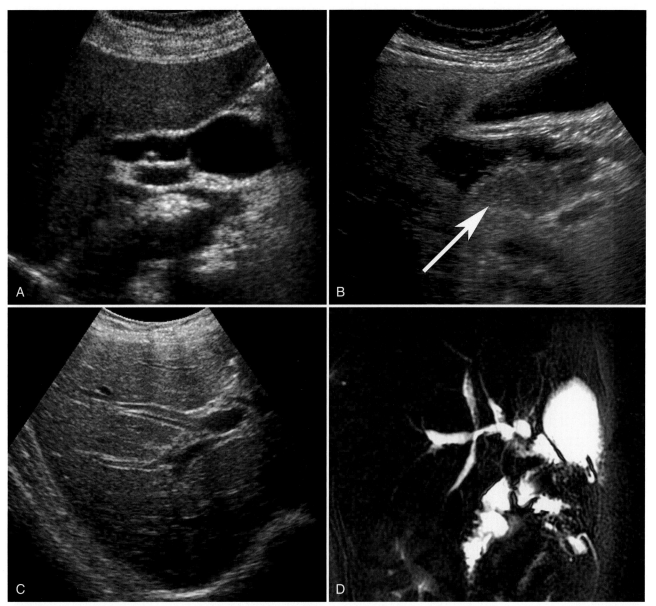

FIGURE 6-7. Choledochal cysts. A, Type I. Fusiform dilation of the common bile duct is seen, but no obstructive lesion is noted. This is the most common type of choledochal cyst. **B,** Type I cyst reveals a cholangiocarcinoma *(arrow)* growing into the cyst (longitudinal view). **C,** Sonogram, and **D,** MRCP, **Type IV.** There is tubular dilation of the more central intrahepatic biliary tree. The dilated extrahepatic ducts have been previously resected.

CAUSES OF BILIARY OBSTRUCTION

BENIGN MISCELLANEOUS
Choledocholithiasis*
Hemobilia*
Congenital biliary diseases
  Caroli's disease*
  Choledochal cysts
Cholangitis
  Infectious
Acute pyogenic cholangitis*
Biliary parasites*
Recurrent pyogenic cholangitis*
HIV cholangiopathy
  Sclerosing cholangitis

*Denotes causes of painful jaundice.

NEOPLASMS
Cholangiocarcinoma
Gallbladder carcinoma
Locally invasive tumors (esp. pancreatic
  adenocarcinoma)
Ampullary tumors
Metastases

EXTRINSIC COMPRESSION
Mirizzi syndrome*
Pancreatitis
Adenopathy

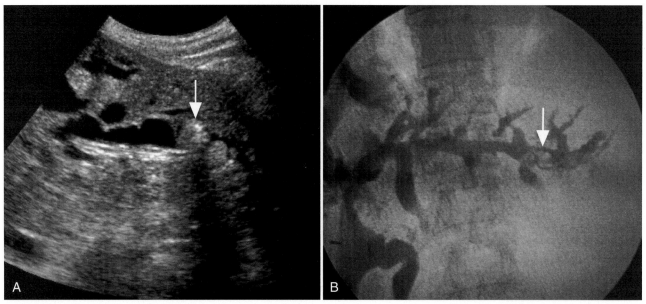

FIGURE 6-8. Caroli's disease. A, Transverse image through the left lobe of the liver demonstrates a dilated duct with sacculations typical of Caroli's disease. Mildly shadowing stones *(arrow)* are seen in the proximal duct. **B,** Corresponding cholangiogram shows the stones *(arrow)* as filling defects.

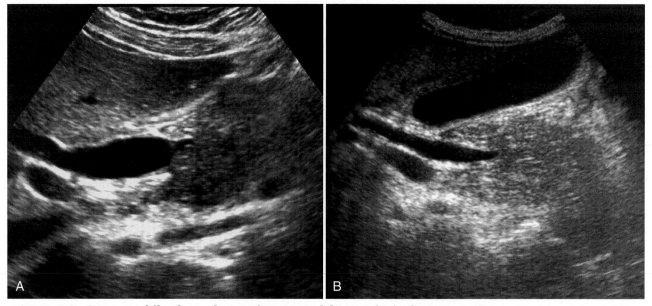

FIGURE 6-9. Common bile duct obstruction caused by extrinsic factors. A, Pancreatic adenocarcinoma. Short transition zone with shouldering, large duct caliber, along with an obstructive mass are typical findings in malignant obstruction. **B, Pancreatitis.** Elongated tapering of the duct suggests a benign cause. Note mild sympathetic gallbladder wall thickening caused by adjacent inflammation.

Choledocholithiasis

Choledocholithiasis may be classified into primary and secondary forms. **Primary choledocholithiasis** denotes de novo formation of stones, often made of calcium bilirubinate (**pigment stones**) within the ducts. The etiologic factors are often related to diseases causing strictures or dilation of the bile ducts, leading to stasis, as follows:

- Sclerosing cholangitis
- Caroli's disease
- Parasitic infections of the liver (e.g., *Clonorchis, Fasciola, Ascaris*)[17]

- Chronic hemolytic diseases, such as sickle cell disease
- Prior biliary surgery, such as biliary-enteric anastomoses

Migration of stones from the gallbladder into the common bile duct constitutes **secondary choledocholithiasis.** Whereas primary choledocholithiasis is relatively rare outside endemic regions (East Asia), secondary choledocholithiasis is quite common, representing the worldwide distribution of gallstone disease. Bile duct stones are found in 8% to 18% of patients with symptomatic gallstones.[18]

Intrahepatic Stones

Harmonic and compound imaging have improved the ability to find small stones within the intrahepatic bile ducts, especially with dilated ducts. Our experience indicates that sonography compares to and occasionally surpasses other biliary imaging methods, including MRCP. However, the current sensitivity of sonography in detecting intrahepatic stones is unknown.

The appearance of stones depends on their size and texture (Fig. 6-10). Most stones are highly echogenic with posterior acoustic shadowing, although. Small (<5 mm) or soft pigment stones in the patient with recurrent pyogenic cholangitis may not show shadowing (see Fig. 6-11, *D*). When the affected ducts are filled with stones, the individual stones may not be appreciated; instead a bright, echogenic linear structure with posterior shadowing is seen. Stones should always be suspected if discrete or linear echogenicities with or without shadowing are seen in the region of the portal triads, paralleling the course of the portal veins within the liver. Harmonic imaging improves both the contrast resolution and the detection of the acoustic shadow and is therefore recommended for routine assessment of the biliary tree.[19]

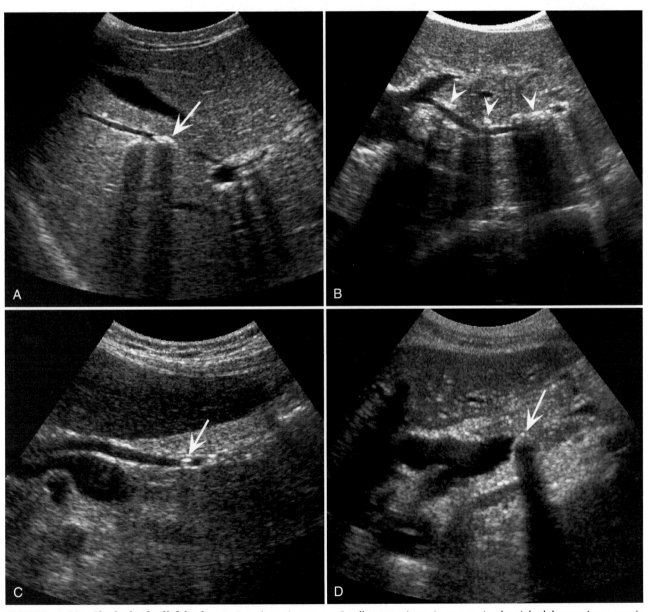

FIGURE 6-10. Choledocholithiasis. A, Intrahepatic stones. Small stones *(arrow)* are seen in the right lobe causing acoustic shadowing. Note the dilated duct proximal to the larger stone. **B, Multiple stone clusters** *(arrowheads)* in the left lobe appearing as echogenic linear structures with shadowing. Both patients (in **A** and **B**) had cystic fibrosis. **C** and **D, Common bile duct (CBD) stones. C,** Small stone *(arrow)* may not show shadowing. **D,** Large stone *(arrow)* has classic findings within a dilated CBD. *(C and D from Ortega D, Burns PN, Hope Simpson D, Wilson SR: Tissue harmonic imaging: is it a benefit for bile duct sonography? AJR Am J Roentgenol 2001;176:653-659.)*

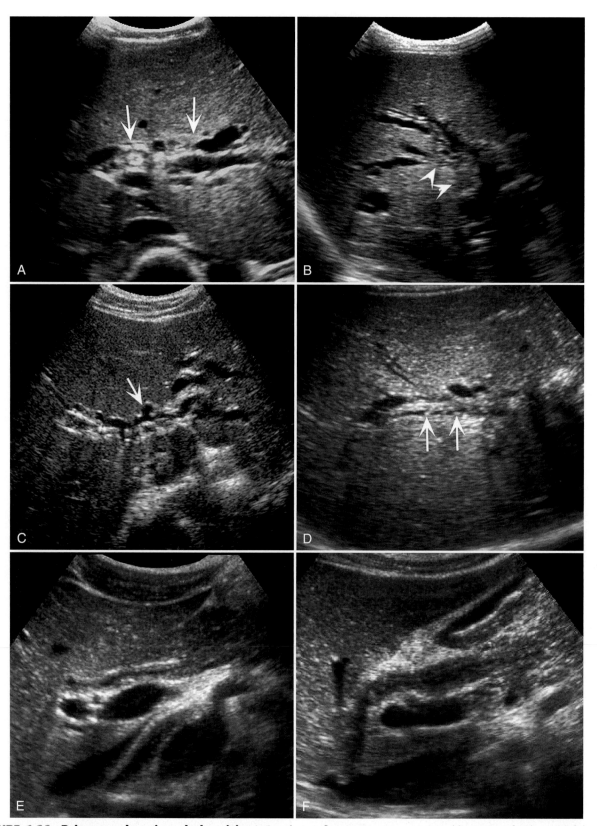

FIGURE 6-11. Primary sclerosing cholangitis. A, Isoechoic inflammatory tissue causing obliteration of right and left hepatic ducts *(arrows)* with proximal dilation. **B,** Dilated intrahepatic ducts "rat-tail" as they extend centrally toward the hepatic hilum. Note the hypoechoic ductal/periductal tissue obstructing the central ducts *(arrowheads).* **C,** Saccular diverticula *(arrow)* of the duct are occasionally seen. Note the variable caliber of the dilated ducts. **D,** Minute intraductal stones *(arrows)* are seen in irregular, mildly dilated ducts. **E** and **F,** Common bile duct wall thickening of moderate and severe degrees, respectively. Note the extremely narrowed, anechoic central lumen.

Common Bile Duct Stones

The majority of stones in the CBD will be in the distal duct right at the ampulla of Vater. Therefore, sonographic evaluation should include assessment of the entire duct, focusing on the periampullary region. Unfortunately, this region is often the most difficult area to see because it may be hidden by bowel gas, making detection of distal CBD stones also difficult. **Optimal technical factors** to improve assessment include the following:

- **Changes in patient position.** The CBD may be examined in supine, left lateral decubitus, and standing positions. The change in the relative position of adjacent organs and bowel gas may allow significantly improved visualization of the distal duct.
- **Choice of sonographic window.** The subcostal view is most useful for the assessment of the porta hepatis and proximal CBD. An epigastric view is best for the distal CBD.
- **Use of compression sonography.** Physically compressing the epigastrium may collapse the superficial bowel and displace the bowel gas that is blocking the view.
- **Detailed assessment of the distal CBD.** The distal intrapancreatic CBD is often best visualized with the probe focused on the pancreatic head in the **transverse** plane. Once the dilated CBD is identified, a slight rocking of the transducer to just "peek" at the point of caliber change will often allow a glimpse of a stone impacted in the distal duct, which is otherwise hidden from sonographic view. Similarly, a **sagittal** view focused on the pancreatic head should show the dilated CBD on the dorsal aspect of the head. Again, slight manipulation of the transducer, focusing on the point of caliber change, is best to see a solitary stone impacted in the distal duct.

The classic appearance of CBD stones is a **rounded echogenic lesion** with **posterior acoustic shadowing** (see Fig. 6-10). Importantly, no fluid rim will be seen around an impacted distal CBD stone because it is compressed against the duct wall. The lateral margins of the stone are therefore not seen, decreasing the conspicuity of the stone, versus a stone seen in the gallbladder or proximal duct, where it is likely to be surrounded by bile. Small stones may lack good acoustic shadows and appear only as a reproducible bright, linear echogenicity, either straight or curved. Awareness of this subtle appearance of CBD stones definitely improves their detection.

Pitfalls in the diagnosis of choledocholithiasis include **blood clot** (hemobilia), **papillary tumors,** and occasionally **biliary sludge**; none of these will shadow. **Surgical clips** in the porta hepatis, mostly from previous cholecystectomy, appear as linear echogenic foci with shadowing.[20] The short length, the relatively high degree of echogenicity, the lack of ductal dilation, and the absence of the gallbladder should allow differentiation of surgical clips from stones.

Mirizzi Syndrome

Mirizzi syndrome describes a clinical syndrome of jaundice with pain and fever resulting from obstruction of the common hepatic duct caused by a stone impacted in the cystic duct. It occurs most often when the cystic duct and CHD run a parallel course. The stone is often impacted in the distal cystic duct, and the accompanying inflammation and edema result in the obstruction of the adjacent CHD. The obstruction of the cystic duct results in recurrent bouts of cholecystitis, and the impacted stone may erode into the CHD, resulting in a cholecysto-choledochal fistula and biliary obstruction.[21] Identification of the fistula complication (called Mirizzi type II) is important because the treatment requires surgical repair of the fistula. Acute cholecystitis, cholangitis, and even pancreatitis may occur.[22]

Mirizzi syndrome should be considered on sonography when biliary obstruction with dilation of the biliary ducts to the CHD level is seen with acute or chronic cholecystitis. Thus the gallbladder has features of acute cholecystitis but may or may not be distended.[2] A stone impacted in the cystic duct with surrounding edema at the level of the obstruction is confirmatory (Fig. 6-12).

Hemobilia

Iatrogenic biliary **trauma,** mostly caused by percutaneous biliary procedures or liver biopsies, accounts for

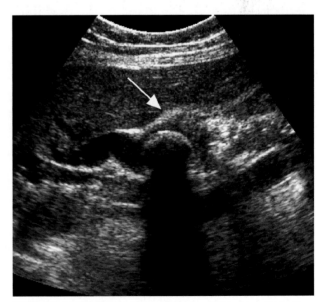

FIGURE 6-12. Mirizzi syndrome. Mirizzi syndrome in a patient with abdominal pain and jaundice. Sagittal sonogram shows a dilated common bile duct obstructed by a large stone impacted in the distal cystic duct. This appearance may be mistaken for a common bile duct stone. There is thickening of the wall of the cystic duct *(arrow).*

approximately 65% of all causes of hemobilia. Other etiologies include cholangitis or cholecystitis (10%), vascular malformations or aneurysms (7%), abdominal trauma (6%), and malignancies, especially hepatocellular carcinoma and cholangiocarcinoma (7%).[23] Pain, bleeding, and biochemical jaundice are the usual complaints at presentation. Apart from the blood loss, which occasionally is severe, complications are rare and include cholecystitis, cholangitis, and pancreatitis.

The appearance of blood within the biliary tree is similar to blood clots encountered elsewhere (Fig. 6-13). Most often, the clot is echogenic or of mixed echogenicity, and retractile, conforming to the shape of the duct. Occasionally, hemobilia may appear tubular with a central hypoechoic area. Acute hemorrhage will appear as fluid with low-level internal echoes. Blood clots may be mobile. Extension into the gallbladder is common. The clinical history is often essential to the diagnosis.

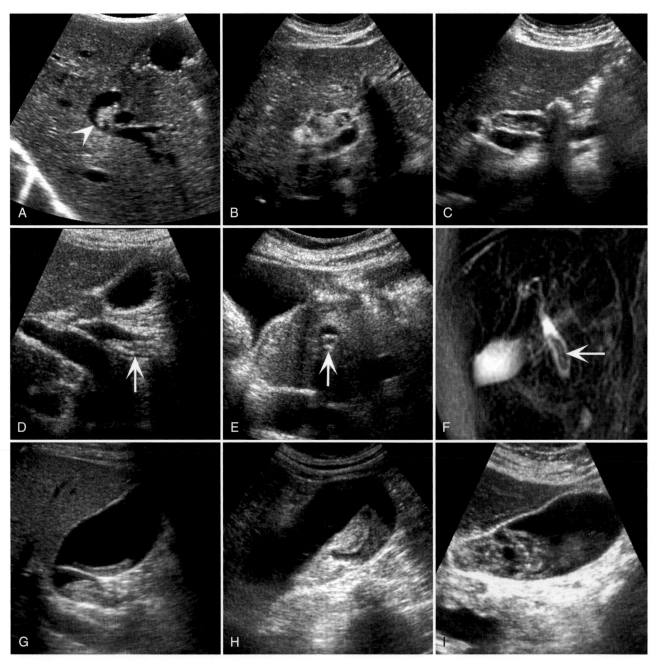

FIGURE 6-13. Hemobilia: spectrum on sonography. A, Echogenic blood clot *(arrowhead)* within a dilated duct, after insertion of biliary drainage catheter. Biliary obstruction was caused by pancreatic tumor. **B** and **C,** Echogenic clot in the common hepatic duct in two patients after liver biopsy. **D** and **E,** Spontaneous hemobilia in patient receiving anticoagulation therapy. Note the tubular appearance of the clot *(arrow)* with central anechoic lumen. **F,** Corresponding MRCP image depicts the same. **G, H,** and **I,** Blood in gallbladder in three different patients. All patients developed pain after liver biopsy. Note the angled edges of the clot in **G,** typical of blood clots.

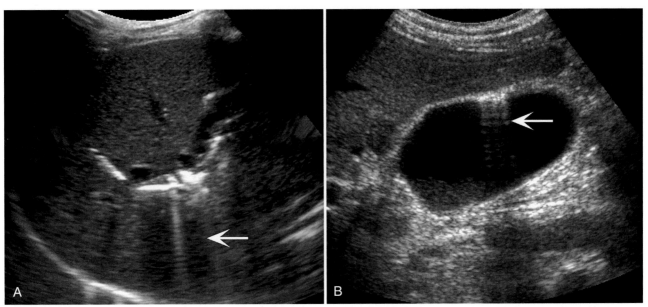

FIGURE 6-14. Pneumobilia. A, Extensive air within the central ducts manifests as linear echogenic structures paralleling the portal veins. Note the dirty shadowing *(arrow)* and reverberation artifact. **B,** Air in the gallbladder. Pneumobilia often extends into the gallbladder. Note the reverberation artifact *(arrow)*.

Pneumobilia

Air within the biliary tree usually results from previous biliary intervention, biliary-enteric anastomoses, or common bile duct stents. In the acute abdomen, pneumobilia may be caused primarily by three entities. **Emphysematous cholecystitis** may lead to pneumobilia; its risk factors and findings are discussed under Acute Cholecystitis. Inflammation caused by an impacted stone in the common bile duct may cause erosion of the duct wall, leading to **choledochoduodenal fistula.** The third entity, prolonged acute cholecystitis, may lead to erosion into an adjacent loop of bowel, most frequently the duodenum or transverse colon, called **cholecystoenteric fistula.** Stones may then pass from the gallbladder into the bowel and can cause a bowel obstruction called **gallstone ileus.**

Air in the bile ducts has a characteristic appearance. Bright, echogenic linear structures following the portal triads are seen, more often in a nondependent position (Fig. 6-14). Posterior "dirty" shadowing and reverberation ("ringdown") artifact are seen with large quantities of air. Movement of the air bubbles, best seen just after changing the patient's position, is diagnostic. Extensive arterial calcifications, seen especially in diabetic patients, can mimic pneumobilia.

Biliary Tree Infection

Acute (Bacterial) Cholangitis

Antecedent **biliary obstruction** is an essential component of bacterial cholangitis, associated in 85% of cases with common bile duct stones.[24] Other causes of obstruction include biliary stricture as a result of trauma or surgery, congenital abnormalities such as choledochal cysts, and partially obstructive tumors. Intrinsic or extrinsic neoplasms causing complete biliary obstruction rarely cause pyogenic cholangitis before biliary intervention.[25] The clinical presentation is usually that of (1) fever (~90%), (2) right upper quadrant (RUQ) pain (~70%), and (3) jaundice (~60%), the classic **Charcot's triad.** There is leukocytosis, or at least a left shift, and elevated levels of serum alkaline phosphatase (ALP) and bilirubin in the great majority of patients. Often, mild serum hepatic transaminitis is present, but occasionally, levels above 1000 are seen early in the disease because of a sudden increase in intrabiliary pressures.[25] The bile is most often infected by gram-negative enteric bacteria, which are often retrieved in blood cultures.

Acute cholangitis is a medical emergency. Sonography is advocated as the first imaging modality to determine the cause and level of obstruction and to exclude other diseases, such as cholecystitis, acute hepatitis, and Mirizzi syndrome. Sonography is more accurate than computed tomography (CT) and more practical than magnetic resonance imaging (MRI), endoscopic ultrasound, and ERCP in the initial assessment of patients with potential acute biliary disease.[26]

The sonographic findings of bacterial cholangitis include the following (Fig. 6-15):

- Dilation of the biliary tree
- Choledocholithiasis and possibly sludge
- Bile duct wall thickening
- Hepatic abscesses

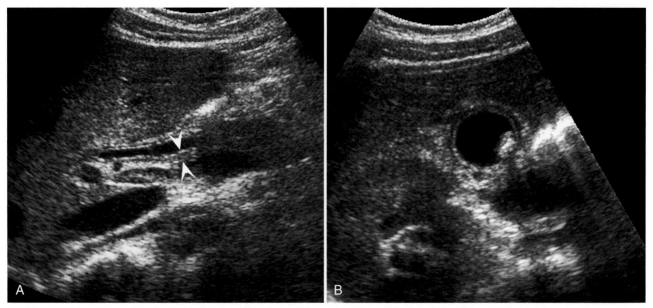

FIGURE 6-15. Acute bacterial cholangitis in a 22-year-old woman. A, Bile duct wall thickening *(arrowheads),* and **B,** gallbladder wall thickening, help to differentiate acute bacterial cholangitis from primary sclerosing cholangitis, where the gallbladder is affected in only 10% to 15% of cases. Note gallstone in the gallbladder.

Dilation of the biliary tree, when present, can be well diagnosed by sonography. A CBD diameter greater than 6 mm is considered abnormal in most patients. Subtle dilation of the intrahepatic biliary tree is a frequently overlooked finding that should be specifically sought. This includes use of subcostal oblique scanning of the porta hepatis to assess the caliber of the right and left hepatic ducts, as well as evaluation of the CBD, which may measure normal but still show a somewhat "tense" or distended morphology. Dilation of the biliary tree is seen in 75% of patients. The obstructive stone is usually lodged in the distal CBD but may be mobile, causing intermittent obstruction. Air is rarely seen within the ducts; thus its presence suggests a choledochoenteric fistula in the absence of previous biliary manipulation. Circumferential thickening of the bile duct wall, similar to other causes of cholangitis, may be present and may extend to the gallbladder. Multiple small hepatic abscesses—sometimes grouped in a lobe or segment of the liver—may be seen but tend to become visible on sonography when they have undergone liquefaction and are a late finding.

Liver Flukes

Fascioliasis. *Fasciola hepatica* infection is unevenly endemic in many regions of the world, including Asia, Europe, Northern Africa, and South America (mainly Peru and Bolivia).[27] Infection is caused by consumption of water or raw vegetables contaminated with the larvae (metacercariae) of the *F. hepatica* fluke. The infection has two stages: the **acute phase,** lasting 3 to 5 months, and the **chronic phase,** which may last several years to

over a decade. The acute phase corresponds to the migration of the immature larvae through the bowel wall, peritoneal cavity, and liver capsule, into the liver parenchyma. Patients may present with acute RUQ pain, hepatomegaly, and prolonged fevers. The final destination of the larvae is the biliary tree, where the parasite matures and produces eggs, indicating the chronic phase of infection. The mature *Fasciola* is the largest of the liver flukes (20-40 mm in length), is flat in shape (1 mm thin), and can be directly seen within the bile ducts. Symptoms then relate to biliary obstruction with intermittent jaundice, fevers, and intrahepatic abscesses. Half the patients are asymptomatic in the chronic phase.[27]

The imaging appearance of fascioliasis depends on the phase of infection. In the acute phase, sonography demonstrates non-specific findings of hepatomegaly, hilar adenopathy, and hypoechoic or mixed echogenicity lesions[28,29] (Fig. 6-16). The liver lesions are often multiple, confluent, subcapsular and ill-defined and are present in ~90% of patients.[29] The specific finding of the migratory tract of the larvae, manifest by small cyst-like clusters in serpiginous tracts in the periphery of the liver are better imaged with CT or MRI.[30] Serial examination may show slowly evolving disease with progressive central migration of lesions and periportal tracking representing lymphangiectasia in the portal triads.[31] Sonography is more useful in the **chronic ductal phase** of the disease, depicting ductal dilation and the flukes in the ducts and gallbladder as flat, sometimes moving, material (Fig. 6-17). The living flukes within the gallbladder were present in 37% of patients in a series of 87 patients.[29]

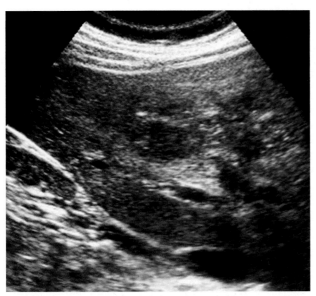

FIGURE 6-16. *Fasciola hepatica* **infection, acute (parenchymal) phase.** Oblique image through the right lobe shows poorly defined hypoechoic lesions in the liver parenchyma. Patients often present with fever and pain. *(Courtesy Dr. Adnan Kabaalioglu, Akdeniz University Hospital, Antalya, Turkey.)*

Clonorchiasis and Opisthorchiasis. *Clonorchis sinensis, Opisthorchis viverrini* and *Opisthorchis felineus* are similar in morphology and life cycle but vary in their geographic distribution. They all present major public health problems to large populations of humans. *C. sinensis* is endemic in East and Southeast Asia; *O. viverrini* in Cambodia, Laos, Thailand, and Vietnam; and *O. felineus* in Central Asia, Russia, and Ukraine.[27] The infection is acquired by ingestion of raw fish (carp) contaminated by the larvae (metacercariae), which migrate through the ampulla of Vater, up the bile duct, then mature and live within the small and medium-sized intrahepatic bile ducts. The mature flukes are smaller than *F. hepatica*, measuring 8 to 15 mm. The acute phase of infection tends to be asymptomatic for *C. sinensis* and *O. viverrini*. The infestation may last for many years or decades.[27]

Ultrasound imaging of *C. sinensis* and *O. viverrini* infestation shows similar findings, which are present in moderate and severe infestation.[32] The principal abnormality is the **diffuse dilation** of the peripheral intrahepatic bile ducts, often with normal or minimally dilated central and extrahepatic ducts (Fig. 6-18). The peripheral dilation results from the predilection of the fluke for these ducts. Active infection is suggested by increased periportal echoes (likely representing edema) and floating echogenic foci in the gallbladder, representing the flukes or debris.[32] The biliary dilation may persist even after treatment. Chronic infection by these flukes has been directly linked to **cholangiocarcinoma** and is postulated as a cause of recurrent pyogenic cholangitis. The imaging of *O. felineus* infestation has not been systematically described.

Recurrent Pyogenic Cholangitis

Recurrent pyogenic cholangitis has been known by other names, including **hepatolithiasis** and **Oriental cholangiohepatitis.** It is a disease characterized by chronic biliary obstruction, stasis, and stone formation, leading to recurrent episodes of acute pyogenic cholangitis. Its incidence is highest in Southeast and East Asia. It is rare and sporadic in other populations. Although liver fluke infections (especially *C. sinensis*), malnutrition, and portal bacteremia have all been implicated, the etiology of recurrent pyogenic cholangitis remains unknown.[33] Any segment of the liver may be affected, but the **lateral segment of the left lobe** is most often involved. Acute complications of the disease, namely sepsis, may be fatal and may need urgent percutaneous biliary decompression or surgery. The chronic stasis and inflammation eventually leads to severe atrophy of the affected segment. Biliary cirrhosis and cholangiocarcinoma are long-term complications. The treatment of hepatolithiasis lies in repeated biliary dilation and stone removal.[34]

Ultrasound is often used for both screening and monitoring of pyogenic cholangitis.[25] The typical appearance on sonography is dilated ducts filled with sludge and stones, confined to one or more segments of the liver (Figs. 6-19 and 6-20). Patients may also present with multiple echogenic masses in the liver, and recognizing that these, in fact, lie within extremely dilated ducts requires care. When dilated ducts are identified, their contents may be hypoechoic or echogenic, and the stones may not show shadowing. With severe atrophy of the affected segment, minimal liver parenchyma may be present, and the crowded, stone-filled ducts may appear as a single, heterogeneous mass.

Ascariasis

Ascaris lumbricoides is a parasitic roundworm estimated to infect up to one quarter of the world's population. It uses a **fecal-oral route** of transmission and is most common in children, presumably because of their lower hygiene levels.[35] The worm is generally 20 to 30 cm long and up to 6 mm in diameter. It is active within the small bowel and may enter the biliary tree retrogradely through the ampulla of Vater, causing acute biliary obstruction. Generally, infected patients are asymptomatic but may present with biliary colic, cholangitis, acalculous cholecystitis, or pancreatitis.

The appearance of biliary ascariasis on sonography depends on the number of worms within the bile ducts at the time of the study. Most often, a single worm is identified that appears as a tube or as parallel echogenic lines within the bile ducts. The appearance is similar to a biliary stent, which should be excluded on clinical history. On the transverse view, the rounded worm surrounded by the duct wall gives a target appearance. The worm may be folded on itself or may occupy any portion

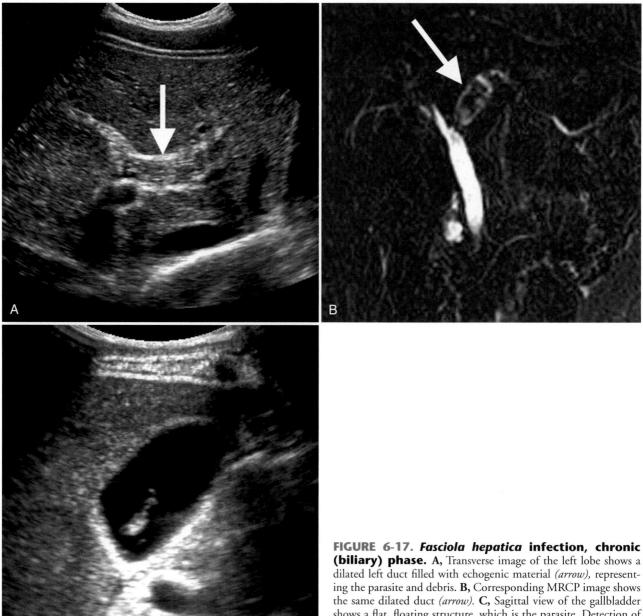

FIGURE 6-17. *Fasciola hepatica* **infection, chronic (biliary) phase. A,** Transverse image of the left lobe shows a dilated left duct filled with echogenic material *(arrow),* representing the parasite and debris. **B,** Corresponding MRCP image shows the same dilated duct *(arrow).* **C,** Sagittal view of the gallbladder shows a flat, floating structure, which is the parasite. Detection of motion of the parasite is pathognomonic. Patients have few or no symptoms in the chronic phase of infection.

of the ductal system, including far into the liver parenchyma, close to the capsule, or within the gallbladder. Movement of the worm during the scan facilitates the diagnosis. When infestation is heavy, multiple worms may lie adjacent to each other within a distended duct, resembling spaghetti. Occasionally, the worms may appear as an amorphous, echogenic filling defect, making the diagnosis more difficult.[35]

HIV Cholangiopathy

Also known as **AIDS cholangitis,** HIV cholangiopathy is an inflammatory process affecting the biliary tree in the advanced stages of human immunodeficiency virus (HIV) infection (AIDS, acquired immunodeficiency syndrome). It is most often caused by an opportunistic infection and therefore occurs in patients with CD4 counts of less than 100. Patients present with severe RUQ or epigastric pain, a nonicteric cholestatic picture, and greatly elevated serum ALP with a normal bilirubin level. In most patients a pathogen is recovered, usually *Cryptosporidium* or less often cytomegalovirus.[36]

Sonography has been advocated as the first imaging test for assessment of HIV cholangiopathy (Fig. 6-21). A negative scan effectively rules out the disease. The findings include the following:

• Bile duct wall thickening of the intrahepatic and extrahepatic biliary tree.

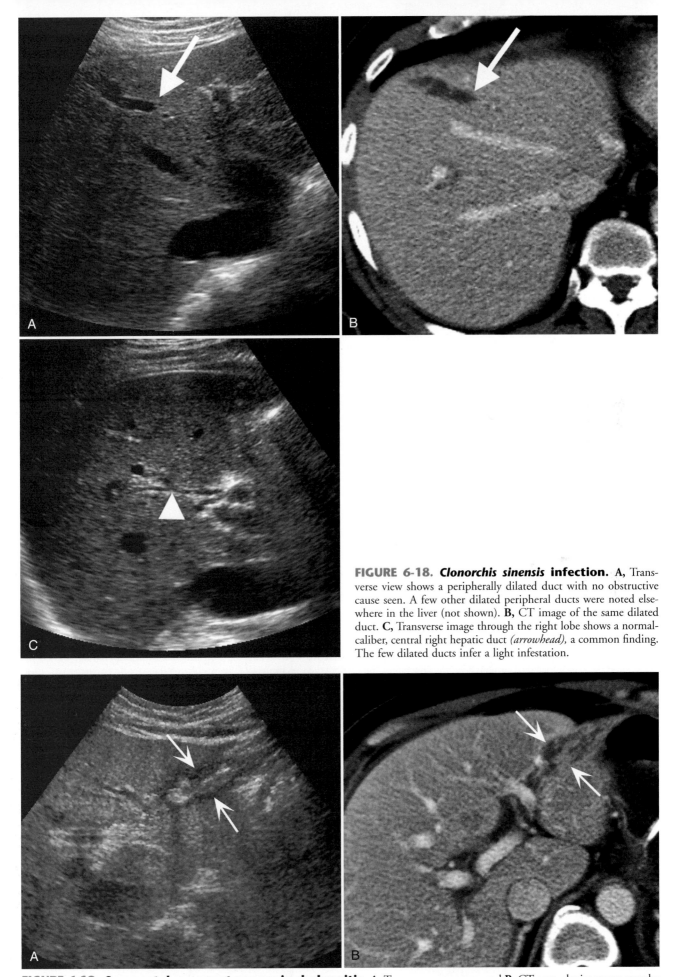

FIGURE 6-18. *Clonorchis sinensis* **infection. A,** Transverse view shows a peripherally dilated duct with no obstructive cause seen. A few other dilated peripheral ducts were noted elsewhere in the liver (not shown). **B,** CT image of the same dilated duct. **C,** Transverse image through the right lobe shows a normal-caliber, central right hepatic duct *(arrowhead),* a common finding. The few dilated ducts infer a light infestation.

FIGURE 6-19. Segmental recurrent pyogenic cholangitis. A, Transverse sonogram, and **B,** CT scan, depict severe atrophy of segment 3 *(arrows)* around abnormal, stone-filled ducts.

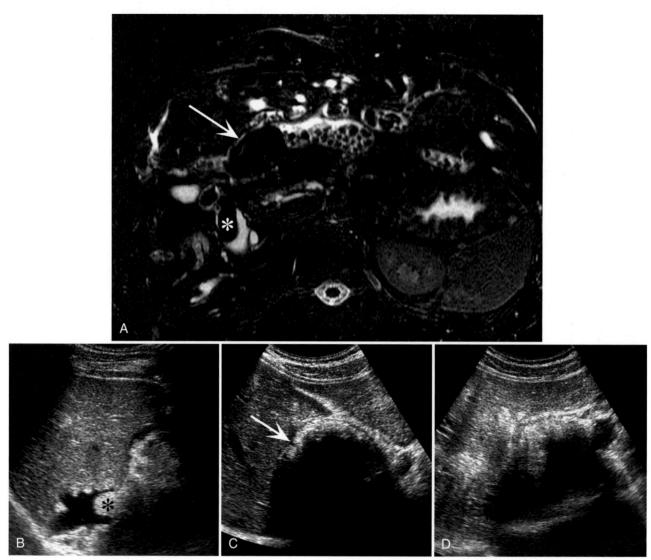

FIGURE 6-20. Recurrent pyogenic cholangitis. A, Axial MRCP view through the liver demonstrates greatly dilated biliary tree filled with stones. **B,** Transverse ultrasound image of the right lobe shows a large stone *(asterisk)* in the dilated right posterior duct, corresponding to abnormality on MRCP view *(asterisk in **A**). **C,** Huge stone in the central duct *(arrow)* with marked posterior acoustic shadowing. **D,** Multiple small stones in the left lobe, which appear as a masslike, echogenic conglomerate on the sonogram. This is the most common appearance of recurrent pyogenic cholangitis, especially when accompanied by atrophy of the hepatic parenchyma.

- Focal strictures and dilations identical to primary sclerosing cholangitis.
- Dilation of the CBD caused by an inflamed and stenosed papilla of Vater (papillary stenosis). The inflamed papilla itself may be seen as an echogenic nodule protruding into the distal duct.[37]
- Diffuse gallbladder wall thickening, seen much more often than in primary sclerosing cholangitis.[38]

Immune-Related Diseases of the Biliary Tree

Primary Biliary Cirrhosis and Autoimmune Cholangitis

Primary biliary cirrhosis and autoimmune cholangitis (also called autoimmune cholangiopathy) affect ducts that are too small to resolve by imaging. Only gross changes in the liver architecture resulting from biliary cirrhosis are detected. Biliary cirrhosis, resulting from any cause of chronic diffuse biliary obstruction, appears as diffusely enlarged liver unless the liver is end-stage.

Primary Sclerosing Cholangitis

Sclerosing cholangitis is a chronic inflammatory disease process affecting the biliary tree. If the etiology of the disease is unknown, the term **primary** sclerosing cholangitis is used.

Primary sclerosing cholangitis is a chronic disease affecting the entire biliary tree. The process involves a fibrosing inflammation of the small and large bile ducts, leading to biliary strictures and cholestasis and eventually biliary cirrhosis, portal hypertension, and hepatic

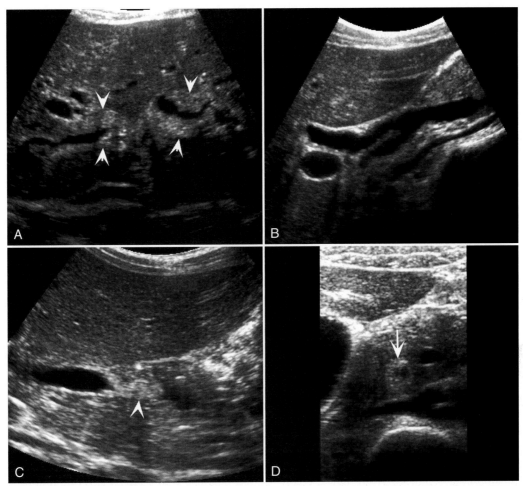

FIGURE 6-21. HIV cholangiopathy. A, Intrahepatic biliary tree. Note the thick rind of echogenic tissue *(arrowheads)* surrounding the central portal triads and causing irregular narrowing of the bile ducts. **B,** Common bile duct (CBD) is dilated, and its wall is minimally irregular. **C,** Papillary stenosis. The dilated CBD abruptly tapers in an echogenic, inflamed ampulla *(arrowhead).* **D,** Transverse view of ampulla *(arrow),* which is enlarged and echogenic, viewed in the caudal aspect of pancreatic head.

CAUSES OF SECONDARY SCLEROSING CHOLANGITIS

IgG4-related sclerosing cholangitis
AIDS cholangiopathy
Bile duct neoplasm*
Biliary tract surgery, trauma
Choledocholithiasis
Congenital abnormalities of biliary tract

Ischemic stricturing of bile ducts
Toxic strictures related to intra-arterial infusion of floxuridine
Posttreatment for hydatid cyst
Primary sclerosing cholangitis

Modified from Narayanan Menon KV, Wiesner RH. Etiology and natural history of primary sclerosing cholangitis. J Hepatobiliary Pancreat Surg 1999;6:343-351.
*Primary sclerosing cholangitis not previously established.

failure.[39,40] It occurs more frequently in men, with median age of 39 years at diagnosis.[35] About 80% of the patients have concomitant **inflammatory bowel disease,** typically ulcerative colitis, but this association occurs less often in a non-Western population. It may also occur with other autoimmune disorders or systemic sclerosing conditions, such as retroperitoneal fibrosis.[33]

Most patients diagnosed with primary sclerosing cholangitis are asymptomatic. Ultrasound is a key component of the multimodality assessment of patients with this disease. The high spatial resolution of ultrasound allows for detection of minute early changes that can be missed with MRCP. Sonographic findings include irregular, circumferential bile duct wall thickening of varying degree, encroaching on and narrowing the lumen (Fig. 6-11). Focal strictures and dilations of the bile ducts ensue. The extrahepatic disease is more easily visible. A high degree of suspicion and careful examination of the portal triads in all hepatic segments is required to detect intrahepatic ductal involvement. **Irregularity of the thickened bile duct mucosa** is a key feature that should be sought. An earlier study suggested false normal appearance of the intrahepatic bile ducts in 25% of patients.[36] The gallbladder and cystic duct are involved in 15% to 20% of patients.[37] **Choledocholithiasis,** once thought to exclude the disease, is now recognized as a complication and is more frequently seen in symptomatic patients.[38] In more advanced cases, findings of cirrhosis are also present.

Cholangiocarcinoma develops in 7% to 30% of patients with primary sclerosing cholangitis and is particularly a difficult diagnosis to make in this setting.[40] Rapid progression of the disease or development of a visible mass is a clue to this complication. Hepatic transplantation is required in the latter stages of the disease. Unfortunately, the disease may recur in the transplanted organ in 1% to 20% of patients.[41]

IgG4-Related Cholangitis

IgG4-related cholangitis is the biliary manifestation of multifocal systemic fibrosclerosis (MSF). The exact etiology of the disease is unknown but is associated with elevation of serum immunoglobulin G and specifically IgG subtype 4 levels in a majority of patients. In the abdomen, the most commonly affected organ is the pancreas, resulting in autoimmune pancreatitis, followed by the biliary tree and gallbladder, the kidneys (interstitial nephritis), and the retroperitoneum (retroperitoneal fibrosis). A history of salivary or lactrimal gland disease is also common. The disease predominates in elderly patients and is more common in males. The disease tends to be **steroid responsive**, as opposed to primary sclerosing cholangitis. IgG4-related cholangitis affects both large and small ducts. There is a lymphoplasmacytic infiltrate about the ducts with associated fibrosis causing strictures; if untreated it can lead to cirrhosis. Given the similarity in imaging appearance to primary sclerosing cholangitis, it has until recently been mistaken for this disease.

There are no systematic studies comparing the cross-sectional imaging appearance of IgG4-related cholangitis to primary sclerosing cholangitis. Several features help the differentiation or at least direct the referring clinicians to further investigations. In IgG4-related disease, the patient is usually older and the disease may spontaneously resolve or improve. In our experience, bile duct wall thickening can be much more pronounced than in PSC and can appear mass-like. Strictures are longer, but mucosal irregularity, which is an important feature of PSC, is difficult to appreciate. Many patients with IgG4-related cholangitis have involvement of other organs, which can be searched for during the scan; pancreatic involvement virtually makes the diagnosis. Many of the changes improve within weeks of commencement of steroid therapy.

Cholangiocarcinoma

Cholangiocarcinoma is an uncommon neoplasm that may arise from any portion of the biliary tree. Its incidence varies geographically and is highest in populations with known risk factors. Overall incidence ranges from 1 to 2 per 100,000 population in the United States, 2 to 6 in other Western countries, 5.5 in Japan, and up to 80 to 130 per 100,000 in northeastern Thailand, where the liver fluke *Opisthorchis viverrini* is endemic.[42,43] The frequency of cholangiocarcinomas increases with age, with the peak incidence in the eighth decade. Most cholangiocarcinomas are sporadic, but several risk factors exist, usually related to chronic biliary stasis and inflammation. **Primary sclerosing cholangitis** is the most common risk factor for cholangiocarcinoma in the Western world; the lifetime risk of developing a clinically detectable cholangiocarcinoma in these patients is about 10%.[44] The most common risk factors in other populations are **recurrent biliary infections** and **stone disease**.

Cholangiocarcinomas are classified based on the anatomic location: **intrahepatic,** also called peripheral (~10%); **hilar,** also called Klatskin's (~60%); and **distal** (~30%).[45] Approximately 90% of cholangiocarcinomas are **adenocarcinomas,** with squamous carcinomas the next most common subtype.[46] Macroscopically, cholangiocarcinomas are divided into three subtypes: sclerosing, nodular, and papillary; the first two subtypes frequently occur together. **Nodular-sclerosing tumors**, the most common subtype, appear as a firm mass surrounding and narrowing the affected duct, with a nodular intraductal component. Most hilar cholangiocarcinomas are of the nodular-sclerosing variety. These tumors incite a prominent desmoplastic reaction and demonstrate a periductal, perineural, and lymphatic pattern of spread along the ducts, as well as subendothelial spread within the ducts. **Papillary cholangiocarcinomas** represent approximately 10% of these tumors and are most common in the distal CBD. Patients present with an intraductal polypoid mass that expands, rather than constricts, the duct.[45,47,48]

The overall prognosis for cholangiocarcinoma is poor. In a large, single-center series, the 5-year survival rate for patients with intrahepatic, hilar, and distal cholangiocarcinoma was 23%, 6%, and 24%, respectively, and improved to only 44%, 11%, and 28% in patients who underwent resection.[49]

Intrahepatic Cholangiocarcinoma

Intrahepatic cholangiocarcinomas, also called **peripheral cholangiocarcinomas,** are the least common location

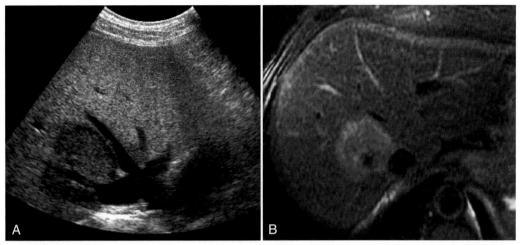

FIGURE 6-22. Peripheral cholangiocarcinoma. A, Ultrasound, and **B,** T2-weighted MR, images depict a solid mass encasing the right hepatic vein. Differentiation from a metastasis is not possible by imaging.

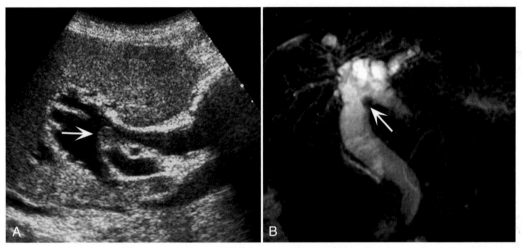

FIGURE 6-23. Intraductal papillary, mucin-producing tumor of bile ducts. A, Ultrasound, and **B,** MRCP, images show papillary tumor arising from the common hepatic duct *(arrow)* and causing diffuse ductal dilation due to excessive mucin production.

for cholangiocarcinomas, but they represent the second most common primary malignancy of the liver. They arise from the second-order or higher-order branches of the biliary tree within the liver parenchyma, and their histologic origin is different than that of extrahepatic ducts. The incidence of intrahepatic cholangiocarcinomas has been dramatically rising in the past two decades, in part because of the increase in numbers of patients with liver cirrhosis and long-term hepatitis C infection.[50] Hepatitis B also has recently been identified as a risk factor.[51] These tumors are associated with a poor prognosis because the mass is often unresectable.[52,53]

The most common manifestation of intrahepatic cholangiocarcinoma is a large hepatic mass. The sonographic appearance is often that of a hypovascular solid mass with heterogeneous echotexture, and it may appear hypoechoic, isoechoic, or hyperechoic (Fig. 6-22). A clue to the differentiation from **hepatocellular carcinoma (HCC)** is a much higher incidence of **ductal obstruc-**

tion, reportedly occurring in 31% of intrahepatic cholangiocarcinomas and only 2% of HCC.[54,55] However, a metastasis to the liver may cause intrahepatic ductal obstruction and therefore may be indistinguishable.[56]

A more unusual manifestation of intrahepatic cholangiocarcinoma is a purely intraductal mass, called **intraductal intrahepatic cholangiocarcinoma.** These polypoid masses distend the affected ducts, often third-order or fourth-order branches, spreading within the duct and filling it with **mucin.** These tumors have a much better prognosis and are thought to be histologically separate from other intrahepatic cholangiocarcinomas, resembling papillary tumors of the extrahepatic bile ducts.[53,57] The most common appearance of the intraductal intrahepatic cholangiocarcinoma is one or more polypoid masses confined to the bile ducts. Abundant mucin production can greatly distend the affected lobar and distal ducts (Fig. 6-23). A less common form may present as a solid mass within a cystic structure,

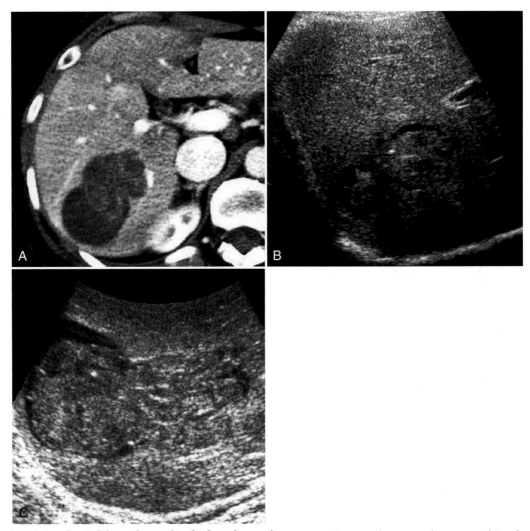

FIGURE 6-24. Intraductal intrahepatic cholangiocarcinoma. A, Computed tomography scan, and **B,** ultrasound view, show a solid and cystic mass in the right lobe of the liver. **C,** Intraoperative sonogram demonstrates the mass to lie entirely within an extremely dilated duct. Low-grade cholangiocarcinoma was found at pathologic examination.

representing tumor within an extremely distended duct that does not communicate with the biliary tree (Fig. 6-24).

Hilar Cholangiocarcinoma

The correct identification and staging of hilar cholangiocarcinoma are challenging with all imaging modalities. This results from the tumor's **desmoplastic** nature (causing fibrous tissue formation), its peribiliary and subendothelial patterns of growth, and the complex anatomy of the porta hepatis, with structures lying just outside the liver and surrounded by connective tissue. Ultrasound plays an important role in both **detection** and **staging** of hilar cholangiocarcinomas because it is often the first modality used in assessment of these tumors. Furthermore, ultrasound is often performed before any biliary manipulation and stent placement. Because biliary intervention often significantly obscures the intraductal disease and causes secondary bile duct thickening, sono-

graphy may be the only cross-sectional modality to assess the unmanipulated ducts. Most patients with hilar cholangiocarcinoma present for a sonographic evaluation with jaundice, pruritus, and elevated cholestatic liver parameters, or with vague symptoms and elevated serum ALP or γ-glutamyl transpeptidase levels.

Patterns of Tumor Growth. Hilar cholangiocarcinomas often begin in either the right or the left bile duct and extend both proximally into higher-order branches and distally into the CHD and contralateral bile ducts. The spread of tumor may be subendothelial, or within the peribiliary connective tissue, leading to obstruction or irregular ductal narrowing. The tumors also extend outside the ducts to involve adjacent portal vein and arteries. Chronic obstruction, especially if accompanied with portal vein involvement, leads to atrophy of the involved lobe. Nodal disease often begins in the porta hepatis and within the hepatoduodenal ligaments (local nodes) and extends to celiac, superior mesenteric, peripancreatic, and posterior pancreatoduodenal stations (distant nodes).[58] Metastases are usually to the liver and peritoneal surfaces.

Treatment and Staging. Curative treatment of cholangiocarcinoma requires surgical resection; the vast majority of patients with unresectable disease die within 12 months of diagnosis.[45] The current surgical approach to patients with hilar cholangiocarcinoma is resection of the involved lobe with extensive hilar dissection to remove tumor extending to the contralateral lobe (extended lobectomy). A biliary-enteric anastomosis is created to allow bile drainage. Currently, no widely used staging systems accurately stratify patients based on surgical resectability. However, Jarnagin et al.[58] proposed a system that allows for preoperative staging of hilar cholangiocarcinoma. Because a lobectomy is performed, the remaining liver parenchyma, its portal vein, hepatic artery, and at least some proximal length of its lobar bile duct (first-order branch of CHD) should ideally be free of disease. The main portal vein and proper hepatic artery should also ideally be disease free. The remaining liver should not have undergone significant atrophy because it may not be able to maintain hepatic function. Although regional nodes may be removed en bloc with the tumor, distant nodal disease precludes resection. Advancements in surgical techniques now allow biliary-enteric anastomoses using second-order ducts and vessel resection with reconstruction; therefore criteria for resectability vary according to the age of the patient and local surgical preferences.

CRITERIA FOR UNRESECTABLE HILAR CHOLANGIOCARCINOMA

Hepatic duct involvement up to secondary biliary radicles bilaterally

Encasement or occlusion of the main portal vein proximal to its bifurcation

Atrophy of one hepatic lobe with encasement of contralateral portal vein branch

Atrophy of one hepatic lobe with contralateral involvement of secondary biliary radicles

Distant metastases (peritoneum, liver, and lung)

From Jarnagin WR. Cholangiocarcinoma of the extrahepatic bile ducts. Semin Surg Oncol 2000;19:156-176.

Assessment by Conventional and Doppler Sonography. An accurate assessment of hilar cholangiocarcinoma requires diligent, hands-on involvement by the responsible physician. The use of various views and patient positions as well as familiarity with biliary anatomy and common variants significantly improves sonographic performance. Once **dilated intrahepatic ducts** have been detected, the following parameters should be assessed:

- Level of the obstruction
- Presence of a mass
- Lobar atrophy
- Patency of main, right, and left portal veins
- Encasement of hepatic artery
- Local and distant adenopathy
- Presence of metastases

Dilation of the higher-order intrahepatic bile ducts with non-union of the right and left ducts is the classic appearance of hilar cholangiocarcinomas[56] (Figs. 6-25 and 6-26). When encountered, dilated ducts should be followed centrally toward the hepatic hilum to determine which order of branching (segmental ducts and higher or right/left hepatic ducts) is involved with tumor. Tumor extension into segmental ducts bilaterally precludes resection.

The obstructing tumor is not always visualized by sonography. Rates of sonographic detection of masses range from 21% to 87%, with more recent studies showing higher rates.[59-61] When a mass is not directly visualized, its presence can be inferred based on the level of obstruction, although this often underestimates the tumor extent.[62] **Lobar atrophy** leads to crowding of the dilated bile ducts and, if long-standing, a shift in the axis of the liver caused by hypertrophy of the contralateral side. The atrophy of the lobe is often accompanied by obliteration of its portal vein and precludes its resection. **Differences in lobar echogenicity**, caused by the varying degree of ductal and vascular obstruction between the two lobes, is an uncommon finding (Fig. 6-27).

The main, right, and left **portal veins** should all be examined with both gray-scale and color Doppler sonography. Narrowing of the right or left portal veins leads to compensatory increased flow in the accompanying hepatic artery; when prominent arterial signal is noted on color Doppler, the portal venous flow should be carefully examined (Fig. 6-27). Tumor encasing, narrowing, or obliterating the main portal vein or the proper hepatic artery renders the tumor unresectable, unless en bloc resection of the vessels is contemplated. Detection of the extrahepatic tumor infiltration and early peritoneal metastases is difficult with sonography, and CT or MRI is recommended as an adjunct for preoperative assessment.

Assessment by Contrast-Enhanced Sonography. Some ultrasound contrast agents persist in the liver parenchyma after a brief intravascular phase. This postvascular, liver-specific phase of enhancement significantly increases the contrast difference between the liver parenchyma and invasive tumors that do not enhance. Therefore the invasive component of cholangiocarcinoma—not seen in a significant minority of patients—becomes visible in most, if not all, cases[62] (Fig. 6-28). The ability to visualize the invasive tumor directly also allows for improved performance of sonography in the staging of hilar cholangiocarcinomas.[62] The liver-specific phase of enhancement results from contrast uptake by Kupffer cells and only occurs with some first- and second-generation contrast agents.[63]

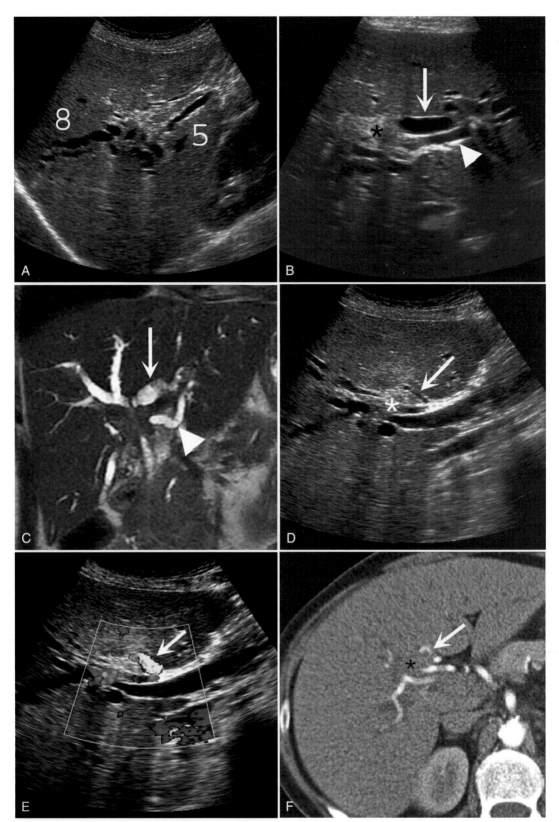

FIGURE 6-25 Resectable hilar cholangiocarcinoma. A, Sagittal image of the right lobe shows an invasive central echogenic tumor with segmental dilation of the ducts of segments 8 and 5, indicating second-order branch involvement. **B,** Transverse view of the central left lobe shows the tumor *(asterisk)* obstructing the distal left hepatic duct *(arrow)* and an aberrant segment 4 duct *(arrowhead)*. **C,** Coronal T2-weighted MR image confirms the ultrasound findings of the central tumor obstructing the left hepatic *(arrow)* and aberrant segment 4 ducts *(arrowhead)*. **D,** Transverse image of the porta hepatis depicts the tumor *(asterisk)* narrowing the right portal vein and displacing branches of the right hepatic artery *(arrow)*. **E,** Doppler image (same plane as **D**) confirms the right hepatic artery involvement. **F,** Corresponding CT image in the arterial phase also shows intimate contact of tumor *(asterisk)* with right hepatic artery branches *(arrow)*. The tumor did not extend deep into the left lobe, and the main and left hepatic arteries and portal vein were not involved; therefore the patient underwent an extended right-sided hepatectomy.

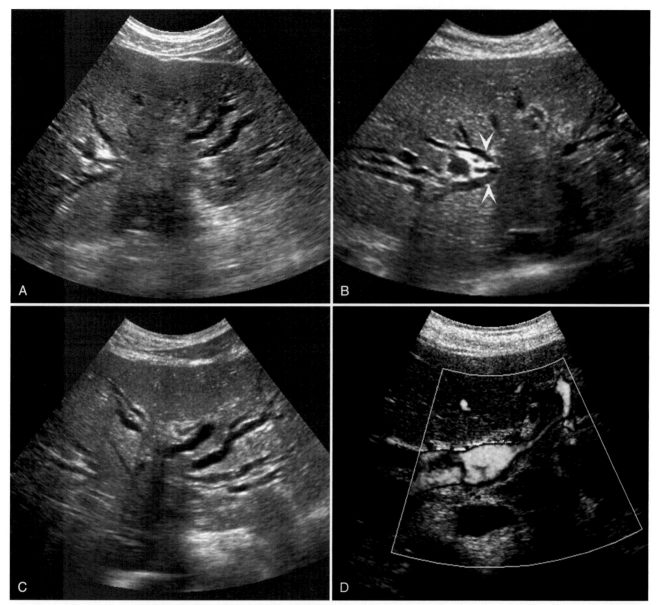

FIGURE 6-26. Unresectable hilar cholangiocarcinoma. A, Dilated right-sided and left-sided intrahepatic ducts with nonunion centrally, as seen here, are hallmarks of hilar cholangiocarcinoma. Determination of the level of obstruction is key in assessing resectability. **B,** In right lobe view, the right anterior and posterior ducts *(arrowheads)* approach each other, but never join to form the right hepatic duct. **C,** In left lobe view, second-order and third-order branches end abruptly, blocked by tumor. Because the tumor completely involves the first-order branches (right and left hepatic ducts) bilaterally, it is unresectable. **D,** Tumor also encases and narrows the left portal vein.

Distal Cholangiocarcinoma

Distal cholangiocarcinomas are clinically indistinguishable from the hilar forms, with progressive jaundice seen in 75% to 90% of patients.[45] Although the nodular-sclerosing subtype still predominates, polypoid masses are seen more frequently. Surgical resection is the most effective therapy, so a careful search for spread that would preclude resection is vital. The tumor may locally extend cranially within the ducts, even involving the cystic and right and left hepatic ducts; therefore the superior extent of the tumor must be clearly defined. The tumor may also extend beyond the duct walls. Patients may present

with a distal obstructive mass with identical appearance to pancreatic adenocarcinoma. The status of the adjacent vascular structures must be determined, including portal and superior mesenteric veins and common hepatic artery. Spread to **lymph nodes** adjacent to the tumor is common. Spread to more distant nodes, such as celiac, superior mesenteric, and periportal regions may preclude resection.[45] Surgical approach to a distal cholangiocarcinoma is a pancreaticoduodenectomy.

On sonography the distal cholangiocarcinoma has a variable appearance. A **polypoid tumor** appears as a duct-expanding, well-defined intraductal mass, often with no internal vascularity (Fig. 6-29). The **nodular-**

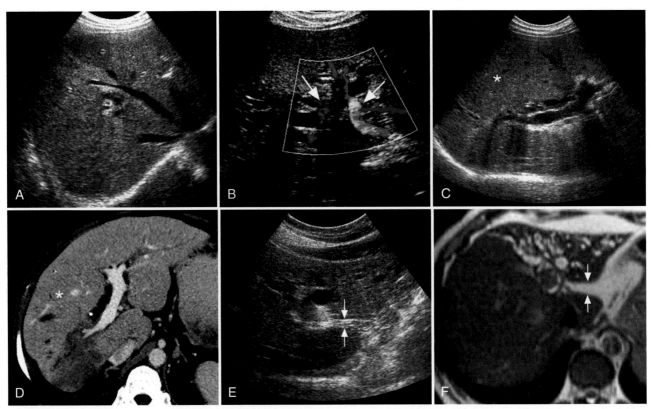

FIGURE 6-27. Secondary findings in hilar cholangiocarcinoma. A, Difference in lobar echogenicity. The right lobe of the liver is demarcated from the left by its increased echogenicity. The right biliary system was obstructed by tumor centrally. **B, Compensatory increased flow in hepatic arteries.** Enlarged hepatic arterial branches *(arrows)* on either side of the ascending branch of the left portal vein are clearly seen, whereas no flow is noted in the portal vein. This finding suggests severe stenosis or obstruction of the portal vein. **C** and **D, Lobar atrophy.** Marked atrophy of the right lobe with compensatory hypertrophy of the left lobe. *Asterisks,* Enlarged medial segment of the left lobe. **E** and **F, Lobar atrophy.** Marked atrophy of the left lobe of the liver. Besides the small size, widening of the fissure for ligamentum venosum *(arrows)* and concave liver margins are secondary clues. **F,** Axial SSFSE T2-weighted MR image shows the same.

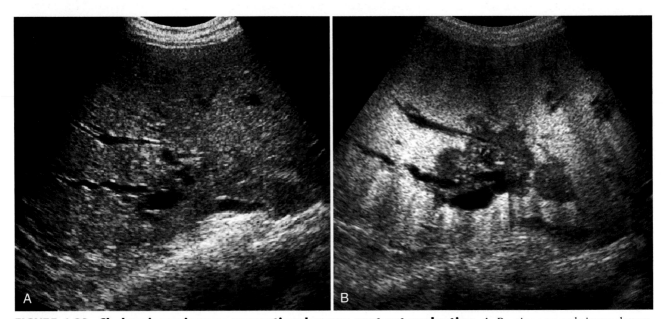

FIGURE 6-28. Cholangiocarcinoma: conventional versus contrast evaluation. A, Routine gray-scale image demonstrates dilated ducts terminating abruptly. The tumor is not visible. **B,** Levovist-enhanced image obtained in the postvascular phase clearly depicts the margins of the unenhancing tumor.

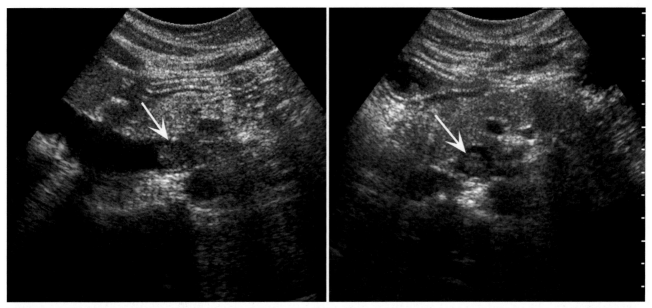

FIGURE 6-29. Distal cholangiocarcinoma. Polypoid solid intraductal mass *(arrows)* within the distal common bile duct, causing ductal obstruction.

sclerosing tumor causes focal irregular ductal constriction and duct wall thickening. In more advanced disease the tumor appears as a hypoechoic, hypovascular mass with poorly defined margins invading adjacent structures.

Metastases to Biliary Tree

Metastases to the biliary tree mimic the varied appearance of cholangiocarcinoma, affecting both the intrahepatic and extrahepatic ducts (Fig. 6-30). The history of past or concurrent malignancy along with multiple lesions should suggest metastases. In our experience the breast, colon, and skin (melanoma) constitute the primary sites of malignancy.

THE GALLBLADDER

Anatomy and Normal Variants

The gallbladder is a pear-shaped organ lying in the inferior margin of the liver, between the right and left lobes (Fig. 6-31). The middle hepatic vein lies in the same anatomic plane and may be used to help find the **gallbladder fossa.** The **interlobar fissure,** the third structure separating the two hepatic lobes, extends from the origin of the right portal vein to the gallbladder fossa. This fissure has been seen in up to 70% of hepatic ultrasound studies[64] and may also be used as a landmark for the gallbladder fossa. The gallbladder is divided into the fundus, body, and neck; the **fundus** is the most anterior, and often inferior, segment. In the region of the gallbladder **neck,** there may be an infundibulum, called **Hartmann's pouch,** which is a common location for impaction of gallstones.[10]

The gallbladder derives as an outpouching from the embryonic biliary tree. The proximal portion of the pouch forms the cystic duct, and the distal portion forms the gallbladder. Within the cystic duct (and sometimes the gallbladder neck) are small mucosal folds called the **spiral valves of Heister;** these are occasionally identified on sonography. During its initial development, the gallbladder lies in an intrahepatic position, but as it migrates to the surface of the liver, it acquires a peritoneal covering (part of liver capsule) over 50% to 70% of its surface.[10] The remainder of the gallbladder surface is covered with adventitial tissue that merges with connective tissue in contiguity with the liver. In generalized edematous processes or local inflammation, this potential space between the gallbladder and liver is a common area for edema. Failure to migrate may lead to an **intrahepatic gallbladder** (or partially intrahepatic), a rare but significant finding that may preclude laparoscopic surgery[65] (Fig. 6-32). Conversely, the gallbladder may become fully enveloped in visceral peritoneum, hanging from a mesentery that extends from the liver. This leads to increased mobility of the gallbladder and appears to be a risk factor in the rare development of **torsion** (volvulus) of the gallbladder.[66]

Failure to identify the gallbladder on sonographic examination most often results from a previous **cholecystectomy.** Occasionally, chronic **cholecystitis** leading to a collapsed and fibrosed gallbladder makes its detection difficult. **Agenesis** of the gallbladder is rare, occurring in up to 0.09% of the population.[67] Although most often incidental, dilation of the bile duct and choledocholithiasis may occur with gallbladder agenesis, leading to attempted cholecystectomy in some patients. In most cases the cystic duct is also absent. The lack of visualization of the gallbladder on sonography in symptomatic

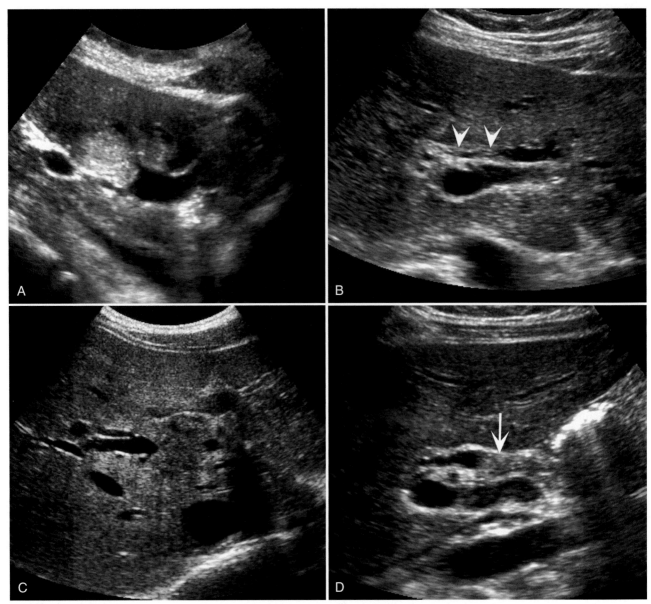

FIGURE 6-30. Metastases to the biliary tree: spectrum of appearances. A, Entirely intraductal echogenic mass obstructing left lobe of liver. **B,** Periductal/duct wall infiltration *(arrowheads)* with obliteration of the left hepatic duct. **C,** Poorly defined hilar tumor with ductal obstruction. **D,** Echogenic intraductal tumor *(arrow)* within the extrahepatic ducts. In all cases, tumor mimics cholangiocarcinoma. The diagnosis in all four images was metastatic breast carcinoma.

CAUSES OF SONOGRAPHIC NONVISUALIZATION OF GALLBLADDER

Previous cholecystectomy
Physiologic contraction
Fibrosed gallbladder duct—chronic cholecystitis
Air-filled gallbladder or emphysematous cholecystitis
Tumefactive sludge
Agenesis of gallbladder
Ectopic location

patients warrants CT or MRCP to avoid an unnecessary surgical procedure. The gallbladder may also lie in **ectopic** positions, including suprahepatic, suprarenal, within the anterior abdominal wall, or in the falciform ligament.[10]

The gallbladder may fold unto itself, the body onto the neck, or the fundus onto the body. The latter is called a **phrygian cap** and has no clinical significance. A **septate gallbladder** is composed of two or more intercommunicating compartments divided by thin septa.[10] This is distinguished from the hourglass gallbladder (see Adenomyomatosis), which has thick septa separating the components. **Duplication** of the gallbladder often

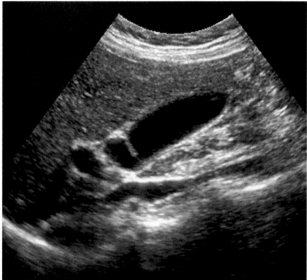

FIGURE 6-31. Normal gallbladder showing a thin fold.

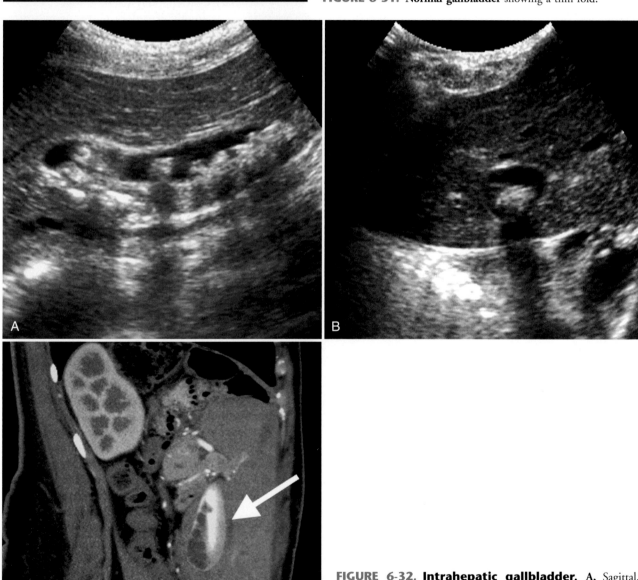

FIGURE 6-32. Intrahepatic gallbladder. A, Sagittal, and **B,** transverse, images through the liver depict a complete rim of liver tissue surrounding the gallbladder. There is extensive cholelithiasis. **C,** Sagittal CT cholangiogram image shows contrast within the gallbladder *(arrow)* with multiple stones. The patient had situs ambiguus with intrahepatic gallbladder and repeat bouts of cholecystitis.

occurs with duplication of the cystic duct and may be diagnosed prenatally. Variations of the cystic duct are discussed in the section on anatomy of the biliary tree.

The gallbladder derives its blood supply from the **cystic artery,** which arises from the right hepatic artery, or less often from the gastroduodenal artery. In acute cholecystitis an enlarged, prominent cystic artery may be identified on sonography.

Sonographic Technique

Evaluation of the gallbladder is usually performed with routine sagittal and transverse sonograms. If the gallbladder is not visualized, however, maneuvers to evaluate the gallbladder fossa are essential to avoid missing gallbladder pathology. This is done primarily with subcostal oblique sonograms, performed with the left edge of the transducer more cephalad than the right edge. The face of the transducer is directed toward the right shoulder. A sweep from cephalad to caudad shows the middle hepatic vein superiorly and the gallbladder fossa inferiorly in a single plane. They form the anatomic boundary separating the right and left liver lobes. The fossa runs from the anterior surface of the right portal vein obliquely to the surface of the liver. It may have a variable appearance, mainly influenced by the state of the gallbladder, and after gallbladder removal the fossa appears as an echogenic line as a result of the remaining connective tissues.

Ingestion of food, particularly fatty food, stimulates the gallbladder to contract. The contracted gallbladder appears thick walled and may obscure luminal or wall abnormalities. Therefore the examination of the gall-bladder should be performed after a minimum of 4 hours of fasting.

Gallstone Disease

Gallstone disease is common worldwide. The prevalence of gallstones is highest in the European and North American populations (~10%) and lowest in the East Asian (~4%) and sub-Saharan African (2%-5%) populations.[68] Common risk factors are increasing age, female gender (but not in Asian populations), fecundity, obesity, diabetes, and pregnancy. Although most patients are asymptomatic, about one in five develops a complication, often biliary colic. The risk of acute cholecystitis or other serious complications of gallstones in patients with a history of biliary colic is about 1% to 2% per year.[69]

Sonography is highly sensitive in the **detection of stones** within the gallbladder. The varying size and number of stones within the gallbladder lead to a variable appearance on sonography (Fig. 6-33, *A*). The large difference in the acoustic impedance of stones and adjacent bile makes them highly reflective, which results in an echogenic appearance with strong posterior acoustic shadowing. Small stones (<5 mm) may not show shadowing but will still appear echogenic. **Mobility** is a key feature of stones, allowing differentiation from polyps or other entities. Various maneuvers may be used to demonstrate mobility of a stone; scanning with the patient in the right or left lateral decubitus or upright standing position may allow the stone to roll within the gallbladder.

Multiple stones may appear as one large stone, producing uniform acoustic shadowing. When the gallblad-

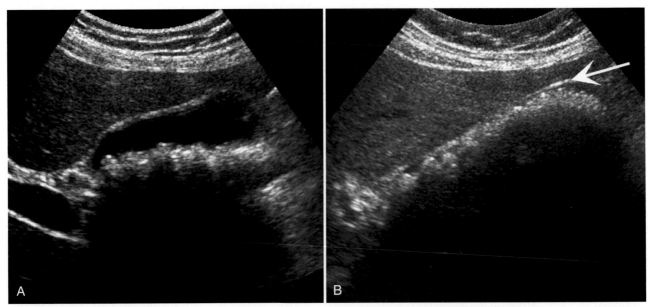

FIGURE 6-33. Gallbladder stones. A, Sagittal image shows multiple dependent stones appearing as echogenic foci with posterior acoustic shadowing. **B,** "Wall-echo-shadow complex" in a gallbladder filled with stones. Gallbladder wall *(arrow)* is thin.

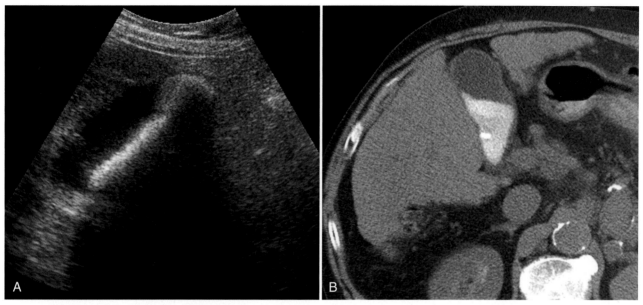

FIGURE 6-34. Milk of calcium bile. A, Sonogram, and **B,** corresponding CT scan, show a bile calcium level.

der is filled with small stones or a single giant stone, the gallbladder fossa will appear as an echogenic line with posterior shadowing. This can be differentiated from air or calcification in the gallbladder wall by analysis of the echoes. With stones the gallbladder *wall* is first visualized in the near field, followed by the bright *echo* of the stone, followed by the acoustic *shadowing,* called the **wall-echo-shadow** (WES) **complex** (Fig. 6-33, *B*). When air or calcification is present, the normal gallbladder wall is not seen, and only the bright echo and the posterior dirty shadowing are seen.

Milk of calcium bile, also known as **limey bile,** is a rare condition in which the gallbladder becomes filled with a pasty, semisolid substance of mainly calcium carbonate.[70] It is often associated with gallbladder stasis and rarely may cause acute cholecystitis or migrate into the bile ducts. The appearance on sonography is highly echogenic material with posterior acoustic shadowing, forming a bile calcium level on various patient positions (Fig. 6-34).

Biliary Sludge

Biliary sludge, also known as **biliary sand** or **micro-lithiasis,** is defined as a mixture of particulate matter and bile that occurs when solutes in bile precipitate. Its existence was first recognized with the advent of sonography. The exact prevalence of sludge is unknown in the general population because most studies have examined high-risk populations. The predisposing factors in development of sludge are pregnancy, rapid weight loss, prolonged fasting, critical illness, long-term total parenteral nutrition (TPN), ceftriaxone or prolonged octreotide therapy, and bone marrow transplantation. In one

study, over a 3-year period, about 50% of cases resolved spontaneously, 20% persisted asymptomatically, 5% to 15% developed gallstones, and 10% to 15% became symptomatic.[71] The complications of biliary sludge are stone formation, biliary colic, acalculous cholecystitis, and pancreatitis.

The sonographic appearance of sludge is that of amorphous, low-level echoes within the gallbladder in a dependent position, with no acoustic shadowing. With a change in patient position, sludge may slowly resettle in the most dependent location. In fasting, critically ill patients, sludge may be present in large quantities and completely fill the gallbladder. Sludge may mimic polypoid tumors, called **tumefactive sludge** (Fig. 6-35). Lack of internal vascularity, potential mobility of the sludge, and a normal gallbladder wall are all clues to the presence of sludge. When doubts persist, lack of contrast enhancement on ultrasound, CT, or MRI allows conservative management. Occasionally, sludge has the same echotexture as the liver, camouflaging the gallbladder; called **hepatization** of the gallbladder, this may be easily recognized by identifying the normal gallbladder wall.

Acute Cholecystitis

Acute cholecystitis is a relatively common disease, accounting for 5% of the patients presenting to the emergency department with abdominal pain and 3% to 9% of hospital admissions.[72] It is caused by gallstones in more than 90% of patients.[73] Impaction of the stones in the cystic duct or the gallbladder neck results in obstruction, with luminal distention, ischemia, superinfection, and eventually necrosis of the gallbladder. In the under-50 age group, women are affected three times more often

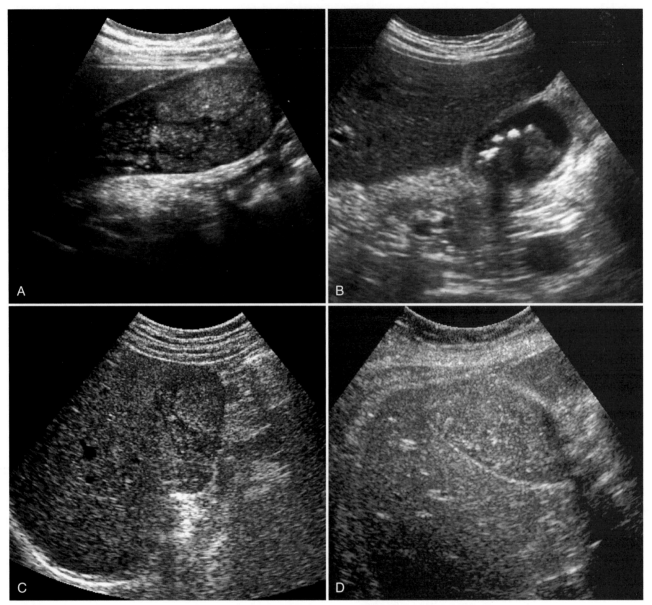

FIGURE 6-35. Tumefactive sludge in three patients. A, Sagittal sonogram shows gallbladder filled with tumorlike sludge. **B,** Transverse image shows a polypoid appearance of sludge on the dependent gallbladder wall, with stones along its margin. **C,** Sagittal, and **D,** subcostal oblique, sonograms of the same patient show "hepatization" of the gallbladder, with internal echoes mimicking the normal liver parenchyma. In all three patients the gallbladder wall was normal. There was no vascularity detected from the tumefactive sludge.

than men, although incidence of acute cholecystitis is similar in older age groups.[69] Clinically, patients present with a prolonged, constant RUQ or epigastric pain associated with RUQ tenderness. Fever, leukocytosis, and increased serum ALP and bilirubin levels may be present.

Sonography is currently the most practical and accurate method to diagnose acute cholecystitis (Figs. 6-36 and 6-37). When adjusted for verification bias, sensitivity and specificity of ultrasound are approximately 88% and 80%, respectively.[74] Cholescintigraphy uses ionizing radiation, cannot be performed at the bedside, and also has a significant false-positive rate.

Although less accurate than sonography in the diagnosis of acute cholecystitis, CT may be useful for depiction of complications.[75] Sonographic findings include the following[76] (Table 6-1):
- Thickening of the gallbladder wall (>3 mm)
- Distention of the gallbladder lumen (diameter >4 cm)
- Gallstones
- Impacted stone in cystic duct or gallbladder neck
- Pericholecystic fluid collections
- Positive sonographic Murphy's sign
- Hyperemic gallbladder wall on Doppler interrogation

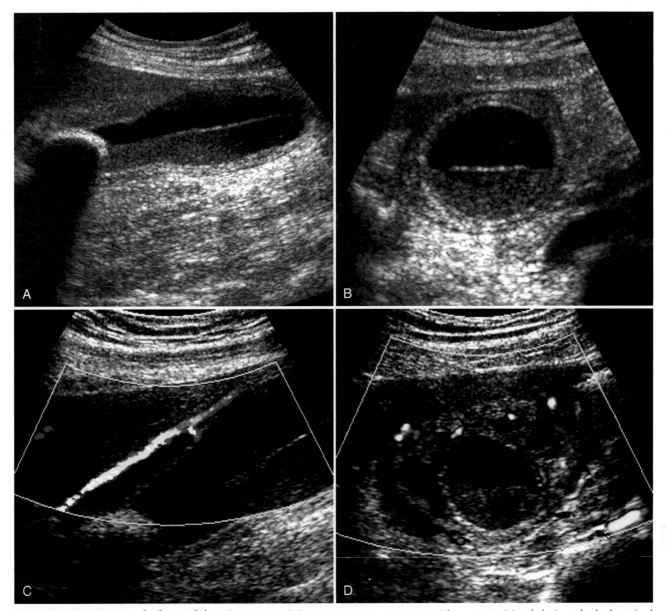

FIGURE 6-36. Acute cholecystitis. Classic acute cholecystitis in a young woman with a negative Murphy's sign who had received narcotic analgesics. **A,** Sagittal, and **B,** transverse, images show a tense gallbladder, wall thickening, fluid-debris level, and an obstructing stone in the gallbladder neck. **C,** Color Doppler image shows a large cystic artery. **D,** Transverse power Doppler image shows pockets of edema fluid within the thickened, hyperemic wall. *(From Wilson SR. Gastrointestinal disease. 6th series. Test and syllabus. Reston, Va, 2004, American College of Radiology.)*

Gallbladder wall thickening has many causes. The appearance of the gallbladder wall in acute cholecystitis is nonspecific, but marked thickening of the wall with visible stratification, as seen in generalized edematous states, is usually not present (Fig. 6-38). Multiple focal, noncontiguous, hypoechoic pockets of edema fluid within the thickened wall are typically observed. The inflamed gallbladder is often significantly distended, unless its wall is perforated. **Gallstones,** including the obstructing stone, and sludge are usually identified. A thin rim of fluid, representing edema, is often seen around much of the organ.

A sonographic **Murphy's sign** is maximal tenderness over the gallbladder when the probe is used to compress the right upper quadrant. It is often better elicited with deep inspiration, which displaces the gallbladder fundus below the costal margin, allowing for direct compression. Sonographic Murphy's sign may be absent in elderly patients, if analgesics were taken before the study, or when prolonged inflammation has led to gangrenous cholecystitis. **Hyperemia** in the gallbladder wall and a **prominent cystic artery** are relatively specific findings in acute cholecystitis (see Fig. 6-36, *D*). Power Doppler has been shown to be superior to color Doppler in

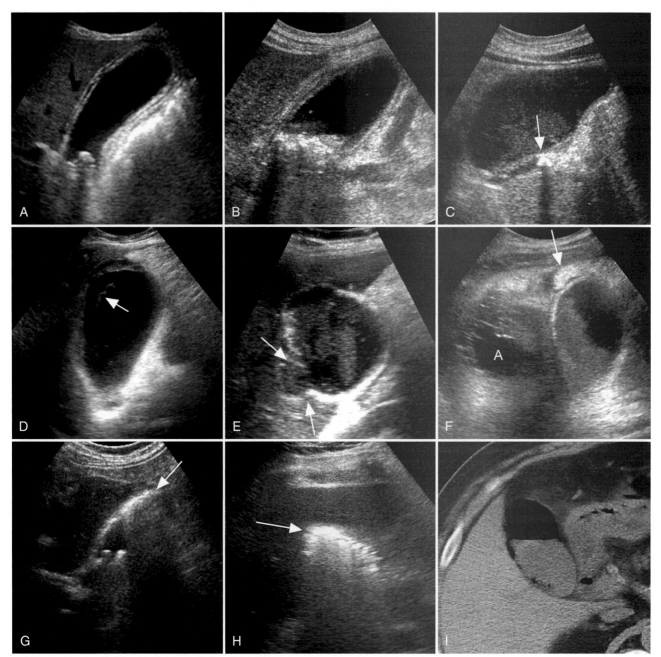

FIGURE 6-37. Acute cholecystitis: spectrum of appearances. A to **C, Uncomplicated acute cholecystitis. A,** Classic appearance with gallbladder distention, mild wall thickening, and gallstones. **B,** Acute cholecystitis. More advanced classic changes with a thicker wall and a larger lumen. There are multiple dependent stones. **C,** Distended gallbladder filled with sludge. After careful scrutiny, a stone *(arrow)* was detected in the cystic duct. **D, Gangrenous cholecystitis.** Sloughed membrane *(arrow)* appearing as a linear intraluminal echo. **E, Perforation,** shown as disruption of the gallbladder wall *(arrows)*. **F, Pericholecystic inflammatory change.** There is echogenic inflamed fat *(arrow)* and an abscess *(A)*. The gallbladder remains large and tense. **G** to **I, Emphysematous cholecystitis. G,** Sagittal sonogram of the gallbladder with a focus of intraluminal air appearing as a bright echogenic focus *(arrow)* with dirty shadowing. **H,** Gallbladder that is filled with air *(arrow)*. The gallbladder is not actually visualized, and knowledge of the location of the gallbladder fossa is essential to avoid mistaking this for bowel gas. **I,** Corresponding CT scan shows air in the gallbladder wall and lumen. *(F courtesy Dr. A.E. Hanbidge, University of Toronto.)*

detecting such hyperemia.[77] Hyperemia is only qualitatively assessed, however, and motion artifact somewhat limits the utility of power Doppler. The latest generation of sonography equipment has highly sensitive Doppler techniques, and detection of flow in the cystic artery of a normal gallbladder is common. In our experience this limits the qualitative assessment of gallbladder wall hyperemia. We rely heavily on the morphologic changes in the gallbladder for the diagnosis of acute cholecystitis but find Doppler ultrasound useful in some equivocal cases.

Although none of the signs just described is pathognomonic of acute cholecystitis, the combination of

CAUSES OF GALLBLADDER WALL THICKENING

GENERALIZED EDEMATOUS STATES
Congestive heart failure
Renal failure
End-stage cirrhosis
Hypoalbuminemia

INFLAMMATORY CONDITIONS
Primary
    Acute cholecystitis
    Cholangitis
    Chronic cholecystitis
Secondary
    Acute hepatitis
    Perforated duodenal ulcer
    Pancreatitis
    Diverticulitis/colitis

NEOPLASTIC CONDITIONS
Gallbladder adenocarcinoma
Metastases

MISCELLANEOUS
Adenomyomatosis
Mural varicosities

TABLE 6-1. ACUTE CALCULOUS CHOLECYSTITIS: PATHOLOGIC-SONOGRAPHIC CORRELATION

PATHOPHYSIOLOGY	SONOGRAPHIC APPEARANCE
Obstruction of cystic duct or neck of gallbladder	Stones in gallbladder, possibly in neck or cystic duct
Continued secretions	Gallbladder distention
Inflammatory cell infiltration *and* Gallbladder wall edema	Thickening of gallbladder wall. Gallbladder wall often striated with pockets of edema fluid. Positive sonographic Murphy's sign (>90%)
Hypervascularity	Hyperemia of gallbladder wall
Gallbladder stasis with bacterial overgrowth by 72 hours	Biliary sludge
Empyema of gallbladder	Heterogeneous luminal contents of variable echogenicity with layering
Increased pressure in gallbladder lumen and wall	Sloughed membranes; hypovascularity
Gangrene	Loss of Murphy's sign
Perforation	Loss of gourd shape; collection in or adjacent to gallbladder fossa

multiple findings should lead to the correct diagnosis. Some patients with acute cholecystitis may not show classic findings, making diagnosis challenging. This occurs in patients with mild inflammation but occurs more often in patients hospitalized for other reasons, not receiving an oral diet, and unable to communicate symptoms. A distended gallbladder in these patients should trigger a high index of suspicion, and careful RUQ scanning is recommended. Perforated duodenal ulcer, acute hepatitis, pancreatitis, colitis or diverticulitis, and even pyelonephritis can demonstrate a Murphy's sign and sympathetic gallbladder wall thickening (Fig. 6-39). Absence of a distended gallbladder and gallstones is often a clue to the nonbiliary origin of the cholecystic process.

Gangrenous Cholecystitis

When acute cholecystitis is especially severe or prolonged, the gallbladder may undergo necrosis. Sonographic findings of gangrenous cholecystitis include nonlayering bands of echogenic tissue within the lumen representing sloughed membranes and blood (see Fig. 6-37, *D*). The gallbladder wall also becomes irregular, with small collections within the wall that may represent abscesses or hemorrhage.[69] Murphy's sign is absent in two thirds of patients,[78] presumably because of necrosis of the nerve supply to the gallbladder. **Hemorrhagic cholecystitis** represents a rare gangrenous process marked by bleeding within the gallbladder wall and lumen. The clinical

symptoms are indistinguishable from gangrenous cholecystitis, and only occasionally does the patient experience a gastrointestinal bleed.

Perforated Gallbladder

Perforation of the gallbladder occurs in 5% to 10% of patients with acute cholecystitis, generally in cases of prolonged inflammation.[69] The focus of perforation, seen as a small defect or rent in the wall of the gallbladder, is often visible (see Fig. 6-37, *E*). Clues to perforation are the deflation of the gallbladder, with loss of its normal gourdlike shape, and a **pericholecystic fluid collection.** The latter is often a small fluid collection around the wall defect, unlike the thin rim of fluid around the entire organ in uncomplicated cholecystitis.[79] The collection may have internal strands typical of abscesses elsewhere (see Fig. 6-37, *F*). Perforation of the gallbladder may extend into the adjacent liver parenchyma, forming an abscess collection. The presence of a cystic liver lesion around the gallbladder fossa should suggest a pericholecystic abscess.

Emphysematous Cholecystitis

Emphysematous cholecystitis represents fewer than 1% of all cases of acute cholecystitis, but it is rapidly progressive and fatal in approximately 15% of patients. Emphysematous cholecystitis differs from acute cholecystitis

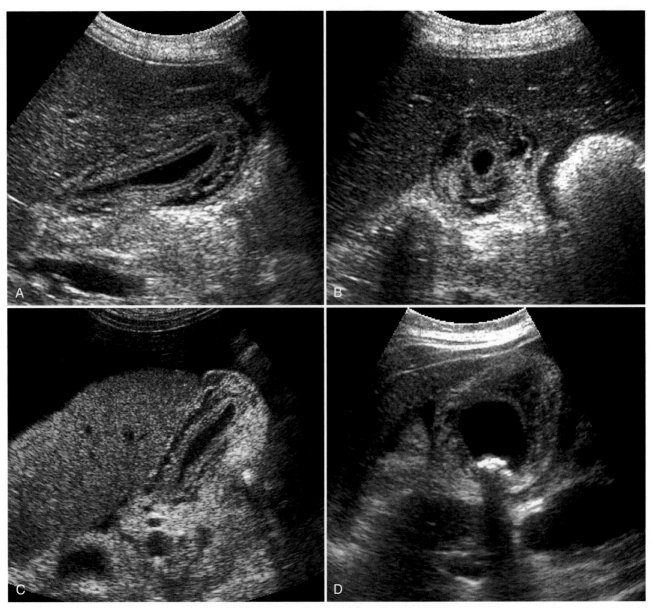

FIGURE 6-38. Systemic causes of gallbladder wall edema. A, Sagittal, and **B,** transverse, images of **hypoalbuminemia** show marked thickening of the gallbladder wall with a small lumen. **C,** Sagittal image of the gallbladder in a patient with **cirrhosis** demonstrating similar changes to those in **A** and **B. D,** Patient with **congestive heart failure,** no pain, and negative Murphy's sign has marked gallbladder wall thickening and incidental gallstones.

in several ways. It is three to seven times more common in men than women; about half of patients have diabetes; and one third to one half have no gallstones.[69,80] The gas is produced by gas-forming bacteria, presumably after an ischemic event affecting the gallbladder.[80] These patients have a much higher incidence of gallbladder perforation than those with typical acute cholecystitis, and urgent surgical treatment is advocated for all patients.

The appearance of emphysematous cholecystitis on sonography depends on the amount of gas present (see Fig. 6-37, *G-I*). The gas is often both within the lumen and the wall of the gallbladder. Small amounts of gas appear as echogenic lines, with posterior dirty shadowing

or reverberation artifact (ringdown artifact). Large amounts of gas can be more difficult to appreciate. The absence of a normal gallbladder is a clue. A bright, echogenic line with posterior dirty shadowing is seen within the entire gallbladder fossa. Movement of gas bubbles is a helpful finding and may be precipitated by compression of the gallbladder fossa. Pneumobilia may also be seen.[80]

Acalculous Cholecystitis

Acalculous cholecystitis may occur in patients with no risk factors but is more common in critically ill patients, who thus have a worse prognosis. Risk factors include

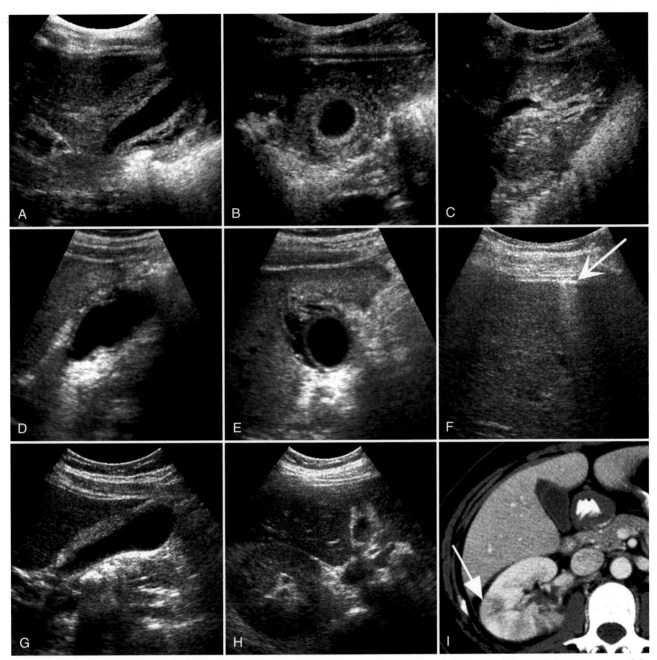

FIGURE 6-39. Sympathetic thickening of the gallbladder wall in three patients with positive sonographic Murphy's sign. A to C, Acute hepatitis. A and **B,** Views of the gallbladder show marked circumferential thickening of the gallbladder wall. The lumen is not distended. **C,** Left lobe of the liver shows periportal cuffing. **D to F, Perforation of a duodenal ulcer. D** and **E,** Asymmetrical, marked thickening of the gallbladder wall. **F,** Free intraperitoneal air. The peritoneal line in the epigastrium *(arrow)* marks a focus of increased brightness (enhancement) with posterior dirty shadowing. **G to I, Acute pyelonephritis. G** and **H,** Asymmetrical thickening of the gallbladder wall. **I,** CT scan shows striated nephrogram *(arrow). (D, E, and F courtesy Dr. A.E. Hanbidge, University of Toronto.)*

major surgery, severe trauma, sepsis, TPN, diabetes, atherosclerotic disease, and HIV infection.[73] In nonhospitalized patients, it is more common in elderly male patients with atherosclerotic disease,[81] who have a much better prognosis.

The diagnosis of acalculous cholecystitis can be difficult because gallbladder distention, wall thickening, internal sludge, and pericholecystic fluid may all be present in critically ill patients without cholecystitis.[82] Patients may be obtunded or receiving analgesics, reducing the sensitivity of Murphy's sign. The combination of findings suggests the diagnosis; the more signs present, the greater is the likelihood of cholecystitis.[83] Nevertheless, cholescintigraphy or percutaneous sampling of the luminal contents should be used more liberally to assist in the diagnosis.

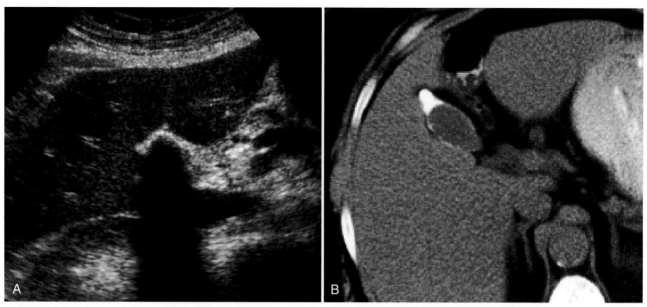

FIGURE 6-40. Porcelain gallbladder. A, Sonogram; **B,** corresponding CT scan. On ultrasound, this appearance could be mistaken for a stone within the gallbladder lumen. There is, however, no gallbladder wall superficial to the echogenic focus.

Torsion (Volvulus) of Gallbladder

Gallbladder torsion is a rare, acute entity. Patients present with symptoms of acute cholecystitis. Volvulus is often seen in elderly women and may be related to a mobile gallbladder with a long suspensory mesentery. The hallmarks on imaging are a massively distended and inflamed gallbladder lying in an unusual horizontal position, with its long axis oriented in a left-to-right direction. A twist of the cystic artery and cystic duct may be visible. If the torsion is greater than 180 degrees, gangrene of the gallbladder ensues; otherwise, obstruction of the cystic duct and acute cholecystitis occur. In either case, treatment is usually surgical.[84]

Chronic Cholecystitis

Chronic cholecystitis is associated with the mere presence of gallstones; therefore patients are usually asymptomatic and have mild disease. Chronic cholecystitis has the same incidence and risk factors as gallstone disease. More advanced cases involve wall thickening and fibrosis, appearing on sonographic examination as a thick-walled gallbladder with gallstones. Differentiation from acute cholecystitis is made by the absence of other signs, namely, gallbladder distention, Murphy's sign, and hyperemia in the wall.[85] Bouts of acute cholecystitis may complicate chronic cholecystitis.

Xanthogranulomatous cholecystitis is a rare form of chronic cholecystitis in which collections of lipid-laden macrophages occur within grayish yellow nodules or streaks in the gallbladder wall. In addition to gallstones, hypoechoic nodules or bands within the thickened wall, representing the lipid-laden xanthogranulomatous nodules, may suggest the diagnosis.[86]

Porcelain Gallbladder

Calcification of the gallbladder wall is termed "porcelain" gallbladder. Its cause is unknown, but it occurs in association with gallstone disease and may represent a form of chronic cholecystitis. This rare entity is seen in up to 0.8% of cholecystectomy specimens, with a female predominance and most often found in the sixth decade of life.[87] Two large studies disputed a high incidence of gallbladder carcinoma in porcelain gallbladder, suggesting the coincidental occurrence of the two entities in 0% to 7% of patients.[88,89] Nevertheless, prophylactic resection is advised.[86]

The degree and pattern of calcification determines the sonographic appearance (Fig. 6-40). When the entire gallbladder wall is thickly calcified, a hyperechoic semilunar line with dense posterior acoustic shadowing is noted. Mild calcification appears as an echogenic line with variable degrees of posterior acoustic shadowing. The luminal contents may be visible. Interrupted clumps of calcium appears as echogenic foci with posterior shadowing.[69] Differential diagnosis includes gallstones and emphysematous cholecystitis. Because the calcifications occur in the wall of the gallbladder, the WES complex is absent (see Gallstone Disease).

Adenomyomatosis (Adenomatous Hyperplasia)

Gallbladder adenomyomatosis is a benign condition caused by exaggeration of the normal invaginations of the luminal epithelium (Rokitansky-Aschoff sinuses) with associated smooth muscle proliferation (Fig. 6-41). The affected areas demonstrate thickening of the gallbladder wall with internal cystic spaces, the key to the

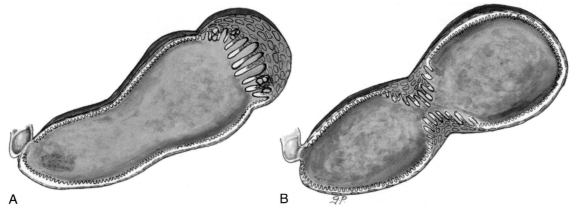

FIGURE 6-41. Segmental adenomyomatosis. A, Fundal adenomyoma. **B,** Hourglass adenomyomatosis. In both cases, note the constricted contour of the gallbladder and thickening of the wall with hypertrophy of the smooth muscle. On sonography, the exaggerated Rokitansky-Aschoff sinuses may appear as cystic spaces or as echogenic foci with comet-tail artifact, possibly caused by cholesterol crystals (depicted here as *yellow particles*) lodged in them.

radiologic diagnosis. The great majority of adenomyomatoses are asymptomatic.[90]

Adenomyomatosis may be **focal** or **diffuse.** The most common appearance on sonography is tiny, echogenic foci in the gallbladder wall that create **comet-tail artifacts,** presumably caused by either the cystic space itself or the internal debris (Fig. 6-42). Prominent masslike focal areas of adenomyomatosis, called **adenomyomas,** are the next most common manifestation. Careful evaluation of the adenomyoma, sometimes requiring higher frequency or linear probes, can show several features that are diagnostic of the entity and allow for differentiation from neoplasm. The most diagnostic finding, although not the most common, is the presence of cystic spaces. Echogenic foci with ringdown or "twinkling" artifact on Doppler examination are also typical. Focal adenomyomatosis is most common in the gallbladder fundus, less often narrowing the midportion of the organ, called **hourglass gallbladder** (Fig. 6-43).

Fundal adenomyomas are often folded onto the body of the gallbladder and can occasionally be mistaken for a pericholecystic or even a hepatic mass. The entire gland wall may be involved, causing collapse of the lumen. The absence of the cystic spaces, echogenic foci, or twinkling artifact or the presence of internal vascularity should prompt further investigation to differentiate from neoplasm. MRI or MRCP allows for improved specificity, with the presence of cystic spaces within the thickened wall leading to the diagnosis.[91]

Polypoid Masses of Gallbladder

Differentiation of benign and malignant polyps is essential because benign masses are common and malignant polyps require early intervention to improve outcome. Multiple masses and size up to 10 mm are the most frequently used criteria for **benignity.** Lesions less than 10 mm are most often benign when resected and do not

change in size when followed.[92] **Malignancy** has been documented in 37% to 88% of resected polyps greater than 10 mm.[93] Other factors that increase the risk of malignancy are age over 60, singularity, gallstone disease, rapid change in size on follow-up sonography, and sessile morphology.[94] Although Doppler ultrasound features of benign and malignant masses overlap, a blood flow velocity greater than 20 cm/sec and resistive index less than 0.65 are more suggestive of malignancy.[95]

COMMON POLYPOID MASSES OF THE GALLBLADDER

Cholesterol polyps* (50%-60%)
Inflammatory polyps* (5%-10%)
Adenoma* (<5%)
Focal adenomyomatosis
Gallbladder adenocarcinoma
Metastases (esp. melanoma)

*Data from Bilhartz LE. Acalculous cholecystitis, cholesterolosis, adenomyomatosis, and polyps of the gallbladder. In Feldman M et al, editors. *Sleisenger & Fordtran's gastrointestinal and liver disease,* 7th ed. New York, 2002, Elsevier Science, pp 1116-1130.

Cholesterol Polyps

Approximately one half of all polypoid gallbladder lesions are cholesterol polyps. These represent the focal form of gallbladder **cholesterolosis,** a common non-neoplastic condition of unknown etiology. Cholesterolosis results in accumulation of lipids within macrophages. The diffuse form, commonly known as "strawberry gallbladder," is not visible on imaging. Cholesterolosis

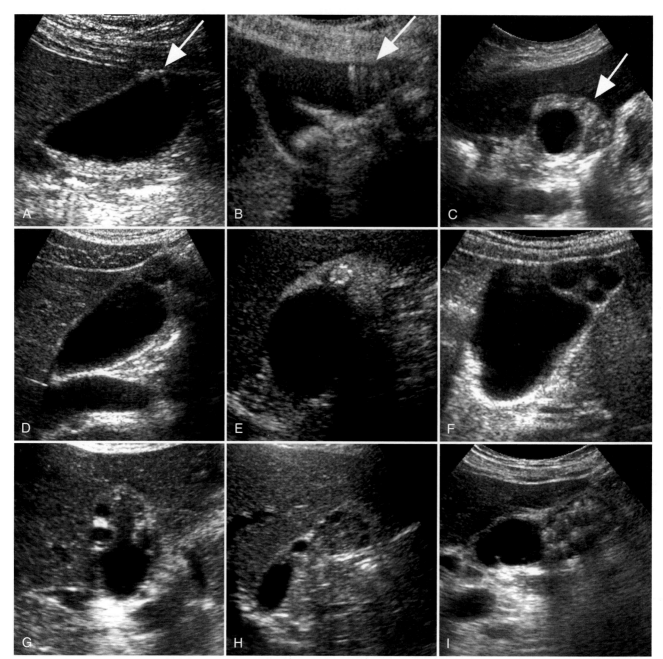

FIGURE 6-42. Adenomyomatosis: spectrum of appearances. A to C, Focal adenomyomatosis, the most common manifestation. **A,** Small focal area of thickening of the anterior fundal wall *(arrow)* with a bright echogenic focus with a distal comet-tail artifact. **B,** Multiple bright foci *(arrow)* with distal artifacts. **C,** Highly echogenic focal thickening of the gallbladder wall *(arrow).* Increased echogenicity is unusual for a malignant tumor that is more likely to appear hypoechoic. **D to F, Fundal adenomyomas. D,** Adenomyoma appears hypoechoic and masslike. **E,** Caplike area with multiple tiny, highly echogenic foci that suggest multiple crystals in the Rokitansky-Aschoff sinuses. **F,** Multiple cystic spaces within the adenomyoma. **G to I, Segmental adenomyomatosis. G and H,** Masslike areas obliterating the gallbladder lumen. Multiple cystic spaces suggest the correct diagnosis. **I,** Multiple echogenic foci suggest crystals in the Rokitansky-Aschoff sinuses.

has the same risk factors as gallstone disease, but the two conditions rarely coexist.[96] Cholesterol polyps usually are 2 to 10 mm, although lesions up to 20 mm have been described.[93] On pathologic series, one fifth are solitary, but the mean number of polyps is eight.[96]

The sonographic appearance of cholesterol polyps is multiple ovoid, nonshadowing lesions attached to the gallbladder wall (Fig. 6-44). Unlike small, nonshadow-

ing stones, polyps are not mobile. Larger lesions may contain a fine pattern of echogenic foci.[97]

Adenomas, Adenomyomas, and Inflammatory Polyps

Adenomas are true benign neoplasms of the gallbladder, with a premalignant potential much lower than for

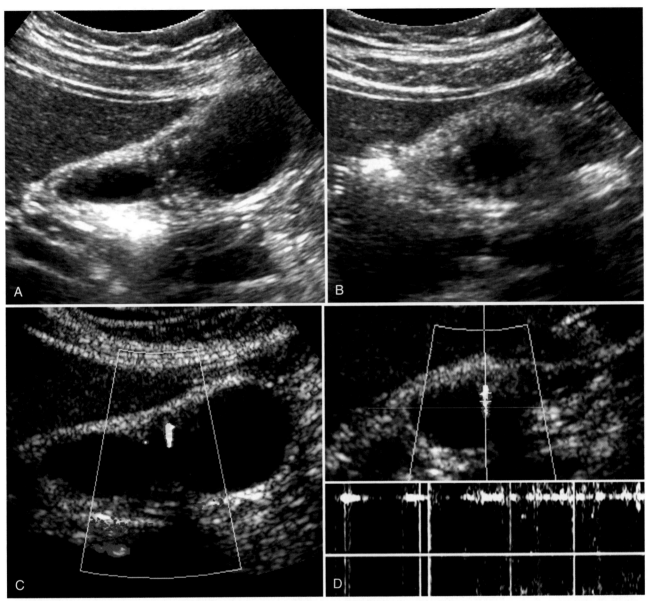

FIGURE 6-43. Hourglass adenomyoma. A, Sagittal, and **B,** transverse, sonograms show thickening of the gallbladder wall, creating an hourglass configuration. At the point of wall thickening, there are innumerable bright echogenic foci with "ringdown" artifact, suggesting cholesterol crystals in Rokitansky-Aschoff sinuses. **C** and **D,** Color and spectral Doppler show "twinkling" artifact without real vascularity, supportive of the correct diagnosis.

colonic adenomas. Adenomas represent less than 5% of gallbladder polyps and occur as a solitary lesion. Adenomas are usually pedunculated, and larger lesions may contain foci of malignant transformation.[96] Adenomas tend to be homogeneously hyperechoic but become more heterogeneous as they increase in size[93] (Fig. 6-45). Thickening of the gallbladder wall adjacent to an adenoma should suggest malignancy. On occasion, an **adenomyoma** may appear as a sessile, polypoid gallbladder lesion. Imaging features, as previously described for adenomyomatosis, should allow differentiation. **Inflammatory polyps** of the gallbladder constitute 5% to 10% of gallbladder polyps and are multiple in half the cases.[96] Inflammatory polyps tend to occur in the background

of gallstone disease and chronic cholecystitis.[98] The sonographic appearance of these lesions has not been systematically studied.

Malignancies

Primary gallbladder adenocarcinomas may appear as a polypoid mass. Melanoma is the cause of 50% to 60% of metastases to the gallbladder. These appear as hyperechoic, broad-based polypoid lesions, potentially multiple and usually more than 10 mm in diameter.[99] Other adenocarcinomas can rarely metastasize to the gallbladder. Advanced hepatocellular carcinoma can directly invade the gallbladder fossa and extend through

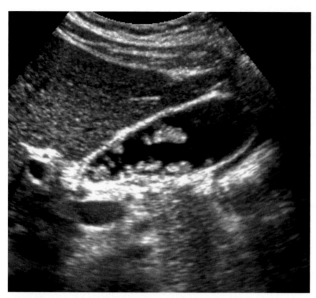

FIGURE 6-44. Gallbladder polyps. Small size (≤10 mm) and multiple tumors are features most suggestive of a benign lesion.

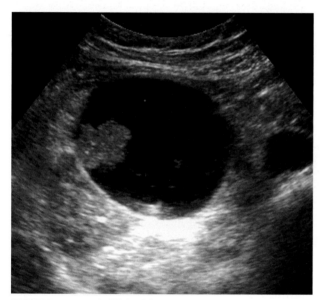

FIGURE 6-45. Gallbladder adenoma. Transverse image through the gallbladder shows a polypoid lesion found incidentally in a patient with mild acute cholecystitis. The lesion was a tubulovillous adenoma on resection.

the gallbladder wall to appear as a luminal mass. The large hepatic component of the mass and its hypervascular nature assist in the diagnosis.

Gallbladder Carcinoma

Gallbladder carcinoma is an uncommon malignancy occurring mainly in the elderly population, with a 3:1 female/male ratio. In a majority of cases, carcinoma is associated with gallstones. Chronic gallstone disease and resultant dysplasia have been cited as a causative factor.[100]

About 98% of gallbladder carcinomas are **adenocarcinomas,** with squamous cell carcinoma and metastases accounting for the rest. The following three patterns of disease have been described:
- Mass arising in the gallbladder fossa, obliterating the gallbladder and invading the adjacent liver (most common pattern)
- Focal or diffuse, irregular wall thickening
- Intraluminal polypoid mass

Patterns of Tumor Spread

Because the gallbladder wall is quite thin and little connective tissue separates it from the liver parenchyma, **contiguous hepatic invasion** is the most common pattern of spread. Gallbladder tumors also extend along the cystic duct into the porta hepatis, where they mimic hilar cholangiocarcinomas. Tumor extension into bile ducts or encasement of the portal vein or hepatic artery may ensue. Direct invasion into adjacent loops of bowel, especially the duodenum or colon, may also occur. A resultant **cholecystoenteric fistula** and inflammation may be mistaken for a benign abscess collection. Metastases to the peritoneum are a common finding.

Lymphatic spread is also a common feature of gallbladder carcinoma and may occur in the absence of invasion of adjacent organs.[101] The first nodes to be affected are in the hilar region. Adenopathy may then extend either down the hepatoduodenal ligament, to affect peripancreatic and mesenteric nodes, or across the gastrohepatic ligament to celiac nodal stations.

Surgical resection is the only chance of cure; however, reported resection rates range from 10% to 30%.[101] If the tumor is not confined to the mucosa, an extended cholecystectomy, involving resection of 3 to 5–cm rim of liver adjacent to the gallbladder fossa, or a formal right hepatectomy is required. Regional lymph nodes of the cystic and common bile ducts are also removed. The presence of noncontiguous hepatic or peritoneal metastases, celiac or peripancreatic nodal disease, or encasement of the main portal vein or hepatic artery renders the patient unresectable and should be carefully sought.

Sonographic Appearance

The appearance on sonography varies depending on the **pattern** of carcinoma (Fig. 6-46). When masses replacing the normal gallbladder fossa are small, it may be difficult to appreciate them because they may blend into the liver. The absence of a normal-appearing gallbladder with no history of cholecystectomy should raise suspicion. A clue to the diagnosis is the common presence of an immobile stone that is engrossed by the tumor, the "trapped stone." On Doppler interrogation the mass may demonstrate internal arterial and venous flow. Diffuse, malignant thickening of the wall differs from other causes in that the wall is irregular with loss of

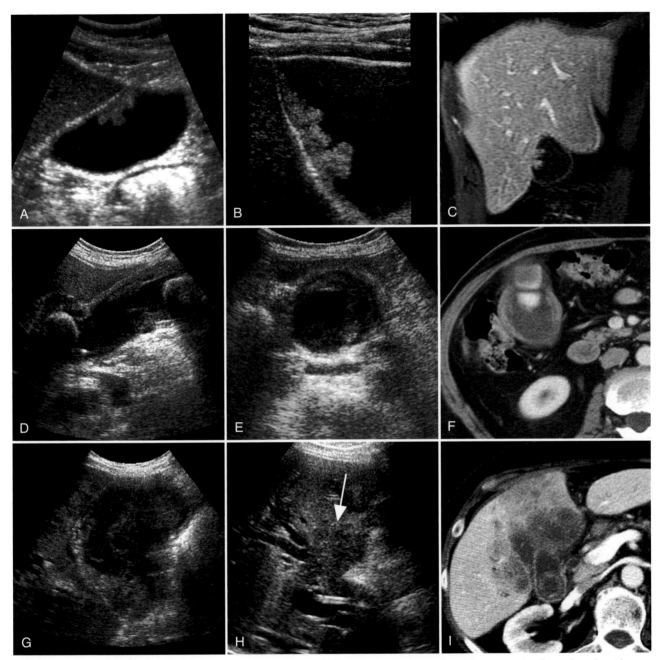

FIGURE 6-46. Gallbladder cancer: spectrum of appearances. A and **B, Polypoid mass. A,** Small, sessile polypoid mass. **B,** Examination with high-frequency linear probe shows no invasion beyond the gallbladder wall. **C,** Corresponding coronal MR image shows the enhancing polyp. **D** to **F, Wall thickening. D** and **E,** Extensive asymmetrical, heterogeneous wall thickening. **F,** Corresponding CT scan. **G** to **I, Invasive gallbladder cancer. G** and **H,** Huge mass replacing the gallbladder fossa and invading the liver. **H,** Biliary obstruction caused by the invasive mass *(arrow).* **I,** Corresponding CT scan.

the normal mural layers. Polypoid intraluminal masses are differentiated from nonneoplastic abnormalities by immobility of the mass, larger size (>1 cm), and prominent internal vascularity. Gallbladder carcinomas may produce large quantities of **mucin,** which distends the gallbladder.

Sonography performs very well in locally staging gallbladder carcinoma. Bach et al.[102] reported 94% sensitivity and 63% accuracy for prediction of resectability compared with surgical findings. However, sonography is often difficult in patients with unresectable disease

because of limited detection of noncontiguous hepatic, lymph node, and especially peritoneal metastases. A CT scan is recommended to improve detection of metastatic gallbladder disease.

References

The Biliary Tree
1. Bret PM, de Stempel JV, Atri M, et al. Intrahepatic bile duct and portal vein anatomy revisited. Radiology 1988;169:405-407.
2. Bressler EL, Rubin JM, McCracken S. Sonographic parallel channel sign: a reappraisal. Radiology 1987;164:343-346.

3. Puente SG, Bannura GC. Radiological anatomy of the biliary tract: variations and congenital abnormalities. World J Surg 1983;7:271-276.

4. Russell E, Yrizzary JM, Montalvo BM, et al. Left hepatic duct anatomy: implications. Radiology 1990;174:353-356.

5. Bowie JD. What is the upper limit of normal for the common bile duct on ultrasound: how much do you want it to be? Am J Gastroenterol 2000;95:897-900.

6. Horrow MM, Horrow JC, Niakosari A, et al. Is age associated with size of adult extrahepatic bile duct? Sonographic study. Radiology 2001;221:411-414.

7. Lamah M, Karanjia ND, Dickson GH. Anatomical variations of the extrahepatic biliary tree: review of the world literature. Clin Anat 2001;14:167-172.

8. Sato M, Ishida H, Konno K, et al. Choledochal cyst due to anomalous pancreatobiliary junction in the adult: sonographic findings. Abdom Imaging 2001;26:395-400.

9. De Vries JS, de Vries S, Aronson DC, et al. Choledochal cysts: age of presentation, symptoms, and late complications related to Todani's classification. J Pediatr Surg 2002;37:1568-1573.

10. Adkins Jr RB, Chapman WC, Reddy VS. Embryology, anatomy, and surgical applications of the extrahepatic biliary system. Surg Clin North Am 2000;80:363-379.

11. Todani T, Watanabe Y, Narusue M, et al. Congenital bile duct cysts: classification, operative procedures, and review of thirty-seven cases including cancer arising from choledochal cyst. Am J Surg 1977;134:263-269.

12. Matsumoto Y, Fujii H, Itakura J, et al. Recent advances in pancreaticobiliary malfunction. J Hepatobiliary Pancreat Surg 2002;9:45-54.

13. Parada LA, Hallen M, Hagerstrand I, et al. Clonal chromosomal abnormalities in congenital bile duct dilatation (Caroli's disease). Gut 1999;45:780-782.

14. Suchy FJ. Anatomy, histology, embryology, developmental anomalies, and pediatric disorders of the biliary tract. In: Feldmen M, et al, editors. Sleisenger & Fordtran's gastrointestinal and liver disease. 7th ed. New York: Elsevier Science; 2002. p. 1033.

15. Fulcher AS, Turner MA, Sanyal AJ. Case 38: Caroli disease and renal tubular ectasia. Radiology 2001;220:720-723.

16. Marchal GJ, Desmet VJ, Proesmans WC, et al. Caroli disease: high-frequency ultrasound and pathologic findings. Radiology 1986;158:507-511.

17. Greenberger NJ, Paumgartner G. Diseases of the gallbladder and bile ducts. In: Braunwald E, et al, editors. Harrison's principles of internal medicine. 15th ed. New York: McGraw-Hill; 2001.

18. Ko CW, Lee SP. Epidemiology and natural history of common bile duct stones and prediction of disease. Gastrointest Endosc 2002;56:S165-S169.

19. Ortega D, Burns PN, Hope Simpson D, Wilson SR. Tissue harmonic imaging: is it a benefit for bile duct sonography? AJR Am J Roentgenol 2001;176:653-659.

20. Baron RL, Tublin ME, Peterson MS. Imaging the spectrum of biliary tract disease. Radiol Clin North Am 2002;40:1325-1354.

21. Turner MA, Fulcher AS. The cystic duct: normal anatomy and disease processes. Radiographics 2001;21:3-22; questionnaire 288-294.

22. Abou-Saif A, Al-Kawas FH. Complications of gallstone disease: Mirizzi syndrome, cholecystocholedochal fistula, and gallstone ileus. Am J Gastroenterol 2002;97:249-254.

23. Green MH, Duell RM, Johnson CD, Jamieson NV. Haemobilia. Br J Surg 2001;88:773-786.

24. Horton JD, Bilhartz LE. Gallstone disease and its complications: clinical manifestations of gallstone disease. In: Feldman M, et al, editors. Sleisenger & Fordtran's gastrointestinal and liver disease. 7th ed. New York: Elsevier Science; 2002. pp. 1065-1087.

25. Hanau LH, Steigbigel NH. Acute (ascending) cholangitis. Infect Dis Clin North Am 2000;14:521-546.

26. Harvey RT, Miller Jr WT. Acute biliary disease: initial CT and follow-up ultrasound versus initial ultrasound and follow-up CT. Radiology 1999;213:831-836.

27. Marcos LA, Terashima A, Gotuzzo E. Update on hepatobiliary flukes: fascioliasis, opisthorchiasis and clonorchiasis. Curr Opin Infect Dis 2008;21:523-530.

28. Cosme A, Ojeda E, Poch M, et al. Sonographic findings of hepatic lesions in human fascioliasis. J Clin Ultrasound 2003;31:358-363.

29. Kabaalioglu A, Ceken K, Alimoglu E, et al. Hepatobiliary fascioliasis: sonographic and CT findings in 87 patients during the initial phase and long-term follow-up. AJR Am J Roentgenol 2007;189:824-828.

30. Lim JH, Kim SY, Park CM. Parasitic diseases of the biliary tract. AJR Am J Roentgenol 2007;188:1596-1603.

31. Han JK, Jang HJ, Choi BI, et al. Experimental hepatobiliary fascioliasis in rabbits: a radiology-pathology correlation. Invest Radiol 1999;34:99-108.

32. Choi D, Hong ST. Imaging diagnosis of clonorchiasis. Korean J Parasitol 2007;45:77-85.

33. Mahadevan U, Bass NM. Sclerosing cholangitis and recurrent pyogenic cholangitis. In: Feldman M, et al, editors. Sleisenger & Fordtran's gastrointestinal and liver disease. 7th ed. New York: Elsevier Science; 2002. pp. 1131-1152.

34. Cosenza CA, Durazo F, Stain SC, et al. Current management of recurrent pyogenic cholangitis. Am Surg 1999;65:939-943.

35. Olsson R, Danielsson A, Jarnerot G, et al. Prevalence of primary sclerosing cholangitis in patients with ulcerative colitis. Gastroenterology 1991;100:1319-1323.

36. Majoie CB, Smits NJ, Phoa SS, et al. Primary sclerosing cholangitis: sonographic findings. Abdom Imaging 1995;20:109-112; discussion 113.

37. Stockbrugger RW, Olsson R, Jaup B, Jensen J. Forty-six patients with primary sclerosing cholangitis: radiological bile duct changes in relationship to clinical course and concomitant inflammatory bowel disease. Hepatogastroenterology 1988;35:289-294.

38. Pokorny CS, McCaughan GW, Gallagher ND, Selby WS. Sclerosing cholangitis and biliary tract calculi: primary or secondary? Gut 1992;33:1376-1380.

39. MacCartney RL. Noncalculous inflammatory disorders of the biliary tract. In: Gore RM, Levine MS, Laufer I, editors. Textbook of gastrointestinal radiology. Philadelphia. Saunders; 1994. pp. 1727-1745.

40. Narayanan Menon KV, Wiesner RH. Etiology and natural history of primary sclerosing cholangitis. J Hepatobiliary Pancreat Surg 1999;6:343-351.

41. Graziadei IW, Wiesner RH, Batts KP, et al. Recurrence of primary sclerosing cholangitis following liver transplantation. Hepatology 1999;29:1050-1056.

42. Darwin PE, Kennedy AS, Bonheur JL. Cholangiocarcinoma. eMedicine 2009. http://www.emedicine.com/med/topic343.htm.

43. Watanapa P, Watanapa WB. Liver fluke–associated cholangiocarcinoma. Br J Surg 2002;89:962-970.

44. De Groen PC, Gores GJ, LaRusso NF, et al. Biliary tract cancers. N Engl J Med 1999;341:1368-1378.

45. Jarnagin WR. Cholangiocarcinoma of the extrahepatic bile ducts. Semin Surg Oncol 2000;19:156-176.

46. Sohn TA, Lillemoe KD. Tumors of the gallbladder, bile ducts, and ampulla. In: Feldman M, et al, editors. Sleisenger & Fordtran's gastrointestinal and liver disease. 7th ed. New York: Elsevier Science; 2002. pp. 1153-1165.

47. Colombari R, Tsui WM. Biliary tumors of the liver. Semin Liver Dis 1995;15:402-413.

48. Gihara S, Kojiro M. Pathology of cholangiocarcinoma. In: Okuda K, Ishak KG, editors. Neoplasms of the liver. Tokyo: Springer Verlag; 1987. pp. 236-301.

49. Nakeeb A, Pitt HA, Sohn TA, et al. Cholangiocarcinoma: a spectrum of intrahepatic, perihilar, and distal tumors. Ann Surg 1996;224:463-473; discussion 473-475.

50. Patel T. Worldwide trends in mortality from biliary tract malignancies. BMC Cancer 2002;2:10.

51. Aishima S, Kuroda Y, Nishihara Y, et al. Proposal of progression model for intrahepatic cholangiocarcinoma: clinicopathologic differences between hilar type and peripheral type. Am J Surg Pathol 2007;31:1059-1067.

52. Maetani Y, Itoh K, Watanabe C, et al. MR imaging of intrahepatic cholangiocarcinoma with pathologic correlation. AJR Am J Roentgenol 2001;176:1499-1507.

53. Sano T, Kamiya J, Nagino M, et al. Macroscopic classification and preoperative diagnosis of intrahepatic cholangiocarcinoma in Japan. J Hepatobiliary Pancreat Surg 1999;6:101-107.

54. Wibulpolprasert B, Dhiensiri T. Peripheral cholangiocarcinoma: sonographic evaluation. J Clin Ultrasound 1992;20:303-314.

55. Lee NW, Wong KP, Siu KF, Wong J. Cholangiography in hepatocellular carcinoma with obstructive jaundice. Clin Radiol 1984;35:119-123.

56. Bloom CM, Langer B, Wilson SR. Role of ultrasound in the detection, characterization, and staging of cholangiocarcinoma. Radiographics 1999;19:1199-1218.
57. Lee JW, Han JK, Kim TK, et al. CT features of intraductal intrahepatic cholangiocarcinoma. AJR Am J Roentgenol 2000;175:721-725.
58. Jarnagin WR, Fong Y, DeMatteo RP, et al. Staging, resectability, and outcome in 225 patients with hilar cholangiocarcinoma. Ann Surg 2001;234:507-517; discussion 517-519.
59. Robledo R, Muro A, Prieto ML. Extrahepatic bile duct carcinoma: ultrasound characteristics and accuracy in demonstration of tumors. Radiology 1996;198:869-873.
60. Hann LE, Greatrex KV, Bach AM, et al. Cholangiocarcinoma at the hepatic hilus: sonographic findings. AJR Am J Roentgenol 1997;168:985-989.
61. Choi BI, Lee JH, Han MC, et al. Hilar cholangiocarcinoma: comparative study with sonography and CT. Radiology 1989;172:689-692.
62. Khalili K, Metser U, Wilson SR. Hilar biliary obstruction: preliminary results with Levovist-enhanced sonography. AJR Am J Roentgenol 2003;180:687-693.
63. Yanagisawa K, Moriyasu F, Miyahara T, et al. Phagocytosis of ultrasound contrast agent microbubbles by Kupffer cells. Ultrasound Med Biol 2007;33:318-325.

The Gallbladder
64. Fried AM, Kreel L, Cosgrove DO. The hepatic interlobar fissure: combined in vitro and in vivo study. AJR Am J Roentgenol 1984;143:561-564.
65. Martin DF, Laasch HL. The biliary tract. In: Grainger RG, Allison DJ, editors. Diagnostic radiology: a textbook of medical imaging. 4th ed. New York: Churchill Livingstone; 2001, p. 1277.
66. Stieber AC, Bauer JJ. Volvulus of the gallbladder. Am J Gastroenterol 1983;78:96-98.
67. Waisberg J, Pinto Jr PE, Gusson PR, et al. Agenesis of the gallbladder and cystic duct. Sao Paulo Med J 2002;120:192-194.
68. Kratzer W, Mason RA, Kachele V. Prevalence of gallstones in sonographic surveys worldwide. J Clin Ultrasound 1999;27:1-7.
69. Gore RM, Yaghmai V, Newmark GM, et al. Imaging benign and malignant disease of the gallbladder. Radiol Clin North Am 2002;40:1307-1323, vi.
70. Naryshkin S, Trotman BW, Raffensperger EC. Milk of calcium bile: evidence that gallbladder stasis is a key factor. Dig Dis Sci 1987;32:1051-1055.
71. Ko CW, Sekijima JH, Lee SP. Biliary sludge. Ann Intern Med 1999;130:301-311.
72. Trowbridge RL, Rutkowski NK, Shojania KG. Does this patient have acute cholecystitis? JAMA 2003;289:80-86.
73. Indar AA, Beckingham IJ. Acute cholecystitis. BMJ 2002;325:639-643.
74. Shea JA, Berlin JA, Escarce JJ, et al. Revised estimates of diagnostic test sensitivity and specificity in suspected biliary tract disease. Arch Intern Med 1994;154:2573-2581.
75. Fidler J, Paulson EK, Layfield L. CT evaluation of acute cholecystitis: findings and usefulness in diagnosis. AJR Am J Roentgenol 1996;166:1085-1088.
76. Wilson SR. Gastrointestinal disease. 6th series. Test and syllabus. Reston, Va: American College of Radiology; 2004.
77. Uggowitzer M, Kugler C, Schramayer G, et al. Sonography of acute cholecystitis: comparison of color and power Doppler sonography in detecting a hypervascularized gallbladder wall. AJR Am J Roentgenol 1997;168:707-712.
78. Simeone JF, Brink JA, Mueller PR, et al. The sonographic diagnosis of acute gangrenous cholecystitis: importance of the Murphy sign. AJR Am J Roentgenol 1989;152:289-290.
79. Sood BP, Kalra N, Gupta S, et al. Role of sonography in the diagnosis of gallbladder perforation. J Clin Ultrasound 2002;30:270-274.
80. Konno K, Ishida H, Naganuma H, et al. Emphysematous cholecystitis: sonographic findings. Abdom Imaging 2002;27:191-195.
81. Ryu JK, Ryu KH, Kim KH. Clinical features of acute acalculous cholecystitis. J Clin Gastroenterol 2003;36:166-169.
82. Boland GW, Slater G, Lu DS, et al. Prevalence and significance of gallbladder abnormalities seen on sonography in intensive care unit patients. AJR Am J Roentgenol 2000;174:973-977.
83. Helbich TH, Mallek R, Madl C, et al. Sonomorphology of the gallbladder in critically ill patients: value of a scoring system and follow-up examinations. Acta Radiol 1997;38:129-134.
84. Ikematsu Y, Yamanouchi K, Nishiwaki Y, et al. Gallbladder volvulus: experience of six consecutive cases at an institute. J Hepatobiliary Pancreat Surg 2000;7:606-609.
85. Schiller VL, Turner RR, Sarti DA. Color Doppler imaging of the gallbladder wall in acute cholecystitis: sonographic-pathologic correlation. Abdom Imaging 1996;21:233-237.
86. Parra JA, Acinas O, Bueno J, et al. Xanthogranulomatous cholecystitis: clinical, sonographic, and CT findings in 26 patients. AJR Am J Roentgenol 2000;174:979-983.
87. Opatrny L. Porcelain gallbladder. CMAJ 2002;166:933.
88. Towfigh S, McFadden DW, Cortina GR, et al. Porcelain gallbladder is not associated with gallbladder carcinoma. Am Surg 2001;67:7-10.
89. Stephen AE, Berger DL. Carcinoma in the porcelain gallbladder: a relationship revisited. Surgery 2001;129:699-703.
90. Bilhartz LE. Acalculous cholecystitis, cholesterolosis, adenomyomatosis, and polyps of the gallbladder. In: Feldman M, et al, editors. Sleisenger & Fordtran's gastrointestinal and liver disease. 7th ed. New York: Elsevier Science; 2002. pp. 1123-1125.
91. Yoshimitsu K, Honda H, Aibe H, et al. Radiologic diagnosis of adenomyomatosis of the gallbladder: comparative study among MRI, helical CT, and transabdominal ultrasound. J Comput Assist Tomogr 2001;25:843-850.
92. Csendes A, Burgos AM, Csendes P, et al. Late follow-up of polypoid lesions of the gallbladder smaller than 10 mm. Ann Surg 2001;234:657-660.
93. Levy AD, Murakata LA, Abbott RM, Rohrmann Jr CA. Benign tumors and tumorlike lesions of the gallbladder and extrahepatic bile ducts: radiologic-pathologic correlation. Archives of Armed Forces Institute of Pathology. Radiographics 2002;22:387-413.
94. Mainprize KS, Gould SW, Gilbert JM. Surgical management of polypoid lesions of the gallbladder. Br J Surg 2000;87:414-417.
95. Hirooka Y, Naitoh Y, Goto H, et al. Differential diagnosis of gallbladder masses using colour Doppler ultrasonography. J Gastroenterol Hepatol 1996;11:840-846.
96. Bilhartz LE. Acalculous cholecystitis, cholesterolosis, adenomyomatosis, and polyps of the gallbladder. In: Feldman M, et al, editors. Sleisenger & Fordtran's gastrointestinal and liver disease. 7th ed. New York: Elsevier Science; 2002. pp. 1116-1130.
97. Sugiyama M, Atomi Y, Kuroda A, et al. Large cholesterol polyps of the gallbladder: diagnosis by means of ultrasound and endoscopic ultrasound. Radiology 1995;196:493-497.
98. Maeyama R, Yamaguchi K, Noshiro H, et al. A large inflammatory polyp of the gallbladder masquerading as gallbladder carcinoma. J Gastroenterol 1998;33:770-774.
99. Holloway BJ, King DM. Ultrasound diagnosis of metastatic melanoma of the gallbladder. Br J Radiol 1997;70:1122-1125.
100. Levy AD, Murakata LA, Rohrmann Jr CA. Gallbladder carcinoma: radiologic-pathologic correlation. Radiographics 2001;21:295-314; questionnaire, 549-555.
101. Curley SA. The gallbladder. In: Abeloff MD, editor. Clinical oncology. 2nd ed. New York: Churchill Livingstone; 2000. pp. 1415-1420.
102. Bach AM, Loring LA, Hann LE, et al. Gallbladder cancer: can ultrasonography evaluate extent of disease? J Ultrasound Med 1998;17:303-309.

CHAPTER 7

The Pancreas

Philip Ralls

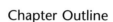

Chapter Outline

For reasons that are not clear, transabdominal sonography of the pancreas has been largely ignored in review articles from the United States,[1,2] although it is often featured prominently in the European literature.[3] This is indicative of radiology practice trends in North America and is not necessarily related to the actual usefulness of sonography compared with other modalities in pancreatic imaging. Several factors have led to the increasing unpopularity of ultrasound for pancreatic imaging in radiology practices, including difficulty in interpreting and especially performing sonography of the pancreas. Other factors are economic, as follows:

1. In the United States, sonography is reimbursed less well than CT or MRI/MRCP.
2. Sonography is perceived as requiring more radiologist time than other modalities.
3. Gastroenterologists are more likely to refer patients with pancreatic disease to modalities performed by gastroenterologists, such as ERCP and endoscopic ultrasound.

Despite these trends and the "research" reflecting these biases, the safety and effectiveness of sonography are evident. Pancreatic sonography can be an efficient and valuable tool in many common diseases, such as pancreatitis and pancreatic neoplasm. Sonography is often the first test used in patients with jaundice or abdominal pain. However, sonography is "technically dependent" and necessitates understanding techniques to optimize pancreatic sonography. Knowledge of sonographic findings in common (and less common) pancreatic diseases is crucial to obtaining good imaging and clinical outcomes in these patients.

ANATOMY AND SONOGRAPHIC TECHNIQUE

Patient preparation is important in pancreatic sonography. My colleagues and I prefer that our patients fast for 8 hours before the study (usually overnight). We allow our patients to drink water and take medicines orally.

There are three key regions of the pancreas: head, body, and tail. The visualization of each requires knowledge of pancreatic anatomy, appropriate patient positioning, and often the use of multiple transducers. The pancreas lies obliquely in the anterior pararenal space of the **retroperitoneum,** with the head caudal to the body and tail. The pancreas is draped over the **spine and aorta;** thus the neck and body are more superficial than the head and tail. The more caudal position of the head often leads to the technical error of not visualizing the entire head on "transverse" scans. This can be avoided by understanding the anatomy and by visualizing the normal uncinate process behind the gastrocolic trunk on

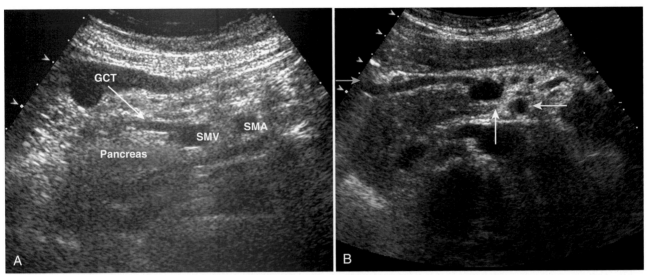

FIGURE 7-1. Normal pancreatic head and gastrocolic trunk. A, Transverse image of the pancreatic head and its ventral landmark, the gastrocolic venous trunk *(GCT)*. The caudal uncinate is dorsal to the GCT. *SMV,* Superior mesenteric vein; *SMA,* superior mesenteric artery. **B**, In another patient, note the triangular point of the uncinate that points medially *(white arrow)* behind the SMV and nearly reaches the SMA *(yellow arrow)*. GCT *(blue arrow)* enters the SMV.

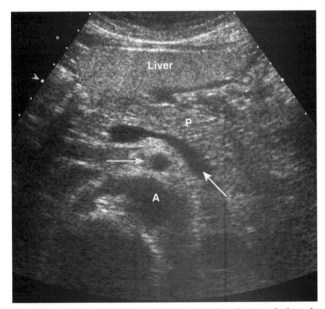

FIGURE 7-2. Normal pancreatic body and land-marks. Transverse image of the pancreatic body and its dorsal landmark, the splenic vein *(white arrow)* and portosplenic confluence. Note the normal parenchymal echogenicity, equal to that of the liver echogenicity. The superior mesenteric artery *(yellow arrow)* is surrounded by a collar of fat. *A,* Aorta; *P,* pancreas.

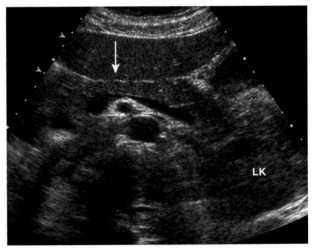

FIGURE 7-3. Normal pancreatic neck and body. Transverse image of pancreatic body. The "neck" of the pancreas *(arrow)* is that part of the body ventral to the superior mesenteric artery and portosplenic confluence. *LK,* Left kidney.

images of the pancreatic head (Fig. 7-1). Knowledge of a few key scanning techniques will optimize imaging of the entire pancreas.

Pancreatic Body

Compression scanning with a "large footprint," curved linear transducer is the key technique in visualizing the body of the pancreas. Compression displaces gas and fluid from the overlying stomach and duodenum and places the transducer closer to the pancreas itself. The key vascular landmarks for the body of the pancreas are the **splenic vein** (SV), its confluence with the **superior mesenteric vein** (SMV), and the **superior mesenteric artery** (SMA) (Fig. 7-2). Some call the region between the body and head of the pancreas the "neck," generally referring to the part of the pancreatic body ventral to the SMA-SMV and portosplenic confluence (Fig. 7-3).

Start scanning with the patient supine. Initially, scan the patient in quiet respiration. Breath holding may cause the patient to contract the abdominal muscles, preventing good compression. Images obtained in various degrees of held inspiration or less often expira-

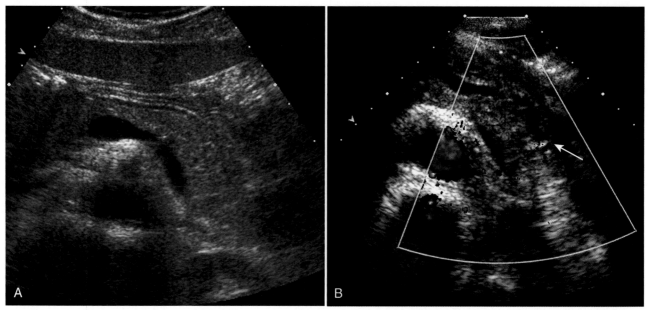

FIGURE 7-4. Pancreatic body and tail. A, Transverse image of the pancreatic body obtained by positioning the transducer to the right of the midline and angling back toward the left. **B,** In another patient, with chronic pancreatitis, the transverse view shows the dilated pancreatic duct with scattered calcifications *(arrow)* at the end of the duct in the pancreatic tail.

tion may facilitate pancreatic visualization. In inspiration the liver may be a useful sonographic window. In some patients a high-riding transverse colon may prevent good visualization of the pancreatic body. Unlike the stomach and duodenum, the contents of which are generally compressible, the colon often contains stool, which contains suspended gas. Stool cannot be compressed and is therefore an impediment to pancreatic sonography. In these patients, scanning caudal to the transverse colon and angling cephalic behind the colon may be useful. The left lateral decubitus position may also be useful, especially to see the left part of the body and more central tail. Position the transducer to the right of the midline and angle "down the barrel" (longitudinal axis) of the pancreatic body and tail (Fig. 7-4).

Other potentially useful techniques include scanning during a Valsalva maneuver and scanning after oral water or contrast administration, sometimes combined with scanning while the patient is standing or sitting, using the fluid-filled stomach as a window.

Pancreatic Head

The head is the key pancreatic structure; common bile duct stones, periampullary neoplasms, and pancreatic/extrahepatic duct obstructions occur here. Failure to adequately visualize the pancreatic head is a common but usually avoidable technical failure. Supine compression imaging is useful but rarely allows demonstration of the periampullary region. Vascular landmarks for the pancreatic head are the **inferior vena cava** (IVC) dorsally, the SMA and (SMV medially, and the **gastroduodenal artery** (GDA) and the **pancreaticoduodenal arcade**

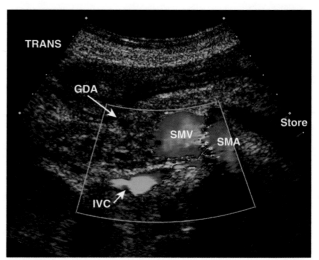

FIGURE 7-5. Normal pancreatic head and vascular landmarks. Transverse sonogram shows vascular landmarks for the pancreatic head: inferior vena cava *(IVC)* dorsally, superior mesenteric artery *(SMA)* and superior mesenteric vein *(SMV)* medially, and gastroduodenal artery *(GDA)*.

anterolaterally (Fig. 7-5). The pancreatic head is usually directly ventral to the IVC. Cephalic to the pancreas, the IVC is adjacent to the portal vein; this location is the entrance into the lesser peritoneal sac, the **epiploic foramen** (foramen of Winslow).

The **uncinate process** (or uncinate) is a portion of the caudal pancreatic head that wraps around behind the SMA and SMV, ending in a point oriented medially. The uncinate process is medial and dorsal to the SMA and SMV (Fig. 7-6; see also Fig 7-1, *B*). The GDA is a

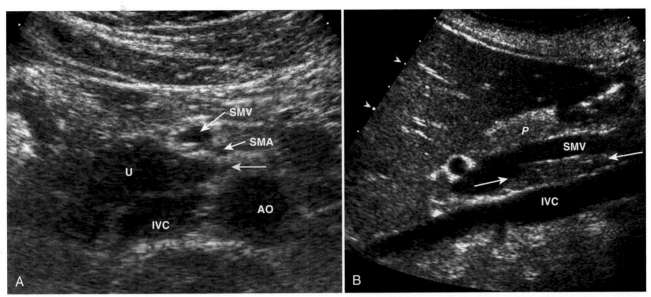

FIGURE 7-6. Normal uncinate process. A, Transverse sonogram showing the uncinate process *(U),* the part of the pancreatic head dorsal to the superior mesenteric vein *(SMV)* and superior mesenteric artery *(SMA).* Note the pointed medial tip of the uncinate *(yellow arrow)* (see also Fig. 7-1, *B*). *IVC,* Inferior vena cava; *AO,* aorta. **B,** Longitudinal sonogram in another patient shows the uncinate process *(arrows)* dorsal to the SMV and ventral to the inferior vena cava *(IVC).* The neck/body of the pancreas *(P)* is ventral to the SMV.

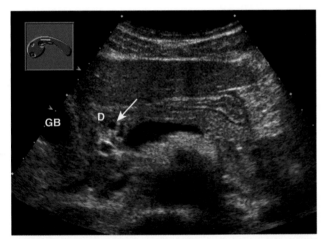

FIGURE 7-7. Normal gallbladder, duodenum, and pancreatic head. Transverse sonogram shows the gastroduodenal artery *(arrow)* as a landmark for the ventrolateral pancreatic head. The GDA courses between the pancreas and the second portion of the duodenum *(D).* The gallbladder *(GB)* is lateral to the duodenum. The image shows the cephalic portion of the pancreatic head.

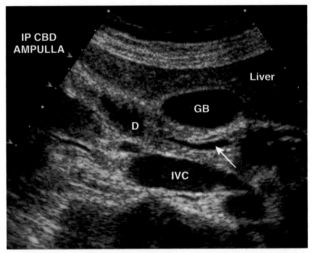

FIGURE 7-8. Normal ampullary area and bile duct. Sonographic scan through the gallbladder and liver, with the patient in the left lateral decubitus position, to visualize the ampullary region shows the normal distal bile duct *(arrow)* as it passes through the pancreatic head and enters the duodenum through the major papilla; *D,* duodenum.

landmark for the ventrolateral pancreatic head; the GDA courses between the pancreas and the second portion of the duodenum (Fig. 7-7).

Another useful vascular landmark for the pancreatic head and uncinate process is the **gastrocolic trunk** (GCT). Several splanchnic veins variably join to form the GCT. These often include the right or middle colic vein, right gastroepiploic vein, and pancreaticoduodenal veins. The GCT enters the right side of the SMV just anterior to the pancreatic head, thus serving as a ventral landmark for the uncinate process[4] (see Fig. 7-1).

The **left lateral decubitus** (LLD) **position** is best to see the pancreas adjacent to the duodenum. In the LLD position, scan in inspiration, and use the gallbladder or liver to either side of the gallbladder to view the rightmost portion of the pancreas and the distal (ampullary) pancreatic and bile ducts (Fig. 7-8).

Pancreatic Tail

It is rarely necessary or helpful for the patient to drink water when scanning the head or body of the pancreas.

The **water-filled stomach**, however, may provide an excellent window for visualizing the pancreatic tail, the most difficult portion of the pancreas to visualize sonographically. To see the tail, place the patient in a right anterior oblique position and scan through the water-filled stomach (Fig. 7-9). Another helpful way to see the

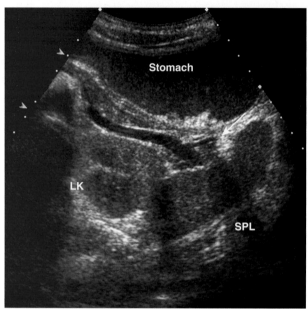

FIGURE 7-9. Normal pancreatic body and tail. Transverse image of the pancreatic body and tail, surrounding the splenic vein, seen through the fluid-filled stomach, with patient in a right anterior oblique position; *LK,* left kidney; *SPL,* spleen.

region of the pancreatic tail is coronal imaging through the spleen and left kidney, with the patient in a right lateral decubitus position (Fig. 7-10). Color Doppler sonography can reveal the splenic artery and vein, facilitating identification of the tail. Scanning through the spleen and left kidney, although not always revealing the normal pancreatic tail itself, may show abnormalities in the region of the tail (e.g., pseudocysts, masses) that are invisible on other views. The view through the left kidney and spleen should be routine in all pancreatic sonograms.

Pancreatic Parenchyma

The sonographic appearance of the normal pancreas varies widely in parenchymal echogenicity and texture, shape, and size. The parenchyma is usually isoechoic or hyperechoic compared with hepatic parenchyma (Fig. 7-11; see also Figs. 7-2 and 7-3). Evidence indicates that pancreatic echogenicity increases with age.[5]

The parenchymal **texture** varies widely from homogeneous to lobular internal architecture (Fig. 7-12). Pancreatic **size** varies considerably from individual to individual. Guerra et al.[6] found that the size of the head of the pancreas ranged from 6 to 28 mm (17.7 ± 4.2 mm), body size from 4 to 23 mm (10.1 ± 3.8 mm), and tail size from 5 to 28 mm (16.4 ± 4.2 mm). Men and women had comparable pancreatic size. The size of the pancreas diminishes with age.[6,7]

The **shape** of the pancreas can also vary considerably.[8] Variations in the shape of the pancreatic head are the most troublesome because they can simulate a pancreatic

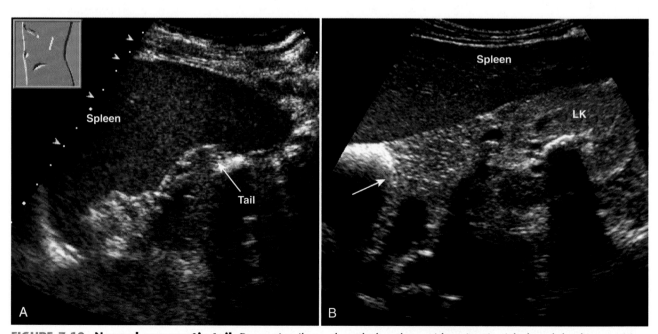

FIGURE 7-10. Normal pancreatic tail. Pancreatic tail seen through the spleen, with patient in right lateral decubitus position. **A,** Longitudinal coronal image shows the normal pancreatic tail *(arrow)* through the spleen. **B,** Transverse image of the normal pancreatic tail *(arrow)*. Note large stone in the left kidney *(LK)* with a conspicuous acoustic shadow.

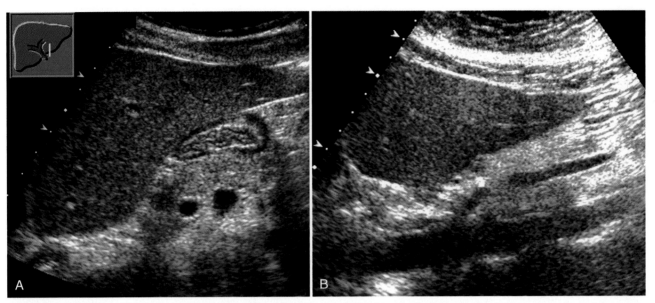

FIGURE 7-11. Normal pancreatic parenchymal echogenicity. Longitudinal sonograms. **A,** Image has echogenicity, somewhat similar to the liver. **B,** Image of another patient has much more echogenic appearance.

head mass, a **pseudomass.** Typically, these bulges extend to the right of the gastroduodenal and superior pancreaticoduodenal arteries (Fig. 7-13). Another common pseudomass is a bulge on the anterior body, often seen where the left lobe of the liver touches the pancreas. Pseudomasses have texture and echogenicity identical to normal pancreas, allowing differentiation from true pancreatic mass lesions. When high-quality images of the pancreas cannot be obtained because of technical difficulties, however, it may be difficult to differentiate a pseudomass from a true neoplasm of the pancreas.

Fatty Pancreas

Because the pancreatic parenchyma can be very echogenic normally, it may be difficult or impossible to diagnose fatty infiltration with sonography. Although the fatty pancreas has been described as being more echogenic than the normal pancreas,[9] this is difficult to judge (see Fig. 7-12). The pancreas can appear sonographically normal with complete fatty replacement[10] (Fig. 7-14). Computed tomography (CT) is sensitive in diagnosing fatty replacement, whereas ultrasound is unreliable. Severe fatty replacement of the pancreatic parenchyma can occur with cystic fibrosis, diabetes, obesity, and occasionally, old age and Shwachman-Diamond syndrome (SDS). SDS is a rare congenital genetic disorder characterized by pancreatic insufficiency, bone marrow dysfunction, and skeletal abnormalities.[11]

An interesting pseudomass can be caused by a relatively hypoechoic pancreatic head or uncinate process (ventral pancreas) compared with the dorsal pancreas (Fig. 7-15). Some evidence suggests that this phenomenon is related to relative fatty sparing in that part of the gland.[12-14] Based on a large prospective study, Coulier[15] found that "hypoechoic ventral embryologic cephalic pancreas" is never found before age 25 and is most common in middle-aged women with a "moderately echoic pancreas."

Embryology and Pancreatic Duct

The embryologic precursors of the adult pancreas develop as two outpouchings ("buds"), called the **dorsal (cranial) pancreatic anlage** and **ventral (caudal) pancreatic anlage**. These embryonic buds arise from opposite sides of the junction of the primitive foregut and midgut (Fig. 7-16). The two pancreatic anlagen (primordia) rotate to be in proximity, typically fusing at 6 to 8 weeks of gestation.[16] The dorsal (cranial) pancreatic bud becomes the body and tail of the pancreas. The ventral (caudal) bud becomes the pancreatic head and uncinate process, ending up in a position caudal to the body and tail. The ventral bud is also the embryologic origin of the gallbladder, bile duct, and liver. The bile duct and pancreatic head sharing a common origin explains the usual fusion (60%-80%) of the pancreatic and bile duct in the ampulla and their common entry into the duodenum through the major papilla.

The pancreatic duct is crucial to the exocrine function of the pancreas, conveying the pancreatic digestive secretions to the duodenum. Most adults have a single, **main pancreatic duct** that originates when portions of the two ducts from each pancreatic anlage fuse. The main pancreatic duct empties into the duodenum via the major papilla, usually after merging with the common bile duct in the ampulla. In 20% to 40% of individuals the ducts do not join—only the bile duct enters the duodenum through the major papilla.[17] The pancreatic duct enters separately, usually near the bile duct.

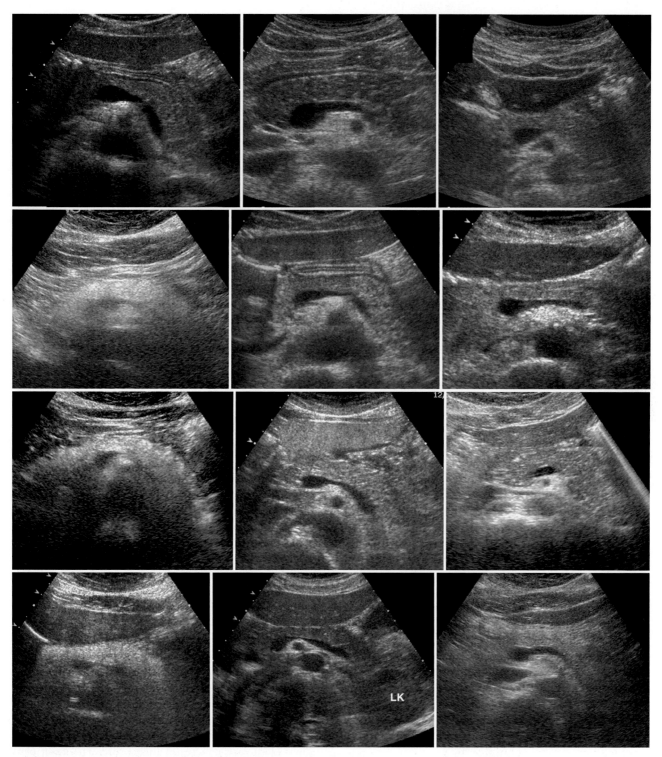

FIGURE 7-12. Normal pancreatic parenchymal echogenicity. Transverse sonograms in 12 normal patients demonstrate the various patterns of normal pancreatic parenchyma. Echogenicity, texture, and size vary considerably.

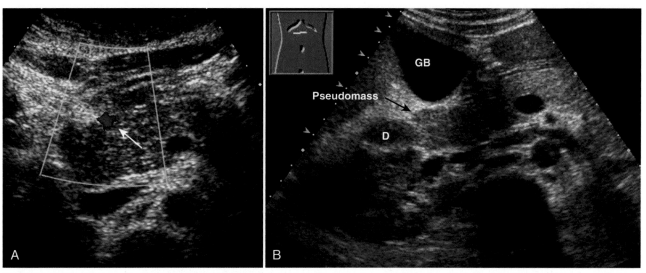

FIGURE 7-13. Normal anatomic variations: pancreatic head pseudomass. Variations in shape of the pancreatic head include bulges to the right of gastroduodenal artery. **A,** Transverse image of a pseudomass that extends to the right of the gastroduodenal artery *(arrow).* **B,** Transverse image of another pseudomass. *D,* Duodenum.

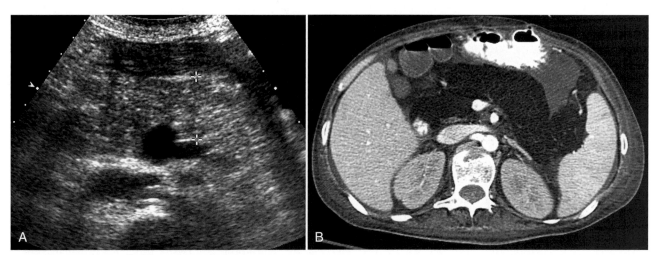

FIGURE 7-14. Fatty infiltration of pancreas. A, In this transverse image, the appearance and echogenicity of the pancreas do not differ substantially from many normal glands (see also Fig. 7-12). **B,** CT scan shows diffuse fatty infiltration. *(Case courtesy Drs. Vinay Duddlewar and Jabi Shiriki.)*

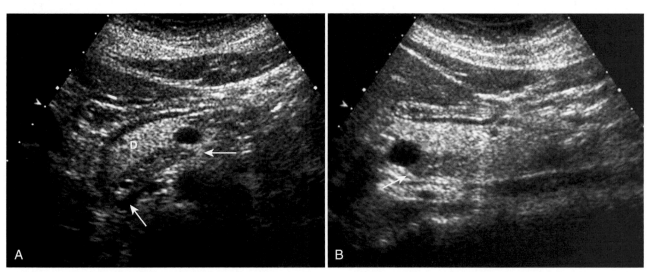

FIGURE 7-15. Hypoechoic ventral pancreas. A, Transverse sonogram of pancreatic head. Note the hypoechoic uncinate *(arrows),* likely related to less fatty change than present in the dorsal component *(D).* **B,** Longitudinal sonogram of pancreas. The more posterior uncinate *(arrow)* is lower in echogenicity than the remainder of the pancreas. *(Case courtesy Stephanie Wilson, MD.)*

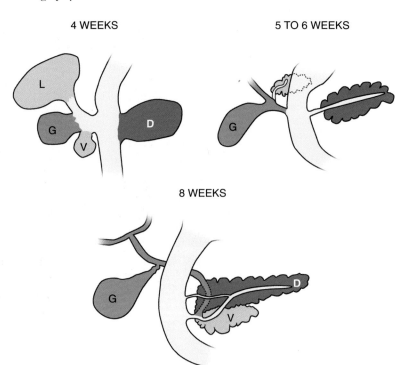

4 WEEKS

5 TO 6 WEEKS

8 WEEKS

FIGURE 7-16. Embryologic development of pancreas. At 4 weeks the embryologic precursors of the adult pancreas develop as two outpouchings ("buds"), called the dorsal (*D, blue*) and ventral (*V, brown*) pancreatic anlage. The ventral bud is also the embryologic origin of the gallbladder *(G)*, bile duct, and liver *(L)*. The embryonic pancreatic buds arise from opposite sides of the junction of the primitive foregut and midgut. **At 5 to 6 weeks** the two pancreatic anlagen rotate into proximity. **At 6 to 8 weeks** the anlagen typically fuse. The dorsal pancreatic bud becomes the body and tail of the pancreas.

The duct in the body and tail (from duct in dorsal pancreatic anlage) fuses with the duct in the head (from duct in ventral pancreatic anlage) to form the main pancreatic duct (Fig. 7-16). A portion of the duct from the body and tail, the **accessory duct** (Fig. 7-17), often persists (~50% in autopsy series) and enters the duodenum through the minor papilla.[18] The minor duodenal papilla is several centimeters proximal to the major papilla.

Usually, only an insignificant amount of the pancreatic secretions drain through the accessory duct. An exception occurs when the accessory duct is the only duct entering the duodenum; the duct from the pancreatic head empties into the dorsal duct, not the duodenum (Fig. 7-18, *A*). This anatomic variant is found in 10% of individuals who have an accessory duct. Another exception is **pancreatic divisum,** in which the ventral and dorsal pancreatic ducts do not fuse (Fig. 7-18, *B*). This results in most of the pancreatic secretions (those secreted by dorsal pancreas) entering the duodenum through the accessory duct via the minor papilla.

The descriptive terminology of the pancreatic ducts is confusing. It is most clear to use the functional description shown in Figure 7-15, *B*—main pancreatic duct and accessory duct. Most authors use the accessory duct and the **duct of Santorini** synonymously. Some define the duct of Santorini as the entire ventral duct, including the accessory duct. The main pancreatic duct is sometimes called the **duct of Wirsung,** whereas others reserve that name for the ventral duct only.

In normal individuals the pancreatic duct diameter is usually 3 mm or less. Hadidi[19] found that the mean duct diameter was 3 mm in the head, 2.1 mm in the body, and 1.6 mm in the tail. The diameter of the duct can vary significantly. In fasting individuals the duct is often seen as a linear structure in the pancreatic body (Fig. 7-19). The diameter increases with age, although 3 mm is still an appropriate upper limit of normal in elderly patients.[5] Using a 2.5-mm upper limit of normal, Wachsberg[20] showed that inspiration could increase duct size to exceed that limit in 12% of patients without pancreatic disease. Secretin injection increases duct size, presumably because of increased pancreatic secretion,[21] which likely explains our and others' observation that pancreatic duct size may increase postprandially in some normal individuals.[7]

Imaging Anatomic Variants

Transabdominal ultrasound plays little role in the diagnosis of anatomic variants of the pancreas, which are generally discovered and evaluated with endoscopic retrograde cholangiopancreatography (ERCP), magnetic resonance cholangiopancreatography (MRCP), and more recently, multidetector CT.[16] Endoscopic ultrasound has been found to be useful in diagnosing pancreas divisum, especially in patients with unexplained pancreatitis.[22] Congenital variants of the pancreas are common, occurring in about 10% of the population. Variants include pancreas divisum, annular pancreas, and partial agenesis. Most

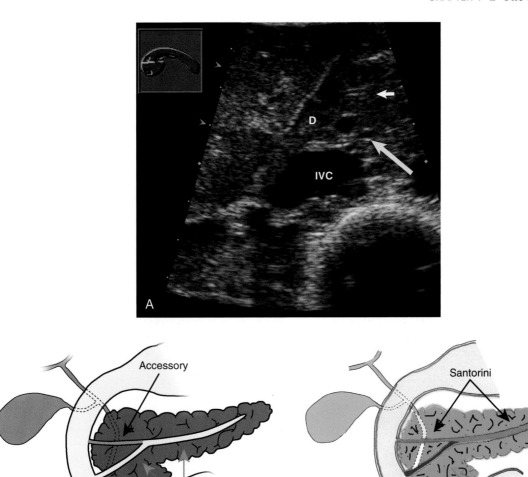

FIGURE 7-17. Pancreatic ductal anatomy. A, Pancreatic head. Transverse sonogram shows the accessory pancreatic duct *(white arrow).* The main pancreatic duct *(yellow arrow)* is seen dorsal and medial to the common bile duct *(red arrow). IVC,* Inferior vena cava; *D,* duodenum **B, Pancreatic ductal system, functional description.** Accessory duct is shown in pink *(black arrow)* and the main duct in brown. The accessory duct *(orange arrows)* persists in only a minority of individuals. **C, Pancreatic ductal system, embryologic origin.** Dorsal component of main adult duct and the accessory duct *(black arrows,* duct of Santorini, *pink)* both originate from the dorsal anlage. Ventral component of main duct *(orange arrow,* duct of Wirsung, *brown)* in pancreatic head arises from the ventral anlage and usually fuses with main duct from pancreatic body (dorsal anlage).

pancreatic variants are of no clinical significance and are found incidentally with imaging, at surgery, or on autopsy. Pancreas divisum, the most common variant, may predispose to pancreatitis, although the literature is unclear about this association.[23] The vast majority of patients (95%) with divisum do not develop pancreatitis.[24]

Peripancreatic Structures

The **intraperitoneal stomach** is generally located immediately ventral to the retroperitoneal pancreatic body, with the collapsed potential space of the lesser peritoneal sac between the two organs (Fig. 7-20). This explains why fluid in the stomach can sometimes be helpful in sonographic visualization of the pancreas. The **lesser peritoneal sac** is situated between the lesser omentum, greater omentum, and the stomach anteriorly and the parietal peritoneum and transverse mesocolon posteriorly (Fig. 7-21).

The **antrum** and **duodenal bulb** are intraperitoneal structures, whereas the **duodenal sweep** (second and third parts of duodenum) is retroperitoneal and hugs the pancreatic head. The third portion of the duodenum is a useful landmark, defining the caudal aspect of the pancreatic head. The transverse colon and hepatic flexure often overlie the pancreas, sometimes obscuring direct visualization.

The **transverse mesocolon** arises from the anterior pancreas and duodenum, formed by the parietal peritoneum that invests the pancreas and duodenum

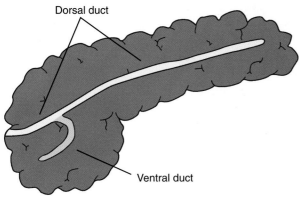

Dorsal duct

Ventral duct

A   Drainage via minor papilla only

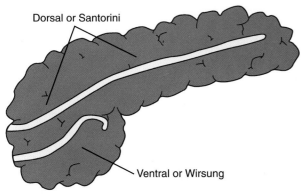

Dorsal or Santorini

Ventral or Wirsung

B   Pancreas divisum

FIGURE 7-18. Pancreatic ductal variants with secretions entering duodenum via minor papilla. A, Minor papilla only. Ventral duct from pancreatic head empties into the dorsal duct instead of the duodenum. **B, Pancreas divisum** lacks formation of the main adult duct because the ducts from each pancreatic anlage did not fuse. The duct from the dorsal anlage remains separate from the main duct in the head. This anatomic variant is present in 5% to 10% of the population.

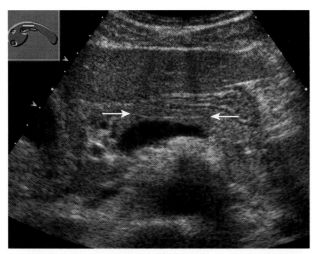

FIGURE 7-19. Normal pancreatic duct. Transverse image of the pancreas shows the appearance of the pancreatic duct as a linear, collapsed structure in the body *(arrows)*.

(Fig. 7-21). The transverse mesocolon invests the transverse colon and forms part of the posterior limits of the lesser peritoneal sac.

The tail of the pancreas lies within the splenorenal ligament and contacts the left kidney, left colic (splenic) flexure, and the hilum of the spleen posteriorly. Thus a portion of the pancreatic tail is intraperitoneal and somewhat mobile.

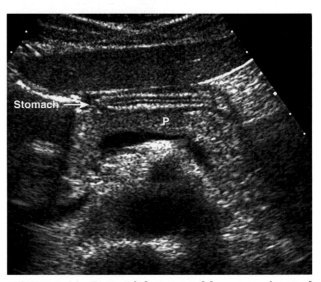

Stomach

P

FIGURE 7-20. Potential space of lesser peritoneal sac. Transverse image is between the stomach *(arrow)* and pancreas *(P)*.

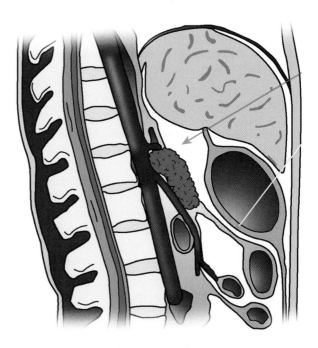

FIGURE 7-21. Peritoneal reflections and transverse mesocolon. Transverse mesocolon *(yellow arrow)* arises from the anterior pancreas and duodenum, formed by the parietal peritoneum that invests the pancreas and duodenum. The transverse mesocolon invests the transverse colon and forms part of the posterior limits of the lesser peritoneal sac *(blue arrow)*.

ACUTE PANCREATITIS

Acute pancreatitis (AP) is defined by the 1992 Atlanta Classification as "an acute inflammatory process of the pancreas with variable involvement of other regional tissues or remote organ systems associated with raised pancreatic enzyme levels in blood and/or urine."[25] More than 200,000 patients are admitted to U.S. hospitals annually with acute pancreatitis. It is difficult to determine the prevalence of acute pancreatitis because mild pancreatitis is often missed. The annual incidence of AP has been reported as 5 to 35 per 100,000 population (0.005%-0.035%).[26]

The clinical spectrum of AP ranges from a benign, self-limited disorder (75% of patients) to severe pancreatitis that may be fulminant and quickly cause death from multiorgan failure.[27] Mild AP generally resolves spontaneously with supportive management. Acute interstitial/edematous pancreatitis results in an enlarged and congested gland without appreciable necrosis or hemorrhage.[28] Banks and Freeman[29] found that the overall mortality of pancreatitis is approximately 5%. AP causes death by two mechanisms: infection and multiorgan failure. Mortality in the first 2 weeks usually results from organ failure, and after that, from infection. Mortality was 3% in patients with nonnecrotic (interstitial) pancreatitis and 17% for those with necrotizing pancreatitis. The same review noted 30% mortality with infected necrosis versus 12% for uninfected necrosis. Organ failure is even more skewed; there was no mortality with no organ failure, 3% with single-organ failure, and 47% mortality with multiorgan failure.[29]

The causes of AP are numerous and diverse. One problem in evaluating and treating AP has been the lack of a universally accepted classification system. The International Symposium on Acute Pancreatitis (Atlanta, 1992) attempted to address these problems by proposing a classification system that is clinically oriented.[30] The predominant causes of AP are gallstones and alcohol abuse, accounting for about 80% of all cases (Table 7-1).[31]

All patients, including known alcoholics, who present with their first episode of AP should have sonography to evaluate the biliary tree for **gallstones.**[32] Evaluation of the biliary tree is crucial in AP patients because chole-

TABLE 7-1. CAUSES OF ACUTE PANCREATITIS (AP)

CAUSE	AP CASES
Gallstones	40%
Alcoholism	40%
Idiopathic	10%
Other	10%

cystectomy with removal of common duct stones prevents recurrence of AP,[33] which can be fatal. Gallstones affect about 15% of the U.S. population,[34] but prevalence varies widely by ethnicity. Among some Native Americans, about 50% of men and 80% of women are affected, the highest prevalence in the world.[35] After a careful search of the gallbladder for stones, the bile duct should be evaluated for choledocholithiasis and obstruction. Reports vary, but the prevalence of **common duct stones** in patients with symptomatic gallstones is likely 10% to 20%. If the ducts are not dilated sonographically, however, the prevalence of common duct stones is probably about 5%.[36] With careful technique, ultrasound can identify common duct stones with a sensitivity of 75%.[37]

When biliary dilation or choledocholithiasis is present sonographically, a stone may be impacted in the distal common duct. It seems reasonable to assume that urgent intervention to relieve the obstruction is necessary in these patients. There is conflicting evidence, however, whether patients benefit from intervention in the acute setting.[38-42] Acosta et al.[43] reported results from a prospective randomized clinical trial of patients with biliary pancreatitis that showed better outcomes with decompression of the duct within 48 hours from the onset of symptoms. It made no difference if the decompression was spontaneous or from surgical treatment or ERCP.

How gallstones cause AP is unknown, although it is somehow related to passage of stones into and through the common duct. Gallstones cause 30% to 50% of AP attacks, whereas only 3% to 7% of patients with gallstones develop pancreatitis.[33] Another important cause of AP is **biliary sludge** (microlithiasis). These cases comprise most of what was previously characterized as "idiopathic" pancreatitis.[44] The myriad other causes of AP include neoplasm,[45,46] infection, pancreas divisum, toxins, drugs, and genetic, traumatic, and iatrogenic (endoscopy, postoperative), factors.[31] From 5% to 7% of patients with pancreaticobiliary tumors, benign or malignant, present with acute pancreatitis.[47]

Approach to Imaging

Abdominal sonography and contrast-enhanced computed tomography (CECT) are the two most useful imaging modalities in patients with AP. Other useful, but usually secondary diagnostic and therapeutic studies include MRCP, magnetic resonance imaging (MRI), ERCP, and endoscopic ultrasound. The choice of modality depends on the clinical situation. Ultrasound should be performed to detect gallstones and bile duct obstruction in all patients in whom biliary AP is possible. CECT is indicated early in the clinical course of patients with severe pancreatitis, mainly to diagnose pancreatic necrosis. Necrosis appears as nonenhancement of the pancreas on CECT.[48] Pancreatic necrosis is considered significant when more than 30% of the gland is affected, or an area larger than 3 cm is present. Patients with pancreatic necrosis must be observed closely for clinical deterioration and treated with prophylactic antibiotics.[49-51] Sharma and Howden[52] found that antibiotic prophylaxis significantly reduced sepsis by 21.1% and mortality by 12.3% compared with no prophylaxis. CT is also the most accurate examination when seeking delayed complications of acute pancreatitis.

IMAGING IN ACUTE PANCREATITIS (AP)

ROLE OF ULTRASOUND
Detect gallstones as a cause of AP.
Detect bile duct dilation and obstruction.
Diagnose unsuspected AP or confirm diagnosis of AP.
Guide aspiration and drainage.

ROLE OF COMPUTED TOMOGRAPHY
Detect pancreatic necrosis (patients with suspected severe pancreatitis).
Detect complications of AP.
Diagnose unsuspected AP or confirm diagnosis of AP.
Diagnose conditions mimicking AP, including gastrointestinal ischemia, ulceration, or perforation and ruptured abdominal aortic aneurysm.
Guide aspiration and drainage.

Magnetic resonance cholangiopancreatography is an accurate means of detecting stones in the gallbladder and bile ducts of patients with AP.[31] Abdominal MRI can provide information similar to CECT, including the diagnosis of pancreatic necrosis.[53,54] Because of expense, MRCP and MRI should generally be reserved for patients in whom CT or ultrasound does not provide adequate information to guide management and for those who have a contraindication to CECT.

Endoscopic ultrasound is more sensitive than abdominal ultrasound for the detection of common bile duct stones and can be useful in suspected gallstone pancreatitis.[55] Endoscopic ultrasound is also valuable in diagnosing microlithiasis and pancreas divisum.[56]

Because of its complications and expense, ERCP, formerly both a diagnostic and a therapeutic modality, is now usually reserved for therapy.[57] Sometimes coupled with endoscopic sphincterotomy (ES) and stone removal, ERCP is a valuable therapeutic modality in choledocholithiasis with jaundice, dilated common bile duct, AP, or cholangitis.[58]

Ultrasound Findings

Evaluation of the gallbladder and bile ducts is the focus of most sonographic examinations performed in patients with acute pancreatitis. Nevertheless, understanding pancreatic and extrapancreatic abnormalities associated with AP is important. The combined use of serum amylase and serum lipase yields sensitivity and specificity of 90% to 95% in diagnosing AP,[59] but mild cases may be missed. In mild AP the patient may present after transient elevated amylase and lipase levels have resolved; thus, no serologic indicators of pancreatitis may be present.[60] In these patients the diagnosis of mild AP is clinical. On the other hand, the diagnosis may be missed in severe pancreatitis because pain is absent or masked by other, more severe symptoms. Analyzing fatal pancreatitis between 1980 and 1985, Lankisch et al.[61] reported that 30.2% of cases were not diagnosed until autopsy. In cases such as these, imaging (CT, sonography, or MRI) may be important in supporting a clinical diagnosis or suggesting an unsuspected diagnosis of acute pancreatitis.

After a careful search of the gallbladder and bile duct for **stones**, the entire pancreas should be scanned. After scanning the pancreas, peripancreatic pathology should be sought in the lesser sac, anterior pararenal spaces, and transverse mesocolon.

The reported prevalence of sonographic abnormality in AP varies from 33% to 91.7%. In a retrospective evaluation of AP patients, Finstad et al.[32] found abnormalities in 91.7% of patients.[32] Pancreatic echogenicity typically decreases in AP because of interstitial edema. In some patients, echogenicity is normal. Rarely, echogenicity may actually increase, possibly because of hemorrhage, necrosis, or fat saponification. Cotton et al.[62] noted that, compared with the liver, the pancreatic echogenicity was increased in 16% of normal individuals and 32% of AP patients. Finstad et al.[32] found no AP patients with globally increased echogenicity, although focal areas of increased echogenicity and inhomogeneity did occur.

Enlargement of the pancreas is almost universal in acute pancreatitis. Unfortunately, enlargement may be difficult to judge, because pancreatic size before the onset of pancreatitis is usually unknown and varies widely. In 1995, Guerra et al.[6] found that the thickness of the body of the normal pancreas in 261 adults was 10.1 mm (±3.8 mm; range, 4-23 mm). In 2005, Finstad et al.[32] found that the mean anteroposterior (AP) measurement of the pancreatic body at the SMA level was 21.1 mm (±6.4 mm; range, 12-45 mm), almost twice the average found in normal individuals by Guerra. It seems reasonable, therefore, to use **22 mm** (mean plus 3 standard deviations) as the upper limit of normal pancreatic thickness, understanding that this is likely to be an insensitive parameter for diagnosing AP (Fig. 7-22).

Using a defined scanning protocol to look for pancreatitis-associated findings, Finstad et al.[32] found that sonography revealed abnormalities in 45 of 48 patients (91.7%) (Table 7-2).

The classic finding of **decreased gland echogenicity** is present in only 44% of patients. In addition, when there is fatty infiltration of the liver, the normal pancreas

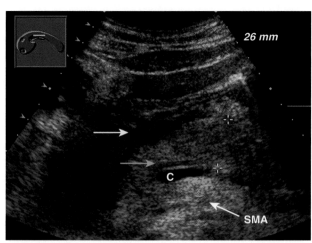

FIGURE 7-22. Enlarged pancreas, acute pancreatitis with inflammation. Transverse image of the pancreas shows 26-mm anteroposterior dimension at the level of the superior mesenteric artery *(SMA).* Note the acute inflammation ventral to the pancreas *(yellow arrow)* and ventral to *(blue arrow)* the splenic vein–superior mesenteric vein confluence *(C).*

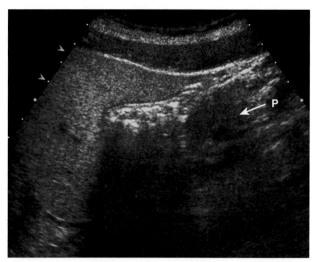

FIGURE 7-23. Pseudopancreatitis. Longitudinal image of pancreas *(P)* and liver shows that the fatty liver is more echogenic than the normal pancreas, simulating a hypoechoic pancreas.

TABLE 7-2. SONOGRAPHIC ABNORMALITIES IN ACUTE PANCREATITIS

ABNORMALITY	NO. OF PATIENTS (48 TOTAL)	PREVALENCE
Peripancreatic inflammation	29	60%
Heterogeneous parenchyma	27	56%
Decreased gland echogenicity	21	44%
Indistinct ventral margin	16	33%
Pancreas enlarged*	13	27%
Focal intrapancreatic echo change	11	23%
Peripancreatic fluid collections	10	21%
Focal mass	8†	17%
Perivascular inflammation	5	10%
Pancreatic duct dilation	2	4%
Venous thrombosis	2	4%

Modified from Finstad TA, Tchelepi H, Ralls PW. Sonography of acute pancreatitis: prevalence of findings and pictorial essay. Ultrasound Q 2005;21:95-104.
*Anteroposterior (AP) dimension ≥23 mm at superior mesenteric artery.
†Five of 8 hypoechoic.

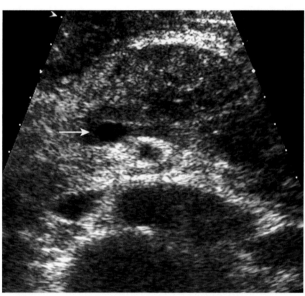

FIGURE 7-24. Heterogeneous pancreas, acute pancreatitis. Transverse image shows that heterogeneity can be a subtle, subjective finding. Arrow indicates the perivascular inflammation and splenic vein–superior mesenteric vein clot.

may appear hypoechoic, a pattern called "pseudopancreatitis" (Fig. 7-23). Pancreatic heterogeneity is a subjective but common finding, present in more than 50% of patients (Fig. 7-24). Focal hypoechoic regions are noted in some patients (Fig. 7-25).

The least subjective, most common, and thus most useful finding is **pancreatitis-associated inflammation**

(Fig. 7-26; see also Figs. 7-22 and 7-24). Extrapancreatic inflammatory changes may be detected even when the pancreatic contour is normal and the pancreas is not obviously enlarged. Pancreatic inflammation is typically hypoechoic or anechoic (Fig. 7-27) and conforms to a known retroperitoneal or peritoneal space **(Video 7-1)**. It may be difficult or impossible to distinguish inflammation from fluid (Fig. 7-28). In contrast to inflammation, fluid collections often have convex margins, are thicker and more localized, may cause a mass effect, and sometimes have through-transmission of sound (Fig. 7-29; **Video 7-2**).

Inflammation is most often seen ventral and adjacent to the pancreas in the **prepancreatic retroperitoneum**

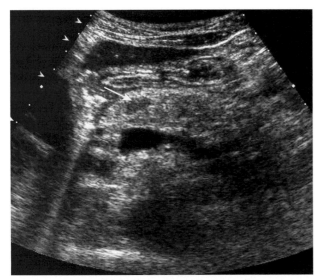

FIGURE 7-25. Focal hypoechoic area, acute pancreatitis. Transverse image shows heterogeneous pancreas with focal hypoechoic area *(arrow)*.

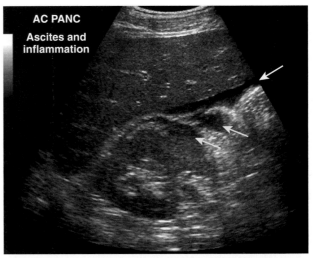

FIGURE 7-27. Inflammation and ascitic fluid, acute pancreatitis. Transverse image of right upper quadrant shows acute inflammation in the anterior pararenal (retroperitoneal) space and the perirenal space *(yellow arrows)*. Ascites is present in the adjacent subhepatic space *(white arrow)*.

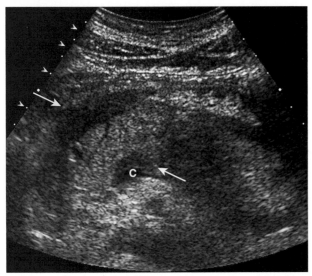

FIGURE 7-26. Inflammation from acute pancreatitis. Transverse image shows acute inflammation ventral to the pancreas *(yellow arrow)* and ventral to *(white arrow)* the splenic vein–superior mesenteric vein confluence *(C)*. The pancreas is enlarged and heterogeneous.

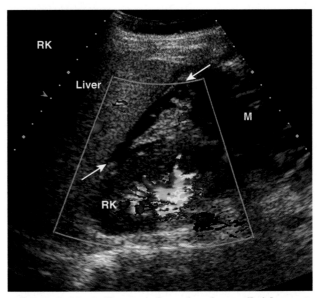

FIGURE 7-28. Inflammation simulates fluid. Longitudinal image of right upper quadrant shows that the acute inflammation *(arrows)* in the anterior pararenal (retroperitoneal) space simulates fluid and might be mistaken for ascites. Note the retroperitoneal inflammatory mass *(M)*. *RK,* Right kidney.

(see Figs. 7-22, 7-26, and 7-28), the right and left anterior pararenal spaces, the perirenal spaces, and the transverse mesocolon. The **anterior pararenal spaces** are best seen through a coronal flank approach (Fig. 7-30). The patient is scanned while in a decubitus position with the transducer angled to achieve a sagittal scan plane through the flank. Areas of inflammation within the anterior pararenal space are often seen immediately adjacent to the echogenic fat within the **perirenal space.** Acute pancreatic inflammation within the anterior pararenal space occasionally outlines Gerota's fascia (Fig. 7-30). Inflammatory masses (formerly called phlegmon) maybe present (Fig. 7-31) (see Fig. 7-28). The **transverse mesocolon**

region can be seen well in most patients on longitudinal scans. Look caudal to the pancreas and behind the stomach (Fig. 7-32; see also Fig. 7-21); inflammation extends caudally and may reach the transverse colon. The transverse colon itself may be difficult to identify; in the transverse plane it lays directly ventral (anterior) to the head and uncinate process of the pancreas. Spread of inflammation along perivascular spaces, especially the splenic vein and splenoportal confluence, is characteristic of AP (Figs. 7-33, 7-34, and 7-35; see also Figs. 7-22, 7-24, and 7-26). This perivascular inflammation may

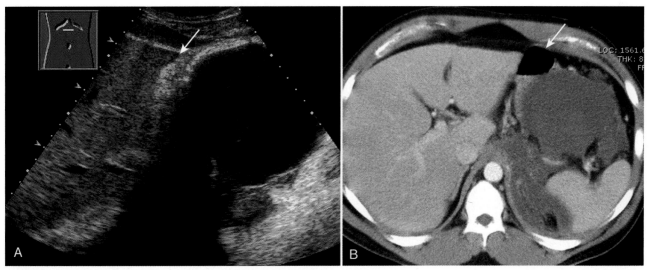

FIGURE 7-29. Pancreatitis-associated fluid collection. A, Transverse sonogram, and **B,** CT image, of a "lesser sac" fluid collection. Such collections are actually in the prepancreatic retroperitoneum. Note the displaced stomach *(arrows).*

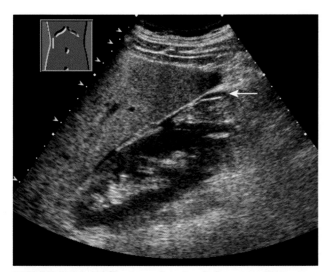

FIGURE 7-30. Inflammation in right anterior pararenal and perirenal spaces. Longitudinal coronal image of right upper quadrant; decubitus position facilitates visualization of the pararenal and perirenal spaces. The inflammation partially outlines the perirenal space *(arrow)*, which is contained by Gerota's fascia.

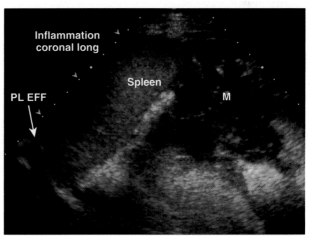

FIGURE 7-31. Inflammatory mass in left anterior pararenal space. Longitudinal coronal image of left upper quadrant shows retroperitoneal inflammatory mass *(M)*. Such masses were formerly called "phlegmons" before this term was proscribed by the 1992 International Symposium on Acute Pancreatitis (Atlanta). *PL EFF,* Left pleural effusion.

explain why some patients develop thrombosis of the portal veins (Figs. 7-36 and 7-37; see also Fig. 7-34). Occasionally, retroperitoneal findings similar to those seen in AP can be seen in patients with ascites, perhaps because of a "leaky" peritoneum.

Complications

Complications of acute pancreatitis can be classified as systemic complications (those related to organ failure) and local complications.[63]

LOCAL COMPLICATIONS OF ACUTE PANCREATITIS

Acute fluid collections
Pseudocysts
Pancreatic abscess
Necrosis
Infected necrosis
Hemorrhage
Venous thrombosis
Pseudoaneurysms

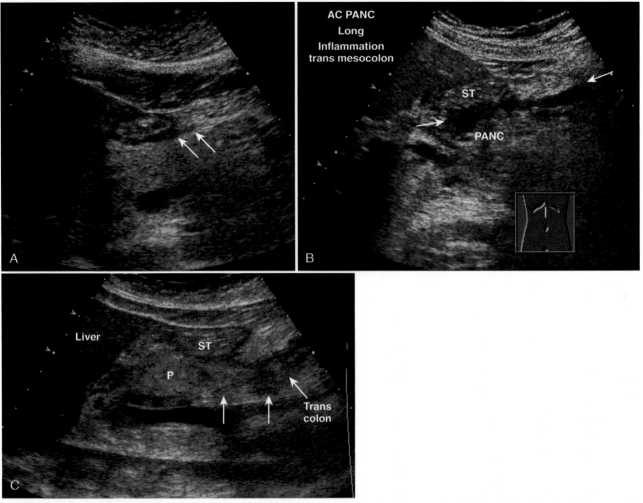

FIGURE 7-32. Inflammation in transverse mesocolon. Longitudinal images. **A,** Subtle, relatively minor inflammation *(arrows).* **B,** More significant inflammation *(arrows).* **C,** Transverse colon, which may be difficult to visualize; mesocolon inflammation is more diffuse *(arrows).*

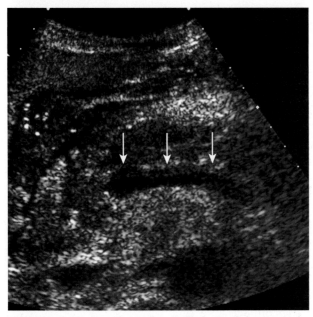

FIGURE 7-33. Perivascular inflammation. Transverse image of the pancreatic body shows hypoechoic inflammation *(arrows)* around the splenic vein.

Acute Fluid Collections

Pancreatitis-associated fluid collections represent a spectrum of disease and thus can be problematic to classify (Figs. 7-38 and 7-39; see also Fig. 7-29). Fluid collections, when they contain debris or necrosis or may be infected, cannot always be categorized. Approximately 40% of patients with AP develop acute fluid collections.[64,65] About half of these appear to resolve spontaneously,[64] with almost 70% resolving in patients with nonnecrotizing pancreatitis.[65] Thus, drainage or other intervention in acute collections is inappropriate, unless a rare superinfection occurs. The Atlanta Classification suggests that the differentiation between acute fluid collection and pseudocyst should be made after 4 weeks from the onset of disease.[25] Others suggest that a fluid collection that persists for 6 weeks can be considered a pseudocyst. The 6-week definition is based on classic surgical management; the pseudocyst wall requires 6 weeks to "mature" to the point where it can be drained surgically.[66]

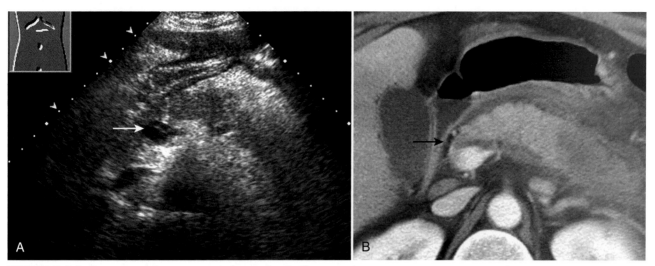

FIGURE 7-34. Pancreatitis causes perivascular inflammation. A, Transverse sonogram, and **B,** CT image, of the pancreas show obvious evidence of perivascular inflammation *(arrows),* hypoechoic on sonogram and low density on CT.

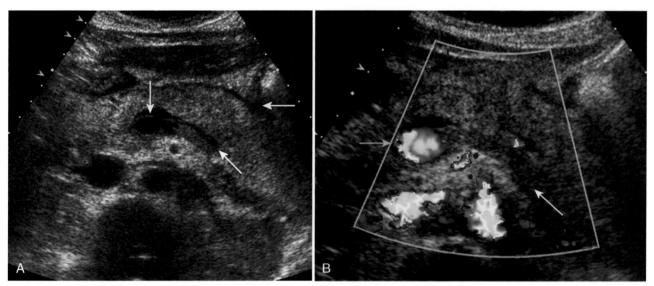

FIGURE 7-35. Perivascular inflammation and clot caused by pancreatitis. A, Transverse sonogram of pancreas shows the confluence free of thrombus. Note the obvious signs of perivascular and pre-pancreatic inflammation *(yellow arrows).* **B,** Transverse color Doppler sonogram confirms splenic vein clot *(yellow arrow)* and the open confluence *(green arrow).*

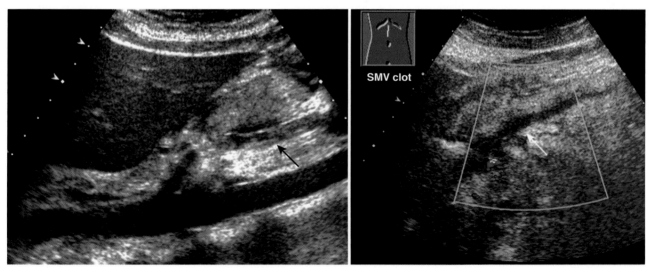

FIGURE 7-36. Superior mesenteric vein clot. Longitudinal sonograms show clot in the superior mesenteric vein *(arrows)* in two patients with acute pancreatitis.

Pseudocysts

Pancreatic pseudocysts are a well-known complication of acute or chronic pancreatitis. Pseudocysts comprise 75%[67] to 90%[68] of all cystic lesions of the pancreas. The "wall" of pancreatic pseudocysts consists of fibrous and granulation tissue. Thus, unlike true cysts or cystic neoplasms, pseudocysts do not have an epithelial lining. Pseudocysts are more common in patients with chronic pancreatitis (CP) than in patients with acute pancreatitis. Pseudocyst prevalence ranges from 5% to 16% in patients with AP. In CP, prevalence varies from 20% to 40%, with the highest rates in alcohol-related CP.[69] On occasion, pseudocysts can be caused by trauma (Fig. 7-40).

The most important issue in diagnosing pseudocysts on images is avoiding confusion with cystic neoplasm, a mistake that can lead to adverse clinical outcomes.[70] Unfortunately, this distinction may be difficult. The major criterion for diagnosing a pseudocyst is a clinical history or imaging evidence of acute or chronic pancreatitis. Failing this, differentiating a pseudocyst from cystic pancreatic lesions becomes problematic. The sonographic findings in pseudocysts are variable. Pseudocysts can range in appearance from almost purely cystic to collections with considerable mural irregularity, septations, and internal echogenicity because of debris (Fig. 7-41) from necrosis, hemorrhage (see Fig. 7-40), or infection. Successful differentiation of cystic neoplasm from pseudocyst thus depends on a high degree of suspicion for possible cystic neoplasm and understanding

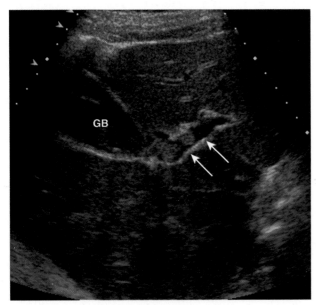

FIGURE 7-37. Left portal vein clot. Transverse sonogram shows clot in the left portal vein *(arrows)* caused by pancreatitis.

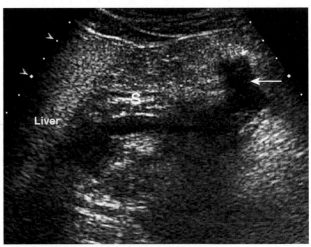

FIGURE 7-38. Acute fluid collection. Longitudinal image shows inflammation and an acute fluid collection *(arrow)* in the transverse mesocolon; *S*, stomach.

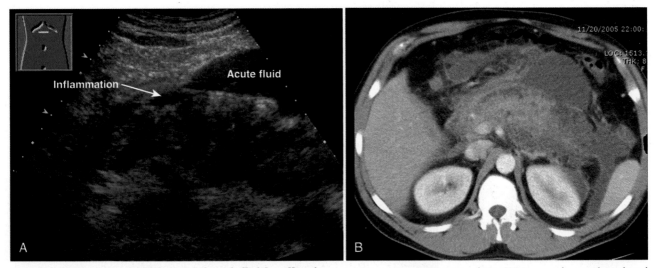

FIGURE 7-39. Pancreatitis-associated fluid collection. A, Transverse sonogram, and **B,** CT image, show enlarged and heterogeneous pancreas, with prominent peripancreatic inflammation and an acute fluid collection that later resolved spontaneously.

findings strongly suggestive of "the usual suspects": serous cystic neoplasm (microcystic adenoma), mucinous cystic neoplasm, solid-pseudopapillary tumor, and intraductal papillary mucinous neoplasm.[71] Characterization of cystic neoplasms by CT or MRI is unreliable, even when the reviewers' diagnostic certainty was 90% or more.[72]

Conservative management of pseudocysts is appropriate unless complications occur. As noted, many pseudocysts resolve spontaneously. Persistent uncomplicated pseudocysts require no intervention and can be safely observed.[73,74] Indications for drainage of a pseudocyst include abdominal pain, usually related to growth of (or

hemorrhage into) the pseudocyst, biliary obstruction (Fig. 7-41), and gastrointestinal obstruction (usually duodenal).[75] Internal or external fistula formation can result in pancreatic ascites or pleural effusion.[76] Inflammation from pancreatitis can digest and dissect through tissue plane boundaries. For example, pseudocysts and inflammatory masses can present in the neck[77] or the groin[78] (Fig. 7-42).

Necrosis and Abscess

Significant pancreatic necrosis is defined by the Atlanta Classification system as nonenhanced pancreatic parenchyma greater than 3 cm or involving more than 30% of the area of the pancreas on CECT (see Fig. 7-35). These patients are at greater risk than patients without necrosis and are treated with prophylactic antibiotics and observed closely. Necrosis cannot be definitively diagnosed by ultrasound, although ultrasound contrast agents may change that situation.

The terminology of the Atlanta Classification is somewhat confusing when describing significant infection associated with pancreatitis. "Pancreatic abscess" is reserved for infected fluid collections, essentially pseudocysts that become infected. **Infected pancreatic necrosis,** a much more serious condition, can also result in pus-filled collections, which might also be called "abscesses" in other clinical settings. Thus it is best to think of **two distinct types of acute pancreatitis-associated abscess,** as follows:

1. The Atlanta Classification pancreatic abscess, an infected fluid collection/pseudocyst, which has minimal necrosis.
2. Infected necrosis with a fluid collection, which arises from infection of necrotic pancreatic tissue.

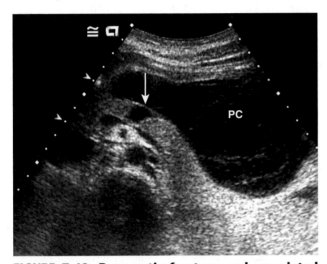

FIGURE 7-40. Pancreatic fracture and associated pseudocyst. Transverse sonogram shows the fracture/laceration *(arrow)* of the pancreatic body. A pseudocyst *(PC)* has developed ventral to the pancreas. Trauma is an uncommon cause of pancreatic pseudocysts. *(Case courtesy Stephanie Wilson, MD.)*

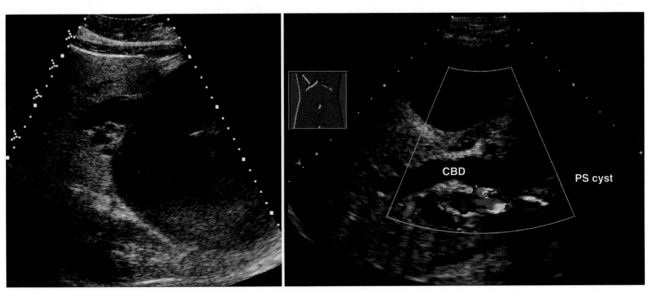

FIGURE 7-41. Pseudocysts causing biliary obstruction. Longitudinal oblique sonograms in two different patients demonstrate bile duct dilation from obstruction. Biliary obstruction is an indication for pseudocyst drainage.

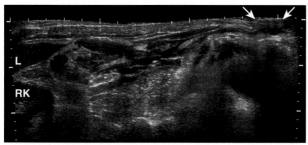

FIGURE 7-42. Inflammation from pancreatitis causing groin mass. Longitudinal extended field of view sonogram from right upper quadrant to right groin. An inflammatory mass *(arrows)* is caudal to the inguinal ligament. Extensive spread of acute inflammation is common in acute pancreatitis. *RK,* Right kidney; *L,* liver.

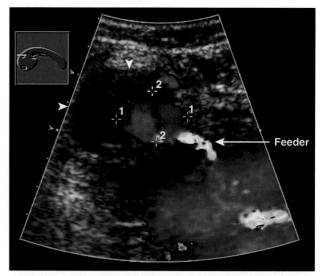

FIGURE 7-43. Pancreatic pseudoaneurysm. Transverse color Doppler sonogram shows AP-associated pseudoaneurysm arising from the gastroduodenal artery. The clotted portion of the pseudoaneurysm *(arrowheads)* is noted. Calipers denote the patent portion of the pseudoaneurysm. Pseudoaneurysm is a rare complication of pancreatitis, much less common than venous thrombosis. Notice the "yin and yang" *(red/blue)* color Doppler appearance representing the blood swirling in the lesion.

Treatment

The major approaches to the treatment of **pseudocysts** include surgery, percutaneous image guided drainage and endoscopic guided drainage. Andrén-Sandberg et al.[66] state:

> There are no randomized studies for the management protocols for pancreatic pseudocysts. … First of all it is important to differentiate acute from chronic pseudocysts for management, but at the same time not miss cystic neoplasias. Conservative treatment should always be considered the first option (pseudocysts should not be treated just because they are there).

It is difficult to determine the best method to treat pseudocysts. The cause of pancreatitis, communication of the pancreatic duct with the pseudocyst, and local technical expertise must be considered when choosing a treatment method. Although the data are unclear, **percutaneous drainage** (PCD) of pseudocysts likely is overall less successful than surgical or endoscopic drainage.[79] Nevertheless, PCD can be used as a first option with other techniques reserved for PCD failures. In the large subset of patients WITH normal duct anatomy and no communication of the pseudocyst with the pancreatic duct, PCD is successful in more than 80%. On the other hand, PCD failed in 77% to 91% of patients who had duct obstruction or strictures.[75] Therefore, ERCP,[80] and in some cases MRCP,[53,69] may be useful in the selection of treatment technique.

Pancreatic abscess (infected fluid collections without significant necrosis) is often best treated by PCD.[81] PCD can also be used in **infected necrosis,** for which it is curative in some patients[82] and is a useful temporizing technique in others.[79] Although management of infection in pancreatitis is evolving,[25] therapy for infected pancreatic necrosis remains surgical debridement.

Vascular Complications

Vascular complications occur in both acute and chronic pancreatitis. **Pseudoaneurysms** and **venous thrombosis** are the most significant vascular complications. Most clinically insignificant hemorrhagic pancreatitis is related to venous and small vessel disease, whereas potentially fatal hemorrhage is usually related to enzymatic digestion or pseudoaneurysm of major vessels, including the splenic, gastroduodenal (Fig. 7-43), and superior pancreaticoduodenal arteries. The prevalence of hemorrhage in pseudocyst patients is 5%, but with up to 40% mortality.[83] Vascular erosion can produce a sudden, painful expansion of the cyst or gastrointestinal (GI) bleeding caused by bleeding into the pancreatic duct ("hemosuccus pancreaticus").[84] Thrombosis of the portal venous system may occur in both acute and chronic pancreatitis;[63] **splenic vein thrombosis** is most common (Fig. 7-44). Agarwal et al.[85] reported a 22% prevalence of splenic vein thrombosis in patients with chronic pancreatitis. Bernades et al.[86] reported the prevalence of **portal vein thrombosis** as 5.6% (15/266). Splenic vein thrombosis may result in upper GI bleeding from gastric varices, called "sinistral" (left-sided) portal hypertension.

CHRONIC PANCREATITIS

The prevalence of chronic pancreatitis ranges from 3.5 to 10 per 100,000 in the population. CP is characterized by intermittent pancreatic inflammation with progressive, irreversible damage to the gland. Histologically, the key features are fibrosis, acinar atrophy, chronic inflammation, and distorted and blocked ducts.[87] CP ultimately leads to permanent structural change and deficient endocrine and exocrine function. Some lasting morphologic

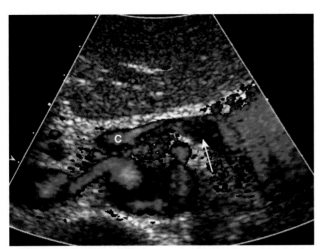

FIGURE 7-44. Splenic vein clot. Transverse power Doppler image shows partial splenic vein clot *(arrow)* caused by chronic pancreatitis. *C,* Confluence of splenic and superior mesenteric veins.

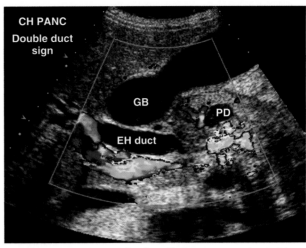

FIGURE 7-45. "Double duct" sign. Longitudinal oblique image shows dilation from obstruction of the pancreatic duct *(PD)* and extrahepatic bile duct *(EH).* Chronic pancreatitis often causes the double-duct sign. *GB,* Gallbladder.

changes include alterations in parenchymal texture, glandular atrophy, glandular enlargement, focal masses, dilation and beading of the pancreatic duct (often with intraductal calcifications), and pseudocysts.

Alcoholism is the predominant cause of chronic pancreatitis (70%-90% in Occidental countries).[88] Other causes include **pancreatic duct obstruction** caused by strictures, **hypertriglyceridemia, hypercalcemia, autoimmune pancreatitis, tropical pancreatitis,** and other genetic mutations.[89]

Chronic pancreatitis is characterized clinically by pain, malabsorption, and diabetes. Treatment of uncomplicated CP is usually conservative, with the major aim to improve the patient's quality of life by alleviating pain and mitigating malabsorption and diabetes. Surgical and endoscopic interventions are reserved for complications such as pseudocysts, abscesses, and malignancies.[87] Obstruction and thrombosis of the portal veins may occur (see Fig. 7-37). CP may also lead to obstruction of the pancreatic and bile ducts, sometimes resulting in the "double duct" sign (Fig. 7-45). In my institution, because of a high prevalence of alcoholism, the double-duct sign is caused by CP more often than by periampullary neoplasm.[90] The frequency of common bile duct obstruction in patients hospitalized for CP ranges from 3% to 23% (mean, 6%). The frequency of duodenal obstruction is about 1.2% in hospitalized patients.[91] All these findings occur in various combinations and with differing frequency.[7]

Approach to Imaging

The imaging diagnosis of chronic pancreatitis depends on detecting the structural changes associated with advanced disease. Unfortunately, these changes are rarely present in early disease, decreasing imaging sensitivity.

Consequently imaging is not very useful in early CP. Furthermore, morphologic changes do not correlate well with endocrine or exocrine function.[92]

Despite the common belief that it is diagnostically inferior overall to CECT, MRCP, and endoscopic ultrasound,[93-95] ultrasound is often recommended as the first diagnostic test.[87] Bolondi[7] states that ultrasound diagnosis of CP remains difficult because of "the polymorphism of anatomic changes and the relatively high incidence of false-negative results in early stages of the disease." In clinical practice, however, ultrasound currently is accepted as the first diagnostic step when CP is suspected.

Ultrasound Findings

Sonography can be effective in diagnosing CP, but other tests are generally required if intervention is contemplated. The hallmark of CP is **ductal dilation** (Fig. 7-46) and **calcifications,** which can be in the branch ducts (Fig. 7-47), main duct (Fig. 7-48), or both **(Video 7-3).** When these findings are present in a patient with pain and a history of alcoholism, the diagnosis of CP is secure. CT is superior to sonography in detecting calcifications and ductal dilation. Calcifications are often made much more conspicuous on ultrasound images by looking for the **color comet-tail artifact** (CCTA)[96] (Fig. 7-49; **Video 7-4).**

Areas of increased and decreased echogenicity are related to the effects of patchy fibrosis. These focal areas of altered echogenicity are often subjective and difficult to appreciate.

Pseudocysts

Pseudocysts are more common in patients with chronic (20%-40%) than with acute (5%-16%) pancreatitis

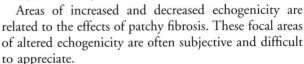

(Figs. 7-50 and 7-51).[69] Pseudocysts may present with various shapes, contain necrotic debris (Fig. 7-52), hemorrhage (~5%) (Fig. 7-53),[67] or even have a completely solid pattern.[7]

Portal and Splenic Vein Thrombosis

Thrombosis of the portal venous system can occur in chronic pancreatitis because of (1) intimal injury from recurrent acute inflammation, (2) chronic fibrosis and inflammation, or (3) compression by either a pseudocyst or an enlarged pancreas.[97] **Splenic vein thrombosis** is relatively common in patients with CP (5%[98] to 40%[97])

(see Fig. 7-44). **Portal vein thrombosis** occurs less frequently. Bernades et al.[86] reported the prevalence of splenoportal vein obstruction as 13.2%, with the splenic vein obstructed in 8%, portal vein in 4%, and superior mesenteric vein in 1%.

Pancreatitis-associated thrombus in the splenic or portal vein often results in collaterals different from those in portal hypertension from liver disease. These collaterals, rather than conveying blood away from the diseased liver, conduct blood *toward* the liver, bypassing the clot. Splenic vein thrombosis will often result in **left sided** ("sinistral") **portal hypertension** (Fig. 7-54). This can result in isolated gastric varices, which can cause

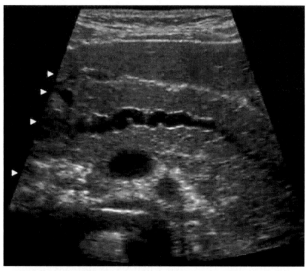

FIGURE 7-46. Dilation of pancreatic duct. Transverse sonogram of the pancreatic body shows a beaded, dilated pancreatic duct, resulting from chronic pancreatitis.

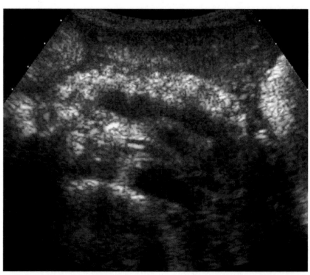

FIGURE 7-47. Dilated pancreatic duct and branch duct calcifications. Ductal calcification is a hallmark of chronic pancreatitis. Transverse sonogram shows many branch duct stones.

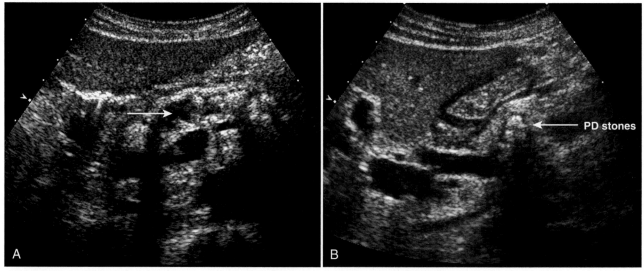

FIGURE 7-48. Dilated pancreatic duct and stones. A, Transverse, and **B,** longitudinal, sonograms show chronic pancreatitis with dilation of the pancreatic duct and multiple stones in the main duct *(arrow).* Branch duct stones are manifest as almost confluent, echogenic parenchymal foci.

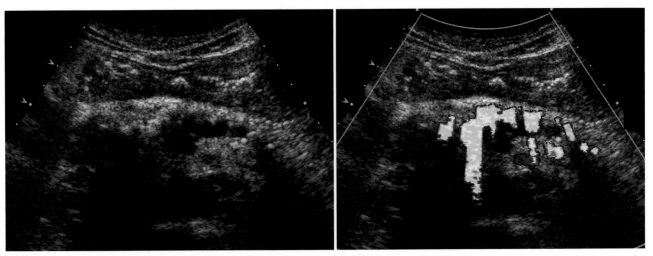

FIGURE 7-49. Calcifications highlighted by color comet-tail artifact (CCTA). Transverse gray-scale and color Doppler sonograms show that CCTA makes the extensive pancreatic calcification much more conspicuous. Patient had chronic pancreatitis.

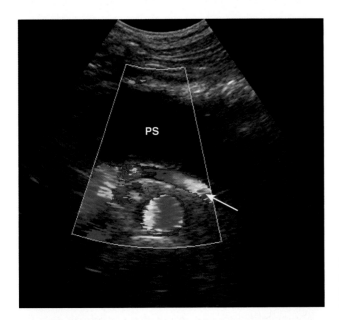

FIGURE 7-50. Pseudocyst in pancreatic body. This pseudocyst *(PS)* is almost free of internal debris. The flow reversal in the splenic vein *(arrow)* is related to cirrhotic portal hypertension. Patient had chronic pancreatitis.

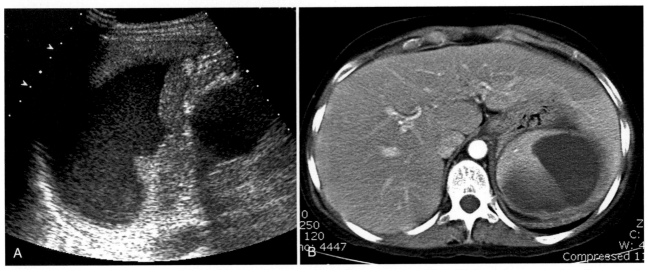

FIGURE 7-51. Hemorrhagic pseudocyst in pancreatic tail. A, Complex, debris-filled pseudocyst seen through pancreatic tail in patient with chronic pancreatitis. **B,** CT shows also shows debris in the pseudocyst.

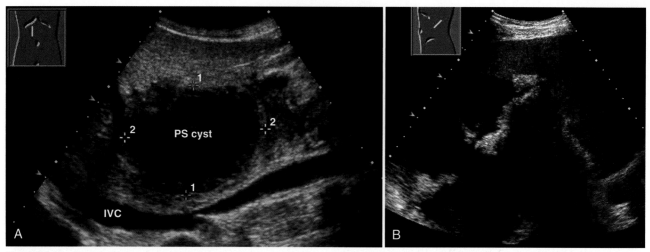

FIGURE 7-52. Chronic pancreatitis in two patients with pseudocysts. A, Longitudinal sonogram shows irregular margins with some internal debris. **B,** Oblique sonogram through the spleen shows massive, complex, debris-filled pseudocyst in the pancreatic tail.

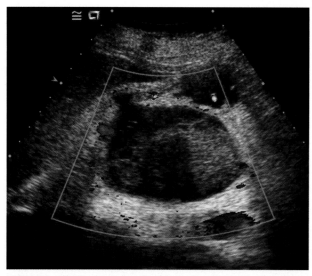

FIGURE 7-53. Hemorrhagic pseudocyst in pancreatic body. Chronic pancreatitis–associated debris-filled pseudocyst; it may be difficult or impossible to distinguish a hemorrhagic pseudocyst from a debris-filled nonhemorrhagic pseudocyst. Normal pancreas is not included.

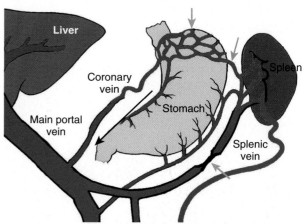

FIGURE 7-54. Splenic vein clot with left-sided ("sinistral") portal hypertension. This can result in isolated gastric varices *(green arrow),* which can cause life-threatening gastrointestinal bleeding. The hepatopetal pathway to bypass the splenic vein clot *(purple arrow)* includes short gastric collaterals *(orange arrows).*

life-threatening GI bleeding. The hepatopetal pathway to bypass the splenic vein clot (Fig. 7-55) includes short gastric collaterals that lead to the **gastric mural varices** (Fig. 7-56), then flow toward the liver in the coronary vein. It may be difficult or impossible to detect splenic vein clot, or even the splenic vein itself. Therefore the diagnosis of splenic vein clot may depend on detection of collaterals, such as short gastric varices or an enlarged coronary vein.[99] When the main portal vein is clotted, blood flows to the liver around the clot. If the portal vein clot persists, these hepatopetal collaterals may enlarge, resulting in cavernous transformation of the portal vein. **Gallbladder wall varices** were present in 30% of patients

with portal vein thrombosis in one study[100] (Fig. 7-57). These can be successfully diagnosed with color Doppler[101] or gray-scale[102] imaging.

Masses Associated with Chronic Pancreatitis

Focal pancreatic masses occur in approximately 30% of CP patients. Carcinoma and pancreatitis related masses are usually easy to differentiate clinically and by imaging (Fig. 7-58). In some patients, however, the distinction may be difficult[103] (Fig. 7-59). Pancreatitis-associated masses are found in a surprisingly large percentage of patients having surgery for suspected pancreatic malignancy (5%-18.4%).[104] In one series, 10.6% (47 patients) of 442 patients undergoing pancreaticoduodenectomy

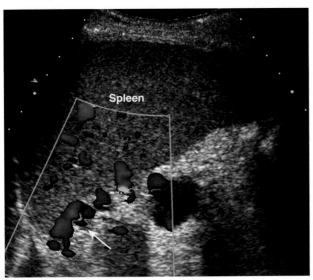

FIGURE 7-55. **Short gastric collaterals from splenic vein clot (arrow).** Longitudinal coronal color Doppler sonogram in patient with left-sided (sinistral) portal hypertension shows blood in the short gastric venous collaterals (arrow) flowing away from the splenic hilum.

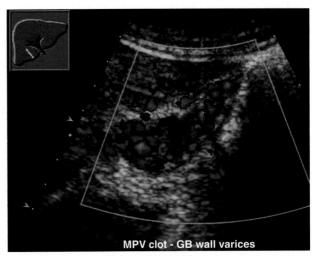

FIGURE 7-57. **Varices and clot.** Oblique color Doppler sonogram shows that main portal vein clot engenders hepatopetal collaterals, including cavernous transformation of the portal vein and, in some patients, gallbladder wall varices.

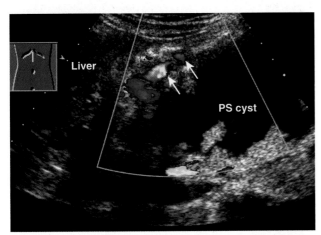

FIGURE 7-56. **Gastric mural varices.** Longitudinal color Doppler sonogram in patient with left-sided portal hypertension. The actual gastric mural varices (arrows) are visualized, unusual in these patients. The pseudocyst that caused the splenic vein clot is compressing the stomach.

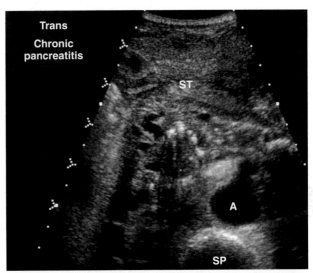

FIGURE 7-58. **Chronic pancreatitis–associated mass, with calcification and dilated ducts.** Transverse sonogram of pancreatic head; when classic findings such as ductal dilation and multiple calcifications are present, the diagnosis of chronic pancreatitis is clear.

(Whipple resection) had benign disease.[105] Of these 47, 40 (9.2%) were resected because of a suspected malignancy.

The presence of calcification within a mass makes the diagnosis of CP likely (Fig. 7-60). Only 4% to 6% of ductal adenocarcinomas have calcifications.[106,107] The pattern of calcification in ductal adenocarcinoma is different from the usual CP patient. In CP calcifications are multiple and ductal. In carcinoma there are generally only one or a few coarse calcifications, usually unrelated to dilated ducts. Hyperechoic masses, even without discrete calcifications, are usually (but not always) related to CP. An uncalcified isoechoic or hypoechoic mass occurring in a patient without clinical or imaging evi-

dence of CP is nonspecific. In this case, other imaging or biopsy is indicated to differentiate carcinoma from CP. As noted, the double-duct sign is nonspecific, occurring in both pancreatitis and pancreatic carcinoma. Finding multiple dilated branch ducts in the pancreatic head is more typical of CP and is rarely found in pancreatic cancer (Fig. 7-61). Pseudocysts are common in CP (20%-40%)[69] and rare in carcinoma,[108] but they occur in both conditions. So-called obstructive pseudocysts that occur with carcinoma usually are peripheral to body or tail lesions. Pancreatitis-associated pseudocysts occur anywhere in the gland, usually arising in areas of necrosis.

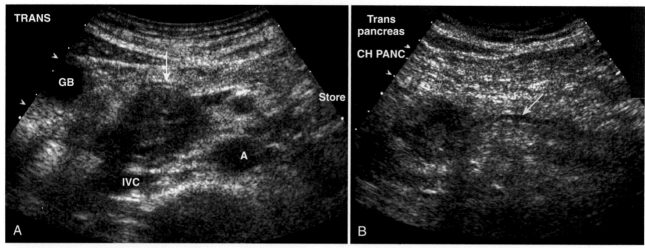

FIGURE 7-59. Chronic pancreatitis–associated masses in pancreatic head simulating carcinoma. Two different patients. **A,** Transverse sonogram reveals a mass *(arrow)* that lacks calcification and other features of chronic pancreatitis, simulating a malignant mass; *A,* aorta; *GB,* gallbladder; *IVC,* inferior vena cava. **B,** Transverse sonogram reveals a mass *(blue arrow)* that simulates a malignancy; *yellow arrow,* pancreatic duct.

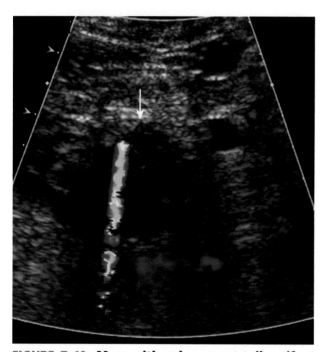

FIGURE 7-60. Mass with color comet-tail artifact from calcification. Transverse sonogram reveals a mass *(arrow).* Calcification, revealed by a prominent CCTA, indicates a likely diagnosis of chronic pancreatitis.

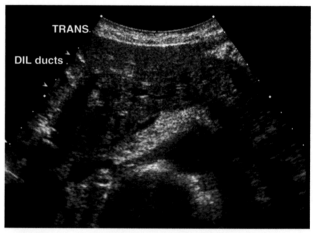

FIGURE 7-61. Many small, dilated ducts. Transverse sonogram shows multiple dilated branch ducts in the pancreatic head, more typical of chronic pancreatitis and rarely found in pancreatic cancer.

Autoimmune pancreatitis (AIP) is a masslike imitator of pancreatic carcinoma[109] (Fig. 7-62). AIP accounts for many cases previously classified as "idiopathic pancreatitis," comprising perhaps 4% to 6% of all patients diagnosed with CP. The AIP terminology is confusing; synonyms include chronic sclerosing pancreatitis, lymphoplasmacytic sclerosing pancreatitis, and tumefactive chronic pancreatitis.[110] About 2% of pancreatic masses resected for suspected malignancy are found instead to be AIP.[111] Although benign masses from the usual causes of CP are more common, AIP masses are much more likely to be confused for carcinoma. In one series, 13 of 19 (68.4%) masses caused by the usual types of CP were resected for a clinical suspicion of malignancy, whereas all 11 (100%) of AIP-related masses were thought to be malignant preoperatively.[105]

Anecdotal experience suggests that when a definite pancreatic mass is seen sonographically, but not imaged on CT, chronic pancreatitis is the likely cause of the mass. Another slightly confounding fact is that CP patients have an increased lifetime risk of developing pancreatic carcinoma (4%)[112] compared with the general population (1%-2%).[113]

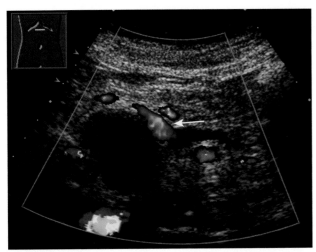

FIGURE 7-62. Mass in pancreatic head. Transverse sonogram shows hypoechoic mass in the pancreatic head from autoimmune pancreatitis (AIP) simulating pancreatic carcinoma. The portal vein *(arrow)* is displaced by the mass.

TABLE 7-3. FIVE-YEAR CANCER SURVIVAL RATES*

SITE	%	RANK*
Pancreas	**5**	**1**
Liver	10.8	2
Lung/bronchus	15	3
Esophagus	15.6	4
Colon/rectum	64	9
Kidney	65.5	10
Uterus/cervix	71.6	11
Thyroid	96.7	17
Prostate	98.4	18

Data from American Cancer Society.
*Worst to best; 18 common neoplasms.

PANCREATIC NEOPLASMS

Periampullary Neoplasm

Periampullary neoplasms are difficult to differentiate from one another and are generally managed identically—by pancreaticoduodenectomy (Whipple resection). **Jaundice** is the most common presentation of these tumors (85%).[114] Tumors in this group include pancreatic ductal adenocarcinoma (about two thirds of periampullary neoplasms), ampullary carcinoma (15%-25%), duodenal carcinoma (10%), and distal cholangiocarcinoma (10%).[114] Survival is best for duodenal and ampullary carcinoma, but only in comparison to the poor survival rates for cholangiocarcinoma and especially pancreatic cancer.

Image evaluation of these tumors is basically the same as that described later for pancreatic ductal adenocarcinoma. The approach varies depending on the clinical presentation and local expertise. Most agree, however, with Ross and Bismar[114]: "The relative availability, economy, and usefulness of the results make transabdominal ultrasound a common initial imaging study for patients with suspected obstructive jaundice."

Pancreatic Carcinoma

Pancreatic ductal adenocarcinoma is the most common primary pancreatic neoplasm, accounting for 85% to 95% of all pancreatic malignancies.[115,116] Ductal adenocarcinoma has a slight male predominance, most frequently affecting patients 60 to 80 years of age. The prevalence of pancreatic carcinoma tripled during the mid-20th century. Mortality for pancreatic cancer has continued to decline since 1975 in men and has leveled off in women after increasing from 1975 to 1984.[117]

Pancreatic cancer represents only 2% of all cancers but is the fourth most common cause of cancer death in the United States. According to 2008 American Cancer Society data, **pancreatic ductal adenocarcinoma is the most lethal malignancy** (Table 7-3). Overall 5-year survival is poor: 2% to 5%. Risk factors include tobacco smoking (twice the risk as for nonsmokers), obesity, chronic pancreatitis, diabetes, cirrhosis, and use of smokeless tobacco. A family history of pancreatic cancer also increases risk.[118] Rare syndromes associated with increased risk include Peutz-Jeghers syndrome.[119]

The selection of imaging techniques in patients with pancreatic cancer requires a rational approach based on grim realities about the disease. Although sophisticated imaging of candidates for resection consumes much time and effort, it is crucial to remember that only a few patients have potentially resectable disease at initial diagnosis. These are the patients who can potentially benefit from sophisticated "resectability" studies. Further, even for that small minority who can be resected with a hope for cure, the prognosis is poor. Most patients with newly diagnosed pancreatic carcinoma have advanced unresectable disease at initial diagnosis. In most studies from major oncology centers, only 10% to 20% of the patients are eligible for curative surgery at diagnosis.[120,121] The initial routine imaging study, whether ultrasound or CT, can usually detect advanced disease.[122]

Although the diagnosis of periampullary tumors and safety of the Whipple procedure have improved over the decades, prognosis for patients with pancreatic cancer remains poor. In a meta-analysis of virtually the entire surgical literature on resection of pancreatic cancer, Gudjonsson[123] found significant errors and exaggerations in the reporting of survival figures, and that the overall survival rate actually was less than 0.4%. The best overall survival rate in detailed surgical studies is only 3.6%, and for a nonsurgical study, 1.7%. In another report, Gudjonsson[124] stated:

PANCREATIC CANCER IMAGING: THREE KEY CONCEPTS

1. The vast majority of patients with pancreatic cancer can be classified as "unresectable for cure," based on the initial ultrasound or CT.
2. Only 10% to 20% of patients require sophisticated "resectability" studies, whether done with CT, MRI, or ultrasound (transabdominal or endoscopic).
3. The survival statistics for patients with pancreatic cancer have been exaggerated in the literature. The usefulness of surgery is questionable in this malignancy.

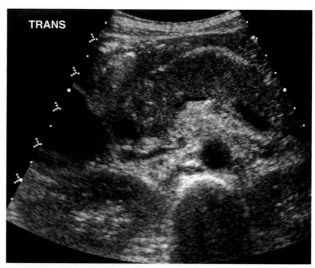

FIGURE 7-63. Diffuse pancreatic carcinoma. Transverse sonogram; fewer than 5% of all ductal adenocarcinomas are diffuse.

Resections for pancreatic cancer have been performed for 65 years, with approximately 20,000 reported. A number of authors claim a 5-year survival rate of 30% to 58%. Review of the literature reveals only about 1,200 5-year survivors; however, 10 times as many individual resected survivors have been reported (in various countries), and nonresected survivors are overlooked. This high survival percentage is obtained by reducing the subset on which calculations are based and by using methods such as the Kaplan-Meier method, which produces higher figures as increasing numbers of patients are lost to follow-up. After adjustments, hardly more than 350 resected survivors could be found. Revision of statistical methods is urgently needed.

Conlon et al.[121] reported that 5-year survival does not equal cure. In their series of 118 resected patients, median survival was 14.3 months. Twelve patients survived 5 years after surgery (10.2% of resected patients), but five of these 12 patients died of pancreatic cancer in the sixth postoperative year. At the time of the report, six patients were alive without evidence of disease, at a median follow-up of 101 months (range, 82-133 months). In periampullary tumors other than ductal adenocarcinoma, 5-year survival is higher, for example, 9% versus 36% in the study by Wade et al.[125]

Despite these grim facts, most surgeons favor an aggressive approach, as expressed by Farnell et al.[126]:

> Significant progress has been made in diagnosis, preoperative staging, and safety of surgery; however, long-term survival after resection is unusual, and cure is rare. That said, the authors maintain their aggressive posture regarding this disease, recognizing that resection offers the only potential for cure.

Because of prevailing surgical opinion, radiologists will continue to be asked to do studies to assess the potential resectability of pancreatic cancer in the 10 to 20% of patients in whom the initial study does not show advanced disease.

Detection of Pancreatic Cancer

Sonography and CT are the primary tools used to detect focal pancreatic disease, especially pancreatic carcinoma and periampullary neoplasms. Sonography often detects pancreatic carcinoma because it is the method of choice to screen patients with jaundice[127] and is frequently used to assess patients with pain. There are few recent U.S. studies of ultrasound in pancreatic carcinoma. Nonetheless, sonography clearly is effective in detecting pancreatic carcinoma,[122,128,129] with sensitivity of 72% to 98%.[63] **Multidetector computed tomography** (MDCT) has a reported sensitivity of 86% to 97% for all pancreatic tumors.[127] CT is less operator dependent than ultrasound, which, along with CT's higher reimbursement, likely accounts for most radiologists' preference for CT in tumor detection. Sonography may be useful to characterize abnormalities noted on CT, such as determining whether a lesion is cystic or solid. MRI, MRCP, ERCP, and endoscopic ultrasound are all comparably sensitive to CT, but reserved for problem solving or special circumstances.[115]

Ultrasound Findings

From 60% to 70% of pancreatic cancers originate from the pancreatic head, 25% to 35% are in the body and tail, and 3% to 5% are diffuse[106,116] (Fig. 7-63). This distribution explains in part the good detection rates of cancer, because the head and body are more easily seen sonographically than the tail. The hallmark of periampullary pancreatic cancer is the double-duct sign, with both bile duct dilation (Fig. 7-64) and pancreatic duct dilation (Fig. 7-65). Pancreatic ductal adenocarcinoma may cause considerable desmoplastic reaction, so even a mass that appears eccentric can cause ductal obstruction (Fig. 7-66). If a mass in the pancreatic head region is found and there is no ductal dilation, lesions other than pancreatic ductal adenocarcinoma should be sought.

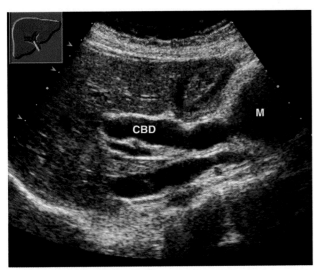

FIGURE 7-64. Large pancreatic carcinoma. Longitudinal oblique sonogram shows large, hypoechoic mass *(M)* obstructing the extrahepatic common bile duct *(CBD)*.

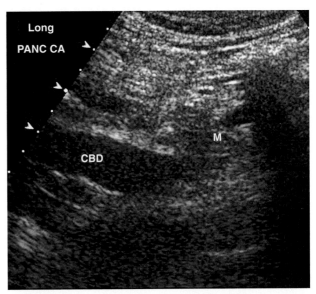

FIGURE 7-66. Eccentric pancreatic ductal adenocarcinoma. Longitudinal oblique sonogram shows that this carcinoma may cause considerable fibrosis (desmoplastic reaction) and obstruct the extrahepatic bile duct. Thus, even this mass *(M)*, which appears somewhat distant from the common bile duct *(CBD)*, can cause ductal obstruction.

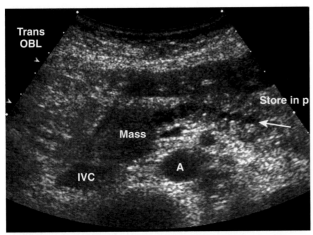

FIGURE 7-65. Pancreatic carcinoma. Transverse sonogram shows hypoechoic mass obstructing the pancreatic duct. Note the "beaded" pattern of the dilated, obstructed duct. *A,* Aorta; *IVC,* inferior vena cava.

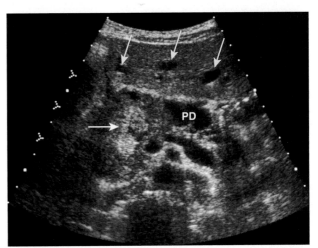

FIGURE 7-67. Heterogeneous, mainly echogenic pancreatic carcinoma. Transverse sonogram shows tumor obstructing the extrahepatic bile duct. Increased echogenicity *(white arrow)* is unusual in pancreatic ductal adenocarcinoma. This heterogeneous cancer causes a double-duct sign with pancreatic duct dilation *(PD)*. The intrahepatic duct dilation is manifest as dilated minor ducts *(yellow arrows)*.

Reviewing findings in 62 patients with pancreatic carcinoma, Yassa et al.[106] found that tumors were ovoid or spherical in 37 patients (60%) and irregular in 25 (40%). Forty tumors (65%) deformed the shape of the gland, whereas six lesions (10%) caused no glandular contour abnormality and were visualized only because tumor echogenicity differed from that of the normal pancreas. Thirty-four tumors (55%) were homogeneously hypoechoic compared with the normal pancreas, 25 (40%) had heterogeneous echotexture (Fig. 7-67), two (3%) were homogeneously hyperechoic, and one (2%) was isoechoic. Many of the heterogeneous tumors were predominantly hypoechoic with areas of varied echogenicity. **Calcifications** were noted in four patients (6%) and **small, intratumoral cystic areas** in nine patients

(15%) (Fig. 7-68; **Video 7-5**). **Postobstructive pseudocysts** were found in four patients (6%) (Fig. 7-69), similar to the 5% to 10% of patients reported in a review article.[130] Such pseudocysts may be caused by obstructive pancreatitis.[131] **Glandular atrophy** may occur from obstruction caused by a tumor. This atrophy is more easily appreciated with CT than ultrasound. It is important to remember that masses caused by chronic pancreatitis can closely simulate periampullary cancers. Very few carcinomas have internal flow that can be imaged on color Doppler.

Resectability Imaging

As the safety of pancreaticoduodenectomy (Whipple procedure) improves, some surgeons have become more aggressive. Also, with advances in surgery, many pancreatic cancers are technically resectable. Unfortunately, the technical ability to resect does not equate to improved outcome (compared to no resection).

Findings that suggest unresectability for cure include **tumor larger than 2 cm, extracapsular extension, vas-**

cular invasion (venous or arterial), **lymphadenopathy,** and **metastatic disease.** Image findings of unresectability are reliable (PPV ≈ 100%). Only rarely can such a tumor be resected for cure at surgery. Conversely, many tumors believed resectable because of their imaging appearance are discovered to be unresectable at surgery. Unfortunately, even "resectable" patients with local disease have 5-year survival of only 10%[121] to 20%.[117]

As noted, only a small percentage of patients who have no evidence of advanced disease on initial imaging studies (10%-20%) require sophisticated resectability studies, whether done with transabdominal ultrasound, CT, MRI, or endoscopic ultrasound.[132,133] In this subset of pancreatic cancer patients, most U.S. radiologists prefer to use CT or MRI rather than ultrasound. Other techniques include endoscopic ultrasound[134] and positron emission tomography (PET).[135] The usefulness of three-dimensional (3-D) workstation–reconstructed thin-section MDCT evaluation of pancreatic tumors, pioneered by Jeffrey and his group at Stanford,[136,137] is unmistakable. No comparative data are available, but these CT images undoubtedly show more abnormalities than transabdominal ultrasound. MDCT has clear advantages for duodenal and retroperitoneal invasion, as well as for detection of malignant lymph nodes. It is unclear, however, how many resectability CT scans would be needed if resectability sonograms were done first. Sonography, especially with color Doppler, can be effective in detecting patients who are unresectable for cure.[129,138-141] Our data showed a predictive value of 100% for unresectability.[139] In the prediction of resectability, however, 40% of patients thought to be potentially resectable at color Doppler ultrasound were found unresectable at surgery. Given these facts, it seems best to use less invasive ultrasound to screen the subgroup of patients needing resectability studies, reserving 3-D MDCT for those with no sonographic signs of advanced disease.[142]

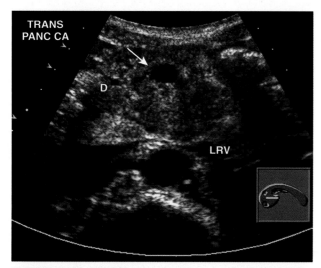

FIGURE 7-68. Cystic area in pancreatic ductal adenocarcinoma. Transverse sonogram shows a complex mass in the pancreatic head. Small, intratumoral cystic areas *(arrow)* are present in about 10% to 15% of pancreatic cancers. These cysts can be seen in chronic pancreatitis as well, rendering this feature unhelpful in differentiating the two conditions. *D,* Duodenum; *LRV,* left renal vein.

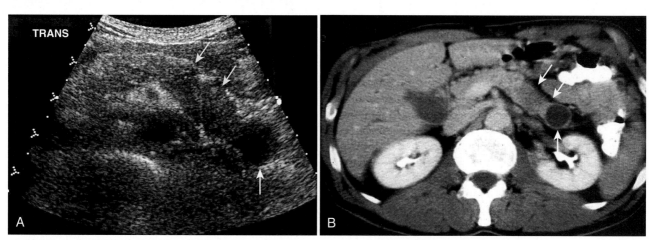

FIGURE 7-69. Pancreatic ductal adenocarcinoma causing "obstructive pseudocyst." A, Transverse sonogram reveals a subtle cancer in the body of the pancreas *(yellow arrows)* with a pseudocyst peripheral to the mass *(white arrow).* **B,** CT image at a similar level shows identical findings.

PANCREATIC CANCER IMAGING: SUGGESTED APPROACH

- Color Doppler ultrasound should be used to screen patients for resectability of pancreatic cancer.
- Multidetector CT or other examinations may then be used in patients with no sonographic evidence of advanced disease.

Color Doppler Ultrasound

We have developed a technique to assess the resectability of pancreatic tumors using color Doppler sonography.[139] Images are obtained with a large-footprint, curved linear array transducer, using compression technique and color Doppler sonography to evaluate the relationship of the tumor mass to critical vessels, including the main portal vein, SMV (Fig. 7-70), splenic vein, left renal vein, and IVC. Arteries evaluated include the aorta, celiac axis (Fig. 7-71), splenic and common hepatic arteries, and SMA (Fig. 7-72; **Video 7-6**). Anatomic variations are noted in the figures. Vessels that are touched or occluded by tumor are categorized according to a **pancreatic color Doppler score**. Other factors affecting resectability (metastasis, enlarged nodes) are recorded (Table 7-4).

Color Doppler flow sonography can correctly predict unresectability in 80% or more of pancreatic carcinoma patients. Most of these patients would then require less CT and subsequent imaging evaluation, thus decreasing expense and the need to use more invasive tests.

Although almost ignored in recent U.S. studies of imaging in pancreatic and periampullary neoplasms, much evidence indicates that color flow sonography can

be very useful in evaluating the resectability of pancreatic neoplasms. Any future evaluation of imaging and management of pancreatic tumors should include color flow sonography. A Polish study found that the diagnostic accuracy of routine, color, and power Doppler and 3-D ultrasound was comparable to that of helical CT in detecting and staging pancreatic carcinoma.[122] The use of ultrasound contrast agents shows some promise to improve the sonographic evaluation of pancreatic tumors,[143] but this is currently an investigational technique.

CYSTIC PANCREATIC LESIONS

Understanding cystic pancreatic lesions is increasingly important because improved imaging techniques result in the detection of progressively more of these lesions,

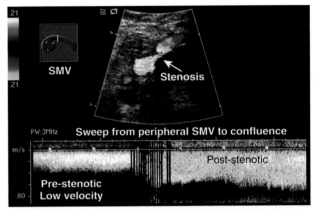

FIGURE 7-70. Pancreatic ductal adenocarcinoma narrowing superior mesenteric vein. Longitudinal oblique spectral Doppler sample volume was swept from the pre-stenotic lower-velocity region to the poststenotic area (high velocity). Color Doppler image reveals the area of stenosis *(arrow)*.

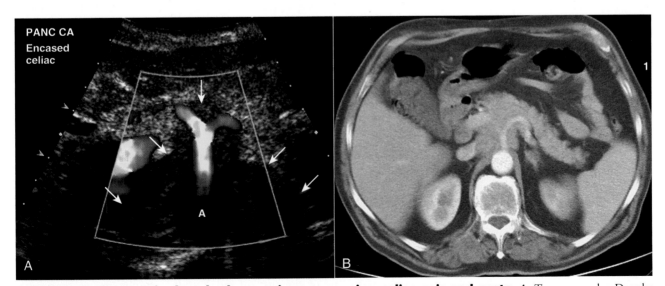

FIGURE 7-71. Pancreatic ductal adenocarcinoma encasing celiac axis and aorta. A, Transverse color Doppler sonogram shows a hypoechoic mass *(arrows)* that encases the aorta *(A)* and celiac axis. **B,** CT image at a similar level shows the same findings. This lesion is clearly unresectable for cure.

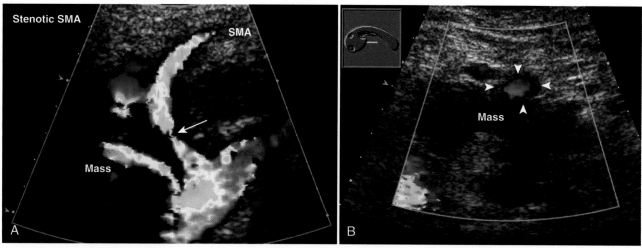

FIGURE 7-72. Pancreatic ductal adenocarcinoma encasing superior mesenteric artery (SMA). A, Longitudinal color Doppler sonogram shows that hypoechoic mass, which also encases the celiac axis, narrows the SMA *(arrow)*. **B,** Transverse color Doppler sonogram in a different patient demonstrates much more subtle encasement *(arrowheads)*. Ductal adenocarcinoma narrows and occludes veins much more frequently than arteries. This narrowing is equivalent to classic angiographic encasement.

TABLE 7-4. PANCREATIC COLOR DOPPLER SCORE (PCDS)

SCORE	DESCRIPTION
PCDS 0	Tumor *does not touch* a vessel.
PCDS 1	Tumor touches, 1%-24% around the vessel circumference.
PCDS 2	Tumor touches, 25%-49% around the vessel circumference.
PCDS 3	Tumor touches, 50%-99% around the vessel circumference.
PCDS 4	Tumor encased, 100% around the vessel circumference.
PCDS 5	Vessel invaded or occluded.

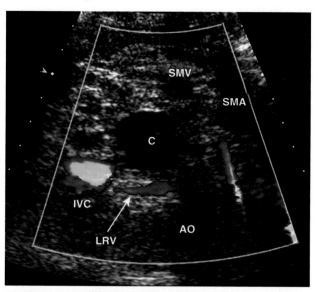

FIGURE 7-73. Benign pancreatic cyst (presumed). Transverse color Doppler sonogram shows 2-cm cyst discovered incidentally on abdominal sonogram and followed for 4 years without a change in size. It is generally safe to follow such lesions. *C,* Cyst; *AO,* aorta; *LRV,* left renal vein; *IVC,* inferior vena cava; *SMA,* superior mesenteric artery; *SMV,* superior mesenteric vein.

often as incidental findings.[67,144,145] New concepts and pathologic definitions of cystic neoplasms, especially mucinous and intraductal papillary forms, have altered the approach to diagnosis and management of these lesions.

Although the number of cystic lesions of the pancreas detected is increasing because of improved imaging techniques,[144,145] pancreatic pseudocyst remains the most common, accounting for 75% or more of all cystic lesions.[67] A careful history must be obtained to rule out previous acute or chronic pancreatitis, so as to minimize the chance of confusing pseudocyst with other cystic masses. Nonpseudocyst lesions include simple cysts and cystic neoplasms. Although certain image features may be helpful, the differential diagnosis of cystic lesions, especially when small, is unreliable by CT or MRI. Visser et al.[72] found that, even when their diagnostic certainty was 90% or greater, characterization was unreliable.

Fortunately, it appears safe to follow unilocular pancreatic cystic lesions with a diameter 3 cm or less[67] (Fig. 7-73). Sahani et al.[146] reported that 35 of 36 unilocular pancreatic cystic lesions 3 cm or less were benign. Internal septations were associated with borderline or in situ malignancy in 10 of 50 cases (20%). Other surgeons believe that resection of these lesions is a better approach.[68,147] The usefulness of tumor markers and cyst fluid cytology is debated.[68,148-150] Most agree that high-risk patients and features should be managed more aggressively, including symptomatic patients, growth of the cyst on serial studies, tumor greater than 3 cm in diameter, internal soft tissue, and mural or septal thickening.

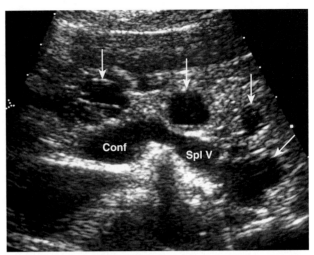

FIGURE 7-74. Von Hippel–Lindau (VHL) disease with multiple pancreatic cysts. Transverse sonogram shows multiple simple pancreatic cysts *(arrows)*, which should suggest the diagnosis of VHL because simple cysts are rare and usually single, and multiple cysts in polycystic disease are also rare.

Simple Pancreatic Cysts

Simple pancreatic cysts are rare in the general population, with a prevalence of 0.2%[151] to 1.2%.[147] These low percentages may be underestimated because imaging[152] and autopsy[153] studies have recorded a substantially higher prevalence, about 20% and 24.3%, respectively. Our experience suggests that the lower prevalence rates are closer to the actual experience in clinical imaging. Detecting a simple pancreatic cyst should raise suspicion of an inherited disease that has a high prevalence of cysts, such as **autosomal dominant polycystic kidney disease (ADPKD)**[154] or **von Hippel–Lindau (VHL) disease**.[155] Multiple pancreatic cysts can also occur in cystic fibrosis.[156]

Multiple pancreatic cysts are more common in VHL disease than in ADPKD. Prevalence of pancreatic cysts in VHL patients ranges from 50% to 90%, making pancreatic cysts the most common lesion in VHL disease.[155] Thus, multiple simple pancreatic cysts should suggest the diagnosis of VHL (Figs. 7-74 and 7-75). In addition to simple cysts, other pancreatic lesions associated with VHL include serous cystic neoplasm and pancreatic endocrine tumors, with a slightly increased risk of ductal adenocarcinoma.[155]

Cystic Neoplasms

Cystic tumors of the pancreas account for about 10% of cystic pancreatic lesions. Although most solid tumors are ductal adenocarcinomas with a poor prognosis, cystic tumors are usually either benign lesions or low-grade malignancies. Malignant cystic tumors account for about 1% of all pancreatic malignancies.[68] Mucinous tumors (IPMN, MCN) are often malignant. The risk of malignancy is greater in older individuals. Reliable prevalence data are difficult to find.[157] Table 7-5 lists the most common tumors in order of prevalence.

Serous Cystic Neoplasm

Serous cystic neoplasm (SCN), previously known as "microcystic adenoma," is a benign tumor, although a few invasive, malignant examples have been reported.[68,157] SCN occurs more frequently in women and is most often found in the pancreatic head.[150] These lesions are composed of myriad tiny cysts, generally too small to be individually resolved sonographically (Fig. 7-76, *A*). The multiple reflective interfaces caused by the walls of the tiny cysts leads to an echogenic appearance, analogous to that of infantile polycystic kidney disease. Through-transmission is usual. On CT, SCN appears as water density (mean density of cysts). Larger cysts (1-3 cm in diameter) often are present at the periphery of the lesion (Fig. 7-76, *B*). A radially oriented, fibrous pattern occurs in a minority of patients,[145] and a central calcification is often present (30%-50%) (Fig. 7-77). Small lesions (<2 cm) may appear identical to simple cysts. This pattern is common in the serous oligocystic adenoma variant.[150]

Intraductal Papillary Mucinous Neoplasm

Intraductal papillary mucinous neoplasm (IPMN) was unreported before 1982;[158] other names include intraductal papillary mucinous tumor (IPMT), intraductal mucin-hypersecreting neoplasm, and ductectatic mucinous neoplasm.[150] Unlike MCN, IMPN arises from the pancreatic ducts, usually in the head of the pancreas. IMPN occurs in an older population than with MCN and affects men and women equally.

Mucin is secreted into the ducts, causing prominent dilation (Fig. 7-78) and sometimes mucin extrusion from the ampulla of Vater.[157] IPMN often presents as acute pancreatitis. Both benign and malignant lesions can cause bile duct obstruction[159] (Fig. 7-79). IPMN ranges from a benign to an overtly malignant lesion. Invasive adenocarcinoma is seen in approximately 30% of resected cases. Invasive or in situ carcinomas are likely present in about 70% of patients.[145] The overall 5-year survival for patients with a resected IPMN is

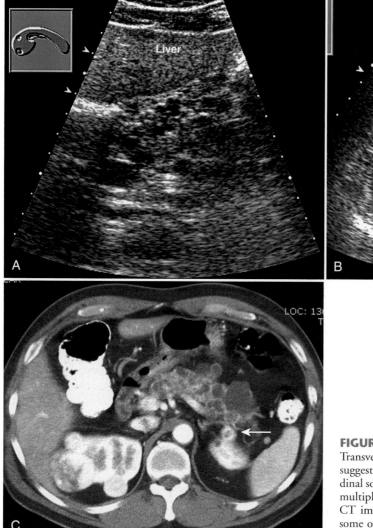

FIGURE 7-75. Multiple pancreatic cysts in VHL. A, Transverse sonogram of pancreas shows multiple pancreatic cysts, suggesting the diagnosis von Hippel–Lindau disease. **B,** Longitudinal sonogram of the right kidney shows associated VHL lesions: multiple renal cell carcinomas *(RCC)* and a large renal cyst. **C,** CT image at a similar level shows myriad pancreatic cysts and some of the right-sided RCCs. A small, left-sided RCC is noted *(arrow).*

TABLE 7-5. PREVALENCE OF CYSTIC PANCREATIC LESIONS

RANK*	NEOPLASM
1	Serous cystic neoplasm (microcystic adenoma)
2	Intraductal papillary mucinous neoplasm (IPMN)
3	Mucinous cystic neoplasm (MCN)
4	Solid-pseudopapillary tumor (SPT)
5	Other cystic tumors

*Subjective estimate based on author's experience.

over 70%.[157] Controversy surrounds the evolving management of these patients. Some believe that asymptomatic patients or those with lesions of branch duct origin can be observed or treated with segmental pancreatectomy.[160]

The hallmark of IPMN on ultrasound is **ductal dilation** (Fig. 7-80; also Figs. 7-78 and 7-79). Findings include lobulated multicystic dilation of the branch ducts, diffuse dilation of the main pancreatic duct, and intraductal papillary tumors.[161] Because mucin has a sonographic appearance that may be similar to debris or sludge **(Video 7-7),** the degree and extent of ductal dilation may be more difficult to appreciate on ultrasound than on CT or T2-weighted MRI. Calcification is rare.

Mucinous Cystic Neoplasm

Mucinous cystic neoplasms (MCNs) arise as de novo cystic tumors, unlike IPMNs, which arise from the pancreatic ducts. MCNs occur most often in the pancreatic body but may occur anywhere in the gland.[160] MCNs may be unilocular and simulate a simple cyst but generally have up to six internal loculations. Internal

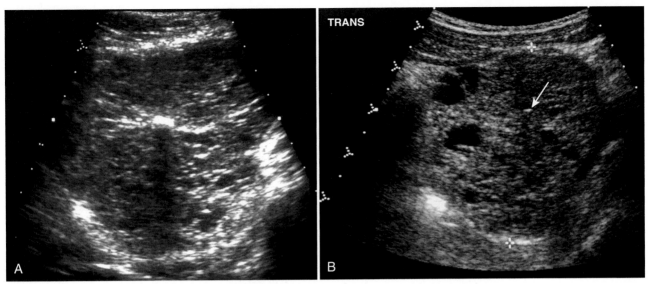

FIGURE 7-76. Serous cystic neoplasm (SCN). A, Oblique sonogram shows classic SCN findings, with many tiny cysts, radial architecture, and a central calcification. No normal pancreas is shown. **B,** Transverse sonogram shows classic SCN findings, including many tiny cysts; a small, central calcification *(arrow)*; and a few larger, more peripheral cysts. No normal pancreas is shown. *(Case courtesy of R. Brooke Jeffrey, MD.)*

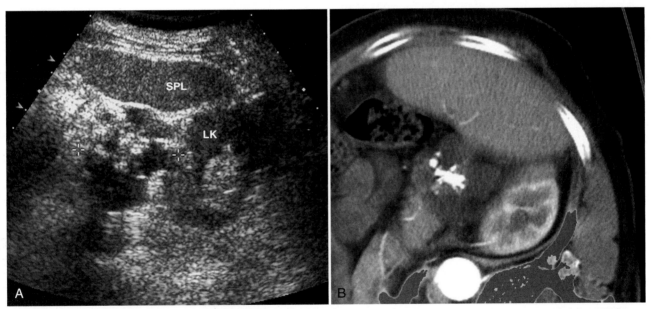

FIGURE 7-77. Serous cystic neoplasm. A, Transverse sonogram shows lesion through the spleen and left kidney. Calcifications and some larger peripheral cysts are noted. *SPL,* Spleen; *LK,* left kidney. **B,** CT image, rotated and cropped to match the ultrasound image, shows the dense calcifications to advantage.

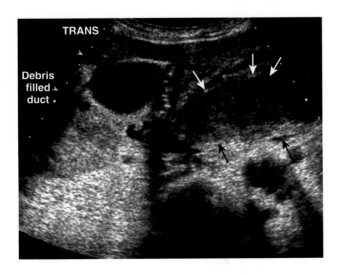

FIGURE 7-78. Intraductal papillary mucinous neoplasm (IPMN). Transverse sonogram shows massively dilated main pancreatic duct *(arrows)* filled with mucin, characteristic of main duct IMPN.

septations may be few or many, quite thin or thick, and papillary; internal debris is common (Fig. 7-81). Calcifications, usually linear and peripheral, occur in about 15% to 20% of lesions. MCN is found in perimenopausal women as thick-walled multilocular cystic masses, usually in the tail of the pancreas[157] **(Video 7-8).**

The MCN is the lesion most likely to be confused with pseudocyst because of their similar appearance in some cases. MCN shares histologic and prognostic similarities with mucinous ovarian cystic tumors. Because of the newer pathologic definition that requires the presence of ovarian stroma in MCN, these tumors are now rarely diagnosed in men.[157,162] Mucinous tumors, previously classified as MCNs in men, would likely now be considered IPMNs. The MCN may be benign, may have "low malignant potential," or may be overtly malignant. Thus, MCNs are generally best managed as malignant lesions.

Solid-Pseudopapillary Tumor

Solid-pseudopapillary tumor (SPT) is the most recent name advocated by the World Health Organization[163] and is found most frequently in young female patients. Previous names include solid and cystic tumor, solid and papillary epithelial neoplasm, papillary-cystic neoplasm, papillary cystic epithelial neoplasm, papillary cystic tumor, and Franz tumor. Franz first described SPT in 1959.[164] About 15% of SPTs are malignant. The likelihood of malignancy increases with patient age.[150] Resection is generally curative.

The SPT occurs most often in the tail of the pancreas. SPTs are usually round, encapsulated masses[165] with variable amounts of necrotic, cystic-appearing areas and soft tissue foci (Fig. 7-82). The cavities in SPTs are not "true" cysts but rather necrotic regions containing blood and debris.[157] Central and rim calcifications have been reported in 29% of patients.[150] Buetow et al.[166] described 31 cases studied with ultrasound, CT, and MRI and noted variable echotexture; anechoic and hypoechoic areas were seen centrally. Through-transmission was seen in all cases in which internal cystic areas were grossly depicted, regardless of the echotexture.

Rare Cystic Tumors

Virtually any imaginable histology has been reported as a "necrotic" or "cystic" lesion of the pancreas.[156,167-169] In general, there is no characteristic ultrasound appearance for these rare tumors.

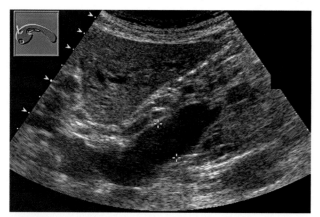

FIGURE 7-79. Intraductal papillary mucinous neoplasm. Longitudinal oblique sonogram shows IPMN causing massive bile duct obstruction. Both benign and malignant IMPTs can cause bile duct obstruction.

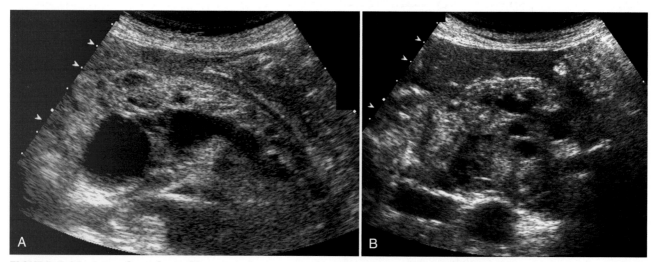

FIGURE 7-80. Intraductal papillary mucinous neoplasm. IPMN with main and branch duct involvement. **A,** Transverse sonogram shows lobulated dilation of the branch ducts and diffuse dilation of the main pancreatic duct. **B,** Transverse sonogram of pancreatic head and proximal body shows dilation of branch ducts in the enlarged head.

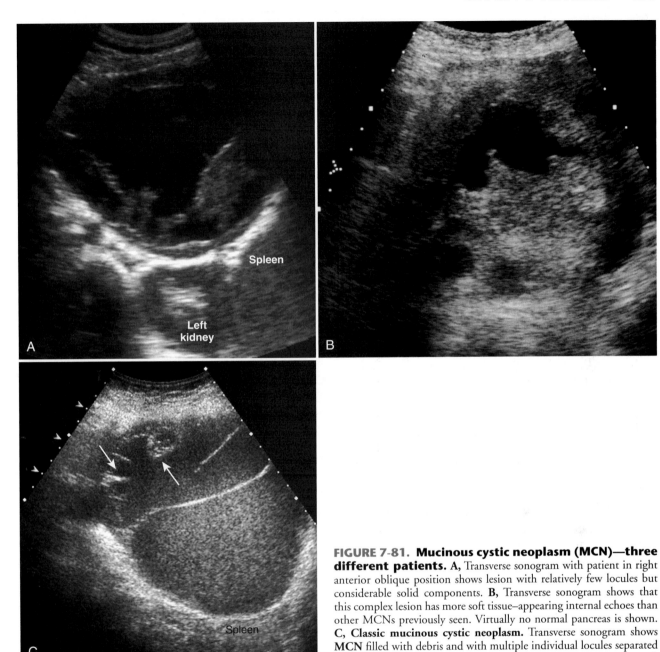

FIGURE 7-81. Mucinous cystic neoplasm (MCN)—three different patients. A, Transverse sonogram with patient in right anterior oblique position shows lesion with relatively few locules but considerable solid components. **B,** Transverse sonogram shows that this complex lesion has more soft tissue–appearing internal echoes than other MCNs previously seen. Virtually no normal pancreas is shown. **C, Classic mucinous cystic neoplasm.** Transverse sonogram shows **MCN** filled with debris and with multiple individual locules separated by thin septations. A few peripheral calcifications are present *(arrows)*.

OTHER PANCREATIC MASSES

Pancreatic Endocrine Tumors

Pancreatic endocrine tumors (PETs) are a small but important group of pancreatic neoplasms, previously called "islet cell tumors" or neuroendocrine tumors. Formerly thought to arise from pancreatic islets, these tumors are now believed to originate from neuroendocrine stem cells in the duct epithelium.[170] PETs are rare, with an annual incidence of approximately 5 cases per million.[171] PETs constitute 1% to 5% of pancreatic neoplasms.[172] The two different presentations depend on whether there is endocrine hyperfunction.[173] **Hyperfunctioning** lesions tend to present clinically when the

RARE CYSTIC TUMORS
Acinar cell cystadenocarcinoma
Cystic choriocarcinoma
Cystic lymphangioma
Cystic teratoma
Cystic pancreatic endocrine tumor
Metastases, other

tumor is small; that is, the endocrine manifestations cause clinical symptoms before the tumor grows enough to cause problems because of its size, invasion, or metastasis. About 90% of PETs are hyperfunctioning. **Nonhyperfunctioning** tumors cause no endocrine-related

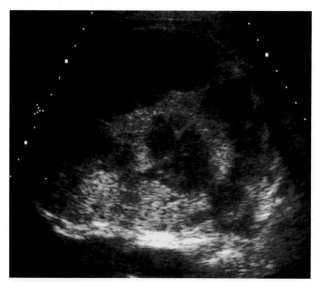

FIGURE 7-82. Large solid-pseudopapillary tumor (SPT). Transverse sonogram shows a large SPT in the pancreatic tail, the most common location for these tumors. SPTs are usually round with variable amounts of necrotic, cystic-appearing areas and soft tissue foci. The cavities in SPTs are not "true" cysts but rather necrotic regions containing blood and debris.

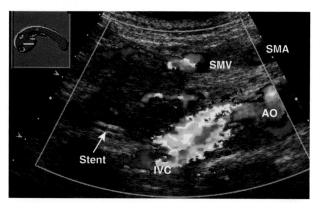

FIGURE 7-83. Pancreatic endocrine tumor (PET), nonhyperfunctioning. Longitudinal oblique color Doppler sonogram shows 5-cm, hypoechoic malignant tumor large enough to cause bile duct obstruction, requiring stenting. Internal color flow is typical with PETs.

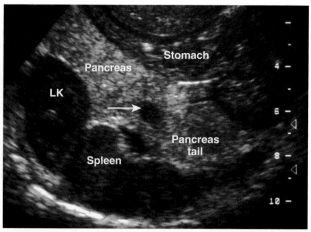

FIGURE 7-84. Small, nonhyperfunctioning PET. Transverse sonogram shows 9-mm hypoechoic nonhyperfunctioning pancreatic endocrine tumor discovered incidentally during an abdominal ultrasound. Distal pancreatectomy was performed.

TABLE 7-6. PANCREATIC ENDOCRINE TUMORS (PETS)

TUMOR TYPE	LOCATED IN PANCREAS	SIZE	All PETs
	Hyperfunctioning		
Insulinoma	90%-100%	2-3 cm	45%
Gastrinoma	40%-60%	1-2 cm	35%
Others			10%
VIPoma	90%		
Glucagonoma	100%		
Somatostatinoma	50%-60%		
Carcinoid PET	100%		
	Nonhyperfunctioning		
All tumors		5+ cm	10%

VIP, Vasoactive intestinal polypeptide.

symptoms. Therefore, these tumors must be larger to present clinically—because of pain,[174] mass effect, or if malignant, invasion and metastasis[114] (Fig. 7-83). Incidental detection of smaller, nonhyperfunctioning tumors is becoming more frequent (Figs. 7-84 and 7-85).

Insulinomas and gastrinomas are the most common hyperfunctioning PETs (about 80% of all PETs); others are rare (Table 7-6). Hyperfunctioning PETs tend to be small and, with the exception of insulinoma, malignant. When a hyperfunctioning PET is suspected, preoperative localization is appropriate. Choice of modality depends on institutional preference and includes trans-abdominal ultrasound, CT, or endoscopic ultrasound.[175] MDCT is superior to sonography in detecting small endocrine tumors,[174] but sometimes ultrasound shows lesions that are occult on CT. It is difficult to image PETs with conventional transabdominal sonography; they are usually small when the patient presents with hormonal abnormalities. Insulinomas and gastrinomas are frequently less than 2 cm in diameter. Sensitivity of detection with ultrasound varies. Detection rates for insulinomas range from 9%[176] to 65%.[175] The sensitivity of ultrasound in the detection of gastrinoma is only 20% to 30%.[177] Sonographically, most **hyperfunctioning** PETs are small (1-3 cm), round or oval, hypoechoic masses with smooth margins. Intraoperative sonography is the most sensitive and accurate means of evaluating these neoplasms (Fig. 7-86). Many consider it mandatory in the surgical treatment of hyperfunctioning PETs.[175]

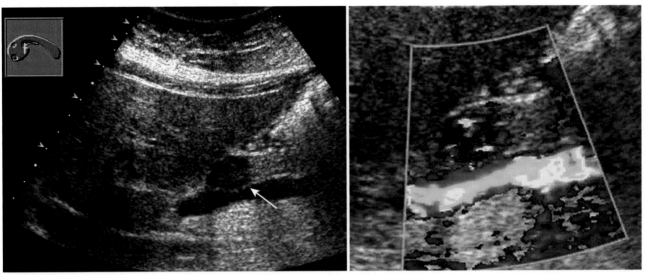

FIGURE 7-85. Small, nonhyperfunctioning PET. Longitudinal sonogram and magnified color Doppler sonogram, show 2-cm pancreatic endocrine tumor indenting the superior mesenteric artery *(arrow)*. PET is hypervascular on color Doppler.

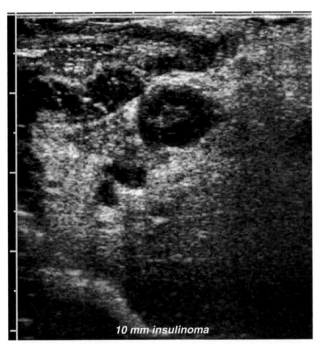

10 mm insulinoma

FIGURE 7-86. Insulinoma on intraoperative ultrasound. This 10-mm lesion was discovered because of hyperinsulinism. Functional pancreatic endocrine tumors are typically found when smaller than nonhyperfunctioning lesions because of the presenting endocrine symptoms. Intraoperative ultrasound is considered mandatory in many institutions for the surgical management of PETs. *(Courtesy Dr. Hisham Tchelepi.)*

Sonographically, the larger, **nonhyperfunctioning** PETs are usually well defined and round or oval (see Figs. 7-83 and 7-85). They generally appear hypoechoic compared to the normal parenchyma. These tumors may have cystic changes and calcification.[177] The larger, nonhyperfunctioning PETs may be difficult to differentiate

from the more common pancreatic ductal adenocarcinoma. Sonographic findings that suggest the diagnosis are (1) prominent internal color flow (rare in carcinoma) **(Video 7-9)**, (2) lack of biliary or pancreatic ductal dilation in a pancreatic head lesion, and (3) lack of progression or metastasis on serial imaging.[115]

Unusual and Rare Pancreatic Neoplasms

On ultrasound, many histologic variants of pancreatic ductal adenocarcinoma are indistinguishable from tumors with the usual histologic features. These include adenosquamous cell carcinoma, anaplastic carcinoma, and pleomorphic giant cell carcinoma. Acinar center cell carcinoma and pleomorphic giant cell carcinoma, although often indistinguishable from ductal adenocarcinoma, may be larger and may exhibit central necrosis. Primary pancreatic lymphoma is prohibitively rare, although adenopathy or diffuse involvement from more generalized disease occurs with some frequency.[115] Other rare pancreatic tumors include connective tissue origin tumors (sarcomas), pancreaticoblastomas, dysontogenetic cysts, and metastases.[178,179]

Lipoma

In contrast to the usual echogenic appearance of fat and fatty lesions, pancreatic lipomas are usually **hypoechoic**[180,181] (Fig. 7-87). Other lipomas may have a mixed appearance, with a variable amount of internal echoes, or may appear hyperechoic. The cause of hypoechoic fat is not known but may involve the number of blood vessels, amount and thickness of connective tissue stroma, number of fibrous septae that separate fat lobules, and amount of water content in the fat.[180,182]

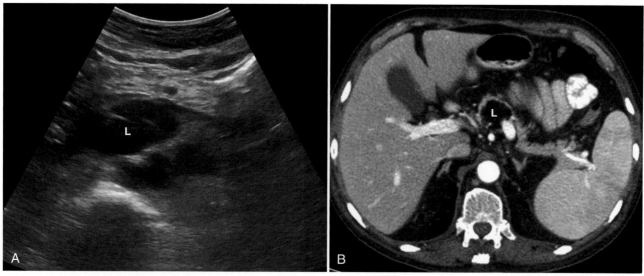

FIGURE 7-87. Pancreatic lipoma. A, Transverse sonogram of almost anechoic pancreatic lipoma *(L).* In contrast to the usual echogenic appearance of fat and fatty lesions, pancreatic lipomas are usually hypoechoic. **B,** CT image confirms the fatty nature of the lesion. *(Case courtesy Dr. Vinay Duddlewar.)*

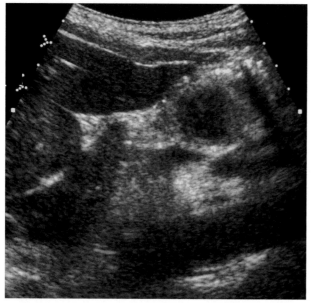

FIGURE 7-88. Lung carcinoma metastasis to pancreas. Longitudinal sonogram shows typical hypoechoic metastasis. Pancreatic metastases are the most common pancreatic neoplasm in autopsy series but are rarely found clinically because they generally occur late with widespread metastatic disease.

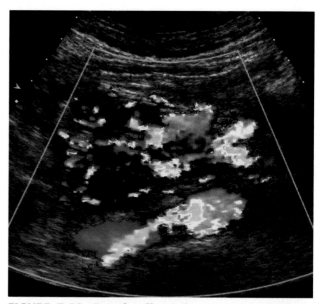

FIGURE 7-89. Renal cell carcinoma metastasis to pancreas. Longitudinal color Doppler sonogram shows hypervascular metastasis. Differentiation from a hypervascular pancreatic endocrine tumor may be difficult in these cases.

Metastatic Tumors

In autopsy series, metastasis is the most common pancreatic neoplasm, found about four times as often as pancreatic cancer.[179] Clinical discovery of metastasis was rare until the advent of modern imaging.[183] Pancreatic metastases are rarely clinically significant because they generally occur late in patients with widespread metastatic disease. Primary tumors that most often metastasize to the pancreas include **renal cell carcinoma** (RCC), **breast carcinoma, lung carcinoma** (Fig. 7-88), **melanoma, colon carcinoma,** and **stomach carcinoma.**[115,179,183]

With metastasis to the pancreas, there may be a long interval between initial diagnosis of the primary lesion and discovery of the metastasis. This is especially true of RCC and, to a lesser degree, melanoma. Klein et al.[183] found that the mean delay between discovery of the primary RCC and metastasis was 10 years; the longest interval was more than 24 years. A classic scenario is the discovery of a hypervascular mass (or masses) in the pancreas of a patient who had a remote, presumably cured RCC (Fig. 7-89). Differential diagnosis from a hypervascular PET may be difficult in such cases.

CONTRAST-ENHANCED ULTRASOUND

Contrast-enhanced ultrasound (CEUS) shows promise as a technique that will be beneficial in both endoscopic ultrasound and transabdominal ultrasound of the pancreas. At present, CEUS is best considered an experimental technique.[94,184] CEUS might be helpful in diagnosing pancreatic necrosis in patients with severe acute pancreatitis.[143]

References

1. Kalra MK, Maher MM, Sahani DV, et al. Current status of imaging in pancreatic diseases. J Comput Assist Tomogr 2002;26:661-675.
2. Wray CJ, Ahmad SA, Matthews JB, Lowy AM. Surgery for pancreatic cancer: recent controversies and current practice. Gastroenterology 2005;128:1626-1641.
3. Merkle EM, Gorich J. Imaging of acute pancreatitis. Eur Radiol 2002;12:1979-1992.

Anatomy and Sonographic Technique
4. Mori H, McGrath FP, Malone DE, Stevenson GW. The gastrocolic trunk and its tributaries: CT evaluation. Radiology 1992;182:871-877.
5. Glaser J, Stienecker K. Pancreas and aging: a study using ultrasonography. Gerontology 2000;46:93-96.
6. Guerra M, Gutierrez L, Carrasco R, Arroyo A. [Size and echogenicity of the pancreas in Chilean adults: echo tomography study in 261 patients]. Rev Med Chil 1995;123:720-726.
7. Bolondi L, Li Bassi S, Gaiani S, Barbara L. Sonography of chronic pancreatitis. Radiol Clin North Am 1989;27:815-833.
8. Mortele KJ, Rocha TC, Streeter JL, Taylor AJ. Multimodality imaging of pancreatic and biliary congenital anomalies. Radiographics 2006;26:715-731.
9. Daneman A, Gaskin K, Martin DJ, Cutz E. Pancreatic changes in cystic fibrosis: CT and sonographic appearances. AJR Am J Roentgenol 1983;141:653-655.
10. So CB, Cooperberg PL, Gibney RG, Bogoch A. Sonographic findings in pancreatic lipomatosis. AJR Am J Roentgenol 1987;149:67-68.
11. Coccia P, Ruggerio A, Attina G, et al. Shwachman-Diamond syndrome: an emergency challenge. Signa Vitae 2007;2:10-13.
12. Marchal G, Verbeken E, Van Steenbergen W, et al. Uneven lipomatosis: a pitfall in pancreatic sonography. Gastrointest Radiol 1989;14:233-237.
13. Donald JJ, Shorvon PJ, Lees WR. A hypoechoic area within the head of the pancreas: a normal variant. Clin Radiol 1990;41:337-338.
14. Atri M, Nazarnia S, Mehio A, et al. Hypoechogenic embryologic ventral aspect of the head and uncinate process of the pancreas: in vitro correlation of ultrasound with histopathologic findings. Radiology 1994;190:441-444.
15. Coulier B. [Hypoechogenic aspects of the ventral embryonic cephalic pancreas: a large prospective clinical study]. J Belge Radiol 1996;79:120-124.
16. Yu J, Turner MA, Fulcher AS, Halvorsen RA. Congenital anomalies and normal variants of the pancreaticobiliary tract and the pancreas in adults. Part 2. Pancreatic duct and pancreas. AJR Am J Roentgenol 2006;187:1544-1553.
17. Misra SP, Dwivedi M. Pancreaticobiliary ductal union. Gut 1990;31:1144-1149.
18. Dawson W, Langman J. An anatomical-radiological study on the pancreatic duct pattern in man. Anat Rec 1961;139:59-68.
19. Hadidi A. Pancreatic duct diameter: sonographic measurement in normal subjects. J Clin Ultrasound 1983;11:17-22.
20. Wachsberg RH. Respiratory variation of the diameter of the pancreatic duct on sonography. AJR Am J Roentgenol 2000;175:1459-1461.
21. Glaser J, Hogemann B, Krummenerl T, et al. Sonographic imaging of the pancreatic duct. New diagnostic possibilities using secretin stimulation. Dig Dis Sci 1987;32:1075-1081.
22. Petrone MC, Arcidiacono PG, Testoni PA. Endoscopic ultrasonography for evaluating patients with recurrent pancreatitis. World J Gastroenterol 2008;14:1016-1022.
23. Delhay M, Matos C, Deviere J. Acute relapsing pancreatitis: congenital variants—diagnosis, treatment, outcome. JOP 2001;2:373-381.
24. Klein SD, Affronti JP. Pancreas divisum: an evidence-based review. Part I. Pathophysiology. Gastrointest Endosc 2004;60:419-425.

Acute Pancreatitis
25. Bollen TL, van Santvoort HC, Besselink MG, et al. The Atlanta Classification of acute pancreatitis revisited. Br J Surg 2008;95:6-21.
26. Vege SS, Yadav D, Chari ST. Pancreatitis. In: Talley NJ, Locke GR, Saito YA, editors. Gastrointestinal epidemiology. Malden, Mass: Blackwell; 2007.
27. Tenner S, Sica G, Hughes M, et al. Relationship of necrosis to organ failure in severe acute pancreatitis. Gastroenterology 1997;113:899-903.
28. Swaroop VS, Chari ST, Clain JE. Severe acute pancreatitis. JAMA 2004;291:2865-2868.
29. Banks PA, Freeman ML. Practice guidelines in acute pancreatitis. Am J Gastroenterol 2006;101:2379-2400.
30. Bradley 3rd EL. A clinically based classification system for acute pancreatitis. Summary of the International Symposium on Acute Pancreatitis, Atlanta, 1992. Arch Surg 1993;128:586-590.
31. Topazian M, Gorelick FS. Acute pancreatitis. In: Yamada T, Alpers DH, Kaplowitz N, et al, editors. Textbook of gastroenterology. Philadelphia: Lippincott–Williams & Wilkins; 2003. p. 2026.
32. Finstad TA, Tchelepi H, Ralls PW. Sonography of acute pancreatitis: prevalence of findings and pictorial essay. Ultrasound Q 2005;21:95-104; quiz 150, 153-154.
33. Riela A, Zinsmeister AR, Melton LJ, DiMagno EP. Etiology, incidence and survival of acute pancreatitis in Olmsted County, Minnesota. Gastroenterology 1991;100:A296.
34. Everhart JE, Khare M, Hill M, Maurer KR. Prevalence and ethnic differences in gallbladder disease in the United States. Gastroenterology 1999;117:632-639.
35. Sampliner RE, Bennett PH, Comess LJ, et al. Gallbladder disease in Pima Indians: demonstration of high prevalence and early onset by cholecystography. N Engl J Med 1970;283:1358-1364.
36. Collins C, Maguire D, Ireland A, et al. A prospective study of common bile duct calculi in patients undergoing laparoscopic cholecystectomy: natural history of choledocholithiasis revisited. Ann Surg 2004;239:28-33.
37. Dong B, Chen M. Improved sonographic visualization of choledocholithiasis. J Clin Ultrasound 1987;15:185-190.
38. Kelly TR, Wagner DS. Gallstone pancreatitis: a prospective randomized trial of the timing of surgery. Surgery 1988;104:600-605.
39. Neoptolemos JP, Carr-Locke DL, London NJ, et al. Controlled trial of urgent endoscopic retrograde cholangiopancreatography and endoscopic sphincterotomy versus conservative treatment for acute pancreatitis due to gallstones. Lancet 1988;2:979-983.
40. Fan ST, Lai EC, Mok FP, et al. Early treatment of acute biliary pancreatitis by endoscopic papillotomy. N Engl J Med 1993;328:228-232.
41. Nowak A, Nowakowska-Dulawa E, Marek TA, et al. Final results of the prospective, randomized controlled study on endoscopic sphincterotomy versus conventional management in acute biliary pancreatitis. Gastroenterology 1995;108:380.
42. Folsch UR, Nitsche R, Ludtke R, et al. Early ERCP and papillotomy compared with conservative treatment for acute biliary pancreatitis. German Study Group on Acute Biliary Pancreatitis. N Engl J Med 1997;336:237-242.
43. Acosta JM, Katkhouda N, Debian KA, et al. Early ductal decompression versus conservative management for gallstone pancreatitis with ampullary obstruction: a prospective randomized clinical trial. Ann Surg 2006;243:33-40.
44. Lee SP, Nicholls JF, Park HZ. Biliary sludge as a cause of acute pancreatitis. N Engl J Med 1992;326:589-593.
45. Kinney TP, Freeman ML. Approach to acute, recurrent, and chronic pancreatitis. Minn Med 2008;91:29-33.

46. Lin A, Feller ER. Pancreatic carcinoma as a cause of unexplained pancreatitis: report of ten cases. Ann Intern Med 1990;113:166-170.

47. Levy MJ, Geenen JE. Idiopathic acute recurrent pancreatitis. Am J Gastroenterol 2001;96:2540-2555.

48. Johnson CD, Stephens DH, Sarr MG. CT of acute pancreatitis: correlation between lack of contrast enhancement and pancreatic necrosis. AJR Am J Roentgenol 1991;156:93-95.

49. Pederzoli P, Bassi C, Vesentini S, Campedelli A. A randomized multicenter clinical trial of antibiotic prophylaxis of septic complications in acute necrotizing pancreatitis with imipenem. Surg Gynecol Obstet 1993;176:480-483.

50. Banks PA. Acute pancreatitis: medical and surgical management. Am J Gastroenterol 1994;89:S78-S85.

51. Dambrauskas Z, Gulbinas A, Pundzius J, Barauskas G. Meta-analysis of prophylactic parenteral antibiotic use in acute necrotizing pancreatitis. Medicina (Kaunas) 2007;43:291-300.

52. Sharma VK, Howden CW. Prophylactic antibiotic administration reduces sepsis and mortality in acute necrotizing pancreatitis: a meta-analysis. Pancreas 2001;22:28-31.

53. Miller FH, Keppke AL, Dalal K, et al. MRI of pancreatitis and its complications. Part 1. Acute pancreatitis. AJR Am J Roentgenol 2004;183:1637-1644.

54. Arvanitakis M, Delhaye M, De Maertelaere V, et al. Computed tomography and magnetic resonance imaging in the assessment of acute pancreatitis. Gastroenterology 2004;126:715-723.

55. Chak A, Hawes RH, Cooper GS, et al. Prospective assessment of the utility of EUS in the evaluation of gallstone pancreatitis. Gastrointest Endosc 1999;49:599-604.

56. Kimmey MB, Vilmann P. Endoscopic ultrasonography. In: Yamada T, Alpers DH, Kaplowitz N, et al, editors. Textbook of gastroenterology. 4th ed. Philadelphia: Lippincott–Williams & Wilkins; 2003.

57. Baillie J. Endoscopic therapy in acute recurrent pancreatitis. World J Gastroenterol 2008;14:1034-1037.

58. National Institutes of Health. Endoscopic retrograde cholangiopancreatography (ERCP) for diagnosis and therapy. NIH Consens State Sci Statements 2002;19:1-26.

59. Nam JH, Murthy S. Acute pancreatitis: the current status in management. Expert Opin Pharmacother 2003;4:235-241.

60. Clavien PA, Robert J, Meyer P, et al. Acute pancreatitis and normoamylasemia: not an uncommon combination. Ann Surg 1989; 210:614-620.

61. Lankisch PG, Schirren CA, Kunze E. Undetected fatal acute pancreatitis: why is the disease so frequently overlooked? Am J Gastroenterol 1991;86:322-336.

62. Cotton PB, Lees WR, Vallon AG, et al. Gray-scale ultrasonography and endoscopic pancreatography in pancreatic diagnosis. Radiology 1980;134:453-459.

63. Martinez-Noguera A, D'Onofrio M. Ultrasonography of the pancreas. 1. Conventional imaging. Abdom Imaging 2007;32:136-149.

64. Kourtesis G, Wilson SE, Williams RA. The clinical significance of fluid collections in acute pancreatitis. Am Surg 1990;56:796-799.

65. Lenhart DK, Balthazar EJ. MDCT of acute mild (nonnecrotizing) pancreatitis: abdominal complications and fate of fluid collections. AJR Am J Roentgenol 2008;190:643-649.

66. Andrén-Sandberg A, Ansorge C, Eiriksson K, et al. Treatment of pancreatic pseudocysts. Scand J Surg 2005;94:165-175.

67. Garcea G, Ong SL, Rajesh A, et al. Cystic lesions of the pancreas: a diagnostic and management dilemma. Pancreatology 2008;8:236-251.

68. Gasslander T, Arnelo U, Albiin N, Permert J. Cystic tumors of the pancreas. Dig Dis 2001;19:57-62.

69. Aghdassi A, Mayerle J, Kraft M, et al. Diagnosis and treatment of pancreatic pseudocysts in chronic pancreatitis. Pancreas 2008;36: 105-112.

70. Singhal D, Kakodkar R, Sud R, Chaudhary A. Issues in management of pancreatic pseudocysts. JOP 2006;7:502-507.

71. Kim YH, Saini S, Sahani D, et al. Imaging diagnosis of cystic pancreatic lesions: pseudocyst versus nonpseudocyst. Radiographics 2005;25:671-685.

72. Visser BC, Yeh BM, Qayyum A, et al. Characterization of cystic pancreatic masses: relative accuracy of CT and MRI. AJR Am J Roentgenol 2007;189:648-656.

73. Yeo CJ, Bastidas JA, Lynch-Nyhan A, et al. The natural history of pancreatic pseudocysts documented by computed tomography. Surg Gynecol Obstet 1990;170:411-417.

74. Cheruvu CV, Clarke MG, Prentice M, Eyre-Brook IA. Conservative treatment as an option in the management of pancreatic pseudocyst. Ann R Coll Surg 2003;85:313-316.

75. Bergman S, Melvin WS. Operative and nonoperative management of pancreatic pseudocysts. Surg Clin North Am 2007;87:1447-1460, ix.

76. Gupta R, Munoz JC, Garg P, et al. Mediastinal pancreatic pseudocyst: a case report and review of the literature. MedGenMed 2007;9:8.

77. Wechalekar M, Falodia S, Gamanagatti S, Makharia GK. An extension of pancreatic pseudocysts in the neck. Pancreas 2007;34:171-173.

78. Erzurum VZ, Obermeyer R, Chung D. Pancreatic pseudocyst masquerading as an incarcerated inguinal hernia. South Med J 2000; 93:221-222.

79. Lang EK, Paolini RM, Pottmeyer A. The efficacy of palliative and definitive percutaneous versus surgical drainage of pancreatic abscesses and pseudocysts: a prospective study of 85 patients. South Med J 1991;84:55-64.

80. Nealon WH, Walser E. Main pancreatic ductal anatomy can direct choice of modality for treating pancreatic pseudocysts (surgery versus percutaneous drainage). Ann Surg 2002;235:751-758.

81. Bhattacharya D, Ammori BJ. Minimally invasive approaches to the management of pancreatic pseudocysts: review of the literature. Surg Laparosc Endosc Percutan Tech 2003;13:141-148.

82. Baril NB, Ralls PW, Wren SM, et al. Does an infected peripancreatic fluid collection or abscess mandate operation? Ann Surg 2000; 231:361-367.

83. Flati G, Salvatori F, Porowska B, et al. Severe hemorrhagic complications in pancreatitis. Ann Ital Chir 1995;66:233-237.

84. Risti B, Marincek B, Jost R, et al. Hemosuccus pancreaticus as a source of obscure upper gastrointestinal bleeding: three cases and literature review. Am J Gastroenterol 1995;90:1878-1880.

85. Agarwal AK, Raj Kumar K, Agarwal S, Singh S. Significance of splenic vein thrombosis in chronic pancreatitis. Am J Surg 2008;196: 149-154.

86. Bernades P, Baetz A, Levy P, et al. Splenic and portal venous obstruction in chronic pancreatitis: a prospective longitudinal study of a medical-surgical series of 266 patients. Dig Dis Sci 1992;37:340-346.

Chronic Pancreatitis

87. Witt H, Apte MV, Keim V, Wilson JS. Chronic pancreatitis: challenges and advances in pathogenesis, genetics, diagnosis, and therapy. Gastroenterology 2007;132:1557-1573.

88. Behrman SW, Fowler ES. Pathophysiology of chronic pancreatitis. Surg Clin North Am 2007;87:1309-1324, vii.

89. Etemad B, Whitcomb DC. Chronic pancreatitis: diagnosis, classification, and new genetic developments. Gastroenterology 2001;120:682-707.

90. Ralls PW, Halls J, Renner I, Juttner H. Endoscopic retrograde cholangiopancreatography (ERCP) in pancreatic disease: a reassessment of the specificity of ductal abnormalities indifferentiating benign from malignant disease. Radiology 1980;134:347-352.

91. Vijungco JD, Prinz RA. Management of biliary and duodenal complications of chronic pancreatitis. World J Surg 2003;27:1258-1270.

92. Kim DH, Pickhardt PJ. Radiologic assessment of acute and chronic pancreatitis. Surg Clin North Am 2007;87:1341-1358, viii.

93. Del Frate C, Zanardi R, Mortele K, Ros PR. Advances in imaging for pancreatic disease. Curr Gastroenterol Rep 2002;4:140-148.

94. Kinney TP, Freeman ML. Recent advances and novel methods in pancreatic imaging. Minerva Gastroenterol Dietol 2008;54:85-95.

95. Rizk MK, Gerke H. Utility of endoscopic ultrasound in pancreatitis: a review. World J Gastroenterol 2007;13:6321-6326.

96. Tchelepi H, Ralls PW. Color comet-tail artifact: clinical applications. AJR Am J Roentgenol 2009;192:11-18.

97. Sakorafas GH, Tsiotou AG. Splenic vein thrombosis complicating chronic pancreatitis. Scand J Gastroenterol 1999;34:1171-1177.

98. Rosch W, Lux G, Riemann JF, Hoh L. [Chronic pancreatitis and the neighboring organs]. Fortschr Med 1981;99:1118-1121.

99. Miller FH, Keppke AL, Wadhwa A, et al. MRI of pancreatitis and its complications. Part 2. Chronic pancreatitis. AJR Am J Roentgenol 2004;183:1645-1652.

100. Chawla Y, Dilawari JB, Katariya S. Gallbladder varices in portal vein thrombosis. AJR Am J Roentgenol 1994;162:643-645.

101. Ralls PW, Mayekawa DS, Lee KP, et al. Gallbladder wall varices: diagnosis with color flow Doppler sonography. J Clin Ultrasound 1988;16:595-598.

102. Rosen IE, Wilson SR. Varices of the gallbladder. J Can Assoc Radiol 1980;31:73-74.

103. DelMaschio A, Vanzulli A, Sironi S, et al. Pancreatic cancer versus chronic pancreatitis: diagnosis with CA 19-9 assessment, US, CT, and CT-guided fine-needle biopsy. Radiology 1991;178:95-99.

104. Yadav D, Notahara K, Smyrk TC, et al. Idiopathic tumefactive chronic pancreatitis: clinical profile, histology, and natural history after resection. Clin Gastroenterol Hepatol 2003;1:129-135.

105. Abraham SC, Wilentz RE, Yeo CJ, et al. Pancreaticoduodenectomy (Whipple resections) in patients without malignancy: are they all "chronic pancreatitis"? Am J Surg Pathol 2003;27:110-120.

106. Yassa NA, Yang J, Stein S, et al. Gray-scale and color flow sonography of pancreatic ductal adenocarcinoma. J Clin Ultrasound 1997;25:473-480.

107. Shawker TH, Garra BS, Hill MC, et al. The spectrum of sonographic findings in pancreatic carcinoma. J Ultrasound Med 1986;5:169-177.

108. Kimura W, Sata N, Nakayama H, et al. Pancreatic carcinoma accompanied by pseudocyst: report of two cases. J Gastroenterol 1994;29:786-791.

109. Weber SM, Cubukcu-Dimopulo O, Palesty JA, et al. Lymphoplasmacytic sclerosing pancreatitis: inflammatory mimic of pancreatic carcinoma. J Gastrointest Surg 2003;7:129-137; discussion 137-139.

110. Zandieh I, Byrne MF. Autoimmune pancreatitis: a review. World J Gastroenterol 2007;13:6327-6332.

111. Toomey DP, Swan N, Torreggiani W, Conlon KC. Autoimmune pancreatitis. Br J Surg 2007;94:1067-1074.

112. Lowenfels AB, Maisonneuve P, Cavallini G, et al. Pancreatitis and the risk of pancreatic cancer. International Pancreatitis Study Group. N Engl J Med 1993;328:1433-1437.

113. Lowenfels AB, Maisonneuve P. Risk factors for pancreatic cancer. J Cell Biochem 2005;95:649-656.

Pancreatic Neoplasms

114. Ross WA, Bismar MM. Evaluation and management of periampullary tumors. Curr Gastroenterol Rep 2004;6:362-370.

115. Faria SC, Tamm EP, Loyer EM, et al. Diagnosis and staging of pancreatic tumors. Semin Roentgenol 2004;39:397-411.

116. Elsayes KM, Narra VR, Abou El Abbass HA, et al. Pancreatic tumors: diagnostic patterns by 3D gradient-echo post contrast magnetic resonance imaging with pathologic correlation. Curr Probl Diagn Radiol 2006;35:125-139.

117. American Cancer Society. Cancer facts & figures. Atlanta: ACS; 2008.

118. Canto MI, Goggins M, Hruban RH, et al. Screening for early pancreatic neoplasia in high-risk individuals: a prospective controlled study. Clin Gastroenterol Hepatol 2006;4:766-781; quiz 665.

119. Klein AP, Hruban RH, Brune KA, et al. Familial pancreatic cancer. Cancer J 2001;7:266-273.

120. Wilkowski R, Thoma M, Bruns C, et al. Chemoradiotherapy with gemcitabine and continuous 5-FU in patients with primary inoperable pancreatic cancer. JOP 2006;7:349-360.

121. Conlon KC, Klimstra DS, Brennan MF. Long-term survival after curative resection for pancreatic ductal adenocarcinoma: clinicopathologic analysis of 5-year survivors. Ann Surg 1996;223:273-279.

122. Klek S, Kulig J, Popiela T, et al. The value of modern ultrasonographic techniques and computed tomography in detecting and staging pancreatic carcinoma. Acta Chir Belg 2004;104:659-667.

123. Gudjonsson B. Carcinoma of the pancreas: critical analysis of costs, results of resections, and the need for standardized reporting. J Am Coll Surg 1995;181:483-503.

124. Gudjonsson B. Survival statistics gone awry: pancreatic cancer, a case in point. J Clin Gastroenterol 2002;35:180-184.

125. Wade TP, el-Ghazzawy AG, Virgo KS, Johnson FE. The Whipple resection for cancer in US Department of Veterans Affairs hospitals. Ann Surg 1995;221:241-248.

126. Farnell MB, Nagorney DM, Sarr MG. The Mayo Clinic approach to the surgical treatment of adenocarcinoma of the pancreas. Surg Clin North Am 2001;81:611-623.

127. Tamm EP, Bhosale PR, Lee JH. Pancreatic ductal adenocarcinoma: ultrasound, computed tomography, and magnetic resonance imaging features. Semin Ultrasound CT MR 2007;28:330-338.

128. Karlson BM, Ekbom A, Lindgren PG, et al. Abdominal US for diagnosis of pancreatic tumor: prospective cohort analysis. Radiology 1999;213:107-111.

129. Campbell JP, Wilson SR. Pancreatic neoplasms: how useful is evaluation with US? Radiology 1988;167:341-344.

130. Freeny PC. Radiologic diagnosis and staging of pancreatic ductal adenocarcinoma. Radiol Clin North Am 1989;27:121-128.

131. Kosmahl M, Pauser U, Anlauf M, Kloppel G. Pancreatic ductal adenocarcinomas with cystic features: neither rare nor uniform. Mod Pathol 2005;18:1157-1164.

132. Pappas S, Federle MP, Lokshin AE, Zeh 3rd HJ. Early detection and staging of adenocarcinoma of the pancreas. Gastroenterol Clin North Am 2007;36:413-429, x.

133. Gress FG, Hawes RH, Savides TJ, et al. Role of EUS in the preoperative staging of pancreatic cancer: a large single-center experience. Gastrointest Endosc 1999;50:786-791.

134. Boujaoude J. Role of endoscopic ultrasound in diagnosis and therapy of pancreatic adenocarcinoma. World J Gastroenterol 2007;13:3662-3666.

135. Kalra MK, Maher MM, Mueller PR, Saini S. State-of-the-art imaging of pancreatic neoplasms. Br J Radiol 2003;76:857-865.

136. Nino-Murcia M, Tamm EP, Charnsangavej C, Jeffrey Jr RB. Multidetector-row helical CT and advanced postprocessing techniques for the evaluation of pancreatic neoplasms. Abdom Imaging 2003;28:366-377.

137. Vargas R, Nino-Murcia M, Trueblood W, Jeffrey Jr RB. MDCT in pancreatic adenocarcinoma: prediction of vascular invasion and resectability using a multiphasic technique with curved planar reformations. AJR Am J Roentgenol 2004;182:419-425.

138. Angeli E, Venturini M, Vanzulli A, et al. Color Doppler imaging in the assessment of vascular involvement by pancreatic carcinoma. AJR Am J Roentgenol 1997;168:193-197.

139. Ralls PW, Wren SM, Radin R, et al. Color flow sonography in evaluating the resectability of periampullary and pancreatic tumors. J Ultrasound Med 1997;16:131-140.

140. Tomiyama T, Ueno N, Tano S, et al. Assessment of arterial invasion in pancreatic cancer using color Doppler ultrasonography. Am J Gastroenterol 1996;91:1410-1416.

141. Wren SM, Ralls PW, Stain SC, et al. Assessment of resectability of pancreatic head and periampullary tumors by color flow Doppler sonography. Arch Surg 1996;131:812-817; discussion 817-818.

142. Ishida H, Konno K, Hamashima Y, et al. Assessment of resectability of pancreatic carcinoma by color Doppler sonography. Abdom Imaging 1999;24:295-298.

143. Rickes S, Malfertheiner P. Echo-enhanced sonography: an increasingly used procedure for the differentiation of pancreatic tumors. Dig Dis 2004;22:32-38.

Cystic Pancreatic Lesions

144. Fernandez-del Castillo C, Targarona J, Thayer SP, et al. Incidental pancreatic cysts: clinicopathologic characteristics and comparison with symptomatic patients. Arch Surg 2003;138:427-423; discussion 433-434.

145. Edirimanne S, Connor SJ. Incidental pancreatic cystic lesions. World J Surg 2008;32:2028-2037.

146. Sahani DV, Saokar A, Hahn PF, et al. Pancreatic cysts 3 cm or smaller: how aggressive should treatment be? Radiology 2006;238:912-919.

147. Spinelli KS, Fromwiller TE, Daniel RA, et al. Cystic pancreatic neoplasms: observe or operate. Ann Surg 2004;239:651-657; discussion 657-659.

148. Maker AV, Lee LS, Raut CP, et al. Cytology from pancreatic cysts has marginal utility in surgical decision making. Ann Surg Oncol 2008;15:3187-3192.

149. Belsley NA, Pitman MB, Lauwers GY, et al. Serous cystadenoma of the pancreas: limitations and pitfalls of endoscopic ultrasound-guided fine-needle aspiration biopsy. Cancer 2008;114:102-110.

150. Megibow AJ. Update in imaging of cystic pancreatic masses for gastroenterologists. Clin Gastroenterol Hepatol 2008;6:1194-1197.

151. Ikeda M, Sato T, Morozumi A, et al. Morphologic changes in the pancreas detected by screening ultrasonography in a mass survey, with special reference to main duct dilatation, cyst formation, and calcification. Pancreas 1994;9:508-512.

152. Zhang XM, Mitchell DG, Dohke M, et al. Pancreatic cysts: depiction on single-shot fast spin-echo MR images. Radiology 2002; 223:547-553.
153. Kimura W, Nagai H, Kuroda A, Muto T, Esaki Y. Analysis of small cystic lesions of the pancreas. Int J Pancreatol 1995;18:197-206.
154. Chang MY, Ong AC. Autosomal dominant polycystic kidney disease: recent advances in pathogenesis and treatment. Nephron Physiol 2008;108:1-7.
155. Leung RS, Biswas SV, Duncan M, Rankin S. Imaging features of von Hippel–Lindau disease. Radiographics 2008;28:65-79; quiz 323.
156. Cahill ME, Parmentier JM, Van Ruyssevelt C, Pauls CH. Pancreatic cystosis in cystic fibrosis. Abdom Imaging 1997;22:313-314.
157. Adsay NV. Cystic neoplasia of the pancreas: pathology and biology. J Gastrointest Surg 2008;12:401-404.
158. Ohashi KM, Maruyama Y. Four cases of mucin-producing cancer of the pancreas: specific findings in the ampulla of Vater [Japanese]. Prog Dig Endosc 1982;20:348-351.
159. Zamora C, Sahel J, Cantu DG, et al. Intraductal papillary or mucinous tumors (IPMT) of the pancreas: report of a case series and review of the literature. Am J Gastroenterol 2001;96:1441-1447.
160. Sarr MG, Kendrick ML, Nagorney DM, et al. Cystic neoplasms of the pancreas: benign to malignant epithelial neoplasms. Surg Clin North Am 2001;81:497-509.
161. Lim JH, Lee G, Oh YL. Radiologic spectrum of intraductal papillary mucinous tumor of the pancreas. Radiographics 2001;21:323-337; discussion 337-340.
162. Suzuki M, Fujita N, Onodera H, et al. Mucinous cystic neoplasm in a young male patient. J Gastroenterol 2005;40:1070-1074.
163. Klimstra DS, Wenig BM, Heffess CS. Solid-pseudopapillary tumor of the pancreas: a typically cystic carcinoma of low malignant potential. Semin Diagn Pathol 2000;17:66-80.
164. Choi JY, Kim MJ, Kim JH, et al. Solid pseudopapillary tumor of the pancreas: typical and atypical manifestations. AJR Am J Roentgenol 2006;187:W178-W186.
165. Sidden CR, Mortele KJ. Cystic tumors of the pancreas: ultrasound, computed tomography, and magnetic resonance imaging features. Semin Ultrasound CT MR 2007;28:339-356.
166. Buetow PC, Buck JL, Pantongrag-Brown L, et al. Solid and papillary epithelial neoplasm of the pancreas: imaging-pathologic correlation on 56 cases. Radiology 1996;199:707-711.
167. Tucci G, Muzi MG, Nigro C, et al. Dermoid cyst of the pancreas: presentation and management. World J Surg Oncol 2007;5:85.
168. Demos TC, Posniak HV, Harmath C, et al. Cystic lesions of the pancreas. AJR Am J Roentgenol 2002;179:1375-1388.
169. Koenig TR, Loyer EM, Whitman GJ, et al. Cystic lymphangioma of the pancreas. AJR Am J Roentgenol 2001;177:1090.

Other Pancreatic Masses

170. Kloppel G, Heitz PU. Pancreatic endocrine tumors. Pathol Res Pract 1988;183:155-168.
171. Phan GQ, Yeo CJ, Hruban RH, et al. Surgical experience with pancreatic and peripancreatic neuroendocrine tumors: review of 125 patients. J Gastrointest Surg 1998;2:472-482.
172. Shah S, Mortele KJ. Uncommon solid pancreatic neoplasms: ultrasound, computed tomography, and magnetic resonance imaging features. Semin Ultrasound CT MR 2007;28:357-370.
173. O'Grady HL, Conlon KC. Pancreatic neuroendocrine tumours. Eur J Surg Oncol 2008;34:324-332.
174. Horton KM, Hruban RH, Yeo C, Fishman EK. Multi-detector row CT of pancreatic islet cell tumors. Radiographics 2006;26:453-464.
175. Grant CS. Insulinoma. Best Pract Res Clin Gastroenterol 2005; 19:783-798.
176. Doppman JL, Chang R, Fraker DL, et al. Localization of insulinomas to regions of the pancreas by intra-arterial stimulation with calcium. Ann Intern Med 1995;123:269-273.
177. Buetow PC, Miller DL, Parrino TV, Buck JL. Islet cell tumors of the pancreas: clinical, radiologic, and pathologic correlation in diagnosis and localization. Radiographics 1997;17:453-472; quiz 72A-72B.
178. Degen L, Wiesner W, Beglinger C. Cystic and solid lesions of the pancreas. Best Pract Res Clin Gastroenterol 2008;22:91-103.
179. Cubilla AL, Fitzgerald PJ. Cancer of the exocrine pancreas: the pathologic aspects. CA Cancer J Clin 1985;35:2-18.
180. Ryan MF, Hamilton PA, Smith AJ, Khalifa M. Radiologic features of pancreatic lipoma. Can Assoc Radiol J 2003;54:41-44.
181. Barutcu O, Cihangiroglu M, Yildirim T, et al. Fat containing unusual tumor of the pancreas. Eur Radiol 2002;12:770-773.
182. Spencer GM, Rubens DJ, Roach DJ. Hypoechoic fat: a sonographic pitfall. AJR Am J Roentgenol 1995;164:1277-1280.
183. Klein KA, Stephens DH, Welch TJ. CT characteristics of metastatic disease of the pancreas. Radiographics 1998;18:369-378.

Contrast-Enhanced Ultrasound

184. D'Onofrio M, Zamboni G, Faccioli N, et al. Ultrasonography of the pancreas. 4. Contrast-enhanced imaging. Abdom Imaging 2007;32:171-181.

CHAPTER **8**

The Gastrointestinal Tract

Stephanie R. Wilson

Chapter Outline

Gastrointestinal tract sonography is frequently frustrating and always challenging. Gas content within the gut lumen can make visibility difficult or even impossible; intraluminal fluid may mimic cystic masses; and fecal material may create a variety of artifacts and pseudotumors. Nevertheless, normal gut has a reproducible pattern, or gut signature, and a variety of gut pathologies create recognizable sonographic abnormalities. Also, in a few conditions, such as acute appendicitis and acute diverticulitis, sonography may play a primary investigative role. Further, endosonography, performed with high-frequency transducers in the gut lumen, is an increasingly popular technique for assessing the esophagus, stomach, and rectum.

ANATOMY AND SONOGRAPHIC TECHNIQUE

The Gut Signature

The gut is a continuous hollow tube with **four concentric layers** (Fig. 8-1). From the lumen outward, these layers are (1) mucosa, which consists of an epithelial lining, loose connective tissue (or lamina propria), and muscularis mucosa; (2) submucosa; (3) muscularis propria, with inner circular and outer longitudinal fibers; and (4) serosa, or adventitia. These histologic layers correspond with the sonographic appearance[1-3] (Table 8-1) and are referred to as the **gut signature,** where up to **five layers** may be visualized (Fig. 8-2). The sonographic layers appear alternately echogenic and hypoechoic; the first, third, and fifth layers are echogenic, and the second and fourth layers are hypoechoic. This relationship of the histologic layering with the sonographic layering is best remembered by recognition that the muscular components of the gut wall—the muscularis mucosa and the muscularis propria—constitute the hypoechoic layers on sonography.

On routine sonograms, the gut signature may vary from a "bull's-eye" in cross section, with an echogenic central area and a hypoechoic rim, to full depiction of the five sonographic layers. The quality of the scan and the resolution of the transducer determine the degree of layer differentiation. The normal gut wall is uniform and compliant, with an average thickness of 3 mm if

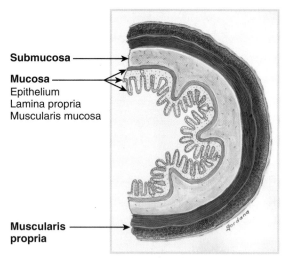

FIGURE 8-1. Schematic depiction of the histologic layers of the gut wall.

HISTOLOGIC LAYERS OF THE GUT

- Mucosa
  Consists of an epithelial lining, loose connective tissue or *lamina propria,* and *muscularis mucosa*
- Submucosa
- Muscularis propria
  Consists of inner circular and outer longitudinal fibers
- Serosa or adventitia

TABLE 8-1. GUT SIGNATURE: HISTOLOGIC-SONOGRAPHIC CORRELATION

HISTOLOGY	SONOGRAPHY
Superficial mucosa/interface	Echogenic
Muscularis mucosa	Hypoechoic
Submucosa	Echogenic
Muscularis propria	Hypoechoic
Serosa/interface	Echogenic

distended and 5 mm if not. Other morphologic features that allow recognition of specific portions of the gut include the gastric rugae, valvulae conniventes (plicae circulares), and colonic haustrations (Fig. 8-3).

Real-time sonography allows assessment of the **content** and **diameter** of the gastrointestinal lumen and the motility of the gut. Hypersecretion, mechanical obstruction, and ileus are implicated when gut fluid is excessive.

Peristalsis is normally seen in the small bowel and stomach. Activity may be increased with mechanical obstruction and inflammatory enteritides. Decreased activity is seen with paralytic ileus and in the end stages of mechanical bowel obstruction.

Gut Wall Pathology

Evaluation of thickened gut on sonography is far superior to the evaluation of normal gut for two important reasons. Thick gut, particularly if associated with abnormality of the perienteric soft tissues, creates a **mass effect,** which is easily seen on sonography. In addition, thickened gut is frequently relatively gasless, improving its sonographic evaluation.[4] Gut wall pathology creates characteristic sonographic patterns (Fig. 8-4; **Video 8-1**). The most familiar, the **target pattern**, was first described by Lutz and Petzoldt[5] in 1976 and later by Bluth et al.,[6] who referred to the pattern as a "pseudokidney," noting that a pathologically significant lesion was found in more than 90% of patients with this pattern. In both descriptions the hypoechoic external rim corresponds to thickened gut wall, whereas the echogenic center relates to residual gut lumen or mucosal ulceration. The target and pseudokidney are the abnormal equivalents of the gut signature created by normal gut.

Identification of thickened gut on sonography may be related to a variety of pathologies.[4] Diagnostic possibilities are predicted by determining the (1) extent and location of disease, (2) preservation or destruction of wall layering, and (3) concentricity or eccentricity of wall involvement. **Benignancy** is favored by long segment involvement with concentric thickening and wall layer preservation. The classic benign pathology showing gut wall thickening is *Crohn's disease.* **Malignancy** is favored by short segment involvement with eccentric disease and wall layer destruction. The classic malignant pathology showing gut wall thickening is *adenocarcinoma* of the stomach or colon. These are guidelines rather than rules, because chronically thickened gut in Crohn's disease may show layer destruction related to fibrotic change, and infiltrative adenocarcinoma may show some wall layer preservation. Lymphadenopathy and hyperemia of the thickened gut wall may be seen in association with both malignant and benign gut wall thickening.

Gut wall masses, as distinguished from thickened gut wall, may be intraluminal, mural, or exophytic, all with or without ulceration (Fig. 8-4). Intraluminal gut masses and mucosal masses may have a variable appearance on sonography but are frequently hidden by gas or luminal content. In contrast, gut pathology creating an exophytic mass without or with mucosal involvement or ulceration may form masses that are more readily visualized. These may be difficult to assign to a gastrointestinal tract origin if typical gut signatures, targets, or pseudokidneys are not seen on sonography. Consequently, intraperitoneal masses of varying morphology, which do not clearly arise

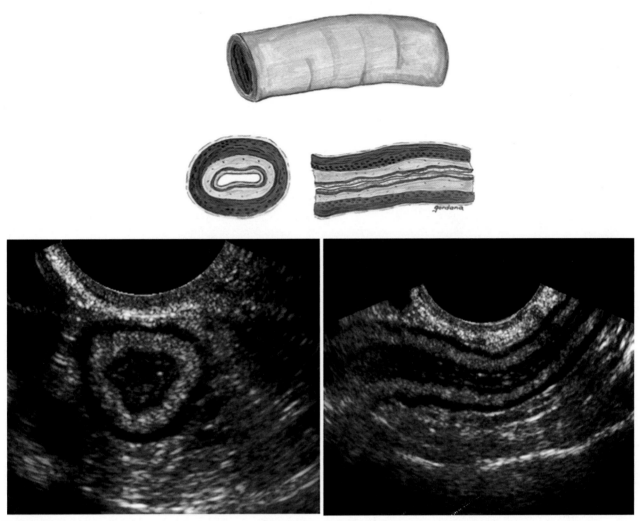

FIGURE 8-2. Gut signature: schematic-sonographic correlation. Schematic and corresponding ultrasound images in a patient with mild gut thickening caused by Crohn's disease. The muscle layers *(blue)* are black or hypoechoic on the sonogram. The submucosa and superficial mucosa layers *(yellow)* are hyperechoic. There is a small amount of fluid and air in the gut lumen on the sonogram.

from the solid abdominal viscera or the lymph nodes, should be considered to have a potential gut origin.

Imaging Technique

Routine sonograms are best performed when the patient has fasted. A real-time survey of the entire abdomen is performed with a 3.5-MHz and/or a 5-MHz transducer, and any obvious masses or gut signatures are observed. The pelvis is scanned before and after the bladder is emptied because the full bladder facilitates visualization of pathologic conditions in some patients and displaces abdominal bowel loops in others. Areas of interest then receive detailed analysis, including compression sonography[7] (Fig. 8-5). Although this technique was initially described using high-frequency linear probes, 5-MHz and 9-MHz convex linear probes and some sector probes work extremely well. The critical factor is a transducer with a short focal zone, allowing optimal resolution of structures close to the skin.

Slow, graded pressure is applied. Normal gut will be compressed and gas pockets displaced away from the region of interest. In contrast, thickened abnormal loops of bowel and obstructed noncompressible loops will remain unchanged. Patients with peritoneal irritation or local tenderness will usually tolerate the slow, gentle increase in pressure of compression sonography, whereas they show a marked painful response if rapid, uneven scanning is performed. In women, **transvaginal sonography** is invaluable for evaluation of the portions of the gut within the true pelvis, particularly the rectum and sigmoid colon. On occasion, oral fluid or a fluid enema are helpful aids to sonography, if the clinician is attempting to determine the origin of a documented fluid collection. Further, oral fluid and a Fleet enema may improve localization and diagnosis of

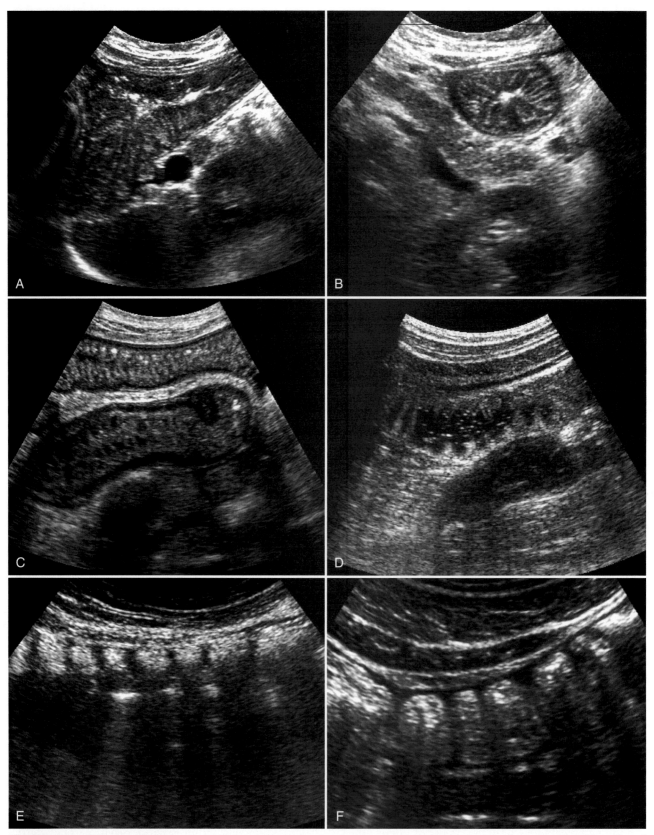

FIGURE 8-3. Gut recognition. A, Sagittal, and **B,** cross-sectional, views of the stomach show normal gastric rugae. The collapsed stomach shows variable wall thickness. **C** and **D,** Valvulae conniventes (plicae circulares) of the small bowel. These are more easily seen when there is fluid in the lumen of the bowel **(C)** or if the valvulae are edematous **(D). E** and **F,** Variations in the appearance of the colonic haustrations in two normal persons.

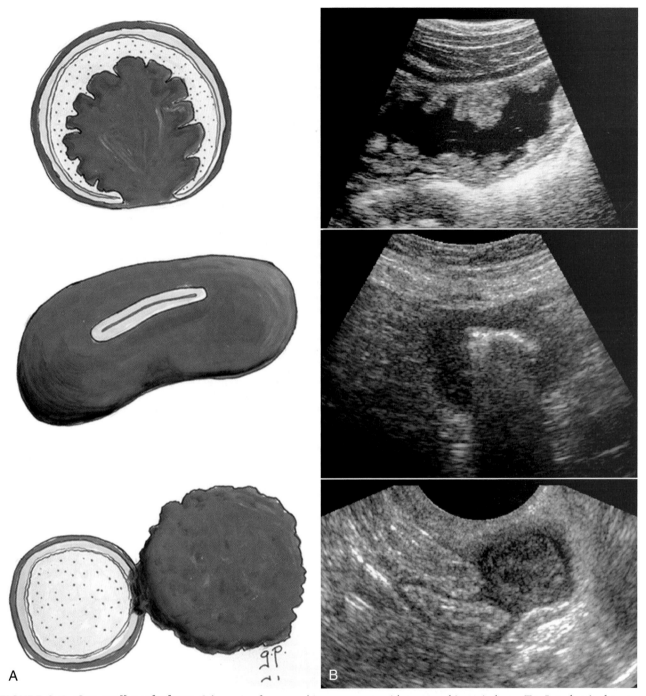

FIGURE 8-4. Gut wall pathology. Schematic of sonographic appearances with sonographic equivalents. *Top,* **Intraluminal mass.** Inflammatory pseudopolyp on sonogram. *Middle,* **Pseudokidney sign,** with symmetrical wall thickening and wall layer destruction. Carcinoma of the colon on sonogram. *Bottom,* **Exophytic mass.** Serosal seed on visceral peritoneum of the gut on sonogram. *(From Wilson SR. The bowel wall looks thickened: what does that mean? In Cooperberg PL, editor. Radiologic Society of North America categorical course syllabus. Chicago, 2002, RSNA, pp 219-228.)*

intraluminal or intramural gastric masses and rectal masses, respectively.

Doppler Evaluation of Gut Wall

Normal gut shows little signal on conventional color Doppler because interrogation is difficult in a normal and mobile bowel loop. Both **neoplasia** and **inflamma-tory disease** show increased vascularity compared with the normal gut wall (Fig. 8-6), whereas ischemic and edematous gut tends to be relatively hypovascular. The addition of color and spectral Doppler ultrasound evaluation to the study of the gut wall provides supportive evidence that gut wall thickening is caused by either ischemic or inflammatory change in the patient with acute abdominal pain. Teefey et al.[8] examined 35

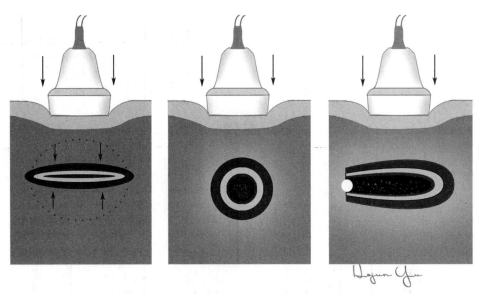

FIGURE 8-5. Schematic of compression sonography. *Left,* Normal gut is compressed. *Middle,* Abnormally thickened gut, or *right,* an obstructed loop, such as that seen in acute appendicitis, will be noncompressible. *(Based on Puylaert JB. Acute appendicitis: ultrasound evaluation using graded compression. Radiology 1986;158:355-360.)*

patients and found absent or barely visible blood flow on color Doppler and absence of arterial signal to be suggestive of ischemia. In contrast, readily detected color Doppler flow and a resistive index less than 0.6 were consistent with inflammation (Fig. 8-6). In my group's experience, we have found color Doppler to be of great value in confirming our suspicion of an inflammatory gut process.

GASTROINTESTINAL TRACT NEOPLASMS

The role of sonography in the evaluation of gastrointestinal (GI) tract neoplasms is similar to that of computed tomography (CT) scan. Visualization is rarely obtained in early mucosal lesions or with small intramural nodules, whereas tumors growing to produce an exophytic mass, a thickened segment of gut with or without ulceration (see Fig. 8-4), or a sizable intraluminal mass (Fig. 8-7) may all be seen. Sonograms are frequently performed early in the diagnostic workup of patients with GI tract tumors, often before their initial identification. Vague abdominal symptomatology, abdominal pain, a palpable abdominal mass, and anemia are common indications for these scans. Appreciation of the typical morphologies associated with GI tract neoplasia may lead to accurate recognition, localization, and even staging of disease, with the opportunity for directing appropriate further investigation, including sonography-guided aspiration biopsy.

Adenocarcinoma

Adenocarcinoma is the most common malignant tumor of the GI tract. It accounts for 80% of all malignant gastric neoplasms. These tumors arise most often in the prepyloric region, the antrum, and the lesser curve, which are the most optimally assessed portions of the stomach on sonography. Grossly, adenocarcinoma has variable growth patterns, including infiltrative, polypoid (Fig. 8-7, *E* and *F*), fungating, and ulcerated tumors. Infiltration may be superficial or transmural, the latter creating a linitis plastica, or "leather bottle," stomach.

Adenocarcinoma occurs much less frequently in the small bowel than in the stomach or large bowel. It accounts for approximately 50% of the small bowel tumors found, 90% of them arising in either the proximal jejunum (Fig. 8-8, *A* and *B*) or the duodenum.[9] Crohn's disease is associated with a significantly increased incidence of adenocarcinoma that usually develops in the ileum. Small bowel adenocarcinomas are generally annular in gross morphology, frequently with ulceration.

Colon carcinoma is very common, its incidence surpassed only by lung and breast cancer. Colon carcinoma accounts for virtually all malignant colorectal neoplasms. Colorectal adenocarcinoma grows with two major gross morphologic patterns: **polypoid intraluminal tumors,** which are most prevalent in the cecum and ascending colon, and **annular constricting lesions** (see Fig. 8-7, *C* and *D*), which are most common in the descending and sigmoid colon. Rarely, infiltrative tumors similar to those seen in the stomach may occur in the colon (Fig. 8-8, *C* and *D*).

Most GI tract mucosal cancers are not visualized on sonography. However, large masses, either intraluminal (see Fig. 8-7) or exophytic, and annular tumors (see Fig. 8-7, *B* and *C*) create sonographic abnormalities.[10,11] Tumors of variable length may thicken the gut wall in either a concentric symmetrical or an asymmetrical pattern. A target or pseudokidney morphology may be

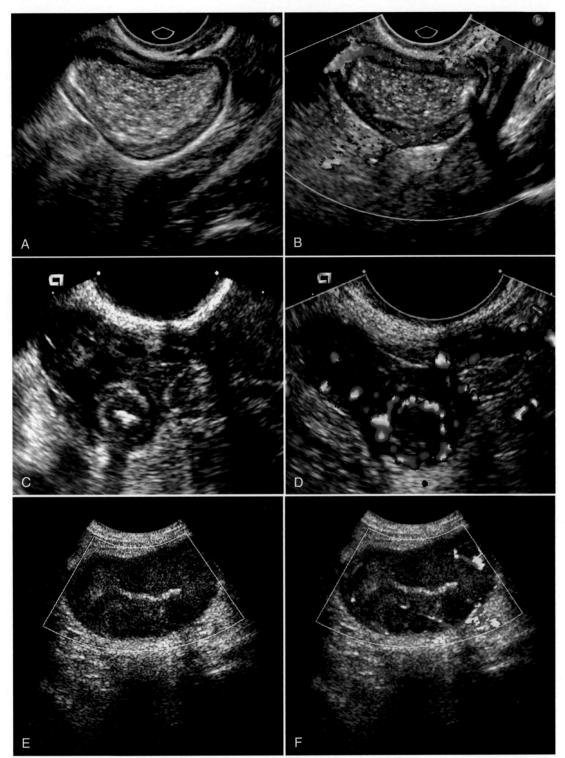

FIGURE 8-6. Contribution of Doppler to gut assessment in three patients. A and **B,** Cross-sectional images of the ileum proximal to an obstructing lesion. The lumen is distended with fluid. The wall is slightly thick. **B,** Color Doppler image shows marked hyperemia of the gut wall as a reflection of its inflammation. **C** and **D,** Transvaginal views in a young woman with right lower quadrant pain show the appendix as a round, tubular structure adjacent to the ovary. **D,** Color Doppler image shows that appendix is hyperemic, consistent with inflammation **E** and **F,** Transverse images of the ascending colon show wall thickening with total layer destruction related to **invasive colon carcinoma.** Neoplastic tumors of the gut invariably show vascularity as here.

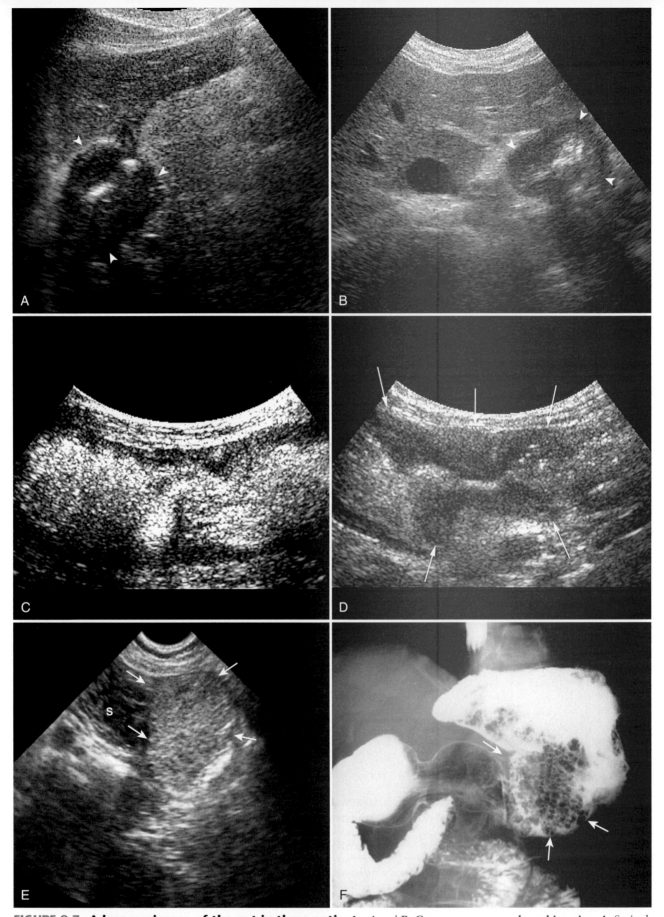

FIGURE 8-7. Adenocarcinoma of the gut in three patients. A and **B, Cancer at gastroesophageal junction. A,** Sagittal, and **B,** transverse, sonograms of the upper abdomen show a pseudokidney *(arrowheads)* adjacent to the left lobe of the liver. **C** and **D, Carcinoma of transverse colon. C,** Long-axis image of the colon shows a dilated lumen filled with echogenic particulate fluid. **D,** Distally, there is a black, circumferential mass *(arrows)* with an "apple core" appearance. An enlarged hypoechoic lymph node is just deep to the tumor. **E** and **F, Intraluminal villous adenocarcinoma of stomach. E,** Transverse sonogram after fluid ingestion shows a relatively well-defined, inhomogeneous, echogenic mass *(arrows)* within body of stomach. Fluid is in the stomach lumen *(S).* **F,** Confirmatory barium swallow shows the villous tumor *(arrows).*

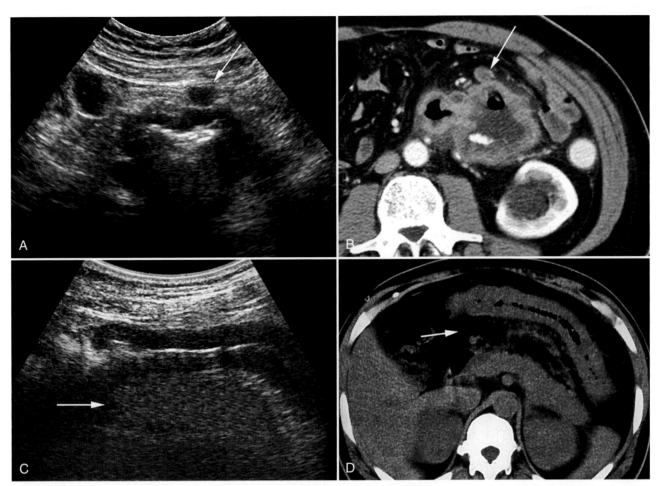

FIGURE 8-8. Adenocarcinoma of bowel: sonographic-CT correlation. A, Sonogram, and **B,** CT scan, show large, necrotic, left upper quadrant mass with enlargement of the perienteric lymph nodes *(arrow)* in a 60-year-old man who presented with abdominal discomfort and blood loss. **C** and **D,** Infiltrative carcinoma of transverse colon in a 42-year-old black man who presented to the emergency department with acute abdominal pain. **C,** Transverse sonogram of the epigastrium shows a featureless segment of thick gut with total loss of wall layering in the location of the transverse colon. Deep to the gut is a diffuse echogenic mass effect *(arrow)* suggesting infiltrated or inflamed fat. **D,** Confirmatory CT scan. Neoplasia was not suspected on the basis of either imaging test or at surgery.

created (see Fig. 8-4, *middle*). Air in mucosal ulcerations typically produces linear echogenic foci, often with "ringdown" artifact, within the bulk of the mass. Tumors are usually, but not invariably, hypoechoic. Annular lesions may produce gut obstruction with dilation, hyperperistalsis, and increased luminal fluid of the gut proximal to the tumor site.[11] Evidence of direct invasion, regional lymph node enlargement, and liver metastases should be specifically sought in all cases.

Gastrointestinal Stromal Tumors

Of the mesenchymal tumors affecting the gut, those of smooth muscle origin are the most common and account for about 1% of all GI tract neoplasms. These gastrointestinal stromal tumors (GISTs) are found most often in the stomach and the small bowel. Colonic tumors are the least common and occur most often in the rectum. Although GISTs may be found as an incidental observation at surgery, sonography, or autopsy, these vascular

tumors frequently become very large and may undergo ulceration, degeneration, necrosis, and hemorrhage.[12]

On sonography, smooth muscle (stromal) tumors typically produce round mass lesions of varying size and echogenicity, often with central cystic areas[13] related to hemorrhage or necrosis (Fig. 8-9). Their gut origin is not always easily determined, but if ulceration is present, pockets of gas in an ulcer crater may suggest their origin. Smooth muscle tumors of gut origin should be considered in the differential diagnosis of incidentally noted, indeterminate abdominal masses in asymptomatic patients, particularly if they show central cystic or necrotic change (Fig. 8-9, *E* and *F*). These tumors are very amenable to sonographic-guided aspiration biopsy.

Lymphoma

The gut may be involved with lymphoma in two basic forms: as widespread dissemination in stage III or IV lymphoma of any cell type or, more often, as primary

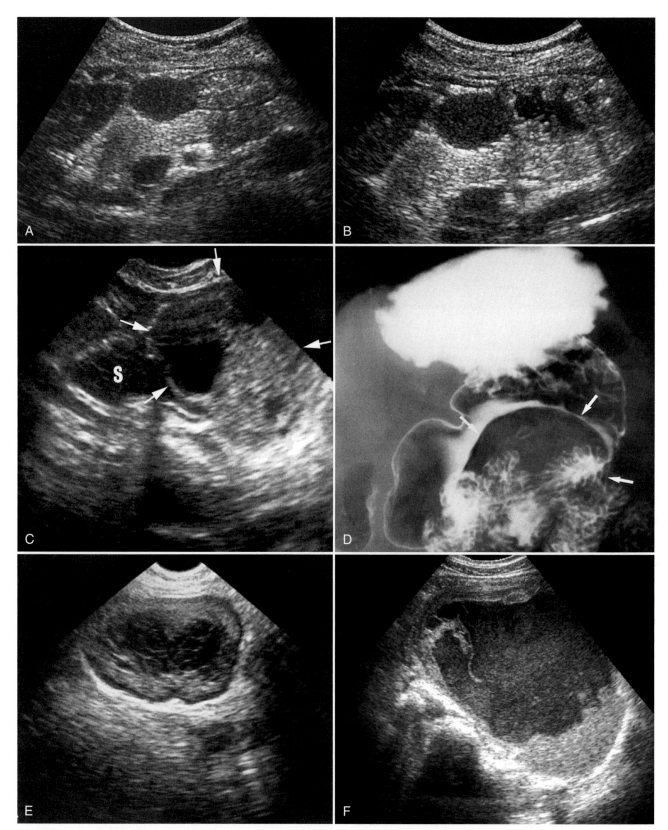

FIGURE 8-9. Gastrointestinal stromal tumors (GISTs) in four patients. A and **B,** Exophytic gut mass, a **gastric leio-myoma,** analogous to Figure 8-4. **A,** Transverse sonogram of epigastrium shows the normal gastric gut signature and the focal exophytic mass. **B,** After water ingestion, the lumen contains fluid that appears black. The solid mass is now clearly seen. **C** and **D, Gastric leio-myosarcoma. C,** Transverse sonogram after fluid ingestion shows a complex, smooth intramural mass *(arrows)* projecting into the fluid-filled stomach lumen *(S).* **D,** Confirmatory barium swallow shows the intramural tumor *(arrows).* **E** and **F,** Two patients presented with a large, upper abdominal, complex and necrotic-appearing mass on sonography. Although the gut origin of the masses is not evident on the images, the correct diagnosis of GIST was suggested based on the appearance. The jejunum is the origin of the tumor in **E** and the stomach in **F.**

lymphoma of the GI tract, which is virtually always a non-Hodgkin's lymphoma. Primary tumors constitute only 2% to 4% of all GI tract malignant tumors[12] but account for 20% of those found in the small bowel. **Three predominant growth patterns** are observed: nodular or polypoid, carcinoma-like ulcerations, and infiltrating tumor masses that frequently invade the adjacent mesentery and lymph nodes.[9]

GROWTH PATTERNS OF LYMPHOMA

Nodular or polypoid
Carcinoma-like ulcerative lesions
Infiltrating tumor masses

Small, submucosal nodules may be easily overlooked on sonography. However, many patients have large, easily visible, very hypoechoic, ulcerated masses in the stomach or small bowel[14,15] (Fig. 8-10). Long, linear, high-amplitude echoes with **ringdown artifacts,** indicating gas in the residual lumen or ulcerations, are

common observations. This particular pathology has been recognized as one of the more frequent presentations of patients with acquired immunodeficiency syndrome (AIDS)–related lymphoma, compared with other lymphoma populations. Regional lymph node enlargement may be visualized, although generalized lymph node abnormality is uncommon.

Metastases

Malignant melanoma and primary tumors of the lung and breast are the tumors most likely to have secondary involvement of the GI tract[16] (Fig. 8-11). In order of frequency, the stomach, small bowel, and colon are involved. Secondary neoplasm affecting the omentum and peritoneum may cause **ascites,** tiny or confluent superficial secondary nodules on the gut surface, or extensive **omental cakes** that virtually engulf the involved gut loops[17,18] (Fig. 8-12). Metastases to the peritoneum most often arise from primary tumors in the ovary or the gut. A **drop metastasis** in the pelvic pouch of Douglas shows as a small, solid, peritoneal nodule without obvious origin from the pelvic viscera.

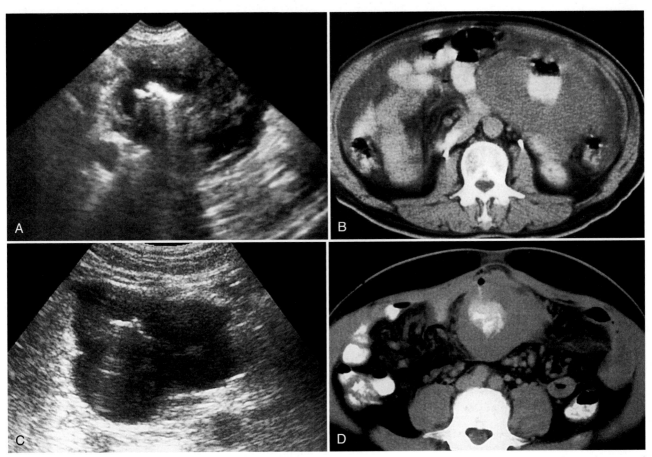

FIGURE 8-10. Small bowel lymphoma in two patients. A, Transverse left paramedian sonogram shows a hypoechoic round mass lesion. Central echogenicity with "ringdown" gas artifact suggests its gut origin. **B,** Confirmatory CT scan shows large, soft tissue mass with corresponding residual gut lumen. **C** and **D,** AIDS patient. **C,** Sonogram shows a focal midabdominal, very hypoechoic *(black)* mass with no wall layer definition, which is classic for gut lymphoma. The luminal gas appears as central bright echogenicity with dirty shadowing. **D,** Confirmatory CT scan.

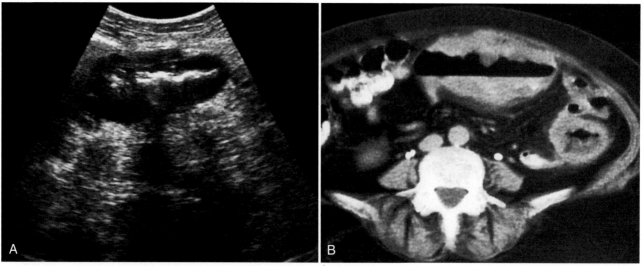

FIGURE 8-11. Metastatic malignant melanoma to small bowel. A, Transverse paraumbilical sonogram shows well-defined, hypoechoic mass with central irregular echogenicity with gas artifact suggesting, correctly, its gut origin. **B,** Confirmatory CT scan.

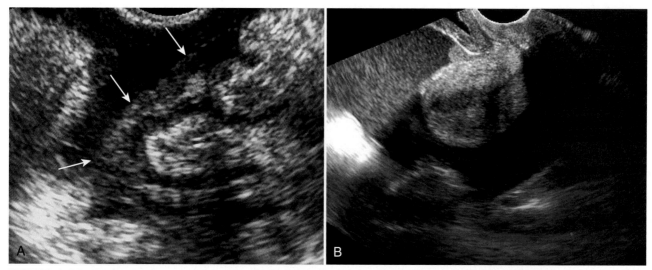

FIGURE 8-12. Peritoneal metastases in two patients. A, Transvaginal image shows ascites and visceral peritoneal plaque from metastatic ovarian cancer as a plaque of soft tissue *(arrows)* on the surface of the small bowel loop. **B,** Transvaginal scan of peritoneal drop metastasis from stomach primary shows grossly particulate ascites. There is a tiny seed in the vesicouterine angle.

On sonography, small submucosal nodules that tend to ulcerate are rarely seen, whereas large, diffusely infiltrative tumors with large ulcerations are common, particularly in the small bowel (see Fig. 8-11), where they create hypoechoic, well-defined masses that often have bright, specular echoes with ringdown artifacts in areas of ulceration. Particulate ascites, omental thickening, and visceral/parietal peritoneal nodules and plaques all should suggest metastatic disease.

INFLAMMATORY BOWEL DISEASE: CROHN'S DISEASE

Inflammatory bowel disease (IBD) comprises Crohn's disease and ulcerative colitis. **Ulcerative colitis** is a mucosal inflammation of the colon that shows minimal sonographic change, even with acute or long-standing disease. **Crohn's disease,** by comparison, is a chronic, transmural, granulomatous inflammatory process affecting all layers of the gut wall, also showing frequent changes in the perienteric soft tissue. Because of this unique gross pathology, Crohn's disease provides the major source of IBD patients referred for sonographic examination.

Crohn's disease is a complex process of unknown etiology. It most often affects the terminal ileum and the colon, although any portion of the gut may be involved. Grossly, the gut wall in Crohn's disease is typically very thick and rigid with secondary luminal narrowing. Discrete or continuous ulcers and deep fissures are characteristic, frequently leading to fistula formation.

Mesenteric lymph node enlargement and matting of involved loops are common. The mesentery may be greatly thickened and fatty, creeping over the edges of the gut to the antimesenteric border. Recurrence after surgery and perianal disease are classic features.

Characterized by frequent exacerbations and remissions, with disease onset often in young adults, the chronic nature of Crohn's disease is well assessed by a noninvasive, sensitive modality, such as sonography. Although barium study and endoscopy remain the major tools to evaluate mucosal and luminal abnormality, sonography, similar to CT, offers valuable additional information about the gut wall, lymph nodes, mesentery, and regional soft tissues. Baseline examination determines the extent and activity of disease by assessing the **classic features** of Crohn's disease: gut wall thickening, creeping fat, hyperemia, mesenteric lymphadenopathy, strictures, and mucosal abnormalities. Sonography also predicts **complications:** inflammatory masses (phlegmon or abscess), fistulas, obstruction, perforation, and appendicitis.[19] Further, ultrasound detects postoperative recurrence and identifies patients who require more invasive imaging techniques.[19] Radiation exposure is significant in the younger population with Crohn's disease, if a CT scan is performed with each exacerbation. Sonography is therefore our routine evaluation technique for patients with this diagnosis.

CROHN'S DISEASE: SONOGRAPHIC FEATURES

CLASSIC FEATURES
Gut wall thickening
Creeping fat
Hyperemia
Strictures
Mesenteric lymphadenopathy
Mucosal abnormalities

COMPLICATIONS
Inflammatory masses
Fistula
Obstruction
Perforation
Appendicitis

Classic Features

Gut Wall Thickening

The most frequently observed abnormality in patients with Crohn's disease, demonstration of gut wall thickening on sonography is the basis for initial detection, for detection of recurrence,[20] and for determining the extent of disease. In a meta-analysis on the accuracy of sonography in detecting Crohn's disease, Fraquelli et al.[21]

showed sensitivity and specificity of 88% and 93%, respectively, when a bowel wall thickness threshold greater than 3 mm was used, and 75% and 97% with a threshold greater than 4 mm. In another meta-analysis comparing different modalities for diagnosis of IBD, mean sensitivity estimates for the diagnosis on a per-patient basis were high and not significantly different among the imaging modalities: 89.7%, 93.0%, 87.8%, and 84.3% for ultrasound, magnetic resonance imaging (MRI), scintigraphy, and CT, respectively.[22]

Gut wall thickening in Crohn's disease is most frequently concentric and may be marked.[23,24] Wall echogenicity varies depending on the degree of inflammatory infiltration and fibrosis. Stratification with retention of the gut layers is typical (Fig. 8-13, A and B; see also Fig. 8-2). A target or pseudokidney appearance is possible in acute disease or long-standing fibrotic disease as the gut wall layering is progressively lost (Fig. 8-13, C and D). Long-standing and often burnt-out disease may also show subtle wall thickening with fat deposition in the submucosa, which appears as increased echogenicity of this layer (Fig. 8-13, E and F). Actively involved gut typically appears rigid and fixed, with decreased or absent peristalsis. Skip areas are frequent. Involved segments vary in length from a few millimeters to many centimeters.

Creeping Fat

Mesenteric edema and fibrosis are also characteristic of Crohn's disease, producing a mass in the mesentery adjacent to the diseased gut that may creep over the border of the abnormal gut or completely engulf it. Fat creeping onto the margins of the involved gut creates a uniform echogenic halo around the mesenteric border of the gut, with a thyroid-like appearance in cross section (Fig. 8-14). It may become more heterogeneous and even hypoechoic in long-standing disease. Creeping fat is the most common cause of gut loop separation seen on gastrointestinal contrast studies.[19] It is also the most striking and detectable abnormality on sonography of patients with perienteric inflammatory processes (Fig. 8-15). Therefore, detection of creeping fat should lead to a detailed evaluation of the regional gut.

Lymphadenopathy

Tender and enlarged mesenteric and perienteric nodes are common features of the active phase of inflammation with Crohn's disease (Fig. 8-16). Lymphadenopathy is observed much less in the inactive phase. The nodes appear as focal hypoechoic masses circumferentially surrounding the gut and in the expected location of the mesenteric attachment. Nodes are frequently quite round and typically lose the normal linear echogenic streak from the nodal hilum. Similar to the gut, the lymph nodes show hyperemia as a reflection of their

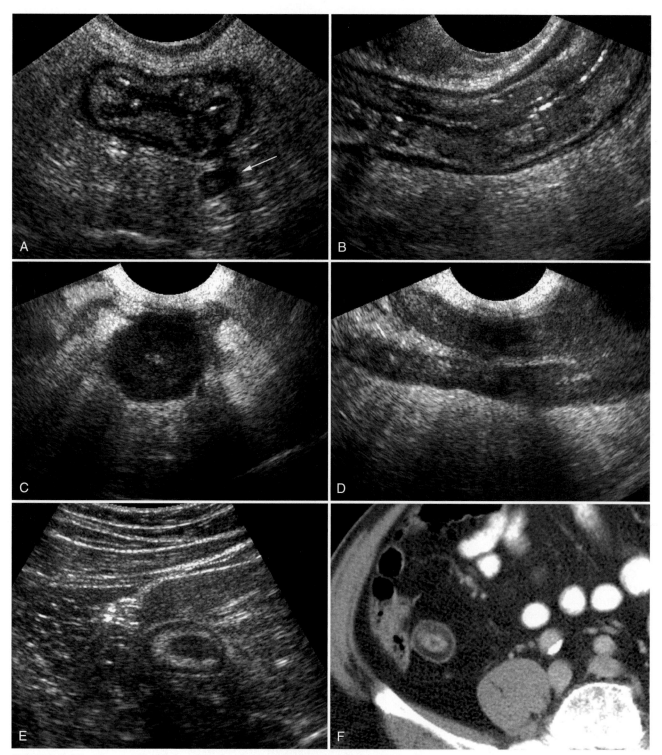

FIGURE 8-13. Gut wall thickening in three patients with Crohn's disease. A, Cross-sectional, and B, sagittal, views showing the typical thickening in active disease with wall layer retention; *arrow,* lymph node. C, Cross-sectional, and D, sagittal, views show complete loss of wall layering, as seen with very active disease. E, Sonogram, and F, corresponding CT image, of the terminal ileum in a patient with burnt-out disease and fatty deposition in the submucosa, which appears echogenic on the sonogram. *(C and D from Wilson SR. The bowel wall looks thickened: what does that mean? In Cooperberg PL, editor. Radiologic Society of North America categorical course syllabus. Chicago, 2002, RSNA, pp 219-228.)*

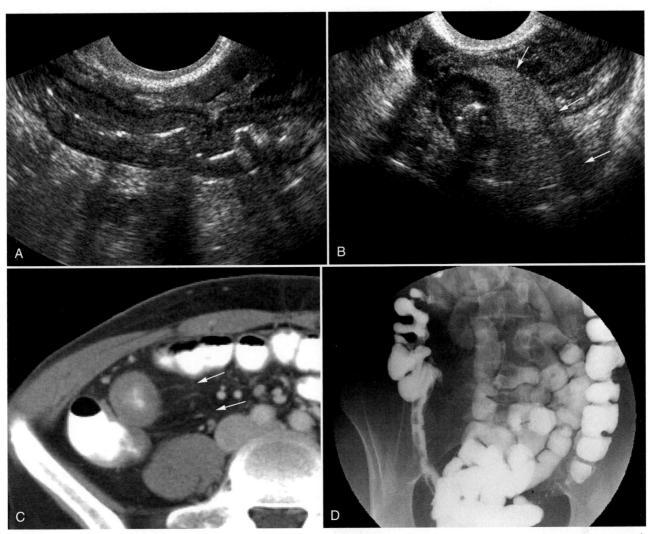

FIGURE 8-14. Creeping fat in Crohn's disease. A, Long-axis view of thickened terminal ileum (TI). Wall layering is preserved. **B,** Cross-sectional view of TI shows a hyperechoic mass effect *(arrows)* along the medial border of the gut representing creeping fat. **C,** Confirmatory CT scan shows both the thick wall of the TI and the streaky fat *(arrows).* **D,** Subsequent barium study shows separation of loops of small bowel in the same location. Creeping fat is the most common explanation for this bowel separation.

inflammation. Nodes are usually of moderate size. Larger nodes, over 3 cm in diameter, suggest a malignant complication of Crohn's disease.

Hyperemia

Evaluation of blood flow is a useful tool to monitor inflammatory activity and response to therapy. Activity of inflammatory change is shown to correlate with hyperemia, as seen on **color Doppler evaluation**[25] (Fig. 8-17). Although subjective, this addition of color Doppler to gray-scale sonography is valuable supportive evidence of inflammatory change in the gut and adjacent inflamed fat[19] (see Fig. 8-6, *A-D;* **Video 8-2**). Further, van Oostayen et al.[26] showed that blood flow measurement in the superior mesenteric artery also correlated with disease activity; blood flow values were significantly higher (826 ± 407 mL/min) in 15 patients with active disease than in 14 patients without active disease (323 ± 103 mL/min)

($p < .05$). More recently, Serra et al.[27] showed that **contrast-enhanced ultrasound** (CEUS) performed with a second-generation microbubble contrast agent is a more sensitive and reproducible technique than Doppler. CEUS allows both qualitative and quantitative evaluation of hyperemia of the bowel wall by looking at the pattern of enhancement, as well as the ratio between the major thickness of the enhanced layer on CEUS and the thickness of the entire wall section, as shown on gray-scale sonography (Fig. 8-17, *C;* **Video 8-3**).

Strictures

Strictures relate to rigid narrowing of the gut lumen and fixed acute angulations. The luminal surfaces of involved segments of gut most often appear to be in fixed constant apposition, with the lumen appearing as a linear echogenic central area within a thickened gut loop (Figs. 8-18 and 8-19; **Video 8-2**). This is in contrast to thickened

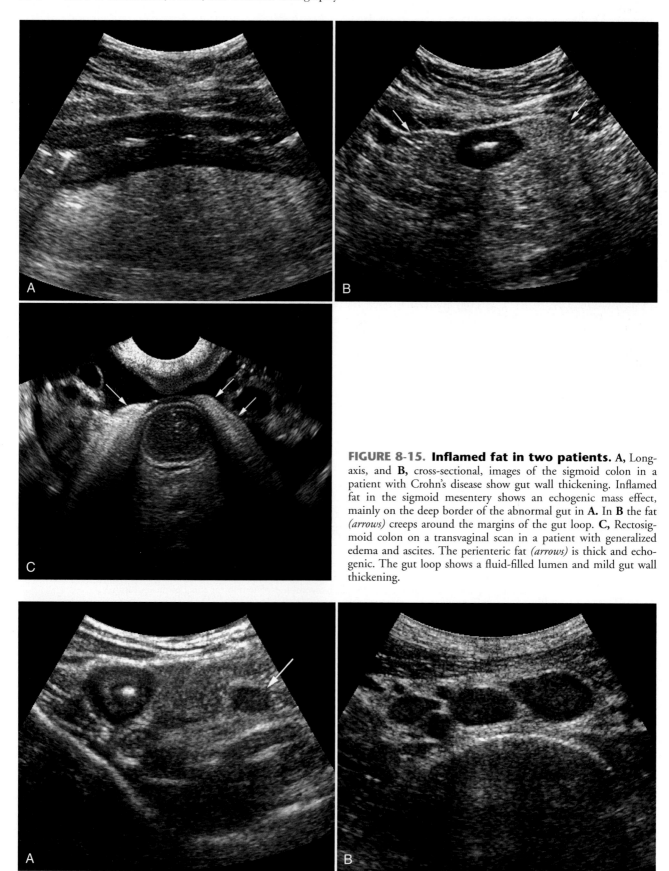

FIGURE 8-15. Inflamed fat in two patients. A, Long-axis, and **B,** cross-sectional, images of the sigmoid colon in a patient with Crohn's disease show gut wall thickening. Inflamed fat in the sigmoid mesentery shows an echogenic mass effect, mainly on the deep border of the abnormal gut in **A.** In **B** the fat *(arrows)* creeps around the margins of the gut loop. **C,** Rectosigmoid colon on a transvaginal scan in a patient with generalized edema and ascites. The perienteric fat *(arrows)* is thick and echogenic. The gut loop shows a fluid-filled lumen and mild gut wall thickening.

FIGURE 8-16. Lymphadenopathy in two patients with Crohn's disease. A, Transverse image in the right lower quadrant shows a thick terminal ileum in cross section. There is inflamed fat in the location of the mesentery. A mesenteric node *(arrow)* shows as a small, solid, hypoechoic mass within the fat. **B,** Multiple mesenteric nodes of varying size show as hypoechoic soft tissue masses within the mesentery, optimally shown in an oblique plane between the region of the ileocecal valve and the aortic bifurcation.

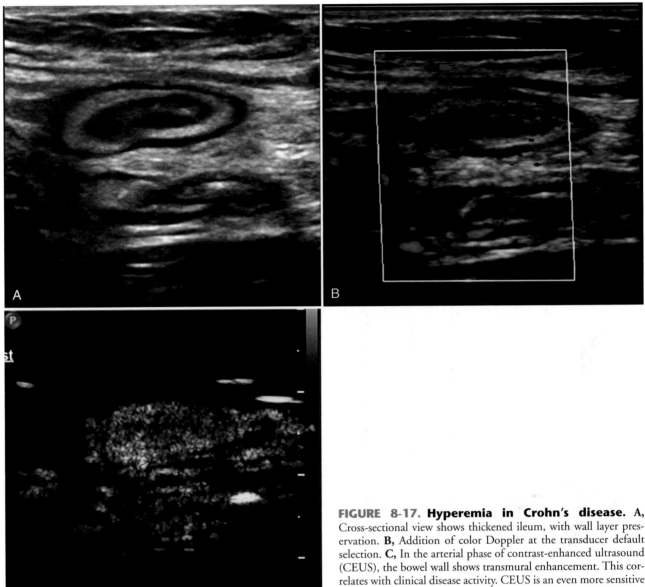

FIGURE 8-17. Hyperemia in Crohn's disease. A, Cross-sectional view shows thickened ileum, with wall layer preservation. **B,** Addition of color Doppler at the transducer default selection. **C,** In the arterial phase of contrast-enhanced ultrasound (CEUS), the bowel wall shows transmural enhancement. This correlates with clinical disease activity. CEUS is an even more sensitive method to show transmural enhancement of the bowel wall at the peak of arterial phase enhancement. See also Video 8-3.

sections, where the luminal diameter may be maintained (Fig. 8-20). Incomplete mechanical obstruction may be inferred if dilated, hyperperistaltic segments are seen proximal to a stricture. Peristaltic waves from the obstructed gut, proximal to a narrowed segment, may produce visible movement through the strictured segment **(Video 8-4).** Less often, involved segments of gut may show luminal dilation with sacculation, as well as narrowing, and the retained lumen may be of variable caliber **(Video 8-5).** Concretions and bezoars may develop in gut between strictured segments. Parente et al.[28] showed that bowel ultrasound is an accurate technique for detecting small bowel strictures, especially in patients with severe disease who are candidates for surgery.

Mucosal Abnormalities

Conglomerate masses may be related to clumps of matted bowel, inflamed edematous mesentery, increased fat deposition in the mesentery, and infrequently, mesenteric lymphadenopathy. Involved loops may demonstrate angulation and fixation resulting from retraction of the thickened fibrotic mesentery.

Complications

In experienced hands, sonography is an accurate method for the detection of intestinal complications in Crohn's disease. It is therefore an excellent first choice at times of acute exacerbation in this patient population.[29]

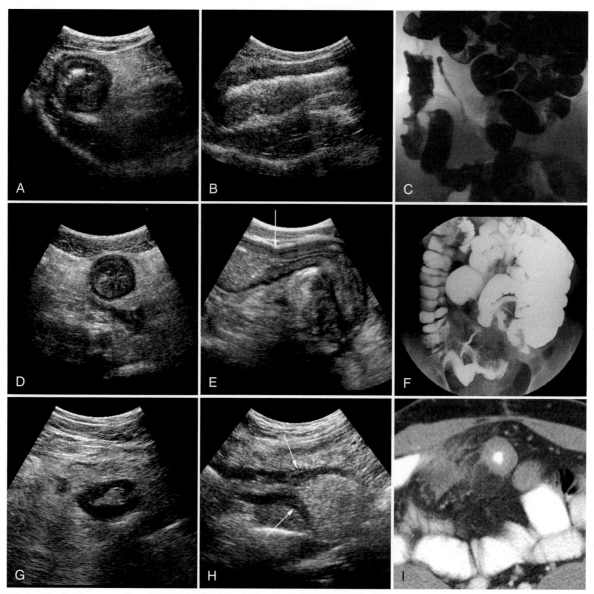

FIGURE 8-18. Strictures in three patients with Crohn's disease. A, Long-axis, and B, short-axis, sonograms show a diffusely thickened loop of gut, the ileum proximal to the ileocecal valve, and narrowing of the central echogenic lumen. Mesenteric fat is inflamed. C, Confirmatory fluoroscopic image from a small bowel enema shows the long, tight stricture in the ileum. D, Long-axis, and E, short-axis, sonograms of the terminal ileum show an abrupt transition in the caliber of the gut *(arrow)*. The gut proximal to the arrow is dilated and fluid filled. The distal gut has a stricture, confirmed on F, the small bowel enema. G, Long-axis image of the neoterminal ileum shows a thickened, featureless wall with a caliber alteration *(arrows)*. H, Short-axis image through the stricture shows the thickened wall and surrounding inflamed fat. I, Confirmatory CT scan.

Inflammatory Masses

Inflammatory masses involving the fibrofatty mesentery are the most common complication of Crohn's disease, although the development of abscesses with drainable pus occurs infrequently. Before the stage of liquefaction, **phlegmonous change** may be noted as poorly defined, hypoechoic zones without fluid content in areas of inflamed fat (Fig. 8-21). **Abscess formation** results in a complex or fluid-filled mass (Fig. 8-21, *G* and *H*). Gas content within an abscess is helpful in both suggesting

an abscess and being a potential source of sonographic error, particularly if large quantities are present. Abscesses may be intraperitoneal or extraperitoneal or may be in remote locations such as the liver, abdominal wall (Fig. 8-21, *H* and *I*), and psoas muscles.

Fistula Formation

This characteristic complication of Crohn's disease occurs most often at the proximal end of a thickened, strictured segment of bowel **(Video 8-6)**. Although

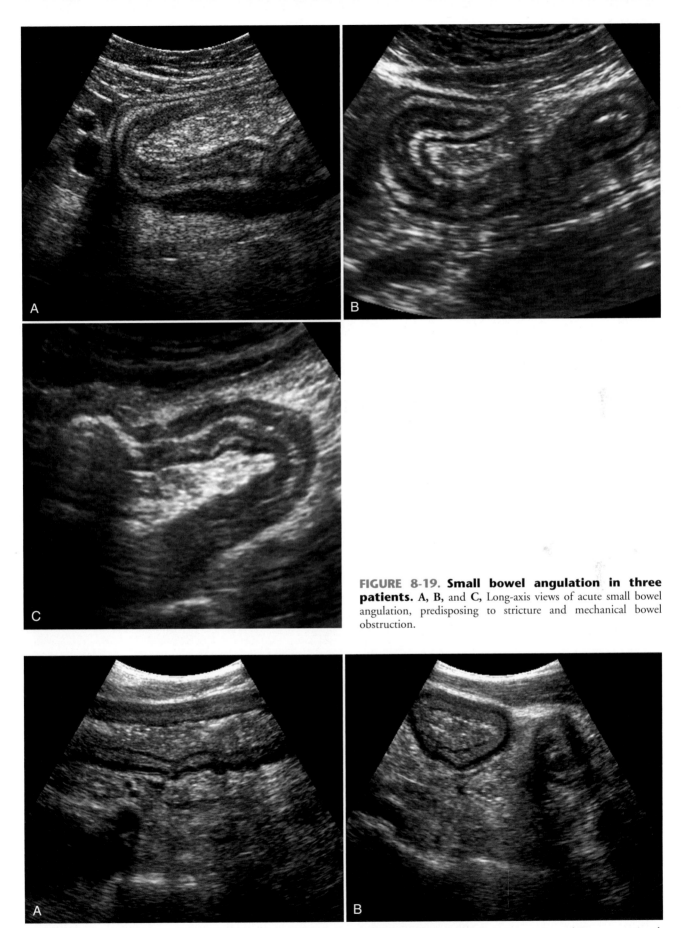

FIGURE 8-19. Small bowel angulation in three patients. A, B, and C, Long-axis views of acute small bowel angulation, predisposing to stricture and mechanical bowel obstruction.

FIGURE 8-20. Segment of involved gut proximal to a strictured segment. A, Long-axis, and B, cross-sectional, images show thickening of the gut wall with layer preservation in a patient with Crohn's disease. The lumen is fluid filled and substantial in caliber.

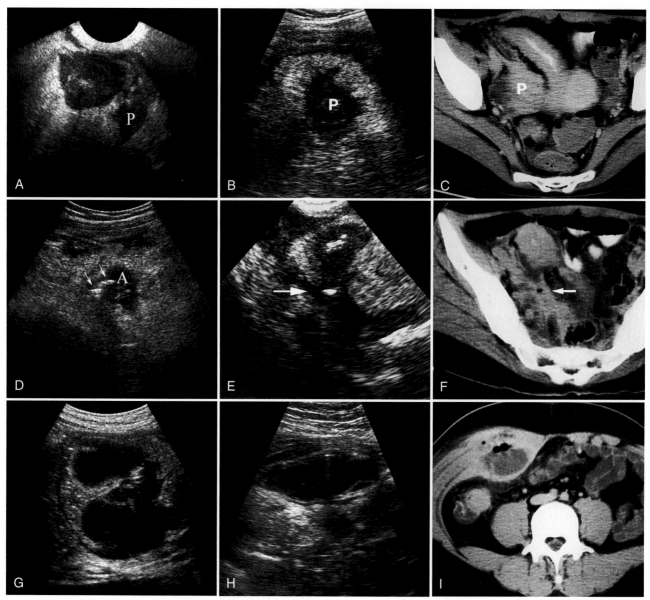

FIGURE 8-21. Inflammatory masses in Crohn's disease. *Top row,* **Phlegmons** *(P).* **A,** Loop of thick sigmoid colon is seen in cross section. Adjacent to the margin is a poorly defined, hypoechoic zone within extensive inflamed fat. **B,** Transverse sonogram in the right lower quadrant shows a thick terminal ileum superficially. Within the extensive inflamed fat is a poorly defined, hypoechoic zone representing the phlegmon. **C,** Confirmatory CT scan. *Middle row,* **Inflammatory masses,** with air but no drainable pus. **D,** Transverse image of the right lower quadrant shows abundant inflamed fat. Centrally, there is a small fluid collection or abscess *(A)* with small, echogenic shadowing foci *(arrows)* caused by air bubbles. **E,** Cross-sectional sonogram through the terminal ileum shows gut thickening, echogenic inflamed fat, and a poorly defined, focal hypoechoic area deep to the gut. Bubbles of gas outside the gut are seen as bright, echogenic foci *(arrow)* on sonography. **F,** Confirmatory CT scan. *Bottom row,* **Drainable abscesses. G,** Large, interloop fluid collection. **H,** Sonogram, and **I,** confirmatory CT scan, show a superficial fluid collection with small gas bubbles in the anterior abdominal wall. *(B, E, F, H, and I from Sarrazin J, Wilson SR. Manifestations of Crohn disease at ultrasound. Radiographics 1996;16:499-520.)*

mucosal ulcerations are not well assessed on sonography, deep fissures in the gut wall appear as echogenic linear areas penetrating deeply into the wall beyond the margin of the gut lumen (Figs. 8-22 and 8-23). With fistula formation, linear bands of varying echogenicity can be seen extending from segments of abnormal gut to the skin (Fig. 8-23, *C*), bladder (Fig. 8-23, *A*), vagina, or other abnormal loops. If there is gas or movement in the fistula during the sonographic study, the fistula will usually appear bright or echogenic, with or without ring-down artifact related to air in the tract. Conversely, if the tract is empty or partially closed, the fistula may appear as a black or hypoechoic tract (Fig. 8-23, *B* and *C*). Palpation of the abdomen during the examination may produce movement of fluid or air through the fistula, assisting in its identification.

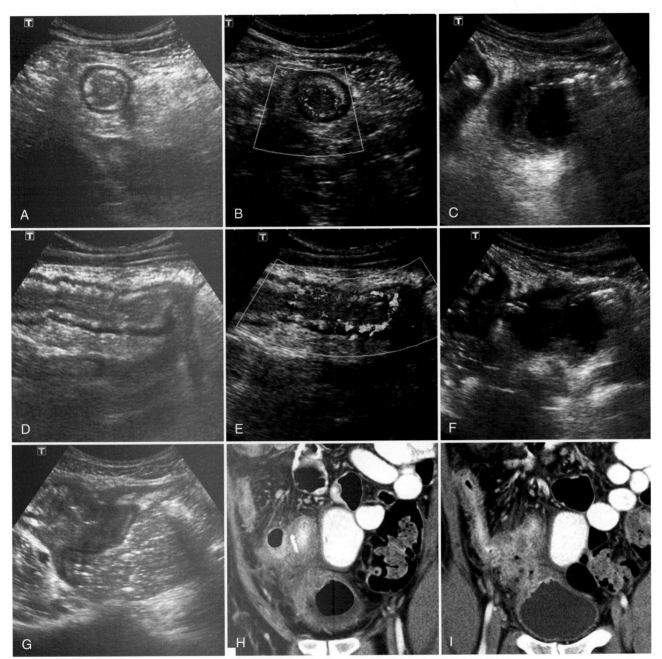

FIGURE 8-22. Enterovesical fistula in Crohn's disease. A and **B,** Cross-sectional images of the terminal ileum show wall thickening and hyperemia. **C,** Air in the bladder appears as nondependent bright echoes with dirty shadowing. **D** and **E,** Long-axis views of the ileum show the hyperemia and the constant luminal apposition, consistent with stricture. **F,** Bladder with the luminal air and an air-containing tract from the bladder to the adjacent bowel. **G,** Dilated, fluid-filled bowel proximal to the thickening, suggesting incomplete mechanical bowel obstruction. **H** and **I,** Coronal CT images confirming that the bladder air and inflammatory mass are related to the bladder dome. See also Video 8-6.

Localized Perforation

Although free perforation of the bowel is rare in Crohn's disease, localized perforation with phlegmonous masses contained within the surrounding perienteric inflammatory fat is common. Spiking of the border of acutely inflamed gut is characteristic (Fig. 8-24). On occasion, an air-containing tract may be identified, traversing the bowel wall into the perienteric fat. Phlegmonous masses

should alert the sonographer to possible underlying localized perforation.

Perianal Inflammatory Problems

Perianal inflammation is a frequent and debilitating complication of Crohn's disease. Highly complex, transsphincteric tracts may extend to involve the deep tissues of the buttocks (Fig. 8-25), perineum, scrotum (men),

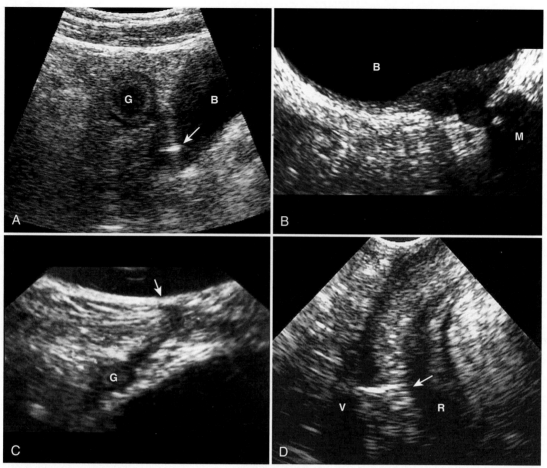

FIGURE 8-23. Fistulas in four patients with Crohn's disease. A and **B, Enterovesical fistulas. A,** Image shows a tract between the abnormal gut *(G)* and the bladder *(B)*. An air bubble within shows as a bright, echogenic focus *(arrow)*. **B,** Hypoechoic tract connects an inflammatory mass *(M)* to the bladder *(B)*. **C, Enterocutaneous fistula.** Hypoechoic tract runs from a loop of abnormal gut *(G)* to the skin surface *(arrow)*. **D, Rectovaginal fistula** on transvaginal sonogram appears as a bright, air-containing tract *(arrow)* coursing from the rectum *(R)* to the vagina *(V)*.

and labia and vagina (women). Unlike commonly encountered perianal fistulas based on the cryptoglandular theory, fistulas in Crohn's disease have no predilection for the location of the internal openings and are highly complex. **Transrectal ultrasound** (TRUS) is often requested in patients with rectal Crohn's disease or perianal pathology and may successfully show abscesses and fistulous tracts. However, we have not had uniform success with this procedure, which is often painful and noncontributory in this particular population. In contrast, in patients of either gender, we have found **transperineal scanning** to be a more comfortable and often more informative technique, alone or in combination with TRUS.[30] Further, in women, transvaginal scan contributes greatly to our assessment of rectal and perirectal disease. It is also ideal for showing enterovesical, enterovaginal, and rectovaginal fistulas.[31] If bladder symptoms are present, we recommend that transvaginal sonography be performed with a partially full bladder. Rectal involvement in Crohn's disease is characterized by (1) thickening of the rectal wall with wall layer preservation, (2) inflammation of the perirectal fat, and (3) enlargement

of the perirectal lymph nodes The principles of interpretation of perianal inflammatory disease are discussed later under Endosonography.

ACUTE ABDOMEN

Sonography is a valuable imaging tool in patients who may have specific gastrointestinal disease, such as acute appendicitis or acute diverticulitis.[32] However, its contribution to the assessment of patients with possible GI tract disease is less certain. Seibert et al.[33] emphasized the value of ultrasound in assessing the patient with a distended and gasless abdomen and detecting ascites, unsuspected masses, and abnormally dilated, fluid-filled loops of small bowel. In my experience, sonography has been helpful not only in the gasless abdomen, but also in a variety of other situations. Sonography may add greatly to diagnostic acumen if used in conjunction with plain radiography, CT, and other imaging modalities. The real-time aspect of sonographic study allows for direct patient-sonographer/physician interaction, with confirmation of palpa-

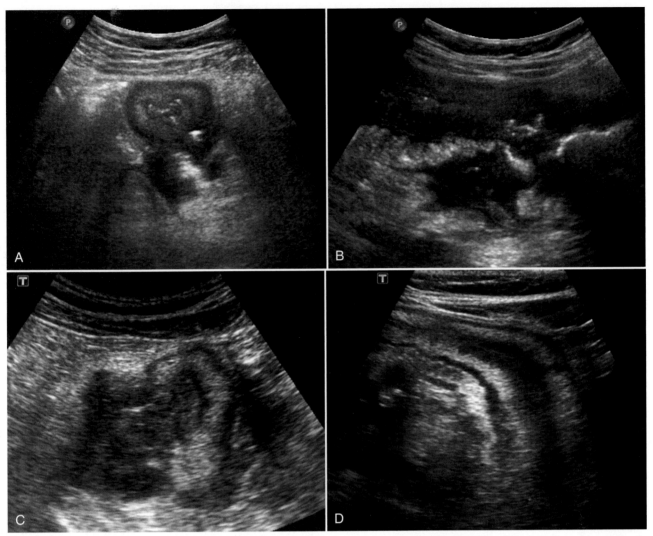

FIGURE 8-24. Localized perforation with phlegmon. *Two young women with acute flare of Crohn's disease symptoms. In first patient,* **A,** *cross sectional, and* **B,** *long-axis, images of the bowel show wall thickening and a deep hypoechoic mass with fingerlike projections into the surrounding perienteric fat, suggesting phlegmon. Also, on* **A,** *air appears as a bright focus extending beyond the lumen of the bowel into the bowel wall, suggesting localized perforation. In second patient,* **C,** *Cross sectional image of the ileum shows a large area of disruption of the bowel wall, an adjacent hypoechoic phlegmon, and an air tract from localized perforation.* **D,** *Long-axis image of loop of ileum shows that the wall is uniformly thickened with layer preservation. The phlegmon is on the margin of the bowel and not shown in the longitudinal view.*

ble masses and focal points of tenderness. The doctrine "scan where it hurts" is invaluable and has led sonographers to describe the value of the sonographic equivalent to clinical examination with such descriptors as a sonographic Murphy's sign or sonographic McBurney's sign. Similar to the radiographic approach to plain film interpretation, a systematic approach is essential in the sonographic assessment of the abdomen in a patient with an acute abdomen of uncertain etiology.

The abdominal ultrasound evaluation should include visible gas and fluid (to determine their luminal or extraluminal location), the perienteric soft tissues, and the GI tract itself. Identification of gas in a location where it is not usually found is a clue to many important diagnoses. The gas itself may appear as a bright, echo-

genic focus, but the identification of the *artifacts* associated with the gas pockets usually leads to their detection. These include both ringdown artifacts and "dirty" shadowing. Extraluminal gas may be intraperitoneal or retroperitoneal, and its presence should suggest either hollow viscus perforation (Fig. 8-26, *A* and *B*) or infection with gas-forming organisms[34] (*C* and *D*). Nonluminal gas may be easily overlooked, particularly if the collection is large. Gas in the wall of the GI tract, **pneumatosis intestinalis,** with or without gas in the portal veins, raises the possibility of ischemic gut.

Free intraperitoneal gas may be difficult to detect on sonography, and suspicion of its presence should prompt a recommendation for further imaging. The potential for large artifacts from gas to obscure visualization of part

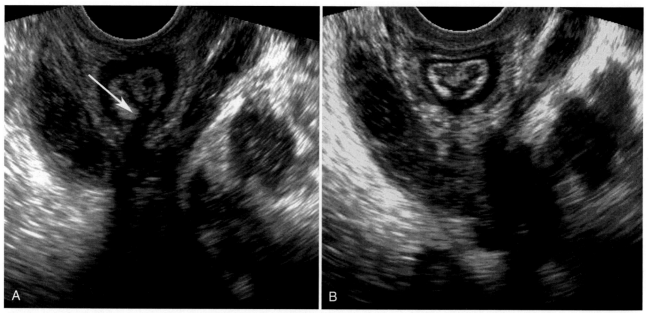

FIGURE 8-25. Perianal inflammatory Crohn's disease. A, Axial image of the anal canal shows an internal opening *(arrow)* posteriorly at 6 o'clock. A transphincteric fistula runs to a large, horseshoe-shaped posterior abscess more optimally shown in **B,** which also shows deeper collections in the left buttock.

ACUTE ABDOMEN: SONOGRAPHIC APPROACH

Gas
Intraluminal
Extraluminal
  Intraperitoneal
  Retroperitoneal
  Gut wall
  Gallbladder/biliary
    ducts
  Portal veins

Fluid
Intraluminal
  Normal caliber gut
  Dilated gut
Extraluminal
  Free
  Loculated

Masses
Neoplastic
Inflammatory

Perienteric Soft Tissues
Inflamed fat
Lymph nodes

Gut
Wall
Caliber
Peristalsis

Clinical Interaction
Palpable mass
Maximal tenderness
Sonographic
  Murphy's sign
  McBurney's sign

or all of a sonographic image leads many to avoid the challenge of ultrasound interpretation, with a preference for CT scan. However, there are valuable clues to the presence of intraperitoneal gas on sonography.

The likelihood of gas artifacts between the abdominal wall and the underlying liver to be related to free intraperitoneal gas was well described by Lee et al.[34] In my group's work, we have found that the peritoneal stripe

appears as a bright, continuous, echogenic line, and that air adjacent to the peritoneal stripe produces enhancement of this layer, because the gas has a higher acoustic impedance to sound waves than does the peritoneum itself (Fig. 8-26, *A* and *B*). Careful peritoneal assessment is best done with a 5-MHz probe or even a 7.5-mHz probe, with the focal zone set at the expected level of the peritoneum. In a clinical situation, enhancement of the peritoneal stripe is a highly specific but insensitive sign to detect pneumoperitoneum.[35]

Loculated **fluid collections** can mimic portions of the GI tract. Left upper quadrant and pelvic collections suggestive of the stomach and rectum may be clarified by adding fluid orally and rectally. Assessing peristaltic activity and wall morphology also helps in distinguishing luminal from extraluminal collections. Interloop and flank collections are aperistaltic and tend to correspond in contour to the adjacent abdominal wall or intestinal loops, frequently forming acute angles, which are rarely seen with intraluminal fluid.

The appearance of the **perienteric soft tissues** is frequently the first and most obvious clue to abdominal pathology on abdominal sonograms. Inflammation of the perienteric fat shows as a hyperechoic mass effect (see Fig. 8-15), often without the usual appearance of normal gut and its contained small pockets of gas. Neoplastic infiltration of the perienteric fat is often indistinguishable from inflammatory infiltration on ultrasound (see Fig. 8-8, *C* and *D*).

Mesenteric adenopathy is another manifestation of both inflammatory and neoplastic processes of the gut that should be specifically sought when performing

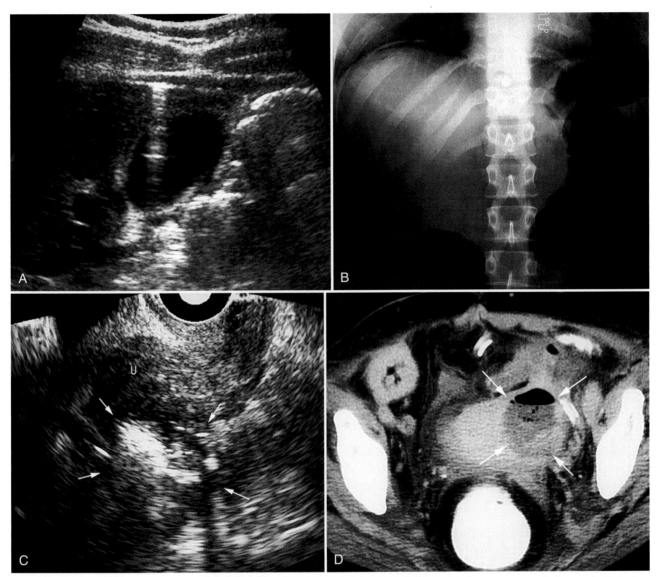

FIGURE 8-26. Value of gas for sonographic diagnosis in two patients. A and **B, Pneumoperitoneum A,** Sonogram shows a bright, echogenic focus representing free air between the abdominal wall and liver. Also shown is enhancement of the peritoneal stripe. **B,** Confirmatory plain film. **C** and **D, Unsuspected gas-containing abscess,** secondary to acute diverticulitis in a renal transplant recipient. **C,** Transvaginal image shows a large, gas-containing mass *(arrows)* posterior to the uterus. **D,** CT scan confirms gas-containing abscess. This type of abscess may be very difficult to appreciate on suprapubic scan. *(B from Muradali D, Wilson S, Burn PN, et al. A specific sign of pneumoperitoneum on sonography: enhancement of the peritoneal stripe. AJR Am J Roentgenol 1999; 17:1257-1262.)*

abdominal sonography. As elsewhere, lymph nodes tend to change in size and shape when replaced by abnormal tissue. A normal, oval or flattened lymph node with a normal linear hilar echo becomes increasingly round and hypoechoic with either inflammatory or neoplastic replacement. In contrast to the sonographic appearance of loops of gut, mesenteric lymph nodes typically appear as focal, discrete hypoechoic masses of varying size (see Fig. 8-16). Their identification on sonography suggests enlargement because they are not usually seen on routine examinations. Abnormal masses related to or causing a GI tract abnormality should also be sought; these most often are neoplastic or inflammatory in origin.

Right Lower Quadrant Pain

Acute Appendicitis

Acute appendicitis is the most common explanation for the "acute abdomen presentation" to an emergency department. Patients typically have right lower quadrant (RLQ) pain, tenderness, and leukocytosis. A mass may also be palpable. The patient with a classic presentation usually has an appendectomy without preoperative imaging. This approach often becomes complicated when a normal appendix is removed in a patient with symptomatology caused by other factors. On the other hand, surgery may be delayed in some patients with acute appendicitis if the presentation is atypical. This approach may lead to perforation before the surgery, making it a complicated and difficult procedure, often followed by abscess formation. In the clinical literature, laparotomy resulting in removal of normal, noninflamed appendices is reported in 16% to 47% of cases (mean, 26%).[36,37] Also, perforation may occur in up to 35% of patients.[38] It is a balance between this negative laparotomy rate and the perforation rate at surgery that motivates cross-sectional imaging before initiating treatment for the patient who presents with acute RLQ pain. For a patient with suspected appendicitis, the sonographic objectives are to identify the patient with acute appendicitis, to identify the patient without acute appendicitis, and in this latter population, to identify an alternate explanation for the RLQ pain.

Symptoms of appendicitis overlap with a variety of other gastrointestinal conditions, including acute typhlitis, acute mesenteric adenitis, variations of Crohn's disease, right-sided diverticulitis, acute segmental infarction of the omentum, and in women, acute gynecologic conditions.[39] It is important to recognize that not only can other conditions suggest acute appendicitis, but that acute appendicitis may also suggest other diagnoses, particularly acute **pelvic inflammatory disease** (PID). This occurs most often when the appendix is located in the true pelvis, in which case acute inflammatory change may implicate the uterine cervix and ovaries on clinical examination. The appendix is usually located caudal to the base of the cecum. It may also be retrocecal and retroileal. In a minority of patients, the appendix may be located in the true pelvis; this is the situation that causes diagnostic confusion, most often mistaken diagnosis with gynecologic disease.

From a retrospective review of 462 patients with suspected appendicitis who underwent appendectomy, Bendeck et al.[40] found that women in particular benefit most from preoperative imaging, with a statistically significant, lower negative appendectomy rate than women with no preoperative imaging. No similar improvement was found in the negative appendectomy rate for girls, boys, or men.

Both CT and ultrasound provide sensitive and accurate diagnosis of appendicitis. The choice of imaging modality is determined somewhat by local expertise.[41] Some institutions also screen patients on the basis of their weight, sending thin patients for ultrasound and reserving CT for larger patients. These considerations aside, we recommend **sonographic evaluation of all women**—with the addition of transvaginal scan for all patients whose pain is still not explained after completion of a traditional suprapubic pelvic sonogram.

The pathophysiology of acute appendicitis likely involves obstruction of the appendiceal lumen, with 35% of cases demonstrating a fecalith.[42] Mucosal secretions continue, increasing the intraluminal pressure and

---

ACUTE APPENDICITIS: SONOGRAPHIC DIAGNOSIS

Patient with right lower quadrant (RLQ) pain and elevated white blood cell (WBC) count.

IDENTIFY APPENDIX
Blind ended
Noncompressible
Aperistaltic tube
Gut signature
Arising from base of cecum
Diameter greater than 6 mm

SUPPORTIVE FEATURES
Inflamed perienteric fat
Pericecal collections
Appendicolith

---

compromising venous return. The mucosa becomes hypoxic and ulcerates. Bacterial infection ensues, eventually with gangrene and perforation. A walled-off abscess is more common than free peritoneal contamination.

Acute appendicitis begins with transient, visceral, or referred crampy pain in the periumbilical area associated with nausea and vomiting. Coincident with inflammation of the serosa of the appendix, the pain shifts to the RLQ and may be associated with physical signs of peritoneal irritation. Both clinical and experimental data support the belief that some patients have repeated attacks of appendicitis.[43,44] Surgical specimens have shown chronic inflammatory infiltrate in patients with recurrent attacks of RLQ pain before appendectomy.

In 1986, Puylaert[7] described the value of **graded compression sonography** in the evaluation of 60 consecutive patients suspected of having acute appendicitis. Since then, other investigators have improved the sonographic criteria for diagnosis, firmly establishing the value of sonography in assessing patients with equivocal evidence of appendicitis. The accuracy afforded by sonography should keep negative laparotomy rates at approximately 10%, clearly an improvement over the rate achieved by "instinct" alone.[45]

Puylaert's initial reports of success in diagnosing acute appendicitis with compression sonography depended solely on visualization of the abnormal appendix, a blind-ended, noncompressible, aperistaltic tube arising from the tip of the cecum with a gut signature (Fig. 8-27). However, other investigators reported seeing normal appendices on a sonogram[46,47] (Fig. 8-28). The normal appendix is compressible, with a wall thickness of 3 mm or less.[48] Jeffrey et al.[45] concluded that **size** can differentiate the normal from the acutely inflamed appendix. Threshold levels for the diameter of the appendix, above which acute appendicitis is highly likely, have been set at either 6 mm or 7 mm, with a resultant

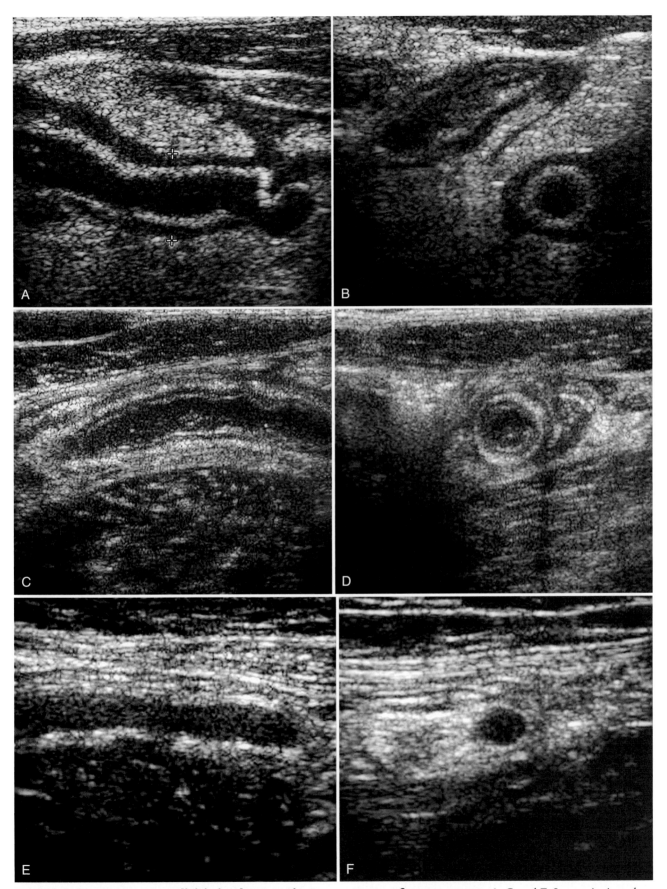

FIGURE 8-27. Acute appendicitis in three patients: spectrum of appearances. A, C, and **E,** Long-axis views show the blind-ended tip of the appendix. **C,** Tip is directed to the left of the image as the appendix ascends cephalad from its origin from the cecum. **B, D,** and **F,** Corresponding cross-sectional views. The appendix looks round in short axis on all cases, and the lumen is distended with fluid. The appendix is surrounded with inflamed fat. The gut signature is preserved in the top two cases *(A-D)*. The bottom case *(E, F)* shows loss of definition of the wall layers, suggesting gangrenous change.

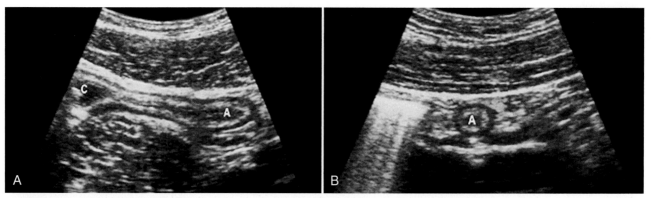

FIGURE 8-28. Normal appendix. A, Long-axis image, and **B,** cross-sectional image, show the normal appendix *(A)* arising from the base of the cecum *(C).* The appendix shows a gut signature, a blind end, and measures 6 mm or less in diameter.

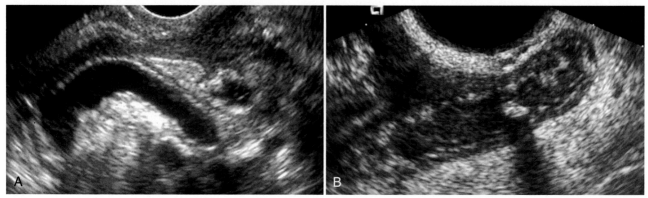

FIGURE 8-29. Value of transvaginal sonography for diagnosis of acute appendicitis. A, Long-axis view of the appendix on transvaginal sonography was the only view to show the blind-ended tip of the fluid-distended appendix. **B,** Appendix is large, fluid-filled, thick-walled structure and shows a shadowing appendicolith.

change in sensitivity and specificity. Sonographic visualization of an appendix with an **appendicolith,** regardless of appendiceal diameter, should also be regarded as a positive test. Rettenbacher et al.[49] added assessment of appendiceal **morphology** in confirming suspicion of appendicitis. A round or partly round appendix had a high correlation with acute appendicitis, whereas an ovoid appendix did not (see Fig. 8-27). Color Doppler is also contributory, showing hyperemia in the appendiceal wall in the acutely inflamed appendix.

Lee et al.[50] described graded compression sonography with adjuvant use of a **posterior manual compression technique** for diagnosis of acute appendicitis. Using graded compression sonography alone, the authors achieved visualization of the vermiform appendix in 485 of 570 patients (85%). Use of a posterior manual compression technique identified the vermiform appendix in an additional 57 of the remaining 85 patients, increasing the number of identified vermiform appendices to 542 (95%).

The appendix positioned in the true pelvis may show subtle evidence of inflammation on a suprapubic scan because the pathology may be deep in the pelvic cavity. In our experience, this occurs most often in women, possibly related to a more capacious pelvis, and the clini-

cal presentation is frequently that of PID. This particular pathology is optimally studied with transvaginal placement of the ultrasound probe because the appendix is often intimately related to either the uterus or the ovaries. The sonographic features required for diagnosis are identical, although the origin of such an appendix from the base of the cecum may be impossible to determine on transvaginal sonography, and compression with the ultrasound probe is often not feasible. Nonetheless, the identification of the blind-ended tip of the appendix with an increased diameter, luminal distention, and inflammation of the surrounding fat is obvious (Fig. 8-29). If rupture of a pelvic appendix has occurred before the sonogram, the identification of a pelvic abscess without identification of the appendix itself may produce an equivocal result as to the source of the pelvic inflammatory problem.

Although the sensitivity of sonography for the diagnosis of appendicitis decreases with **perforation,** features statistically associated with its occurrence include loculated pericecal fluid, phlegmon or abscess, prominent pericecal or periappendiceal fat, and circumferential loss of the submucosal layer of the appendix[51] (Fig. 8-30, *A* and *B*). False-positive diagnosis for acute appendicitis may occur if a normal appendix or a thickened terminal

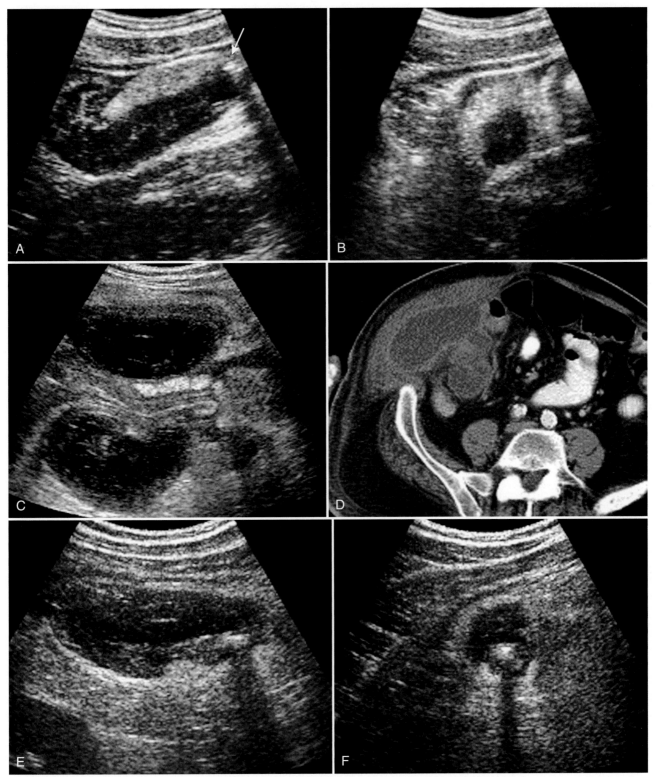

FIGURE 8-30. Perforation of appendix in three patients. A, Long-axis image, and **B,** cross-sectional image, show the blind-ended appendix. There is loss of definition of the wall layers, and the appendix is surrounded by an echogenic mass effect representing inflamed fat in the mesoappendix. In **A,** arrow points to a bubble of extraluminal gas at the tip of the appendix; tip perforation was confirmed at surgery. **C,** Sonogram, and **D,** CT scan, show a periappendiceal fluid collection, or abscess. The decompressed appendix is seen centrally on the sonogram. **E,** Long-axis, and **F,** transverse, images in the right lower quadrant show an abscess with an escaped appendicolith with acoustic shadowing. The appendix is no longer visible. (*C from Birnbaum BA, Wilson SR. Appendicitis at the millennium. Radiology 2000;215:337-348.*)

SONOGRAPHY OF APPENDICEAL PERFORATION

- Loculated pericecal fluid
  Phlegmon
  Abscess
- Prominent pericecal fat
- Circumferential loss of submucosal layer of the appendix

ileum is mistaken for an inflamed appendix. Awareness of the diagnostic criteria stated previously, particularly appendiceal diameter and morphology, should minimize these errors.

Clinical misdiagnosis of appendicitis occurs most frequently in young women with gynecologic conditions, especially acute PID, rupture or torsion of ovarian cysts, and postpartum ovarian vein thrombosis. As noted, Bendeck et al.[40] confirmed that women with suspected appendicitis benefit most from preoperative CT or ultrasound, with a statistically significant, lower negative appendectomy rate than women who undergo no preoperative imaging. They concluded that preoperative imaging should be part of the routine evaluation of women with suspected acute appendicitis.

Diseases other than those of gynecologic origin may also be misdiagnosed as acute appendicitis. Gastrointestinal illnesses include acute terminal ileitis with mesenteric adenitis,[52] acute typhlitis, acute diverticulitis (especially of cecal tip diverticulum), and Crohn's disease in the ileocecal area or involving the appendix itself.[53] Urologic disease, especially stone-related and right-sided segmental omental infarction, may also mimic acute appendicitis. Addressing the value of sonography in establishing an alternative diagnosis in patients with suspected acute appendicitis, Gaensler et al.[54] found that 70% of patients with another diagnosis had abnormalities visualized on the sonogram.

Crohn's Appendicitis

Patients with Crohn's disease may present with acute appendicitis caused by inflammatory bowel involvement of the appendix, in contrast to acute suppurative appendicitis. The wall of the appendix typically is extremely thickened and hyperemic with wall layer preservation, and the luminal surfaces are often in apposition[53] (Fig. 8-31). This appearance contrasts with that in suppurative appendicitis, where luminal distention is the expectation and wall thickening is moderate at best.

Crohn's appendicitis is a self-limited process,[55,56] and treatment may be conservative if the appropriate diagnosis can be established with noninvasive techniques. In a small number of the patients for whom we have suggested this diagnosis, follow-up sonograms have shown resolution of the sonographic findings with no disease

progression. Patients with Crohn's disease who present with Crohn's appendicitis account for about 10% of total presentations. This patient population typically has a more benign course. If the appendix is removed surgically in the mistaken belief that the patient has acute suppurative appendicitis, recurrence or progression of Crohn's disease is rare.

Right-Sided Diverticulitis

Acute inflammation of a right-sided diverticulum is distinct from the more common diverticulitis that is encountered in the left hemicolon. These diverticula occur more often in women than in men and have a predilection for Asian populations. Most patients are young adults. Right-sided diverticula are usually solitary and are congenital in origin. They are **true** diverticula and therefore have all layers of the gut wall. Their inflammation is associated with RLQ pain, tenderness, and leukocytosis, with a mistaken diagnosis of appendicitis in virtually all cases.

On sonography, acute diverticulitis is associated with inflammation of the pericolonic fat. The diverticula may be located in the cecum or the adjacent ascending colon. When inflamed, they may have one of two appearances.[57] Most often, the diverticulum may show as a pouch or saclike structure arising from the colonic wall[58] (Fig. 8-32). Wall layers are continued into the wall of the congenital diverticulum. Hyperemia of the diverticulum and the inflamed fat is typical. If a fecalith is present within the diverticulum, it may show as a bright, echogenic focus located within or beyond a segment of thickened colonic wall. Occasionally, the culprit diverticulum may not be evident, and the only observations may be the inflamed fat and the focal thickening of the colonic wall. In the appropriate clinical milieu, this is highly suspicious for acute diverticulitis.

Treatment of acute diverticulitis is conservative and not surgical, emphasizing the importance of preoperative imaging in patients with RLQ pain attributed to this condition.

Acute Typhlitis

Immunocompromised patients are most often affected with acute typhlitis, with **AIDS** patients and those with **acute myelogenous leukemia** accounting for the overwhelming majority of cases. **Cytomegalovirus** (CMV) and Cryptosporidium are the pathogens isolated most often in patients with typhlitis and colitis, although other organisms have been implicated. Sonographic study most often shows striking concentric, uniform thickening of the colon wall, usually localized to the cecum and the adjacent ascending colon[59] (Fig. 8-33). The colon wall may be several times the normal thickness, reflecting inflammatory infiltration throughout the gut wall.[60,61] Acute abdominal catastrophe in patients

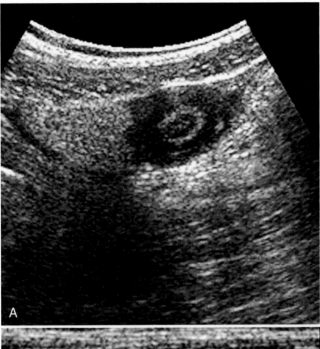

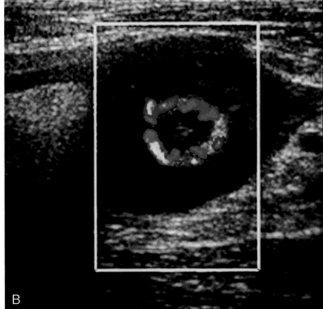

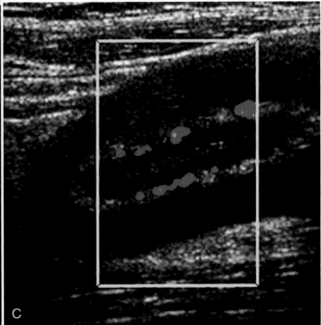

FIGURE 8-31. Crohn's appendicitis. A, Transverse sonogram in the right lower quadrant shows a thick-walled loop of gut surrounded by inflamed fat. **B,** Cross-sectional, and **C,** long-axis, high-frequency linear images of this loop of gut show that it is blind ended. There is massive mural thickening and hyperemia. The luminal surfaces are in apposition. All changes resolved completely with conservative management. *(From Wilson SR. The bowel wall looks thickened: what does that mean? In Cooperberg PL, editor.* Radiologic Society of North America categorical course syllabus. *Chicago, 2002, RSNA, pp 219-228.)*

with AIDS is usually a complication of CMV colitis with deep ulceration and may result in hemorrhage, perforation, and peritonitis.[62] **Tuberculous colitis** may similarly affect the right colon and is frequently associated with lymphadenopathy (particularly involving the mesenteric and omental nodes), splenomegaly, intrasplenic masses, ascites, and peritoneal masses, all of which may be assessed using sonography.

Mesenteric Adenitis with Terminal Ileitis

Mesenteric adenitis, in association with acute terminal ileitis, is the most frequent gastrointestinal cause of

misdiagnosis of acute appendicitis. Patients typically have RLQ pain and tenderness. On the sonographic examination, enlarged mesenteric lymph nodes and mural thickening of the terminal ileum are noted. *Yersinia enterocolitica* and *Campylobacter jejuni* are the most common causative agents.[52,63]

Right-Sided Segmental Omental Infarction

Right-sided segmental infarction of the omentum is a rare condition invariably mistaken clinically for acute appendicitis.[64] Of unknown etiology, it is postulated to occur with an anomalous and fragile blood supply to the

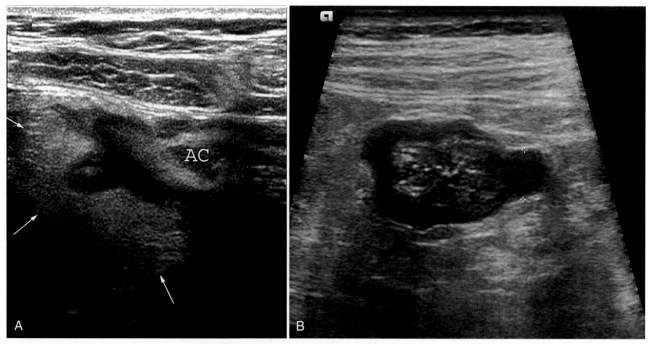

FIGURE 8-32. Right-sided diverticulitis in two patients. Transverse sonograms through the ascending colon *(AC)* show a hypoechoic pouchlike projection, representing the inflamed diverticulum, which arises from **A,** the lateral wall of the gut, and **B,** the medial border of the gut. Both are surrounded by inflamed fat *(arrows).*

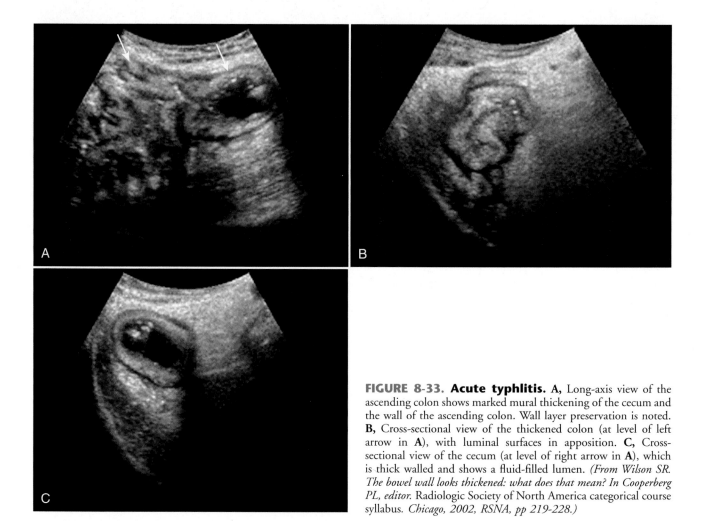

FIGURE 8-33. Acute typhlitis. A, Long-axis view of the ascending colon shows marked mural thickening of the cecum and the wall of the ascending colon. Wall layer preservation is noted. **B,** Cross-sectional view of the thickened colon (at level of left arrow in **A**), with luminal surfaces in apposition. **C,** Cross-sectional view of the cecum (at level of right arrow in **A**), which is thick walled and shows a fluid-filled lumen. *(From Wilson SR. The bowel wall looks thickened: what does that mean? In Cooperberg PL, editor.* Radiologic Society of North America categorical course syllabus. *Chicago, 2002, RSNA, pp 219-228.)*

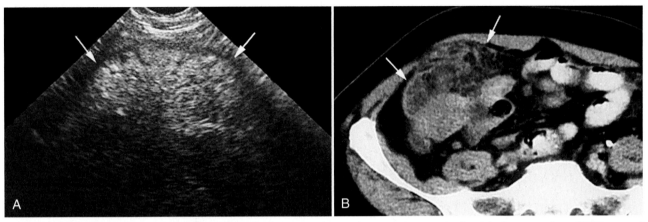

FIGURE 8-34. Acute omental infarction. A, Sonogram shows a large, tender mass in the right lower quadrant (RLQ; *arrows)* in elderly man with acute RLQ pain. The mass is uniformly echogenic and attenuating, with an ultrasound appearance suggesting inflamed fat. **B,** Confirmatory CT scan.

right lower omentum, making it susceptible to painful infarction.[65] Patients present with RLQ pain and tenderness and are diagnosed clinically with acute appendicitis. On sonography, a plaque or cakelike area of increased echogenicity, suggesting inflamed or infiltrated fat, is seen superficially in the right flank with adherence to the peritoneum[64] (Fig. 8-34). No underlying gut abnormality is shown. Because segmental infarction is a self-limited process, its correct diagnosis will prevent unnecessary surgery. CT scan is confirmatory, showing streaky fat in a masslike configuration in the right side of the omentum.

Left Lower Quadrant Pain

The sonographic evaluation of the patient with left lower quadrant (LLQ) pain is less problematic than that of the patient with pain on the right side. The potential causes for RLQ pain are not present for LLQ pain, and acute diverticulitis is the explanation for the overwhelming majority of cases for which a valid explanation for the pain is found. The diagnostic features of **acute diverticulitis** are also less variable than those for acute appendicitis, making a suspicion of diverticulitis a good indication for the use of sonographic examination.

Acute Diverticulitis

Diverticula of the colon are usually acquired deformities and are found most frequently in Western urban populations.[66] The incidence of diverticula increases with age,[67] affecting approximately half the population by the ninth decade. Muscular dysfunction and hypertrophy are constant associated features. Diverticula are usually multiple, and their most common location is the sigmoid and left colon. Acute diverticulitis and **spastic diverticulosis** may both be associated with a classic triad of presentation: LLQ pain, fever, and leukocytosis. Diverticula may also be found singly and in the right colon, where no

association with muscular hypertrophy or dysfunction has been established.

Inspissated fecal material is believed to incite the initial inflammation in the apex of the diverticulum leading to acute diverticulitis.[68] Spread to the peridiverticular tissues and microperforation or macroperforation may follow. Localized abscess formation occurs more often than peritonitis. Fistula formation, with communication to the bladder, vagina, skin, or other bowel loops, is present in a minority of cases. Surgical specimens demonstrate shortening and thickening of the involved segment of colon, associated with muscular hypertrophy. The peridiverticular inflammatory response may be minimal or extensive.

Sonography appears to be of value in early assessment of patients thought to have acute diverticulitis.[69,70] **Classic features** include segmental thickened gut and inflamed diverticula and inflamed perienteric fat. A negative scan combined with a low clinical suspicion is usually a good indication to stop investigation. However, a negative scan in a patient with a highly suggestive clinical picture justifies a CT scan. Similarly, demonstration of extensive pericolonic inflammatory changes on the sonogram may be appropriately followed by CT scan to define better the nature and extent of the pericolonic disease before surgery or other intervention.

Because diverticula and smooth muscle hypertrophy of the colon are so prevalent, it seems likely that they would be frequently seen on routine sonography, but this is not the usual experience. However, with the development of acute diverticulitis, both the inflamed diverticulum and the thickened colon become evident. Presumably, the impacted fecalith, with or without microabscess formation, accentuates the diverticulum, whereas smooth muscle spasm, inflammation, and edema accentuate the gut wall thickening. Identification of diverticula on the sonogram strongly indicates diverticulitis.[71]

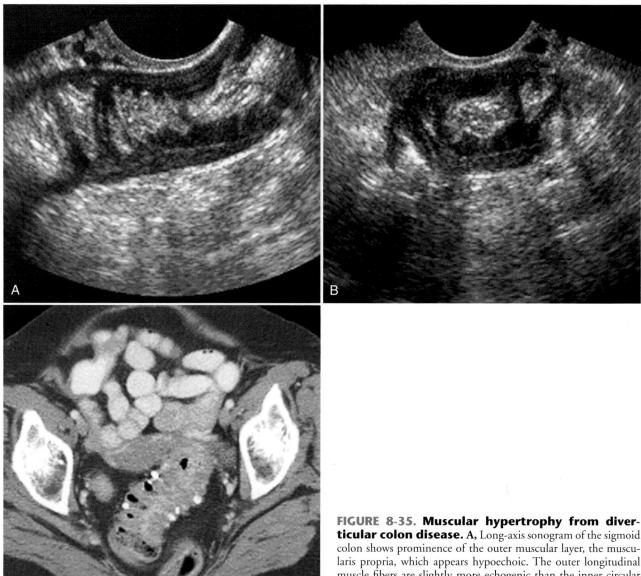

FIGURE 8-35. Muscular hypertrophy from diverticular colon disease. A, Long-axis sonogram of the sigmoid colon shows prominence of the outer muscular layer, the muscularis propria, which appears hypoechoic. The outer longitudinal muscle fibers are slightly more echogenic than the inner circular muscle fibers. **B,** Cross-sectional view. **C,** Characteristic CT scan shows the effects of the smooth muscle hypertrophy.

Diverticula are arranged in parallel rows along the margins of the teniae coli, so careful technique is required to make their identification. After demonstration of a thickened loop of gut, the long axis of the loop should be determined (Fig. 8-35). Slight tilting of the transducer to the margins of the loop will increase visualization of the diverticula, because they may be on the lateral and medial edges of the loop rather than directly anterior or posterior. Cross-sectional views are then obtained along the entire length of the thickened gut. Abnormalities must be confirmed on both views. Errors related to overlapping gut loops, in particular, can be virtually eliminated with this careful technique. Identification of diverticula on sonography is correlated highly with inflammation, because it is unusual to show the diverticula in the absence of inflammation (Fig. 8-36).

Failure to identify gas-containing abscesses or interloop abscesses is the major source of error when using sonography to evaluate patients with suspected diverticulitis. The meticulous technique of following involved thickened segments of colon in long-axis and transverse section will help detect even small amounts of extraluminal gas.

Sonographic features of diverticulitis include segmental concentric thickening of the gut wall that is frequently strikingly hypoechoic, reflecting the predominant thickening in the muscle layer (see Fig. 8-35); inflamed diverticula, seen as bright, echogenic foci with acoustic shadowing or ringdown artifact within or beyond the thickened gut wall (Fig. 8-37); acute inflammatory changes in the pericolonic fat, seen as poorly defined hyperechoic zones without obvious gas or fluid content

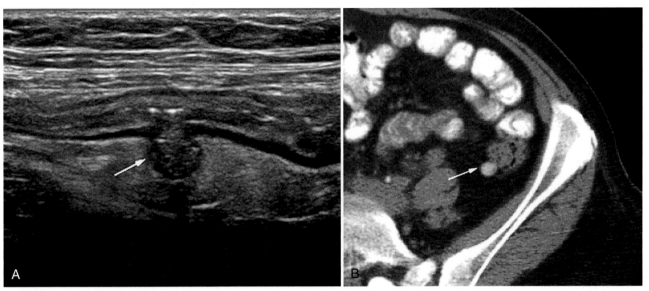

FIGURE 8-36. Diverticulum of colon. A, Long-axis sonogram, and **B,** correlative CT scan, show a small pouch *(arrows)* arising from the wall of the descending colon. There is mild inflammatory change in the perienteric fat.

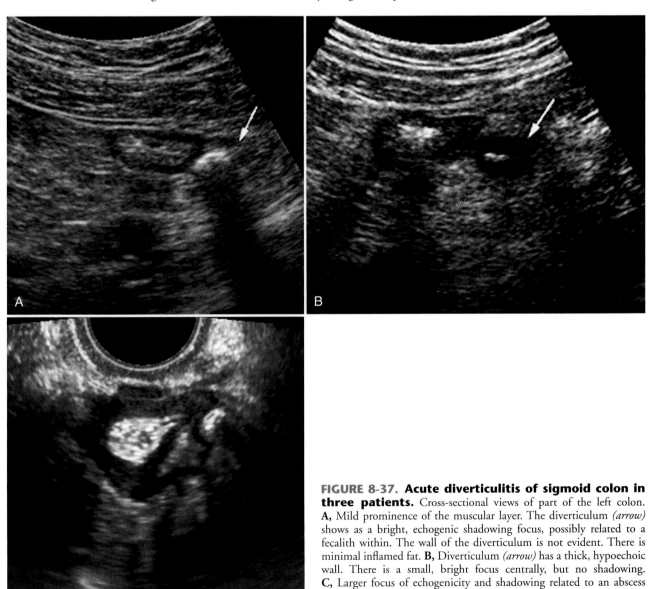

FIGURE 8-37. Acute diverticulitis of sigmoid colon in three patients. Cross-sectional views of part of the left colon. **A,** Mild prominence of the muscular layer. The diverticulum *(arrow)* shows as a bright, echogenic shadowing focus, possibly related to a fecalith within. The wall of the diverticulum is not evident. There is minimal inflamed fat. **B,** Diverticulum *(arrow)* has a thick, hypoechoic wall. There is a small, bright focus centrally, but no shadowing. **C,** Larger focus of echogenicity and shadowing related to an abscess that formed at the base of the inflamed diverticulum *(arrow).* Diverticula frequently show optimally on the cross-sectional images.

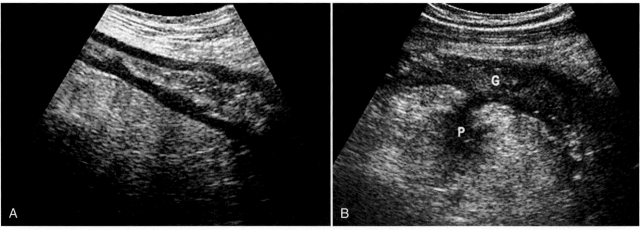

FIGURE 8-38. Pericolonic changes with diverticulitis in two patients. A, Long-axis view of descending colon shows a long segment of thickened gut with prominent muscularis propria. Edema of the perienteric fat is striking and shows as a homogeneous echogenic mass effect deep to the gut. **B,** Similarly inflamed fat; phlegmonous change (P) shows as a hypoechoic zone centrally within the fat; G, gut.

SONOGRAPHY OF DIVERTICULITIS

GUT
- Segmental concentric thickening of wall
  Hypoechoic reflecting muscular hypertrophy

INFLAMED DIVERTICULA
- Echogenic foci within or beyond gut wall
- Intramural sinus tracts
  High-amplitude linear echoes within gut wall
  Acoustic shadowing or "ringdown" artifact

PERIENTERIC SOFT TISSUE
- Inflammation of pericolonic fat
  Hyperechoic mass effect
- Thickening of the mesentery
- Abscess formation
  Loculated fluid collection
  Often with gas component
- Fistulas
  Linear tracts from gut to bladder, vagina, or
    adjacent loops
  Hypoechoic or hyperechoic

(Fig. 8-38); and abscess formation, seen as loculated fluid collections in an intramural, pericolonic, or remote location. With the development of extraluminal inflammatory masses, the diverticulum may no longer be identified on sonography, presumably being incorporated into the inflammatory process. Therefore, demonstration of a thickened segment of colon with an adjacent inflammatory mass may be consistent with diverticulitis, but also with neoplastic or other inflammatory disease. Intramural sinus tracts appear as high-amplitude, linear echoes, often with ringdown artifact, within the gut wall. Typically, the tracts are deep, between the muscularis propria and the serosa. Fistulas appear as linear tracts that extend from the involved segment of gut to the bladder, vagina, or

adjacent loops. Their echogenicity depends on their content, usually gas or fluid. Thickening of the mesentery and inflamed mesenteric fat may also be seen (Fig. 8-38).

The sonographic and clinical features of diverticulitis are more specific than those of acute appendicitis, and errors of diagnosis occur less often. However, torsion of appendices epiploicae (omentales) may produce a sonographic appearance so closely resembling acute diverticulitis that differentiation may be difficult.[71] The inflamed or infarcted fat of the appendix shows as shadowing of increased echogenicity related to the margin of the colon, mimicking an inflamed diverticulum. However, regional perienteric inflammatory change is usually minimal, with fewer systemic symptoms. The noninflamed colonic appendices epiploicae are not visible, except with ascites, where they are seen as uniformly spaced, echogenic foci along the margins of the colon.

OTHER ABNORMALITIES

Occlusion of the GI tract lumen producing obstruction may be either **mechanical,** where an actual physical impediment to the progression of the luminal content exists, or **functional,** where paralysis of the intestinal musculature impedes progression (paralytic ileus).[72]

Mechanical Bowel Obstruction

Mechanical bowel obstruction (MBO) is characterized by (1) dilation of the GI tract proximal to the site of luminal occlusion, (2) accumulation of large quantities of fluid and gas, and (3) hyperperistalsis as the gut attempts to pass the luminal content beyond the obstruction. If the process is prolonged, exhaustion and overdistention of the bowel loops may occur, with a secondary decrease in peristaltic activity. There are three broad categories of mechanical obstruction: **obturation**

obstruction, related to blockage of the lumen by material in the lumen; **intrinsic abnormalities of the gut wall** associated with luminal narrowing; and **extrinsic bowel lesions,** including adhesions. **Strangulation** obstruction develops when the circulation of the obstructed intestinal loop becomes impaired.

Sonography in patients with suspected MBO is usually not helpful because **adhesions,** the most common cause of intestinal obstruction, are not visible on the sonogram. Also, the presence of abundant **gas** in the intestinal tract, characteristic of most patients with obstruction, frequently produces sonograms of nondiagnostic quality. However, in the minority of patients with MBO who do not have significant gaseous distention, sonography may be helpful. In a prospective study of 48 patients, Meiser and Meissner[73] found that ultrasound was positive in 25% of patients with a "normal" plain film. Ultrasound alone allowed complete diagnosis of the cause of obstruction in six patients in a retrospective study of sonography on 26 patients with known colonic obstruction; it also correctly predicted the location of colonic obstruction in 22 cases (85%) and the etiology of the obstruction in 21 cases (81%).[11] Of 13 patients ultimately confirmed to have adenocarcinoma, five had a mass on sonography, five had segmental thickening, and 11 others showed a target sign of intussusception.

Sonographic study of potential MBO should include assessment of the following:
- Gastrointestinal tract **caliber** from the stomach to the rectum, noting any point at which the caliber alters (Fig. 8-39; see also Video 8-5).
- **Content** of any dilated loops, with special attention to their fluid and gaseous nature (Fig. 8-40; see also Video 8-7).
- **Peristaltic activity** within the dilated loops, which is typically greatly exaggerated and abnormal, frequently producing a to-and-fro motion of the luminal content. With strangulation, peristalsis may decrease or cease.

- **Site of obstruction** for *luminal* (large gallstones, bezoars,[74] foreign bodies, intussusception, occasional polypoid tumors), *intrinsic* (segmental gut wall thickening and stricture formation from Crohn's disease, annular carcinomas), and *extrinsic* (abscesses, endometriomas) abnormality as a cause of the obstruction.
- **Location of gut loops,** noting any abnormal position. Obstruction associated with external hernias is ideal for sonographic detection in that dilated loops of gut may be traced to a portion of the gut with normal caliber but abnormal location (Fig. 8-41). Spigelian and inguinal hernias are the types most frequently seen on sonograms.

Unique sonographic features are seen in the closed-loop and afferent loop obstructions, intussusception, and midgut malrotation. **Closed-loop obstruction** occurs if the bowel lumen is occluded at two points along its length, a serious condition that facilitates strangulation and necrosis. As the obstructed loop is closed off from the more proximal portion of the GI tract, little or no gas is present within the obstructed segments, which may become dilated and fluid filled. Consequently, the abdominal radiograph may be unremarkable (Fig. 8-42, *A*), and sonography may be most helpful by showing the dilated involved segments (Fig. 8-42, *B*) and often the normal-caliber bowel distal to the point of obstruction. The features of closed-loop obstruction are well described on ultrasound and include dilated small bowel, a C- or U-shaped bowel loop (Fig. 8-42, *C*), a whirl sign, and two adjacent collapsed loops.[75,76] This last important observation is difficult to observe on ultrasound, in contrast to CT scan. However, we have correctly suspected closed-loop obstruction in many patients on the basis of virtually normal plain films, small bowel dilation, and a U- or C-shaped bowel loop, especially if there is gut wall thickening or pneumatosis intestinalis suggesting gut infarction.

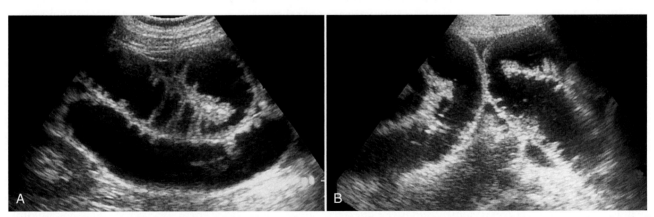

FIGURE 8-39. Mechanical small bowel obstruction. A, Sagittal image of right flank shows multiple, adjacent, long loops of dilated, fluid-filled small bowel with the classic morphology for a distal mechanical small bowel obstruction. **B,** Transverse image in the left lower quadrant confirms the multiplicity of dilated loops involved in the process. A small amount of ascites is seen between the dilated loops.

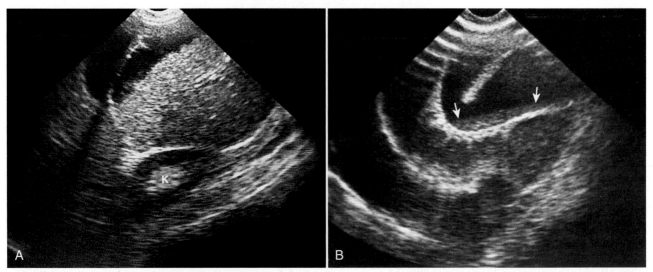

FIGURE 8-40. Dilated hypoperistaltic segments. A, Sagittal sonogram in the right flank of a patient with a Crohn's stricture shows gross dilation of the ascending colon. A long, fluid-sediment level is seen as a reflection of the hypoperistalsis of this segment of obstructed gut. *K,* Kidney. **B,** Sagittal sonogram in a patient with paralytic ileus shows extensive small bowel dilation. Loops are fluid filled and quiet with fluid-fluid level *(arrowheads)*. *(A from Sarrazin J, Wilson SR. Manifestations of Crohn disease at ultrasound. Radiographics 1996;16:499-520.)*

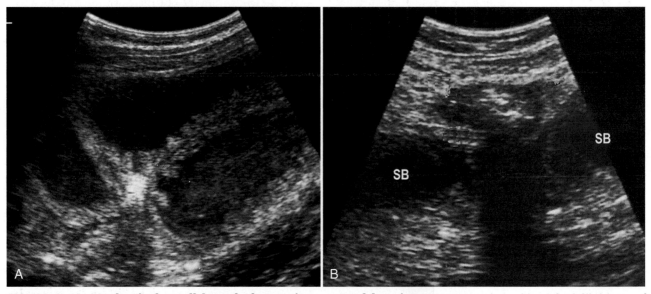

FIGURE 8-41. Mechanical small bowel obstruction: ventral hernia. A, Sonogram shows dilated fluid-filled loops of small bowel with edematous valvulae conniventes. **B,** Transverse paraumbilical sonogram shows normal-caliber gut lying in abnormal superficial location between two dilated loops of small bowel *(SB)*.

Afferent loop obstruction is an uncommon complication of subtotal gastrectomy, with Billroth II gastrojejunostomy, that may occur by twisting at the anastomosis, internal hernias, or anastomotic stricture. Again, a gasless, dilated loop may be readily recognized on sonography in a location consistent with the enteroenteric anastomosis coursing from the right upper quadrant across the midline. Its detection, location, and shape should allow for correct sonographic diagnosis of afferent loop obstruction.[77]

Intussusception, invagination of a bowel segment (the intussusceptum) into the next distal segment (the

intussuscipiens), is a relatively infrequent cause of MBO in the adult, usually associated with a tumor as a lead point. In our experience, this is often a lipoma that appears as a highly echogenic, intraluminal mass related to its fat content. A sonographic appearance of multiple concentric rings, related to the invaginating layers of the telescoped bowel and seen in cross section, is virtually pathognomonic[78] (Fig. 8-43, *A*). Occasionally, only a target appearance may be seen.[79] The longitudinal appearance suggesting a "hay fork"[80] is not as reliably detected. In both projections, the mesenteric fat invaginating with the intussusceptum will show as an eccentric

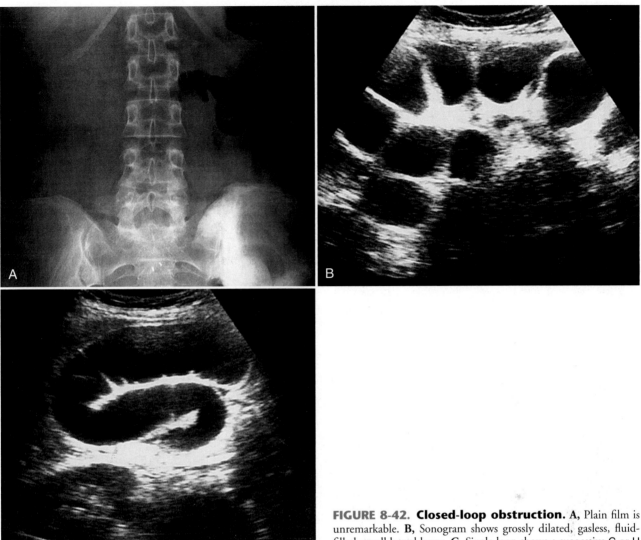

FIGURE 8-42. **Closed-loop obstruction. A,** Plain film is unremarkable. **B,** Sonogram shows grossly dilated, gasless, fluid-filled, small bowel loops. **C,** Single loop shows a suggestive C or U shape.

area of increased echogenicity. A lipoma, as a lead point, similarly shows as a focus of increased echogenicity (Fig. 8-43, *B* and *C*).

Midgut malrotation predisposes to MBO and infarction. It is infrequently encountered in adults. A sonographic abnormality related to the superior mesenteric vessels suggests malrotation.[81] On transverse sonograms, the superior mesenteric vein is seen on the left ventral aspect of the superior mesenteric artery, a reversal of the normal relationship.

Paralytic Ileus

Paralytic ileus is a type of bowel obstruction related to adynamic function of the bowel wall. Paralysis of the intestinal musculature, in response to general or local insult, may impede the progression of luminal contents. Although the lumen remains patent, no progression occurs. Sonography is usually of little value because these patients characteristically have poor-quality sonograms

resulting from large quantities of gas in the intestinal tract. However, on rare occasions, the sonogram may demonstrate dilated, fluid-filled, very quiet, or aperistaltic loops of intestine **(Video 8-7).** A fluid-fluid level in a dilated loop is characteristic of paralytic ileus, reflecting lack of movement of the intestinal contents (see Fig. 8-40, *B*).

Gut Edema

Patients with **acute vasculitis** of various etiologies may present with acute abdominal pain and ascites, with massive edema of the small bowel wall seen as the major abnormality on imaging. Hypoalbuminemia, congestive heart failure, and spontaneous venous thrombosis may also show diffuse edema of the gut wall. Prominent, thickened, hypoechoic valvulae conniventes[82] (Fig. 8-44) and gastric rugae are relatively easy to recognize on the sonographic study, which should also include Doppler evaluation of the mesenteric and portal veins.

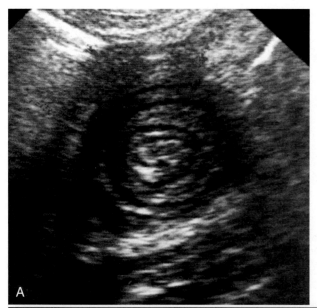

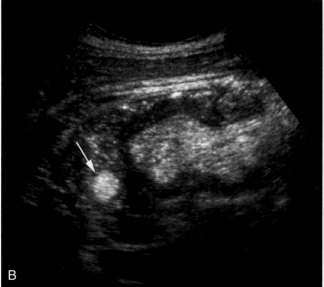

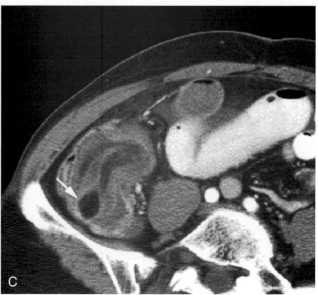

FIGURE 8-43. Intussusception in two patients. A, Sonogram shows multiple concentric rings representative of the invaginating intussuscipiens and the intussusceptum. Submucosal metastatic nodule as lead point. **B,** Sonogram of the right lower quadrant shows a highly echogenic lead point related to a lipoma *(arrow).* The invaginating fat in the mesentery is also echogenic. **C,** Confirmatory CT scan for image **B.** *(B and C from Wilson SR. The bowel wall looks thickened: what does that mean? In Cooperberg PL, editor.* Radiologic Society of North America categorical course syllabus. *Chicago, 2002, RSNA, pp 219-228.)*

Gastrointestinal Tract Infections

Although fluid-filled, actively peristaltic gut may be seen with infectious viral or bacterial gastroenteritis, most affected patients do not demonstrate a sonographic abnormality. However, some pathogens, notably *Yersinia enterocolitica, Mycobacterium tuberculosis,* and *Campylobacter jejuni,* produce highly suggestive sonographic abnormalities in the ileocecal area, as described earlier. Certain high-risk populations, such as those with AIDS and neutropenia,[59] appear to be susceptible to **acute typhlitis** and **colitis,** which also have a highly suggestive sonographic appearance.

AIDS Patients

Patients with AIDS are at increased risk for development of both GI tract neoplasia, especially lymphoma (see Fig.

8-10, *C* and *D*), and unusual opportunistic infections, most often *Candida* esophagitis and CMV colitis.[60,61] The relative incidence of infection compared with neoplasia is about 4:1 or 5:1. Acute typhlitis is described earlier (see Fig. 8-33). The frequent symptom of watery diarrhea, associated with a variety of small bowel pathogens, often shows nothing on sonography apart from an active and fluid-filled small bowel of normal thickness. Currently, with the use of triple-drug therapy, clinicians seldom encounter patients with AIDS-related gastrointestinal disease.

Pseudomembranous Colitis

Pseudomembranous colitis is a necrotizing inflammatory bowel condition that may occur as a response to a heterogeneous group of insults. At present, antibiotic therapy with effects from the toxin of *Clostridium diffi-*

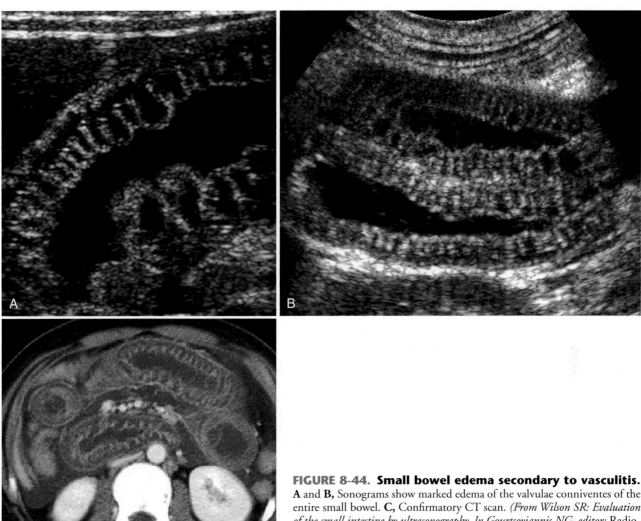

FIGURE 8-44. Small bowel edema secondary to vasculitis. **A** and **B,** Sonograms show marked edema of the valvulae conniventes of the entire small bowel. **C,** Confirmatory CT scan. *(From Wilson SR: Evaluation of the small intestine by ultrasonography. In Gourtsoyiannis NC, editor:* Radiological imaging of the small intestine. *Heidelberg, 2002, Springer-Verlag, pp 73-86.)*

cile, a normal inhabitant of the GI tract, is most often implicated.[83] Watery diarrhea is the most common symptom and usually occurs during antibiotic therapy but may be quite remotely associated, occurring up to 6 weeks later. Endoscopic demonstration of pseudomembranous exudative plaques on the mucosal surface of the gut and culture of the enterotoxin of *C. difficile* are diagnostic. Superficial ulceration of the mucosa is associated with inflammatory infiltration of the lamina propria and the submucosa, which may be thickened to many times the normal size.[84]

Sonography is frequently performed before pseudomembranous colitis is diagnosed, often based on a history of fever, abdominal pain, and watery diarrhea. Sonographic features have only rarely been described[85,86] but are suggestive of pseudomembranous colitis. Usually the entire colon is involved in a process that may produce striking thickening of the colon wall. Exaggerated haustral markings and a nonhomogeneous thickened submucosa, with virtual apposition of the mucosal surfaces of the thickened walls, are characteristic[58] (Fig. 8-45). Pseu-

domembranous colitis should be suspected in any patient with diffuse colonic wall thickening but without a previous history of IBD. Because the history of concurrent or prior antibiotic therapy is not always given, direct questioning of the patient is frequently helpful.

Congenital Cysts

Duplication cysts, characterized by the presence of the normal layers of the gut wall, may occur in any portion of the GI tract. These cysts may be visualized on sonogram, either routine or endoscopic, and should be considered as diagnostic possibilities whenever unexplained abdominal cysts are seen. **Tailgut cysts** are variants of abdominal cysts that are seen in the presacral region and are related to the rectum (Fig. 8-46).

Ischemic Bowel Disease

Ischemic bowel disease most often affects the colon and is most prevalent in elderly persons with arteriosclerosis.

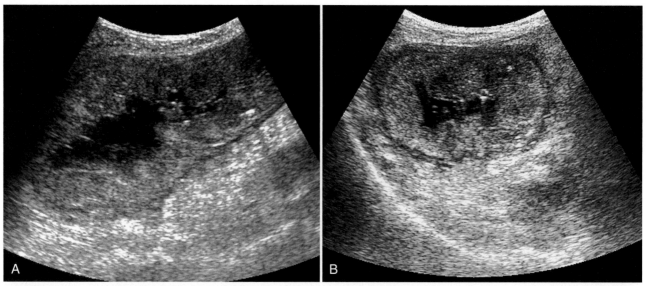

FIGURE 8-45. Pseudomembranous colitis. A, Long-axis view, and **B,** cross-sectional view, of the ascending colon show striking mural thickening of the gut wall. *(From O'Malley ME, Wilson SR. Ultrasound of gastrointestinal tract abnormalities with CT correlation. Radiographics 2003;23:59-72.)*

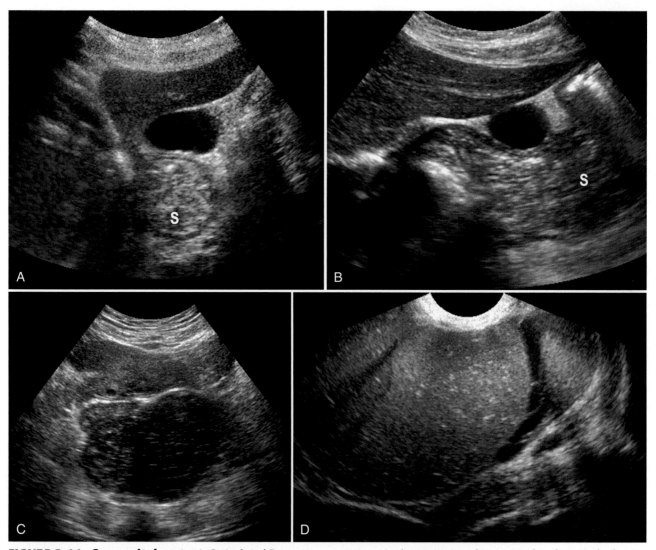

FIGURE 8-46. Congenital cysts. A, Sagittal, and **B,** transverse, sonograms in the epigastrium show an incidental gastric duplication cyst adjacent to the lesser curve of the stomach(s). **C,** Suprapubic, and **D,** transvaginal, pelvic scans show a complex, presacral pelvic mass, an incidental tailgut cyst.

In younger patients, it may complicate cardiac arrhythmia, vasculitis, coagulopathy, embolism, shock, or sepsis.[12] Sonographic features of ischemic bowel disease have been poorly described, although gut wall thickening may be encountered. Pneumatosis intestinalis may complicate gut ischemia with a characteristic sonographic appearance.

Pneumatosis Intestinalis

Pneumatosis intestinalis is a relatively rare condition in which intramural pockets of gas are found throughout the GI tract. It has been associated with a wide variety of underlying conditions, including chronic obstructive pulmonary disease, collagen vascular disease, IBD, traumatic endoscopy, and post–jejunoileal bypass. In many situations, affected patients are asymptomatic and the observation is incidental. However, its demonstration is of great clinical significance when necrotizing enterocolitis or ischemic bowel disease is present. Both conditions are associated with mucosal necrosis in which gas from the lumen passes to the gut wall.

Sonographic description of pneumatosis intestinalis is limited to isolated case reports. High-amplitude echoes may be demonstrated in the gut wall, with typical air artifact or shadowing[87,88] (Fig. 8-47). Gut wall thickening may be noted if the pneumatosis is associated with underlying IBD. If gut ischemia is suspected, careful evaluation of the liver is recommended to look for evidence of portal venous air.

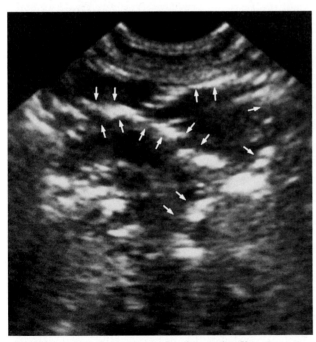

FIGURE 8-47. Pneumatosis intestinalis. Sonogram shows three loops of gut with bright, high-amplitude echoes (arrows) originating within the gut wall.

Mucocele of Appendix

Mucocele of the appendix is relatively uncommon; occurring in 0.25% of 43,000 appendectomy specimens in one series. Many patients with this condition are asymptomatic. A mass may be palpated in approximately 50% of cases. **Benign** and **malignant** varieties occur in a ratio of approximately 10:1.[89] In the benign form the appendiceal lumen is obstructed by either inflammatory scarring or fecaliths. The glandular mucosa in the isolated segment continues to secrete sterile mucus. The neoplastic variety of mucocele is associated with primary mucous **cystadenoma** or **cystadenocarcinoma** of the appendix. Although the gross morphology of the appendix may be similar in the benign and malignant varieties, the malignant form is often associated with pseudomyxoma peritonei if rupture occurs.[90]

On sonography, **mucoceles** typically produce large, hypoechoic, well-defined RLQ cystic masses with variable internal echogenicity, wall thickness, and wall calcification (Fig. 8-48). The internal contents often show a laminated or whorled appearance. These masses are frequently retrocecal and may be mobile. Although their sonographic appearance is not always specific, the diagnostic possibility of mucocele should be considered when an elongated oval cystic mass is found in the right lower quadrant in any patient with an appendix.[91]

Gastrointestinal Tract Hematoma

Blunt abdominal trauma, complicated by duodenal hematoma and rectal trauma, either sexual or iatrogenic after rectal biopsy, are the major causes of local hematomas seen on sonography. Hematoma is usually localized to the submucosa. Larger or more diffuse hematomas may complicate anticoagulation therapy or bleeding disorders associated with leukemia. If hematomas are large, diffuse gut wall thickening may be seen on sonograms.

Peptic Ulcer

Peptic ulcer, a defect in the epithelium to the depth of the submucosa, may be seen in either **gastric** or **duodenal** locations. Although rarely visualized, peptic ulcer has a fairly characteristic sonographic appearance. A gas-filled ulcer crater is seen as a bright, echogenic focus with ringdown artifact, either in a focal area of wall thickening or beyond the wall, depending on the depth of penetration (Fig. 8-49). **Edema** in the acute phase and **fibrosis** in the chronic phase may produce localized wall thickening and deformity.

Bezoars

Bezoars are masses of foreign material or food, typically found in the stomach after surgery for peptic ulcer disease (**phytobezoars**) or after ingestion of indigestible

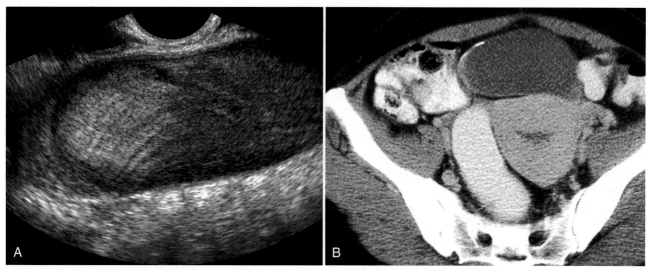

FIGURE 8-48. Mucocele of the appendix. A, Sonogram, and **B,** CT scan, show a large, mucus-filled appendix as an incidental observation. The whorled appearance on the sonogram is characteristic. There is a fleck of calcification in the wall on the CT scan.

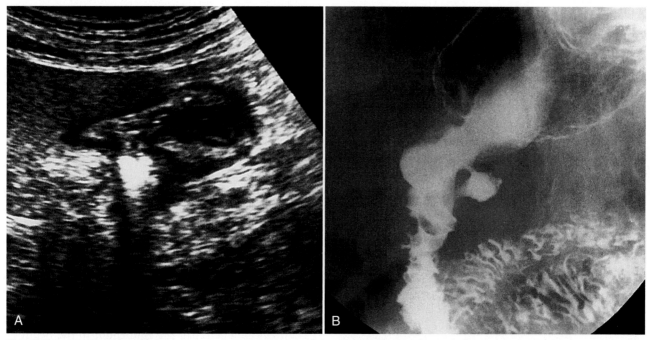

FIGURE 8-49. Peptic ulcer. A, Cross-sectional sonogram of the stomach shows a hypoechoic eccentric mass with a bright, central echogenic focus representing air in the ulcer crater. **B,** Confirmatory scan with barium swallow.

organic substances such as hair **(trichobezoars).** These masses may produce shadowing intraluminal densities on the sonogram and have been documented as a rare cause of small bowel obstruction.[74] They may also form in the small bowel in association with chronic stasis.

Intraluminal Foreign Bodies

Large foreign bodies, including bottles, candles, sexual vibrators, contraband, tools, and food, may be identified in the GI tract, particularly in the rectum and sigmoid colon, where they produce fairly sharp, distinct specular echoes with sharp, acoustic shadows. Their recognition is enhanced by suspicion of their presence.

Celiac Disease

Undiagnosed adult patients with celiac disease are encountered infrequently in general ultrasound departments. Nonetheless, I have occasionally seen patients in whom sonography is the first test to suggest the correct diagnosis. Sonographic observations include abnormal fluid-filled small intestine with moderate dilation of the involved loops. Abnormal morphology is observed, which Dietrich et al.[92] describe as a reduction in Kerckring's plicae circulares (valvulae conniventes) with loss of density and uniformity. Peristalsis is increased above normal. An increase in the caliber of the superior mesenteric artery and portal vein may also be seen.[93] I have also observed frequent intermittent intussusception in this patient population.

Cystic Fibrosis

Aggressive treatment of the pulmonary problems of cystic fibrosis (CF) increases the likelihood of encountering adult patients in a general ultrasound department that performs abdominal sonography. Thickening of the gut wall, particularly of the right hemicolon and to a lesser extent the left colon and small bowel, may be seen in association with infiltration of both the pericolonic and the mesenteric fat.[94] These may often be incidental observations without significant associated symptomatology. In advanced CF, a fibrosing colonopathy with stricture may be seen.[95,96] The culture of *C. difficile* is also documented in some patients with CF and colon wall thickening, without the accompanying symptoms of abdominal pain and diarrhea.[97] However, positive stool culture is not the rule in CF patients with detectable colon wall thickening.

ENDOSONOGRAPHY

Endoscopic sonography, performed with high-frequency transducers in the lumen of the gut, allows for detection of mucosal abnormality, delineation of the layers of the gut wall, and definition of the surrounding soft tissues to a depth of 8 to 10 cm from the transducer crystal. Thus, tumors hidden below normal mucosa, tumor penetration into the layers of the gut wall, and tumor involvement of surrounding vital structures or lymph nodes may be well evaluated. Staging of previously identified mucosal tumors is one of the major applications of endosonographic technique.

Upper Gastrointestinal Tract

Rotating, high-frequency transducers, using 7.5-MHz crystals fitted into a fiberoptic endoscope, are most suitable for endosonography of the esophagus, stomach, and duodenum. Light sedation of the patient is usually required. The patient is placed in the left lateral decubitus position and the endoscope inserted to the desired location. Intraluminal gas is aspirated, and a balloon covering the transducer crystal is inflated with deaerated water. Localization is determined from the distance of insertion from the teeth and identification of anatomic landmarks, such as the spleen, liver, pancreas, and gall-bladder. Rotation and deflection of the transducer tip allow scanning of visualized lesions in different planes.[98]

Identification, localization, and characterization of benign masses are possible with endosonography. **Varices** are seen as compressible hypoechoic or cystic masses deep to the submucosa or in the outer layers of the esophagus, gastroesophageal junction, or gastric fundus.[99] Benign tumors such as **fibromas** or **leiomyomas** are well-defined, solid masses without mucosal involvement that can be localized to the layer of the wall from which they arise, usually the submucosa and the muscularis propria, respectively. Peptic ulcer typically produces marked thickening of all layers of the gastric wall, with a demonstrated ulcer crater. Ménétrier's disease produces thickening of the mucosal folds.

Staging of **esophageal carcinoma** involves assessment of depth of tumor invasion and evaluation of involvement of the local lymph nodes and adjacent vital structures.[100] Constricting lesions that do not allow passage of the endoscope may produce technically unsatisfactory or incomplete examinations.

Gastric lymphoma is typically very hypoechoic; its invasion is along the gastric wall or horizontal, and involvement of extramural structures and lymph nodes is less than with gastric carcinoma. Thus, localized mucosal ulceration with extensive infiltration of the deeper layers suggests lymphoma, which may also grow with a polypoid pattern or as a diffuse infiltration without ulceration.[101] **Gastric carcinoma,** in contrast, arises from the gastric mucosa, is usually more echogenic, tends to invade vertically or through the gastric wall, and frequently involves the perigastric lymph nodes at diagnosis.

Rectum: Tumor Staging of Rectal Carcinoma

Transrectal (endorectal) sonography is an established modality for the staging of rectal carcinoma. Its resolution of the layers of the rectum surpasses the performance of both CT and MRI (Fig. 8-50). Although a variety of pathologic conditions may be assessed with endorectal sonography, the **staging of previously detected rectal carcinoma** is its major role. Patients are scanned in the left lateral decubitus position following a cleansing enema. Both axial and sagittal images are obtained. A variety of rigid intrarectal probes are now commercially available, using a range of transducer technologies with phased array, mechanical sector, and rotating crystals. In our laboratory, a rigid biplane probe now replaces the traditional probe with a mechanical rotating crystal, which demonstrates the rectum on axial imaging as a multilayered circle.

Further, we have also been routinely evaluating women with rectal carcinoma using a transvaginal probe placed in the vagina after a Fleet enema. This technique is excellent, especially for larger tumors, because the

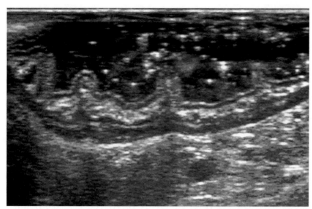

FIGURE 8-50. Normal rectal endosonogram. This patient had a Fleet enema, and there is fluid within the rectal lumen. The wall layers are well depicted. Muscle layers are hypoechoic, and submucosa is the dominant echogenic layer. Perirectal fat appears echogenic or white. A small, normal node is shown in the perirectal fat as a around small, hypoechoic nodule. *(From Berton F, Gola G, Wilson SR. Perspective on the role of transrectal and transvaginal sonography of tumors of the rectum and anal canal. AJR Am J Roentgenol 2008;190:1495-1504.)*

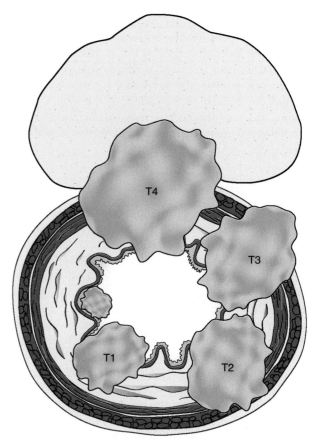

FIGURE 8-51. Schematic of tumor (T) component of TNM staging of rectal cancer on sonography. Tumors *(red)* exhibit progressively deeper invasion beginning at 10 o'clock, where T superficial noninvasive lesion involves only superficial layers of intestinal wall. At 7 o'clock, T1 lesion invades submucosa *(yellow)*. At 5 o'clock, T2 lesion invades muscularis propria *(blue)*. At 2 o'clock, T3 lesion exhibits full-thickness invasion through layers of rectal wall, with invasion of surrounding perirectal fat. In directly anterior aspect (12 o'clock), T4 lesion exhibits invasion of prostate gland. *(From Berton F, Gola G, Wilson SR. Perspective on the role of transrectal and transvaginal sonography of tumors of the rectum and anal canal. AJR Am J Roentgenol 2008;190:1495-1504.)*

rectovaginal septum, the tumor, and the lymph nodes in the mesorectum are more optimally seen.[102]

Tumors are staged according to the Astler-Coller modification[103] of the Dukes Classification, or more simply with the **primary tumor** component of the Union Internationale Contre le Cancer (UICC) **TNM classification**,[104] where **T** represents the primary tumor, **N** the nodal involvement, and **M** the distant metastases (Fig. 8-51).

Rectal carcinoma arises from the mucosal surface of the gut. Tumors appear as relatively hypoechoic masses that may distort the rectal lumen. Invasion of the deeper layers, the submucosa, the muscularis propria, and the perirectal fat produces discontinuity of these layers on the sonogram (Figs. 8-52 and 8-53). Superficial ulceration or crevices that allow small bubbles of gas to be trapped deep to the crystal surface may demonstrate ringdown artifact and shadowing, with loss of layer definition deep to the ulceration. Lymph nodes appear as round or oval, hypoechoic masses in the perirectal fat. Color Doppler is an excellent addition to transrectal probes, showing the extent of tumors on the basis of their hypervascularity (Fig. 8-54). Sonographically, many visible nodes may be **reactive** rather than neoplastic, and normal-sized nodes may have microscopic invasion (see Fig. 8-52). Infrequently, actual deposits may be shown within enlarged nodes (see Fig. 8-53). Therefore, definitive staging requires pathologic assessment of both the tumor and the regional nodes.

Wang et al.[105] studied six normal and 16 neoplastic colorectal specimens in vitro with an 8.5-MHz ultrasound transducer. They accurately demonstrated invasion of the submucosa in 92.5% and invasion of the muscularis propria in 77%. Invasive tumors with exten-

sion beyond the muscularis propria were accurately predicted 90% of the time. In vivo studies support this excellent result.[106,107] Comparing preoperative transrectal ultrasound and CT staging in 102 consecutive patients, Rifkin et al.[108] found transrectal sonography superior to CT in assessment of tumor extent and in the detection of lymph node involvement.

Limitations of rectal sonography include the following:

1. Inability to identify microscopic tumor invasion
2. Inability to image stenotic tumors
3. Inability to image tumors greater than 15 cm from the anal verge
4. Inability to distinguish nodes involved with tumor from those with reactive change
5. Inability to identify normal-sized nodes with microscopic tumor invasion

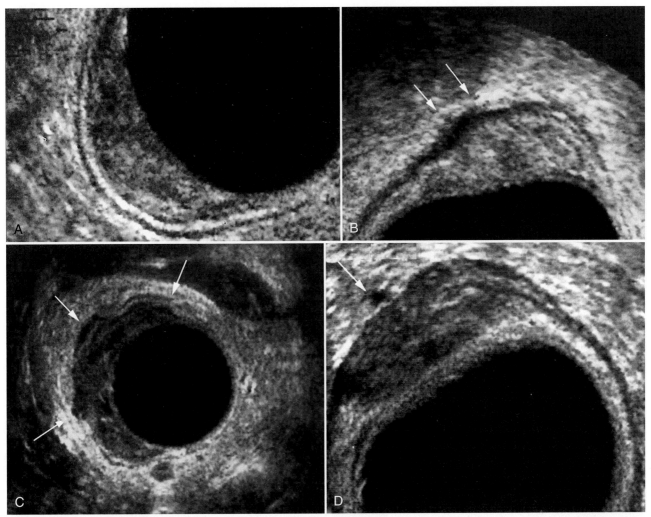

FIGURE 8-52. Rectal tumors seen at transrectal sonography. A, Rectal carcinoma: **T1.** Hypoechoic mass between 6 o'clock and 8 o'clock is noted. The submucosa—the echogenic line—and the muscularis propria—the external hypoechoic line—are intact. **B, Rectal carcinoma: T2.** Tumor is seen anteriorly. The muscularis propria *(arrows)* is the hypoechoic line that is thickened and nodular, consistent with tumor involvement. **C, Rectal carcinoma: T3.** A large tumor involves the entire right lateral wall of the rectum. Invasion of the perirectal fat *(arrows)* is noted in several locations. A large node is seen at the 6 o'clock position; smaller nodes are seen at 5 o'clock and 8 o'clock. **D, Metastatic carcinoma to rectal wall.** Hypoechoic mass is seen between 10 o'clock and 1 o'clock. It involves the deep layers of the rectal wall and not the rectal mucosa. There is a small lymph node *(arrow).*

Despite these limitations, endorectal ultrasound appears to be an excellent imaging tool for preoperative staging of accessible rectal cancers.

Cancer of the anal canal is a very rare tumor that is well shown on anal sonography (Fig. 8-55).

Recurrent rectal cancer after local resection is usually extraluminal, involving the resection margin secondarily. Serial transrectal sonography may be used in conjunction with serum carcinoembryonic antigen (CEA) levels to detect these recurrences. A pericolic hypoechoic mass or local thickening of the rectal wall, in either deep or superficial layers, is taken as evidence of recurrence. Previous radiation treatment may produce a diffuse thickening of the entire rectal wall, usually of moderate or high echogenicity, with an appearance that is usually easily differentiated from the focal hypoechoic appearance of recurrent cancer. Sonographic-guided biopsy of a

detected abnormality facilitates histologic differentiation of recurrence from postoperative, inflammatory, or postradiation change.

Prostatic carcinoma may invade the rectum directly, or more remote tumors may involve the rectum, usually as a result of seeding to the posterior peritoneal pouch. Because these tumors initially involve the deeper layers of the rectal wall, with mucosal involvement occurring as the disease progresses, their sonographic appearance is distinct from that of primary rectal carcinoma (see Fig. 8-52, *D*).

Benign mesenchymal tumors, especially of smooth muscle origin, are uncommon in the rectum. When seen, their sonographic features are the same as elsewhere (Fig. 8-56). **Mucous retention cysts,** resulting from obstruction of mucous glands, produce cystic masses of varying size that are located deep in the rectal wall.

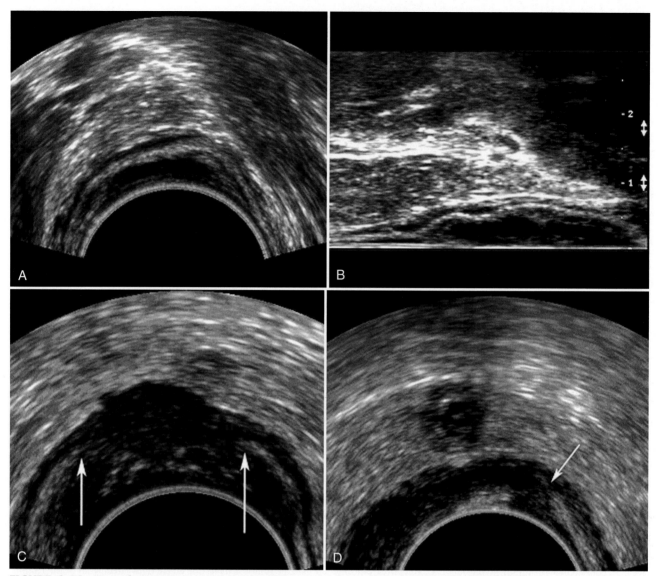

FIGURE 8-53. Rectal tumors on transrectal sonography, using biplane technology. A and B, **Superficial T1 cancer** in 42-year-old woman with a small, palpable mass on digital rectal examination. Curved axial (**A**) and linear sagittal (**B**) images show hypoechoic tumor with subtle involvement of the echogenic submucosa. **C, T3 rectal carcinoma** on an axial image in 56-year-old man. Gross extension of tumor into perirectal fat is evident. Echogenic margins *(arrows)* of remaining submucosa are present on each side of invasive tumor. **D,** Extensive **T3 mucinous rectal adenocarcinoma** in 64-year-old man. Axial image shows destruction of submucosa, the echogenic edge *(arrow)* of which is evident on right side of image. Enlarged, round perirectal node shows a hypoechoic tumor deposit. *(From Berton F, Gola G, Wilson SR. Perspective on the role of transrectal and transvaginal sonography of tumors of the rectum and anal canal. AJR Am J Roentgenol 2008;190:1495-1504.)*

Anal Canal

Fecal Incontinence

Anal endosonography, performed with the addition of a hard cone attachment to a radial 7.5-MHz probe, allows accurate assessment of the anal canal, including the internal and external sphincters.[109] Performed primarily for assessment of fecal incontinence, this test shows the integrity of the sphincters with documentation of the degree and size of muscle defects.

Young women, following traumatic obstetric delivery, are most often afflicted with fecal incontinence. We, and others, have found transvaginal assessment of the anal sphincter—performed with a side-firing transvaginal probe close to the introitus—to be as equally effective as a transanal approach.[31,108,110-112]

The internal anal sphincter, in continuity with the muscularis propria of the rectum above, is seen as a circular hypoechoic or black ring just deep to the convoluted mucosal echoes (Fig. 8-57). The external anal sphincter, in contrast, is less well defined and more echogenic, appearing gray on the ultrasound examination, and in continuity with fibers from the puborectalis sling. Traumatic disruption of the muscle layers will show as defects in the continuity of the normal muscle texture, most often anterior (Fig. 8-58). Posttraumatic scarring may be associated with a change of shape of the anal canal from round to oval (see Fig. 8-57).

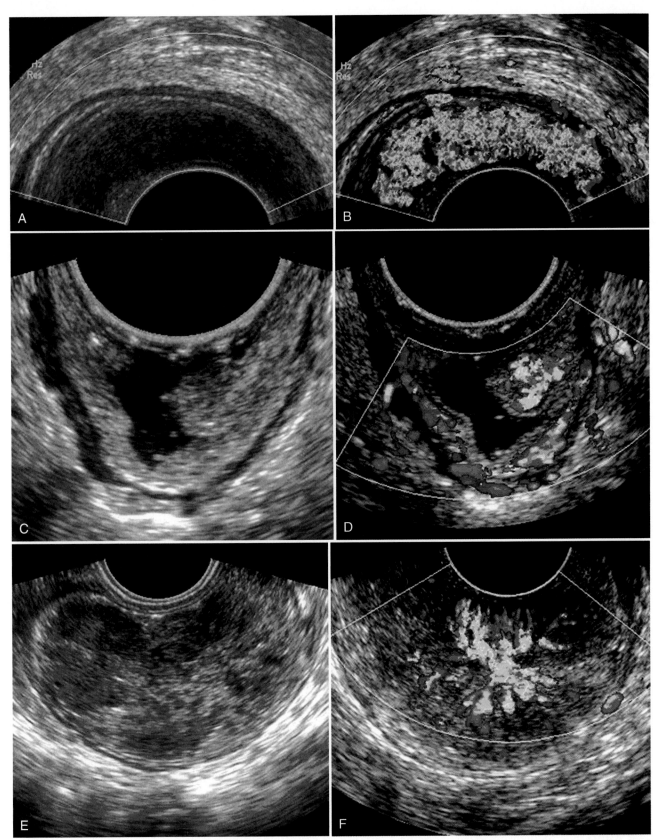

FIGURE 8-54. Contribution of Color Doppler at transrectal sonography to staging and diagnosis of rectal cancer. A and **B, T2 rectal cancer** in 58-year-old man. **A,** Axial image shows hypoechoic tumor. Destruction of submucosa is evident with involvement of muscularis propria on right side of image. **B,** Color Doppler at default setting shows typical hypervascularity. Color demarcates tumor from normal rectal wall on left side of image. **C** and **D,** Small **rectal adenocarcinoma** originating in adenomatous polyp in 55-year-old man. **C,** Axial image shows an isoechoic polypoid mass with a broad base surrounded by fluid within the rectal lumen. Mass involves the submucosal layer only. **D,** Color Doppler image shows profuse vascularity and vascular stalk of the polypoid mass. **E** and **F,** tubulovillous adenoma in 58-year-old woman. **E,** Axial transvaginal image shows a mixed-echogenic mass that seems to fill the lumen of the rectum. **F,** Color Doppler frequently shows this type of stellate, branching vascularity in tubulovillous tumors. *(From Berton F, Gola G, Wilson SR. Perspective on the role of transrectal and transvaginal sonography of tumors of the rectum and anal canal. AJR Am J Roentgenol 2008;190:1495-1504.)*

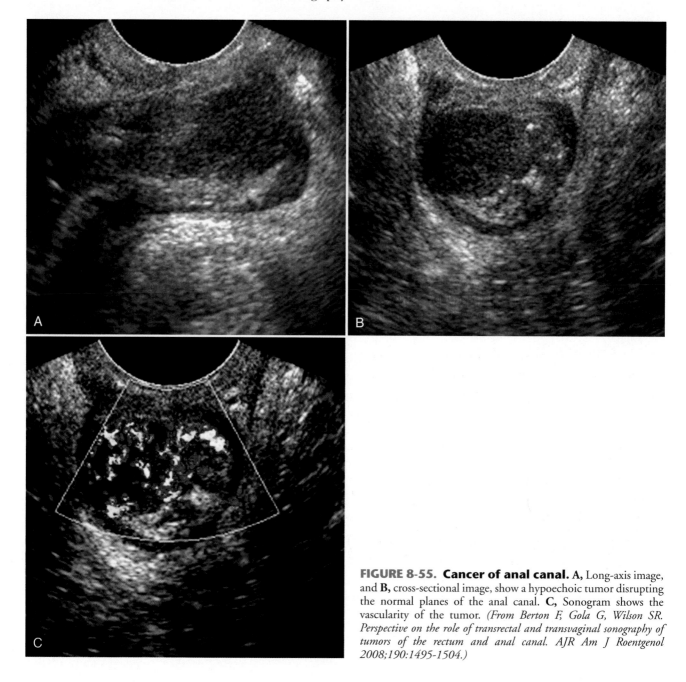

FIGURE 8-55. Cancer of anal canal. A, Long-axis image, and **B,** cross-sectional image, show a hypoechoic tumor disrupting the normal planes of the anal canal. **C,** Sonogram shows the vascularity of the tumor. *(From Berton F, Gola G, Wilson SR. Perspective on the role of transrectal and transvaginal sonography of tumors of the rectum and anal canal. AJR Am J Roentgenol 2008;190:1495-1504.)*

Perianal Inflammatory Disease

Perianal inflammatory disease is seen in two distinct patient populations: (1) those with **Crohn's disease** who develop perianal inflammation as part of their disease and (2) those who develop a **perianal abscess** or **perianal fistula** as a spontaneous event. The first group is described earlier in the section on Crohn's disease. In other patients, perianal infection arises in small, intersphincteric anal glands predominantly located at the dentate line. This occurs most frequently in young adult men. Documentation of fluid collections and the relationship of inflammatory tracts to the sphincter mechanism are important for surgical treatment.

Transanal sonography for assessment of perianal inflammatory disease is limited because placement of the rigid probe into the anal canal does not allow assessment of disease in the perineal region. We prefer transvaginal sonography in conjunction with transperineal sonography in women and transperineal sonography in men for evaluation of this problem.

Scans are performed with curved and high-frequency linear probes placed firmly on the skin of the perineum between the introitus and the anal canal in women and between the scrotum and the anal canal in men.[110] Firm pressure on the transducer is required to afford good visualization of the anal canal. We begin the procedure with the transducer in the transverse plane relative to the

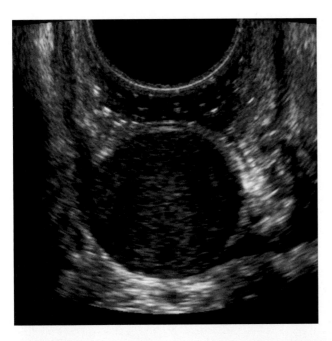

FIGURE 8-56. Gastrointestinal stromal tumor (GIST) of rectum. Transrectal sonographic image shows solid, well-defined, round mass arising from muscularis propria layer in 59-year-old woman with asymptomatic palpable mass found at routine physical examination. Tumor is growing with submucosal pattern, and mucosal surface bulges into fluid-filled lumen.

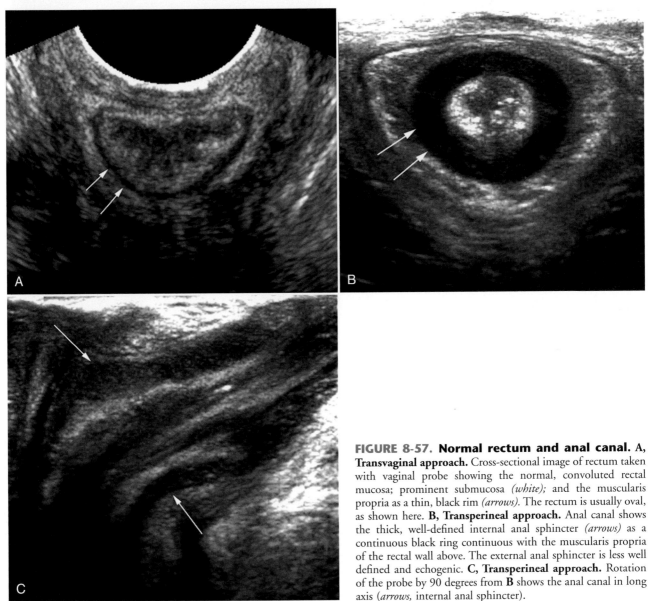

FIGURE 8-57. Normal rectum and anal canal. **A, Transvaginal approach.** Cross-sectional image of rectum taken with vaginal probe showing the normal, convoluted rectal mucosa; prominent submucosa *(white);* and the muscularis propria as a thin, black rim *(arrows).* The rectum is usually oval, as shown here. **B, Transperineal approach.** Anal canal shows the thick, well-defined internal anal sphincter *(arrows)* as a continuous black ring continuous with the muscularis propria of the rectal wall above. The external anal sphincter is less well defined and echogenic. **C, Transperineal approach.** Rotation of the probe by 90 degrees from **B** shows the anal canal in long axis *(arrows, internal anal sphincter).*

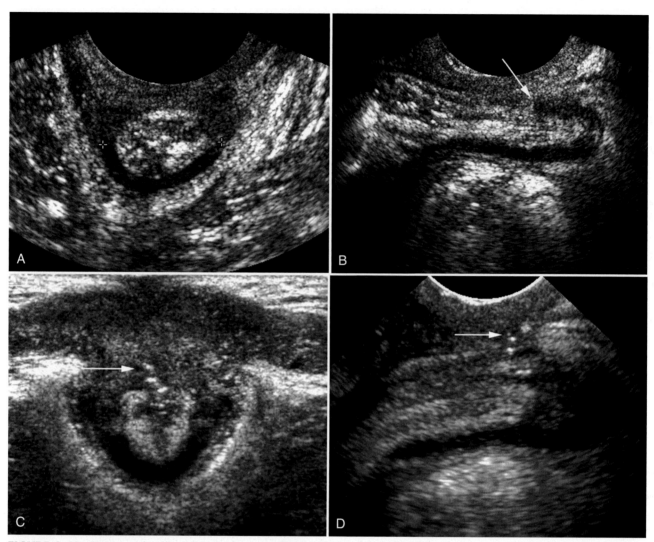

FIGURE 8-58. Traumatic disruption of anal sphincter in two patients. A, Cross-sectional, and **B,** long-axis, views of the anal canal from a transvaginal approach show disruption of the sphincter anteriorly from 9 to 3 o'clock. The arrow on the sagittal image shows the cephalad extent of the internal anal sphincter. **C,** Cross-sectional, and **D,** long-axis, views of the anal canal show full-thickness disruption of the anterior anal canal between 11 and 1 o'clock. The arrow in each image shows air bubbles within an anovaginal fistula.

SONOGRAPHY OF PERIANAL INFLAMMATORY DISEASE

- Internal opening in the anal canal or rectum
- Tracts and their relationship to anal sphincter
- External openings
- Fluid collections

body. The transducer should be directed cephalad and anterior to the plane of the anal canal, then angled slowly through the plane of the anal canal, which will show it in cross section from the anorectal junction to the external anal opening. Rotation of the transducer by 90 degrees will allow for imaging in the longitudinal plane. Tracts and collections in the perineum, buttocks,

scrotum, and labia can also be assessed and followed in a retrograde direction to their connection with the anal canal.

Perianal inflammatory tracts and masses are classified according to Parks et al.[113] Their classification provides an anatomic description of fistulous tracts, which acts as a guide to operative treatment. The four main subtypes are **intersphincteric** (between internal and external sphincter), **transsphincteric** (crossing both internal and external anal sphincter into ischiorectal or ischioanal fossa), **suprasphincteric,** and **extrasphincteric.** In each patient, we also document the internal opening and the external openings, as possible. Tracts show on the ultrasound scan as hypoechoic linear areas or fluid-containing tubular areas, depending on their size and activity (Fig. 8-59). As with fistulas elsewhere, air bubbles within the tract show as bright, echogenic foci that may move during the scan, helping with their identification. In our

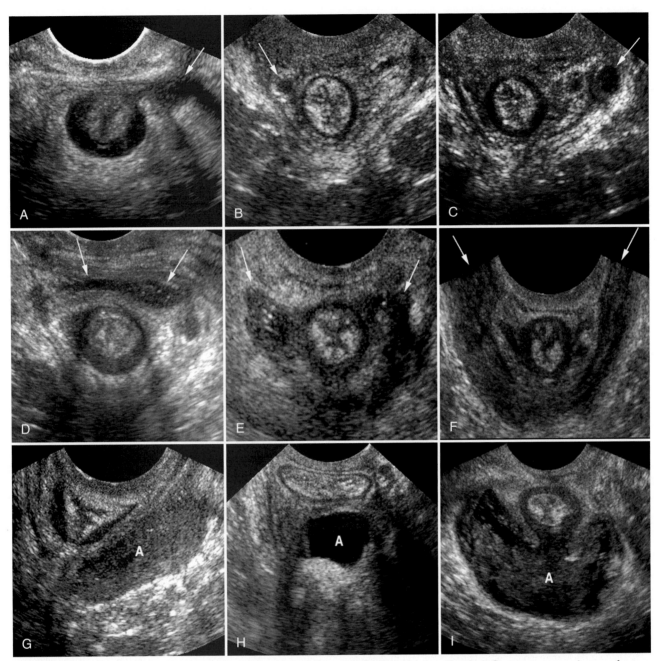

FIGURE 8-59. Perianal inflammatory disease in nine patients. *Top row,* **Simple inflammatory openings and tracts** *(arrows).* Cross-sectional images of the anal canal show internal opening at 1 o'clock with **A,** transsphincteric tract running to a small collection; **B,** intersphincteric tract; **C,** larger extrasphincteric tract. *Middle row,* **More complex tracts** *(arrows).* **D,** Anterior extrasphincteric tract shows fluid within. **E,** Bilateral, complex, intersphincteric tracts and collections show bright, echogenic foci representing extraluminal air. **F,** Boomerang, or horseshoe, tract surrounds the anal canal posteriorly and laterally. There are internal openings at 2, 4, and 9 o'clock. *Bottom row,* **Perianal abscesses** *(A).* **G,** Abscess on left posterolateral aspect of the anal canal is particle filled. **H,** Large, posterior abscess is complex, with a dependent debris level. **I,** Large, posterior abscess shows a large internal opening posteriorly at 6 o'clock.

initial experience with 54 patients with perianal inflammatory masses, sonographic findings were confirmed in 22 of 26 patients (85%) who underwent surgical treatment for their disease.

Acknowledgment

The author would like to acknowledge Gordana Popovich for her artwork.

References

Anatomy and Sonographic Technique
1. Bolondi L, Caletti G, Casanova P, et al. Problems and variations in the interpretation of the ultrasound feature of the normal upper and lower GI tract wall. Scand J Gastroenterol Suppl 1986;123:16-26.
2. Heyder N, Kaarmann H, Giedl J. Experimental investigations into the possibility of differentiating early from invasive carcinoma of the stomach by means of ultrasound. Endoscopy 1987;19:228-232.
3. Kimmey MB, Martin RW, Haggitt RC, et al. Histologic correlates of gastrointestinal ultrasound images. Gastroenterology 1989;96:433-441.

4. Wilson SR. The bowel wall looks thickened: what does that mean? In: Cooperberg PL, editor. Radiologic Society of North America categorical course syllabus. Chicago: RSNA; 2002. p. 219-228.

5. Lutz HT, Petzoldt R. Ultrasonic patterns of space occupying lesions of the stomach and the intestine. Ultrasound Med Biol 1976; 2:129-132.

6. Bluth EI, Merritt CR, Sullivan MA. Ultrasonic evaluation of the stomach, small bowel, and colon. Radiology 1979;133:677-680.

7. Puylaert JB. Acute appendicitis: ultrasound evaluation using graded compression. Radiology 1986;158:355-360.

8. Teefey SA, Roarke MC, Brink JA, et al. Bowel wall thickening: differentiation of inflammation from ischemia with color Doppler and duplex ultrasound. Radiology 1996;198:547-551.

Gastrointestinal Tract Neoplasms

9. Winawer SJ, Sherlock P. Malignant neoplasms of the small and large intestine. In: Sleisenger MH, Fordtran JS, editors. Gastrointestinal disease: pathophysiology, diagnosis, management. 3rd ed. Philadelphia: Saunders; 1983.

10. Lim JH. Colorectal cancer: sonographic findings. AJR Am J Roentgenol 1996;167:45-47.

11. Lim JH, Ko YT, Lee DH, et al. Determining the site and causes of colonic obstruction with sonography. AJR Am J Roentgenol 1994;163:1113-1137.

12. Fenoglio-Preiser CM, Lantz PE, Listrom M, et al, editors. Gastrointestinal pathology: an atlas and text. 2nd ed. New York: Lippincott-Raven; 1999.

13. Kaftori JK, Aharon M, Kleinhaus U. Sonographic features of gastrointestinal leiomyosarcoma. J Clin Ultrasound 1981;9:11-15.

14. Derchi LE, Banderali A, Bossi C, et al. The sonographic appearances of gastric lymphoma. J Ultrasound Med 1984;3:251-256.

15. Salem S, Hiltz CW. Ultrasonographic appearance of gastric lymphosarcoma. J Clin Ultrasound 1978;6:429-440.

16. Telerman A, Gerard B, van den Heule B, Bleiberg H. Gastrointestinal metastases from extra-abdominal tumors. Endoscopy 1985; 17:99-101.

17. Rubesin SE, Levine MS. Omental cakes: colonic involvement by omental metastases. Radiology 1985;154:593-596.

18. Yeh HC. Ultrasonography of peritoneal tumors. Radiology 1979; 133:419-424.

Inflammatory Bowel Disease: Crohn's Disease

19. Sarrazin J, Wilson SR. Manifestations of Crohn disease at ultrasound. Radiographics 1996;16:499-520.

20. DiCandio G, Mosca F, Campatelli A, et al. Sonographic detection of postsurgical recurrence of Crohn disease. AJR Am J Roentgenol 1986;146:523-526.

21. Fraquelli M, Colli A, Casazza G, et al. Role of ultrasound in detection of Crohn disease: meta-analysis. Radiology 2005;236: 95-101.

22. Horsthuis K, Bipat S, Bennink RJ, Stoker J. Inflammatory bowel disease diagnosed with ultrasound, MR, scintigraphy, and CT: meta-analysis of prospective studies. Radiology 2008;247:64-79.

23. Dubbins PA. Ultrasound demonstration of bowel wall thickness in inflammatory bowel disease. Clin Radiol 1984;35:227-231.

24. Worlicek H, Lutz H, Heyder N, Matek W. Ultrasound findings in Crohn's disease and ulcerative colitis: a prospective study. J Clin Ultrasound 1987;15:153-163.

25. Spalinger J, Patriquin H, Miron MC, et al. Doppler ultrasound in patients with crohn disease: vessel density in the diseased bowel reflects disease activity. Radiology 2000;217:787-791.

26. Van Oostayen JA, Wasser MN, van Hogezand RA, et al. Doppler sonography evaluation of superior mesenteric artery flow to assess Crohn's disease activity: correlation with clinical evaluation, Crohn's disease activity index, and alpha$_1$-antitrypsin clearance in feces. AJR Am J Roentgenol 1997;168:429-433.

27. Serra C, Menozzi G, Labate AM, et al. Ultrasound assessment of vascularization of the thickened terminal ileum wall in Crohn's disease patients using a low–mechanical index real-time scanning technique with a second-generation ultrasound contrast agent. Eur J Radiol 2007;62:114-121.

28. Parente F, Maconi G, Bollani S, et al. Bowel ultrasound in assessment of Crohn's disease and detection of related small bowel strictures: a prospective comparative study versus x ray and intraoperative findings. Gut 2002;50:490-495.

29. Gasche C, Moser G, Turetschek K, et al. Transabdominal bowel sonography for the detection of intestinal complications in Crohn's disease. Gut 1999;44:112-117.

30. Stewart LK, McGee J, Wilson SR. Transperineal and transvaginal sonography of perianal inflammatory disease. AJR Am J Roentgenol 2001;177:627-632.

31. Damani N, Wilson SR. Nongynecologic applications of transvaginal ultrasound. Radiographics 1999;19 Spec No:179-200; quiz 65-66.

Acute Abdomen

32. Puylaert JB. Ultrasound of acute GI tract conditions. Eur Radiol 2001;11:1867-1877.

33. Seibert JJ, Williamson SL, Golladay ES, et al. The distended gasless abdomen: a fertile field for ultrasound. J Ultrasound Med 1986; 5:301-308.

34. Lee DH, Lim JH, Ko YT, Yoon Y. Sonographic detection of pneumoperitoneum in patients with acute abdomen. AJR Am J Roentgenol 1990;154:107-109.

35. Muradali D, Wilson S, Burns PN, et al. A specific sign of pneumoperitoneum on sonography: enhancement of the peritoneal stripe. AJR Am J Roentgenol 1999;173:1257-1262.

36. Kazarian KK, Roeder WJ, Mersheimer WL. Decreasing mortality and increasing morbidity from acute appendicitis. Am J Surg 1970; 119:681-685.

37. Pieper R, Forsell P, Kager L. Perforating appendicitis: a nine-year survey of treatment and results. Acta Chir Scand Suppl 1986; 530:51-57.

38. Van Way 3rd CW, Murphy JR, Dunn EL, Elerding SC. A feasibility study of computer aided diagnosis in appendicitis. Surg Gynecol Obstet 1982;155:685-688.

39. Berry Jr J, Malt RA. Appendicitis near its centenary. Ann Surg 1984;200:567-575.

40. Bendeck SE, Nino-Murcia M, Berry GJ, Jeffrey Jr RB. Imaging for suspected appendicitis: negative appendectomy and perforation rates. Radiology 2002;225:131-136.

41. Birnbaum BA, Wilson SR. Appendicitis at the millennium. Radiology 2000;215:337-348.

42. Shaw RE. Appendix calculi and acute appendicitis. Br J Surg 1965;52:451-459.

43. Dachman AH, Nichols JB, Patrick DH, Lichtenstein JE. Natural history of the obstructed rabbit appendix: observations with radiography, sonography, and CT. AJR Am J Roentgenol 1987;148:281-284.

44. Savrin RA, Clausen K, Martin Jr EW, Cooperman M. Chronic and recurrent appendicitis. Am J Surg 1979;137:355-357.

45. Jeffrey Jr RB, Laing FC, Lewis FR. Acute appendicitis: high-resolution real-time ultrasound findings. Radiology 1987;163:11-14.

46. Abu-Yousef MM, Bleicher JJ, Maher JW, et al. High-resolution sonography of acute appendicitis. AJR Am J Roentgenol 1987; 149:53-58.

47. Jeffrey Jr RB, Laing FC, Townsend RR. Acute appendicitis: sonographic criteria based on 250 cases. Radiology 1988;167:327-329.

48. Rioux M. Sonographic detection of the normal and abnormal appendix. AJR Am J Roentgenol 1992;158:773-778.

49. Rettenbacher T, Hollerweger A, Macheiner P, et al. Ovoid shape of the vermiform appendix: a criterion to exclude acute appendicitis: evaluation with ultrasound. Radiology 2003;226:95-100.

50. Lee JH, Jeong YK, Hwang JC, et al. Graded compression sonography with adjuvant use of a posterior manual compression technique in the sonographic diagnosis of acute appendicitis. AJR Am J Roentgenol 2002;178:863-868.

51. Borushok KF, Jeffrey Jr RB, Laing FC, Townsend RR. Sonographic diagnosis of perforation in patients with acute appendicitis. AJR Am J Roentgenol 1990;154:275-278.

52. Puylaert JB, Lalisang RI, van der Werf SD, Doornbos L. *Campylobacter* ileocolitis mimicking acute appendicitis: differentiation with graded-compression ultrasound. Radiology 1988;166:737-740.

53. Agha FP, Ghahremani GG, Panella JS, Kaufman MW. Appendicitis as the initial manifestation of Crohn's disease: radiologic features and prognosis. AJR Am J Roentgenol 1987;149:515-518.

54. Gaensler EH, Jeffrey Jr RB, Laing FC, Townsend RR. Sonography in patients with suspected acute appendicitis: value in establishing alternative diagnoses. AJR Am J Roentgenol 1989;152:49-51.

55. Higgins MJ, Walsh M, Kennedy SM, et al. Granulomatous appendicitis revisited: report of a case. Dig Surg 2001;18:245-248.
56. Roth T, Zimmer G, Tschantz P. [Crohn's disease of the appendix]. Ann Chir 2000;125:665-667.
57. Chou YH, Chiou HJ, Tiu CM, et al. Sonography of acute right side colonic diverticulitis. Am J Surg 2001;181:122-127.
58. O'Malley ME, Wilson SR. Ultrasound of gastrointestinal tract abnormalities with CT correlation. Radiographics 2003;23:59-72.
59. Teefey SA, Montana MA, Goldfogel GA, Shuman WP. Sonographic diagnosis of neutropenic typhlitis. AJR Am J Roentgenol 1987; 149:731-733.
60. Balthazar EJ, Megibow AJ, Fazzini E, et al. Cytomegalovirus colitis in AIDS: radiographic findings in 11 patients. Radiology 1985; 155:585-589.
61. Frager DH, Frager JD, Brandt LJ, et al. Gastrointestinal complications of AIDS: radiologic features. Radiology 1986;158:597-603.
62. Teixidor HS, Honig CL, Norsoph E, et al. Cytomegalovirus infection of the alimentary canal: radiologic findings with pathologic correlation. Radiology 1987;163:317-323.
63. Puylaert JB. Mesenteric adenitis and acute terminal ileitis: ultrasound evaluation using graded compression. Radiology 1986;161: 691-695.
64. Puylaert JB. Right-sided segmental infarction of the omentum: clinical, ultrasound, and CT findings. Radiology 1992;185:169-172.
65. Bender MD, Ockner RK. Diseases of the peritoneum, mesentery and diaphragm. In: Sleisenger MH, Fordtran JS, editors. Gastrointestinal disease: pathophysiology, diagnosis, management. 5th ed. Philadelphia: Saunders; 1993. p. 2004-2011
66. Painter NS, Burkitt DP. Diverticular disease of the colon, a 20th century problem. Clin Gastroenterol 1975;4:3-21.
67. Parks TG. Natural history of diverticular disease of the colon. Clin Gastroenterol 1975;4:53-69.
68. Fleischner FG, Ming SC. Revised concepts on diverticular disease of the colon. II. So-called diverticulitis: diverticular sigmoiditis and perisigmoiditis; diverticular abscess, fistula, and frank peritonitis. Radiology 1965;84:599-609.
69. Parulekar SG. Sonography of colonic diverticulitis. J Ultrasound Med 1985;4:659-666.
70. Wilson SR, Toi A. The value of sonography in the diagnosis of acute diverticulitis of the colon. AJR Am J Roentgenol 1990;154:1199-1202.
71. Derchi LE, Reggiani L, Rebaudi F, Bruschetta M. Appendices epiploicae of the large bowel: sonographic appearance and differentiation from peritoneal seeding. J Ultrasound Med 1988;7:11-14.

Other Abnormalities
72. Jones RS. Intestinal obstruction, pseudo-obstruction, and ileus. In: Sleisenger MH, Fordtran JS, editors. Gastrointestinal disease: pathophysiology, diagnosis, management. 5th ed. Philadelphia: Saunders; 1993. p. 898-903.
73. Meiser G, Meissner K. [Sonographic differential diagnosis of intestinal obstruction–results of a prospective study of 48 patients]. Ultraschall Med 1985;6:39-45.
74. Tennenhouse JE, Wilson SR. Sonographic detection of a small-bowel bezoar. J Ultrasound Med 1990;9:603-605.
75. Balthazar EJ, George W. Holmes Lecture: CT of small-bowel obstruction. AJR Am J Roentgenol 1994;162:255-261.
76. Siewert B, Raptopoulos V. CT of the acute abdomen: findings and impact on diagnosis and treatment. AJR Am J Roentgenol 1994; 163:1317-1324.
77. Lee DH, Lim JH, Ko YT. Afferent loop syndrome: sonographic findings in seven cases. AJR Am J Roentgenol 1991;157:41-43.
78. Parienty RA, Lepreux JF, Gruson B. Sonographic and CT features of ileocolic intussusception. AJR Am J Roentgenol 1981;136: 608-610.
79. Weissberg DL, Scheible W, Leopold GR. Ultrasonographic appearance of adult intussusception. Radiology 1977;124:791-792.
80. Alessi V, Salerno G. The "hay-fork" sign in the ultrasonographic diagnosis of intussusception. Gastrointest Radiol 1985;10:177-179.
81. Gaines PA, Saunders AJ, Drake D. Midgut malrotation diagnosed by ultrasound. Clin Radiol 1987;38:51-53.
82. Wilson SR. Evaluation of the small intestine by ultrasonography. In: Gourtsoyiannis NC, editor. Radiological imaging of the small intestine. Heidelberg: Springer; 2002. p. 73-86.
83. Bartlett J. The pseudomembranous enterocolitides. In: Sleisenger MH, Fordtran JS, editors. Gastrointestinal disease: pathophysiology, diagnosis, management. 5th ed. Philadelphia: Saunders; 1993. p. 1174-1189.
84. Totten MA, Gregg JA, Fremont-Smith P, Legg M. Clinical and pathological spectrum of antibiotic-associated colitis. Am J Gastroenterol 1978;69:311-319.
85. Bolondi L, Ferrentino M, Trevisani F, et al. Sonographic appearance of pseudomembranous colitis. J Ultrasound Med 1985;4:489-492.
86. Downey DB, Wilson SR. Pseudomembranous colitis: sonographic features. Radiology 1991;180:61-64.
87. Sigel B, Machi J, Ramos JR, et al. Ultrasonic features of pneumatosis intestinalis. J Clin Ultrasound 1985;13:675-678.
88. Vernacchia FS, Jeffrey RB, Laing FC, Wing VW. Sonographic recognition of pneumatosis intestinalis. AJR Am J Roentgenol 1985;145:51-52.
89. Cotran RS, Kumar V, Collins T, Robbins SL, editors. Robbins pathologic basis of disease. 6th ed. Philadelphia: Saunders; 1999.
90. Young RH, Gilks CB, Scully RE. Mucinous tumors of the appendix associated with mucinous tumors of the ovary and pseudomyxoma peritonei: a clinicopathological analysis of 22 cases supporting an origin in the appendix. Am J Surg Pathol 1991;15:415-429.
91. Horgan JG, Chow PP, Richter JO, et al. CT and sonography in the recognition of mucocele of the appendix. AJR Am J Roentgenol 1984;143:959-962.
92. Dietrich CF, Brunner V, Seifert H, et al. [Intestinal B-mode sonography in patients with endemic sprue: intestinal sonography in endemic sprue]. Ultraschall Med 1999;20:242-247.
93. Rettenbacher T, Hollerweger A, Macheiner P, et al. Adult celiac disease: ultrasound signs. Radiology 1999;211:389-394.
94. Pickhardt PJ, Yagan N, Siegel MJ, et al. Cystic fibrosis: CT findings of colonic disease. Radiology 1998;206:725-730.
95. Connett GJ, Lucas JS, Atchley JT, et al. Colonic wall thickening is related to age and not dose of high-strength pancreatin microspheres in children with cystic fibrosis. Eur J Gastroenterol Hepatol 1999;11:181-183.
96. Haber HP, Benda N, Fitzke G, et al. Colonic wall thickness measured by ultrasound: striking differences in patients with cystic fibrosis versus healthy controls. Gut 1997;40:406-411.
97. Welkon CJ, Long SS, Thompson Jr CM, Gilligan PH. *Clostridium difficile* in patients with cystic fibrosis. Am J Dis Child 1985;139: 805-808.

Endosonography
98. Shorvon PJ, Lees WR, Frost RA, Cotton PB. Upper gastrointestinal endoscopic ultrasonography in gastroenterology. Br J Radiol 1987; 60:429-438.
99. Strohm WD, Classen M. Benign lesions of the upper GI tract by means of endoscopic ultrasonography. Scand J Gastroenterol Suppl 1986;123:41-46.
100. Takemoto T, Ito T, Aibe T, Okita K. Endoscopic ultrasonography in the diagnosis of esophageal carcinoma, with particular regard to staging it for operability. Endoscopy 1986;18(Suppl 3):22-25.
101. Bolondi L, Casanova P, Caletti GC, et al. Primary gastric lymphoma versus gastric carcinoma: endoscopic ultrasound evaluation. Radiology 1987;165:821-826.
102. Berton F, Gola G, Wilson SR. Perspective on the role of transrectal and transvaginal sonography of tumors of the rectum and anal canal. AJR Am J Roentgenol 2008;190:1495-1504.
103. Astler VB, Coller FA. The prognostic significance of direct extension of carcinoma of the colon and rectum. Ann Surg 1954;139: 846-852.
104. Spiessl B, editor. TNM atlas: illustrated guide to the TNM/PTNM classification of malignant tumors. 3rd ed. Heidelberg: Springer-Verlag; 1992.
105. Wang KY, Kimmey MB, Nyberg DA, et al. Colorectal neoplasms: accuracy of ultrasound in demonstrating the depth of invasion. Radiology 1987;165:827-829.
106. Hildebrandt U, Feifel G. Preoperative staging of rectal cancer by intrarectal ultrasound. Dis Colon Rectum 1985;28:42-46.
107. Yamashita Y, Machi J, Shirouzu K, et al. Evaluation of endorectal ultrasound for the assessment of wall invasion of rectal cancer: report of a case. Dis Colon Rectum 1988;31:617-623.

108. Rifkin MD, Ehrlich SM, Marks G. Staging of rectal carcinoma: prospective comparison of endorectal ultrasound and CT. Radiology 1989;170:319-322.
109. Law PJ, Bartram CI. Anal endosonography: technique and normal anatomy. Gastrointest Radiol 1989;14:349-353.
110. Berton F, Gola G, Wilson SR. Sonography of benign conditions of the anal canal: an update. AJR Am J Roentgenol 2007;189: 765-773.

111. Stewart LK, Wilson SR. Transvaginal sonography of the anal sphincter: reliable, or not? AJR Am J Roentgenol 1999;173:179-185.
112. Sudakoff GS, Quiroz F, Foley WD. Sonography of anorectal, rectal, and perirectal abnormalities. AJR Am J Roentgenol 2002;179: 131-136.
113. Parks AG, Gordon PH, Hardcastle JD. A classification of fistula-in-ano. Br J Surg 1976;63:1-12.

CHAPTER 9

The Kidney and Urinary Tract

Mitchell Tublin, Wendy Thurston, and Stephanie R. Wilson

Chapter Outline

*T*he prime function of the kidney is excretion of metabolic waste products. The kidneys do this by converting more than 1700 liters of blood per day into 1 liter of highly concentrated urine.[1] The kidney is an endocrine organ that secretes many hormones, including erythropoietin, renin, and prostaglandins. The kidneys also function to maintain homeostasis by regulating water-salt and acid-base balance. The renal collecting system, ureters, and urethra function as conduits and the bladder serves as a reservoir for urinary excretion.

EMBRYOLOGY

Development of the Kidneys and Ureter

Three sets of kidneys develop in human embryos: the pronephros, mesonephros, and metanephros (definitive or permanent kidney).[2] The **pronephroi** appear early in the fourth embryologic week and are rudimentary and nonfunctioning. The **mesonephroi** form late in the fourth week and function as interim kidneys until the developing metanephroi begin to function (ninth week). The **metanephroi** (permanent kidneys) develop from two sources: the **ureteric bud** and **metanephrogenic blastema.**[2] The ureteric bud forms the ureter, renal pelvis, calices, and collecting ducts, interacting with and penetrating the metanephrogenic blastema. This interaction is necessary to initiate ureteric bud branching and differentiation of nephrons within the blastema (Fig. 9-1). Initially, the permanent kidneys are found in the pelvis. With fetal growth, the kidneys come to lie in the upper retroperitoneum. With ascent, the kidneys rotate medially 90 degrees so that the renal pelvis is directed anteromedially. The kidneys are in their adult location and position by the ninth gestational week. As the kidneys ascend, they derive their blood supply from nearby vessels; adult blood supply is from the abdominal aorta.

Development of the Bladder

In the seventh gestational week the urorectal septum fuses with the cloacal membrane, dividing it into a ventral **urogenital sinus** and a dorsal **rectum.** The bladder develops from the urogenital sinus. Initially, the bladder is continuous with the allantois, which eventually becomes a fibrous cord called the **urachus,** the adult median umbilical ligament. As the bladder enlarges, the

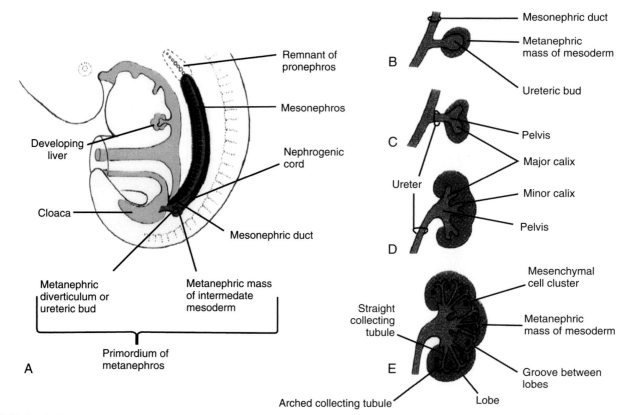

FIGURE 9-1. Embryology of the kidney and ureter. A, Lateral view of a 5-week embryo shows the three embryologic kidneys. **B** to **E,** Successive stages of development of the ureteric bud (fifth to eighth week) into the ureter, pelvis, calices, and collecting tubules. *(From The urogenital system. In Moore KL, Persaud TVN, editors:* The developing human: clinically oriented embryology. *5th ed. Philadelphia, 1993, Saunders, pp 265-303.)*

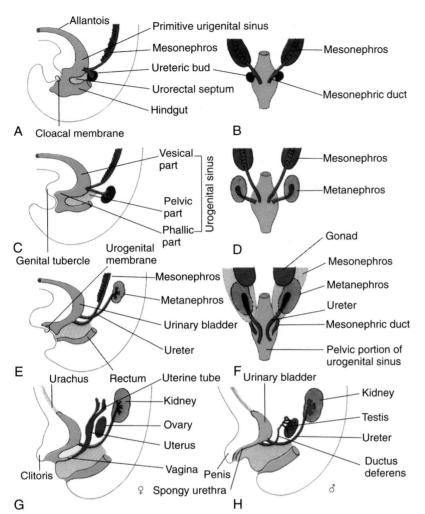

A   Cloacal membrane

B

C   Genital tubercle   Urogenital membrane

D

E

F

G   ♀ Spongy urethra

H   ♂

FIGURE 9-2. Embryology of the bladder and urethra. Diagrams show division of the cloaca into the urogenital sinus and rectum; absorption of the mesonephric ducts; development of the urinary bladder, urethra, and urachus; and change in location of the ureters; **A** and **B,** 5-week embryo; **C** to **H,** 7- to 12-week embryo (**A, C, E,** and **G,** female; **B, D, F,** and **H,** male). *(From The urogenital system. In Moore KL, Persaud TVN, editors:* The developing human. *5th ed. Philadelphia, 1993, Saunders, pp 265-303.)*

distal portion of the mesonephric ducts is incorporated as connective tissue into the bladder trigone. At the same time, the ureters come to open separately into the bladder.[2] In infants and children the bladder is an abdominal organ; it is not until after puberty that it becomes a true pelvic structure[2] (Fig. 9-2).

Development of the Urethra

The epithelium of most of the male urethra and the entire female urethra is derived from the endoderm of the urogenital sinus. The urethral connective tissue and smooth muscle form from adjacent splanchnic mesenchyme.[2]

ANATOMY

The Kidney

In the adult, each kidney measures approximately 11 cm long, 2.5 cm thick, and 5 cm wide and weighs 120 to 170 grams.[3] Emamian et al.[4] demonstrated that the parenchymal volume of the right kidney is smaller than that of the left kidney, possibly because of a relatively

larger potential space for left renal growth (growth of right kidney inhibited by liver) or relatively increased left renal blood flow (left renal artery typically shorter than right renal artery). Renal length correlates best with body height, and renal size decreases with advancing age because of parenchymal reduction.

The left kidney usually lies 1 to 2 cm higher than the right kidney.[3] The kidneys are mobile and will move depending on body position. In the supine position, the superior pole of the left kidney is at the level of the 12th thoracic vertebra, and the inferior pole is at the level of the third lumbar vertebra.

The **normal adult kidney** is bean shaped with a smooth, convex contour anteriorly, posteriorly, and laterally. Medially, the surface is concave; the medial surface is known as the **renal hilum.** The renal hilum is continuous with a central cavity called the **renal sinus.** Within the renal sinus are the major branches of the renal artery, major tributaries of the renal vein, and the collecting system.[3] The remainder of the renal sinus is packed with fat. The collecting system (renal pelvis) lies posterior to the renal vessels in the renal hilum (Fig. 9-3).

Renal parenchyma is composed of cortex and medullary pyramids. The **renal medullary pyramids** are hypoechoic relative to the renal cortex and can be identified in most normal adults (Fig. 9-4). Normal **renal cortex** is typically less echogenic than adjacent liver and spleen. Platt et al.[5] found that 72% of 153 patients with renal cortical echogenicity equal to that of the liver had normal renal function. Greater renal echogenicity than liver echogenicity showed a specificity and a positive predictive value for abnormal renal function of 96% and 67%, respectively. However, the sensitivity of this ultrasound criterion was poor (20%).

During normal development, two parenchymal masses called **ranunculi** partially fuse. Parenchymal junctional

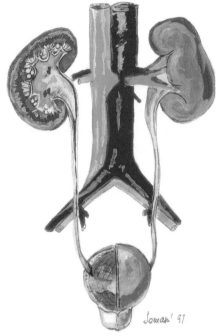

FIGURE 9-3. Anatomy of the kidney, ureter, and bladder.

defects occur at the site of fusion and must not be confused with pathologic processes (e.g., renal scar, angiomyolipoma). The **junctional parenchymal defect** is most often located anteriorly and superiorly and can be traced medially and inferiorly into the renal sinus. Usually, it is oriented more horizontally than vertically and therefore it is best appreciated on sagittal scans[6] (Fig. 9-5). Junctional cortical defects are more often shown within the right kidney, although left junctional cortical defects may be detected with favorable acoustic windows.

A **hypertrophied column of Bertin** (HCB) is a normal variant; it represents unresorbed polar parenchyma from one or both of the two subkidneys that fuse to form the normal kidney.[7] Sonographic features that may aid in the demarcation of HCB include indentation of the renal sinus laterally and a border formed by the junctional parenchymal defect. Hypertrophied columns are usually located at the junction of the upper and middle thirds of the kidney and contain renal cortex that is continuous with the adjacent renal cortex of the same subkidney. Columns contain renal pyramids and usually measure less than 3 cm[7,8] (Fig. 9-6). The echogenicity of HCB and adjacent renal cortex depend on the scan plane. Alterations in tissue orientation produce different acoustic reflectivity.[7] The echoes of the HCB are brighter than those of adjacent renal cortex when seen en face[7] (Fig. 9-6). It may be difficult to differentiate a small, avascular tumor from an HCB; however, demonstration of arcuate arteries by color Doppler ultrasound indicates an HCB rather than a tumor. Occasionally, contrast-enhanced computed tomography (CT) may be necessary to differentiate between an HCB and a non–border-deforming renal lesion.

Renal duplication artifact can result from sound beam refraction between the lower portion of the spleen or liver and adjacent fat.[9] Middleton and Melson[9] found that duplication artifact mimicked collecting system

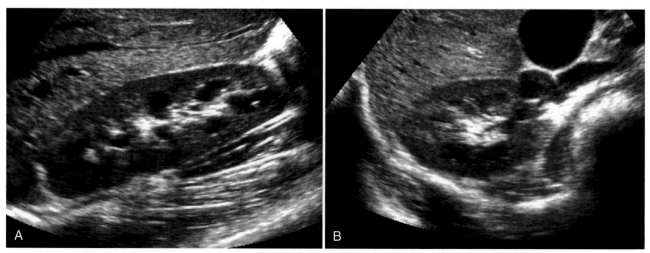

FIGURE 9-4. Normal kidney. A, Sagittal, and **B,** transverse, sonograms of normal anatomy with corticomedullary differentiation show relatively hypoechoic medullary pyramids, with cortex slightly less echogenic than the liver and spleen.

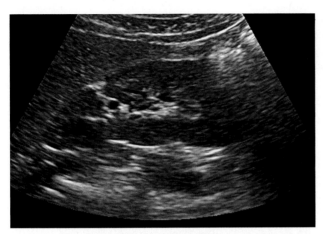

FIGURE 9-5. Anterior junction line. Sagittal sonogram demonstrates an echogenic line that extends from the renal sinus to perinephric fat. The defect is typically located at the junction of the upper and middle thirds of the kidney, as in this example.

SONOGRAPHIC CRITERIA FOR HYPERTROPHIED COLUMN OF BERTIN

Indentation of renal sinus laterally
Bordered by junctional parenchymal defect
Location at junction of upper and middle thirds
Continuous with adjacent renal cortex
Contains renal pyramids
Less than 3 cm in size

---

duplication, suprarenal masses, and upper-pole renal cortical thickening. This artifact is seen most frequently in the left kidney and in obese patients. Changing the transducer position or using deep inspiration so that the liver and spleen are interposed as an acoustic window will eliminate the false impression.

The kidney has a thin, fibrous true **capsule.** The capsule is surrounded by perirenal fat. Perirenal fat is encased anteriorly by **Gerota fascia** and posteriorly by **Zuckerkandl fascia.**[10] The right perirenal space opens superiorly at the bare area of the liver, and both perirenal spaces communicate with the pelvic peritoneal space.[11] Right and left perirenal spaces communicate with each other across the midline at the level of the third to fifth lumbar vertebrae (L3-L5).[11]

The Ureter

The ureter is a long (30-34 cm), mucosal-lined conduit that delivers urine from the renal pelvis to the bladder. Each ureter varies in diameter from 2 to 8 mm.[3] As it enters the pelvis, the ureter passes anterior to the common (external) iliac artery. The ureter has an oblique course through the bladder wall (see Fig. 9-3).

The Bladder

The bladder is positioned in the pelvis, inferior and anterior to the peritoneal cavity and posterior to the pubic bones.[3] Superiorly, the peritoneum is reflected over the anterior aspect of the bladder. Within the bladder, the ureteric and urethral orifices demarcate an area known as the **trigone;** the urethral orifice also marks the **bladder neck.** The bladder neck and trigone remain constant in shape and position; however, the remainder of the bladder will change shape and position depending on the volume of urine within it. Deep to the peritoneum covering the bladder is a loose, connective tissue layer of subserosa that forms the adventitial layer of the bladder wall. Adjacent to the adventitia are three muscle layers: the outer (longitudinal), middle (circular), and internal longitudinal layers. Adjacent to the muscle, the innermost layer of the bladder is composed of mucosa. The bladder wall should be smooth and of uniform thickness. The wall thickness depends on the degree of bladder distention.

SONOGRAPHIC TECHNIQUE

The ability to visualize organs of the genitourinary tract by ultrasound depends on the patient's body habitus, operator experience, and scanner platform. The patient should fast a minimum of 6 hours before the examination to limit bowel gas. High-frequency probes should be used for patients with a favorable body habitus (see Chapter 1). Harmonic imaging is often useful for difficult-to-scan patients (e.g., obese patients); additional recent software advances, including compound imaging and speckle reduction, may increase lesion conspicuity and decrease artifacts.

The Kidney

The kidneys should be assessed in the transverse and coronal plane. Optimal patient positioning varies; supine and lateral decubitus positions often suffice, although oblique and occasionally prone positioning may be necessary (e.g., obese patients). Usually, a combination of subcostal and intercostal approaches is required to evaluate the kidneys fully; the upper pole of the left kidney may be particularly difficult to image without a combination of approaches.

The Ureter

The proximal ureter is best visualized using a coronal oblique view with the kidney as an acoustic window. The ureter is followed to the bladder, maintaining the same approach. A nondilated ureter may be impossible to visualize because of overlying bowel gas. Transverse scanning of the retroperitoneum often demonstrates a dilated

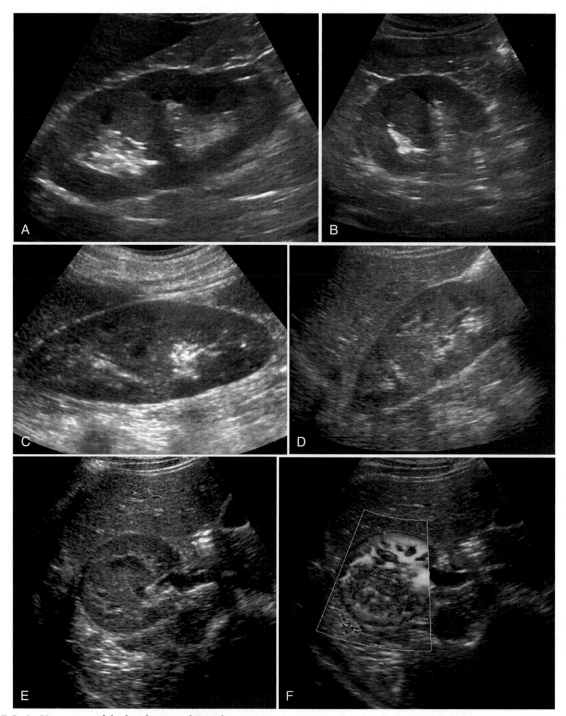

FIGURE 9-6. Hypertrophied column of Bertin. A, Sagittal, and **B,** transverse, sonograms show classic appearance of the column of Bertin. **C,** Medullary pyramids can be seen within the hypertrophied column of Bertin. **D,** Echogenicity of the column may vary based on orientation. **E,** Transverse sonogram, and **F,** corresponding power Doppler image, confirm a hypertrophied column.

ureter, which can then be followed caudally with both transverse and sagittal imaging. In women, a dilated distal ureter is well seen with transvaginal scanning.

The Bladder and Urethra

The **bladder** is best evaluated when it is moderately filled; an overfilled bladder causes patient discomfort. The bladder should be scanned in the transverse and sagittal planes. To better visualize the bladder wall in women, transvaginal scanning may be helpful. If the nature of a large, fluid-filled mass in the pelvis is uncertain, voiding or insertion of a Foley catheter will clarify the location and appearance of the bladder relative to the fluid-filled mass. The **urethra** in a woman can be scanned with transvaginal, transperineal, or translabial sonography[12] (Fig. 9-7). The posterior or the prostatic urethra in men is best visualized with endorectal probes (Fig. 9-8).

CONGENITAL ANOMALIES

Anomalies Related to Renal Growth

Hypoplasia

Renal hypoplasia is a renal parenchymal anomaly in which there are too few nephrons. Renal function depends on the mass of the kidney. True hypoplasia is a rare anomaly. Many patients with **unilateral** hypoplasia are asymptomatic; the condition is typically an incidental finding. Patients with **bilateral** hypoplasia often have evidence of renal insufficiency. Hypoplasia is believed to result from the ureteral bud making contact with the most caudal portion of the metanephrogenic blastema. This can occur with delayed development of the ureteric bud, or from delayed contact of the bud with the cranially migrating blastema. Hypoplasia is established when fewer but otherwise histologically normal renal lobules are identified.[13] At ultrasound, the kidney is small but otherwise appears normal.

Fetal Lobation

Fetal lobation is usually present until 4 or 5 years of age; however, persistent lobation is seen in 51% of adult kidneys.[14] There is infolding of the cortex without loss of cortical parenchyma. At ultrasound, sharp clefts are shown overlying the columns (septa) of Bertin.[15]

Compensatory Hypertrophy

Compensatory hypertrophy may be diffuse or focal. It occurs when existing healthy nephrons enlarge to allow healthy renal parenchyma to perform more work. The **diffuse** form is seen with contralateral nephrectomy, renal agenesis, renal hypoplasia, renal atrophy, and renal dysplasia. The **focal** form is seen when residual islands of normal tissue enlarge in an otherwise diseased kidney; focal compensatory hypertrophy may be particularly prominent in the setting of reflux nephropathy. Diffuse compensatory hypertrophy is suggested at ultrasound when an enlarged but otherwise normal-appearing kidney is identified. Focal compensatory hypertrophy may be more problematic at ultrasound. Large areas of nodular but normal renal tissue identified between scars may mimic a solid renal mass.[5]

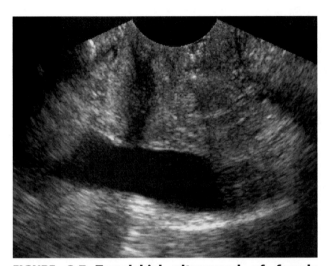

FIGURE 9-7. Translabial ultrasound of female urethra. Sagittal sonogram shows the tubular hypoechoic urethra extending from the bladder to the skin surface.

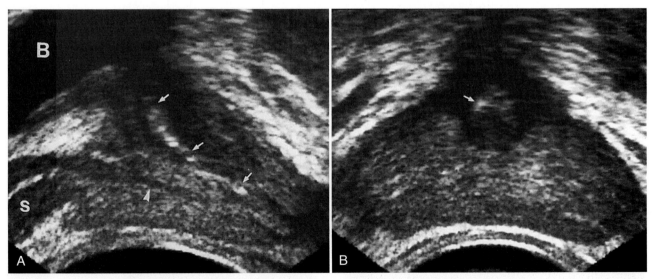

FIGURE 9-8. Transrectal ultrasound of male urethra. A, Sagittal, and **B,** transverse, sonograms show the urethra with calcifications in the urethral glands *(arrows)* surrounded by the echo-poor muscle of the internal urethral sphincter; B, bladder; *arrowhead*, ejaculatory duct; S, seminal vesicles. *(Courtesy Ants Toi, MD, The Toronto Hospital.)*

Anomalies Related to Ascent of Kidney

Ectopia

Failure of the kidney to ascend during embryologic development results in a **pelvic kidney;** prevalence is 1 in 724 pediatric autopsies.[15] These kidneys are often small and abnormally rotated. Fifty percent of pelvic kidneys have decreased function.[15] The ureters are often short; poor drainage and collecting system dilation predispose pelvic kidneys to infection and stone formation. The blood supply is often complex; multiple arteries may be derived from regional arteries (typically, internal iliac or common iliac). If the kidney ascends too high, it may pass through the foramen of Bochdalek and become a true **thoracic kidney;** this is usually of no clinical significance. A search for a pelvic kidney should immediately be performed if the kidney is not identified within renal fossae (Fig. 9-9). If the kidney has ascended too high, ultrasound is helpful to determine if the diaphragm is intact.

Crossed Renal Ectopia

In crossed renal ectopia, both kidneys are found on the same side. In 85% to 90% of cases, the ectopic kidney will be fused to the other kidney. The upper pole of the ectopic kidney is usually fused to the lower pole of the other kidney, although fusion may occur anywhere. The incidence is 1:1000 to 1:1500 at autopsy.[14] Fusion of metanephrogenic blastema does not allow proper rotation or ascent; thus both kidneys are more caudally located, although the ureterovesical junctions are located normally. At sonography, both kidneys are on the same side and are typically fused (Fig. 9-10). In patients with renal colic, knowing that the ureterovesi-

cal junctions are in the normal location is particularly important.

Horseshoe Kidney

The incidence of horseshoe kidneys in the general population is 0.01% to 0.25%. Horseshoe kidneys occur when metanephrogenic blastema fuse prior to ascent; fusion is usually at the lower poles (95%). Typically, the isthmus is composed of functioning renal tissue, although rarely it is made up of fibrous tissue. The horseshoe kidney sits anterior to the abdominal great vessels and derives its blood supply from the aorta and other regional vessels, such as inferior mesenteric, common iliac, internal iliac, and external iliac arteries. Abnormal rotation of renal pelves often results in ureteropelvic junction obstruction; the horseshoe kidney is thus predisposed to infection and stone formation. Additional associated anomalies include vesicoureteral reflux, collecting system duplication, renal dysplasia, retrocaval ureter, supernumerary kidney, anorectal malformation, esophageal atresia, rectovaginal fistula, omphalocele, and cardiovascular and skeletal abnormalities.

At sonography, horseshoe kidneys are usually lower than normal, and the lower poles project medially. Transverse imaging of the retroperitoneum will demonstrate the renal isthmus crossing the midline anterior to abdominal great vessels (Fig. 9-11). Hydronephrosis (pyelocaliectasis) and collecting system calculi may be evident.

Anomalies Related to Ureteral Bud

Renal Agenesis

Renal agenesis may be unilateral or bilateral. **Bilateral** renal agenesis is a rare anomaly that is incompatible with

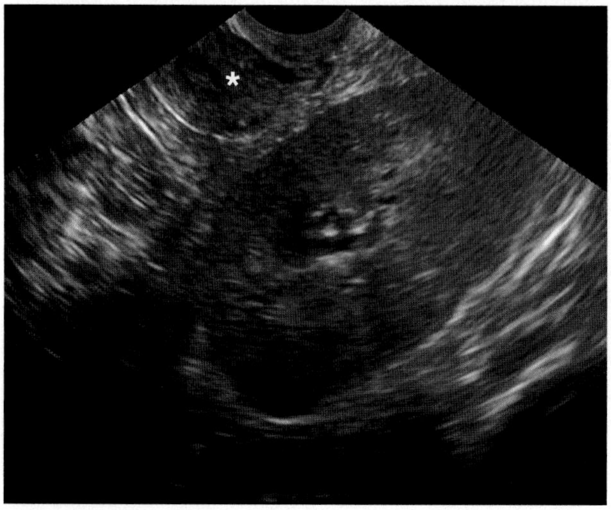

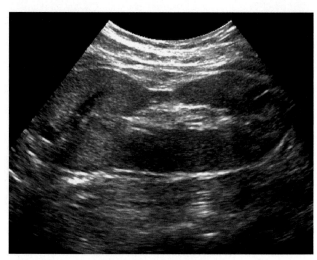

FIGURE 9-9. Pelvic kidney. Transverse sonogram demonstrates a left pelvic kidney posterior to the uterus *(asterisk)*.

FIGURE 9-10. Cross-fused ectopia. Sagittal sonogram demonstrates two kidneys fused to each other.

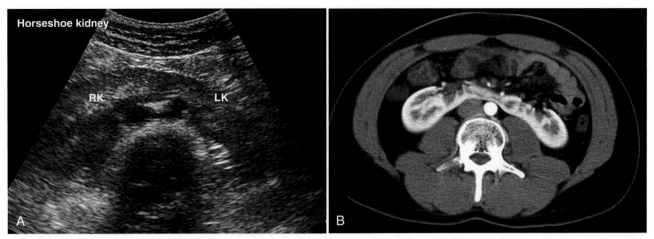

FIGURE 9-11. Horseshoe kidney. A, Transverse sonogram shows the isthmus crossing anterior to the retroperitoneal great vessels, with the renal parenchyma of each limb of the horseshoe draping over the spine. **B,** Confirmatory contrast-enhanced CT examination.

life. The prevalence rate of bilateral agenesis at autopsies is 0.04%. The condition has a 3 : 1 male predominance.[14] **Unilateral** renal agenesis is usually an incidental finding; the contralateral kidney of these patients may be quite large secondary to compensatory hypertrophy. Renal agenesis occurs when there is (1) absence of the metanephrogenic blastema, (2) absence of ureteral bud development, or (3) absence of interaction and penetration of the ureteral bud with the metanephrogenic blastema. Renal agenesis is associated with genital tract anomalies, which are often cystic pelvic masses in both men and women. Other associated anomalies include skeletal abnormalities, anorectal malformations, and cryptorchidism.

At ultrasound, although the kidney is absent, a normal adrenal gland is usually found. The adrenal gland will be absent in 8% to 17% of patients with renal agenesis.[15] It may be difficult to differentiate between renal agenesis and a small, hypoplastic or dysplastic kidney. With all these conditions, the contralateral kidney will be enlarged as a result of compensatory hypertrophy. Usually, the colon falls into the empty renal bed. Care should be taken not to confuse a loop of gut with a normal kidney.

Supernumerary Kidney

Supernumerary kidney is an exceedingly rare anomaly. The supernumerary kidney is usually smaller than normal and can be found above, below, in front of, or behind the normal kidney. The supernumerary kidney often has only a few calices and a single infundibulum. The formation of a supernumerary kidney is likely caused by the same mechanism that gives rise to a duplex collecting system.[14] Two ureteric buds reach the metanephrogenic blastema, which then divides, or alternatively, there are initially two blastema. On sonography, an extra kidney will be found.

Duplex Collecting System and Ureterocele

Duplex collecting system is the most common congenital anomaly of the urinary tract, with a reported incidence of 0.5% to 10% of all live births.[14] The degree of duplication is variable. Duplication is complete when there are two separate collecting systems and two separate ureters, each with their own ureteral orifice. Duplication is incomplete when the ureters join and enter the bladder through a single ureteral orifice. Ureteropelvic duplication arises when two ureteral buds form and join with the metanephrogenic blastema or when there is division of a single ureteral bud early in embryogenesis. Normally during embryologic development, the ureteral orifice migrates superiorly and laterally to become part of the bladder trigone. With complete duplication, the ureter from the lower pole of the kidney migrates to assume its normal location, whereas the ureter draining the superior pole of the kidney migrates abnormally to a more medial and inferior ureteral orifice. Patients have an increased incidence of ureteropelvic junction obstruction and uterus didelphys (duplex uterus).[15]

In complete duplication, the ureter draining the lower pole has a more perpendicular course through the bladder wall, making it more prone to reflux. The ectopic ureter from the upper pole is prone to obstruction, reflux, or both (Fig. 9-12). Obstruction can result in cystic dilation of the intramural portion of the ureter, giving rise to a ureterocele. **Ureteroceles** may be unilateral or bilateral and may occur in normal, duplicated, or ectopic ureters. Ureteroceles may result in ureteral obstruction and give rise to recurrent or persistent urinary tract infections (UTIs). If large, they may block the contralateral ureteral orifice and the urethral orifice at the bladder neck. Treatment of these symptomatic ureteroceles is surgical. However, most ureteroceles are transient, incidental, and clinically insignificant.

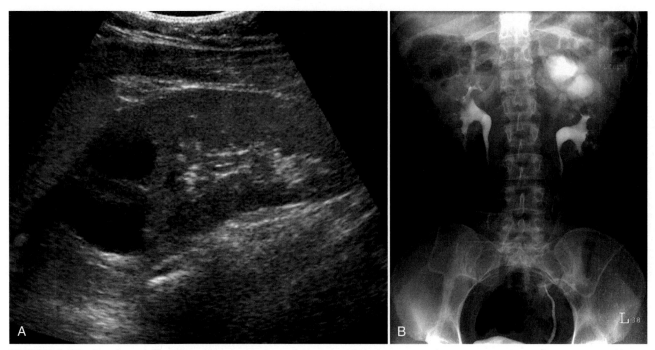

FIGURE 9-12. Duplex collecting system. A, Sagittal sonogram shows an upper-pole cystic mass. Note collecting system dilation and cortical thinning. **B,** Delayed intravenous urogram shows duplicated left collecting system and dilated upper-pole moiety.

At ultrasound, a duplex collecting system is seen as two central echogenic renal sinuses with intervening, bridging renal parenchyma. Unfortunately, this sign is insensitive and is only seen in 17% of duplex kidneys.[16] Hydronephrosis of the upper-pole moiety and visualization of two distinct collecting systems and ureters are diagnostic. The bladder should always be carefully evaluated for the presence of a ureterocele. A ureterocele will appear as a round, cystlike structure within the bladder (Fig. 9-13). Occasionally, it may be large enough to occupy the entire bladder and will cause obstruction of the bladder neck. In female patients, transvaginal sonography can be helpful to identify small ureteroceles[17] (Fig. 9-14). These ureteroceles may be transient. Madeb et al.[18] demonstrated that transvaginal sonography with color Doppler and spectral analysis can provide additional information about flow dynamics, eliminating the need for invasive procedures.

Ureteropelvic Junction Obstruction

Ureteropelvic junction (UPJ) obstruction is a common anomaly with a 2:1 male predominance. The left kidney is affected twice as frequently as the right kidney. UPJ obstruction is bilateral in 10% to 30% of cases.[19] Most adult patients present with chronic, vague, back or flank pain. Symptomatic patients and those with complications, including superimposed infection, stones, or impaired renal function, should be treated. Patients have an increased incidence of contralateral multicystic dysplastic kidney and renal agenesis. Most idiopathic UPJ obstructions are thought to be **functional** rather than anatomic.[19] Histologic evaluation of affected resected specimens has demonstrated excessive collagen between muscle bundles, deficient or absent muscle, and excessive longitudinal muscle.[19] Occasionally, intrinsic valves, true luminal stenosis, and aberrant arteries are the cause of obstruction. At ultrasound, hydronephrosis is present to the level of the UPJ (Fig. 9-15). Marked ballooning of the renal pelvis is often shown, and if long-standing, there will be associated renal parenchymal atrophy. The caliber of the ureter, on the other hand, is normal. Careful evaluation of the contralateral kidney should be performed to exclude associated anomalies.

Congenital Megacalices

Congenital megacalices refer to typically unilateral, non-obstructive enlargement of the calices. It is nonprogressive; overlying parenchyma and renal function are maintained. Infection and stone formation are increased because of caliceal enlargement. The exact pathogenesis is speculative; the most common association is with primary megaureter.[20] At ultrasound, numerous enlarged clubbed calices are shown. Papillary impressions are absent, and cortical thickness is maintained.

Congenital Megaureter

Megaureter (congenital megaureter, megaloureter) results in functional ureteric obstruction. The most distal

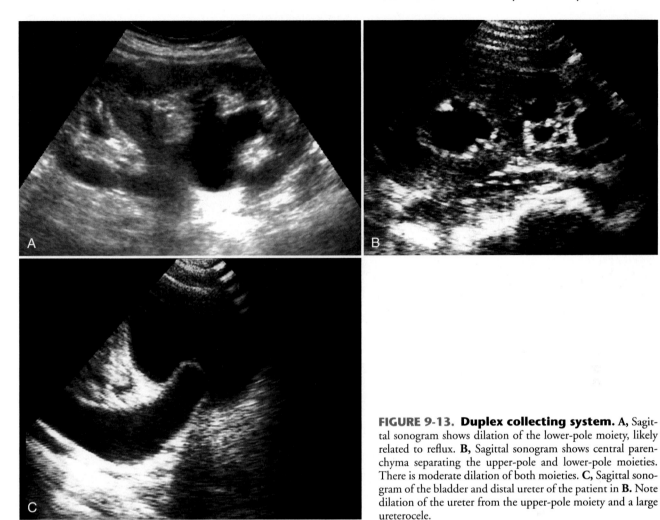

FIGURE 9-13. Duplex collecting system. A, Sagittal sonogram shows dilation of the lower-pole moiety, likely related to reflux. **B,** Sagittal sonogram shows central parenchyma separating the upper-pole and lower-pole moieties. There is moderate dilation of both moieties. **C,** Sagittal sonogram of the bladder and distal ureter of the patient in **B.** Note dilation of the ureter from the upper-pole moiety and a large ureterocele.

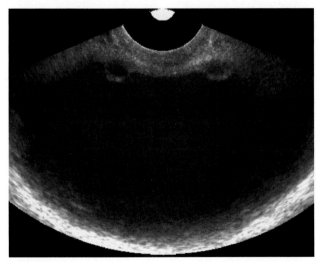

FIGURE 9-14. Small bilateral ureteroceles. Transverse transvaginal sonogram demonstrates two small cystic structures related to the bladder wall. With the probe in the vagina, the bladder trigone and the ureteric orifices are shown in the near field of the transducer.

segment of ureter is aperistaltic: Focal ureteral lack of peristalsis results in a wide spectrum of findings, from insignificant distal ureterectasis to progressive hydronephrosis/hydroureter. As with UPJ obstructions, men are affected more often, and the left ureter is typically involved.[19] Bilateral involvement has been demonstrated in 8% to 50% of patients. The classic finding at ultrasound is **fusiform dilation** of the distal third of the ureter (Fig. 9-16). Depending on the severity, associated pyelocaliectasis may or may not be present. Calculi may form just proximal to the adynamic segment.

Anomalies Related to Vascular Development

Aberrant Vessels

As it ascends during embryologic development, the kidney derives its blood supply from successively higher levels of the aorta. Aberrant renal arteries will be present

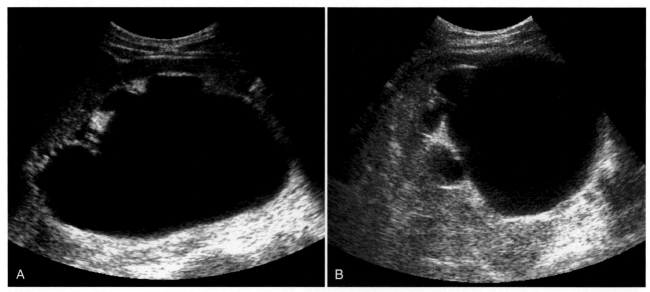

FIGURE 9-15. Ureteropelvic junction obstruction. A, Sagittal, and **B,** transverse, sonograms demonstrate marked ballooning of the renal pelvis with associated proximal caliectasis.

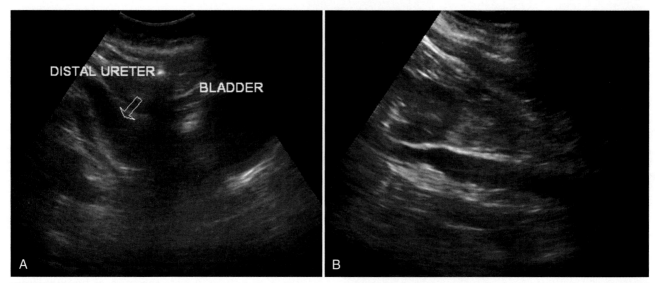

FIGURE 9-16. Congenital megaureter. A, Sagittal sonogram shows marked dilation of the distal ureter up to the ureterovesical junction. **B,** Sagittal sonogram shows moderate midregion ureterectasis.

if the vascular supply from the lower levels of the aorta persists. Aberrant vessels can compress the ureter anywhere along its course. Color Doppler ultrasound may be useful to identify obstructing vessels crossing at the ureteropelvic junction.

Retrocaval Ureter

Retrocaval ureter is a rare but well-recognized congenital anomaly with a 3:1 male predominance. Most patients present with pain in the second to fourth decade of life. Normally, the infrarenal inferior vena cava (IVC) develops from the supracardinal vein; if it develops from the *subcardinal* vein, the ureter will pass posterior to the IVC. The ureter then passes medially and anteriorly

between the aorta and IVC to cross the right iliac vessels. It then enters the pelvis and bladder in a normal manner. Sonography shows collecting system and proximal ureteral dilation. In easy-to-scan patients the compressed retrocaval ureter may be identified.

Anomalies Related to Bladder Development

Bladder Agenesis

Bladder agenesis is a rare anomaly. Most infants with bladder agenesis are stillborn; virtually all surviving infants are female.[21] Many associated anomalies are often present. At ultrasound, the bladder is absent.

Bladder Duplication

Bladder duplication is divided into three types, as follows[15]:

Type 1: A complete or incomplete peritoneal fold separates the two bladders.

Type 2: An internal septum divides the bladder. The septum may be complete or incomplete and may be oriented in a sagittal or coronal plane. There may be multiple septa.

Type 3: A transverse band of muscle divides the bladder into two unequal cavities.

Bladder Exstrophy

Bladder exstrophy occurs in 1 in 30,000 live births, with a 2:1 male predominance.[15] Failure in development of the mesoderm below the umbilicus leads to absence of the lower abdominal and anterior bladder wall. There is a high incidence of associated musculoskeletal, gastrointestinal, and genital tract anomalies. These patients have an increased (200-fold) incidence of bladder carcinoma (adenocarcinoma in 90%).[15]

Urachal Anomalies

Normally, the urachus closes in the last half of fetal life.[15] The four types of congenital urachal anomalies, in order of frequency, are as follows[15,22,23] (Fig. 9-17):
1. Patent urachus (50%)
2. Urachal cyst (30%)
3. Urachal sinus (15%)
4. Urachal diverticulum (5%)

There is a 2:1 predominance in males. A **patent urachus** is usually associated with urethral obstruction and serves as a protective mechanism to allow normal fetal development. A **urachal cyst** forms if the urachus closes at the umbilical and bladder ends but remains patent in between. The cyst is usually situated in the lower third of the urachus. There is an increased incidence of adenocarcinoma. At ultrasound, a midline cyst with or without internal echoes is seen superior to the bladder. A **urachal sinus** forms when the urachus closes at the bladder end but remains patent at the umbilicus. A **urachal diverticulum** forms if the urachus closes at the umbilical end but remains patent at the bladder. Urachal diverticula are usually incidentally found. There is an increased incidence of carcinoma and stone formation.

Anomalies Related to Urethral Development: Diverticula

The majority of urethral diverticula are acquired secondary to injury or infection, although congenital diverticula occur rarely. Most urethral diverticula in women form as a result of infection of the periurethral glands; some may be related to childbirth. Most diverticula are found in the midurethra and are bilateral. Often, a fluctuant anterior vaginal mass is felt. Stones may develop because of urinary stasis. Transvaginal or translabial scanning may demonstrate a simple or complex cystic structure communicating with the urethra through a thin neck (Fig. 9-18).

GENITOURINARY INFECTIONS

Pyelonephritis

Acute Pyelonephritis

Acute pyelonephritis is a tubulointerstitial inflammation of the kidney. Two routes may lead to inflammation: ascending infection (85%; e.g., *Escherichia coli*) and hematogenous seeding (15%; e.g., *Staphylococcus aureus*). Women age 15 to 35 years are most often affected;[24] 2% of pregnant women will develop acute pyelonephritis.[25] Most adults present with flank pain and fever and can be diagnosed clinically with the aid of laboratory studies (bacteriuria, pyuria, and leukocytosis). With appropriate antibiotics, both clinical and laboratory findings show rapid improvement. Imaging is only necessary when symptoms and laboratory abnormalities persist: Imaging is useful to identify potential causes of insufficiently treated infection, including renal and perirenal abscesses, calculi, and urinary obstruction. the Society of Uroradiology proposed using acute **pyelonephritis** to describe acutely infected kidneys, eliminating the need for terms such as bacterial nephritis, lobar nephronia, renal cellulitis, lobar nephritis, renal phlegmon, and renal carbuncle.[26]

At **ultrasound**, the majority of kidneys with acute pyelonephritis appear normal. However, ultrasound findings of pyelonephritis include the following (Fig. 9-19):
- Renal enlargement
- Compression of the renal sinus
- Decreased echogenicity (secondary to edema) or increased echogenicity (potentially from hemorrhage)
- Loss of corticomedullary differentiation

ACUTE PYELONEPHRITIS ON SONOGRAPHY

Renal enlargement
Compression of renal sinus
Abnormal echotexture
Loss of corticomedullary differentiation
Poorly marginated mass(es)
Gas within renal parenchyma

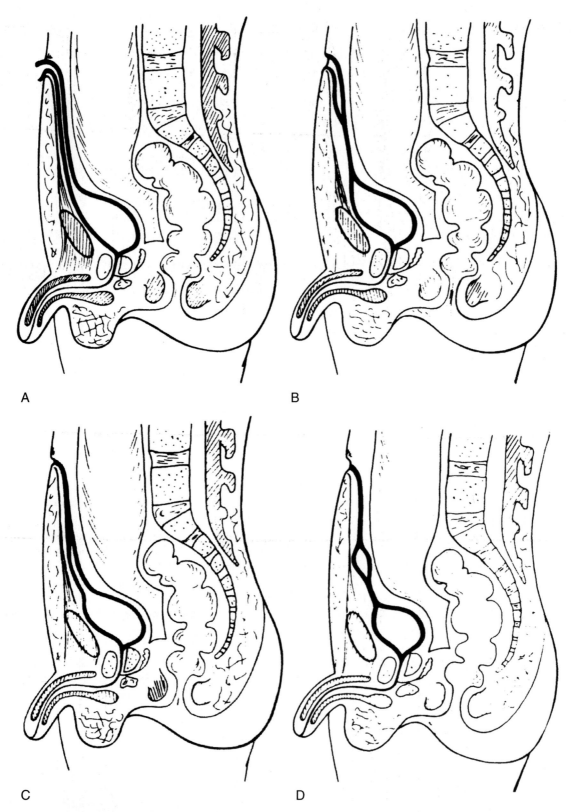

FIGURE 9-17. Congenital urachal anomalies. A, Patent urachus extends from the bladder to the umbilicus. **B,** Urachal sinus. **C,** Urachal diverticulum. **D,** Urachal cyst. *(Modified from Schnyder PA, Candarjia G. Vesicourachal diverticulum: CT diagnosis in two adults. AJR Am J Roentgenol 1981;137:1063-1065.)*

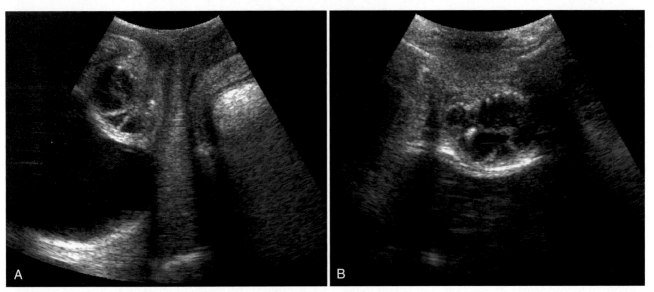

FIGURE 9-18. Urethral diverticulum in young woman with palpable vaginal mass. A, Sagittal, and **B,** transverse, translabial sonograms show a complex cystic mass adjacent to the anterior urethra.

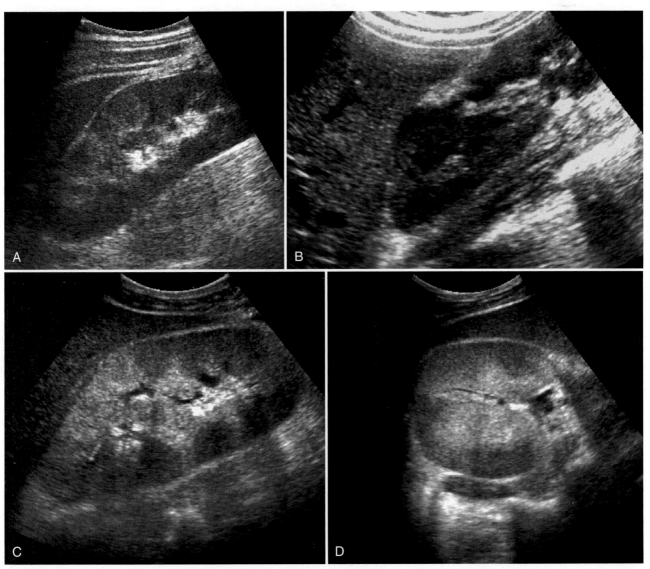

FIGURE 9-19. Acute pyelonephritis in three patients. A, Subtle focal increased echogenic areas are seen in the anterior cortex of the right kidney. **B,** Single focal hypoechoic area is seen in the upper pole of the kidney in another patient. **C,** Sagittal, and **D,** transverse, sonograms in a third patient show a swollen and edematous kidney with focal altered echogenicity and loss of corticomedullary differentiation. The renal sinus fat is attenuated by swollen parenchyma.

- Poorly marginated mass(es)
- Gas within the renal parenchyma[25,26]
- Focal or diffuse absence of color Doppler perfusion corresponding to the swollen inflamed areas

If the pyelonephritis is **focal,** the poorly marginated masses may be echogenic, hypoechoic, or of mixed echogenicity. **Echogenic masses** may be the most common appearance of focal pyelonephritis.[27]

Sonography, including power Doppler, is less sensitive than CT, magnetic resonance imaging (MRI), or technetium-99m single-photon emission computed tomography (^{99m}Tc-DMSA SPECT) renal cortical scintigraphy for demonstrating changes of acute pyelonephritis. However, ultrasound is more accessible and less expensive and thus an excellent screening modality for monitoring and follow-up of complications,[28] as well as in the assessment of pregnant patients with acute pyelonephritis because of its lack of ionizing radiation.[25,26]

A unique renal infection known as **alkaline-encrusted pyelitis** has been described in renal transplants and native kidneys of debilitated and immunocompromised patients.[29] This entity is most frequently caused by *Corynebacterium urealyticum,* a urea-splitting microorganism. Urothelial stone encrustation develops in the kidney and bladder. If the kidney is affected, the patient may present with hematuria, stone passage, or an ammonium odor to the urine. Dysuria and suprapubic pain are the most common clinical signs if the bladder is involved. Treatment is with antibiotics and local acidification of the urine. On sonography, alkaline-encrusted pyelitis may be suggested if thickened, calcified urothelium is identified.[29] The calcification can be thin and smooth or thick and irregular. Care should be taken to distinguish urothelial calcification from layering of collecting system calculi.[29]

Renal and Perinephric Abscess

Untreated or inadequately treated acute pyelonephritis may lead to parenchymal necrosis and abscess formation. Patients at increased risk for **renal abscesses** include those with diabetes, compromised immunity, chronic debilitating diseases, urinary tract obstruction, infected renal calculi, and intravenous (IV) drug abuse.[25,30] Renal abscesses tend to be solitary and may spontaneously decompress into the collecting system or perinephric space. **Perinephric abscesses** also a complication of pyonephrosis, may result from direct extension of peritoneal or retroperitoneal infection or interventions.[23] Small abscesses may be treated conservatively with antibiotics, whereas larger abscesses often require percutaneous drainage and, if drainage is unsuccessful, surgery.

At ultrasound, renal abscesses appear as a round, thick-walled, hypoechoic complex masses that may have good through-transmission (Fig. 9-20). Internal mobile debris and septations may be seen. Occasionally, "dirty shadowing" may be noted posterior to gas within the abscess. The differential diagnosis includes (1) hemorrhagic or infected cysts, (2) parasitic cysts, (3) multiloculated cysts, and (4) cystic neoplasms. Although not as accurate as CT in determining the presence and extent of perinephric abscess extension,[25] sonography is an excellent modality for following conservatively treated patients with abscesses to document resolution.

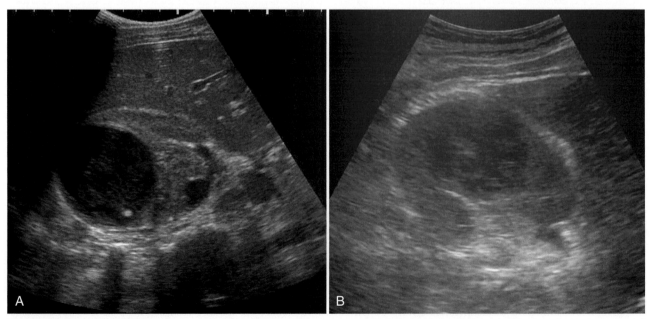

FIGURE 9-20. Renal abscess. Two patients with clinically apparent renal abscesses successfully treated with catheter drainage and antibiotics. **A,** Transverse sonogram shows a large cystic lesion with minimal layering debris. **B,** Transverse sonogram in second patient shows a smaller complex abscess.

Pyonephrosis

Pyonephrosis implies purulent material in an obstructed collecting system. Depending on the level of obstruction, any portion of the collecting system, including the ureter, can be affected. Early diagnosis and treatment are crucial to prevent development of bacteremia and life-threatening septic shock. The mortality rate of bacteremia and septic shock is 25% and 50%, respectively;[31] 15% of patients are asymptomatic at presentation.[32] In the young adult, UPJ obstruction and calculi are the most frequent cause of pyonephrosis, whereas malignant ureteral obstruction is typically the predisposing factor in elderly patients.[25] Pyonephrosis is suggested when ultrasound shows mobile collecting system debris (with or without a fluid-debris level), collecting system gas, and stones (Fig. 9-21).

Emphysematous Pyelonephritis

Emphysematous pyelonephritis (EPN) is an uncommon, life-threatening infection of the renal parenchyma characterized by gas formation.[33] Most patients are women (2:1) and diabetic (90%), with a mean age of 55 years. In diabetic patients, EPN tends to occur in nonobstructed collecting systems; the reverse is true in nondiabetic patients. Bilateral disease occurs in 5% to 10% of EPN patients. *Escherichia coli* is the offending organism in 62% to 70% of cases; *Klebsiella* (9%), *Pseudomonas* (2%) *Proteus, Aerobacter,* and *Candida* are additional causative organisms.[25,30] At presentation, most patients are extremely ill with fever, flank pain, hyperglycemia, acidosis, dehydration, and electrolyte imbalance;[34] 18% present only with fever of unknown origin (FUO).[35]

Wan et al.[36] retrospectively studied 38 patients with EPN and identified two types of disease: **EPN1,** characterized by parenchymal destruction and streaky or mottled gas, and **EPN2,** characterized as renal or perirenal fluid collections, with bubbly or loculated gas or with gas in the collecting system. Mortality rate for EPN1 and EPN2 was 69% and 18%, respectively. The authors postulated that the different clinical outcomes of EPN1 and EPN2 result from the patient's immune status and the vascular supply of the affected kidney. Emergency nephrectomy is the treatment of choice for EPN1, whereas percutaneous drainage is recommended for EPN2. CT is the preferred method to image patients with EPN, to determine the location and extent of renal and perirenal gas. Sonographic evaluation of EPN1 or EPN2 may be difficult because dirty shadowing from parenchymal gas will obscure deeper structures; shadowing might also prompt an erroneous interpretation of renal calculi or bowel gas[37] (Fig. 9-22).

Emphysematous Pyelitis

Emphysematous pyelitis refers to gas localized within the urinary collecting system.[33] This disease entity is seen most often in women with diabetes or obstructing stone disease; a mortality rate of 20% has been reported. It is important to exclude iatrogenic causes of gas within the collecting system. At ultrasound, nondependent linear echogenic lines with dirty distal posterior acoustic shadowing, indicative of gas, are seen within the collecting system (Fig. 9-23). As with EPN, CT is often required to identify emphysematous pyelitis because dirty acoustic shadowing from gas at ultrasound may obscure the exact extent of renal and perirenal disease.

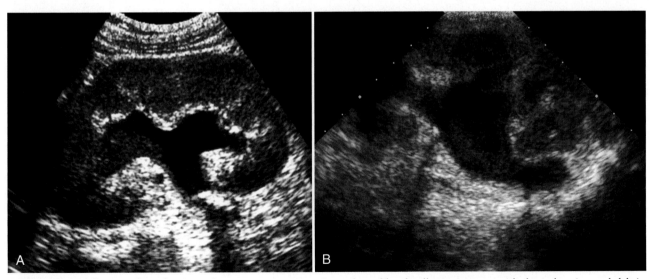

FIGURE 9-21. Pyonephrosis. Sagittal sonograms in two patients show dilated collecting systems with dependent internal debris. **A,** Obstructing stone in ureteropelvic junction. **B,** Layering debris within the dilated collecting system of elderly woman with a malignant distal ureteral obstruction.

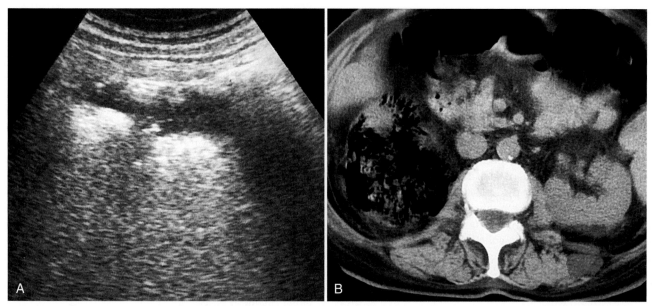

FIGURE 9-22. Emphysematous pyelonephritis type 1 (EPN1). A, Sagittal sonogram of right renal fossa shows extensive shadowing from gas obscuring the underlying kidney. **B,** CT scan demonstrates diffuse parenchymal destruction of the right kidney with extensive mottled gas. Caution must be exercised to avoid missing EPN1 altogether on ultrasound. Failure to see a kidney in a septic patient should prompt alternative cross-sectional imaging.

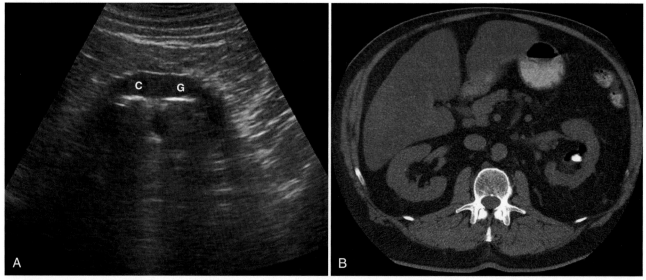

FIGURE 9-23. Emphysematous pyelitis. A, Transverse sonogram of left kidney shows "clean" shadowing posterior to a renal calculus *(C)* and "dirty" shadowing posterior to nondependent collecting system gas *(G).* **B,** Confirmatory unenhanced CT image shows both a calculus and gas within the left collecting system.

Chronic Pyelonephritis

Chronic pyelonephritis is an interstitial nephritis often associated with vesicoureteric reflux. **Reflux nephropathy** is believed to cause 10% to 30% of all cases of **end-stage renal disease** (ESRD)[38] (Fig. 9-24). Chronic pyelonephritis usually begins in childhood and is more common in women. The renal changes may be unilateral or bilateral but usually are asymmetrical. Reflux into the collecting tubules occurs when the papillary duct orifices are incompetent. This reflux occurs more often in com-pound papillae, which are typically found at the poles of the kidneys. Cortical scarring therefore tends to occur over polar calyces. There is associated papillary retraction with caliceal clubbing. At ultrasound, a dilated blunt calix is seen, associated with overlying **cortical scar** or **cortical atrophy**[39] (Fig. 9-25). These changes may be multicentric and bilateral. If the disease is unilateral, there may be compensatory hypertrophy of the contralateral kidney. If the disease is multicentric, compensatory hypertrophy of normal intervening parenchyma may create an island of normal tissue simulating a tumor.

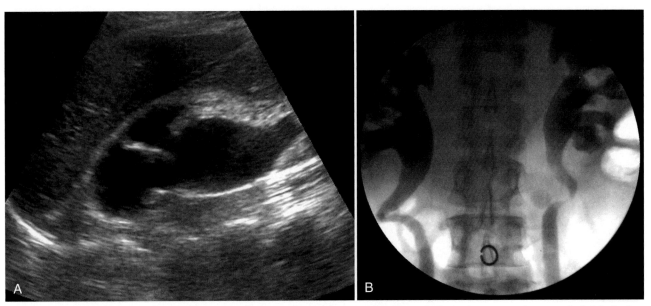

FIGURE 9-24. Reflux nephropathy: renal transplantation evaluation. A, Sagittal sonogram shows marked right hydronephrosis and absence of overlying cortex. **B,** Cystogram confirms massive bilateral ureteral reflux.

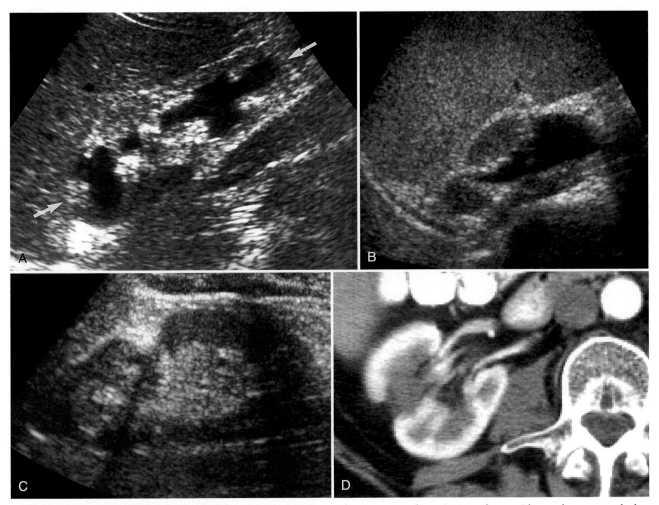

FIGURE 9-25. Chronic pyelonephritis. A, Sagittal sonogram demonstrates echogenic parenchyma with atrophy most marked at the renal poles *(arrows)*. Dilation of the collecting system is from chronic vesicoureteric reflux. **B,** Sagittal sonogram shows an atrophic kidney with scarring and dilation of the collecting system caused by reflux. **C,** Sagittal sonogram shows an echogenic wedge-shaped scar in the midpole of the kidney; **D,** confirmatory CT scan.

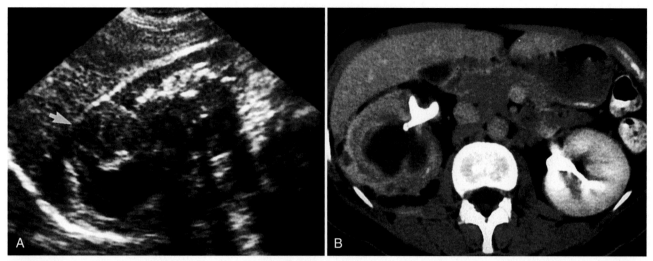

FIGURE 9-26. Xanthogranulomatous pyelonephritis. A, Sagittal sonogram demonstrates a large central mass with calcification. Caliceal dilation with purulent debris is noted *(arrow).* **B,** Confirmatory CT image shows a large staghorn calculus with proximal hydronephrosis and multiple intrarenal abscesses.

Xanthogranulomatous Pyelonephritis

Xanthogranulomatous pyelonephritis (XGP) is a chronic, suppurative renal infection in which destroyed renal parenchyma is replaced with lipid-laden macrophages. XGP is typically unilateral and may be diffuse, segmental, or focal. XGP is typically associated with nephrolithiasis (70%) and obstructive nephropathy.[40-42] The disease most commonly occurs in middle-aged women and diabetic patients.[42] Presenting signs are nonspecific: pain, mass, weight loss, and UTI (*Proteus* or *E. coli*).[40] The diffusely involved kidney is usually nonfunctional. Ultrasound findings of diffuse XGP include renal enlargement, maintenance of a reniform shape and lack of corticomedullary differentiation. Multiple hypoechoic areas correspond to dilated calices or inflammatory parenchymal masses.[40] Through-transmission is variable and depends on the degree of liquefaction of the parenchymal masses. Occasionally, the large, complex cystic masses may mimic pyonephrosis. A **staghorn calculus** will result in extensive shadowing from the central renal sinus (Fig. 9-26). Perinephric extension may occur, but this is often best appreciated with CT. **Diffuse** XGP has no specific sonographic features but is suggested when parenchymal thinning, hydronephrosis, stones, debris in a dilated collecting system, and perinephric fluid collections are present.[43] **Segmental** XGP will be seen as one or more hypoechoic masses, often associated with a single calyx.[40,44] An obstructing calculus may be seen near the papilla. **Focal** XGP arises in the renal cortex and does not communicate with the renal pelvis. It cannot be distinguished sonographically from tumor or abscess.[40]

Papillary Necrosis

Causative factors implicated in the ischemia that leads to papillary necrosis include analgesic abuse, diabetes,

UTI, renal vein thrombosis, prolonged hypotension urinary tract obstruction, dehydration, sickle cell anemia, and hemophilia.[45] Initially, the papilla swells, then a communication with the caliceal system occurs. The central aspect of the papilla cavitates and may slough. Occasionally, a necrotic papilla may calcify. The sonographic findings parallel the pathologic changes. Swollen pyramids may be seen but can be difficult to recognize (Fig. 9-27). With papillary cavitation, ultrasound shows cystic collections within the medullary pyramids. If the papilla sloughs, the affected adjacent calyx will be clubbed. The sloughed papilla can be seen in the collecting system as an echogenic nonshadowing structure. If the sloughed papilla calcifies, distal acoustic shadowing simulating medullary nephrocalcinosis will be seen.[46] Hydronephrosis may develop if the sloughed papilla obstructs the ureter.

SONOGRAPHIC FINDINGS OF PAPILLARY NECROSIS

Swollen pyramids
Papillary cavitation
Adjacent clubbed calix
Sloughed papilla in collecting system that can calcify and simulate a stone
Sloughed papilla may cause obstruction

Tuberculosis

Urinary tract tuberculosis (TB) occurs with hematogenous seeding of the kidney by *Mycobacterium tuberculosis* from an extraurinary source (typically lung). Urinary tract TB usually manifests 5 to 10 years after the initial pulmonary infection. Chest radiographs may be normal

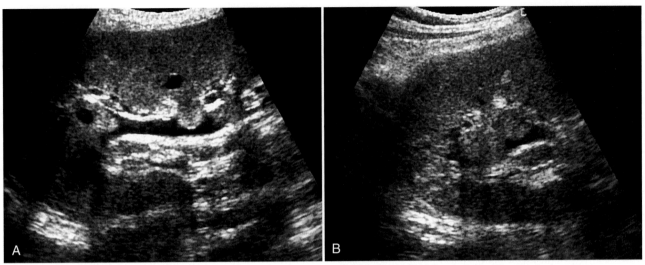

FIGURE 9-27. Papillary necrosis. A, Sagittal, and **B,** transverse, sonograms show swollen bulbous papillae.

(35%-50%) or may show active TB (10%) or inactive healed TB (40%-55%). Most patients present with lower urinary tract signs and symptoms that include frequency, dysuria, nocturia, urgency, and gross or microscopic hematuria; 10% to 20% of patients will be asymptomatic.[47] Urinalysis findings suggestive of urinary tract TB include sterile pyuria, microscopic hematuria, and acid pH. TB is definitively diagnosed with acid-fast bacilli urine cultures; however, this usually requires 6 to 8 weeks for growth.

Although both kidneys are seeded initially, clinical manifestations of urinary tract TB are typically unilateral. The early or acute changes include development of multiple small bilateral tuberculomas. Das et al.[48] found that the most frequently encountered sonographic abnormality was **focal renal lesions.** Small focal lesions (5-15 mm) were echogenic or were hypoechoic with an echogenic rim. Larger, mixed-echogenicity focal lesions (>15 mm) were poorly defined. Bilateral disease was noted in 30% of patients. Most tuberculomas will heal spontaneously or after antituberculous therapy. At some later date (perhaps years later), one or more of the tubercles may enlarge. With enlargement, cavitation and communication with the collecting system will occur. The resultant pathologic changes resemble papillary necrosis; papillary involvement is noted when a sonolucent linear tract is shown extending from the involved calix into the papilla. Soft tissue caliceal masses representing sloughed papilla may be seen. After rupture into the collecting system, *M. tuberculosis* bacilluria develops and allows the spread of the renal infection to other parts of the urinary tract. Spasm or edema in the region of the ureterovesical junction may occur, giving rise to hydronephrosis and hydroureter. Ureteric linear ulcers may also occur, typically within the distal ureter. Bladder involvement is seen in 33% of patients with genitourinary tract TB.[48] Early bladder manifestations include mucosal edema and ulceration. Early clinical symptoms (dysuria and

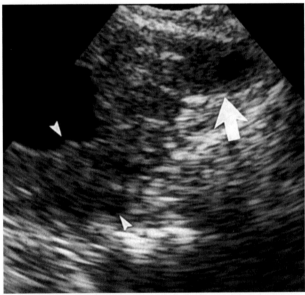

FIGURE 9-28. Acute urinary bladder tuberculosis. Transverse transvaginal sonogram shows marked urothelial thickening of the left bladder wall *(arrowheads)* and of the distal left ureter at the ureterovesical junction *(arrow).*

frequency) are also nonspecific. If edema occurs at the bladder trigone, ureteric obstruction may occur. At ultrasound, early bladder involvement will appear as focal or diffuse wall thickening; the thickening can be quite extensive (Fig. 9-28).

The later or more chronic changes of genitourinary tract TB include fibrotic strictures, extensive cavitation, calcification, mass lesions, perinephric abscesses, and fistulas.[47] The chronic changes, in particular those related to fibrotic strictures, result in significant functional renal damage. Strictures may occur anywhere in the intrarenal collecting system and ureter. The obstruction then results in proximal collecting system dilation and pressure atrophy of the renal parenchyma (Fig. 9-29). With

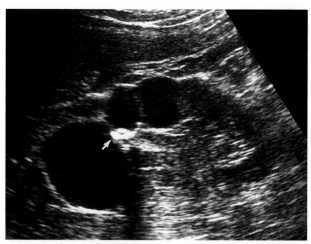

FIGURE 9-29. Chronic renal tuberculosis. Sagittal sonogram shows upper-pole and midpole caliceal clubbing with marked overlying parenchymal atrophy. A focal area of calcification (*arrow*) in the region of the upper-pole infundibulum is noted.

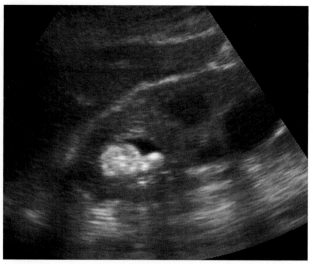

FIGURE 9-30. Fungus ball. Sagittal sonogram shows an echogenic soft tissue mass within a dilated upper-pole cortex.

time, calcification in the areas of caseation or sloughed papilla may occur. If renal infection ruptures into the perinephric space, an abscess may develop. Perinephric abscesses may ultimately result in fistulas to adjacent viscera. The hallmark of chronic, upper tract renal TB is a small, nonfunctional, calcified kidney, the "putty" kidney. In the bladder, chronic infection and fibrosis results in a thickened, small-capacity bladder.[47] Speckled or curvilinear calcification of the bladder wall may rarely occur.[49]

Most cases of genitourinary tract TB can be diagnosed with a combination of intravenous/retrograde urography, ultrasound, CT, and CT urography.[50] Premkumar et al.[51] demonstrated in 14 patients with advanced urinary tract TB that detailed morphologic information and functional renal status are best assessed with CT and urography. Das et al.[52] reported that ultrasound-guided, fine-needle aspiration (1) may be diagnostic in patients with negative urine cultures and (2) may confirm a diagnosis of upper genitourinary tract TB in those patients with suspicious lesions and positive cultures.

Fungal Infections

Patients with a history of diabetes mellitus, chronic indwelling catheters, malignancy, hematopoietic disorders, chronic antibiotic or steroid therapy, transplantation, and IV drug abuse are at risk for developing fungal infections of the urinary tract.[53]

Candida albicans

Candida albicans is the most common fungal agent that affects the urinary tract. Renal parenchymal involvement, typically manifested by small parenchymal abscesses, occurs in the context of diffuse systemic

involvement. The abscesses may calcify over time.[54] Extension into the perinephric space is also possible. Invasion of the collecting system ultimately results in fungus balls. Collecting system mycetomas may be differentiated from blood clots, radiolucent stones, transitional cell tumors, sloughed papillae, fibroepithelial polyps, cholesteatomas, and leukoplakia based on clinical history and urine cultures.[55-57] On sonography, **candidal microabscesses** are typically small, hypoechoic cortical lesions; the appearance is similar to other bacterial abscesses. **Fungus balls** appear as echogenic, nonshadowing soft tissue masses within the collecting system[58] (Fig. 9-30). Fungus balls are mobile and may cause obstruction and hydronephrosis.

Parasitic Infections

A wide variety of parasitic infections are common in developing countries, but sonographers should be familiar with three parasitic infections of the urinary tract: schistosomiasis, echinococcal (hydatid) disease, and filariasis.

Schistosomiasis

Schistosoma haematobium is the most common agent to affect the urinary tract. The worms enter the human host by penetrating the skin. They are then carried via the portal venous system to the liver, where they mature into their adult form. *S. haematobium* likely enters the perivesical venous plexus from the hemorrhoidal plexus.[59] The female worm then deposits eggs into the venules of the bladder wall and ureter. Granuloma formation and obliterative endarteritis occur. Serologic tests demonstrating ova allow diagnosis. Hematuria is the most frequent complaint.[59]

At sonography, the kidneys are normal until late in the disease. Pseudotubercles develop in the ureter and bladder, and the urothelium becomes thickened (Fig. 9-31). Over time the pseudotubercles calcify; the calcification may be fine, granular and linear, or thick and irregular.[60] If repeated infections occur, the bladder will become small and fibrotic. Bladder stasis results in an increased incidence of ureteral and bladder calculi.[59] Patients with chronic disease also have an increased incidence of squamous cell carcinoma.[59]

Echinococcal (Hydatid) Disease

The two major types of hydatid disease that affect the urinary tract are caused by *Echinococcus multilocularis*

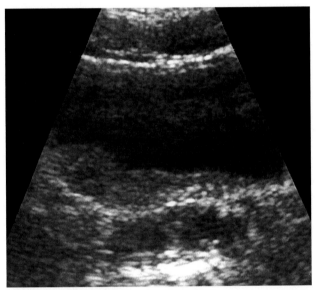

FIGURE 9-31. Bladder schistosomiasis. Sagittal sonogram reveals asymmetrical bladder wall thickening.

and the more common *Echinococcus granulosus.* Renal hydatid disease is found in 2% to 5% of patients with hydatid disease,[59] is usually solitary, and typically involves the renal poles.[61] Hydatid cysts may occur along the ureter or within the bladder. Each hydatid cyst consists of pericyst, ectocyst, and endocyst. Echinococcal disease is often silent until the cyst has grown large enough to rupture or compress adjacent structures.

The ultrasound manifestation of early hydatid disease is an **anechoic cyst** that may have a perceptible wall. Mural nodularity suggests scolices. When **daughter cysts** are present, a multiloculated cystic mass will be shown (Fig. 9-32). The membranes from the endocyst may detach and precipitate to the bottom of the hydatid fluid to become "hydatid sand."[62] Varying patterns of calcification may occur, ranging from eggshell to dense reticular calcification. Ring-shaped calcifications inside a larger, calcified lesion suggest calcified daughter cysts.[59,62] A specific ultrasound diagnosis may be difficult without an appropriate clinical history. However, several features may suggest hydatid disease, including floating membranes, daughter cysts, and thick, double-contour cyst walls.[63]

Filariasis

Most patients with filariasis *(Wuchereria bancrofti)* are infected between 10 and 12 years of age, although the signs and symptoms of elephantiasis, chyluria, and chylous ascites usually do not develop until 5 to 20 years after initial infection. Filariasis is transmitted to humans by mosquitoes, and the worms migrate into the lymphatics.[59] A granulomatous inflammatory reaction occurs. Obstruction of the retroperitoneal lymphatics leads to dilation, proliferation, and subsequent rupture of these lymphatics into the pelvicaliceal (pyelocalyceal) system. Diagnosis is usually made by lymphangiography.[64] Sonography is not helpful.

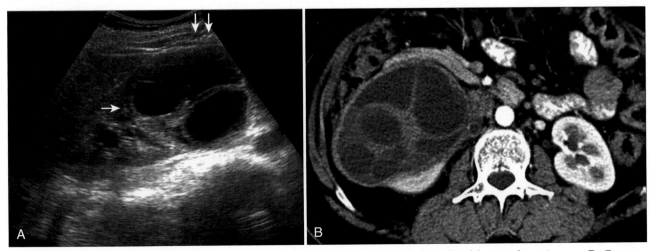

FIGURE 9-32. Renal hydatid cyst. A, Sagittal sonogram shows a complex multiloculated lower-pole cystic mass. **B,** Contrast-enhanced CT shows multiple confluent daughter cysts. *(Case courtesy Drs. Vikram Dogra and Suleman Merchant.)*

Acquired Immunodeficiency Syndrome

The disease course and imaging manifestations of human immunodeficiency virus (HIV) infection, AIDS, and HIV-associated nephropathy have rapidly evolved largely because of advances in the care of HIV-positive patients. Highly active antiretroviral therapy (HAART) has resulted in a decreased incidence of opportunistic infections and improved survival.

Early reports in the radiology literature noted the increased incidence of opportunistic genitourinary infections (cytomegalovirus [CMV], *Candida albicans*, *Cryptococcus*, *Pneumocystis jiroveci* [formerly *P. carinii*], *Mycobacterium avium-intracellulare*, *Mucormycosis*) and tumors (lymphoma, Kaposi's sarcoma) in these immunocompromised patients.[65] The appearance of these infections is often nonspecific (and now rare), but diffuse visceral/renal calcifications may suggest disseminated *P. jiroveci*, CMV, or *M. avium-intracellulare* infections[66-68] (Fig. 9-33). The genitourinary infections that now occur in these patients, including pyelonephritis, renal abscesses, and cystitis, are similar to those seen in non-HIV-infected individuals.

Use of HAART has also changed the spectrum of chronic renal diseases seen in HIV-positive patients. The incidence of ESRD in HIV patients decreased initially after the institution of HAART; however, the increased prevalence of HIV in the U.S. population has resulted in an increased number of patients with **HIV-associated nephropathy** (HIVAN).[69] Renal replacement therapy is a viable long-term option for these patients; several centers have also evaluated the utility of renal transplantation in patients with well-controlled HIV infection.[70] In HIV positive patients, HIVAN is the most common cause of chronic kidney disease; black patients are at particular risk. The histologic hallmark of HIVAN is focal segmental glomerulosclerosis. Nephropathy in HIV-positive patients may also be caused by HIV immune complex disease and HIV thrombotic microangiopathy. However, other disease processes not directly associated with HIV infection (e.g., hypertension, diabetic nephropathy, interstitial nephritis) may result in ESRD in patients successfully treated with HAART.[71] Definitive diagnosis of HIVAN is usually made after renal biopsy. Renal sonography is useful in these patients to exclude obstruction and determine renal size. Early reports also suggested that **greatly increased renal echogenicity** is a fairly specific finding of HIVAN (and heroin nephropathy).[65,72,73] This was also the most common appearance in the largest series performed to date (Fig. 9-34). Other features in this series of 152 HIV-positive patients with renal insufficiency included: globular-appearing kidneys, decreased corticomedullary differentiation, decreased renal sinus fat, and parenchymal heterogeneity.[74]

Cystitis

Infectious Cystitis

Women are at increased risk for cystitis because of colonization of the short female urethra by rectal flora. Bladder outlet obstruction or prostatitis results in cystitis

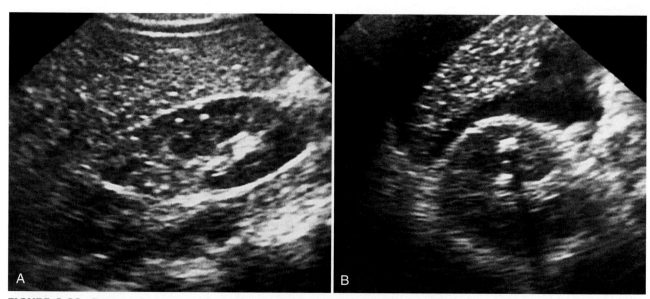

FIGURE 9-33. Proven *Pneumocystis* nephropathy in an AIDS patient. A, Sagittal, and **B,** transverse, sonograms show multiple scattered echogenic foci within the renal parenchyma. Some foci demonstrate the distal acoustic shadowing of calcification. Similar findings are seen in the liver. *(From Spouge AR, Wilson S, Gopinath N, et al. Extrapulmonary* Pneumocystis carinii *in a patient with AIDS: sonographic findings. AJR Am J Roentgenol 1990;155:76-78.)*

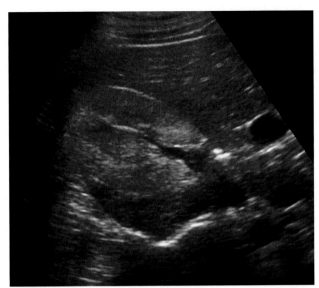

FIGURE 9-34. HIV-associated nephropathy (HIVAN). Transverse sonogram shows greatly increased renal echogenicity. Biopsy confirmed focal segmental glomerulosclerosis.

in men. The most common offending pathogen is *E. coli.*[75] Mucosal edema and decreased bladder capacity are common. Findings may be more prominent at the trigone and bladder neck. Patients will present with bladder irritability and hematuria. The most common finding at sonography is diffuse bladder wall thickening. If cystitis is focal, **pseudopolyps** may form which are impossible to differentiate from tumor[76] (Fig. 9-35).

Malacoplakia

Malacoplakia is a rare granulomatous infection with a predilection for the urinary bladder. The disease is seen more often in women (4:1), with a peak incidence in the sixth decade.[77] The pathogenesis of malacoplakia is not known; however, an association with diabetes mellitus, alcoholic liver disease, mycobacterial infections, sarcoidosis, and transplantation suggests an altered immune response.[78] Patients may present with hematuria and symptoms of bladder irritability. At sonography, single or multiple mucosal-based masses ranging from 0.5 to 3.0 cm are seen, typically at the bladder base. Malacoplakia may be locally invasive[77] (Fig. 9-35, *B*).

Emphysematous Cystitis

Emphysematous cystitis occurs most often in female patients and those with diabetes. Patients present with symptoms of cystitis and occasionally have pneumaturia.[75] The most common offending organism is *E. coli.* Both intraluminal and intramural gas is present, but frank gangrene of the bladder rarely occurs. In these

severely ill patients, the urothelium is ulcerated and necrotic and may slough completely. Emphysematous cystitis may be suggested at sonography when echogenic foci within the bladder wall are associated with "ringdown" artifact or dirty shadowing[79] (Fig. 9-36). Gas may be seen in the lumen as well. The bladder wall is usually thickened and echogenic.[33]

Chronic Cystitis

Chronic inflammation of the bladder may be caused by various agents. Although the histology may also vary, the imaging manifestations, including a small, thickened bladder, are nonspecific. Chronic cystitis may result in invagination of solid "nests" of urothelium into the lamina propria **(Brunn's epithelial nests),** which may result in morphologic changes that mimic neoplasia.[80] If the central portion of a Brunn's nest degenerates, a cyst results **(cystitis cystica).** If chronic irritation persists, the Brunn's nests may develop into glandular structures **(cystitis glandularis).** These may be a precursor of adenocarcinoma.[75] Cystitis cystica and cystitis glandularis may be manifested at ultrasound as bladder wall cysts or solid papillary masses (see Fig. 9-35). Differentiation from malignancy is impossible with imaging, and cystoscopy with biopsy is necessary for diagnostic confirmation.

CAUSES OF BLADDER WALL THICKENING

FOCAL	DIFFUSE
Neoplasm Transitional cell carcinoma Squamous cell carcinoma Adenocarcinoma Lymphoma Metastases	**Neoplasm** Transitional cell carcinoma Squamous cell carcinoma Adenocarcinoma
Infectious/ Inflammatory Tuberculosis (acute) Schistosomiasis (acute) Cystitis Malacoplakia Cystitis cystica Cystitis glandularis Fistula	**Infectious/ Inflammatory** Cystitis Tuberculosis (chronic) Schistosomiasis (chronic)
Medical Diseases Endometriosis Amyloidosis	**Medical Diseases** Interstitial cystitis Amyloidosis
Trauma Hematoma	**Neurogenic Bladder** Detrusor hyperreflexia **Bladder Outlet Obstruction** With muscular hypertrophy

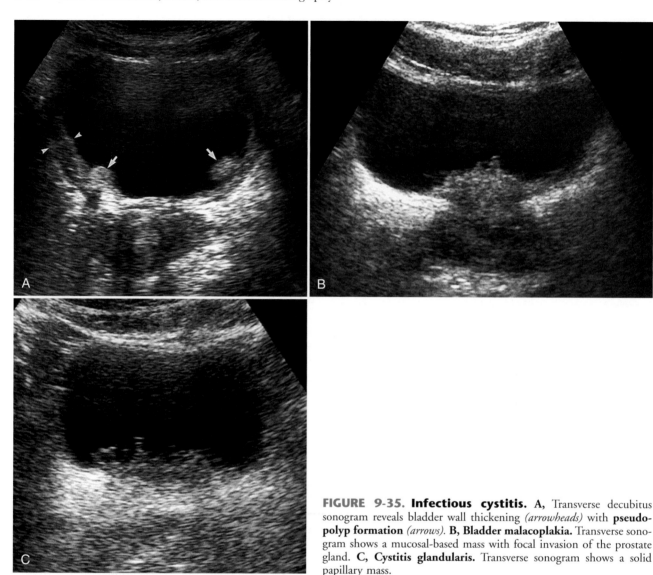

FIGURE 9-35. Infectious cystitis. A, Transverse decubitus sonogram reveals bladder wall thickening *(arrowheads)* with **pseudopolyp formation** *(arrows).* **B, Bladder malacoplakia.** Transverse sonogram shows a mucosal-based mass with focal invasion of the prostate gland. **C, Cystitis glandularis.** Transverse sonogram shows a solid papillary mass.

FISTULAS, STONES (CALCULI), AND CALCIFICATION

Bladder Fistulas

Bladder fistulas may be congenital or acquired. Causes of acquired fistulas include trauma, inflammation, radiation, and neoplasm. Fistula from the bladder to the vagina, gut, skin, uterus, and the ureter may occur. **Vesicovaginal** fistulas are most often related to gynecologic or urologic surgery, bladder carcinoma, and carcinoma of the cervix. **Vesicoenteric** fistulas typically occur as a complication of diverticulitis or Crohn's disease. **Vesicocutaneous** fistulas result from surgery or trauma. **Vesicouterine** fistulas are a rare complication of cesarean section. **Vesicoureteral** fistulas are also rare and usually occur after hysterectomy.[81]

All these fistulas are difficult to identify directly by sonography because the tracts are often thin and short.

Occasionally, linear bands of varying echogenicity may be seen.[82,83] If the bladder communicates with gut, vagina, or skin, an abnormal collection of gas may be seen in the bladder lumen. At ultrasound, this appears as a nondependent linear echogenic focus with distal dirty shadowing. Palpation of the abdomen during scanning may cause gas to percolate through the fistula, enhancing its detection[83] (Fig. 9-36). For depicting often short vesicovaginal fistulas, color Doppler sonographic flow jets may be shown with diluted microbubble contrast agents in the bladder.[84]

Renal Calculi

Renal stones are common, with a reported prevalence of 12% in the general population.[85] Stone disease increases with advancing age, and white men are most often affected. From 60% to 80% of calculi are composed of calcium.[86] Multiple predisposing conditions, including dehydration, urinary stasis, hyperuricemia, hyperpara-

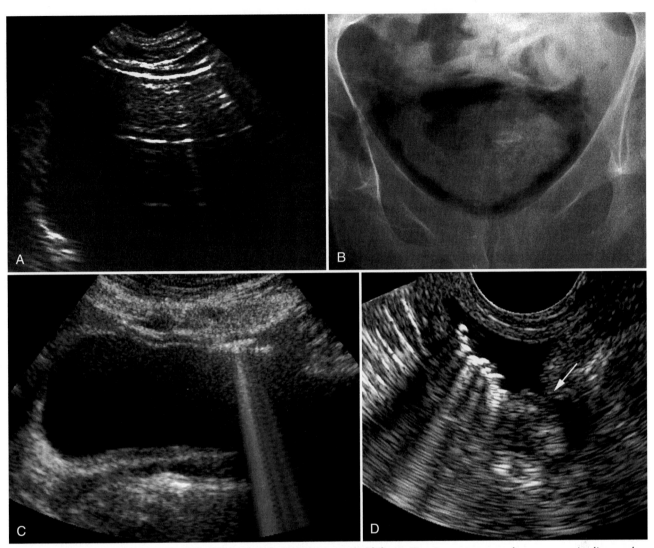

FIGURE 9-36. Gas within the bladder; emphysematous cystitis. A, Transverse sonogram shows an anterior linear echogenic line with dirty shadowing and a multiple posterior reflection artifacts within the bladder. **B,** Confirmatory plain film demonstrates extensive gas in the bladder wall. **C,** Iatrogenic air introduced at cystoscopy appears as a nondependent bright echogenic focus with multiple reflection artifacts. **D,** Enterovesical fistula *(arrow)* showing gas in the bladder as multiple bright echogenic foci on a transvaginal sonogram. *(From Damani N, Wilson S. Nongynecologic applications of transvaginal ultrasound. RadioGraphics 1999;19:S179-S200.)*

thyroidism, and hypercalciuria, may result in renal calculi, but no cause is identified in most patients. **Caliceal calculi** that are nonobstructing are usually asymptomatic. Patients with small caliceal calculi may still have gross or microscopic hematuria and may have colic symptoms despite the lack of imaging findings suggestive of obstruction.[87] A calculus that migrates and causes infundibular or UPJ obstruction often results in clinical signs and symptoms of flank pain. If a stone passes into the ureter, the calculus may lodge in three areas of ureteric narrowing: just past the uteropelvic junction (UPJ); where the ureter crosses the iliac vessels; and at the ureterovesical junction (UVJ). The very small diameter of the UVJ (1-5 mm) accounts for the large percentage of calculi that lodge within the distal ureter.[86] Approximately 80% of stones smaller than 5 mm will pass spontaneously.

Renal calculi can be detected using many different imaging modalities, including plain films, tomography, intravenous urography (IVU), ultrasound, and unenhanced CT. The imaging approach for the detection of calculi, particularly in patients with renal colic, has dramatically changed over the past generation. Even before the introduction of unenhanced CT,[88] the historical "gold standard" for ureteral colic investigation, IVU, had been replaced in many centers with a combination of plain abdominal films and ultrasound. Sensitivities of 12% to 96% for the ultrasound detection of calculi have been reported. This wide discrepancy is a result of differing definitions (renal or ureteral), composition, and sizes of calculi.[89] Middleton et al.[90] reported a 96% ultrasound sensitivity for renal stone detection, which was slightly inferior to the 1988 gold standard of a combination of plain radiography with tomography. Stones greater than 5 mm were detected with 100% sensitivity by ultrasound. Ultrasound with or without plain radiography competes favorably with unenhanced CT in patients with ureteral colic.[91-93] The sensitivity of ultrasound detection of urinary calculi in patients with acute flank pain is 77% to 93%.[94-96] Because of the high negative predictive value of ultrasound in patients with flank pain, some advocate sonography as the initial screening test, particularly for patients with "minor colic."[89]

The growing public awareness of the radiation risks of CT,[97] particularly with repeated exposures, may prompt this more nuanced, cost-effective approach, even in centers with reduced-dosing protocols. However, CT would still be used for (1) patients with severe pain in whom the size and location of ureteral calculi are poorly shown and (2) patients whose initial screening ultrasound examination is negative or equivocal.

Operator technique clearly impacts the ability of ultrasound to depict renal calculi. On sonography, renal calculi are seen as echogenic foci with sharp, distal acoustic shadowing (Fig. 9-37). Even in favorable locations, however, minute urinary tract calculi may be difficult to detect if they have a weak posterior acoustic shadow. The trade-off between tissue penetration and resolution should be considered when selecting probe frequency, with appropriate focal zones applied to maximize signature shadowing. Kimme-Smith et al.[98] showed that annular array transducers are able to demonstrate stone shadowing to better advantage than mechanical sector transducers. Harmonic imaging should also be routinely used, particularly in obese patients. The application of color Doppler may also improve the detection of small, minimally shadowing calculi.[99] Lee et al.[100] demonstrated that most urinary tract stones (83%) show color and power Doppler sonographic **twinkling artifacts,** although the artifact at least partially depends on stone composition[101] (Fig. 9-38).

Several features that mimic renal calculi at ultrasound may result in false-positive examinations, including intrarenal gas (see Fig. 9-23), renal artery calcification (Fig. 9-39), calcified sloughed papilla, calcified transitional cell tumor, alkaline-encrusted pyelitis, and encrusted ureteral stents. Although the ultrasound evaluation of the secondary manifestation of an obstructing ureteral calculus—collecting system dilation—is usually straightforward, pitfalls include (1) evaluation before hydronephrosis develops, leading to a false-negative result, and (2) mistaking parapelvic cysts and nonobstructive pyelocaliectasis as hydronephrosis.[102]

Ureteral Calculi

The search for ureteral calculi may be particularly difficult at sonography because of overlying bowel gas and the deep retroperitoneal location of the ureter (Fig. 9-40). However, **transvaginal** or **transperineal** scanning may be an optimal way to detect and demonstrate distal ureteral calculi that are not seen with a transabdominal suprapubic approach.[83,103,104] When the ureter is dilated, the distal 3 cm will be seen as a tubular hypoechoic structure entering the bladder obliquely. A stone will be identified as an echogenic focus with sharp, distal acoustic shadowing within the ureteric lumen (Fig. 9-41). There may be associated mucosal edema at the bladder trigone. Transabdominal evaluation of the ureteral orifices for jets is helpful to assess for obstruction.[105] At gray-scale ultrasound, a stream of low-level echoes can be seen entering the bladder from the ureteral orifice. The jet is likely shown at ultrasound because of a density difference between the jet and urine in the bladder.[106] Good hydration before the study maximizes the density difference between ureteral and bladder urine. Patients should be instructed not to empty the bladder completely after hydration; the density difference between concentrated urine in the bladder and low–specific gravity urine in the ureter after hydration allows a jet to be seen.[107]

ENTITIES THAT MIMIC RENAL CALCULI

Intrarenal gas
Renal artery calcification
Calcified sloughed papilla
Calcified transitional cell tumor
Alkaline-encrusted pyelitis
Encrusted calcification of ureteric stent

In addition to gray-scale evaluation, Doppler ultrasound improves detection of ureteric jets. **Color Doppler** allows for simultaneous visualization of both ureteral orifices[105] (Fig. 9-42). Depending on the state of hydration, jet frequency may vary from less than one per minute to continuous flow; however, jets should be symmetrical in a healthy individual. Patients with high-grade ureteral obstruction will have either a completely absent jet or a continuous, low-level jet on the symptomatic side. Patients with low-grade obstruction may or may not have **asymmetrical jets**[105] (Fig. 9-42). Semiqualitative assessment of relative jet frequency from the affected side[108] may improve diagnostic accuracy, but this technique has not been widely adopted. Thus, centers that do evaluate ureteral jets with color Doppler use the technique as an adjunct for assessing ureteric obstruction and the possibility of spontaneous ureteral stone passage. Geavlete et al.[109] found that if there was an intravesical ureteric jet on the renal colic side associated with resistive index (RI) values of 0.7 or less and delta RI values of 0.06 or less, spontaneous passage of the stone occurred in 71% of cases.

Initial studies suggested that the addition of renal **duplex Doppler** to the gray-scale ultrasound examination may allow diagnosis of both acute and chronic urinary tract obstruction.[110] Several studies indicated

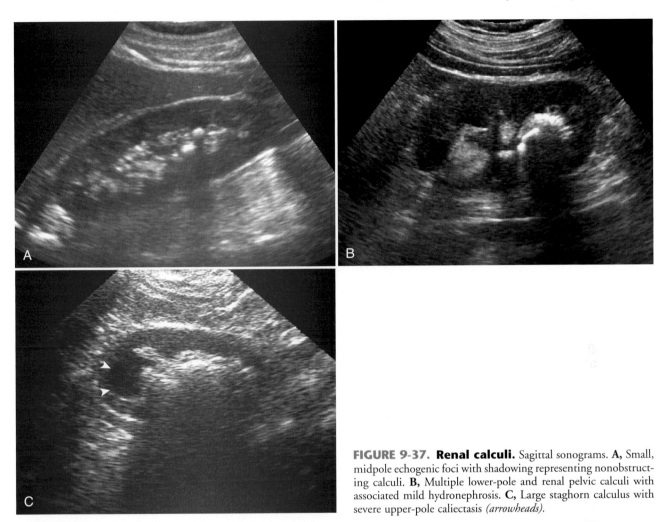

FIGURE 9-37. Renal calculi. Sagittal sonograms. **A,** Small, midpole echogenic foci with shadowing representing nonobstructing calculi. **B,** Multiple lower-pole and renal pelvic calculi with associated mild hydronephrosis. **C,** Large staghorn calculus with severe upper-pole caliectasis *(arrowheads).*

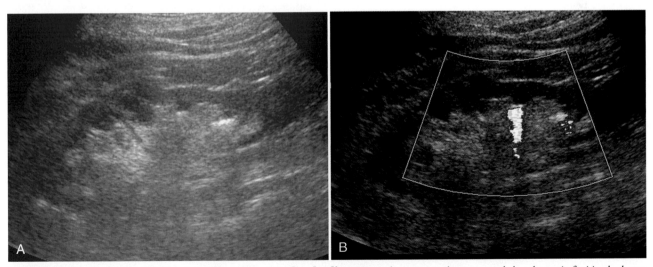

FIGURE 9-38. Twinkle artifacts indicating renal calculi. A, Sagittal sonogram shows two subtle echogenic foci in the lower pole of the kidney. **B,** The addition of color Doppler showing a twinkle artifact confirms calculi.

that the complex hemodynamics that occur with unrelieved obstruction may be semiquantitatively assessed by measuring intrarenal arterial resistive indices (RI = peak systolic velocity – end diastolic velocity/peak systolic velocity). It is believed that with obstruction, renal pelvic

wall tension increases, initially resulting in a short period of prostaglandin-mediated vasodilation.[111] With prolonged obstruction, many hormones, including renin-angiotensin, kallikrein-kinin, and prostaglandin-thromboxane, reduce vasodilation and produce diffuse vasoconstriction. Platt et al.[110] used a threshold RI of greater than 0.70 to indicate obstruction, noting a difference in RI of 0.08 to 0.1 when comparing the patients' obstructed and nonobstructed kidneys. Initial reports advocating the Doppler assessment of renal obstructive physiology were tempered by a series of less promising studies.[102,111] Suggested factors accounting for these discouraging results included (1) a marginal elevation of RI with partial obstruction; (2) a decreased vasoconstricting response to obstruction in patients treated with nonsteroidal anti-inflammatory drugs (NSAIDs); and (3) a generalized vasoconstricting response to iodinated contrast material used for the gold standard, IVU. Follow up studies using in vitro and ex vivo models also suggested that the initial view of the RI as a surrogate for renal vascular resistance was flawed. The RI is largely dependent upon tissue/vascular compliance (diminished compliance results in elevated RI, and vice versa) and driving pulse pressures.[112-115]

Bladder Calculi

Bladder calculi most often result from migration from the kidney or bladder stasis. Urinary stasis is usually related to a bladder outlet obstruction, cystocele, neurogenic bladder, or a foreign body in the bladder. Bladder calculi may be asymptomatic. If symptomatic, patients will complain of bladder pain or foul-smelling urine with or without hematuria. At sonography, a mobile, echogenic focus with distal acoustic shadowing will be seen (Fig. 9-43). If the stone is large, edema of the ureteral orifices and thickening of the bladder wall may be shown. Occasionally, stones can adhere to the bladder wall because of adjacent inflammation; these calculi are known as "hanging" bladder stones.

Nephrocalcinosis

Nephrocalcinosis refers to renal parenchymal calcification. The calcification may be dystrophic or metastatic. With **dystrophic calcification,** there is deposition of calcium in devitalized (ischemic or necrotic) tissue.[116] This type of parenchymal calcification occurs in tumors, abscesses, and hematomas. **Metastatic nephrocalcinosis** occurs most often with hypercalcemic states

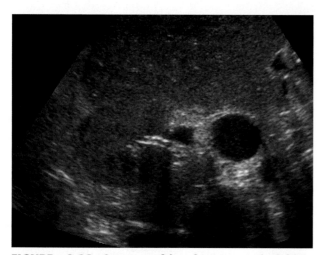

FIGURE 9-39. Sonographic feature mimicking renal calculus. Transverse sonogram shows a linear distal renal artery calcification.

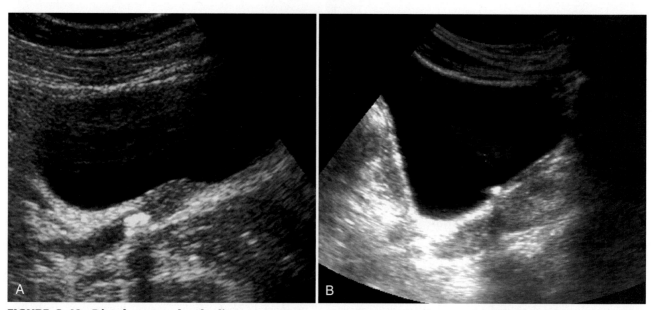

FIGURE 9-40. Distal ureteral calculi. Sagittal sonograms of the distal ureters in two patients. **A,** Calculus is 1 cm from the ureterovesical junction (UVJ), with extensive edema of the distal ureteric mucosa. **B,** Tiny calculus at UVJ with no obvious edema. Note posterior acoustic shadowing.

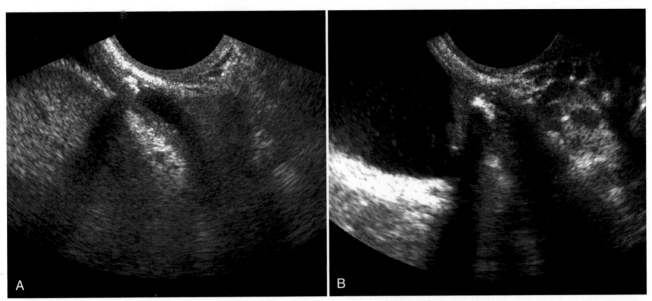

FIGURE 9-41. Ureterovesical calculus. Transvaginal sonograms in two patients show the value of this technique. **A,** Small calculus obstructs a mildly dilated ureter at UVJ. **B,** Larger calculus with extensive surrounding ureteric edema.

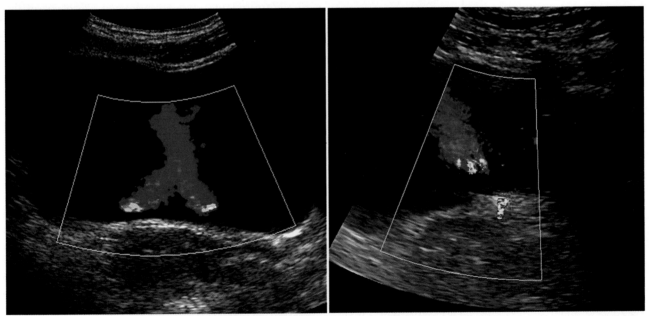

FIGURE 9-42. Color Doppler evaluation of ureteral colic. Transverse images of the bladder in two patients. **A,** Normal symmetrical bilateral ureteral jets. **B,** Persistent left ureteral jet distal to a partially obstructing left UVJ calculus. Note twinkle artifact posterior to ureteral calculus.

caused by hyperparathyroidism, renal tubular acidosis, and renal failure. Metastatic nephrocalcinosis can be further categorized by the location of calcium deposition as cortical or medullary. Causes of **cortical nephrocalcinosis** include acute cortical necrosis, chronic glomerulonephritis, chronic hypercalcemic states, ethylene glycol poisoning, sickle cell disease, and rejected renal transplants. Causes of **medullary nephrocalcinosis** include hyperparathyroidism (40%), renal tubular acidosis (20%), medullary sponge kidney, bone metastases, chronic pyelonephritis, Cushing's syndrome, hyperthyroidism, malignancy, renal papillary necrosis, sarcoidosis, sickle cell disease, vitamin D excess, and Wilson's disease.[116]

The Anderson-Carr-Randall theory of stone progression postulates that the concentration of calcium is high

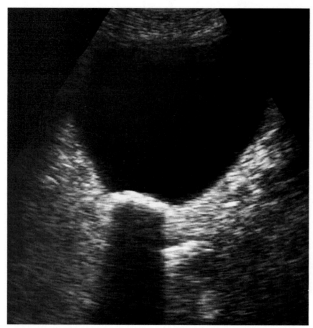

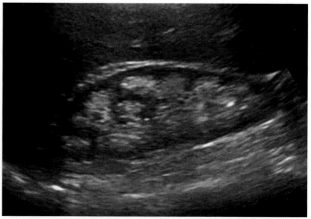

FIGURE 9-44. Medullary sponge kidney. Sagittal sonogram shows greatly increased renal medullary echogenicity ("medullary rings").

FIGURE 9-43. Bladder calculus. Transverse sonogram shows a dependent echogenic focus with posterior sharp acoustic shadowing.

in the fluid around the renal tubules. The calcium is removed by lymphatics, and if the amount exceeds lymphatic capacity, deposits of calcium in the fornical tips and margins of the medulla will result. The ultrasound manifestation of early medullary calcification may be nonshadowing echogenic rims surrounding medullary pyramids.[117] However, increased medullary echogenicity may also be caused by medullary sponge kidney[118] (Fig. 9-44); it may be a normal transient finding in neonates.[119] Further calcium deposition results in acoustic shadowing at ultrasound (Fig. 9-45). The calcifications may perforate the calix and form a nidus for further stone growth.[120]

Although the physiology of cortical nephrocalcinosis differs from medullary nephrocalcinosis, its ultrasound manifestations are similar; early cortical calcification may be suggested by increased cortical echogenicity. With progressive calcification, a continuous, shadowing calcified rim develops.

GENITOURINARY TUMORS

Renal Cell Carcinoma

Renal cell carcinoma (RCC) accounts for approximately 3% of all adult malignancies and 86% of all primary malignant renal parenchymal tumors.[121] There is a 2:1 male predominance, and peak age is 50 to 70 years. The etiology is unknown, although weak associations with

smoking,[122] chemical exposure, asbestosis, obesity, and hypertension have been shown. The vast majority of RCCs are sporadic, but an estimated 4% occur in the context of inherited syndromes.[123,124] These "inherited" RCCs occur at an earlier age, are multifocal and bilateral, and affect men and women equally.[123] **Von Hippel–Lindau** (VHL) disease is the most well-known inherited RCC syndrome; 24% to 45% of VHL patients will develop RCC (see later discussion). Most of these lesions are multicentric and bilateral, and all are clear cell carcinomas.[125-127] Other inherited renal cancer syndromes include hereditary papillary renal cancer, Birt-Hogg-Dubé syndrome, hereditary leiomyoma RCC, familial renal oncocytoma, hereditary nonpolyposis colon cancer, and medullary RCC. An increased incidence of RCC in patients with tuberous sclerosis has also been reported.[124] Another important, but nonsyndromic risk factor for RCC is the **acquired cystic kidney disease** (ACKD) that occurs in patients receiving long-term hemodialysis or peritoneal dialysis. The RCCs in these patients are small and hypovascular and tend to be relatively less aggressive.[128,129]

Histologic subtypes of RCC include **clear cell** (70%-75%), **papillary** (15%), **chromophobe** (5%), **oncocytic** (2%-3%), and **collecting duct** or **medullary** (<1%) tumors. Patients with papillary, chromophobe, and oncocytic tumors have a much better prognosis than those with clear cell and collecting duct tumors. Attempts have been made to differentiate histologic subtypes at imaging, largely based on enhanced-CT kinetics, but to date, overlapping patterns have precluded attempts at preoperative imaging classification. However, potentially relevant features may be shown at ultrasound; for example, lack of necrosis and the presence of calcification appear to be associated with a better prognosis (papillary and chromophobe subtypes).[130]

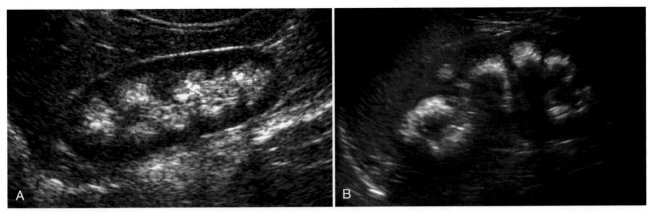

FIGURE 9-45. Medullary nephrocalcinosis in two patients. A, Anderson-Carr kidney. Sagittal sonogram demonstrates increased echogenicity in a rimlike pattern around all medullary pyramids and several punctate, shadowing calculi. **B**, Sagittal sonogram shows extensive medullary calcification in a patient with renal tubular acidosis.

The natural history of RCC has dramatically changed with the advent of modern cross-sectional imaging. Before the advent of imaging, most patients with RCC presented with advanced metastatic disease. The **classic diagnostic triad** of flank pain, gross hematuria, and palpable renal mass was seen in only 4% to 9% of patients at presentation.[131] Systemic symptoms (e.g., anorexia, weight loss) were common with advanced disease. Manifestations reported secondary to hormone production include erythrocytosis (erythropoietin), hypercalcemia (parathormone, vitamin D metabolites, prostaglandins), hypokalemia (ACTH), galactorrhea (prolactin), hypertension (renin), and gynecomastia (gonadotropin). RCC metastases to virtually every organ in the body have been described. Spontaneous regression of the primary tumor may occur, although the mechanism is unclear.[132]

Imaging and Treatment Approaches

With the superior technology of current cross-sectional imaging techniques, sonographers are able to detect smaller renal masses. The prevalence rate of **incidentally discovered occult renal cell carcinoma** on CT is 0.3%.[133] Before the advent of CT, renal tumors less than 3 cm represented 5% of lesions, whereas now these small lesions represent 9% to 38% of all renal tumors.[134] Warshauer et al.[135] demonstrated the relative insensitivity of the prior cross-sectional imaging gold standard—excretory urography/linear tomography—for the identification of renal masses less than 3 cm in diameter and of ultrasound for masses less than 2 cm. Jamis-Dow et al.[136] found that CT was more sensitive than ultrasound for the detection of small renal masses (<1.5 cm), and that both ultrasound and CT could equally characterize a mass larger than 1 cm. They also demonstrated that a combination of ultrasound and CT allowed accurate characterization of a lesion larger than 1.0 cm in 95% of cases. Neither method could accurately characterize

lesions less than 1 cm in diameter. Therefore a combination of ultrasound and CT is superior to either alone. With the advent of helical CT, respiratory misregistration and partial volume averaging can be eliminated. Nephrographic-phase helical CT scans enable better lesion detection and characterization.[137-140] With combined ultrasound and helical CT, other imaging is usually unnecessary in the evaluation of most renal masses.

Magnetic resonance imaging for renal mass characterization has improved significantly with the development of phased array multicoils, fast breath-hold imaging, and gadopentetate dimeglumine contrast enhancement. MRI has assumed an increasingly important niche in the detection and characterization of some renal masses.[141,142] A particular role is in the characterization of high-attenuation renal masses.[143] Most centers, however, still reserve renal MRI for patients with (1) an allergy to iodinated contrast, (2) CT-indeterminate renal masses, or (3) extent of vascular involvement inadequately determined by ultrasound and CT. Previously, renal MRI was also performed to assess lesional enhancement in patients with renal insufficiency. However, recognition of the central role of gadolinium in the development of nephrogenic systemic fibrosis (NSF) highlighted the potential risks in these patients.[144] Thus, ultrasound has again assumed a preeminent role for mass characterization in patients with renal insufficiency at risk for nephropathy after iodinated contrast exposure at CT or for NSF after gadolinium exposure at MRI.

The increased detection of smaller, incidental lesions and better understanding of the natural history of these tumors have led to less aggressive approaches to RCCs. The traditional surgical approach, radical nephrectomy, is now usually reserved for larger, central lesions. The greater likelihood of small, benign, solid lesions in elderly patients[145] and the limited metastatic potential of small (<3 cm) lesions[146] have prompted a "watchful waiting" approach, particularly in elderly or ill patients.[147] Nephron-sparing surgery (open/laparoscopic partial

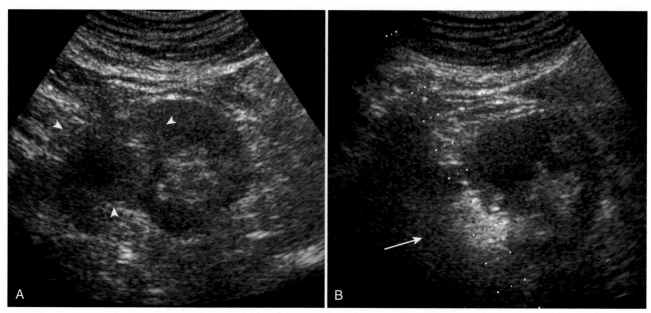

FIGURE 9-46. Ultrasound-guided radiofrequency ablation of renal cell carcinoma. A, Transverse sonogram shows small (<3 cm), subtle, slightly echogenic renal cell carcinoma *(arrowheads)*. **B,** Transverse sonogram during treatment shows ablation cloud *(arrow)*.

nephrectomy, laparoscopic cryoablation, percutaneous radiofrequency ablation/cryoablation) may be offered to younger patients or elderly patients unwilling or unable to undergo imaging surveillance. Primary/secondary efficacy and long-term survival rates with these techniques are likely comparable to traditional nephrectomy.[148] Gervais et al.[149] found that radiofrequency ablation (RFA) of exophytic RCCs up to 5 cm in size can be performed successfully (Fig. 9-46). Tumors with a component in the renal sinus are more difficult to treat.

Sonographic Appearance

Most RCCs are solid at ultrasound. Tumors may be hypoechoic, isoechoic, or hyperechoic (Fig. 9-47). An early ultrasound series reported that the majority of RCCs are isoechoic (86%), whereas the minority are hypoechoic (10%) or echogenic (4%).[150] Later series noted the ultrasound appearance of the smaller RCCs that are now often depicted with cross-sectional imaging. These smaller RCCs (<3 cm) are often echogenic compared with surrounding renal parenchyma; Forman et al.[151] found that 77% of smaller RCCs were echogenic, and Yamashita et al.,[152,153] reported 61% as echogenic.

The small, echogenic RCC may be difficult to differentiate from a benign angiomyolipoma (AML) at ultrasound. Yamashita et al.[153] emphasized the overlap in RCC/AML imaging appearance, was although several distinguishing characteristics were reported. A thin, hypoechoic rim, thought to be a pseudocapsule at histology, was reported in 84% of RCCs and no AMLs. Small,

intralesional cystic spaces were shown exclusively in several echogenic renal cell carcinomas (Fig. 9-47). Weak shadowing posterior to AMLs and hypoechoic halos or cystic spaces in RCCs were also thought to be characteristic features.[154] Nonetheless, imaging overlap should prompt definitive characterization by either MRI or CT.[155]

The exact pathologic basis for the hyperechoic appearance of RCC is not understood, but increased echogenicity has been reported in RCCs with papillary, tubular, or microcystic architecture and in tumors with minute calcification, necrosis, cystic degeneration, or fibrosis.[134] Macroscopic calcification may be identified in 8% to 18% of RCCs. This calcification may be punctate, curvilinear, diffuse (rare), central, or peripheral.[156-160] Daniels et al.[159] showed that central calcification was associated with a malignant tumor in 87% of cases. When posterior rim shadowing or diffuse calcification make it impossible to characterize a renal lesion by ultrasound, CT is needed to identify additional features of malignancy (e.g., enhancement of associated soft tissue mass).[161]

Papillary tumors account for 15% of all RCCs.[130,162] The papillary type is characterized by slower growth, a lower stage at presentation, and a better prognosis.[163] Papillary tumors also tend to be hypoechoic or isoechoic, although no consistent sonographic pattern exists, because some may also be hyperechoic.[162]

From 5% to 7% of all RCCs are **cystic** tumors.[164] Four histologic growth patterns within cystic RCCs have been described: multilocular, unilocular, necrotic (cystic necrosis), and tumors originating in a simple cyst[165]

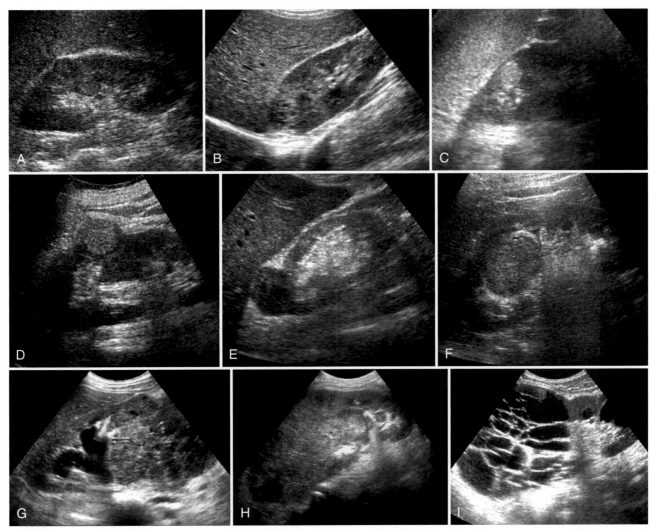

FIGURE 9-47. **Sonographic appearances of renal cell carcinoma on sagittal sonograms. A,** Tiny incidental hypoechoic tumor. **B,** Small echogenic tumor with central cystic spaces. **C,** Small echogenic nodule simulating an angiomyolipoma. **D,** Exophytic echogenic midpole renal mass. **E,** Exophytic hypoechoic upper-pole renal mass. **F,** Large central renal sinus mass with no associated caliectasis. **G,** Large solid heterogeneous mass in the lower pole of the kidney compressing the renal pelvis with upper-pole caliectasis. **H,** Large infiltrative renal mass with maintenance of reniform shape. **I,** Large upper-pole cystic mass showing numerous thick internal septations.

(Figs. 9-48 and 9-49). Recognition of subtypes may have clinical significance because the multilocular and unilocular subtypes seem to be less aggressive.[164] At sonography, **multilocular** cystic RCC will appear as a cystic mass with internal septations. These septations may be thick (>2 mm), nodular, and may contain calcification (see Fig. 9-47). The characteristic ultrasound appearance of a **unilocular** cystic RCC is a debris-filled mass with thick, irregular walls that may be calcified. The appearance of **necrotic** RCCs at ultrasound depends on the degree of tumor necrosis. Tumors originating in a **simple cyst** are rare (excluding VHL patients). At ultrasound, a mural tumor nodule will be found at the base of a simple cyst. Helical CT with ultrasound usually allows accurate characterization of the internal nature of most cystic renal lesions.[166]

The use of **Doppler ultrasound**[167] for detection of tumor vascularity has been reported for malignant lesions in the liver, kidneys, adrenal glands, and pancreas. Most malignant renal tumors (70%-83%) have Doppler shift frequency of 2.5 kHz.[167-171] Similar changes may be noted with inflammatory masses; however, patients with renal infection should be clinically apparent. Unfortunately, the absence of high-frequency Doppler shift does not exclude malignancy.[170] Confirmation of blood flow within malignant solid and cystic renal tumors has also recently been performed with microbubble contrast agents and low–mechanical index (MI) pulse inversion sonography. Criteria for neovascularity used with CT or MRI for mass characterization—septal and nodular enhancement—can also be used with stable, second-generation ultrasound contrast agents[172,173] (Fig. 9-50).

However, lack of U.S. Food and Drug Administration (FDA) approval, reimbursement issues, and logistics associated with technologist/radiologist-intensive, contrast-enhanced sonography protocols have hindered widespread adoption of this technique.

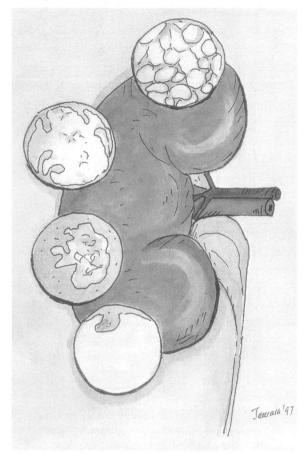

FIGURE 9-48. Cystic growth patterns of renal cell carcinoma. *Upper pole,* Multilocular; *upper lateral,* unilocular; *lower lateral,* cystic necrosis; *lower pole,* origin in the wall of a simple cyst. *(From Yamashita Y, Watanabe O, Miyazaki H, et al. Cystic renal cell carcinoma. Acta Radiologica 1994;35:19-24.)*

Biopsy and Prognosis

In the classic imaging paradigm, there was little role for percutaneous biopsy in the patient with a solitary, solid renal mass and no other known malignancy. Previously, ultrasound- or CT-guided biopsy was reserved for patients in whom renal lymphoma or metastases were considered and those in whom tissue confirmation of metastatic RCC was necessary.[134,166,174] The dogma that "good radiologic imaging is virtually diagnostic in all cases" may not hold true in the era of ubiquitous helical CT scanning. Recent pathologic and biopsy series of small (<3 cm), solid enhancing renal masses have shown that a surprising number of these lesions are benign (i.e., fat-containing AMLs, oncocytomas, metanephric adenomas). Moreover, image-directed needle biopsy (aspiration or core) has been shown to be a relatively safe and usually conclusive procedure.[175-179] Further advances in immunohistology and greater acceptance of percutaneous ablation techniques will likely increase the role of imaging-directed, particularly ultrasound-guided, renal mass biopsy in the near future (Fig. 9-51).

For patients with imaging findings (or biopsy results) definitive for RCC, the **stage at diagnosis** directly impacts prognosis. The Robson staging classification for RCC follows:

I: Tumor confined within renal capsule.
II: Tumor invasion of perinephric fat.
III: Tumor involvement of regional lymph nodes or venous structures.
IV: Invasion of adjacent organs or distant metastases.

Five-year survival rates for patients with Robson stages I, II, III, and IV are 67%, 51%, 33.5%, and 13.5%, respectively.[180] Patients with stage I and stage II disease are treated surgically (partial or radical nephrectomy). Patients with stage III disease, with extensive metastatic lymphadenopathy, are often treated

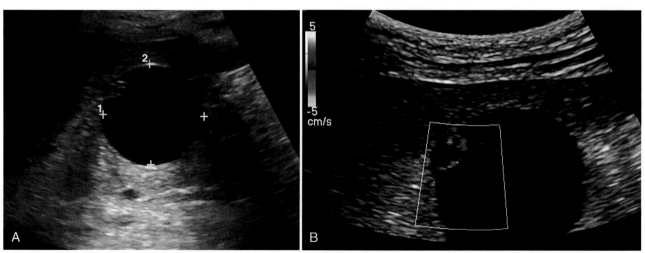

FIGURE 9-49. Renal cell carcinoma within cyst. A, Complex cyst with mural nodule. **B,** Color Doppler shows flow within septation. *(Case courtesy Vikram Dogra, MD.)*

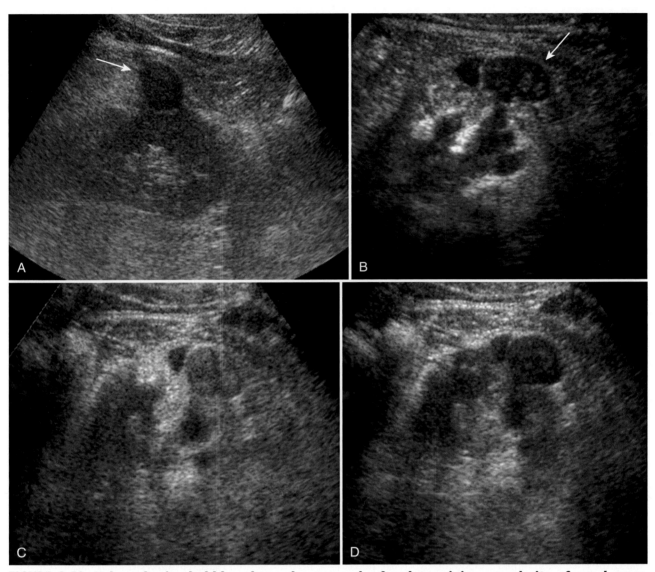

FIGURE 9-50. Value of microbubble-enhanced sonography for determining vascularity of renal mass.
A, Baseline transverse sonogram of exophytic hypoechoic midpole renal mass *(arrow).* **B,** Arterial phase enhancement immediately follow-ing bolus injection of microbubbles. There are small linear vessels in the mass *(arrow).* **C,** Nephrographic phase image shows enhancement of both normal kidney and relatively hypovascular renal cell carcinoma. **D,** Delayed phase image shows de-enhancement of renal cell carcinoma. *(Case courtesy Ed. Grant, MD.)*

palliatively. Patients with stage III disease and tumor thrombus are treated with radical nephrectomy and thrombectomy. Patients with stage IV disease usually receive palliative treatment only,[181] although greater understanding of the molecular biology of RCC has led to clinical trials of novel, small-molecule-targeted inhibi-tors and monoclonal antibodies.[182]

Pitfalls in Interpretation

Ultrasound is inferior to CT and MRI for staging RCC. Unfortunately, obesity and overlying bowel gas often make it difficult to assess for lymphadenopathy or vas-cular involvement. In thin patients and in those with minimal bowel gas, however, the renal veins and retro-peritoneum can be well assessed with ultrasound, which should be done in all patients with a renal mass. Sonog-raphy is excellent for assessment of the intrahepatic IVC and for determination of the cephalad extent of venous tumor thrombus with RCC (Fig. 9-52). Habboub et al.[183] found the accuracy of detecting renal vein and IVC involvement at sonography was 64% and 93%, respectively. The addition of color Doppler sonography improved accuracy for diagnosing both renal vein and IVC thrombus to 87% and 100%, respectively. It is crucial to determine the location and extent of vascular

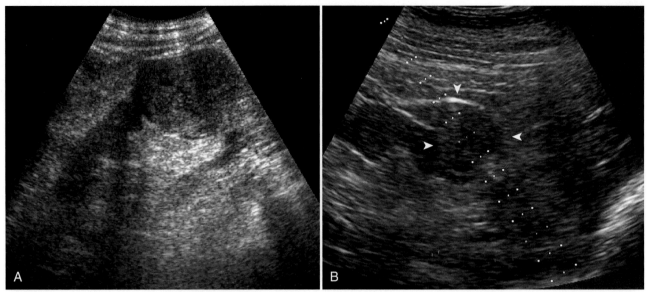

FIGURE 9-51. Renal oncocytoma. A, Sagittal sonogram shows a large, isoechoic, partially exophytic renal mass that cannot be differentiated from renal cell carcinoma. **B,** Ultrasound-guided biopsy of an isoechoic renal lesion *(arrowheads)* in another patient, performed before possible cryoablation, confirms an oncocytoma.

tumor thrombus to plan the surgical approach. However, staging limitations shared by ultrasound, CT, and MRI include (1) detection of microscopic tumor invasion of the renal capsule, (2) detection of metastatic tumor deposits in normal-size lymph nodes, and (3) differentiation of inflammatory hyperplastic nodes from neoplastic nodes.

Transitional Cell Carcinoma

Transitional cell carcinoma (TCC) of the renal pelvis accounts for 7% of all primary renal tumors.[184] **Renal TCC** is two to three times more common than **ureteral** neoplasms. **Bladder** TCC, because of its large surface area, is 50 times more common than renal pelvic TCC.[185] The multifocal and bilateral nature of TCC requires accurate diagnosis and staging to allow appropriate surgical planning. Yousem et al.[186] reviewed 645 cases of TCC of the bladder, ureter, and kidney and found that 3.9% of patients with bladder cancer developed an upper tract lesion (mean, within 61 months); 13% of patients with ureteral TCC and 11% of those with renal TCC developed **metachronous tumors** (mean, within 28 and 22 months, respectively). **Synchronous TCC** was present in 2.3% of patients with bladder TCC, 39% with ureteral TCC, and 24% with renal TCC. Upper tract disease surveillance has traditionally been performed using a combination of IVU, retrograde pyelography, and urine cytology. Recent reports indicate the utility of CT urography and potentially MR urography.[187] Bladder TCC is effectively screened at cystoscopy. Patients at increased risk for development of TCC may require closer surveillance regimens and include

those with Balkan nephritis, vesicoureteric reflux, multifocal recurrent bladder TCC, high-grade bladder tumors, carcinoma in situ of distal ureters after cystectomy, analgesic abuse, heavy smoking habit, exposure to carcinogens, or cyclophosphamide therapy.[186]

Transitional cell carcinomas may be papillary or nonpapillary. **Papillary** TCCs are exophytic polypoid lesions attached to the mucosa by a stalk. This type of tumor tends to be lower grade at presentation; polypoid TCC typically infiltrates slowly and metastasizes late in the disease. **Nonpapillary,** sessile TCCs present as nodular or flat tumors; the mucosal thickening that is a hallmark of sessile TCC may be difficult to depict even at CT. These tumors are usually high grade and infiltrating.[185]

Renal Tumors

Transitional cell tumors of the kidney are more common in men than women (4:1). Renal TCC is typically seen in elderly patients; the mean age at diagnosis is 65 years.[185] About 75% of patients with renal pelvic tumors present with gross or microscopic hematuria; 25% have flank pain. Renal TCC is discovered incidentally in less than 5% of patients.[185]

Unfortunately, the sonographic assessment of the **renal sinus** poses unique problems and is a challenge to evaluate for pathologic processes because of its variable appearance. Fat within the renal sinus can appear as a hypoechoic mass and can simulate a solid TCC (Fig. 9-53). In uncertain cases, confirmation with IVU or CT urography is recommended to rule out neoplasm, particularly in patients with hematuria (Fig. 9-54).

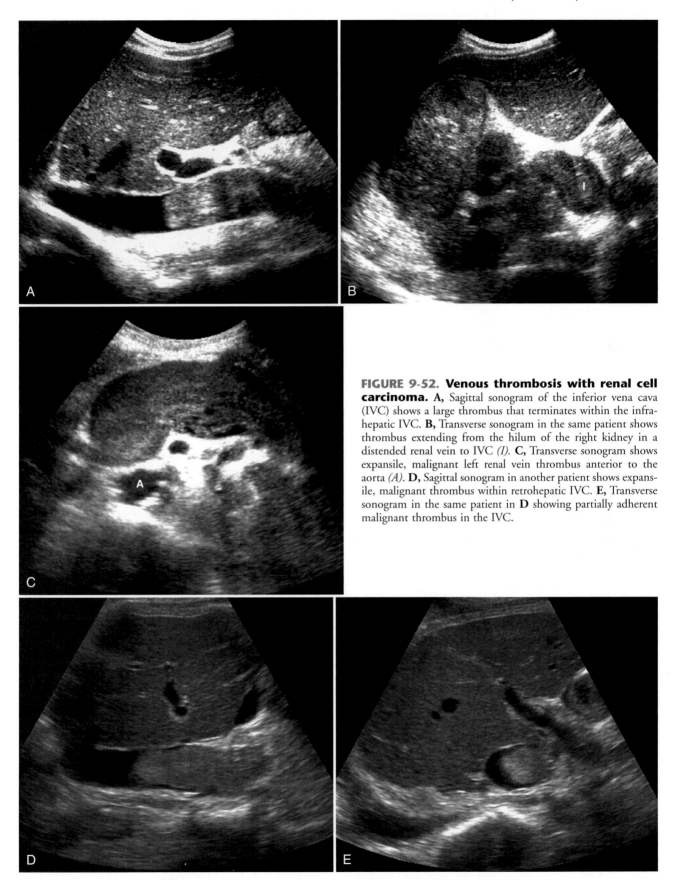

FIGURE 9-52. Venous thrombosis with renal cell carcinoma. A, Sagittal sonogram of the inferior vena cava (IVC) shows a large thrombus that terminates within the infrahepatic IVC. **B,** Transverse sonogram in the same patient shows thrombus extending from the hilum of the right kidney in a distended renal vein to IVC *(I)*. **C,** Transverse sonogram shows expansile, malignant left renal vein thrombus anterior to the aorta *(A)*. **D,** Sagittal sonogram in another patient shows expansile, malignant thrombus within retrohepatic IVC. **E,** Transverse sonogram in the same patient in **D** showing partially adherent malignant thrombus in the IVC.

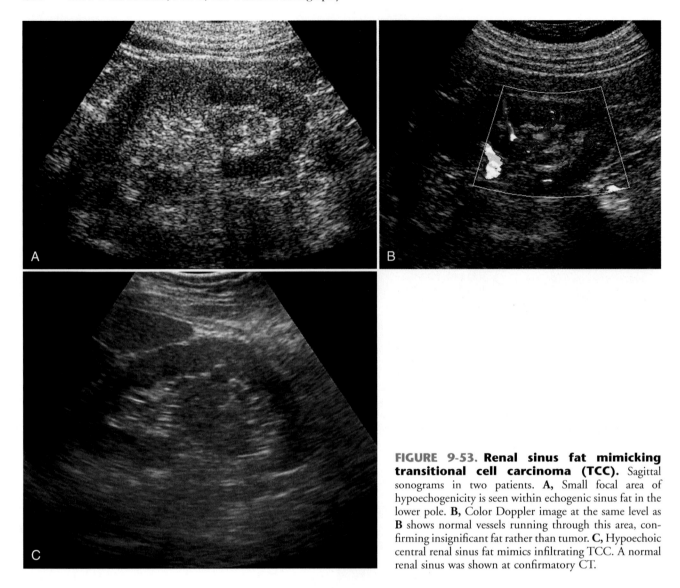

FIGURE 9-53. Renal sinus fat mimicking transitional cell carcinoma (TCC). Sagittal sonograms in two patients. **A,** Small focal area of hypoechogenicity is seen within echogenic sinus fat in the lower pole. **B,** Color Doppler image at the same level as **B** shows normal vessels running through this area, confirming insignificant fat rather than tumor. **C,** Hypoechoic central renal sinus fat mimics infiltrating TCC. A normal renal sinus was shown at confirmatory CT.

The sonographic appearance of renal TCC is variable and depends on the morphology of the lesion (papillary, nonpapillary, or infiltrative), location, size, and the presence or absence of hydronephrosis (Fig. 9-55). Small, nonobstructing tumors may be impossible to visualize at ultrasound. With growth, **papillary tumors** will be seen as discrete, solid, central, hypoechoic renal sinus masses with or without associated proximal caliectasis (Fig. 9-56). The differential diagnosis includes blood clots, sloughed papillae, and fungus balls.

Tumor infiltration within the renal pelvis or renal parenchyma may be subtle. Findings suggestive of infiltrating TCC are distortion and enlargement of the kidney and maintenance of an overall reniform shape (Fig. 9-56). Sessile lesions are particularly difficult to image directly by ultrasound, but the secondary finding of an obstructing lesion (caliectasis, pelviectasis) is usually easily depicted. A small subset of both sessile and papillary TCCs may have dystrophic calcifications, which makes it difficult to differentiate tumor from a sloughed, calcified papilla.[188] TCC rarely invades the renal vein.[189]

Ureteral Tumors

Transitional cell carcinoma of the ureter accounts for 1% to 6% of all upper urinary tract cancers.[185,190] Men are affected more often than women (3:1). As with renal TCC, ureteral lesions are usually identified in elderly patients; peak prevalence of ureteral TCC is between the fifth and seventh decades.[185] The majority of tumors are found in the lower third of the ureter (70%-75%).[185,190] About 60% of ureteral TCCs are papillary and 40% nonpapillary.[185] The most common symptoms are hematuria, frequency, dysuria, and pain.[190] The traditional imaging modalities of choice for evaluation of ureteral TCC have included IVU or retrograde pyelography, but the advantages of multidetector CT urography (ability to detect and stage even small urothelial lesions) have been

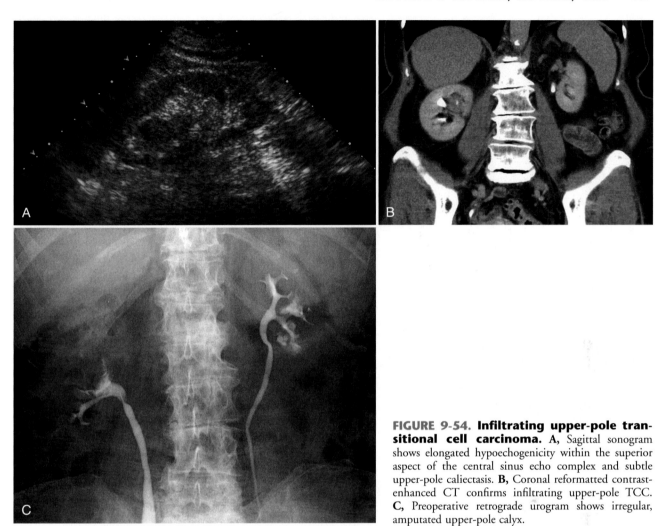

FIGURE 9-54. Infiltrating upper-pole transitional cell carcinoma. A, Sagittal sonogram shows elongated hypoechogenicity within the superior aspect of the central sinus echo complex and subtle upper-pole caliectasis. **B,** Coronal reformatted contrast-enhanced CT confirms infiltrating upper-pole TCC. **C,** Preoperative retrograde urogram shows irregular, amputated upper-pole calyx.

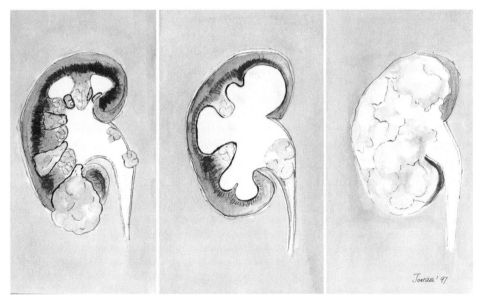

FIGURE 9-55. Morphologic growth patterns of renal transitional cell carcinoma.

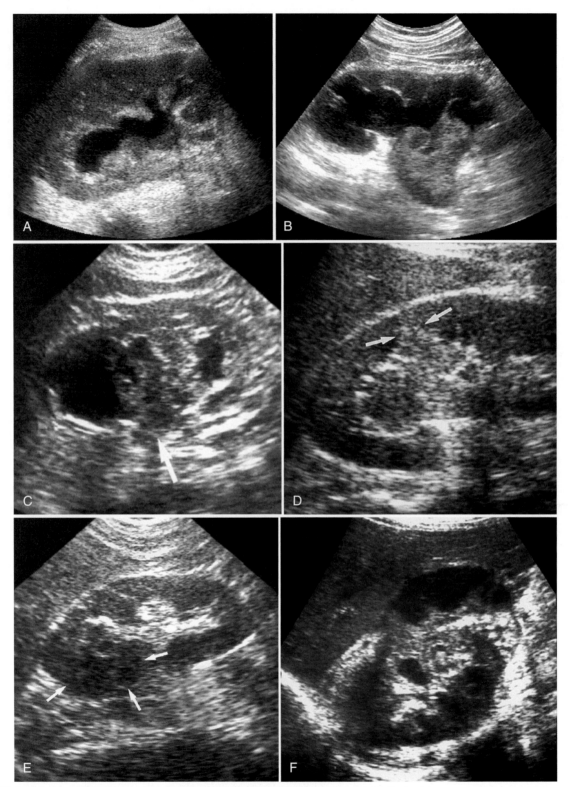

FIGURE 9-56. Transitional cell carcinoma of the kidney. A, B, and **C,** Sagittal sonograms in three different patients showing hydronephrosis related to large, central, solid pelvic tumors *(arrow* in **C**). **D,** Infiltrative TCC in the upper pole extends from the calix into the renal parenchyma *(arrows).* **E,** Large, lobulated, solid parenchymal infiltrative mass *(arrows)* with no associated caliectasis. **F,** Perirenal tumor extension.

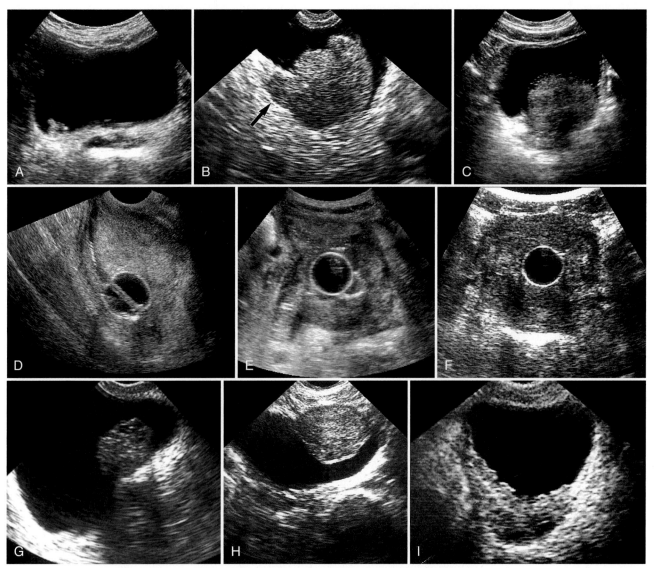

FIGURE 9-57. Bladder masses with many origins: imaging spectrum. A, Small polypoid transitional cell carcinoma (TCC). **B,** Invasive TCC involving the perivesical fat *(arrow).* **C,** Benign prostatic hypertrophy simulating a large invasive bladder wall mass. **D,** Diffuse TCC on a transvaginal sagittal image; Foley catheter is in place. **E,** Diffuse invasive TCC on suprapubic scan. **F,** Interstitial cystitis closely simulates diffuse tumor. **G,** Endometrioma appearing as a solid mass with small cystic spaces. **H,** Pheochromocytoma presenting as an anterior bladder wall submucosal mass. **I,** Lymphoma of the posterior bladder wall.

documented.[191,192] At sonography, hydronephrosis and hydroureter are seen, and occasionally a solid ureteral mass.[190]

Bladder Tumors

Transitional cell carcinoma of the bladder is a common malignant tumor. Bladder TCCs occur more often in men (3 : 1), with a peak incidence in the sixth and seventh decades. They occur most frequently at the trigone and along the lateral and posterior walls of the bladder. Approximately 70% of bladder cancers are superficial; the remaining 30% are invasive. Patients typically present with hematuria, although they may also complain of frequency, dysuria, and suprapubic pain. Sonographic

detection of **polypoid bladder tumors** is excellent (≥95%).[193] The appearance is that of a nonmobile focal mass or of urothelial thickening (Fig. 9-57). Ultrasound appearances are nonspecific, however, and the differential diagnosis is extensive, including cystitis, wall thickening caused by bladder outlet obstruction, postradiation/ postoperative change, adherent blood clot, invasive prostatic carcinoma, lymphoma, metastasis, endometriosis, and neurofibromatosis. Some papillary bladder tumors may also calcify. Cystoscopy and biopsy are necessary for diagnosis. Both transvaginal and transrectal ultrasound may also be used to assess a bladder wall mass if suprapubic visualization is compromised (Fig. 9-57).

Transitional cell (and squamous cell) carcinomas may also arise within **urinary bladder diverticula.** Many diverticula have narrow necks, making them inaccessible for cystoscopic examination, so imaging plays an important role in the detection of these tumors. The periureteric and posterolateral wall locations of most bladder diverticula allow for adequate sonographic visualization.[194] At ultrasound, diverticular tumors are moderately echogenic, nonshadowing masses. Although ultrasound is good for tumor detection, staging is still best performed clinically in combination with CT or contrast-enhanced MRI.[195]

Squamous Cell Carcinoma

Squamous cell carcinoma (SCC) is rare but is the second most common malignant urothelial tumor after TCC. SCC accounts for 6% to 15% of renal pelvic tumors and 5% to 8% of all bladder tumors.[196,197] Chronic infection, irritation, and stones lead to squamous metaplasia and leukoplakia of the urothelium. Leukoplakia is thought to be premalignant. SCC tends to be a solid, flat, infiltrating lesion with extensive ulceration. Distant metastases are usually present at diagnosis. As with other infiltrating renal lesions, renal SCC appears at sonography as a diffusely enlarged kidney that has maintained its reniform shape. Normal renal echotexture is destroyed, and often a stone (47%-58%)[196] will be present. It thus may be impossible to differentiate renal SCC from xanthogranulomatous pyelonephritis. Often, perinephric tumor extension and metastases are present. Ureteral SCC is rare; hydronephroureterectasis proximal to the tumor mass will be apparent. Occasionally, the lesion is seen as a poorly defined, irregular, solid mass. Associated stones are often present. Bladder SCCs tend to be large, solid, and infiltrating. SCCs may also arise within bladder diverticula.[194] Ultrasound may be an effective modality for detecting pedunculated bladder SCC, but CT or MRI are more appropriate modalities for detecting perivesical invasion, regional adenopathy, and distant metastases.

Adenocarcinoma

Adenocarcinoma of the renal pelvis, ureter, and bladder is rare. Almost all patients with adenocarcinoma of the renal pelvis have a history of chronic UTI,[198] and two thirds have a stone, typically a staghorn calculus. Clinicians must be careful to differentiate adenocarcinoma of the bladder from adenocarcinoma of the rectum, uterus, or prostate that has invaded the bladder. The prognosis is poor. At sonography, a renal pelvic, ureteric, or bladder mass is seen, occasionally with calcification. An associated stone is often present.

Oncocytoma

Oncocytes are large, epithelial cells. The characteristic granular eosinophilic cytoplasm in these cells results from extensive cytoplasmic mitochondria. Oncocytomas may occur in the parathyroid glands, thyroid, adrenal glands, salivary glands, and kidneys. Oncocytomas account for 3.1% to 6.6% of all renal tumors.[199,200] They occur more often in men (1.7 : 1), with a peak incidence in the sixth and seventh decades.[201] Most patients are asymptomatic.[199] Oncocytomas may be small or extremely large (mean, 3-8 cm) and may be multicentric (5%-10%) or bilateral (3%). Bilateral tumors are seen particularly in hereditary syndromes (Birt-Hogg-Dubé, hereditary oncocytosis).[200,202] Hemorrhage and calcification are uncommon. These tumors histologically may have a benign or a more malignant appearance. Differentiation between oncocytomas and chromophobe RCCs may be difficult,[203] and hybrid lesions consisting of both oncocytic and chromophobe RCC elements have been reported (see Fig. 9-51).

Not surprisingly, oncocytoma and renal cell carcinoma cannot be differentiated by imaging. Davidson et al.[204] demonstrated that CT homogeneity and a central stellate "scar" are poor predictors in differentiating oncocytomas from RCCs. In earlier surgical series, oncocytomas represented about 5% of all tumors originally diagnosed as RCC on imaging.[205] A higher percentage of benign oncocytomas will likely be documented in future series of smaller, incidental lesions sampled before nephron-sparing procedures.

No distinctive ultrasound appearance of oncocytomas has been shown. These lesions have differing echo patterns and may be homogeneous or heterogeneous with a distinct or poorly demarcated wall, depending on its size.[206] A central scar, central necrosis, or calcification may be seen, although these features may also be identified with RCC (see Fig. 9-51). The lack of specificity of CT and ultrasound features of oncocytomas typically prompts surgical resection, although as mentioned previously, recent improvements in immunohistochemistry may prompt imaging surveillance for patients with biopsy results consistent with benign oncocytomas.

Angiomyolipoma

Angiomyolipomas (AMLs) are benign renal tumors composed of varying proportions of adipose tissue, smooth muscle cells, and blood vessels. AMLs may occur sporadically or may be found in patients with **tuberous sclerosis.** In patients without stigmata of tuberous sclerosis, AMLs are typically unilateral and discovered in middle-aged women. Up to 50% of patients with AMLs will have clinical stigmata of tuberous sclerosis (mental retardation, epilepsy, facial sebaceous adenomas), and up to 80% of patients with tuberous sclerosis will have one or more AMLs.[207] AMLs associated with tuberous sclerosis are usually small, multiple, bilateral tumors, with no gender predilection. **Sporadic** AMLs are histologically identical to those associated with tuberous sclerosis. It is unusual for small tumors (<4 cm)[208] to be symptomatic; with growth, however, these tumors may

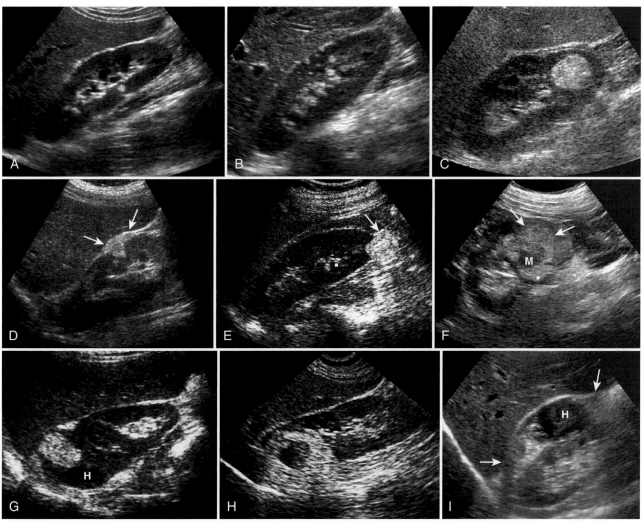

FIGURE 9-58. Imaging spectrum of angiomyolipomas (AMLs). A, Classic small hyperechoic intraparenchymal tumor.
B, Multiple small echogenic foci in the anterior cortex of the midpole. **C,** Solitary, large, highly echogenic mass in the lower pole.
D, Exophytic echogenic mass involves the cortex and the perirenal space *(arrows)*. The flat appearance suggests a compliant soft tumor.
E, Large exophytic lower-pole echogenic mass *(arrow)*. The echogenicity of the mass may be very similar to the perirenal fat. **F,** Large,
complex intrarenal mass *(arrows)* is mildly echogenic and has a hypoechoic component representing myomatous elements *(M)*. **G, H,** and
I, Hemorrhagic AMLs. **G,** Exophytic ruptured upper-pole AML with a perirenal hematoma *(H)*. **H,** Echogenic mass with central
hypoechoic hemorrhage. **I,** Large, predominantly exophytic AML. The kidney below the mass appears normal. The mass *(arrows)* shows
increased echogenicity from the fat in the AML and a large hypoechoic hemorrhage *(H)*.

hemorrhage, with symptoms such as hematuria, flank
pain, and palpable flank mass.

At sonography, the echo pattern of AMLs depends on
the proportions of fat, smooth muscle, vascular elements,
and hemorrhage. These tumors may be located within
renal parenchyma or may be exophytic (Fig. 9-58). If
muscle, hemorrhage, or vascular elements predominate,
the tumor may be hypoechoic. Siegel et al.[154] showed
that the multiple fat and nonfat interfaces in the more
typical AMLs, along with the large acoustic impedance
differences at these interfaces, causes scattering and
attenuation of sound waves. This histology leads to the
classic ultrasound appearance of an AML: an **echogenic
lesion with detectable shadowing.** As mentioned
earlier, although several distinguishing features have
been suggested, there is significant imaging overlap

between classic AMLs and small, echogenic RCCs.
Involvement of regional lymph nodes and extension of
AMLs into the IVC have also been described.[209] Further,
it may be difficult to differentiate a large, exophytic AML
from a large, retroperitoneal **liposarcoma** (Fig. 9-59).
Helpful features that may allow differentiation from
liposarcomas include (1) a defect in the renal parenchyma where the tumor originates and (2) the presence
of enlarged vessels and other associated AMLs.[210] The
blood vessels in an AML lack normal elastic tissue and
are prone to aneurysm formation and hemorrhage.[211]
Color flow Doppler sonography appears to be the best
imaging modality to detect an intratumoral pseudoaneurysm in a hemorrhagic AML.[212]

Small, asymptomatic AMLs may be followed for
growth; if large, symptomatic, or hemorrhaged, surgery

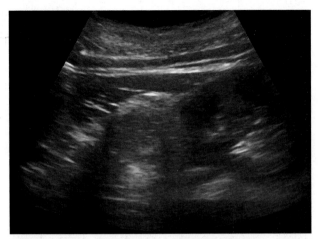

FIGURE 9-59. Exophytic angiomyolipoma. Sagittal sonogram shows a large, exophytic, echogenic AML.

is often performed. If possible, renal-sparing surgery is preferable, because these tumors are benign or may be multiple. Embolization may also be used to treat actively bleeding AMLs.[213]

Lymphoma

Kidney

The kidney does not contain lymphoid tissue. Thus, lymphomatous involvement of the kidney occurs from either hematogenous dissemination or contiguous extension of retroperitoneal disease. Renal involvement occurs more often in the setting of non-Hodgkin's lymphoma than Hodgkin's lymphoma. By the time renal disease is evident, disseminated disease is usually apparent. Urinary tract symptoms are uncommon. Occasionally, flank pain, a flank mass, or hematuria may occur. Nonetheless, at autopsy, renal involvement will be found in one third of lymphoma patients,[214] and bilateral renal disease is more common than unilateral disease. Isolated renal disease may be seen in patients undergoing treatment.

The sonographic appearance of **renal lymphoma** depends on the pattern of involvement. Four patterns are recognized: (1) focal parenchymal involvement, (2) diffuse infiltration, (3) invasion from a retroperitoneal mass, and (4) perirenal involvement. **Focal parenchymal involvement** may appear as solitary or multiple nodules. These masses appear homogeneous and hypoechoic or anechoic (Fig. 9-60). They may simulate cysts; however, increased through-transmission is absent.[215,216] As with other infiltrating renal tumors, **infiltrating lymphoma** is manifested by maintenance of a reniform shape despite disruption of renal architecture. The kidney may be enlarged (Fig. 9-61). Tumor may invade the renal sinus and destroy the echogenic, central echo complex.[217] **Direct invasion** of the kidney by large retroperitoneal **lymph node masses** may occur with associated vascular and ureteral encasement. Large, ret-

roperitoneal, hypoechoic conglomerate adenopathy may extend into the renal pelvis and cause hydronephrosis. The absence of renal venous invasion, despite extensive retroperitoneal and renal sinus tumor, may help in differentiating renal lymphoma from RCC. Rarely, **perirenal predominant tumor** may be depicted at ultrasound as a surrounding hypoechoic perirenal mass or rind. Tumor may be confused with hematoma or extramedullary hematopoiesis[218,219] (Fig. 9-62).

Ureter

The ureter may be either encased or displaced by surrounding retroperitoneal lymphoma. Ureteral displacement by periureteral tumor is more common; actual invasion of the ureteral wall occurs in only one third of cases.[190] The result is usually dilation of the intrarenal collecting system and ureter to the level of the retroperitoneal mass. This is usually easily appreciated on sonography.

Bladder

Primary bladder lymphoma arises from lymphoid follicles in the submucosa. Submucosal tumor usually does infiltrate the other layers of the bladder wall.[220] Most patients with primary bladder lymphoma are 40 to 60 years of age, and women are affected more than men. At sonography, a bladder wall mass is seen, usually covered by intact epithelium. If the mass is large, ulceration may occur (Fig. 9-63).

Leukemia

Leukemic involvement of the kidney may be **diffuse** or **focal**. In autopsy series, renal leukemic infiltration has been reported in 65% of patients.[221] Despite this, renal leukemia may be extremely difficult to identify at ultrasound.

The classic appearance of **renal leukemia** at ultrasound is **bilateral renal enlargement.** However, 15% of patients with leukemia will have nonspecific renomegaly without leukemic infiltration.[222] Renal leukemia may also be manifested as a coarsened renal echo pattern with distortion of the central sinus echo complex.[223] Alternatively, the kidneys may be diffusely echogenic. Focal masses may be single or multiple.[224] These patients are prone to renal, subcapsular, or perinephric hemorrhage.

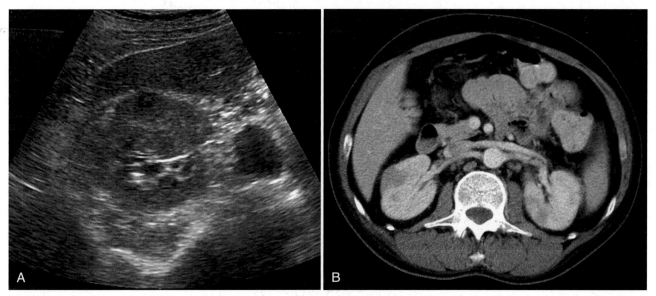

FIGURE 9-60. Renal lymphoma. A, Transverse sonogram shows a subtle right midpole contour deformity and vague hypoechoic lesion. **B,** Contrast-enhanced CT confirms mildly border-deforming renal lesion and shows contralateral lesions.

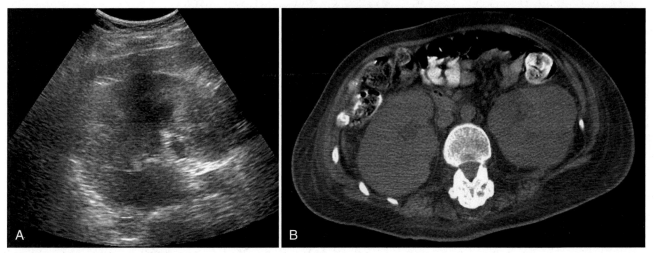

FIGURE 9-61. Renal lymphoma. A, Transverse sonogram shows enlarged, echogenic globular kidney. **B,** Non-contrast-enhanced CT shows marked bilateral renomegaly.

Metastases

Kidney

Renal metastases are typically clinically occult, but autopsy series done before cross-sectional imaging documented an incidence of 2% to 20%.[225] Literature before cross-sectional imaging also suggested that the kidney is the fifth most common site of metastases, after the lung, liver, bone, and adrenal gland.[226,227] The true prevalence of renal metastases in the era of cross-sectional imaging is unknown, but the prevalence of subclinical, imaging-apparent renal involvement is likely greater than estimated by gross autopsy.

Spread to the kidneys is by a hematogenous route. The most **common primary tumors** giving rise to renal metastases are (1) lung carcinoma, (2) breast carcinoma, and (3) renal cell carcinoma of the contralateral kidney.[121] Other tumors that may produce renal metastases include colon, stomach, cervix, ovary, pancreas, and prostate.[121] Renal metastatic spread may manifest as a solitary mass, multiple masses, or a diffusely infiltrating mass that enlarges the kidney. Choyke et al.[228] evaluated 27 patients with renal metastases and found that metastases are usually multifocal; however, large, solitary tumors may occur that are otherwise indistinguishable from primary RCC. Also, a new renal lesion in a patient with advanced cancer is more likely a metastatic than a

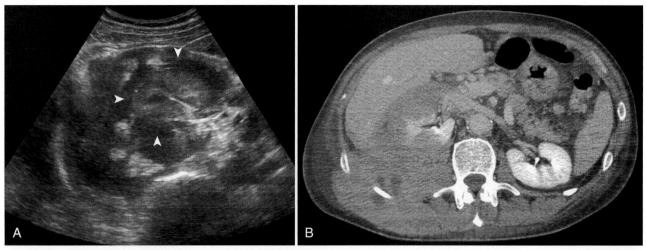

FIGURE 9-62. Perirenal Burkitt's lymphoma. A, Transverse sonogram shows extensive, poorly defined perirenal tumor. The kidney *(arrowheads)* is compressed and invaded by tumor. **B,** Contrast-enhanced CT shows bulky perirenal tumor. Tumor involves both the kidney and the overlying flank musculature.

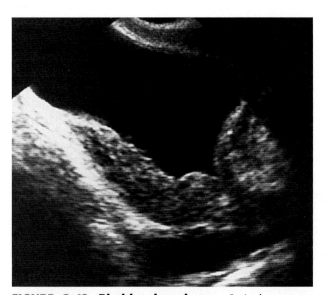

FIGURE 9-63. Bladder lymphoma. Sagittal transverse sonogram shows extensive bladder wall thickening with intact overlying mucosa.

primary tumor. If a single renal lesion is discovered synchronously in a patient with a known primary tumor, or with a tumor in remission with no evidence of other metastases, renal biopsy is necessary to differentiate a primary RCC from a renal metastasis.

Contrast-enhanced CT is the best radiographic technique for detecting renal metastasis, although ultrasound is almost as sensitive.[228] At sonography, the appearance will depend on the **pattern of involvement.** A solitary metastasis will be seen as a solid mass indistinguishable from RCC; this often occurs with colon carcinoma.[228] Central necrosis, hemorrhage, and calcification may be evident. Multiple metastases usually appear as small, poorly marginated, hypoechoic masses. Involvement of the perinephric space is possible, particularly with malig-

nant melanoma and lung cancer.[228] Infiltrating renal metastases may be particularly subtle at ultrasound; as with other infiltrating processes, the only manifestation at sonography may be an enlarged, but still reniform, kidney (Fig. 9-64).

Ureter

Ureteral metastases are rare; evidence of diffuse metastases elsewhere is seen in 90% of cases.[229] Metastatic disease to the ureter occurs by hematogenous or lymphatic dissemination. Tumors that may secondarily involve the ureter include melanoma, bladder, colon, breast, stomach, lung, prostate, kidney, and cervical lesions. Three types of ureteral involvement occur: (1) infiltration of the periureteral soft tissues, (2) transmural involvement of the ureteral wall, and (3) submucosal nodules. With the first two types, imaging may demonstrate strictures with or without an associated mass. Intraluminal lesions may be shown with the third type.[190] At sonography, the site of tumor involvement may be seen if a mass is present. Usually, however, the only manifestation of ureteral involvement is secondary hydronephrosis.

Bladder

Although rare, metastases to the bladder may occur with malignant melanoma, lung, gastric, or breast cancer. The appearance at ultrasound is nonspecific; a solid mass may be seen in the bladder wall (Fig. 9-65).

Urachal Adenocarcinoma

The urachus measures 3 to 10 cm in length and represents the obliterated remnant of the allantois. It is lined by transitional epithelium. The urachal remnant is

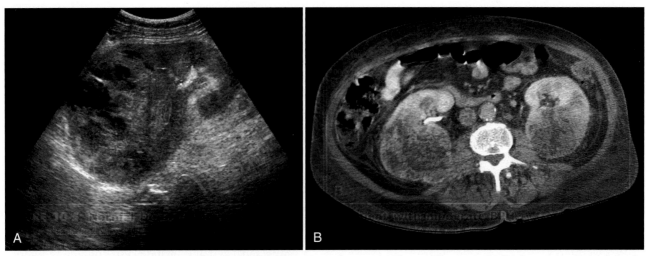

FIGURE 9-64. Renal metastases (lung primary). A, Sagittal sonogram shows infiltrating, mixed-echogenicity tumor throughout the upper pole of the kidney. **B,** Contrast-enhanced CT demonstrates bilateral infiltrating metastases.

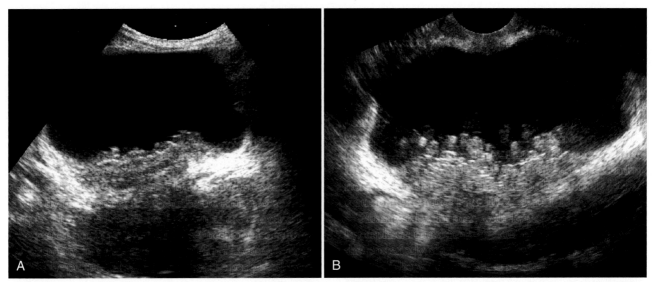

FIGURE 9-65. Bladder metastasis from gastric adenocarcinoma. A, Transverse suprapubic sonogram shows a papillary solid intraluminal mass with obvious bladder wall involvement. **B,** Confirmatory transvaginal scan shows the papillary nature of the tumor to better advantage.

divided into supravesical, intramural, and intramucosal portions. Urachal neoplasms are rare, usually arising in the upper part of the intramural portion of the urachal remnant or in the lower part of the extravesical portion of the bladder.[230] Urachal cancers represent 0.01% of all adult cancers, 0.17% to 0.34% of all bladder cancers, and 20% to 39% of all primary bladder adenocarcinomas.[231] About 75% of urachal cancers occur in men.[232] Most tumors arise at the bladder dome at the vesicourachal junction. Urachal tumors have a poor prognosis and tend to invade the anterior abdominal wall. Most patients present with hematuria, although other common symptoms include frequency, dysuria, and mucosuria.[232] At sonography, a bladder dome mass is seen, often calcified (50%-70%). The mass may be solid, cystic, or complex cystic-solid. Tumor extension into the perivesical fat,

space of Retzius, and the abdominal wall is common. Local recurrence after resection is common.

Rare Neoplasms

Kidney

Juxtaglomerular tumors are rare benign tumors that most frequently affect women. Renin secretion by these lesions results in hypertension. At sonography, they are usually small, solid, and hyperechoic.[233] Excision will alleviate the hypertension. **Leiomyomas** are benign tumors that arise from the renal capsule. They are usually discovered incidentally but may grow large enough to become clinically evident. On sonography, a solid, well-defined peripheral mass is seen. **Carcinoid tumor** is a rare renal tumor that tends to be solid, with peripheral or central calcification.[234] Other benign tumors that have been described include **lipomas** and **hemangiomas**.

Renal sarcomas account for approximately 1% of all malignant renal tumors. **Leiomyosarcoma** is the most common, representing 58% of all renal sarcomas. **Hemangiopericytoma** represents 20%. At sonography, these tumors cannot be distinguished from RCC. **Liposarcoma** accounts for 20% of all renal sarcomas. Depending on the amount of mature fat present, these tumors can be quite hyperechoic and indistinguishable from an AML. Less common sarcomas include rhabdomyosarcoma, fibrosarcoma, and osteogenic sarcoma. Wilms' tumor may rarely occur in adults and cannot be differentiated radiologically from RCC. All renal sarcomas are aggressive tumors.

Bladder

Mesenchymal bladder tumors also are rare, accounting for about 1% of all bladder tumors. **Leiomyoma** is the most common benign bladder tumor. Most leiomyomas arise from the submucosa near the bladder trigone.[235] These tumors may show intravesical (63%), intramural (7%), or extravesical (30%) growth.[235] At sonography, a well-defined, round or oval, solid mass will be seen. Cystic degeneration may occur. **Neurofibromas** of the bladder may be seen as an isolated finding or may occur with diffuse systemic disease. These tumors are similar to leiomyomas at ultrasound. **Cavernous hemangiomas** are most often found in the dome and posterolateral bladder wall.[236] At sonography, two types have been described: (1) a round, well-defined, solid, hyperechoic, intraluminal mass that is highly vascular on color Doppler ultrasound and (2) diffuse wall thickening with multiple hypoechoic spaces and calcification.[236] Bladder **pheochromocytomas** are rare; they account for only 1% of all pheochromocytomas.[235] Patients may have symptoms that include headaches, sweating, and tachycardia related to bladder distention or voiding. Pheochromocytomas arise in the submucosa and may be found anywhere in the bladder, but usually at the dome. At ultrasound, a well-defined, solid, intramural bladder wall mass will be seen (Fig. 9-66). Malignant mesenchymal bladder tumors are rare; the most common are **leiomyosarcomas** and **rhabdomyosarcomas.** At sonography, a large, infiltrative mass is seen.

RENAL CYSTIC DISEASE

Cortical Cysts

Simple renal cysts are benign and fluid filled. Their exact pathogenesis is unknown, although they are probably acquired lesions. They likely originate from distal convoluted or collecting ducts.[237] Incidence of simple cysts increases with advancing age, and they are found in at least 33% of persons over age 60.[238] Most cysts are asymptomatic. Patients with large cysts, however, may present with flank pain or hematuria. A cyst is confidently characterized at sonography when it (1) is anechoic; (2) has a sharply defined, imperceptible back wall; (3) is round or ovoid; and (4) enhances sound transmission.

If all these sonographic criteria are met, further evaluation or follow-up of the cyst is not required (Fig. 9-67). If a renal cyst is large and symptomatic, cyst puncture, aspiration, and sclerosis using a variety of agents may be performed. Several simple cysts may be found in both kidneys, and rarely, several simple cysts may involve only one kidney or a localized portion of one kidney.

Complex renal cysts do not meet the strict criteria of a simple renal cyst and include cysts containing internal echoes, septations, calcifications, perceptible defined walls, and mural nodularity (Fig. 9-68). Depending on the degree of abnormality, most complex renal cysts require further imaging with CT. A combination of ultrasound and contrast-enhanced CT (or MRI) helps determine whether a complex cystic lesion is more likely benign or malignant.

APPROACH TO COMPLEX RENAL CYST DISCOVERED ON SONOGRAPHY

Internal Echoes
Follow up with ultrasound if no other features of malignancy are present.
Perform computed tomography (CT) if associated features of malignancy are present (perceptible thickened wall, multiple or thick septations, or extensive septal calcification).

Septations
Follow up with ultrasound if septations are few and thin (≤1 mm).
Perform CT if there is septal irregularity and nodularity, multiple complex septations, or solid elements at septal wall attachment.

Calcification
Follow up with ultrasound if there is a small amount of calcium or milk of calcium without an associated soft tissue mass.
Perform CT if thick, irregular, or amorphous calcification.
Perform CT if calcification obscures adequate sonographic visualization.

Perceptible Defined Wall or Mural Nodularity
If presumed malignant, perform CT.
Use ultrasound-CT combination to analyze the internal features of a complex renal cyst to determine if more likely benign or malignant.
- Benign-type lesions can be followed with serial imaging.
- Malignant-type lesions will require surgical removal.

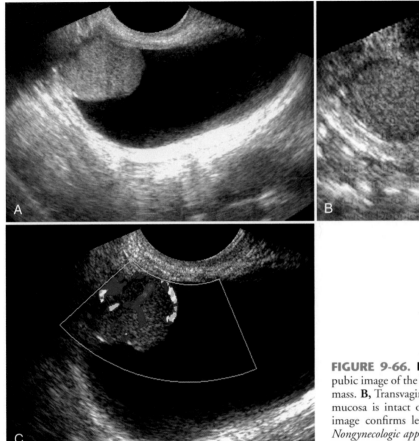

FIGURE 9-66. Bladder pheochromocytoma. A, Suprapubic image of the bladder shows a smooth surface to a solid bladder mass. **B,** Transvaginal scan with partial bladder emptying shows the mucosa is intact over the submucosal nodule. **C,** Color Doppler image confirms lesional vascularity. *(From Damani N, Wilson S. Nongynecologic applications of transvaginal ultrasound. RadioGraphics 1999;19:S179-S200.)*

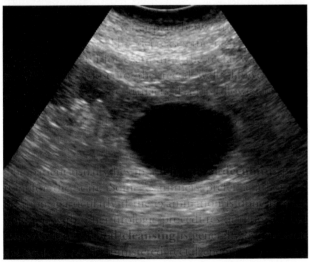

FIGURE 9-67. Renal cyst. Classic features of a renal cyst include a smooth wall, an echo-free center, and posterior acoustic enhancement caused by increased through-transmission.

Internal echoes within a cyst are usually the result of hemorrhage or infection. Approximately 6% of cysts are complicated by hemorrhage.[239] Infection of a cyst may occur by hematogenous seeding, by vesicoureteric reflux, or as a complication of cyst puncture or surgical manipu-

lation. A thickened cyst wall and a debris-fluid or gas-fluid level may suggest an infected cyst at ultrasound. Cysts that are thought to be hemorrhagic at ultrasound (i.e., cysts that contain low-level echoes but otherwise fulfill criteria for a benign cyst) may be followed with serial ultrasound. Infected cysts require aspiration and drainage for diagnosis and treatment.

Septations may be seen within a renal cyst, often the result of hemorrhage, infection, or percutaneous aspiration. Occasionally, two adjacent cysts sharing a wall may appear as a large, septated cyst. If septa are thin or barely perceptible, smooth, and attach to the cyst wall without thickened elements, a benign cyst can be diagnosed[240] (Fig. 9-68, *C*). Complex cysts with irregular, thickened (>1 cm) septa, or with septa that have solid elements at the wall attachment, should be viewed with concern. Cyst aspiration is not indicated in these multiseptated cystic lesions.[240] Ultrasound is often better than CT in defining the internal characteristics of a cystic lesion.

Calcification of renal cysts may be fine and linear or amorphous and thick. Thin wall or septal calcification suggests a complicated cyst rather than malignancy, if all other features of a benign cyst are shown at ultrasound, with no associated soft tissue mass enhancement at CT.[241] Thick, irregular, amorphous calcification is more worrisome, however, and should prompt resection, par-

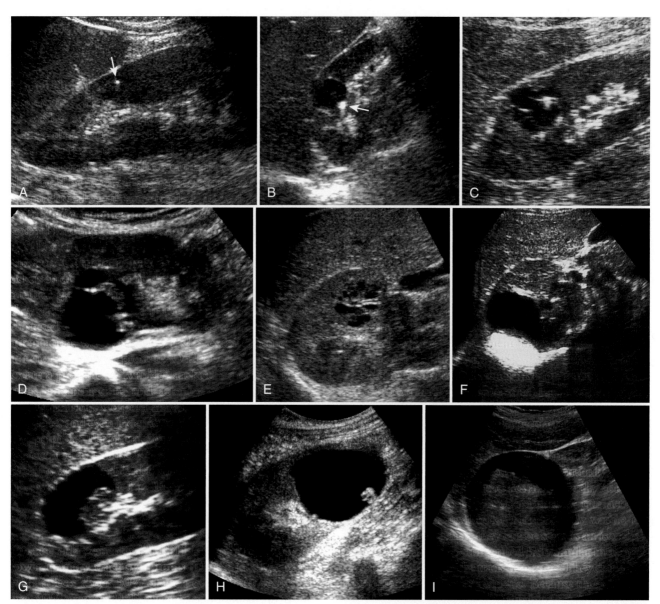

FIGURE 9-68. Complex renal cysts. A, Tiny renal cyst *(arrow)* in the anterior cortex is not resolved. A bright echogenic focus with "ringdown" artifact is the only visible abnormality. **B,** Discernible cyst shows a bright echogenic focus *(arrow)* with ringdown artifact. This echogenicity does not represent calcification. **C,** Complex benign cyst with a few thin septations. Ringdown artifact originates from the septations and the cyst wall. **D,** Complex cyst shows thick nodular septations. **E,** Cyst shows numerous internal thick and thin septations. **F,** Renal cyst with milk of calcium shown as dependent echogenic material that was mobile on real-time examination. **G** and **H,** Cyst with mural nodules. **I,** Large hemorrhagic cyst shows extensive internal debris within an otherwise simple-appearing cyst.

ticularly if there are solid, enhancing components at CT.[241] On the other hand, layering milk of calcium within a cyst is a benign finding (Fig. 9-68, *F*). Mimicking cyst wall calcification, the bright, echogenic foci with ringdown artifact are frequently seen in septa and cyst walls at ultrasound (Fig. 9-68, *A*). These foci are of no consequence, and no corresponding calcification is shown at CT. Perceptible, defined, thickened walls or mural nodularity essentially excludes a diagnosis of a benign cyst (Fig. 9-68, *G* and *H*). These lesions all require surgical removal to exclude malignancy.

The assessment of the **malignant potential** of renal cysts based on complexity at imaging was the basis of the classification introduced in 1991 by Bosniak.[174] Many sonographers attempt to classify cyst complexity using Bosniak terminology. It should be emphasized, however, that Bosniak criteria are primarily based on CT, and sonography is considered to be a useful adjunct. Nonetheless, the criteria are helpful for describing the malignant potential of renal cystic lesions at ultrasound.

The **Bosniak category 1 cystic lesion** has all the benign features of a simple cyst at ultrasound at contrast-enhanced CT. The **Bosniak category 2 cystic lesion** is more complicated and may have thin septa and calcification at CT. A high-attenuation (proteinaceous or hemorrhagic) cyst, that is, with an attenuation of less than 60 Hounsfield units (HU) that enhances less than 10 HU after contrast administration, may often appear as a simple cyst at ultrasound. Malignancy risk assessment may be flawed, however, if the sonographer arbitrarily uses ultrasound features of more complex lesions to assign Bosniak grades. Minimally complex (Bosniak 2) lesions at CT can have a much more malignant appearance at ultrasound. High levels of protein with cyst fluid may appear at ultrasound as low-level echoes, an appearance that might erroneously suggest a solid "malignant" lesion. In addition, thin septations within a Bosniak type 2 cyst at CT will often appear much more ominous at ultrasound. It is this sonographic-CT discrepancy that often prompts a category 2 "F" classification (i.e., a probably benign lesion that nonetheless should be followed by imaging). The risk of malignancy in a cystic lesion appropriately classified as **Bosniak 2F** (by CT) is estimated to be 5%.[242]

The **Bosniak category 3 cystic lesion** is indeterminate at CT. Thick, irregular septations, calcifications, and wall nodularity increase the risk of malignancy, regardless of the imaging modality used. Although surgery is often advocated, imaging follow-up is done in the appropriate clinical setting, as when a renal abscess is suspected in a patient with fever, leukocytosis, and pyuria, or in elderly patients with comorbidities. Other lesions in this category include highly complex hemorrhagic cysts, multilocular cystic nephroma, localized cystic disease, and cystic RCC. CT enhancement of septa, mural nodules, and solid components within highly complex cysts significantly increases the risk of malignancy in the **Bosniak category 4 cystic lesion.**

Ultrasound has played a largely adjunct role in risk stratification of more complex renal cystic lesions because it does not readily demonstrate renal tumor neovascularity. Wall or septal enhancement that is obvious at CT may be rarely depicted at ultrasound as focally increased color or power Doppler flow (see Fig. 9-49). However, microbubble contrast agents may increase the importance of ultrasound in renal mass characterization (see Fig. 9-50). Renal lesion enhancement using continuous, low-MI pulse inversion imaging (or an equivalent) may mimic the enhancement shown at contrast-enhanced CT or MRI.[172,243] The ability of contrast-enhanced ultrasound to show neovascularity may be particularly relevant for patients with renal insufficiency and may assist in assessing adequacy of ablation.[244] Nonetheless, significant obstacles remain. The techniques are labor and time intensive; enhancement is qualitative; and the agents have not been approved by the FDA for noncardiac imaging.

Parapelvic Cysts

Parapelvic cysts do not communicate with the collecting system. They may originate from lymphatics or embryologic rests.[245] Most are asymptomatic, although rarely parapelvic cysts may cause hematuria, hypertension, or hydronephrosis; may become infected; or may bleed.[246] At sonography, parapelvic cysts appear as well-defined, anechoic, renal sinus masses (Fig. 9-69). If they have hemorrhaged, internal echoes will be seen in the cysts. It may be difficult to differentiate multiple parapelvic cysts from hydronephrosis (Fig. 9-69). Optimized technique and real-time examination usually suffice to distinguish between multiple noncommunicating, haphazard parapelvic cysts and the communicating, dilated calices and renal pelvis that are the hallmark of hydronephrosis. If differentiation is not possible with sonography, delayed contrast-enhanced CT will resolve the dilemma.

Medullary Cysts

Medullary Sponge Kidney

Medullary sponge kidney (MSK) is defined as dilated, ectatic collecting tubules. It may be focal or diffuse. The etiology is unknown. The incidence of MSK in the general population is not known, but it is found in up to 12% of patients with renal calculi.[220,247] Associations with hemihypertrophy, Ehlers-Danlos syndrome, congenital hypertrophic pyloric stenosis, hyperparathyroidism, Caroli's disease, and autosomal recessive polycystic disease have been reported.[220] Uncomplicated MSK is usually not associated with symptoms; with stone formation, however, renal colic, hematuria, dysuria, and flank pain may occur.[248] The onset of symptomatic MSK is usually in the third to fourth decades of life.[220]

Tubular ectasia may be difficult to impossible to recognize at ultrasound (see Fig 9-44). When nephrocalcinosis is present, multiple echogenic shadowing foci are seen localized to the medullary pyramids (see Fig. 9-45). Erosion of a calcification into the collecting system may result in obstruction.

Medullary Cystic Disease

Familial juvenile nephronophthisis and medullary cystic disease are both characterized by small cysts at the corticomedullary junction and medulla. The kidneys are small or normal sized. Tubointerstitial fibrosis is a hallmark of both entities.[249] Juvenile nephronophthisis is an autosomal recessive condition. Patients present with polyuria, salt wasting, and ultimately ESRD. **Medullary cystic disease,** on the other hand, is an autosomal dominant condition. Patients with this disease present in the third or fourth decade of life with similar renal symptoms as nephronophthisis.[250] At sonography, small

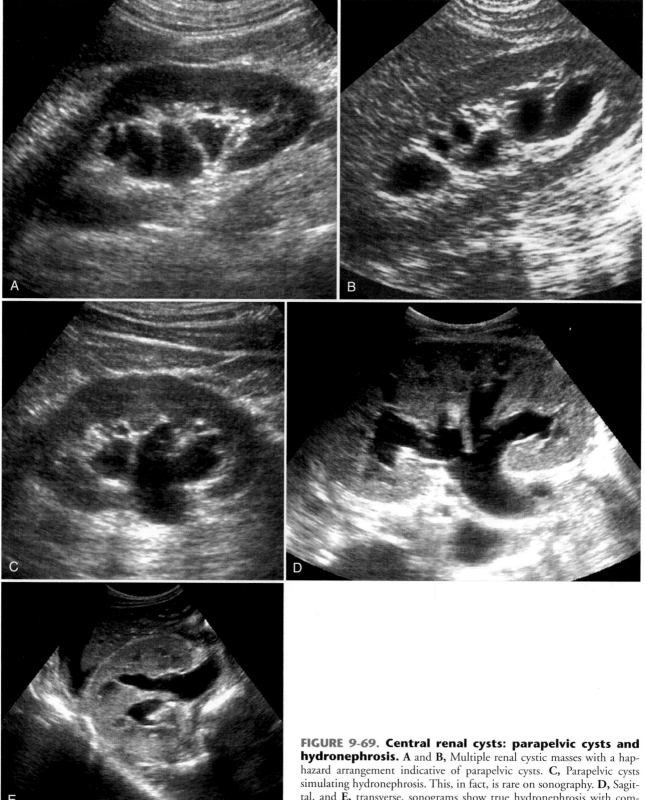

FIGURE 9-69. Central renal cysts: parapelvic cysts and hydronephrosis. A and **B,** Multiple renal cystic masses with a haphazard arrangement indicative of parapelvic cysts. **C,** Parapelvic cysts simulating hydronephrosis. This, in fact, is rare on sonography. **D,** Sagittal, and **E,** transverse, sonograms show true hydronephrosis with communication of the central cystic components.

echogenic kidneys with medullary cysts (0.1-1.0 cm) are seen.

Polycystic Kidney Disease

Autosomal recessive polycystic kidney disease (ARPKD) is divided into four types—perinatal, neonatal, infantile, and juvenile—depending on the patient's age at the onset of clinical manifestations. ARPKD is characterized pathologically as a spectrum of dilated renal collecting tubules, hepatic cysts, and periportal fibrosis. Younger patients present predominantly with renal insufficiency. Hepatic involvement is typically dominant in older patients with ARPKD. ARPKD occurs in 1:6000 to 1:14,000 live births. Patients with perinatal disease will have massively enlarged kidneys, hypoplastic lungs, and oligohydramnios. Death usually results from renal failure and pulmonary hypoplasia. Older children will present with manifestations of portal hypertension. Ultrasound features of renal-dominant ARPKD include a lack of corticomedullary differentiation and massively enlarged, echogenic kidneys (Fig. 9-70). Occasionally, macroscopic cysts will be noted.

Autosomal dominant polycystic kidney disease (ADPKD) results in a large number of bilateral cortical and medullary renal cysts. The cysts may vary in size and are often asymmetrical. ADPKD is the most common hereditary renal disorder and has no gender predilection. Its incidence is 1:500 to 1:1000, and ADPKD accounts for 10% to 15% of patients receiving dialysis. Up to 50% of patients have no family history. Seemingly sporadic involvement is caused by variable expression and spontaneous mutations. Signs and symptoms of palpable masses, pain, hypertension, hematuria, and UTI usually do not develop until the fourth or fifth decade. Renal failure develops in 50% of patients and is usually present by age 60.[251] Complications of ADPKD include infection, hemorrhage, stone formation, cyst rupture, and obstruction. Stone formation tends to occur in patients with more and significantly larger cysts.[252] Associated anomalies include liver cysts (30%-60%); pancreatic cysts (10%); splenic cysts (5%); cysts in thyroid, ovary, endometrium, seminal vesicles, lung, brain, pituitary gland, breast, and epididymis; cerebral berry aneurysms (18%-40%); abdominal aortic aneurysm; cardiac lesions; and colonic diverticula. Patients with ADPKD who are not receiving dialysis do not have an increased incidence of RCC.[251]

At sonography, the kidneys are enlarged and replaced by multiple bilateral, asymmetrical cysts of varying size (Fig. 9-71). Cysts complicated by hemorrhage or infection will have thick walls, internal echoes, and/or fluid-debris levels. Dystrophic calcification within cyst walls or stones may be seen as echogenic foci with sharp, distal acoustic shadowing.

Renal cysts in patients under age 30 are rare. Ravine et al.[253] modified the criteria of Bear et al.[254] and reported that patients age 30 or younger with a family history of ADPKD require two renal cysts (unilateral or bilateral) to have the diagnosis of ADPKD disease. For patients age 30 to 59, two cysts in both kidneys are required, and for those age 60 or older, four cysts in each kidney are needed. These criteria were recently modified to account for the relatively later onset of disease in patients with type 2 polycystic kidney disease, but fewer than two renal cysts in at-risk individuals over age 40 was still sufficient to exclude the disease.[255]

Ultrasound is the most studied initial imaging modality available for screening families of patients with ADPKD, as well as for routine follow-up of patients. Renal volume and blood flow assessment by MRI may ultimately help predict disease progression. In a recent MRI study by the Consortium for Radiologic Imaging Studies of Polycystic Kidney Disease (CRISP), renal blood flow reduction paralleled kidney volume increases.[256] Both were independent predictors of glomerular filtration rate (GFR) decline. However, this MRI-based prognostic approach has not been widely adopted outside of select research centers.

Multicystic Dysplastic Kidney

Multicystic dysplastic kidney (MCDK) is a nonhereditary developmental anomaly also known as **renal dysplasia, renal dysgenesis,** and **multicystic kidney.** The kidney is small, malformed, and composed of multiple cysts with little, if any, normal renal parenchyma. It functions poorly if at all. The dysplastic change is usually

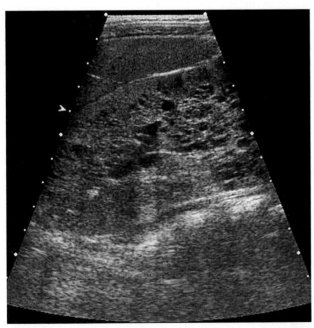

FIGURE 9-70. Autosomal recessive polycystic kidney disease. Two-year-old patient with renal insufficiency. Sagittal sonogram shows marked renal enlargement and innumerable microcysts.

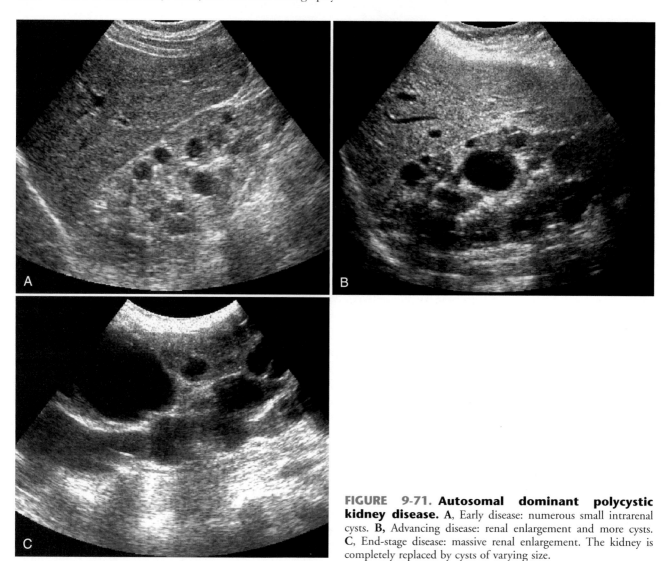

FIGURE 9-71. **Autosomal dominant polycystic kidney disease. A,** Early disease: numerous small intrarenal cysts. **B,** Advancing disease: renal enlargement and more cysts. **C,** End-stage disease: massive renal enlargement. The kidney is completely replaced by cysts of varying size.

unilateral and involves the entire kidney, although rarely it may be bilateral, segmental, or focal. If unilateral, MCDK is asymptomatic. If bilateral, it is incompatible with life. Men and women are equally affected, as are both sides. Up to 30% of patients have a contralateral UPJ obstruction. The exact pathogenesis is obscure. However, 90% of cases are associated with some form of urinary tract obstruction during embryogenesis. The severity of the malformation and the age of the patient at diagnosis account for the varying manifestations of MCKD, from a large, multicystic mass present at birth to a kidney with smaller cysts not discovered until adulthood.

Ultrasound findings of MCKD include (1) multiple noncommunicating cysts, (2) absence of both normal parenchyma and normal renal sinus, and (3) focal echogenic areas representing primitive mesenchyma or tiny cysts[257] (Fig. 9-72). In adults a small, cystic renal fossa mass is shown, and cyst wall calcification is appreciated as echogenic foci with shadowing. Calcification may be so extensive that ultrasound visualization is impossible,

and CT is required to make the diagnosis. Segmental disease is usually seen in duplex kidneys, and if the cysts are tiny, the mass may appear solid and echogenic.

Multilocular Cystic Nephroma

Multilocular cystic nephroma (MLCN) is an uncommon benign cystic neoplasm composed of multiple noncommunicating cysts contained within a well-defined capsule. Occasionally, sarcomatous stroma is present, making this a more malignant lesion. MLCN has no predilection for side, and occasionally, bilateral tumors are seen. These tumors are found in male patients less than 4 years of age and in female patients ages 4 to 20 or 40 to 60 years.[258] Most children present with an abdominal mass. Adults may be asymptomatic or may present with abdominal pain, hematuria, hypertension, and UTI.

The ultrasound appearance of MLCN is variable and depends on the number and size of the locules. With multiple large locules, noncommunicating cysts will be seen within a well-defined mass (Fig. 9-73). If the locules are tiny, a more solid-appearing nonspecific echogenic mass will be present. Calcification of the capsule and septa is uncommon. With either appearance, it is impossible with imaging to differentiate MLCN from cystic RCC.

Localized Cystic Disease

Localized cystic disease is a rare, benign, nonhereditary entity that may mimic autosomal polycystic kidney disease (APKD) and MLCN. In localized cystic disease, multiple closely opposed cysts occupy either a portion of kidney or an entire kidney—thus the previous description of "unilateral polycystic disease."[259] At ultrasound, localized cystic disease appears a conglomerate mass of multiple cysts of varying size separated by normal or

atrophic renal parenchyma (Fig. 9-74). The lack of cysts within other organs (or the contralateral kidney) and the absence of an appropriate family history of APKD might prompt the ultrasound diagnosis of localized cystic disease, although CT/MRI confirmation is typically needed. In addition, CT (or MRI) better shows the thick, fibrous, encapsulating capsule characteristic of MLCN.[260]

Neoplasm-Associated Renal Cystic Disease

Acquired Cystic Kidney Disease

Acquired cystic kidney disease (ACKD) occurs in the native kidneys of patients with **renal failure** undergoing either hemodialysis or peritoneal dialysis. ACKD affects 40% to 90% of these patients, depending on the duration of dialysis.[128,129,250,261] Renal cell carcinoma occurs in 4% to 10% of patients with ACKD.[261] The pathogenesis of ACKD is speculative. Epithelial hyperplasia caused by tubular obstruction resulting from toxic substances plays some role in the development of both cysts and tumors.[261] Pathologically, multiple small cysts (0.5-3 cm) involving both renal cortex and medulla are found. Hemorrhage into cysts is common. Ultrasound, CT, and MRI are useful in the evaluation and follow-up of patients with ACKD and its complications.[128,129,262] Current data suggest that ACKD and tumor development persist even after successful renal transplantation. ACKD and tumors may develop in renal allografts during dialysis therapy.[263]

At sonography, finding three to five cysts in each kidney in a patient with chronic renal failure is diagnostic.[263] The cysts are usually small, as are the kidneys, which typically are quite echogenic (Fig. 9-75). Internal echoes are seen in cysts that have hemorrhaged. Tumors are solid or cystic with mural nodules.

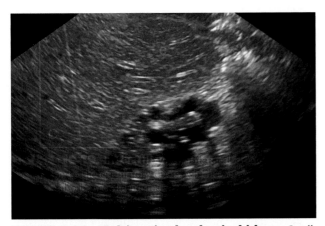

FIGURE 9-72. Multicystic dysplastic kidney. Small, malformed kidney containing multiple cysts. *(Case courtesy Deborah Rubens, MD.)*

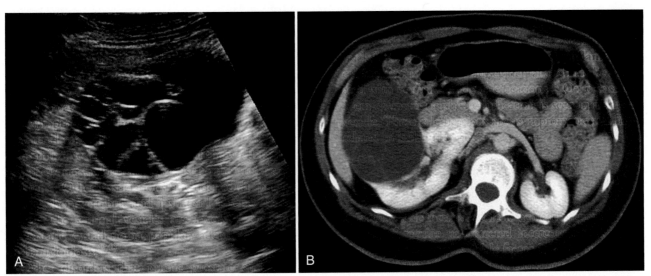

FIGURE 9-73. Multilocular cystic nephroma. A, Transverse sonogram demonstrates a multiseptated, exophytic, complex cystic mass with noncommunicating locules. **B,** Confirmatory contrast-enhanced CT.

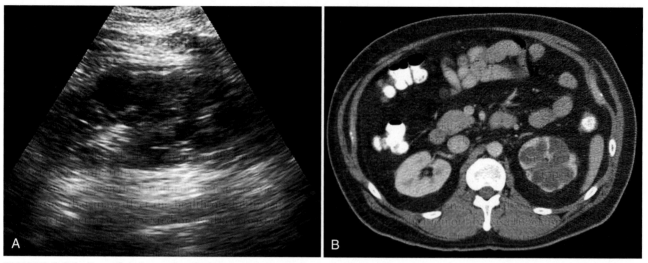

FIGURE 9-74. Localized cystic disease. A, Sagittal sonogram shows multiple, closely opposed, various-sized cysts throughout the kidney. **B,** Contrast-enhanced CT confirms replacement of the left kidney by cysts.

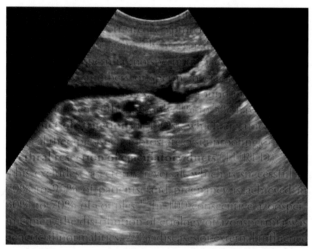

FIGURE 9-75. Acquired cystic kidney disease. Sagittal sonogram demonstrates an echogenic small kidney containing multiple cysts. A small amount of intraperitoneal dialysate fluid is seen.

Von Hippel–Lindau Disease

Von Hippel–Lindau (VHL) disease is transmitted as an autosomal dominant gene with variable expression and moderate penetrance. Its incidence is 1:35,000.[251] The predominant significant abnormalities include **retinal angiomatosis,** central nervous system (CNS) **hemangioblastomas, pheochromocytomas,** and **renal cell carcinoma** (40%). RCC in VHL patients usually is multifocal (75%-90%) and bilateral (75%). These patients are often offered nephron-sparing surgery. In addition, renal cysts, the most common finding in VHL disease, are found in 76% of patients.[264] Cysts range from 0.5 to 3.0 cm in size and are mostly cortical based. Ultrasound may be used as an initial screening test for VHL disease. However, CT or MRI is better for detection of the small, multifocal, bilateral tumors found in VHL disease

and are the preferred modalities for surveillance after nephron-sparing surgery (Fig. 9-76).

Tuberous Sclerosis

Tuberous sclerosis (TS) is a genetically transmitted disease characterized by mental retardation, seizures, and adenoma sebaceum. Some cases are transmitted in an autosomal dominant manner, although many result from spontaneous mutation. The incidence ranges from 1:9000 to 1:170,000.[265] Associated renal lesions include cysts, AML, and RCC (1%-2%).[251] The renal cysts vary in size from microscopic to 3 cm. At sonography, if only cysts are present, it may be difficult to differentiate TS from ADPKD. The presence of cysts and multiple AMLs confirmed with CT suggests TS (Fig. 9-77). Periodic CT screening is recommended to assess for AML growth and tumor development.

TRAUMA

Renal Injuries

Traumatic injury to the kidney may be blunt or penetrating. Most forms of **blunt** trauma to the kidney are relatively minor and heal without treatment. **Penetrating** injuries are usually the result of gunshot or stab wounds. Kidneys with cysts, tumors, and hydronephrosis are more prone to injury. Renal injuries are classified into the following four categories[266]:

I: Minor injury (75%-85%): contusions, subcapsular hematoma, small cortical infarct and lacerations that do not extend into the collecting system

II: Major injury (10%): renal lacerations that may extend into the collecting system and segmental renal infarct

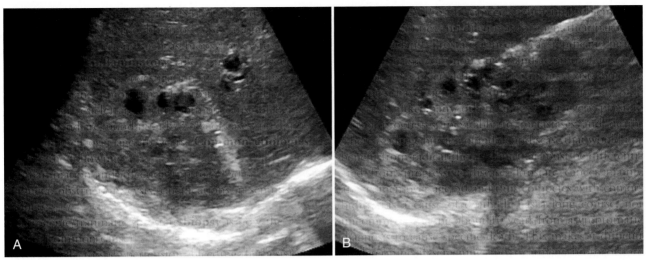

FIGURE 9-76. Von Hippel–Lindau Disease. A, Transverse, and **B,** sagittal, sonograms show multiple small, complex cystic lesions.

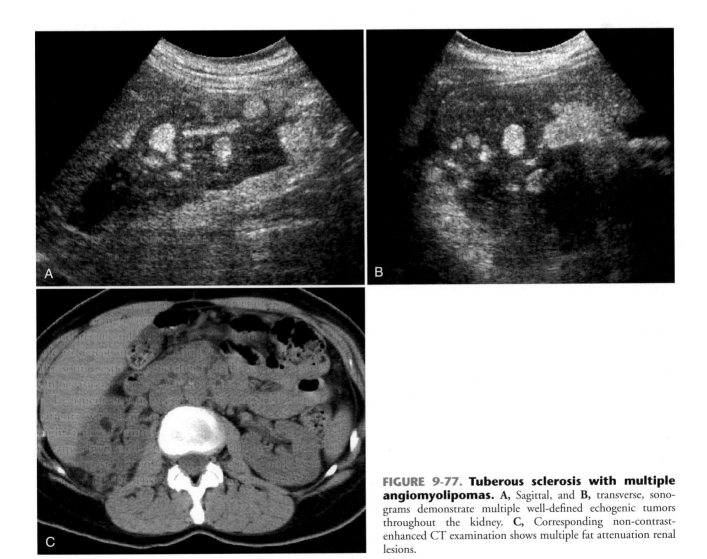

FIGURE 9-77. Tuberous sclerosis with multiple angiomyolipomas. A, Sagittal, and **B,** transverse, sonograms demonstrate multiple well-defined echogenic tumors throughout the kidney. **C,** Corresponding non-contrast-enhanced CT examination shows multiple fat attenuation renal lesions.

III: Catastrophic injury (5%): vascular pedicle injury and shattered kidney

IV: Uteropelvic junction avulsion

Category I lesions are treated conservatively, whereas category III and IV lesions require urgent surgery. Category II lesions will be treated conservatively or surgically depending on severity.[266,267]

Computed tomography is regarded as the premier imaging modality for the evaluation of suspected renal trauma.[266] Because renal trauma is frequently accompanied by injuries to other organs, CT has the advantage of multiorgan imaging. Theoretically, sonography has the capability of evaluating traumatized kidneys; in reality, technical limitations usually hinder an adequate examination. Sonography does not provide information regarding renal function and is probably best used in the follow-up of patients with known renal parenchymal trauma. **Renal hematomas** may be hypoechoic, hyperechoic, or heterogeneous. **Lacerations** are seen as linear defects that may extend through the kidney if a fracture is present (Fig. 9-78). Associated **perirenal collections** consisting of blood and urine will be present if the kidney is fractured. **Subcapsular hemorrhage** may be seen as a perirenal fluid collection that flattens the underlying renal contour (Fig. 9-79). A **shattered kidney** consists of multiple fragments of disorganized tissue with associated hemorrhage and urine collection in the renal bed. Color Doppler sonography may be helpful in the assessment of **vascular pedicle injuries.** Recent reports also suggest a role for contrast-enhanced sonography in the initial bedside assessment and follow-up of renal injuries in critically ill patients.[268,269]

Ureteral Injuries

Traumatic injury of the ureter is most often a complication of either gynecologic (70%) or urologic (30%) surgery.[270] Blunt and penetrating injuries are much less common. The treatment of these injuries is controversial. Many urologists suggest nephrostomy and ureteral stenting as an initial approach, if possible. Ureteral stents are left for 8 to 12 weeks to allow the ureter to heal.[271] Sonography is not useful in the assessment of these injuries, except to detect sizable fluid collections and hydronephrosis.

Bladder Injuries

Bladder injury may be the result of blunt, penetrating, or iatrogenic trauma. Bladder injury may result in extraperitoneal or intraperitoneal rupture, or a combination. Sonography is usually not helpful in the assessment of these injuries, except to identify large fluid collections or free intraperitoneal fluid.

VASCULAR ABNORMALITIES

Renal Vascular Doppler Sonography

The number and size of arteries supplying a kidney are quite variable. Duplex and color Doppler imaging are able to demonstrate both normal and abnormal renal blood flow. Normal flow within the renal artery and its branches has a "low resistance" perfusion pattern, with continuous forward blood flow during diastole. Several Doppler parameters have been used to describe changes in Doppler arterial spectra that may accompany renal disease. The most common parameter is the resistive index (RI = peak systolic frequency − end diastolic frequency/peak systolic frequency). RI is an easily calculated, angle-independent measurement. Calculation software is available on even lower-level ultrasound plat-

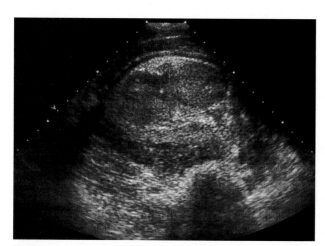

FIGURE 9-78. Renal laceration. Transverse sonogram shows capsular disruption and mixed-echogenicity perirenal hematoma. *(Case courtesy John McGahan, MD.)*

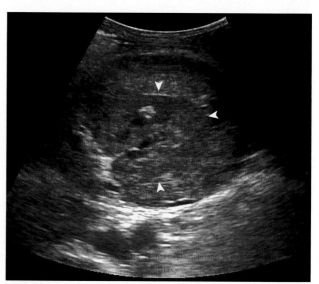

FIGURE 9-79. Subcapsular hematoma after renal biopsy. Note compression of kidney *(arrowheads)* by large, hyperechoic subcapsular hematoma.

forms. However, Keogan et al.[272] recommend averaging a number of RI measurements in a kidney before a single representative average is reported. Most sonographers consider an RI of 0.7 to be the upper threshold of normal in adults, although renal RIs greater than 0.7 may be seen in children under 4 years of age and in elderly patients, despite normal renal function.[273-275] Mostbeck et al.[276] also showed how the RI varies with heart rate and can range from 0.57 ± 0.06 (pulse, 120/min) to 0.70 ± 0.06 (pulse, 70/min).

Despite this variability, early literature indicated the potential of Doppler for improving the sonographic assessment of **renal dysfunction.** Changes in intrarenal spectra (quantified using RI) were associated with acute or chronic urinary obstruction, several intrinsic native renal diseases, renal transplant rejection, and renal vascular disease. Less favorable results in follow-up studies and discouraging clinical experience prompted most radiologists to abandon the RI. A review indicated that this failed promise may have been caused by a lack of understanding of the hemodynamic changes that influence Doppler spectra.[112] Indeed, although the terms "RI" and "renal vascular resistance" were used interchangeably in initial articles, follow-up studies using in vitro and ex vivo models have convincingly shown that the resistive index is largely independent of vascular resistance. These studies show that the RI varies as a result of **driving pulse pressures,** which explains Mostbeck's observation of rate-dependent changes in RIs, as well as changes in vascular/interstitial compliance.[113-115]

Color Doppler sonography is based on mean Doppler frequency shift, whereas power Doppler relies on the integrated Doppler power spectrum, which is related to the number of erythrocytes producing the Doppler shift. Power Doppler is subject to significant flash artifact. However, Bude et al.[277] showed that in normal cooperative individuals, power Doppler is superior to conventional color Doppler in the demonstration of normal intrarenal vessels. Power Doppler also has the advantage of not being subject to aliasing and angle dependence. However, direction and velocity of motion are apparent only with color Doppler ultrasound.

Renal Artery Occlusion and Infarction

Renal artery occlusion may be caused by either emboli or in situ thrombosis. The degree of renal insult depends on the size and location of the occluded vessel. If the main renal artery is occluded, the entire kidney will be affected, whereas segmental and focal infarction may occur with peripherally located vascular occlusion. The acutely infarcted kidney is often normal appearing at gray-scale sonography. However, no flow within the kidney is shown at duplex and color Doppler examination. Segmental or focal infarction may appear as a wedge-shaped mass indistinguishable from acute pyelonephritis (Fig. 9-80). With time, an echogenic mass[278] or scar may form. With chronic occlusion, a small, scarred, end-stage kidney will be seen.

Arteriovenous Fistula and Malformation

Abnormal arteriovenous communications may be acquired (75%) or congenital (25%). **Acquired** lesions are usually iatrogenic, although spontaneous abnormal arteriovenous communications may occur with eroding tumors. Most acquired lesions consist of a single, dominant feeding artery and a single, dominant draining vein. **Congenital** malformations consist of a tangle of small, abnormal vessels. Gray-scale sonography may reveal no abnormality. The addition of duplex and color Doppler imaging has been helpful in defining these lesions.[279] Duplex Doppler demonstrates increased flow velocity, a decreased RI (0.3-0.4), and turbulent diastolic flow in

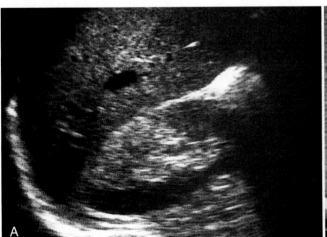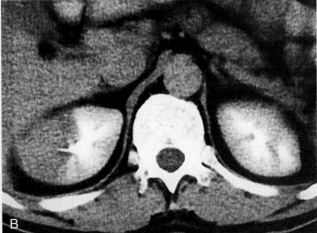

FIGURE 9-80. Renal infarct. A, Sagittal sonogram shows a wedge-shaped echogenic mass in the anterolateral renal cortex. **B,** Confirmatory contrast-enhanced CT image shows segmental infarction.

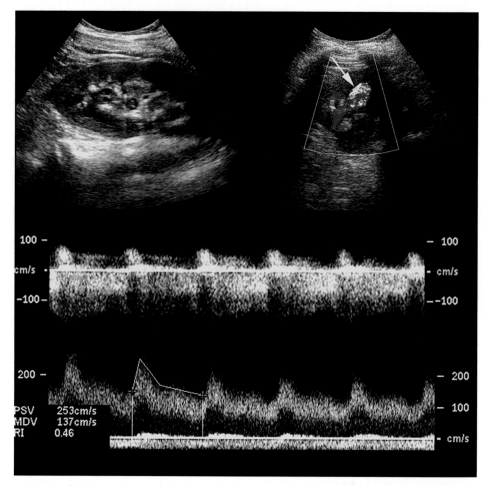

FIGURE 9-81. Renal arteriovenous malformation (AVM). Top: *Left image,* Normal sagittal sonogram of the kidney. *Right image,* Focus of color aliasing *(arrow).* **Middle:** Spectral waveform shows a high-velocity draining vein. **Bottom:** Spectral waveform shows an arterial signal from within the AVM. Note high-velocity, low "resistance" flow (RI = 0.46).

the arterial limb. Arterial pulsations in the draining vein are also observed. Spectral broadening is present. Color Doppler sonography may demonstrate a tangle of tortuous vessels with multiple colors, indicative of the haphazard orientation and turbulent flow within the malformation (Fig. 9-81).

Renal Artery Stenosis

Hypertension may be **primary** (95%-99%) or **secondary** (1%-5%). The vast majority of patients with secondary hypertension have renovascular disease. **Renovascular disease** is most frequently caused by atherosclerosis (66%), and the majority of the remaining cases largely result from fibromuscular dysplasia.[280] Many different imaging techniques have been used in an effort to detect patients with renovascular hypertension. These include intravenous and intra-arterial digital subtraction angiography, captopril renal scintigraphy, duplex and color Doppler ultrasound, and magnetic resonance angiography.

Numerous studies and clinical experience in ultrasound laboratories have indicated the utility of **Doppler ultrasound** as an initial screening examination for renal

vascular hypertension. Despite this, use of this method remains controversial. The screening approach may involve (1) detection of abnormal Doppler signals at or just distal to the stenosis or (2) detection of abnormal Doppler signals in the intrarenal vasculature. Evaluation of the main renal arteries in their entirety is usually impossible. It is estimated that the main renal arteries are not seen in up to 42% of patients.[281] In addition, approximately 14% to 24% of patients will have accessory renal arteries that are usually not detected sonographically. Therefore, evaluation of the main renal arteries as a screening approach for renal artery stenosis often fails, particularly in difficult-to-scan patients. The second approach is to interrogate the intrarenal vasculature, which can be identified in virtually all patients. Normally, there is a steep upstroke in systole with a second small peak in early systole. A **tardus-parvus waveform** downstream from a stenosis refers to a slowed systolic acceleration with low amplitude of the systolic peak (Fig. 9-82). To evaluate the delayed upstroke, two measurements must be taken:

- **Acceleration time:** Time from start of systole to peak systole.
- **Acceleration index:** Slope of the systolic upstroke.

An acceleration time greater than 0.07 second and a slope of systolic upstroke less than 3 m/s^2 are suggested as thresholds to assess for renal artery stenosis.[281] Simple recognition of the change in pattern may be adequate[282] (Fig. 9-83). Pharmacologic manipulation with captopril[283] may enhance the waveform abnormalities in patients with renal artery stenosis. Doppler sonography remains a controversial technique for the detection of native renal artery stenosis. The use of intravascular contrast agents increases the technical success rate for the evaluation of renal artery stenosis.[284] It may also play a role in the assessment and follow-up of patients undergoing renal artery angioplasty and stent placement.[285]

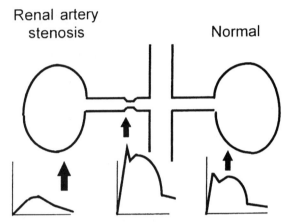

Renal artery stenosis   **Normal**

FIGURE 9-82. Schematic diagram of renal artery Doppler tracings. *Right side,* Tracing from a normal renal artery. Note early systolic peak. *Middle,* Tracing shows high-velocity flow measured at the stenosis. *Left side,* Tracing shows the dampened tardus-parvus waveform downstream from the stenosis. *(From Mitty HA, Shapiro RS, Parsons RB, et al. Renovascular hypertension. Radiol Clin North Am 1996;34:1017-1036.)*

Renal Artery Aneurysm

Renal artery aneurysms are saccular or fusiform dilations of the renal artery or one of its branches. The incidence of renal artery aneurysm is 0.09% to 0.3%.[286] The etiology may be congenital, inflammatory, traumatic, atherosclerotic, or related to fibromuscular disease. If large (>2.5 cm), noncalcified, or associated with pregnancy, the possibility of rupture increases and treatment is recommended. At gray-scale sonography, a cystic mass may be seen. The addition of duplex and color Doppler imaging will readily demonstrate arterial flow within the cystic mass (Fig. 9-84).

Renal Vein Thrombosis

Renal vein thrombosis (RVT) usually results from an underlying abnormality of the kidney, dehydration, or hypercoagulability. Tumors of the kidney and left adrenal gland may grow into the veins, resulting in RVT. Extrinsic compression related to tumors, retroperitoneal fibrosis, pancreatitis, and trauma may cause RVT by attenuating the vessel and slowing flow. In adults the most common etiology is membranous glomerulonephritis; 50% of patients with this disease will have RVT. If thrombosis is acute, the patient may present with flank pain and hematuria. Venous collaterals may develop with more chronic occlusion; patients with chronic RVT thus are often asymptomatic.

The sonographic features of acute RVT are nonspecific and include an enlarged, edematous, hypoechoic kidney with loss of normal corticomedullary differentiation[287,288] (Fig. 9-85). Occasionally, thrombus will be seen within the renal vein, but acutely, it may be anechoic and invisible. The use of duplex and color Doppler ultra-

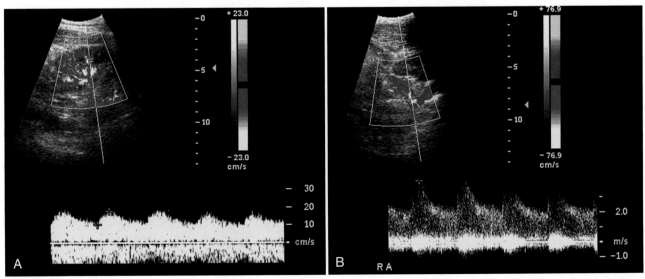

FIGURE 9-83. Renal artery stenosis. A, Intrarenal spectral waveform shows a tardus-parvus signal with a prolonged acceleration time and low resistive index (RI). **B,** Waveform at the origin of the renal artery from the aorta shows a high peak velocity of 410 cm/sec with an RI of 0.43.

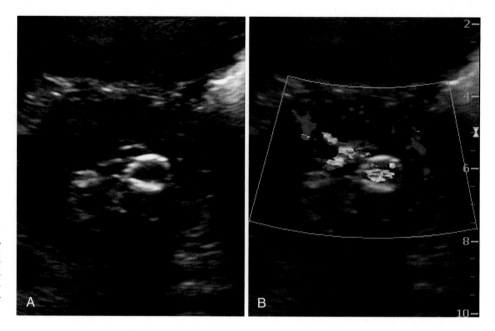

FIGURE 9-84. Renal artery aneurysm. A, Gray-scale, and **B,** color Doppler, ultrasound images show flow within a peripherally calcified, distal renal artery aneurysm.

sound may help; however, the inability to detect flow within renal veins does not necessarily indicate RVT. Extremely slow flow often will not be detected in difficult-to-scan patients despite optimized technique. Absent or reversed end diastolic flow in the intraparenchymal native renal arteries may be a secondary sign of RVT. Platt et al.[289] evaluated 20 native kidneys in 12 patients with clinical findings suggestive of acute RVT. They found that normal arterial Doppler studies should not prevent further workup if RVT is suspected, and that absent or reversed diastolic signals should not be considered highly suggestive of RVT. If findings are equivocal, MRI should be performed. Chronic RVT usually results in a small, end-stage, echogenic kidney.

Ovarian Vein Thrombosis

Ovarian vein thrombosis is seen in postpartum women, but it may also be seen as a result of pelvic inflammatory disease, Crohn's disease, or after gynecologic surgery. The right side is affected more often than the left. Gray-scale, duplex, and color Doppler sonography may reveal a long, tubular structure filled with thrombus extending from the region of the renal vein to deep within the pelvis. Patients are usually treated with anticoagulation and antibiotics.

MEDICAL GENITOURINARY DISEASES

Patients presenting with elevated creatinine levels are often sent to the ultrasound department for an initial screening test. The purpose is to rule out an underlying mechanical obstruction. If obstruction is not found, this often indicates a renal parenchymal abnormality—thus the terms "medical renal disease" or "renal parenchymal disease." The acutely injured kidney may hyperechoic, echogenic, or normal appearing at ultrasound; a thin rim of perirenal fluid is often shown in the acute setting.[290,291] The chronically diseased kidney is small and echogenic (Fig. 9-86). Unfortunately, it is usually impossible to distinguish between the numerous causes of intrinsic renal disease based on the appearance of the kidney at ultrasound, although renal size is a clinically relevant parameter used to distinguish between acute and chronic processes. Thus, percutaneous biopsy is often necessary when clinical features and history are inconclusive.

Acute Tubular Necrosis

Acute tubular necrosis (ATN) is the most common cause of acute reversible renal failure and is related to deposition of cellular debris within the renal collecting tubules. Both ischemic and toxic insults will cause tubular damage. Initiating factors include hypotension, dehydration, drugs, heavy metals, and solvent exposure. The sonographic appearance of ATN depends on the underlying etiology. Hypotension-causing ATN will often produce no sonographic abnormality, whereas drugs, metals, and solvents will cause enlarged, echogenic kidneys. Prerenal disease and ATN account for 75% of all patients presenting with acute renal failure.

Acute Cortical Necrosis

Acute cortical necrosis (ACN) is a rare cause of acute renal failure resulting from ischemic necrosis of the cortex with sparing of the medullary pyramids. The outermost aspect of cortex remains viable as a result of capsular

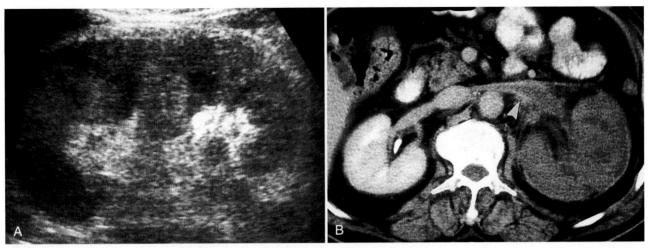

FIGURE 9-85. Renal vein thrombosis. A, Sagittal sonogram demonstrates a diffusely enlarged, edematous left kidney with loss of corticomedullary differentiation. **B,** Confirmatory contrast-enhanced CT shows a large, poorly perfused left kidney and thrombus in the left renal vein *(arrowhead).*

blood supply. ACN occurs in association with sepsis, burns, severe dehydration, snakebite, and pregnancy complicated by placental abruption or septic abortion. The exact etiology is uncertain, although it is likely related to a transient episode of intrarenal vasospasm, intravascular thrombosis, or glomerular capillary endothelial damage. At sonography, the renal cortex is initially hypoechoic[292] (Fig. 9-87). With time (mean, 2 months), both kidneys atrophy and the cortex may calcify.

Glomerulonephritis

Necrosis and mesangial proliferation of the glomerulus are the hallmarks of **acute glomerulonephritis.** Systemic diseases that also have acute glomerulonephritis as a feature include polyarteritis nodosa, systemic lupus erythematosus, Wegener's granulomatosis, Goodpasture's syndrome, thrombocytopenic purpura, and hemolytic uremic syndrome. Patients often present with hematuria, hypertension, and azotemia. At sonography, both kidneys are affected; the size of the kidneys may be normal, but renomegaly is often encountered. The echo pattern of the cortex is altered; renal cortex may be normal, echogenic, or hypoechoic, but the medulla is spared (see Fig. 9-86). With treatment, the kidneys may revert to a normal size and echogenicity. **Chronic glomerulonephritis** occurs with unabated acute disease over weeks to months following an acute episode. Profound, global, symmetrical parenchymal loss occurs. The calices and papillae are normal, and the amount of peripelvic fat increases (see Fig. 9-86). Small, smooth, echogenic kidneys are seen, with prominence of the central echo complex.

Acute Interstitial Nephritis

Acute interstitial nephritis (AIN) is an acute hypersensitivity reaction of the kidney most often related to drugs.

Penicillin, methicillin, rifampin, sulfa drugs, NSAIDs, cimetidine, furosemide, and thiazides have been implicated. Usually, renal failure will resolve with cessation of drug therapy. At sonography, enlarged echogenic kidneys are noted.

Diabetes Mellitus

Diabetes mellitus is the most common cause of **chronic renal failure.** Diabetic nephropathy is believed to be related to glomerular hyperfiltration. Renal hypertrophy occurs. With time, diffuse intercapillary glomerulosclerosis develops, causing a progressive decrease in renal size. At sonography, the kidneys are initially enlarged but, with time and progressive renal insufficiency, the kidneys decrease in size and increase in cortical echogenicity, and corticomedullary junctions are preserved. With end-stage disease, the kidneys become smaller and more echogenic, and the medulla becomes as echogenic as the cortex.[293]

Amyloidosis

Amyloidosis may be primary or secondary and usually is a systemic disease; 10% to 20% of cases may be localized to one organ system.[294] Patients with amyloidosis often present with renal failure. Patients with primary disease are more often men, with a mean age of 60 years. Causes of secondary amyloidosis include **multiple myeloma** (10%-15%), **rheumatoid arthritis** (20%-25%), **tuberculosis** (50%), **familial Mediterranean fever** (26%-40%), **renal cell carcinoma,** and **Hodgkin's disease.**[294] During the acute phase, the kidneys may be symmetrically enlarged. With disease progression, the kidneys shrink; cortical atrophy and increased echogenicity are shown at ultrasound. Focal renal masses, amorphous calcification, a central renal pelvic mass that may be a

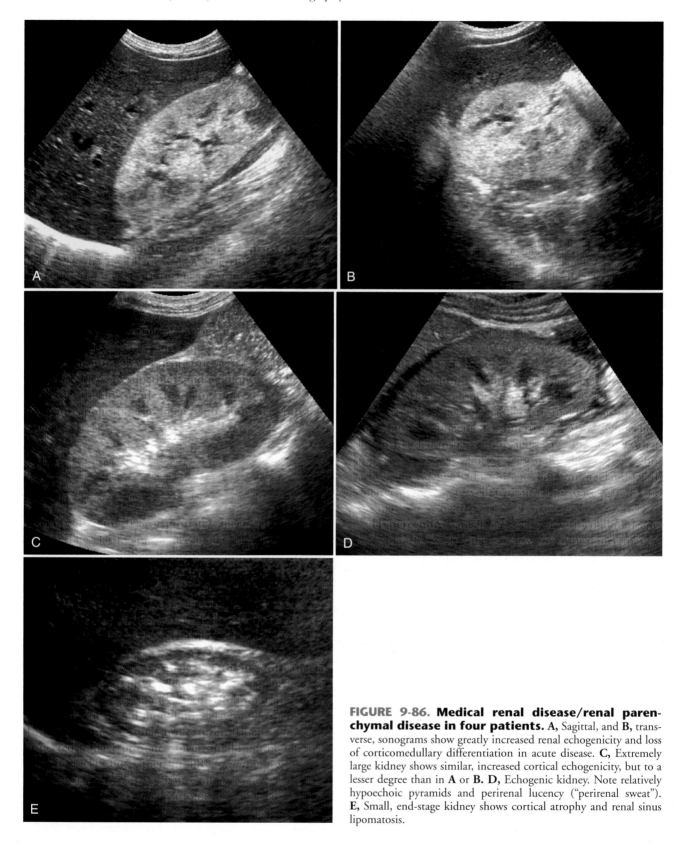

FIGURE 9-86. Medical renal disease/renal parenchymal disease in four patients. A, Sagittal, and **B,** transverse, sonograms show greatly increased renal echogenicity and loss of corticomedullary differentiation in acute disease. **C,** Extremely large kidney shows similar, increased cortical echogenicity, but to a lesser degree than in **A** or **B. D,** Echogenic kidney. Note relatively hypoechoic pyramids and perirenal lucency ("perirenal sweat"). **E,** Small, end-stage kidney shows cortical atrophy and renal sinus lipomatosis.

hemorrhage or amyloid deposit, and perirenal soft tissue masses may be seen. Similarly, involvement of the ureter and bladder may be localized or diffuse. Wall thickening or masses with or without calcification may be demonstrated. The diagnosis is made with biopsy.

Endometriosis

Endometriosis occurs when endometrial tissue is found outside the uterus in women during the reproductive years. Patients typically present with pain, infertility, dysmenorrhea, dyspareunia, and menorrhagia. Approximately 1% of women with pelvic endometriosis will have urinary tract involvement, most frequently in the bladder. Patients with bladder endometriosis will present with hematuria. Bladder endometriosis may be focal or diffuse. Less often the ureter and rarely the kidney are affected. At sonography, patients with bladder endometriosis may present with a mural or intraluminal cyst, or a complex or solid lesion. Diagnosis is usually made cystoscopically with biopsy (Fig. 9-88).

Interstitial Cystitis

Interstitial cystitis is a chronic inflammation of the bladder wall of unknown etiology. It usually affects middle-aged women and has been associated with other systemic diseases, including systemic lupus erythematosus, rheumatoid arthritis, and polyarteritis.[75] Irritative voiding symptoms predominate, and hematuria (30%) may occur.[295] At sonography, a small-capacity, thick-walled bladder is seen (Fig. 9-89). Ureteric obstruction may be present. In some cases it may be impossible to differentiate interstitial cystitis from diffuse transitional cell carcinoma of the bladder; patients should have cystoscopy with biopsy for confirmation.

NEUROGENIC BLADDER

Voiding is a well-coordinated neurologic process controlled by areas within the cerebral cortex. These areas

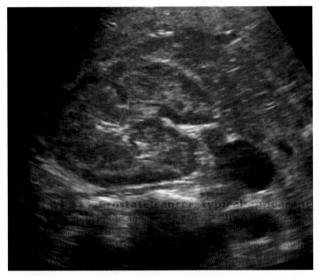

FIGURE 9-87. **Acute cortical necrosis.** Transverse sonogram shows a rim of cortical hypoechogenicity.

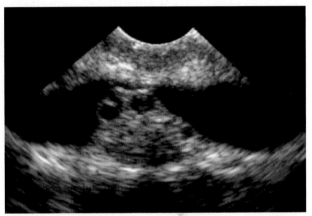

FIGURE 9-88. **Bladder endometrioma.** Transvaginal scan demonstrates cystic components in a mural mass that are typical for an endometrioma. *(From Damani N, Wilson S. Nongynecologic applications of transvaginal ultrasound. RadioGraphics 1999;19:S179-S200.)*

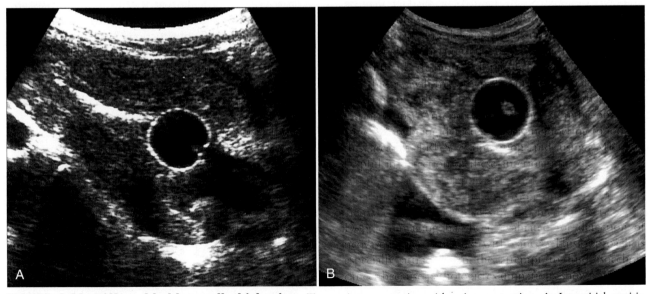

FIGURE 9-89. **Diffuse bladder wall thickening.** Two patients presenting with urinary retention. **A,** Interstitial cystitis. **B,** Diffuse transitional cell carcinoma in second patient. Both sonograms show marked circumferential bladder wall thickening after Foley catheterization. Cystoscopy and biopsy are required for differentiation.

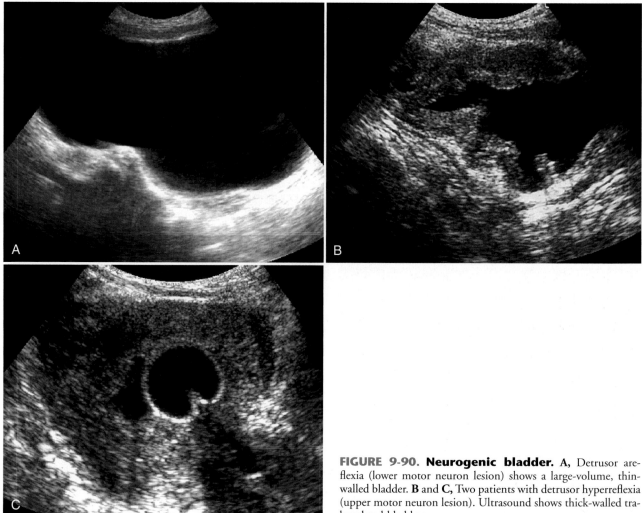

FIGURE 9-90. Neurogenic bladder. A, Detrusor areflexia (lower motor neuron lesion) shows a large-volume, thin-walled bladder. **B** and **C,** Two patients with detrusor hyperreflexia (upper motor neuron lesion). Ultrasound shows thick-walled trabeculated bladders.

control the detrusor muscle of the bladder as well as both the internal and the external urethral sphincter. For simplicity, lesions causing neurogenic bladder may be divided into those causing either detrusor **areflexia**—a lower motor neuron lesion—or detrusor **hyperreflexia**—lesions above the sacral reflex arc.

At sonography, detrusor areflexia results in a smooth, large-capacity, thin-walled bladder. The bladder may extend high into the abdomen (Fig. 9-90, *A*). Detrusor hyperreflexia produces a thick-walled, vertical, trabeculated bladder, often with associated upper tract dilation (Fig. 9-90, *B* and *C*). A large, postvoid residual will be seen.[296] If neurogenic bladder dysfunction is not properly diagnosed and treated, rapid deterioration of renal function may occur.

BLADDER DIVERTICULA

Bladder diverticula may be congenital or acquired. Congenital diverticula are known as **Hutch diverticula** and are located near the ureteral orifice. Most acquired diverticula result from bladder outlet obstruction. Bladder mucosa herniates through weak areas in the wall that are

typically located posterolaterally near the ureteral orifices. The diverticular neck may be narrow or wide. It is the narrow-neck diverticula that lead to urinary stasis and give rise to complications, including infection, stones, tumors, and ureteral obstruction. Tumors arising in a diverticulum have a poorer prognosis than tumors arising within the bladder. Diverticula are composed only of mucosa and submucosa, without the muscularis layer present. Tumors therefore grow and invade much more quickly into the surrounding perivesical fat.

At sonography, diverticula appear as an outpouching sac from the bladder. The internal echogenicity of the diverticulum varies depending on its contents. The neck is often easily appreciated (Fig. 9-91). Urine may be seen flowing into and out of the diverticulum.

POSTSURGICAL EVALUATION

Nephrectomy

Vascularized retroperitoneal fat is often placed with partial nephrectomy defects. The fat may simulate a renal mass at both CT and ultrasound. At sonography,

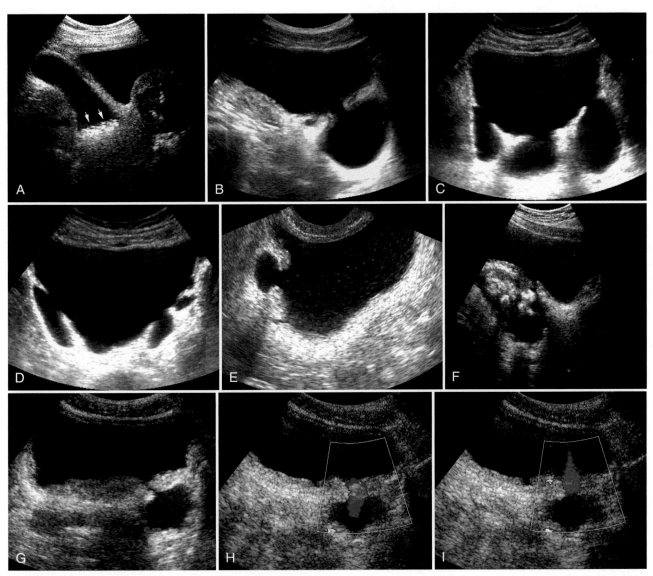

FIGURE 9-91. Bladder diverticula: imaging spectrum. A, Large bladder diverticulum containing multiple calculi *(arrows)*. **B,** Posterolateral Hutch diverticulum. **C,** Multiple wide-neck diverticula. **D,** Multiple diverticula of varying size. **E,** Transvaginal sonogram shows an unusual diverticulum in a woman, with debris in the bladder lumen. **F,** Large transitional cell carcinoma with extensive calcification fills the diverticulum. **G to I,** Patient with a narrow-neck diverticulum **(G). H** and **I,** Urine flow into and out of the diverticulum.

the mass may be hyperechoic or isoechoic.[297,298] Surgical history correlation and an awareness of this potential mimic should obviate additional, unnecessary imaging evaluation.

Urinary Diversion

Urinary diversions, or **ileal conduits,** are constructed for patients with nonfunctioning bladders or for postcystectomy patients. Recently, the trend has been to form continent urinary diversions. A portion of bowel is used to create a pouch that can mimic normal bladder function. The pouch may attach to the abdominal wall (cutaneous pouch) or urethra (orthotopic pouch). Postoperative complications are similar for both and include urine extravasation, reflux, fistula formation, abscess, urinoma, hematoma, deep-vein thrombosis, ileus, and small bowel

obstruction. The role of sonography is mostly for detecting complications rather than for evaluating the pouch itself. If the pouch is urine filled, sonographic assessment is possible (Fig. 9-92). Often, thickened or irregularly shaped bowel wall, pseudomasses, intraluminal mucus collections, and intussuscepted bowel segments can be seen.[299] Stone formation in a pouch may occur.

CONCLUSION

Despite dramatic improvements in MRI and CT over the past generation, sonography continues to occupy a central role in the evaluation of renal, ureteral, and bladder anatomy and disease processes. The ability of ultrasound to identify and characterize genitourinary disease is an ongoing imaging success story.

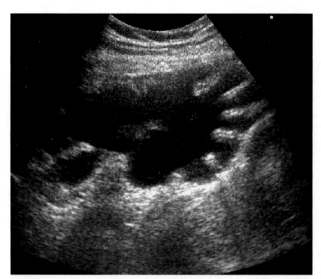

FIGURE 9-92. Ileal conduit (urinary diversion). Ultrasound image of the conduit may show gut wall signature and variable filling.

Acknowledgment

The authors would like to thank Dr. Jenny Tomashpolskaya for her wonderful illustrations.

References

1. Cotran RS, Kumar V, Robbins SL. Robbins pathologic basis of disease. 5th ed. Philadelphia: Saunders; 1994.

Embryology
2. Moore KL, Persaud TVN. The developing human: clinically oriented embryology. 5th ed. Philadelphia: Saunders; 1993.

Anatomy
3. Netter FH. Anatomy, structure, and embryology. In: The CIBA collection of medical illustrations, vol. 6. Kidneys, ureters, and urinary bladder. CIBA Pharmaceutical; 1987. p. 2-35.
4. Emamian SA, Nielsen MB, Pedersen JF, Ytte L. Kidney dimensions at sonography: correlation with age, sex, and habitus in 665 adult volunteers. AJR Am J Roentgenol 1993;160:83-86.
5. Platt JF, Rubin JM, Bowerman RA, Marn CS. The inability to detect kidney disease on the basis of echogenicity. AJR Am J Roentgenol 1988;151:317-319.
6. Carter AR, Horgan JG, Jennings TA, Rosenfield AT. The junctional parenchymal defect: a sonographic variant of renal anatomy. Radiology 1985;154:499-502.
7. Yeh HC, Halton KP, Shapiro RS, et al. Junctional parenchyma: revised definition of hypertrophic column of Bertin. Radiology 1992;185:725-732.
8. Leekam RN, Matzinger MA, Brunelle M, et al. The sonography of renal columnar hypertrophy. J Clin Ultrasound 1983;11:491-494.
9. Middleton WD, Melson GL. Renal duplication artifact in ultrasound imaging. Radiology 1989;173:427-429.
10. Chesbrough RM, Burkhard TK, Martinez AJ, Burks DD. Gerota versus Zuckerkandl: the renal fascia revisited. Radiology 1989;173:845-846.
11. Bechtold RE, Dyer RB, Zagoria RJ, Chen MY. The perirenal space: relationship of pathologic processes to normal retroperitoneal anatomy. Radiographics 1996;16:841-854.

Sonographic Technique
12. Martensson O, Duchek M. Translabial sonography in evaluating the lower female urogenital tract. AJR Am J Roentgenol 1996;166:1327-1331.

Congenital Anomalies
13. Netter FH. Congenital and hereditary disorders. In: The CIBA collection of medical illustrations, vol. 6. Kidneys, ureters, and urinary bladder. CIBA Pharmaceutical; 1987, p. 223-249.
14. Congenital anomalies of the urinary tract. In: Elkin M, editor. Radiology of the urinary system. Boston: Little Brown; 1980.
15. Friedland GW, Devries PA, Nino-Murcia M, et al. Congenital anomalies of the urinary tract. In: Pollack HM, editor. Clinical urography: an atlas and textbook of urologic imaging. Philadelphia: Saunders; 1990. p. 559-787.
16. Horgan JG, Rosenfield NS, Weiss RM, Rosenfield AT. Is renal ultrasound a reliable indicator of a nonobstructed duplication anomaly? Pediatr Radiol 1984;14:388-391.
17. Shimoya K, Shimizu T, Hashimoto K, et al. Diagnosis of ureterocele with transvaginal sonography. Gynecol Obstet Invest 2002;54:58-60.
18. Madeb R, Shapiro I, Rothschild E, et al. Evaluation of ureterocele with Doppler sonography. J Clin Ultrasound 2000;28:425-429.
19. Talner LB. Specific causes of obstruction. In: Pollack HM, editor. Clinical urography: an atlas and textbook of urological imaging. Philadelphia: Saunders; 1990. p. 1629-1751.
20. Vargas B, Lebowitz RL. The coexistence of congenital megacalyces and primary megaureter. AJR Am J Roentgenol 1986;147:313-316.
21. Tortora Jr FL, Lucey DT, Fried FA, Mandell J. Absence of the bladder. J Urol 1983;129:1235-1237.
22. Spataro RF, Davis RS, McLachlan MS, et al. Urachal abnormalities in the adult. Radiology 1983;149:659-663.
23. Schnyder P, Candardjis G. Vesicourachal diverticulum: CT diagnosis in two adults. AJR Am J Roentgenol 1981;137:1063-1065.

Genitourinary Infections
24. Piccirillo M, Rigsby CM, Rosenfield AT. Sonography of renal inflammatory disease. Urol Radiol 1987;9:66-78.
25. Papanicolaou N, Pfister RC. Acute renal infections. Radiol Clin North Am 1996;34:965-995.
26. Talner LB, Davidson AJ, Lebowitz RL, et al. Acute pyelonephritis: can we agree on terminology? Radiology 1994;192:297-305.
27. Farmer KD, Gellett LR, Dubbins PA. The sonographic appearance of acute focal pyelonephritis 8 years experience. Clin Radiol 2002;57:483-487.
28. Majd M, Nussbaum Blask AR, Markle BM, et al. Acute pyelonephritis: comparison of diagnosis with 99mTc-DMSA, SPECT, spiral CT, MR imaging, and power Doppler ultrasound in an experimental pig model. Radiology 2001;218:101-108.
29. Thoumas D, Darmallaicq C, Pfister C, et al. Imaging characteristics of alkaline-encrusted cystitis and pyelitis. AJR Am J Roentgenol 2002;178:389-392.
30. Lowe LH, Zagoria RJ, Baumgartner BR, Dyer RB. Role of imaging and intervention in complex infections of the urinary tract. AJR Am J Roentgenol 1994;163:363-736.
31. Brun-Buisson C, Doyon F, Carlet J, et al. Incidence, risk factors, and outcome of severe sepsis and septic shock in adults: a multicenter prospective study in intensive care units. French ICU Group for Severe Sepsis. JAMA 1995;274:968-974.
32. Yoder IC, Pfister RC, Lindfors KK, Newhouse JH. Pyonephrosis: imaging and intervention. AJR Am J Roentgenol 1983;141:735-740.
33. Grayson DE, Abbott RM, Levy AD, Sherman PM. Emphysematous infections of the abdomen and pelvis: a pictorial review. Radiographics 2002;22:543-561.
34. Patel NP, Lavengood RW, Fernandes M, et al. Gas-forming infections in genitourinary tract. Urology 1992;39:341-345.
35. Michaeli J, Mogle P, Perlberg S, et al. Emphysematous pyelonephritis. J Urol 1984;131:203-208.
36. Wan YL, Lee TY, Bullard MJ, Tsai CC. Acute gas-producing bacterial renal infection: correlation between imaging findings and clinical outcome. Radiology 1996;198:433-438.
37. Joseph RC, Amendola MA, Artze ME, et al. Genitourinary tract gas: imaging evaluation. Radiographics 1996;16:295-308.
38. Bhathena DB, Weiss JH, Holland NH, et al. Focal and segmental glomerular sclerosis in reflux nephropathy. Am J Med 1980;68:886-892.
39. Kay CJ, Rosenfield AT, Taylor KJ, Rosenberg MA. Ultrasonic characteristics of chronic atrophic pyelonephritis. AJR Am J Roentgenol 1979;132:47-49.

40. Hartman DS, Davis Jr CJ, Goldman SM, et al. Xanthogranuloma-tous pyelonephritis: sonographic-pathologic correlation of 16 cases. J Ultrasound Med 1984;3:481-488.

41. Anhalt MA, Cawood CD, Scott Jr R. Xanthogranulomatous pyelo-nephritis: a comprehensive review with report of 4 additional cases. J Urol 1971;105:10-17.

42. Gammill S, Rabinowitz JG, Peace R, et al. New thoughts concerning xanthogranulomatous pyelonephritis (X-P). Am J Roentgenol Radium Ther Nucl Med 1975;125:154-163.

43. Tiu CM, Chou YH, Chiou HJ, et al. Sonographic features of xan-thogranulomatous pyelonephritis. J Clin Ultrasound 2001;29:279-285.

44. Cousins C, Somers J, Broderick N, et al. Xanthogranulomatous pyelonephritis in childhood: ultrasound and CT diagnosis. Pediatr Radiol 1994;24:210-212.

45. Davidson AJ. Chronic parenchymal disease. In: Pollack HM, editor. Clinical urography: an atlas and textbook of urological imaging. Philadelphia: Saunders; 1990. p. 2277-2288.

46. Hoffman JC, Schnur MJ, Koenigsberg M. Demonstration of renal papillary necrosis by sonography. Radiology 1982;145:785-787.

47. Elkin M. Urogenital tuberculosis. In: Pollack HM, editor. Clinical urography: an atlas and textbook of urological imaging. Philadel-phia: Saunders; 1990. p. 1020-1052.

48. Das KM, Indudhara R, Vaidyanathan S. Sonographic features of genitourinary tuberculosis. AJR Am J Roentgenol 1992;158:327-329.

49. Pollack HM, Banner MP, Martinez LO, Hodson CJ. Diagnostic considerations in urinary bladder wall calcification. AJR Am J Roentgenol 1981;136:791-797.

50. Jung YY, Kim JK, Cho KS. Genitourinary tuberculosis: comprehen-sive cross-sectional imaging. AJR Am J Roentgenol 2005;184:143-150.

51. Premkumar A, Lattimer J, Newhouse JH. CT and sonography of advanced urinary tract tuberculosis. AJR Am J Roentgenol 1987;148:65-69.

52. Das KM, Vaidyanathan S, Rajwanshi A, Indudhara R. Renal tuber-culosis: diagnosis with sonographically guided aspiration cytology. AJR Am J Roentgenol 1992;158:571-573.

53. Spring D. Fungal diseases of the urinary tract. In: Pollack HM, editor. Clinical urography: an atlas and textbook of urological imaging. Philadelphia: Saunders; 1990. p. 987-998.

54. Shirkhoda A. CT findings in hepatosplenic and renal candidiasis. J Comput Assist Tomogr 1987;11:795-798.

55. Vazquez-Tsuji O, Campos-Rivera T, Ahumada-Mendoza H, et al. Renal ultrasonography and detection of pseudomycelium in urine as means of diagnosis of renal fungus balls in neonates. Mycopatho-logia 2005;159:331-337.

56. Mindell HJ, Pollack HM. Fungal disease of the ureter. Radiology 1983;146:46.

57. Boldus RA, Brown RC, Culp DA. Fungus balls in the renal pelvis. Radiology 1972;102:555-557.

58. Stuck KJ, Silver TM, Jaffe MH, Bowerman RA. Sonographic dem-onstration of renal fungus balls. Radiology 1982;142:473-474.

59. Palmer P, Reeder MM. Parasitic disease of the urinary tract. In: Pollack HM, editor. Clinical urography: an atlas and textbook of urological imaging. Philadelphia: Saunders; 1990. p. 999-1019.

60. Buchanan WM, Gelfand M. Calcification of the bladder in urinary schistosomiasis. Trans R Soc Trop Med Hyg 1970;64:593-596.

61. Diamond HM, Lyon ES, Hui NT, De Pauw AP. Echinococcal disease of the kidney. J Urol 1976;115:742-744.

62. King D. Ultrasonography of echinococcal cysts. J Clin Ultrasound 1976:64-67.

63. Turgut AT, Odev K, Kabaalioglu A, et al. Multitechnique evaluation of renal hydatid disease. AJR Am J Roentgenol 2009;192:462-467.

64. Sabnis RB, Punekar SV, Desai RM, et al. Instillation of silver nitrate in the treatment of chyluria. Br J Urol 1992;70:660-662.

65. Pastor-Pons E, Martinez-Leon MI, Alvarez-Bustos G, et al. Isolated renal mucormycosis in two patients with AIDS. AJR Am J Roent-genol 1996;166:1282-1284.

66. Spouge AR, Wilson SR, Gopinath N, et al. Extrapulmonary Pneu-mocystis carinii in a patient with AIDS: sonographic findings. AJR Am J Roentgenol 1990;155:76-78.

67. Towers MJ, Withers CE, Hamilton PA, et al. Visceral calcification in patients with AIDS may not always be due to Pneumocystis carinii. AJR Am J Roentgenol 1991;156:745-747.

68. Falkoff GE, Rigsby CM, Rosenfield AT. Partial, combined cortical and medullary nephrocalcinosis: ultrasound and CT patterns in AIDS-associated MAI infection. Radiology 1987;162:343-344.

69. Schwarz E, Szcech LA, Ross MJ, et al. Highly active antiretroviral therapy and the epidemic of HIV-positive end-stage renal disease. J Am Soc Nephrol 2005;16:2412-2420.

70. Wyatt CM, Murphy B. Kidney transplantation in HIV-infected patients. Semin Dial 2005;18:495-498.

71. De Silva TI, Post FA, Griffin MD, Dockrell DH. HIV-1 infection and the kidney: an evolving challenge in HIV medicine. Mayo Clin Proc 2007;82:1103-1116.

72. Hamper UM, Goldblum LE, Hutchins GM, et al. Renal involve-ment in AIDS: sonographic-pathologic correlation. AJR Am J Roentgenol 1988;150:1321-1325.

73. Schaffer RM, Schwartz GE, Becker JA, et al. Renal ultrasound in acquired immune deficiency syndrome. Radiology 1984;153:511-513.

74. Di Fiori JL, Rodrigue D, Kaptein EM, Ralls PW. Diagnostic sonog-raphy of HIV-associated nephropathy: new observations and clinical correlation. AJR Am J Roentgenol 1998;171:713-716.

75. Clayman RV, Weyman PJ, Bahnson RR. Inflammation of the bladder. In: Pollack HM, editor. Clinical urography: an atlas and textbook of urological imaging. Philadelphia: Saunders; 1990. p. 902-924.

76. Stark GL, Feddersen R, Lowe BA, et al. Inflammatory pseudotumor (pseudosarcoma) of the bladder. J Urol 1989;141:610-612.

77. Kenney P, Breatnach ES, Stanley RJ. Chronic inflammation. In: Pollack HM, editor. Clinical urography: an atlas and textbook of urological imaging. Philadelphia: Saunders; 1990. p. 822-843.

78. Lewin KJ, Fair WR, Steigbigel RT, et al. Clinical and laboratory studies into the pathogenesis of malacoplakia. J Clin Pathol 1976;29:354-363.

79. Kauzlaric D, Barmeir E. Sonography of emphysematous cystitis. J Ultrasound Med 1985;4:319-320.

80. Wiener DP, Koss LG, Sablay B, Freed SZ. The prevalence and significance of Brunn's nests, cystitis cystica and squamous metapla-sia in normal bladders. J Urol 1979;122:317-321.

Fistulas, Stones (Calculi), and Calcification

81. Lang EK, Fritzsche P. Fistulas of the genitourinary tract. In: Pollack HM, editor. Clinical urography: an atlas and textbook of urological imaging. Philadelphia: Saunders; 1990. p. 2579-2593.

82. Wilson S. The gastrointestinal tract. In: Rumack CM, Wilson SR, Charboneau JW, editors. Diagnostic ultrasound. St Louis: Mosby–Year Book; 1991. p. 181-207.

83. Damani N, Wilson SR. Nongynecologic applications of transvaginal ultrasound. Radiographics 1999;19 Spec No:179-200; quiz 165-166.

84. Volkmer BG, Kuefer R, Nesslauer T, et al. Colour Doppler ultra-sound in vesicovaginal fistulas. Ultrasound Med Biol 2000;26:771-775.

85. Sierakowski R, Finlayson B, Landes RR, et al. The frequency of urolithiasis in hospital discharge diagnoses in the United States. Invest Urol 1978;15:438-441.

86. Spirnak JP, Resnick M, Banner MP. Calculus disease of the urinary tract: general considerations. In: Pollack HM, editor. Clinical urog-raphy: an atlas and textbook of urological imaging. Philadelphia: Saunders; 1990. p. 1752-1758.

87. Furlan A, Federle MP, Yealy DM, et al. Nonobstructing renal stones on unenhanced CT: a real cause for renal colic? AJR Am J Roent-genol 2008;190:w125-127.

88. Smith RC, Levine J, Dalrymple NC, et al. Acute flank pain: a modern approach to diagnosis and management. Semin Ultrasound CT MR 1999;20:108-135.

89. Ripolles T, Errando J, Agramunt M, Martinez MJ. Ureteral colic: ultrasound versus CT. Abdom Imaging 2004;29:263-266.

90. Middleton WD, Dodds WJ, Lawson TL, Foley WD. Renal calculi: sensitivity for detection with ultrasound. Radiology 1988;167:239-244.

91. Katz DS, Lane MJ, Sommer FG. Unenhanced helical CT of ureteral stones: incidence of associated urinary tract findings. AJR Am J Roentgenol 1996;166:1319-1322.

92. Smith RC, Rosenfield AT, Choe KA, et al. Acute flank pain: com-parison of non-contrast-enhanced CT and intravenous urography. Radiology 1995;194:789-794.

93. Smith RC, Verga M, McCarthy S, Rosenfield AT. Diagnosis of acute flank pain: value of unenhanced helical CT. AJR Am J Roentgenol 1996;166:97-101.

94. Catalano O, Nunziata A, Altei F, Siani A. Suspected ureteral colic: primary helical CT versus selective helical CT after unenhanced radiography and sonography. AJR Am J Roentgenol 2002;178: 379-387.

95. Patlas M, Farkas A, Fisher D, et al. Ultrasound vs CT for the detection of ureteric stones in patients with renal colic. Br J Radiol 2001;74:901-904.

96. Ripolles T, Agramunt M, Errando J, et al. Suspected ureteral colic: plain film and sonography vs unenhanced helical CT: a prospective study in 66 patients. Eur Radiol 2004;14:129-136.

97. Zagoria RJ, Dixon RL. Radiology of urolithiasis: implications of radiation exposure and new imaging modalities. Adv Chronic Kidney Dis 2009;16:48-51.

98. Kimme-Smith C, Perrella RR, Kaveggia LP, et al. Detection of renal stones with real-time sonography: effect of transducers and scanning parameters. AJR Am J Roentgenol 1991;157:975-980.

99. Rubens DJ, Bhatt S, Nedelka S, Cullinan J. Doppler artifacts and pitfalls. Radiol Clin North Am 2006;44:805-835.

100. Lee JY, Kim SH, Cho JY, Han D. Color and power Doppler twinkling artifacts from urinary stones: clinical observations and phantom studies. AJR Am J Roentgenol 2001;176:1441-1445.

101. Chelfouh N, Grenier N, Higueret D, et al. Characterization of urinary calculi: in vitro study of "twinkling artifact" revealed by color-flow sonography. AJR Am J Roentgenol 1998;171:1055-1060.

102. Cronan JJ, Tublin ME. Role of the resistive index in the evaluation of acute renal obstruction. AJR Am J Roentgenol 1995;164:377-378.

103. Laing FC, Benson CB, DiSalvo DN, et al. Distal ureteral calculi: detection with vaginal US. Radiology 1994;192:545-548.

104. Hertzberg BS, Kliewer MA, Paulson EK, Carrol BA. Distal ureteral calculi: detection with transperineal sonography. AJR Am J Roentgenol 1994;163:1151-1153.

105. Burge HJ, Middleton WD, McClennan BL, Hildebolt CF. Ureteral jets in healthy subjects and in patients with unilateral ureteral calculi: comparison with color Doppler ultrasound. Radiology 1991;180: 437-442.

106. Price CI, Adler RS, Rubin JM. Ultrasound detection of differences in density: explanation of the ureteric jet phenomenon and implications for new ultrasound applications. Invest Radiol 1989;24:876-883.

107. Baker SM, Middleton WD. Color Doppler sonography of ureteral jets in normal volunteers: importance of the relative specific gravity of urine in the ureter and bladder. AJR Am J Roentgenol 1992; 159:773-775.

108. De Bessa Jr J, Denes FT, Chammas MC, et al. Diagnostic accuracy of color Doppler sonographic study of the ureteric jets in evaluation of hydronephrosis. J Pediatr Urol 2008;4:113-117.

109. Geavlete P, Georgescu D, Cauni V, Nita G. Value of duplex Doppler ultrasonography in renal colic. Eur Urol 2002;41:71-78.

110. Platt JF, Rubin JM, Ellis JH. Acute renal obstruction: evaluation with intrarenal duplex Doppler and conventional ultrasound. Radiology 1993;186:685-688.

111. Tublin ME, Dodd 3rd GD, Verdile VP. Acute renal colic: diagnosis with duplex Doppler ultrasound. Radiology 1994;193:697-701.

112. Tublin ME, Bude RO, Platt JF. The resistive index in renal Doppler sonography: where do we stand? AJR Am J Roentgenol 2003;180: 885-892.

113. Tublin ME, Tessler FN, Murphy ME. Correlation between renal vascular resistance, pulse pressure, and the resistive index in isolated perfused rabbit kidneys. Radiology 1999;213:258-264.

114. Murphy ME, Tublin ME. Understanding the Doppler resistive index (RI): impact of renal arterial distensibility on the RI in a hydronephrotic ex vivo rabbit kidney model. J Ultrasound Med 2000;19:303-314.

115. Bude RO, Rubin JM. Relationship between the resistive index and vascular compliance and resistance. Radiology 1999;211:411-417.

116. Banner M. Nephrocalcinosis. In: Pollack HM, editor. Clinical urography: an atlas and textbook of urological imaging. Philadelphia: Saunders; 1990. p. 1768-1775.

117. Al-Murrani B, Cosgrove DO, Svensson WE, Blaszczyk M. Echogenic rings: an ultrasound sign of early nephrocalcinosis. Clin Radiol 1991;44:49-51.

118. Patriquin HB, O'Regan S. Medullary sponge kidney in childhood. AJR Am J Roentgenol 1985;145:315-319.

119. Khoory BJ, Andreis IA, Vino L, Fanos V. Transient hyperechogenicity of the renal medullary pyramids: incidence in the healthy term newborn. Am J Perinatol 1999;16:463-468.

120. Patriquin H, Robitaille P. Renal calcium deposition in children: sonographic demonstration of the Anderson-Carr progression. AJR Am J Roentgenol 1986;146:1253-1256.

Genitourinary Tumors

121. Bennington JL, Beckwith JB. Tumors of the kidney, renal pelvis, and ureter. Washington, DC: US Armed Forces Institute of Pathology; 1975.

122. Bennington JL, Laubscher FA. Epidemiologic studies on carcinoma of the kidney. I. Association of renal adenocarcinoma with smoking. Cancer 1968;21:1069-1071.

123. Cohen AJ, Li FP, Berg S, et al. Hereditary renal-cell carcinoma associated with a chromosomal translocation. N Engl J Med 1979; 301:592-595.

124. Choyke PL, Glenn GM, Walther MM, et al. Hereditary renal cancers. Radiology 2003;226:33-46.

125. Choyke PL, Glenn GM, Walther MM, et al. Von Hippel–Lindau disease: genetic, clinical, and imaging features. Radiology 1995; 194:629-642.

126. Choyke PL, Glenn GM, Walther MM, et al. The natural history of renal lesions in von Hippel–Lindau disease: a serial CT study in 28 patients. AJR Am J Roentgenol 1992;159:1229-1234.

127. Linehan WM, Vasselli J, Srinivasan R, et al. Genetic basis of cancer of the kidney: disease-specific approaches to therapy. Clin Cancer Res 2004;10:6282S-6289S.

128. Takase K, Takahashi S, Tazawa S, et al. Renal cell carcinoma associated with chronic renal failure: evaluation with sonographic angiography. Radiology 1994;192:787-792.

129. Levine E, Grantham JJ, Slusher SL, et al. CT of acquired cystic kidney disease and renal tumors in long-term dialysis patients. AJR Am J Roentgenol 1984;142:125-131.

130. Kim JK, Kim TK, Ahn HJ, et al. Differentiation of subtypes of renal cell carcinoma on helical CT scans. AJR Am J Roentgenol 2002;178:1499-1506.

131. Skinner DG, Colvin RB, Vermillion CD, et al. Diagnosis and management of renal cell carcinoma: a clinical and pathologic study of 309 cases. Cancer 1971;28:1165-1177.

132. Sufrin G, Murphy GP. Renal adenocarcinoma. Urol Surv 1980;30:129-144.

133. Raval B, Lamki N. Computed tomography in detection of occult hypernephroma. J Comput Tomogr 1983;7:199-207.

134. Curry NS. Small renal masses (lesions smaller than 3 cm): imaging evaluation and management. AJR Am J Roentgenol 1995;164: 355-362.

135. Warshauer DM, McCarthy SM, Street L, et al. Detection of renal masses: sensitivities and specificities of excretory urography/linear tomography, ultrasound, and CT. Radiology 1988;169:363-365.

136. Jamis-Dow CA, Choyke PL, Jennings SB, et al. Small (≤3-cm) renal masses: detection with CT versus ultrasound and pathologic correlation. Radiology 1996;198:785-788.

137. Szolar DH, Kammerhuber F, Altziebler S, et al. Multiphasic helical CT of the kidney: increased conspicuity for detection and characterization of small (<3 cm) renal masses. Radiology 1997;202:211-217.

138. Urban BA. The small renal mass: what is the role of multiphasic helical scanning? Radiology 1997;202:22-23.

139. Birnbaum BA, Jacobs JE, Ramchandani P. Multiphasic renal CT: comparison of renal mass enhancement during the corticomedullary and nephrographic phases. Radiology 1996;200:753-758.

140. Zeman RK, Zeiberg A, Hayes WS, et al. Helical CT of renal masses: the value of delayed scans. AJR Am J Roentgenol 1996;167: 771-776.

141. Campeau NG, Johnson CD, Felmlee JP, et al. MR imaging of the abdomen with a phased-array multicoil: prospective clinical evaluation. Radiology 1995;195:769-776.

142. Semelka RC, Hricak H, Stevens SK, et al. Combined gadolinium-enhanced and fat-saturation MR imaging of renal masses. Radiology 1991;178:803-809.

143. Silverman SG, Mortele KJ, Tuncali K, et al. Hyperattenuating renal masses: etiologies, pathogenesis, and imaging evaluation. Radiographics 2007;27:1131-1143.

144. Shellock FG, Spinazzi A. MRI safety update 2008. Part 1. MRI contrast agents and nephrogenic systemic fibrosis. AJR Am J Roentgenol 2008;191:1129-1139.

145. Lane BR, Babineau D, Kattan MW, et al. A preoperative prognostic nomogram for solid enhancing renal tumors 7 cm or less amenable to partial nephrectomy. J Urol 2007;178:429-434.

146. Pahernik S, Ziegler S, Roos F, et al. Small renal tumors: correlation of clinical and pathological features with tumor size. J Urol 2007; 178:414-417; discussion 416-417.

147. Bosniak MA, Birnbaum BA, Krinsky GA, Waisman J. Small renal parenchymal neoplasms: further observations on growth. Radiology 1995;197:589-597.

148. Deane LA, Clayman RV. Review of minimally invasive renal therapies: needle-based and extracorporeal. Urology 2006;68:26-37.

149. Gervais DA, McGovern FJ, Arellano RS, et al. Renal cell carcinoma: clinical experience and technical success with radio-frequency ablation of 42 tumors. Radiology 2003;226:417-424.

150. Charboneau JW, Hattery RR, Ernst 3rd EC, et al. Spectrum of sonographic findings in 125 renal masses other than benign simple cyst. AJR Am J Roentgenol 1983;140:87-94.

151. Forman HP, Middleton WD, Melson GL, McClennan BL. Hyperechoic renal cell carcinomas: increase in detection at ultrasound. Radiology 1993;188:431-434.

152. Yamashita Y, Takahashi M, Watanabe O, et al. Small renal cell carcinoma: pathologic and radiologic correlation. Radiology 1992; 184:493-498.

153. Yamashita Y, Ueno S, Makita O, et al. Hyperechoic renal tumors: anechoic rim and intratumoral cysts in ultrasound differentiation of renal cell carcinoma from angiomyolipoma. Radiology 1993;188: 179-182.

154. Siegel CL, Middleton WD, Teefey SA, McClennan BL. Angiomyolipoma and renal cell carcinoma: ultrasound differentiation. Radiology 1996;198:789-793.

155. Farrelly C, Delaney H, McDermott R, Malone D. Do all non-calcified echogenic renal lesions found on ultrasound need further evaluation with CT? Abdom Imaging 2008;33:44-47.

156. Sniderman KW, Krieger JN, Seligson GR, Sos TA. The radiologic and clinical aspects of calcified hypernephroma. Radiology 1979; 131:31-35.

157. Phillips TL, Chin FG, Palubinskas AJ. Calcification in renal masses: an eleven-year survey. Radiology 1963;80:786-794.

158. Kikkawa K, Lasser EC. "Ring-like" or "rim-like" calcification in renal cell carcinoma. Am J Roentgenol Radium Ther Nucl Med 1969;107:737-742.

159. Daniel Jr WW, Hartman GW, Witten DM, et al. Calcified renal masses: a review of ten years experience at the Mayo Clinic. Radiology 1972;103:503-508.

160. Onitsuka H, Murakami J, Naito S, et al. Diffusely calcified renal cell carcinoma: CT features. J Comput Assist Tomogr 1992;16: 654-656.

161. Weyman PJ, McClennan BL, Lee JK, Stanley RJ. CT of calcified renal masses. AJR Am J Roentgenol 1982;138:1095-1099.

162. Press GA, McClennan BL, Melson GL, et al. Papillary renal cell carcinoma: CT and sonographic evaluation. AJR Am J Roentgenol 1984;143:1005-1009.

163. Mancilla-Jimenez R, Stanley RJ, Blath RA. Papillary renal cell carcinoma: a clinical, radiologic, and pathologic study of 34 cases. Cancer 1976;38:2469-2480.

164. Yamashita Y, Watanabe O, Miyazaki T, et al. Cystic renal cell carcinoma: imaging findings with pathologic correlation. Acta Radiol 1994;35:19-24.

165. Hartman DS, Davis Jr CJ, Johns T, Goldman SM. Cystic renal cell carcinoma. Urology 1986;28:145-153.

166. Zagoria RJ. Imaging of small renal masses: a medical success story. AJR Am J Roentgenol 2000;175:945-955.

167. Ramos IM, Taylor KJ, Kier R, et al. Tumor vascular signals in renal masses: detection with Doppler ultrasound. Radiology 1988;168: 633-637.

168. Taylor KJ, Ramos I, Carter D, et al. Correlation of Doppler ultrasound tumor signals with neovascular morphologic features. Radiology 1988;166:57-62.

169. Taylor KJ, Ramos I, Morse SS, et al. Focal liver masses: differential diagnosis with pulsed Doppler ultrasound. Radiology 1987;164: 643-647.

170. Kier R, Taylor KJ, Feyock AL, Ramos IM. Renal masses: characterization with Doppler ultrasound. Radiology 1990;176:703-707.

171. Kuijpers TJ, Obdeijn AI, Kruyt RH, Oudkerk M. Solid breast neoplasms: differential diagnosis with pulsed Doppler ultrasound. Ultrasound Med Biol 1994;20:517-520.

172. Ascenti G, Mazziotti S, Zimbaro G, et al. Complex cystic renal masses: characterization with contrast-enhanced ultrasound. Radiology 2007;243:158-165.

173. Quaia E, Bertolotto M, Cioffi V, et al. Comparison of contrast-enhanced sonography with unenhanced sonography and contrast-enhanced CT in the diagnosis of malignancy in complex cystic renal masses. AJR Am J Roentgenol 2008;191:1239-1249.

174. Bosniak MA. The small (≤3.0 cm) renal parenchymal tumor: detection, diagnosis, and controversies. Radiology 1991;179:307-317.

175. Silverman SG, Gan YU, Mortele KJ, et al. Renal masses in the adult patient: the role of percutaneous biopsy. Radiology 2006;240: 6-22.

176. Caoili EM, Bude RO, Higgins EJ, et al. Evaluation of sonographically guided percutaneous core biopsy of renal masses. AJR Am J Roentgenol 2002;179:373-378.

177. Johnson PT, Nazarian LN, Feld RI, et al. Sonographically guided renal mass biopsy: indications and efficacy. J Ultrasound Med 2001; 20:749-753; quiz 755.

178. Shannon BA, Cohen RJ, de Bruto H, Davies RJ. The value of preoperative needle core biopsy for diagnosing benign lesions among small, incidentally detected renal masses. J Urol 2008;180:1257-1261; discussion 1261.

179. Beland MD, Mayo-Smith WW, Dupuy DE, et al. Diagnostic yield of 58 consecutive imaging-guided biopsies of solid renal masses: should we biopsy all that are indeterminate? AJR Am J Roentgenol 2007;188:792-797.

180. McNichols DW, Segura JW, DeWeerd JH. Renal cell carcinoma: long-term survival and late recurrence. J Urol 1981;126:17-23.

181. Zagoria RJ, Bechtold RE, Dyer RB. Staging of renal adenocarcinoma: role of various imaging procedures. AJR Am J Roentgenol 1995;164:363-370.

182. Chowdhury S, Larkin JM, Gore ME. Recent advances in the treatment of renal cell carcinoma and the role of targeted therapies. Eur J Cancer 2008;44:2152-2161.

183. Habboub HK, Abu-Yousef MM, Williams RD, et al. Accuracy of color Doppler sonography in assessing venous thrombus extension in renal cell carcinoma. AJR Am J Roentgenol 1997;168:267-271.

184. Buckley JA, Urban BA, Soyer P, et al. Transitional cell carcinoma of the renal pelvis: a retrospective look at CT staging with pathologic correlation. Radiology 1996;201:194-198.

185. Leder RA, Dunnick NR. Transitional cell carcinoma of the pelvicalices and ureter. AJR Am J Roentgenol 1990;155:713-722.

186. Yousem DM, Gatewood OM, Goldman SM, Marshall FF. Synchronous and metachronous transitional cell carcinoma of the urinary tract: prevalence, incidence, and radiographic detection. Radiology 1988;167:613-618.

187. Silverman SG, Leyendecker JR, Amis Jr ES. What is the current role of CT urography and MR urography in the evaluation of the urinary tract? Radiology 2009;250:309-323.

188. Dinsmore BJ, Pollack HM, Banner MP. Calcified transitional cell carcinoma of the renal pelvis. Radiology 1988;167:401-404.

189. Hartman DS, Pyatt RS, Dailey E. Transitional cell carcinoma of the kidney with invasion into the renal vein. Urol Radiol 1983;5: 83-87.

190. Winalski CS, Lipman JC, Tumeh SS. Ureteral neoplasms. Radiographics 1990;10:271-283.

191. Caoili EM, Cohan RH, Korobkin M, et al. Urinary tract abnormalities: initial experience with multi-detector row CT urography. Radiology 2002;222:353-360.

192. Caoili EM, Cohan RH, Inampudi P, et al. MDCT urography of upper tract urothelial neoplasms. AJR Am J Roentgenol 2005; 184:1873-1881.

193. Dershaw DD, Scher HI. Sonography in evaluation of carcinoma of bladder. Urology 1987;29:454-457.

194. Dondalski M, White EM, Ghahremani GG, Patel SK. Carcinoma arising in urinary bladder diverticula: imaging findings in six patients. AJR Am J Roentgenol 1993;161:817-820.

195. Barentsz JO, Ruijs SH, Strijk SP. The role of MR imaging in carcinoma of the urinary bladder. AJR Am J Roentgenol 1993;160: 937-947.

196. Narumi Y, Sato T, Hori S, et al. Squamous cell carcinoma of the uroepithelium: CT evaluation. Radiology 1989;173:853-856.

197. Blacher EJ, Johnson DE, Abdul-Karim FW, Ayala AG. Squamous cell carcinoma of renal pelvis. Urology 1985;25:124-126.

198. Mirone V, Prezioso D, Palombini S, Lotti T. Mucinous adenocarcinoma of the renal pelvis. Eur Urol 1984;10:284-285.

199. Merino MJ, Livolsi VA. Oncocytomas of the kidney. Cancer 1982;50:1852-1856.

200. Honda H, Bonsib S, Barloon TJ, Masuda K. Unusual renal oncocytomas: pathologic and CT correlations. Urol Radiol 1992;14:148-154.

201. Hartman GW, Hattery RR. Benign neoplasms of the renal parenchyma. In: Pollack HM, editor. Clinical urography: an atlas and textbook of urological imaging. Philadelphia: Saunders; 1990. p. 1193-1215.

202. Prasad SR, Surabhi VR, Menias CO, et al. Benign renal neoplasms in adults: cross-sectional imaging findings. AJR Am J Roentgenol 2008;190:158-164.

203. Kuroda N, Toi M, Hiroi M, Enzan H. Review of chromophobe renal cell carcinoma with focus on clinical and pathobiological aspects. Histol Histopathol 2003;18:165-171.

204. Davidson AJ, Hayes WS, Hartman DS, et al. Renal oncocytoma and carcinoma: failure of differentiation with CT. Radiology 1993;186:693-696.

205. Goiney RC, Goldenberg L, Cooperberg PL, et al. Renal oncocytoma: sonographic analysis of 14 cases. AJR Am J Roentgenol 1984;143:1001-1004.

206. Tikkakoski T, Paivansalo M, Alanen A, et al. Radiologic findings in renal oncocytoma. Acta Radiol 1991;32:363-367.

207. Gentry LR, Gould HR, Alter AJ, et al. Hemorrhagic angiomyolipoma: demonstration by computed tomography. J Comput Assist Tomogr 1981;5:861-865.

208. Oesterling JE, Fishman EK, Goldman SM, Marshall FF. The management of renal angiomyolipoma. J Urol 1986;135:1121-1124.

209. Arenson AM, Graham RT, Shaw P, et al. Angiomyolipoma of the kidney extending into the inferior vena cava: sonographic and CT findings. AJR Am J Roentgenol 1988;151:1159-1161.

210. Israel GM, Bosniak MA, Slywotzky CM, Rosen RJ. CT differentiation of large exophytic renal angiomyolipomas and perirenal liposarcomas. AJR Am J Roentgenol 2002;179:769-773.

211. Yamakado K, Tanaka N, Nakagawa T, et al. Renal angiomyolipoma: relationships between tumor size, aneurysm formation, and rupture. Radiology 2002;225:78-82.

212. Lapeyre M, Correas JM, Ortonne N, et al. Color-flow Doppler sonography of pseudoaneurysms in patients with bleeding renal angiomyolipoma. AJR Am J Roentgenol 2002;179:145-147.

213. Earthman WJ, Mazer MJ, Winfield AC. Angiomyolipomas in tuberous sclerosis: subselective embolotherapy with alcohol, with long-term follow-up study. Radiology 1986;160:437-441.

214. Richmond J, Sherman RS, Diamond HD, Craver LF. Renal lesions associated with malignant lymphomas. Am J Med 1962;32:184-207.

215. Horii SC, Bosniak MA, Megibow AJ, et al. Correlation of CT and ultrasound in the evaluation of renal lymphoma. Urol Radiol 1983;5:69-76.

216. Heiken JP, Gold RP, Schnur MJ, et al. Computed tomography of renal lymphoma with ultrasound correlation. J Comput Assist Tomogr 1983;7:245-250.

217. Gregory A, Behan M. Lymphoma of the kidneys: unusual ultrasound appearance due to infiltration of the renal sinus. J Clin Ultrasound 1981;9:343-345.

218. Jafri SZ, Bree RL, Amendola MA, et al. CT of renal and perirenal non-Hodgkin lymphoma. AJR Am J Roentgenol 1982;138:1101-1105.

219. Deuskar V, Martin LF, Leung W. Renal lymphoma: an unusual example. Can Assoc Radiol J 1987;38:133-135.

220. Binkovitz LA, Hattery RR, LeRoy AJ. Primary lymphoma of the bladder. Urol Radiol 1988;9:231-233.

221. Kirshbaum JD. Leukemia: A clinical and pathological study of 123 fatal cases in 14,400 necropsies. Arch Intern Med 1943;71:777.

222. Sternby NH. Studies on enlargement of leukaemic kidneys. Acta Haematol 1955;14:354-362.

223. Kumari-Subaiya S, Lee WJ, Festa R, et al. Sonographic findings in leukemic renal disease. J Clin Ultrasound 1984;12:465-472.

224. Araki T. Leukemic involvement of the kidney in children: CT features. J Comput Assist Tomogr 1982;6:781-784.

225. Pascal RR. Renal manifestations of extrarenal neoplasms. Hum Pathol 1980;11:7-17.

226. Mitnick JS, Bosniak MA, Rothberg M, et al. Metastatic neoplasm to the kidney studied by computed tomography and sonography. J Comput Assist Tomogr 1985;9:43-49.

227. Lucke B, Schlumberger HG. Tumors of the kidney, renal pelvis and ureter. Washington, DC: National Research Council, US Armed Forces Institute of Pathology; 1957.

228. Choyke PL, White EM, Zeman RK, et al. Renal metastases: clinicopathologic and radiologic correlation. Radiology 1987;162:359-363.

229. Ambos MA, Bosniak MA, Megibow AJ, Raghavendra B. Ureteral involvement by metastatic disease. Urol Radiol 1979;1:105-112.

230. Mengiardi B, Wiesner W, Stoffel F, et al. Case 44: adenocarcinoma of the urachus. Radiology 2002;222:744-747.

231. Rao BK, Scanlan KA, Hinke ML. Abdominal case of the day. AJR Am J Roentgenol 1986;146:1074-1079.

232. Brick SH, Friedman AC, Pollack HM, et al. Urachal carcinoma: CT findings. Radiology 1988;169:377-381.

233. Dunnick NR, Hartman DS, Ford KK, et al. The radiology of juxtaglomerular tumors. Radiology 1983;147:321-326.

234. McKeown DK, Nguyen GK, Rudrick B, Johnson MA. Carcinoid of the kidney: radiologic findings. AJR Am J Roentgenol 1988;150:143-144.

235. Chen M, Lipson SA, Hricak H. MR imaging evaluation of benign mesenchymal tumors of the urinary bladder. AJR Am J Roentgenol 1997;168:399-403.

236. Kogan MG, Koenigsberg M, Laor E, Bennett B. Ultrasound case of the day: cavernous hemangioma of the bladder. Radiographics 1996;16:443-447.

Renal Cystic Disease

237. Baert L, Steg A. Is the diverticulum of the distal and collecting tubules a preliminary stage of the simple cyst in the adult? J Urol 1977;118:707-710.

238. Laucks SJ, McLauchlan MSF. Aging and simple renal cysts of the kidney. Br J Radiolol 1982;54:12-15.

239. Jackman RJ, Stevens GM. Benign hemorrhagic renal cyst: nephrotomography, renal arteriography, and cyst puncture. Radiology 1974;110:7-13.

240. Bosniak MA. The current radiological approach to renal cysts. Radiology 1986;158:1-10.

241. Israel GM, Bosniak MA. Calcification in cystic renal masses: is it important in diagnosis? Radiology 2003;226:47-52.

242. Israel GM, Bosniak MA. Follow-up CT of moderately complex cystic lesions of the kidney (Bosniak category IIF). AJR Am J Roentgenol 2003;181:627-633.

243. Park BK, Kim B, Kim SH, et al. Assessment of cystic renal masses based on Bosniak classification: comparison of CT and contrast-enhanced ultrasound. Eur J Radiol 2007;61:310-314.

244. Meloni MF, Bertolotto M, Alberzoni C, et al. Follow-up after percutaneous radiofrequency ablation of renal cell carcinoma: contrast-enhanced sonography versus contrast-enhanced CT or MRI. AJR Am J Roentgenol 2008;191:1233-1238.

245. Hidalgo H, Dunnick NR, Rosenberg ER, et al. Parapelvic cysts: appearance on CT and sonography. AJR Am J Roentgenol 1982;138:667-671.

246. Chan JC, Kodroff MB. Hypertension and hematuria secondary to parapelvic cyst. Pediatrics 1980;65:821-823.

247. Ginalski JM, Portmann L, Jaeger P. Does medullary sponge kidney cause nephrolithiasis? AJR Am J Roentgenol 1990;155:299-302.

248. Goldman S, Hartman DS. Medullary sponge kidney. In: Pollack HM, editor. Clinical urography: an atlas and textbook of urological imaging. Philadelphia: Saunders; 1990. p. 1167-1177.

249. Resnick JS, Hartman DS. Medullary cystic disease of the kidney. In: Pollack HM, editor. Clinical urography: an atlas and textbook of urological imaging. Philadelphia: Saunders; 1990. p. 1178-1184.

250. Bisceglia M, Galliani CA, Senger C, et al. Renal cystic diseases: a review. Adv Anat Pathol 2006;13:26-56.

251. Choyke PL. Inherited cystic diseases of the kidney. Radiol Clin North Am 1996;34:925-946.

252. Grampsas SA, Chandhoke PS, Fan J, et al. Anatomic and metabolic risk factors for nephrolithiasis in patients with autosomal dominant polycystic kidney disease. Am J Kidney Dis 2000;36:53-55.

253. Ravine D, Gibson RN, Walker RG, et al. Evaluation of ultrasonographic diagnostic criteria for autosomal dominant polycystic kidney disease 1. Lancet 1994;343:824-827.

254. Bear JC, McManamon P, Morgan J, et al. Age at clinical onset and at ultrasonographic detection of adult polycystic kidney disease: data for genetic counselling. Am J Med Genet 1984;18:45-53.

255. Pei Y, Obaji J, Dupuis A, et al. Unified criteria for ultrasonographic diagnosis of ADPKD. J AM Soc Nephrol 2009;20:205-212.

256. Torres VE, King BF, Chapman AB, et al. Magnetic resonance measurements of renal blood flow and disease progression in autosomal dominant polycystic kidney disease. Clin J Am Soc Nephrol 2007;2:112-120.

257. Sanders RC, Hartman DS. The sonographic distinction between neonatal multicystic kidney and hydronephrosis. Radiology 1984;151:621-625.

258. Madewell JE, Goldman SM, Davis Jr CJ, et al. Multilocular cystic nephroma: a radiographic-pathologic correlation of 58 patients. Radiology 1983;146:309-321.

259. Lee JK, McClennan BL, Kissane JM. Unilateral polycystic kidney disease. AJR Am J Roentgenol 1978;130:1165-1167.

260. Slywotzky CM, Bosniak MA. Localized cystic disease of the kidney. AJR Am J Roentgenol 2001;176:843-849.

261. Master U, Cruz C, Schmidt R, et al. Renal malignancy in peritoneal dialysis patients with acquired cystic kidney disease. Adv Perit Dial 1992;8:145-149.

262. Taylor AJ, Cohen EP, Erickson SJ, et al. Renal imaging in long-term dialysis patients: a comparison of CT and sonography. AJR Am J Roentgenol 1989;153:765-767.

263. Levine E. Acquired cystic kidney disease. Radiol Clin North Am 1996;34:947-964.

264. Levine E, Collins DL, Horton WA, Schimke RN. CT screening of the abdomen in von Hippel–Lindau disease. AJR Am J Roentgenol 1982;139:505-510.

265. Kuntz N. Population studies. In: Gomez MR, editor. Tuberous sclerosis. 2nd ed. New York: Raven Press; 1988. p. 214.

Trauma

266. Kawashima A, Sandler CM, Corl FM, et al. Imaging of renal trauma: a comprehensive review. Radiographics 2001;21:557-574.

267. Federle MP. Evaluation of renal trauma. In: Pollack HM, editor. Clinical urography: an atlas and textbook of urological imaging. Philadelphia: Saunders; 1990. p. 1472-1494.

268. Regine G, Atzori M, Miele V, et al. Second-generation sonographic contrast agents in the evaluation of renal trauma. Radiol Med 2007;112:581-587.

269. McGahan JP, Horton S, Gerscovich EO, et al. Appearance of solid organ injury with contrast-enhanced sonography in blunt abdominal trauma: preliminary experience. AJR Am J Roentgenol 2006;187:658-666.

270. Lang EK. Utereral injuries. In: Pollack HM, editor. Clinical urography: an atlas and textbook of urological imaging. Philadelphia: Saunders; 1990. p. 1495-1504.

271. Titton RL, Gervais DA, Boland GW, Mueller PR. Renal trauma: radiologic evaluation and percutaneous treatment of nonvascular injuries. AJR Am J Roentgenol 2002;178:1507-1511.

Vascular Abnormalities

272. Keogan MT, Kliewer MA, Hertzberg BS, et al. Renal resistive indexes: variability in Doppler US measurement in a healthy population. Radiology 1996;199:165-169.

273. Platt JF, Ellis JH, Rubin JM. Examination of native kidneys with duplex Doppler ultrasound. Semin Ultrasound CT MR 1991;12:308-318.

274. Bude RO, DiPietro MA, Platt JF, et al. Age dependency of the renal resistive index in healthy children. Radiology 1992;184:469-473.

275. Terry JD, Rysavy JA, Frick MP. Intrarenal Doppler: characteristics of aging kidneys. J Ultrasound Med 1992;11:647-651.

276. Mostbeck GH, Gossinger HD, Mallek R, et al. Effect of heart rate on Doppler measurements of resistive index in renal arteries. Radiology 1990;175:511-513.

277. Bude RO, Rubin JM, Adler RS. Power versus conventional color Doppler sonography: comparison in the depiction of normal intrarenal vasculature. Radiology 1994;192:777-780.

278. Erwin BC, Carroll BA, Walter JF, Sommer FG. Renal infarction appearing as an echogenic mass. AJR Am J Roentgenol 1982;138:759-761.

279. Takebayashi S, Aida N, Matsui K. Arteriovenous malformations of the kidneys: diagnosis and follow-up with color Doppler sonography in six patients. AJR Am J Roentgenol 1991;157:991-995.

280. Hillman BJ. Imaging advances in the diagnosis of renovascular hypertension. AJR Am J Roentgenol 1989;153:5-14.

281. Mitty HA, Shapiro RS, Parsons RB, Silberzweig JE. Renovascular hypertension. Radiol Clin North Am 1996;34:1017-1036.

282. Stavros AT, Parker SH, Yakes WF, et al. Segmental stenosis of the renal artery: pattern recognition of tardus and parvus abnormalities with duplex sonography. Radiology 1992;184:487-492.

283. Rene PC, Oliva VL, Bui BT, et al. Renal artery stenosis: evaluation of Doppler ultrasound after inhibition of angiotensin-converting enzyme with captopril. Radiology 1995;196:675-679.

284. Dowling RJ, House MK, King PM, et al. Contrast-enhanced Doppler ultrasound for renal artery stenosis. Australas Radiol 1999;43:206-209.

285. Sharafuddin MJ, Raboi CA, Abu-Yousef M, et al. Renal artery stenosis: duplex ultrasound after angioplasty and stent placement. Radiology 2001;220:168-173.

286. Fleshner NE, Johnston KW. Repair of an autotransplant renal artery aneurysm: case report and literature review. J Urol 1992;148:389-391.

287. Rosenfield AT, Zeman RK, Cronan JJ, Taylor KJ. Ultrasound in experimental and clinical renal vein thrombosis. Radiology 1980;137:735-741.

288. Braun B, Weilemann LS, Weigand W. Ultrasonic demonstration of renal vein thrombosis. Radiology 1981;138:157-158.

289. Platt JF, Ellis JH, Rubin JM. Intrarenal arterial Doppler sonography in the detection of renal vein thrombosis of the native kidney. AJR Am J Roentgenol 1994;162:1367-1370.

Genitourinary Diseases

290. Haddad MC, Medawar WA, Hawary MM, et al. Perirenal fluid in renal parenchymal medical disease ("floating kidney"): clinical significance and sonographic grading. Clin Radiol 2001;56:979-983.

291. Yassa NA, Peng M, Ralls PW. Perirenal lucency ("kidney sweat"): a new sign of renal failure. AJR Am J Roentgenol 1999;173:1075-1077.

292. Sty JR, Starshak RJ, Hubbard AM. Acute renal cortical necrosis in hemolytic uremic syndrome. J Clin Ultrasound 1983;11:175-178.

293. Rodriguez-de-Velasquez A, Yoder IC, Velasquez PA, Papanicolaou N. Imaging the effects of diabetes on the genitourinary system. Radiographics 1995;15:1051-1068.

294. Urban BA, Fishman EK, Goldman SM, et al. CT evaluation of amyloidosis: spectrum of disease. Radiographics 1993;13:1295-1308.

295. Gomes CM, Sanchez-Ortiz RF, Harris C, et al. Significance of hematuria in patients with interstitial cystitis: review of radiographic and endoscopic findings. Urology 2001;57:262-265.

Neurogenic Bladder

296. Amis Jr ES, Blaivas JG. Neurogenic bladder simplified. Radiol Clin North Am 1991;29:571-580.

Postsurgical Evaluation

297. Papanicolaou N, Harbury OL, Pfister RC. Fat-filled postoperative renal cortical defects: sonographic and CT appearance. AJR Am J Roentgenol 1988;151:503-505.

298. Millward SF, Lanctin HP, Lewandowski BJ, Lum PA. Fat-filled postoperative renal pseudotumour: variable appearance in ultrasonography images. Can Assoc Radiol J 1992;43:116-119.

299. Ng C, Amis Jr ES. Radiology of continent urinary diversion. Radiol Clin North Am 1991;29:557-570.

CHAPTER 10

The Prostate

Ants Toi

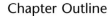

Chapter Outline

BACKGROUND

Role of Transrectal Prostate Ultrasound

In the early 1980s, **transrectal ultrasound** (TRUS) of the prostate was thought to be the pivotal imaging test of the prostate for benign and malignant conditions (e.g., benign hyperplasia, obstructive infertility) and for cancer evaluation, including screening, diagnosis, biopsy, staging, and monitoring of response to therapy. With experience and development of new techniques such as magnetic resonance imaging (MRI), the strengths and limitations of TRUS and other prostate imaging modalities have become better defined.[1,2] Most patients currently are referred for TRUS for examination related to prostate cancer evaluation, biopsy, and guidance of therapeutic procedures.[1,3] TRUS was initially considered a primary *screening* test for prostate cancer. This role has now been replaced by prostate-specific antigen (PSA) and digital rectal examination (DRE).[4,5] Occasional patient referrals relate to infertility and prostatitis. TRUS guidance can also be used to biopsy any accessible lesion in the pelvis in both men and women.

History of Prostate Ultrasound

Initially, the prostate was (and continues to be) assessed by a transabdominal, transvesical approach. The **transvesical** approach is useful for gross prostate and bladder evaluation. Transvesicle assessment is limited to prostate size, shape, and weight. However, detail is inadequate for prostate cancer detection. Also, most prostate cancers occur posteriorly, where transvesical scanning cannot see them. As a result, current interest in ultrasonographic prostatic imaging follows the development of small, intracorporeal transducers that can be employed with **transrectal** techniques.

In the 1960s and 1970s, Japanese investigators published their experience with a radial scanner situated on a chair.[6,7] They installed this device in a van called the "Dolphin," which was used as a mobile screen for prostate cancer in Japan. Since then the technique has evolved, with the development of smaller probes; grayscale, real-time imaging; improved transducer crystal design; and attachment of biopsy guidance devices. An additional breakthrough was the development of the "biopsy gun" by Lindgren in Sweden.

In addition to color flow Doppler, other, newer ultrasound imaging techniques include **contrast-enhanced**

ultrasound, 3D ultrasound, and **elastography.**[8-10] It has become apparent that TRUS, especially for the evaluation of cancer, should not be performed in isolation. It is important to have appropriate history, DRE results, and PSA results available before starting the examination.

ANATOMY

General Structures

Original textbook anatomic descriptions of the prostate referred to **lobar anatomy,** describing anterior, posterior, lateral, and median lobes. Although the concept of a median lobe bulging into the bladder may be useful in the evaluation of patients with benign prostatic hypertrophy (hyperplasia), this lobar anatomy has not been useful in identification of carcinoma of the prostate.[11] Detailed anatomic dissections of the prostate reveal **zonal anatomy,** with the prostate divided into the following four glandular zones surrounding the prostatic urethra:

- Peripheral zone
- Transition zone
- Central zone
- Anterior fibromuscular zone

These zones have differing embryologic origins and susceptibilities to disease (Fig. 10-1). In the normal young man's gland, however, sonography can rarely identify these zones separately unless a pathologic condition is present (Fig. 10-2). On sonography, it is more useful to consider the prostate as having a peripheral or **outer** gland (peripheral zone + central zone) and **inner** gland (transition zone + anterior fibromuscular stroma + internal urethral sphincter)[11-13] (Fig. 10-3).

The **peripheral zone,** the largest of the glandular zones, contains approximately 70% of the prostatic glandular tissue in a young man before the onset of **benign prostatic hyperplasia** (BPH) and is the site for about 70% of prostate cancers[12,14] (Fig. 10-4). It surrounds the distal urethral segment and is separated from the transition zone and central zone by the **surgical capsule,** which is usually seen as a hypoechoic line but may be rendered hyperechoic by the frequent accumulation

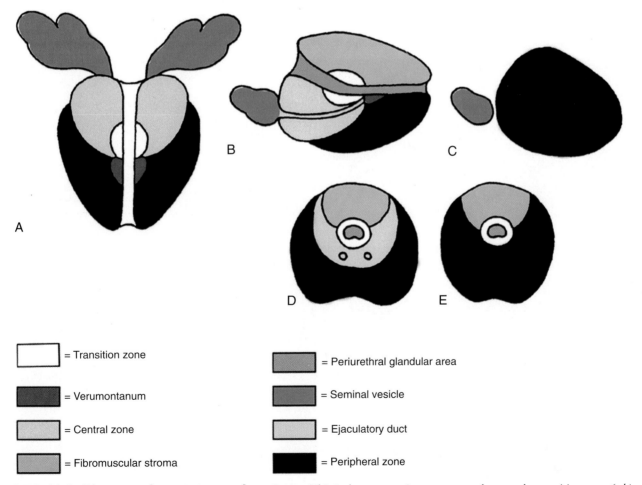

□ = Transition zone

■ = Verumontanum

▨ = Central zone

▨ = Fibromuscular stroma

▨ = Periurethral glandular area

▨ = Seminal vesicle

▨ = Ejaculatory duct

■ = Peripheral zone

FIGURE 10-1. Diagram of prostate zonal anatomy. This is the anatomy in a young man because the transition zone *(white areas)* is small. The transition zone will undergo marked enlargement in older men with benign prostatic hyperplasia. **A,** Coronal section at midprostate level. **B,** Sagittal midline section. **C,** Parasagittal section. **D,** Axial section through base. **E,** Axial section through apex.

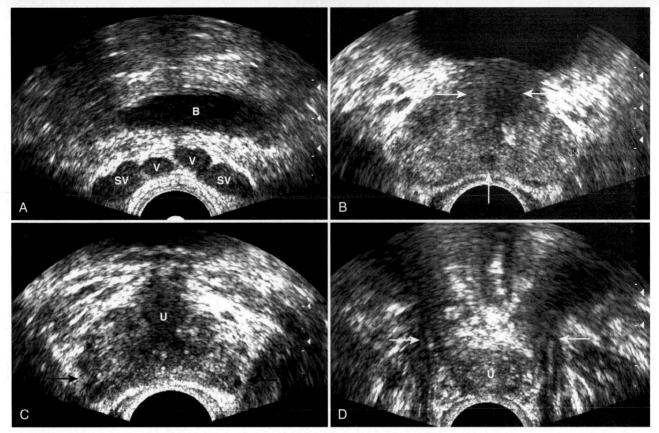

FIGURE 10-2. Axial sonograms of prostate. A, Transverse image above base shows the seminal vesicles *(SV)* and vas deferens *(V); B,* bladder. **B,** Axial scan at midgland level. Note the normal hypoechoic muscular internal urethral sphincter *(horizontal arrows)* and the ejaculatory ducts *(vertical arrow).* **C,** Axial scan at lower third of prostate shows hypoechoic urethra *(U).* Most of the visible gland at this level is peripheral zone. Note the irregular outline at the posterolateral aspects *(arrows),* resulting from the entrance of the neurovascular bundles. **D,** Axial scan just below apex of prostate shows cross section of distal urethra *(U).* Pelvic sling muscles are visible *(arrows).*

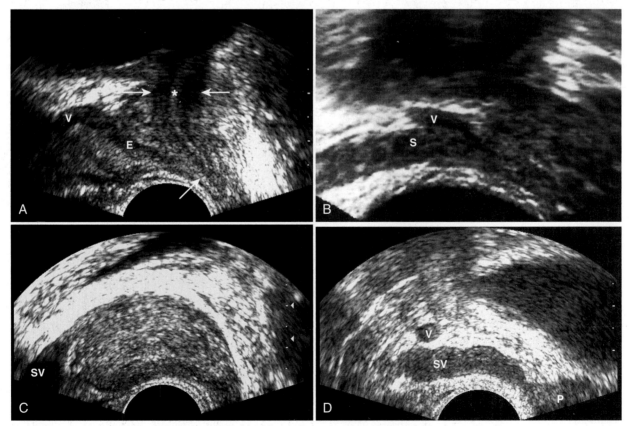

FIGURE 10-3. Sagittal views of prostate. A, Midsagittal view shows internal urethral sphincter *(white arrows),* which contains the echogenic collapsed urethra (*). The ejaculatory ducts *(E)* course from the vas deferens *(V)* to the verumontanum *(oblique arrow).* **B,** Midsagittal view at base shows the vas deferens *(V)* and adjacent seminal vesicles *(S)* as they enter the prostate. **C,** Parasagittal view shows the lateral prostate, which is homogeneous and isoechoic and composed almost totally of peripheral zone tissue; *SV,* seminal vesicle. **D,** Parasagittal view above the prostate shows the normal seminal vesicles *(SV)* and vas deferens *(V)* in cross section above the prostate *(P).*

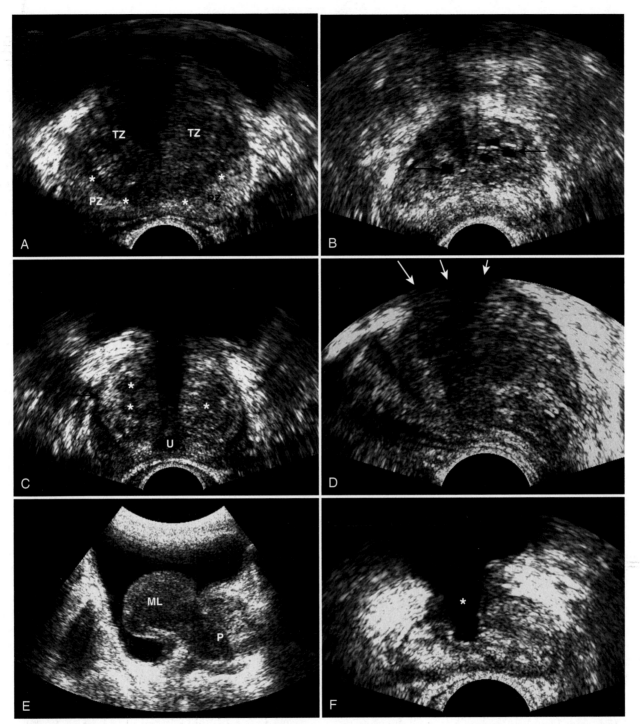

FIGURE 10-4. Benign prostatic hyperplasia (BPH). A, Axial view shows the greatly enlarged, slightly hypoechoic transition zone *(TZ)*, which compresses the more echogenic peripheral zone *(PZ)*. Their interface is the surgical capsule (*). The region inside the surgical capsule (transition zone) is also called the "inner gland" and the region outside the surgical capsule, the "outer gland," which is composed of peripheral zone plus central zone. (Peripheral zone is the "eggcup" holding the "egg" of the central gland.) **B,** Benign degenerative cysts in the transition zone *(arrows)*. These have no clinical significance. The transition zone can become acoustically very inhomogeneous, making cancer diagnosis difficult. **C,** Heterogeneous nature of hyperplasia in the transition zone; *U,* urethra. Both hyperechoic *(black arrow)* and hypoechoic (*) areas are present. This inhomogeneity makes cancer detection difficult. **D,** Sagittal view shows pitfall in transrectal ultrasound (TRUS) imaging of BPH. If the field of view is not deep enough *(arrows)*, prominent median lobe enlargement may be cut off and may escape detection. **E,** Transvesical midsagittal scan shows obvious massive enlargement of the median lobe *(ML)* protruding into the bladder; *P,* prostate. Evaluation for symptoms of prostatism is better done transvesically than transrectally with TRUS. **F,** Axial view of typical transurethral resection of prostate (TURP) surgical defect (*).

of corpora amylacea or calcifications along this line. Traditionally, urologists at the time of suprapubic resection (or transurethral resection of prostate) believed that they dissected to this line; thus the designation "surgical" capsule. The peripheral zone occupies the posterior, lateral, and apical regions of the prostate, extending somewhat anteriorly, resembling an eggcup holding the "egg" of the central gland.

The **transition zone** in a young man contains approximately 5% of the prostatic glandular tissue. It is seen as two small glandular areas positioned like saddlebags adjacent to the proximal urethral sphincter, a muscular tube up to 2 cm in diameter. The transition zone is the site of origin of most BPH and about 20% of prostate cancer.[12,14]

The **central zone** constitutes approximately 25% of the glandular tissue. It is wedge shaped at the prostate base between the peripheral and transition zones. The ducts of the vas deferens and seminal vesicles enter the base of the prostate at the central zone, where they are renamed the **ejaculatory ducts** and pass through it en route to the seminal colliculus (crest), or **verumontanum** (see Figs. 10-1 and 10-2). The central zone is thought to be relatively resistant to disease processes and is the site of origin of only about 5% of prostate cancer.[12,14]

At the base of the prostate is the thick, muscular, continence-providing, **internal urethral sphincter**. Its substantial muscular content can make it appear hypoechoic. It contains periurethral glands that often contain calcifications[11-13] (see Figs. 10-1, 10-2, *B,* and 10-3, *A*).

Vascular and Neural Structures

The prostate is supplied by the prostaticovesical arteries, which arise from the internal iliac arteries on each side. These vessels then gives rise to the prostatic artery and inferior vesical artery. The **prostatic artery** gives rise to the urethral and capsular arteries. The **inferior vesical artery** supplies the bladder base, seminal vesicles, and ureter. The urethral artery supplies about one third of the prostate, and the capsular branches supply the remainder.[15]

With color Doppler ultrasound, particularly using the power mode, the prostate appears mildly to moderately vascular. The capsular and urethral arteries are easily seen, and branches to the inner gland and peripheral zone may be prominent, often in a spokelike radial pattern with the periurethral vessels as the axle (Fig. 10-5). A dense cluster of vessels is often seen capping the base of the prostate, and care must be taken not to mistake these for tumor vascularity.

The **nerve supply** to the prostate has only recently been clarified, and not all textbooks are current.[16-18] Parasympathetic supply is through the S2-S4 sacral roots, and sympathetic supply is through the hypogastric nerve.

These combine in the pelvic plexus just above and lateral to the prostate and give rise to about 6 to 16 small branches that supply the seminal vesicles, prostate, levator ani, and corpora cavernosa. The cavernosal branches are responsible for erections. The nerves and blood vessels travel together as the neurovascular bundle in Denonvilliers (rectoprostatic) fascia at the posterolateral aspect of the prostate, where the vessels are visible with color flow Doppler ultrasound. These nerves are vulnerable to injury during surgery, radiotherapy, and other interventions. Nerve-sparing prostatectomy is designed to spare these nerves and preserve potency.[16-18]

SONOGRAPHIC APPEARANCE

Various scanning orientations have been proposed; the most common matches that for transabdominal sonography and other cross sectional imaging modalities (see Fig. 10-1). The images are displayed as though one stands at the feet of a supine patient and looks headward. The rectum is displayed at the bottom of the screen, with the ultrasound beam emanating from within the rectum. On transverse imaging, the anterior abdominal wall is at the top of the screen, with the right side of the patient on the left side of the image (see Fig. 10-2). In a sagittal plane, the anterior abdominal wall is again located at the top of the screen, and the head of the patient is on the left side of the image (see Fig. 10-3).

Axial Ultrasound Anatomy

Above the prostatic base, the **seminal vesicles** are paired, relatively hypoechoic, multiseptated structures cephalad to the base of the prostate (see Fig. 10-2, *A*). They usually measure about 1 cm front to back, but occasionally are more dilated in normal men. The adjacent vas deferens are visible as uniform muscular tubes measuring about 6 mm in diameter coursing from the internal inguinal ring to lie beside the seminal vesicles and then ultimately enter the prostate at midbase, where they become the **ejaculatory ducts**. The two ejaculatory ducts can be followed to the **verumontanum** (seminal colliculus).

In the axial plane, the urethra between the bladder neck and verumontanum and its surrounding smooth muscle, the internal sphincter, can be quite conspicuous, measuring 2 cm in diameter. Especially in young men, the muscular sphincter can appear so hypoechoic as to mimic the appearance of a transurethral resection defect (see Figs. 10-2, *B,* and 10-3, *A*). Those unfamiliar with transrectal and pelvic ultrasound may mistake the sphincter for tumor because both can be similarly hypoechoic. Such erroneous reports typically state that there is a "2-cm hypoechoic suspicious nodule anteriorly in the prostate." The muscular sphincter ends at the verumontanum, which forms a small bulge pointed ante-

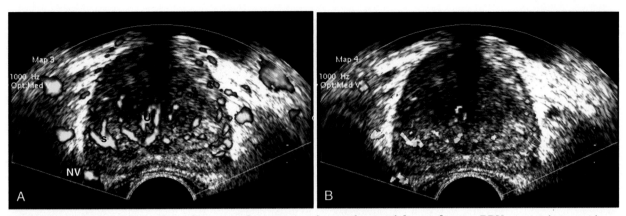

FIGURE 10-5. Normal Doppler ultrasound anatomy in patient with moderate BPH. A, Axial view with power Doppler ultrasound shows the urethral vessels *(U)*, some vessels along the surgical capsule *(S)*, and the neurovascular bundle *(NV)* on one side. This is an average degree of vascularity. Note the large vessels, mostly veins, outside the prostate. Care must be taken when biopsy is performed outside the prostate to avoid injury to these vessels. **B,** Color Doppler flow imaging compared with power Doppler ultrasound. Vascular density is slightly more difficult to evaluate, and degree of color vascularity is more dependent on machine settings than with power Doppler.

riorly, often with a small, conspicuous calcification at its apex, giving it an Eiffel Tower appearance.

The inner transition zone is separated from the peripheral zone by the usually hypoechoic surgical capsule (see Fig. 10-4, *A*). This line becomes obvious as BPH enlarges the transition zone. Often, corpora amylacea, seen as echogenic foci, develop along the surgical capsule (Fig. 10-6, *C*). Frequently, in young men, no clear separating line is seen between the zones (see Fig. 10-2, *B*). The peripheral zone has a uniform, homogeneous texture and is slightly more echogenic than the transition zone. The peripheral zone echogenicity is taken as the standard for echogenicity in the prostate and is defined to be **isoechoic.** Echogenicity in other areas of the gland is compared to that of the peripheral zone. Laterally, the peripheral zone curves anteriorly to enclose the transition zone; this upward curved part was named the "anterior horns" by Dr. Babaian from Texas because it resembled the horns of a steer. The margin of the prostate forms a clear interface with the periprostatic fat except posterolaterally, where vessels enter the prostate and make the margin indistinct, an appearance that can mimic tumor extension through the capsule. Prominent veins of Batson's venous plexus are visible in the periprostatic fat, sometimes containing calcified shadowing phleboliths.[11]

Sagittal Ultrasound Anatomy

On midsagittal view, the muscular internal urethral sphincter can be seen extending from the bladder to verumontanum. When corpora amylacea fill the periurethral glands, they may form a linear hyperechoic configuration (Fig. 10-3, *A*). The anterior fibromuscular zone forms an inconspicuous area anterior to the internal sphincter. At the verumontanum, the distal urethra angles slightly anteriorly and ultimately exits the apex

of the prostate just before it enters the urogenital diaphragm, which is the external urethral sphincter. In the true midline the apex can be difficult to identify because it blends with the urethra. Often, a subtle bulge just at the junction helps to identify it. When measuring the head-to-foot length of the prostate, the scan plane can be shifted minimally to one side of this apical urethra to identify the apex more clearly. In the midplane the ejaculatory ducts are visible as hypoechoic tracts extending from the vas deferens at the base to the centrally located verumontanum (see Figs. 10-2, *A*, and 10-3, *A*).

Parasagittally, in men with hyperplasia, the anterior hyperplastic transition zone can be seen separated from the posteriorly situated peripheral zone by the surgical capsule. The vas deferens and seminal vesicles are visible above the base. Still more laterally, the transition zone ends, leaving only the part of the peripheral zone that curves anteriorly at the sides of the glands (anterior horns). With BPH, the transition zone enlarges anterolaterally and compresses the peripheral zone into a thin, posterior rim[11] (Fig. 10-4, *A*).

Prostate "Capsule"

On transverse and sagittal imaging, the border of the prostate with the periprostatic fat appears sharply defined except at the posterolateral margins, where the neurovascular bundle enters the prostate and makes the margin look ragged (see Fig. 10-2, *C*). Histologically, the prostate does not have a true membranous capsule but rather just condensed connective tissue through which the vessels and nerves course.[19] In addition to the absence of a well-defined capsule, the presence of prominent but normal vessels in the periprostatic soft tissues posterolaterally may make assessment of "capsular" integrity difficult in patients with prostate cancer.

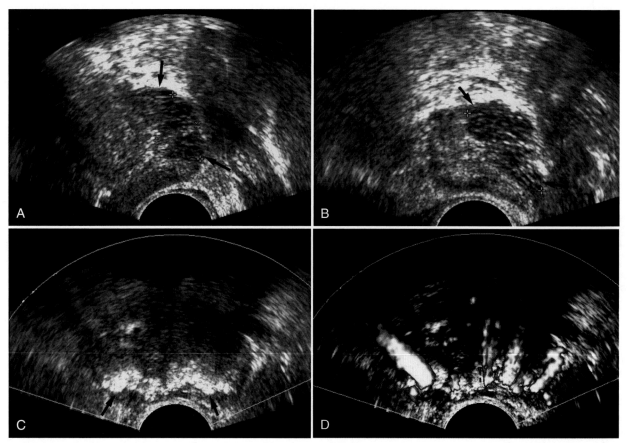

FIGURE 10-6. Normal anatomic variants. A, Axial view with benign glandular ectasia *(arrows)* seen as a peripheral hypoechoic area containing multiple radially oriented tubes. This hypoechoic appearance should not be mistaken for cancer. **B,** Parasagittal view of benign ectatic glands *(arrows)*. **C,** Axial view shows extensive echogenic material, both calcifications and corpora amylacea *(arrows)*, along the surgical capsule and peripheral zone. This has no clinical significance and usually is not palpable. It hinders ultrasonic visibility. **D,** Doppler examination of same patient shows the extensive Doppler noise artifact caused by the calcifications. Virtually all the visible color is artifactual.

EQUIPMENT AND TECHNIQUES

Most modern ultrasound machines have **transrectal probes,** which have been developed to perform ultrasound of the prostate and rectum. Transducer frequency should be at least 5 MHz, and most are as high as 7 or 11 MHz. Probe design and biopsy attachments vary. It is advantageous to use the thinnest probe that provides adequate imaging because some men have "tight" anal sphincters and cannot tolerate large probes.

Crystal arrangements include convex array, linear array, and rotating mechanical configurations. Rotating mechanical transducers allow 360-degree imaging and are superb for evaluating the anus and rectum. Scan plane configurations include end-fire, off-axis end-fire, side-fire axial, and side-fire linear array along the sides of the shaft. Side-fire axial and linear crystals are often combined on the same probe to allow axial and sagittal views without needing to withdraw the probe.

Transducer Design

After initial development of linear array and rotating radial probe designs, manufacturers developed probes for **biplane transrectal prostate scanning** with either a single probe or multiple probes on the same machine. A convenient probe for most biopsy applications is an end-fire transducer, which allows for multiplanar imaging in transverse and axial projections and is well suited for biopsy guidance (Fig. 10-7).

The current trend in probe design emphasizes high midfrequencies (8-10 MHz) and broad bandwidth. This has increased spatial resolution, but at the cost of decreased lesion conspicuity and edge detection. Probes with a center frequency of about 5 MHz were previously shown to provide a good balance between spatial resolution and tissue/cancer contrast. Higher-frequency transducers reduce contrast and result in echo fill-in of lesions.[20]

Probes should be covered with sheaths or condoms during the examination (Fig. 10-7). Sheaths are often

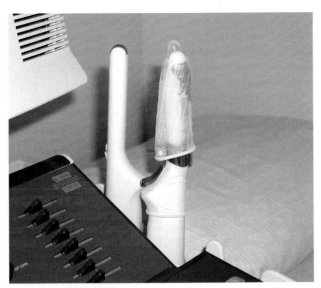

FIGURE 10-7. Typical ultrasound probes for transrectal and intracavitary work. *Left,* Probe is undressed. *Right,* Probe is dressed with inner condom, biopsy guide, and outer condom. Most men come for biopsy, so to save time and avoid additional probe withdrawls and insertions my group starts the examination with the probe dressed and biopsy guide in place.

made of latex, so nonlatex covers should be available for patients with latex allergy. Between uses, the probes are washed and then soaked in an antiseptic solution following manufacturers' recommendations. Care must be taken concerning the depth of safe insertion of the probe into the solution to avoid damaging crystals and electric connections.

Some probes use a water path between the crystal and the rectal mucosa. This decreases the near-field artifact and can be useful for examining the rectal wall itself or the structures close to the rectal wall. However, this water path can create artifacts if air is allowed into the system.

Scanning Technique

The patient usually lies in a **left lateral decubitus** position for the scan. Some examiners prefer a lithotomy position, particularly if the examination is done in conjunction with other urologic procedures or transperineal interventions. **Rectal cleansing** is generally done before the scan. A self-administered rectal enema is preferred, but laxatives can be used in men who cannot administer the enema. Some believe the enema decreases infectious complications of biopsy.[21] It is routine to perform a **digital rectal examination** before probe insertion to ensure no rectal abnormalities interfere with safe probe insertion and to correlate the imaging with palpable abnormalities. Using adequate lubrication, the probe is gently inserted into the rectum. To decrease discomfort, viscous lidocaine (Xylocaine) gel can be used as the lubricant in patients with tight sphincters or anal pathology

such as fissures or inflamed hemorrhoids. End-fire probe insertion may be done under direct vision to facilitate following the curve of the rectal canal and decrease patient discomfort. Recently, Ching et al.[22] suggested that the use of an end-fire probe to guide biopsy also increases cancer detection.

When examining the prostate gland, a **systematic approach** works best (see Figs. 10-2 and 10-3). Typically, the prostate is scanned first in gray scale with representative images taken, starting in the transverse plane, from seminal vesicles at the base to urethra at the apex, then in the sagittal plane, from right to midline to left lobe. Subsequently, the scan is repeated with Doppler flow ultrasound imaging in the transverse plane to allow evaluation of vascular symmetry (see Fig. 10-5).

Measurements are taken as follows: maximal transverse width (W; right to left), anteroposterior plane (AP; anterior midline to rectal surface), length (L; maximal head to foot). Although various sonographic techniques can be used to estimate prostate size,[23,24] **prostate volume** is usually calculated with the "oblate spheroid" formula: volume = $0.5236 \times (W \times AP \times L)$. Volume measurement is only moderately repeatable, and most practitioners are only able to repeat within about $\pm 10\%$ in most cases. Prostate volume can be converted to **prostate weight** because the specific gravity of prostate tissue is about 1, thus 1 cc (mL) of prostate tissue is equivalent to 1 g. More precise and repeatable measurements can be obtained with the "step-section technique," but this is time-consuming and requires special side-fire probes and external stepping equipment.

Color or power Doppler ultrasound is routinely used, particularly when searching for cancer. We find vessel density is more easily evaluated with **power Doppler,** which portrays color more evenly and is three to five times more sensitive than the multicolored Doppler display (see Fig. 10-5). Pulsatility indices have not proved helpful. Halpern et al.[25] suggested that Doppler depiction of prostate vascular density varies with patient position, the dependent side being more vascular; however, this has not been our experience. **Excessively enhanced vascularity is not specific** and can be seen with hypertrophy, inflammation, and cancer. A pitfall for Doppler ultrasound is the normal, high vascular density seen capping the base of the left and right lobes; this should not be mistaken for the enhanced vascularity seen with tumors. Off-axis transverse scans that catch the bases asymmetrically may incorrectly suggest that one side has increased vascularity and lead to suspicion of tumor. It is important to ensure a **true axial orientation** at the base when evaluating these vessels. Even a slightly off axial plane that includes only the vessels on one side can suggest asymmetrically enhanced vascularity suspicious for cancer. Parasagittal views to examine basal vessels are useful to avoid this pitfall.

BENIGN CONDITIONS

Normal Variants

Benign ductal ectasia is seen in older men who develop atrophy and dilation of peripheral prostatic ducts. These are visible as single or grouped, radially oriented, 1 to 2–mm–diameter tubular structures in the peripheral zone, starting at the capsule and radiating toward the urethra. When clustered, dilated ducts can form a hypoechoic area that could be mistaken as prostate cancer. Ductal ectasia has no clinical significance (see Fig. 10-6, *A* and *B*).

Prostatic calcifications and corpora amylacea are normal findings and are more common with advancing age. Both form bright, echogenic foci or clumps in the prostate. **Corpora amylacea** are simply proteinaceous debris in dilated prostatic ducts, most often seen in periurethral glands and along the surgical capsule, although they can occur anywhere in the prostate. When densely clustered, corpora amylacea can cause significant sound attenuation, which prevents TRUS examination of the anterior parts of the prostate. On Doppler imaging they create a prominent "twinkle" artifact. Subclinical infections, inflammation, and atrophy may contribute to their formation. Corpora amylacea have no clinical significance, and even if dense or clumped, they are usually not palpable. Peripheral zone calcifications should not be accepted as a cause for palpable firmness or nodules. Patients with palpable abnormality need further evaluation with biopsy (see Fig. 10-6, *C* and *D*).

Benign Prostatic Hyperplasia

Prostate enlargement with BPH is a common cause of **lower urinary tract symptoms** (LUTS) in older men. BPH affects about 50% of men over age 60 years and over 90% over age 70. The weight of the gland in a young man is approximately 20 g. From age 50, the doubling time of prostate weight is approximately 10 years. Prostates weighing more than 40 g are generally considered enlarged in older men. The etiology of BPH is unclear but probably related to hormonal changes with aging. The process results in hypertrophy and hyperplasia of the fibrous, muscular, and glandular elements, primarily affecting the transition and periurethral zones.[2,12]

Also called **prostatism** and **bladder outlet obstruction**, LUTS can relate to increases in prostate size and muscular tone, both of which result in urethral constriction. Symptoms include frequency, nocturia, weak stream, hesitancy, intermittence, incomplete emptying, and urgency. Symptoms are quantified using the American Urological Association (AUA) symptom index.[12,26] After exclusion of other systemic causes of the symptoms, such as neurologic disease, diabetes, and local urinary conditions, treatment focuses on the prostate. **Transurethral resection of the prostate** (TURP) is considered the standard of care in many patients, but other treatments can include watchful waiting, medical therapy, open surgery, and laser therapy. Many men have a misguided concern about prostate size. The issue is *urinary obstruction,* not prostate size, which correlates only somewhat with obstruction.

The sonographic appearance of BPH varies and depends on underlying histopathologic changes. The typical sonographic feature of BPH is **enlargement of the inner gland** (transition zone). With BPH, the enlarged transition zone can exhibit diffuse enlargement or distinct hypoechoic, isoechoic, or hyperechoic nodules[27] (see Fig. 10-4). The specific echo pattern depends on the admixture of glandular, stromal, and muscular elements and nodules, which may be fibroblastic, fibromuscular, muscular, hyperadenomatous, or fibroadenomatous and may undergo degenerative cavitation.[27,28] BPH nodules tend to have distinct margins, unlike transition zone cancer, which can appear as a diffuse, poorly marginated, usually hypoechoic nodule. Hyperplasia of the periurethral glandular elements results in "median lobe" enlargement manifesting as a bulge into the urinary bladder.

Calcifications and **degenerative or retention cysts** are common in the transition zone (Fig. 10-8, *A,* see also Fig. 10-4, *B*). Because of the distortion of the gland in patients with BPH, some hyperplastic nodules may bulge into the peripheral zone when they actually originate in the transition zone. Hypoechoic, well-circumscribed transition zone nodules are virtually always benign.[29] Although BPH nodules are generally confined to the transition zone, on occasion they can actually (contrary to some textbooks) form entirely within the **peripheral zone,** where they can be seen as an isoechoic nodule with a well-circumscribed halo similar in appearance to those seen in the transition zone. They can create a prominent bulge at the capsule. Because these benign, peripheral zone nodules are palpable as a firm or hard, cancerlike nodule, they should undergo biopsy to confirm their benign nature and obviate continuing concern.[30]

Prostate size correlates poorly with urinary obstruction, and a large prostate is often seen in asymptomatic patients, whereas other patients with severe voiding difficulties caused by prostatic obstruction may have small glands. Also, remember that urinary dysfunction is multifactorial and can arise from abnormalities of the central nervous system, spine, bladder, prostate, and urethra. Patients with urinary dysfunction need evaluation of all these systems, not only the prostate. Investigation of the patient with symptoms of prostatism is best done transvesically. Transvesical ultrasound can adequately assess prostate size, identify median lobe enlargement, and evaluate bladder volume and postvoid residual, bladder wall character, trabeculation, diverticula, tumors, and calculi, as well as evaluate the kidneys and ureters for hydronephrosis and masses[12] (see Fig. 10-4).

Transrectal ultrasound plays only a small role in the assessment of BPH and LUTS. It is used primarily if

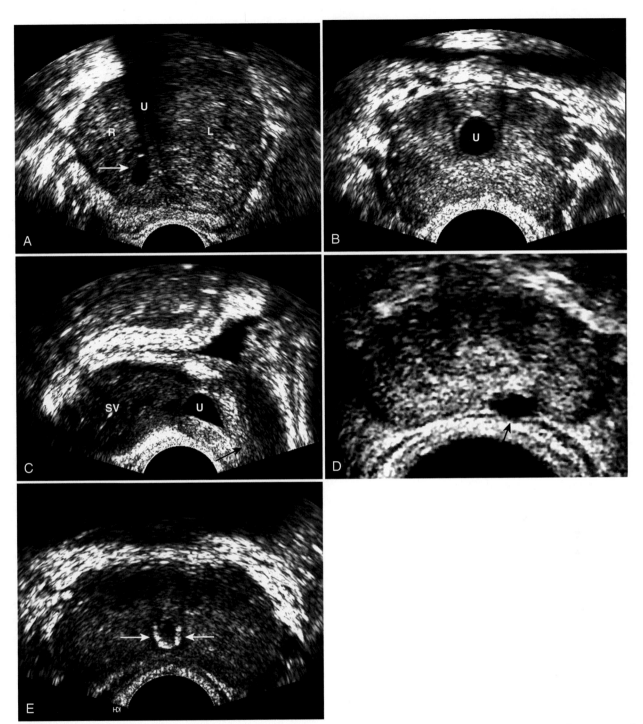

FIGURE 10-8. Prostate cysts. A, Degenerative retention cyst of BPH *(arrow)*. This is the most common type of cyst seen in the prostate and has no clinical significance. Note the marked asymmetry of benign prostatic hyperplasia, with the left transition zone *(L)* much larger than the right *(R)*, and the asymmetrical position of the urethra *(U)*. **B, Utricle cyst** on axial view through the prostate base *(U)*. These cysts are typically in the midline and have a distinct wall. **C,** Midsagittal view shows the **utricle cyst** *(U)* with its characteristic teardrop shape pointing toward the verumontanum *(arrow)*. These cysts can obstruct ejaculatory ducts and result in seminal obstruction and dilation of seminal vesicles *(SV)*, as is seen in this patient. **D, Peripheral zone cyst** *(arrow)*. These cysts are uncommon but may be so tense that they mimic the hardness of cancer at digital rectal examination. Biopsy is needed just to prove that this is not cancer. They disappear after biopsy. **E, Utricle cyst with calcifications along its wall** *(arrows)*. This type of cyst can be related to hematospermia.

there is a clinical concern for prostate cancer (BPH is one cause for PSA elevation) or there is need for precise gland volume determination to help determine and follow appropriate surgical or medical treatments.[11]

Patients who have TURP initially have a large basal surgical defect, but this rapidly decreases in size as the gland collapses into the defect. This can surprise unwary urologists, who may think they have removed considerably more tissue than the visible defect suggests. However, patients are generally symptom free after these procedures, suggesting that the amount of prostatic tissue removed does not necessarily correlate with success (see Fig. 10-4, F).

Prostatitis

Understanding of the condition called "prostatitis" has changed over the years. It is not merely "infection in the prostate." Rather, prostatitis refers to a **chronic pain syndrome** in which, surprisingly, infection, inflammation, and even involvement of the prostate are not always present.[31] Prostatitis and pelvic pain complaints encompass many clinical syndromes and can severely affect the quality of life of many men, who have chronic pain, sexual dysfunction, and LUTS. Patient and physician are often frustrated because diagnosis and treatment can be time-consuming and ineffective. The impact of prostatitis on quality of life has been likened to the morbidity of myocardial infarction, angina, or Crohn's disease. An estimated 9% to 13% of all men in the 40 to 50–year–old age group are affected. About 25% of visits to urologists relate to prostatitis symptoms. In men under 50 years, chronic prostatitis/chronic pelvic pain syndrome is the leading cause of visits to a urologist, and in men over 50, it is the third most common cause, after BPH and cancer.[32,33] The lack of public awareness of this condition likely relates to men's general reluctance to discuss "personal" concerns.

A consensus group at the National Institutes of Health (NIH) in 1999 under the National Institute of Diabetes and Digestive and Kidney Diseases (NIDDK) and the International Prostatitis Collaborative Network established a definition and an NIDDK **classification system for prostatitis** syndromes that includes the following four categories[32-34]:

I. Acute bacterial prostatitis
II. Chronic bacterial prostatitis
III. Chronic prostatitis/chronic pelvic pain syndrome
   A. Inflammatory
   B. Noninflammatory
IV. Asymptomatic inflammatory prostatitis

Acute bacterial prostatitis is the least common form of prostatitis, seen in about 2 of 10,000 office visits; 5% to 10% become chronic.[35] Patients present with symptoms of acute urinary or systemic infection, usually caused by infection with gram-negative organisms such as *Escherichia coli*. Ultrasound findings are seen only in about half of these men and can include edema, prostate enlargement, increased blood flow, venous engorgement, hypoechoic peripheral halo, and altered patchy echo changes that can be decreased or increased, or both[33,36] (Fig. 10-9, *A* and *B*). The diagnosis is mainly clinical. Symptoms should subside promptly with antibiotic therapy, but treatment is continued for 4 to 6 weeks. If symptoms do not quickly subside, abscess formation should be considered. **Abscesses** occur in 0.5% to 2.5% of patients with acute bacterial prostatitis and are more common in those with underlying diabetes mellitus or immunosuppression (including HIV) and after catheterization or instrumentation (Fig. 10-9, *E*). In such patients, TRUS should be promptly employed for diagnosis. Small abscesses may not need drainage, but larger abscesses can be easily drained transrectally or transperineally, using TRUS guidance, or can be unroofed at cystoscopy.[33,37-39] Experience has shown that simple transrectal aspiration can be effective without need for a drainage catheter. Abscesses have resolved even after a single drainage, but repeat aspiration is easily performed if needed.

Chronic bacterial prostatitis is also uncommon. Patients are typically afebrile but have recurrent episodes of bacterial urinary infection–like symptoms. Generally, urine cultures are negative, but some have gram-negative organisms, most often *E. coli*. Empirically, about half of patient with chronic bacterial prostatitis respond to 6- to 12-week courses of antimicrobial therapy.[35] Most have no ultrasound findings.[33]

Chronic prostatitis/chronic pelvic pain (CP/CPP) **syndrome** is the most common form of prostatic inflammation. It accounts for about 90% of cases and affects about 1.9:100 men. It is the most difficult to understand and treat. CP/CPP syndrome is classified into two types, A and B. The **inflammatory type A** is diagnosed by seeing leukocytes in prostate secretions, urine, or semen. In contrast, the **noninflammatory type B** shows no evidence of inflammation and is also called **prostatodynia.** The etiology is unknown, and the CP/CPP name recognizes that the prostate may not be the sole source of discomfort. The symptoms, however, are identical to true prostate infection. Neurologic factors, psychological factors, stress, and genetic predisposition have been implicated, as well as association with other conditions, such as fibromyalgia, irritable bowel syndrome, and chronic fatigue syndrome. No cause is identified in the majority of men with CP/CPP. Patients may respond to antibiotics, alpha blockers, nonsteroidal anti-inflammatory drugs (NSAIDs), and analgesics, which are often used in multimodal fashion.[31,33] In most cases the prostate appears normal at ultrasound. Some sonograms show nonspecific findings such as peripheral hypoechoic areas, calcifications, venous congestion, increased arterial flow, bladder neck thickening, hypoechoic prostatic rim, and periurethral hypogenicity.[33,36,40,41]

Asymptomatic inflammatory prostatitis is diagnosed in men who have no history of genitourinary pain

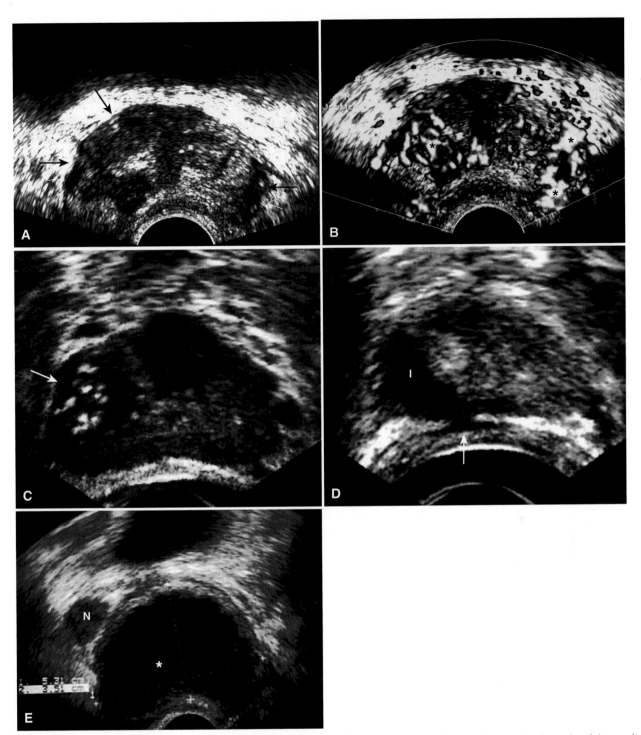

FIGURE 10-9. Prostatitis. Most men with prostatitis have a normal-appearing prostate that can be exceedingly tender if the condition is acute. **A, Biopsy-proven nonacute inflammation.** Multiple geographic hypoechoic areas on both sides *(arrows)* mimic tumor on TRUS and Doppler and are associated with PSA elevation. **B,** Power Doppler ultrasound demonstrates increased vascularity in areas of inflammation (*). **C, BCG noncaseating granulomatous prostatitis** as a mass lesion *(arrow)* in a man whose bladder cancer had been treated with bacille Calmette-Guérin (BCG) instillation. This mimics tumor, but the diagnosis can be suspected from the history. **D, Granulomatous prostatitis** mimics cancer and here appears as a tumor extending beyond the capsule and invading the rectal wall *(arrow); I,* inflammatory mass. **E, Large prostate abscess in AIDS patient.** Virtually the entire prostate is replaced by the abscess collection (*); *N,* node. This patient and other patients with abscess have responded rapidly to one or two TRUS-guided abscess aspirations and antibiotics.

complaints but who are shown to have inflammatory changes at histology. Often, biopsy is done because of PSA elevations that are common with prostate inflammation, even with asymptomatic inflammation.

Diagnostic protocols have attempted to differentiate among the various types of prostatitis using history, physical examination, and urine or other cultures.[32] An issue for TRUS and biopsy is that many of these men have chronically elevated but often fluctuating PSA, even in excess of 10 nanograms per milliliter (ng/mL) and the often-multiple inflammatory areas can mimic cancer at the ultrasound. Biopsy may be needed to exclude cancer. The free/total PSA ratio with inflammatory conditions tends to be higher than seen with cancer[38] (Fig. 10-9, C and D).

Other infectious/inflammatory conditions affecting the prostate do not fit easily into these groups. These include conditions such as malacoplakia, eosinophilic prostatitis, cytomegalovirus (CMV) prostatitis, and granulomatous prostatitis. **Granulomatous prostatitis** is usually idiopathic but also can follow prior instrumentation and may be caused by bacteria (e.g., tuberculosis, brucellosis, syphilis) fungi (e.g., coccidiomycosis, blastomycosis, histoplasmosis, cryptococcosis), and parasites (e.g., schistosomiasis). Cases likely to be seen in North America are caused by bacille Calmette-Guérin (BCG). BCG is commonly instilled into the bladder to treat transitional cell carcinoma. It leaks into the prostate, where it can cause granulomatous inflammation. Granulomatous prostatitis mimics cancer at DRE and TRUS and elevates PSA. A history of BCG instillation can be reassuring, but biopsy generally is needed to exclude cancer[42] (Fig. 10-9, C and D).

The contribution of TRUS is limited in patients with *acute* prostatitis. Physical examination and placing the probe in the rectum are often difficult because of pain. Ultrasound may demonstrate significant abnormality, mimicking carcinoma. In general, inflamed prostates are hypoechoic and often show several strikingly hypoechoic areas and enhanced vascularity.

Prostate and Seminal Vesicle Cysts

Prostate cysts have been grouped into six categories: (1) parenchymal cysts, (2) isolated medial cysts (utricle and müllerian), (3) ejaculatory duct cysts, (4) abscesses, (5) cystic tumors, and (6) cysts related to parasitic disease (schistosomiasis, hydatid disease).[43-45] The most common cysts are **parenchymal degenerative cysts** in hyperplastic nodules in the transition zone. These have no clinical significance but on occasion can become large enough to contribute to urinary or ejaculatory obstruction. Typically, these are seen as unilocular or thinly septated multilocular cysts in a typical BPH nodule in the transition zone (see Fig. 10-8, A). Some patients develop atrophic dilation of prostate ducts, which appear as 1 to 2 mm diameter clusters of radially oriented tubules or cysts. These have no significance.

Retention cysts are focal cysts, often on the surface of the prostate, resulting from duct obstruction. Typically they are small, less than 1 cm. They can be very tense and become palpable as a hard prostate nodule mimicking cancer at DRE, but at ultrasound appear as a typical cyst. They have no significance, but if palpable, my group will aspirate them to confirm their benign nature and to avoid future clinical concern when a hard "nodule" is again palpated (Fig. 10-8, D).

Congenital cysts of the prostate occur in or close to the midline and are related to the wolffian (mesonephric or pronephric [archinephric]) ducts or müllerian (paramesonephric) ducts.[43] Most patients with congenital cystic lesions in the prostate and seminal vesicle will be asymptomatic. Occasionally, these cysts cause symptoms or may become infected, particularly if they are large (see Fig. 10-8, B and C).

Congenital abnormalities are common in and around the prostate and seminal vesicles.[44,46] The müllerian tubercle gives rise to the prostatic utricle, a small, midline blind pouch situated near the summit of the verumontanum. Prostatic **utricle cysts** are caused by dilation of the prostatic utricle (see Fig. 10-8, E). Utricle cysts can be associated with unilateral renal agenesis and rarely, contain spermatozoa. Utricle cysts are always in the midline and are usually small and contained inside the prostate, but occasionally they can become quite large, several centimeters in diameter (see Fig. 10-8, B and C). **Müllerian duct cysts** may arise from remnants of the paramesonephric duct. Müllerian duct cysts are mainly midline but may extend lateral to the midline and can be large and extend above the prostate. They have no other associations and never contain spermatozoa. As with utricle cysts, they have a teardrop shape pointing toward the verumontanum, a thick visible wall, and occasional mural or contained calcifications. In practice, utricle and müllerian cysts appear similarly, and their differentiation is not important. When large, both types may obstruct ejaculatory ducts or develop calcifications and become symptomatic, painful, or infected, and rarely they may develop tumors.

Ejaculatory duct cysts are usually small and probably represent cystic dilation of the ejaculatory duct, possibly as a result of obstruction. Alternatively, they may be diverticula of the duct. They tend to be fusiform in shape and are typically pointed at both ends. Ejaculatory duct cysts contain spermatozoa when aspirated. They can be associated with infertility and may be seen in patients with a low sperm count. Some may cause perineal pain.[43,45,46]

Prostate abscesses form "cysts" that resemble abscesses seen elsewhere as cavities with thick, irregular walls and debris containing fluid (see Fig. 10-9, E). Coliform organisms such as *E. coli* are the most common etiology. Predisposing conditions include diabetes, instrumentation, and immunodeficiency. Transrectal aspiration or TURP drainage can be effective treatments,

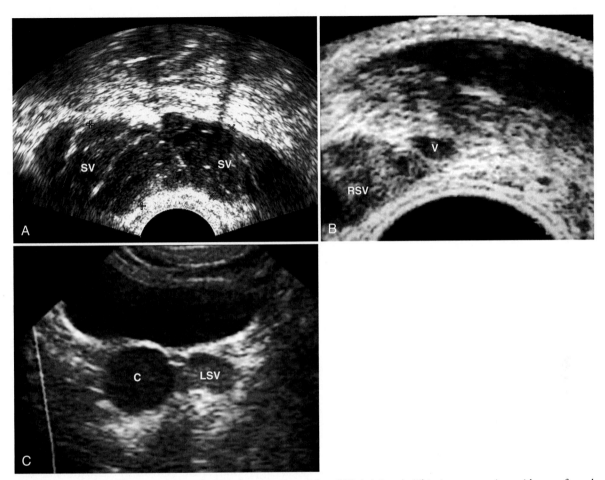

FIGURE 10-10. Infertility. A, Bilateral dilated seminal vesicles *(SV)* (>1.5 cm). This is presumptive evidence of mechanical obstruction to the ejaculatory ducts, which may be the cause of the infertility. The finding is not specific because this degree of enlargement can also be seen in normal, fertile men. **B, Unilateral agenesis of left seminal vesicle and vas deferens** *(V)*. Only the right side is intact; *RSV,* right seminal vesicle; **C, Unilateral right seminal vesicle cyst** *(C);* transvesical scan; *LSV,* left seminal vesicle. This patient also had absence of the ipsilateral right kidney.

in addition to antimicrobial therapy.[43-45] Cysts caused by parasites are rare in Western countries and can result from schistosomiasis (bilharziasis) or hydatid (echinococcal) disease.[44,45]

Cystic neoplasms are rare, but cystadenoma and cystadenocarcinoma have been described.[44,45]

Seminal vesicle cysts are rare and usually solitary (Fig. 10-10, *C*). Most are asymptomatic. Affected patients may benefit from aspiration when cysts are large and symptomatic. They may be associated with ipsilateral renal anomalies, including renal agenesis, because the seminal vesicles are derivatives of the wolffian (mesonephric) ducts, which also give rise to the ureter and vas deferens. Other associations include adult polycystic disease, hemivertebra, and ipsilateral absence of testis. Rarely, the seminal vesicles are involved by tumors, (metastatic, cystadenoma, papillary adenoma), abscesses, and amyloidosis.[47,48]

Other disorders that mimic prostate and seminal vesicle cysts include ectopic ureterocele, Cowper's duct cysts (in urogenital diaphragm below apex of prostate),

and bladder diverticulum. The seminal vesicle is a common site of ectopic insertion of the ureter.[43,47]

Calcification of the vas deferens or seminal vesicles can occur with diabetes or infection. **Diabetic** calcification tends to involve the walls and resembles "tram tracks" on x-ray films, whereas **infectious/inflammatory** calcification is luminal and segmental and may be associated with seminal vesicle calcifications.[48] On occasion, a 1-cm-diameter eggshell calcification is seen in a seminal vesicle. These calcifications are asymptomatic and likely related to inflammation.

Infertility and Transrectal Ultrasound

Infertility is defined as failure to achieve pregnancy after 1 year of regular unprotected intercourse and affects about 15% of couples. Male factor is solely responsible in about 20% of couples and contributory in another 30% to 40%.[49] When present, male infertility is usually, but not always, detected by abnormal semen analysis.

The AUA has defined "best practice" policies for investigating male infertility; both partners should be evaluated simultaneously.[49,50] The **goals of male evaluation** include the following:

1. Identification of potentially correctable conditions.
2. Identification of irreversible conditions for which alternative treatments (e.g., donor insemination) or adoption may be employed, preventing ineffective therapies.
3. Detection of health-threatening conditions underlying infertility.
4. Detection of genetic abnormalities (e.g., cystic fibrosis) that may affect the health of children if affected sperm are harvested or used for assisted reproductive techniques.

Male factors can be categorized as pretesticular, testicular, and posttesticular.[49] **Pretesticular factors** include conditions such as faulty reproductive behavior and genetic abnormalities (e.g., CFTR gene, Y chromosome microdeletions). **Testicular factors** include congenital and acquired intrinsic disorders of spermatogenesis (e.g., infections, trauma, treated cryptorchidism) that, except for varicocele, are generally irreversible. **Posttesticular causes** of azoospermia (no sperm in ejaculate) and oligospermia (low numbers of sperm in ejaculate) generally relate to obstructive issues, and are found in about 40% of infertile men, although only 1% to 5% have **ejaculatory duct obstructions** (EDOs), which are amenable to surgical therapies such as prostate cyst unroofing or **transurethral resection of ejaculatory ducts** (TURED).[49,51,52] This excludes vasectomy reversal, which is successful in 70% to 95% of patients, and pregnancy is achieved in 30% to 70% of couples.[49] In 100 consecutive azoospermic men, the distribution of etiology of azoospermia was genetic abnormalities, 27%; diseases or external influence (orchitis, radiotherapy, infections, surgery, trauma), 22%; corrected cryptorchidism, 27%; and unexplained, 22%.[53] *Campbell-Walsh Urology*[50] lists frequency of causes as varicocele, 38%; idiopathic, 23%; obstruction, 13%; normal, 9%; cryptorchidism and testicular failure, 6%; and all other causes, about 10%. This illustrates the broad spectrum of disorders apart from ejaculatory duct obstructions that relate to azoospermia.

The **role of TRUS** and to a lesser extent MRI[46] is to identify anatomically correctable ejaculatory duct obstructions and anomalies in men who are azoospermic or oligospermic and who have vas deferens by palpation (Fig. 10-10). Of interest, the presence or absence of vas deferens is diagnosed clinically by palpation of the spermatic cord and not through imaging.[49,51,52] Vasography has been used to demonstrate obstruction, but this generally has been discontinued because of the risk of injury to the vas deferens. On occasion, TRUS can be used to inject seminal vesicles with ultrasound or x-ray contrast agents to demonstrate patency of the ejaculatory ducts and to retrieve sperm from the seminal vesicles for assisted reproduction.

There are no specific symptoms associated with **ejaculatory duct obstruction,** although the diagnosis is suggested in infertile males with azoospermia or oligospermia who have low ejaculate volume, normal secondary sex characteristics and testes, pain during or after ejaculation or orgasm, or history of prostatitis. Suggestive imaging findings include midline cysts, dilated seminal vesicles (>1.5 cm) or ejaculatory ducts, and calcifications along the ducts.[51,52] Kuligowska and Fenlon[54] reported the relative frequency of TRUS findings in infertile men with low-volume azoospermia as normal appearance (25%); bilateral absence of vas deferens (34%); bilateral occlusion of the vas deferens, seminal vesicles, and ejaculatory ducts by calcification or fibrosis (16%); unilateral absence of the vas deferens (11%); obstructing cysts of the seminal vesicles, vas ejaculatory ducts, or prostate (9%); and ductal obstruction due to calculi (4%). All these symptoms and findings are also seen in normal, fertile men but are more common in men with obstructive infertility[52] (Fig. 10-10).

The treatment of suspected distal ejaculatory obstruction consists of TURED, used to unroof the ducts or drain obstructing cysts. Of men undergoing TURED, 50% to 100% had improvement in symptoms and 20% to 30% achieved pregnancies.[51,52]

Absence of the vas deferens is a clinical diagnosis made by palpating the spermatic cord. This seems to occur in two groups of men: (1) those with mutation of at least one cystic fibrosis transmembrane regulator (CFTR) gene and (2) genetically normal men with congenital absence of the vas deferens. About 80% to 99% of adult men with cystic fibrosis have congenital bilateral absence of the vas deferens, presumed to occur prenatally. Interestingly, the prevalence is lower in children, suggesting that changes are acquired in some cases. Abnormalities of the vas deferens occur even with only one CFTR mutation in men who have no cystic fibrosis symptoms. Seminal vesicles may be present. Renal anomalies are uncommon in the CFTR group.[55-57]

In general, bilateral absence of vas deferens or seminal vesicle is more likely associated with cystic fibrosis and CFTR gene abnormality (60%-70%) and less likely to have renal agenesis or anomaly. In contrast, unilateral absence of the vas deferens or seminal vesicle is often (91%) associated with renal abnormalities, including agenesis. Remember that since the vas deferens, seminal vesicle, and ureter develop from the mesonephric (wolffian) duct, anomalies may manifest in all the derivatives of this duct.[46,48,57]

Hematospermia

Hematospermia is the macroscopic presence of blood in the semen. In most cases it is a benign, self-limiting condition and typically resolves spontaneously over a few weeks. The incidence is uncertain. Hematospermia causes significant anxiety among men, who fear cancer or sexually transmitted disease (STD). The differential diagnosis list is extensive, but most cases are **iatrogenic** (following interventions such as biopsy or cystoscopy), **infectious,** or **inflammatory** and can be effectively treated with minimal investigation and simple reassurance. Malignant tumors (mainly prostate, but also testis and seminal vesicle) are an uncommon cause of hematospermia and are found in only 3.5% of cases, predominantly in men over age 40 years. **Common etiologies** include the following[58,59]:

- Inflammation and infection (up to 39%)
- Ductal obstruction, cysts, calcifications in seminal ducts
- Iatrogenic/traumatic (prostate **biopsy** is now the most common cause)
- Systemic factors (hypertension, bleeding diathesis)
- Vascular abnormalities (varicosities, arteriovenous malformation)
- Idiopathic (about 15%)

The primary aim of investigation is to allay anxiety, because the great majority of hematospermia cases, especially in younger men, are highly unlikely to be associated with sinister pathology. In addition to history and physical examination, most patients initially undergo evaluation for STD, urinalysis, and urine culture. Men over age 40 should also be assessed for malignancy, especially prostate cancer, even though this is an uncommon etiology.

Imaging may be helpful in unexplained or persistent cases. TRUS is readily available and has shown findings in 74% to 95% of men with persistent hematospermia. Findings include prostate calcifications, ejaculatory duct calculi, dilated ejaculatory ducts, BPH, dilated seminal vesicles, seminal vesicle calcifications, ejaculatory duct cysts, and prostatitis[58-60] (see Figs. 10-8, *E,* and 10-10, *A*). Color Doppler ultrasound may be able to detect the rare vascular malformation. In practice, it can be difficult to establish that a TRUS finding is responsible for hematospermia because similar findings are often seen in asymptomatic men. Fortunately, overall the findings represent benign conditions.

Endorectal coil MRI can also be helpful because it is able to detect sites of bleeding that are not apparent at ultrasound, especially bleeding into the seminal vesicles.[61] On occasion, cystoscopy and urethroscopy are needed.

Treatment beyond reassurance is not needed in most patients with hematospermia because the bleeding is slight and self-limited. Alternatively, therapy is directed to any discovered etiologies, including antimicrobial therapy, cyst unroofing or aspiration, and systemic therapy for hypertension and bleeding diathesis.[58]

PROSTATE CANCER

For optimal patient care, it is important for those using TRUS to evaluate prostate cancer to be aware of the different facets of screening, diagnosis, and management and the role of PSA. Prostate cancer is a difficult problem filled with uncertainties and dilemmas for men, their partners, and physicians. Prostate cancer is a significant health problem; it is a common cancer and a common cause of death from cancer. Effective treatments exist, but the therapies have significant quality of life–altering side effects. Unlike many other cancers, not every prostate cancer progresses inevitably to metastases and death. There is a large burden of indolent disease that would not benefit from radical therapy but that must be differentiated from progressive disease. Prostate cancer mainly affects men over age 50 and thus competes with comorbidities as a cause of death. It has a long course, not uncommonly taking about 10 years from asymptomatic diagnosis to cause-specific death. This makes it difficult to determine if screening and treatment protocols are effective, since trials take more than 10 years, during which diagnostic and therapeutic changes could make study results irrelevant.[62-65]

To complicate matters further, no consensus has emerged for the optimal treatment of **clinically localized disease,** which is the most common presentation (91% of cases) in the United States.[66]

Epidemiology

Prostate adenocarcinoma has become the most frequently diagnosed cancer in men, two to three times more than lung and colorectal cancer. It is a disease seen primarily in men over age 50. After lung cancer, prostate cancer is the second leading cause of cancer deaths in men and in the United States, kills about 45,000 men each year. American men have an about one in six (17%) lifetime risk of developing prostate cancer and about a 1 in 30 mortality risk. The risk is higher in African-American men and those with a family history of prostate cancer.[67-70] It is the fourth most common male malignancy worldwide. The rates are highest in Scandinavia and North America, especially in African Americans (272 per 100,000) and lowest in China (1.9 per 100,000),[12,50] but rates are increasing in those countries.[71] The incidence and stage at diagnosis have been

PROSTATE CANCER: KEY FACTS

- Most common cancer diagnosed in men.
- The second leading cause of cancer deaths in men (after lung cancer).
- The fourth most common male malignancy worldwide.
- Many and varied treatments that are personalized to patient situation.
- Treatments are associated with quality-of-life issues.
- Many men have microscopic tumors that may not affect longevity.

decreasing since the early 1990s, partly because of the introduction of PSA screening. Genetics and environment, including a fatty diet, appear to play roles in prostate cancer incidence.[72] The risk doubles with a single affected relative and is even higher with multiple affected relatives.[70] More than 95% of primary malignant tumors of the prostate are adenocarcinomas. Rarely, a variety of other primary neoplasms involve the prostate, including prostate transitional cell carcinoma, sarcomas, and lymphomas.[50,73] The prostate can be secondarily affected by tumors of regional structures, including bladder and rectum.

Of men with localized untreated cancer, 9% to 68% die in less than 10 years, and the prognosis depends on tumor grade. Metastases precede death by about 3 years. Ten-year mortality with low-grade tumors (Gleason 2-4) is 9% to 13%; intermediate-grade tumors (Gleason 5-7), 13% to 24%; and high-grade tumors (Gleason 8-10), 44% to 66%. Impalpable (T1) and palpable (T2) tumors behave similarly.[65]

Prostate-Specific Antigen

Prostate-specific antigen has been a tremendous advance in the diagnosis and management of prostate cancer.[74-77] PSA is a normally occurring enzyme secreted by the epithelial cells of prostate ducts and functions to liquefy the ejaculate. The prostate is the main source of PSA, and only trace amounts are found in other tissues in men and women. Some PSA leaks into the serum, where it can be measured.[78] Abnormal serum PSA levels result from excessive leakage or excessive production. Cancer is believed to produce on average 10 times as much PSA as a similar volume of benign tissue.[75,79] In the serum, PSA is partly unbound (free) and partly bound to proteins such as alpha-1-antitrypsin. The ratio of free to total PSA (percent free PSA) differs in benign and malignant conditions. With cancer and chronic prostatitis, the ratio tends to be low.[80]

Prostate-specific antigen is probably best considered as a nonspecific test of prostate abnormality or irritation. **Elevated levels** occur with cancer but also variably with benign conditions, including BPH, inflammation, after ejaculation, prostate manipulation, biopsy, and cystoscopy. Digital rectal examination and TRUS without biopsy generally do not elevate PSA significantly, but it is prudent to draw the blood before disturbing the prostate. PSA levels can be artificially reduced by a factor of 2 with antiandrogenic medications such as finasteride (Proscar) and dutasteride (Avodart). Unpredictably reduced levels are found with herbal medications such as saw palmetto and PC SPEC.[74,75,78,81,82]

At least two **PSA standards** are in use, the Hybritech and the World Health Organization (WHO 96/670). Their values differ by about 23%, and there is no way to interconvert. There is a slight diurnal variation. Intersubject variation is 14% to 16%.[81,83] These issues are of importance when PSA is followed serially, as in men under active surveillance or being followed up after therapy. PSA in these men should be done by laboratories using the same standard.

The recommendations for using PSA to direct **biopsy** are changing, and currently there is no longer a general consensus. Previously, **PSA level of 4 mg/mL or less** (and more currently, <2.5 ng/mL) was believed to be "negative" and not needing biopsy; **values over 10 ng/mL** are sufficiently high to recommend biopsy in every case and yield cancer at biopsy exceeding about 50%.[84] The **4 to 10–ng/mL** window was problematic because about 35% to 44% of men in this range have cancer.[85,86] The remainder have benign causes for increased PSA (e.g., BPH) and often undergo unnecessary biopsy (low specificity). Additional tactics involving PSA density, PSA velocity, and age-specific PSA were developed for the 4 to 10–ng/mL group to avoid biopsy when the elevation was likely caused by benign conditions.

PSA Density

Production of PSA by benign prostate tissue (normal and hyperplastic) is generally less than production by cancer. If there is an excess PSA level above that predicted from gland volume measured by TRUS, the patient has an increased risk of cancer. PSA density (PSAd) is defined as PSA/volume (e.g., PSA 6.0 and gland volume 75 cc; PSAd = 6.0/75 = 0.08).[75]

Restricting biopsy in the PSA 4 to 10–ng/mL group to those with PSAd in excess of 0.12 to 0.15 will detect about 80% of those with cancer and avoid some biopsies. In the above example, the PSAd is 0.08, which is less than 0.12. This PSA level is consistent with the prediction from gland volume, and thus biopsy could be avoided at present, with about 80% confidence that cancer is not present. However, 20% of cancers will be missed.[8,79,81,87] PSAd has now also become a marker for prostate cancer aggressiveness to help determine if active surveillance is reasonable for men with low-risk, low-volume cancer at biopsy.[81]

Transition zone (TZ) PSA density is calculated as PSA/TZ volume. It attempts to increase PSA specificity by accounting for the proportion of PSA manufactured by the TZ, which is the site of hyperplasia. Cutoff was estimated at 0.35 ng/mL/cc. This technique has not been reproducible mainly because of difficulties in measuring TZ volume accurately.[75] In our hands, total PSA is more accurate in cancer detection.

Age-Specific PSA

Prostate-specific antigen normally increases with age.[75,82] By using different threshold PSA levels at different ages, it may be possible to make PSA more sensitive in younger men and less sensitive in older men and avoid unneeded referral for biopsy.[75,79,88] Suggested normal ranges are 0.0

to 2.5 ng/mL (40-49 yr), 0.0 to 3.5 ng/mL (50-59 yr), 0.0 to 4.5 ng/mL (60-69 yr), and 0.0 to 6.5 ng/mL (70-79 yr).[88]

We have not found age-specific PSA useful. Although PSA does increase with age, the change related to age alone is very slight.[82] Most of the increase with age is caused by the prostate enlargement with BPH found in older men. Therefore, age-specific PSA is really a surrogate for **prostate volume,** which is better evaluated with TRUS. Also, the suggested age-specific values in the important 50 to 75 age group are about 4.0 ng/mL, which matches most current biopsy recommendations.

PSA Velocity

Over time, PSA levels in men with cancer usually rise more rapidly than in men with BPH. The rate of PSA rise over time is termed **velocity.** In the 4 to 10–ng/mL PSA group, if three PSA tests are done over 2 years and velocity exceeds 0.75 ng/mL/yr, this rapid change distinguishes men with cancer from those with BPH with a specificity of 90%.[75,79,81,87,89] For men up to age 59 and for PSA less than 4 ng/mL, a lower PSA velocity threshold of 0.4 ng/mL/yr could be used.[74,90] Many centers do not wait for 2 years and offer biopsy if there is an unexplained rise in the 4 to 10–ng/mL group of greater than 1 ng/mL between two tests less than 1 year apart.[8,75,79,81,87] Higher velocities are associated with increased cancer aggressiveness.[81]

Free/Total PSA Ratio

Prostate-specific antigen in the blood is partly free and partly bound to proteins, especially alpha-1-antitrypsin. The usual PSA measurement is the sum of free plus bound. For unexplained reasons, the free/total ratio tends to be high with benign conditions and low with cancer.[8,75,79,81,87] In the 4 to 10–ng/mL PSA range, using a free/total ratio of less than 20% detects about 95% of cancers and decreases the number of biopsies by about 30%. However, 5% of clinically significant cancers will be missed. An exact cutoff ratio has not yet been generally accepted.[76]

Current PSA Standards

All the previous techniques using PSA derivatives can decrease the number of biopsies, but at the cost of missing clinically significant cancer. In practice, it is unusual to see PSA greater than 1.5 ng/mL in a healthy man of any age.[82] Many physicians avoid these temporizing tactics and recommend biopsy in any man with unexplained PSA greater than 4 ng/mL and more recently for any man with PSA greater than 2.5 ng/mL.[81,91] The PSA techniques described can be used to guide the urgency of repeat biopsy if the initial biopsy is negative.

Remember also that **not all cancers produce PSA,** and that **20% to 40% of men with clinically significant cancer will have normal PSA.** Biopsy is indicated when there is an obvious suspicious nodule at palpation or ultrasound, even if PSA is normal.[8,84] Although PSA and its variants remain the best serum test for prostate cancer detection, interventional guidance, and therapeutic monitoring,[74] controversy surrounds "normal" values, test characteristics such as sensitivity and specificity,[92] and PSA's value in screening for prostate cancer.[93,94] Previously, 4.0 and more currently 2.5 ng/mL was taken as the upper limit of normal, especially regarding the need for biopsy.[76,81] Most "normal" men at any age have PSA less than about 1.5 ng/mL.[82] Remember that PSA is not a dichotomous "yes/no" or "positive/negative" test, but rather provides a **continuous index of risk** for prostate cancer.[74,76,95,96] There is no level below which cancer is not found, not even at levels less than 0.5 ng/mL. Higher levels imply higher risk of cancer, especially aggressive cancer.[92] A normal PSA should not prevent proceeding to biopsy if the DRE or ultrasound findings are suspicious for cancer.[8,84]

In 2009 the AUA published a new PSA "best practice" statement,[74] taking into consideration the interim results of the ERSPC[94] and PLCO[93] screening studies (see Screening). AUA suggests obtaining a baseline PSA at age 40 (to suggest intensiveness of subsequent screening) and not to use a single threshold PSA value to prompt biopsy. Rather, biopsy decisions should take into account PSA, DRE, and additional factors such as age, family history, prior biopsy and comorbidities, free/total PSA, PSA velocity, and PSA density. In addition, men should be informed of the risks and benefits of cancer screening and the option of active surveillance versus immediate treatment.[74] This guideline is difficult to use to direct biopsy because there is no specific cutoff or trigger point, and need for biopsy is left to the discretion of the patient and physician. Other groups have published different guidelines,[87,93] and updated recommendations are pending.[5]

New serum and molecular genetic tests are being evaluated for their ability to detect and stage prostate cancer and may soon come into active clinical use.[97] In previous years, serum acid phosphatase was used to detect prostate cancer. Acid phosphatase becomes abnormal only when cancer has already metastasized. It is no longer used and has been totally replaced by PSA and imaging tests such as bone scan, CT, and MRI.

Screening

The purpose of screening is to detect clinically significant prostate cancer in asymptomatic men at an early stage, with the intention that curative therapy can be offered that will improve outcomes.[4,68,69,76] The screening tools are PSA and digital rectal examination. Prostate cancer is asymptomatic in its early, curable stages. Symptoms arise when the disease has spread beyond the prostate and has become incurable. In the pre-PSA era, most cancers at initial presentation had already extended beyond the prostate (stage T3 or T4), and only palliative care was possible. The advent of PSA screening has resulted in stage "migration," meaning that most prostate cancer is now being detected at an earlier stage (T1 and T2), when curative therapy is still an option.[12,50,68,98]

However, controversy surrounds prostate cancer screening.[68,98] Prostate cancer is unquestionably a clinically important condition for which therapies can avert symptomatic disease and death.[4,99] However, clinically unimportant microfocal cancer is common, and up to about 30% of men dying from other causes at age 50 have incidental microscopic cancer.[69] Concerns have been raised that screening programs and systematic biopsy protocols will pick up many of these insignificant cancers. This is unlikely, however, especially in younger men, and many detected cancers are likely to cause morbidity and shorten life span. About 16 of every 100 cases of prostate cancer detected through screening would be fatal if left untreated.[50,64]

Prostate cancer is seen in men over 50 years of age and on average takes about 10 years to cause death. At these ages, there are many competing causes for mortality. Therefore, most recommendations suggest **annual screening with DRE and PSA between ages 50 to 75 years,** and also suggest that screening be performed only in reasonably healthy men who have an expected life span of 10 years. Further, screening should be performed only after discussion about benefits and limitations of screening and consequences of diagnostic procedures and therapy.[4,5,64,76,93] Men at **high risk** (African Americans and those with several close relatives with prostate cancer) should consider starting screening at **age 40 to 45 years.** Ending screening at age 75 years acknowledges that the average longevity at age 75 is 10.8 years, so detection and treatment of prostate cancer after that age is less likely to provide health benefits or longevity.[5] Additional variables that increase the likelihood of cancer should be considered before screening (e.g., age, ethnicity, family history, urinary symptoms, PSA, free/total PSA ratio, PSA and DRE, prior negative biopsy). Many nomograms that include these factors are available to help individualize cancer risk before biopsy. These can be found by searching on the Internet under **prostate cancer risk calculator.**[96,100]

To date, the health and mortality benefits of prostate cancer screening in the general population have not been unequivocally established with large, randomized trials. Case studies suggest screening combined with appropriate treatments can improve outcomes. A highly dedicated regional program in Austria using aggressive screening with PSA and its derivatives, sophisticated TRUS and biopsy protocols, and focused, dedicated treatment programs (mainly radical prostatectomy) decreased prostate cancer mortality by 59%, versus 29%

in the rest of Austria.[99] However, the 2009 interim results of two large screening studies (ERSPC and PLCO) had conflicting results.[101]

The European Randomized Study of Screening for Prostate Cancer (ERSPC) reported 9-year results.[94] The study recruited 162,387 men age 55 to 69, half of whom were screened using PSA over an average of 4 years, with biopsy recommended for PSA greater than 3 ng/mL. Treatment protocols were not mandated. Cancer incidence in the screened vs. control patients was 8.2/4.8%. Screening resulted in 20% reduction of prostate cancer–specific mortality (including mortality related to therapy). There was risk of overdiagnosis and overtreatment. The detection of cancers in men who would not have symptoms in their lifetime was estimated at about 50%. They estimated 1410 men would need to be screened and 48 additional cases of cancer treated to prevent one prostate cancer death. These proportions are similar to those seen in breast and colon screening programs.[4] Unresolved issues included cost/benefit analysis, continuing improvements in cancer therapy, and quality of life issues related to investigation and treatment.[94]

The American Prostate, Lung, Colorectal, and Ovarian (PLCO) Cancer Screening Trial reported up to 10-year results.[93] The study recruited 76,693 men age 55 to 74, half of whom were screened with annual DRE and PSA (>4 ng/mL considered positive). At 7 years, prostate cancer detection for screened/control patients was 116/95, giving a significant cancer detection ratio of 1.22. However, the cancer-specific mortality of 2.0/1.7 (ratio 1.13) per 10,000 person-years was not statistically significant, suggesting that screening did not provide survival advantage. Problems with the PLCO study included (1) before recruitment, about 45% of men had already been prescreened with PSA or DRE (i.e., many patients with cancer were removed from the study), and (2) about 52% of the control group was "contaminated" by having PSA testing outside the study.[93] In effect there was no true control group.

The key question remains not whether PSA screening is effective in cancer detection (it is), but rather whether PSA screening overall does more good than harm.[101] Because of this, the risks and benefits of screening and treatment should be discussed with the patient before offering PSA screening, and the decision to proceed is personal and should be made by the patient.[4,5,76]

Staging and Histologic Grading

Tumor stage and histologic grade are important characteristics of prostate cancer to help determine treatment needs and options and provide prognosis.[65] **Staging,** or estimation of tumor spread, is done using the American Joint Committee on Cancer (AJCC) tumor-node-metastasis (TNM) classification, which has international uniformity and ability to integrate clinical, imaging, and pathologic staging information.[102-105] The 2010 edition

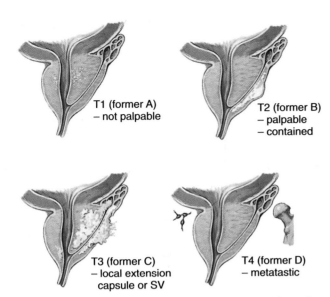

T1 (former A)
– not palpable

T2 (former B)
– palpable
– contained

T3 (former C)
– local extension
capsule or SV

T4 (former D)
– metatastic

FIGURE 10-11. Contemporary prostate cancer staging using the tumor-nodes-metastasis- (TNM) classification.

of the *AJCC Staging Manual* incorporates Gleason score and PSA into staging. Previously, the Jewett and Whitmore classification was used[86,106] (Fig. 10-11 and Table 10-1).

Stage T1 (formerly **A**) tumors are not palpable clinically because they are small, soft, or located in an anterior part of the gland that cannot be reached by palpation. This stage was initially used to describe cancers detected microscopically in chips obtained at TURP. More recently, an additional **T1c** stage was introduced to describe tumors that are impalpable and not visible at TRUS but are found at needle biopsy. An estimated 85% or more of T1c cancers are clinically significant and likely to benefit from treatment.[75,85,107]

Stages T2 (formerly **B**) tumors are palpable as a nodule by DRE and represent cancer confined within the prostate, typically in the peripheral zone. **Stage T3** (formerly **C**) tumors have local extension outside confines of the prostate into the periprostatic soft tissues (**T3a**) or seminal vesicles (**T3b**). **Stage T4** (formerly **D**) tumor is fixed or invades adjacent structures other than seminal vesicles, including the bladder neck, external sphincter, rectum, levator muscles, and pelvic wall.

With **TNM staging** the local tumor T stage is modified with N (node status) and M (non–lymph node distant metastasis).[104,105] Patients with clinical stages T1 to T3 have no evidence of metastatic disease at other imaging techniques (e.g., TRUS, MRI, isotope bone scan, PET). Unfortunately, these other modalities show wide variability in accuracy of local staging, ranging from 50% to 92%.[1,103,108,109] Most clinicians use their clinical acumen or refer to staging calculators on the Internet, such as those by Kattan (www.nomograms.org), to estimate extracapsular or metastatic spread and assign

TABLE 10-1. AMERICAN JOINT COMMITTEE ON CANCER (AJCC) STAGING OF PROSTATE CANCER

STAGE	DESCRIPTION
	Primary Tumor (T)
	Clinical
TX	Primary tumor cannot be assessed
T0	No evidence of primary tumor
T1	Clinically inapparent tumor neither palpable nor visible by imaging
T1a	Tumor incidental histologic finding in 5% or less of tissue resected
T1b	Tumor incidental histologic finding in more than 5% of tissue resected
T1c	Tumor identified by needle biopsy (e.g., because of elevated PSA)
T2	Tumor confined within prostate*
T2a	Tumor involves one-half of one lobe or less
T2b	Tumor involves more than one-half of one lobe but not both lobes
T2c	Tumor involves both lobes
T3	Tumor extends through the prostate capsule†
T3a	Extracapsular extension (unilateral or bilateral)
T3b	Tumor invades seminal vesicle(s)
T4	Tumor is fixed or invades adjacent structures other than seminal vesicles such as external sphincter rectum, bladder, levator muscles, and/or pelvic wall
	Pathologic (pT)‡
pT2	Organ confined
pT2a	Unilateral, one-half of one side or less
pT2b	Unilateral, involving more than one-half of side but not both sides
pT2c	Bilateral disease
pT3	Extraprostatic extension
pT3a	Extraprostatic extension or microscopic invasion of bladder neck§
pT3b	Seminal vesicle invasion
pT4	Invasion of rectum, levator muscles, and/or pelvic wall
	Regional Lymph Nodes (N)
	Clinical
NX	Regional lymph nodes were not assessed
N0	No regional lymph node metastasis
N1	Metastasis in regional lymph nodes(s)
	Pathologic
pNX	Regional nodes not sampled
pN0	No positive regional nodes
pN1	Metastasis in regional node(s)
	Distant Metastasis (M)¶
M0	No distant metastasis
M1	Distant metastasis
M1a	Nonregional lymph node(s)
M1b	Bone(s)
M1c	Other sites with or without bone disease

*Tumor found in one or both lobes by needle biopsy, but not palpable or reliably visible by imaging, is classified as T1c.

†Invasion into the prostatic apex or into (but not beyond) the prostatic capsule classified not as T3 but as T2.

‡There is no pathologic T1 classification.

§Positive surgical margin should be indicated by an R1 descriptor (residual microscopic disease).

¶When more than one site of metastasis is present, the most advanced category is used. pM1c is most advanced

From Edge SB, Byrd DR, Greene FL, et al. AJCC Cancer Staging Manual. 7th ed. New York: Springer-Verlag; 2010.

prognosis.[110-112] Additional pretreatment imaging to detect distant metastases using radionuclide bone scan, CT, or MRI is recommended for cancers with high PSA (>10-20 ng/mL), or with aggressive histology (Gleason score >6 or >7), or with clinical suspicion of extracapsular disease on palpation.[1,109]

In addition to clinical staging, **histologic grading** is done using the Gleason scoring system, which analyzes the microscopic appearance of glandular differentiation and histologic aggressiveness, **grade 1** being well differentiated and **grade 5,** poorly differentiated. Most tumors are not histologically uniform and show different Gleason grades in different parts. Gleason score is assigned by determining the most dominant and the second most dominant grade, then adding the two to obtain a Gleason score between 2 and 10.[113-115] Scores of 1 to 6 are considered well differentiated; 7, moderately differentiated; and 8 to 10, poorly differentiated. Prognosis is worse with higher scores.

Therapy

Once cancer is discovered, determined to be clinically significant, and judged treatable for cure, many treatment options are available, depending on grade, stage, and patient choices. To date, there is no consensus regarding optimal treatment for the most common, clinically localized cancer.[50] Treatment options include established therapies such as radical prostatectomy and radiotherapy (both escalated-dose conformal external beam radiotherapy and brachytherapy) as well as newer emerging but as yet unproven techniques, including active surveillance, cryotherapy, and focal therapies such as high-intensity focused ultrasound, radiofrequency ablation, photodynamic therapy, and highly focused external beam radiation and "boost" brachytherapy. Men with advanced disease can undergo watchful waiting (watching the patient and postponing treatment until symptoms occur) or palliative therapy.[12,50,66]

Cancer control by the established surgical and radiation therapies in men with organ-confined disease exceeds 90% at 10 years in low-risk patients but falls rapidly with higher grade and more extensive disease.[50] All the treatments have side effects of varying degrees that can significantly affect quality of life, including incontinence, erectile dysfunction, and urethral strictures, besides the usual surgical concerns. Patients may select a specific treatment depending on local expertise and the expected complications. High cure rates and long-term survival have made quality of life an important issue when considering treatment.[50,62,63,66,116]

Radical prostatectomy is the "gold standard" of therapy and has a disease-free survival advantage over expectant management.[117] Cure rates in men with low-grade cancer exceed 90% but decrease with advanced grades and stages. For example, when nodes are involved at radical prostatectomy, 10-year survival falls to about 15%. An attempt is made to avoid injury to the neurovascular bundle, if safe for cancer control, to avoid erectile and continence problems (nerve-sparing prostatectomy). In skilled hands, continence is about 90% and erectile function is preserved in 50% to 90%, depending on patient age. Alternatives to the classic open retropubic prostatectomy are laparoscopic surgery and robotic surgery, which have similar outcomes in experienced hands, although postoperative recovery is faster.[50,66]

The two approaches for radiotherapy are external beam and implanted radioactive seeds (brachytherapy). Conformal escalated-dose **external beam radiotherapy** uses image guidance, usually computed tomography (CT), to confine/conform the beam tightly to the prostate. This allows increasing/escalating target dose while minimizing collateral damage to adjacent organs. Usually, fiducial (reference) markers are inserted into the prostate under TRUS guidance to improve planning and to facilitate targeting. Five-year freedom from biochemical recurrence (no PSA rise) is 70% to 85%. Erectile function is preserved in about 50% and continence in 80% of patients.[50,62]

Brachytherapy involves intraoperative placement of radioactive seeds, usually iodine-125, into the prostate using TRUS guidance and a perineal template. Direct radioactive seed placement into the prostate allows higher local radiation doses. The technique is restricted to low-risk patients with PSA less than 10 ng/mL, Gleason score of 6 or less, and gland volume less than 50 cc/mL. Erectile function is preserved in about 50% and continence in about 80% of patients, although urinary stricture and bowel irritation are common.[50,62]

Efficacy has not been firmly established for the following emerging techniques[71,118]:

- **Cryotherapy.** Cryoprobes are inserted under ultrasound control to kill tissue by freezing. The "ice ball" development can be monitored with ultrasound.
- **High-intensity focused ultrasound** (HIFU) heats and destroys tissue. Therapy is monitored by transrectal ultrasound and more recently by MRI.
- **Radiofrequency thermal ablation.** Radiofrequency probes are inserted under transrectal ultrasound control to heat the prostate. The heating may be monitored by MRI.
- **Photodynamic therapy.** Photosensitive agents are injected intravenously. The agents are activated by laser probes inserted into the prostate under ultrasound guidance, and the resulting activation creates reactive chemical radicals that destroy tissue within the illuminated area.

These techniques can be globally applied to the prostate, but now they are also considered for focal therapy of prostate tumors. **Focal therapy** is an attempt to avoid overtreatment and decrease side effects when treating men with low-volume, low-risk disease. In 13% to 38% of men, prostate cancer is essentially unifocal, and in men with multifocal disease, it is felt that the **dominant**

nodule is important and needs treatment, not the secondary foci. New techniques are being developed to better define the primary lesion, including systematic TRUS-mapping biopsy and MRI using enhanced tumor-defining techniques such as MR spectroscopy.[71]

Two new treatment strategies, watchful waiting and active surveillance, are evolving to delay invasive therapy and avoid side effects and possible overtreatment. These approaches are for men who may not tolerate treatment and for men with low volume, possibly clinically insignificant disease. "Clinically insignificant disease" has been defined by Epstein et al.[119] on needle biopsy to mean limited cancer (no core >50% involved, all cores less than Gleason 7, fewer than three positive cores) and PSA density less than 0.15.[119]

Watchful waiting is used in men who have asymptomatic cancer but are unlikely to benefit from therapy because of comorbid conditions. They are monitored until they become symptomatic and then receive palliative care, usually with hormones.[50]

Active surveillance (active monitoring with curative intent) is an increasingly popular "PSA era phenomenon" that is almost unique to prostate cancer. It recognizes that many men with low-risk cancer will never suffer from the cancer and will die from other causes. After initial diagnosis of low-risk disease, they are actively monitored with PSA, DRE, TRUS, and repeat biopsy to detect signs of progression before undergoing therapy. Strict criteria are used to define suitable low-risk patients (PSA <10 ng/mL, Gleason ≤6), stage T1c or T2a, <50% of length of any biopsy core, <3 biopsy cores). These men are regularly monitored with DRE, PSA, and repeat biopsies. **Significant progression** that requires treatment is defined by a rapid rise in PSA (doubling time <2 years) and increase in tumor grade. With this approach in one series after 7 years, 55% of men continued being monitored, 45% needed therapy, actuarial survival was 84%, and disease-specific survival was 99%.[50,120-122]

Role of Transrectal Ultrasound

Unlike originally thought, TRUS has not been pivotal in men suspected to have cancer (e.g., screening, detection, biopsy guidance, staging, therapy guidance, monitoring response to treatment). Experience has shown that all imaging modalities, including TRUS, CT, and MRI, have strengths and limitations in investigating patients.[1,123]

Currently, TRUS has three main roles with prostate cancer: (1) to guide biopsy, (2) to guide therapy, (3) to measure volume. Therapy guidance includes brachytherapy, insertion of fiducial (reference) markers to guide escalated-dose external beam radiotherapy, brachytherapy, cryotherapy, thermotherapy, radiofrequency ablation, and HIFU.[1] Accurate prostate volume measurements are important to determine suitability for brachytherapy and for calculating PSA density, used for staging, monitoring, and following patients under active surveillance.

ROLE OF PROSTATE-SPECIFIC ANTIGEN (PSA)

- Combination of digital rectal examination (DRE) and PSA level constitute the standard of care for identification of prostate cancer.
- PSA level is associated directly with the tumor burden of prostate cancer.
- Not all cancers produce PSA.
- From 20% to 40% of men with clinically significant cancer will have a normal PSA level.
- PSA may be elevated by nonmalignant conditions
- PSA variants are used to improve accuracy
  - PSA density
  - Age-specific PSA
  - Transition zone PSA density
  - PSA velocity
  - Free/total PSA ratio

TRANSRECTAL ULTRASOUND (TRUS) AND PROSTATE CANCER

- At present, TRUS has three main roles related to prostate cancer:
  Guide biopsy
  Guide therapy
  Measure volume
- TRUS is not the primary technique for identification of prostate cancer
- From 50% to 70% of prostate cancer is visible at TRUS
- The classic appearance is that of a hypoechoic nodule in the peripheral zone
- Only about 50% of peripheral zone hypoechoic areas are cancer

Screening is best done with DRE and PSA. Although TRUS is likely as sensitive as or even more sensitive than either DRE or PSA, it is too subjective, intrusive, and expensive to be used for screening. The added value of TRUS over PSA + DRE for cancer detection at screening is about 5%.[124] For cancer diagnosis, biopsy is needed, and this is best done with TRUS guidance. The number of laboratories using TRUS to calculate volume and PSA density to avoid biopsy has been decreasing, but PSAd is being revived to help with active surveillance decisions.

Transrectal ultrasound is not being generally used for staging to detect extracapsular disease. TRUS is moderately accurate for staging but generally is not as accurate as CT and MRI. All these techniques can image macroscopic extension and seminal vesicle involvement, but none can consistently detect microscopic extension and lymph node involvement. As a result, many physicians rely on their clinical acumen or use multifactorial staging nomograms (e.g., Kattan, Partin), which make use of DRE, PSA, Gleason score, and other variables.[110,112] However, some physicians have found meticulous TRUS more accurate than DRE and tables[125] (Fig. 10-12).

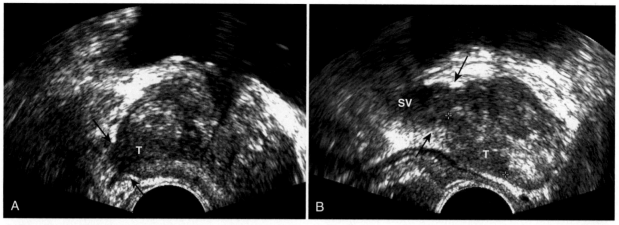

FIGURE 10-12. Staging of extensive prostate cancer. TRUS is about as accurate as CT and MRI for determining the presence of extracapsular extension. **A, Stage T3A cancer** *(T)* has extended outside the prostate at the neurovascular bundle *(arrows)*. Note how difficult it is to differentiate tumor extension from the normal irregularity caused by the neurovascular bundle. **B, Stage T3C** (para-sagittal view) **cancer** *(T)* extending *(arrows)* into the seminal vesicles *(SV)* above the prostate.

Currently, monitoring of therapy is better done with PSA, which is an easier and more objective indicator of total tumor burden and neoplastic activity than TRUS. However, TRUS is superb in guiding biopsy and helping to guide therapy, and these functions have become its main application in men with suspected prostate cancer.

Sonographic Appearance

Gray-Scale Ultrasound

Overall, 50% to 70% of prostate cancers are visible at TRUS. The classic appearance is that of a **hypoechoic nodule** in the **peripheral zone** that cannot be attributed to benign causes typically located in the peripheral zone and abutting the capsule[28,126-128] (Figs. 10-13, 10-14, and 10-15). The sensitivity of this finding is similar to cancer detection by DRE, PSA, and MRI. CT cannot detect cancer until there is gross glandular distortion by extensive tumor growth.

The corollary to this is that **30% to 50% of cancers are not visible at TRUS** (Figs. 10-14, *C,* and 10-15, *A* and *B*). Normal appearances at TRUS do not imply the absence of cancer and should not delay systematic biopsy if there is clinical suspicion of cancer. Patients clinically suspected to have prostate cancer should not be referred only for TRUS but rather for TRUS *and* biopsy.

The sonographic appearance of prostate cancer has been debated extensively. Early investigators incorrectly thought that most prostate cancers were hyperechoic. In 1985, Lee et al.[126] first convincingly demonstrated the **hypoechoic** appearance of cancer. Others subsequently confirmed that a significant portion of peripheral zone cancers are hypoechoic to some extent[28,123,127,129] (see Figs. 10-13 to 10-15). The pathologic basis of this is the replacement of normal loose glandular tissue by a packed mass of tumor cells with fewer reflecting interfaces and thus fewer echoes and hypoechoic appearance. Tumors that grow by infiltration or have a strongly glandular structure will preserve tissue interfaces and echogenicity and thus appear "isoechoic."[28]

When attempting to correlate the echogenicity of neoplasms with the amount of stromal fibrosis, it was found that hypoechoic lesions had less stromal fibrosis than did their more echogenic counterparts. Also, hypoechoic lesions tended to have more aggressive appearances than isoechoic lesions.[129] Further research suggests that echogenicity varies with the presence of tumor glands with enlarged lumina, as well as residual prostatic glands and stroma.[130]

Hyperechoic cancer has been described but occurs infrequently. With large cancers, the appearance may be caused by a desmoplastic response of the surrounding glandular tissue to the presence of the tumor or to infiltration of neoplasm into a BPH background with pre-existing degenerative calcifications.[131,132] Uncommon histologic types of cancer, including the cribriform pattern and comedonecrosis with focal calcifications, can be **echogenic.** The calcifications associated with comedonecrosis are tiny and act as crystals by being highly echogenic, more so than dystrophic calcifications. On scanning they are conspicuous and appear to twinkle, giving a "starry sky" appearance[133] (Fig. 10-15, *C*). A few extensive cancers have a hyperechoic appearance, probably as a result of the infiltration of the neoplasm into a background of BPH. Biopsy of hyperechoic lesions with sonographic guidance is the only way to prove that the lesion seen represents a neoplasm.

A significant number of prostate cancers, about 30%, are difficult or impossible to detect with TRUS because they are **isoechoic** and do not contrast with the surrounding prostate gland (Figs. 10-14, *C,* and 10-15, *A*). When present, an isoechoic tumor can be detected only if secondary signs are appreciated, including glandular asymmetry, capsular bulging, and areas of attenuation.[133] This is often true of transition zone cancer (Figs. 10-14, *E,* and 10-15, *D*).

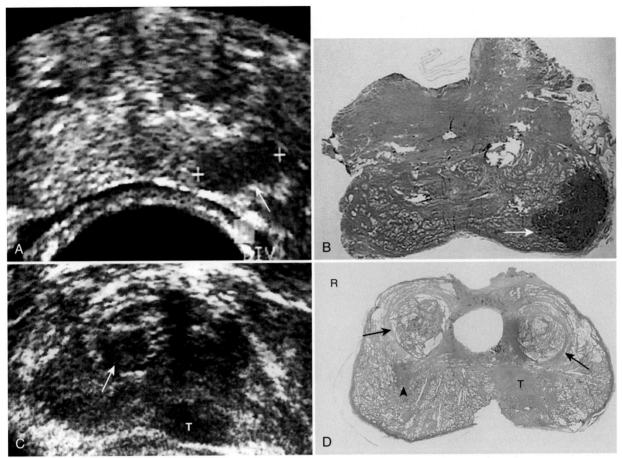

FIGURE 10-13. Prostate cancer: typical appearances. A, Hypoechoic nodule in peripheral zone along the capsule which cannot be attributed to benign causes *(arrow)*. **B,** Giant pathology section of **A** shows the homogeneous solid cellular mass of tumor tissue *(arrow)*, which reflects sound poorly compared with the adjacent prostate, which has the multiple glandular interfaces. **C, Typical hypoechoic peripheral zone cancer nodule** *(T)*. Note also the well-circumscribed hypoechoic BPH nodule in the right transition zone *(arrow)*. **D,** Giant section of **C** for correlation shows the homogeneous tumor mass *(T)*. There is a second small lesion on the right side *(thick arrow)*. Also note the right and left BPH nodules correlating with the TRUS image *(arrows)*.

When the tumor replaces the entire peripheral zone, it often is **less echogenic** than the inner gland, which is a reversal of the normal sonographic relation. When the entire gland is replaced with tumor, on a BPH background, the gland may be diffusely inhomogeneous (Fig. 10-15, *B*).

Only about 50% of **hypoechoic** areas are cancer.[135] Other benign causes of hypoechoic areas seen in the prostate include normal internal sphincter muscle, hyperplasia, prostatitis, cysts, hematoma, vessels, benign glandular ectasia, and cysts.[28]

Fortunately, 70% of prostate cancers arise in the homogeneous **peripheral zone,** which also has a fairly homogeneous ultrasound texture against which cancer is easier to detect. About 20% are in the **transition zone,**[14,136] where prostate cancers are very difficult to find against the heterogeneous and variably vascular background of hyperplasia.[27] Clues to transition zone cancer are the identification of a poorly marginated hypoechoic area that appears different from other BPH nodules and the focal loss of surgical capsule. On occasion, tumors asymmetrically bulge the capsule.[108]

An especially difficult cancer to detect is the **anterior midline** tumor that lies in the fibromuscular area anterior to the urethra, because it is far from the probe and obstructed by the urethra. Anterior midline tumors are also difficult to biopsy. Typically, systematic transition zone biopsy will miss them because of their far anterior location and the deliberate avoidance of the urethra during biopsy. Anterior midline cancers can become very large before being detected. Just remembering to look in this area at TRUS examination and using MRI are helpful in detection of these anterior tumors.[137]

Color and Power Doppler Imaging

Doppler imaging has been evaluated for detection of neovascularity associated with cancer. This approach is especially attractive in the attempt to find isoechoic cancer because pathologic examinations show cancers to have increased microvessel density[136,138] (Fig. 10-14, *B* and *D*). Both color Doppler flow imaging and the three to five times more sensitive power Doppler have been used, but these appear to have similar sensitivity.[137] The

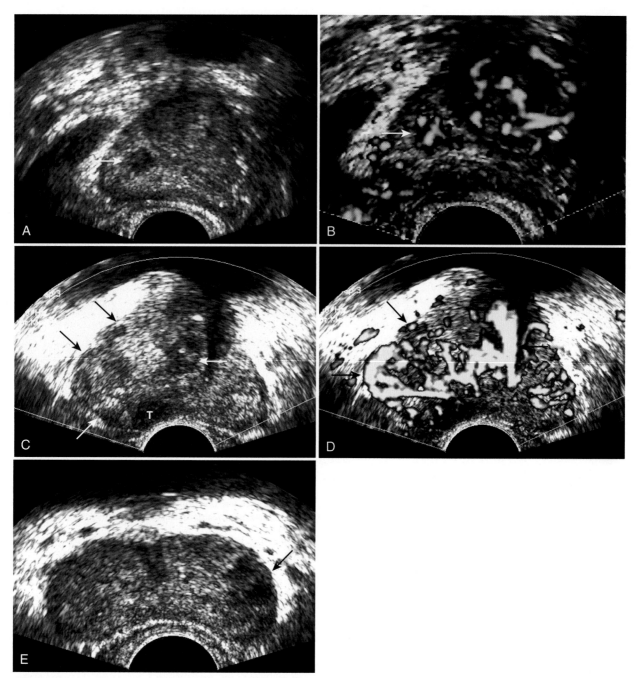

FIGURE 10-14. Prostate cancer: less common appearances. A, Small hypoechoic lesion entirely inside the peripheral zone *(arrow)* proved to be cancer. Digital rectal examination (DRE) was negative but PSA slightly elevated. **B,** Power Doppler scan of **A** shows increased vascularity *(arrow)* in region of the nodule. **C,** Small "tip of the iceberg" lesion visible posteriorly in the right lobe *(T)*. Cancer is filling virtually the entire right lobe *(white and black arrows)*. Most of this tumor is isoechoic and thus not visible on gray-scale imaging. Remember that prostate cancer is typically multifocal and larger than the lesion seen at TRUS. **D,** Power Doppler scan shows large abnormal area of hypervascularity involving not only the small peripheral hypoechoic lesion, but also most of the transition zone *(arrows);* PSA, 265 ng/mL; Gleason score, 7/10. **E,** Multifocal cancer involving both right and left lobes: one hypoechoic, the other isoechoic. DRE was negative; PSA, 4.5 ng/mL with a 14% free/total ratio. In the left lobe there is a suspicious area anteriorly *(arrow)*. The right lobe appears very normal and free of lesions. At biopsy, both lobes had Gleason 6/10 cancer.

results have shown only a 5% to 17% increase in cancer detection over gray-scale imaging.[9,136,138] Suspicious hypoechoic nodules that are also vascular tend to have larger tumor volume and higher Gleason score at biopsy.[136,139] Vascularity may be increased with nonmalignant conditions such as inflammation (Fig. 10-9, *B*).

There is no increased benefit for color flow Doppler in the transition zone because BPH nodules can range from hypovascular to hypervascular.

Doppler appears to be sensitive to patient position. One group has shown that the dependent side of the prostate appears more vascular than the upper side

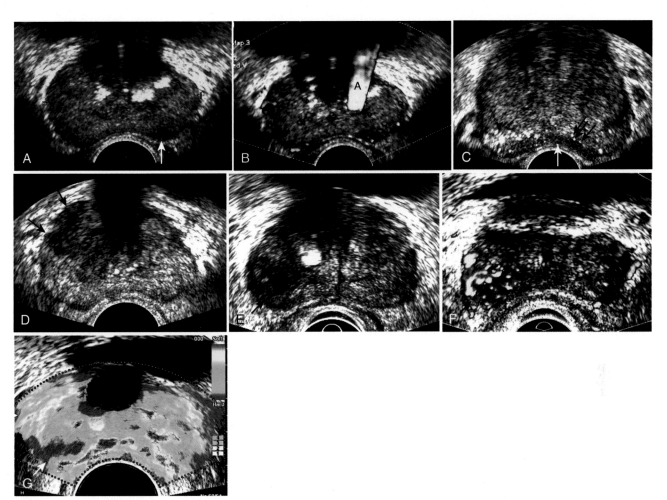

FIGURE 10-15. Prostate cancer: other appearances. A, Almost isoechoic, impalpable **nonvascular cancer.** DRE was normal; PSA, 6.08 ng/mL with 12% free/total ratio. TRUS is only mildly suspicious for cancer at left *(arrow)*. Biopsy showed isoechoic ultrasonically undetectable, Gleason 7/10 cancer in the right side involving 25% of the tissue. On the left, where there is a visible lesion *(arrow)*, the biopsy was only 15% cancer. This highlights the need to do both systematic and targeted biopsy. **B,** Power Doppler shows almost no detectable signal despite **extensive bilateral cancer.** Only about 80% of cancers demonstrate increased vascularity. The strong Doppler color signal anteriorly is all artifactual *(A)*, from calcification. **C, Extensive cancer** with "starry sky" appearance caused by comedonecrosis in the tumor. The malignant nodule extends across the peripheral zone from right to left *(between cursors)*. On the right, the calcified clumps are normal corpora amylacea *(arrowhead)*. On the left, the densities have a different character: small, more scattered, round, and very echogenic, and will "twinkle" on probe movement *(arrows)*. These are highly suggestive of comedonecrosis in tumor. **D,** Isolated **transition zone cancer** visible as an amorphous hypoechoic bulge of the right anterior transition zone *(arrows)*. DRE was negative. Biopsy to investigate PSA of 12.0 ng/mL showed Gleason 6/10 cancer. **E,** Typical hypoechoic **peripheral zone lesion.** Biopsy showed Gleason 8/10 cancer *(arrow)*. **F, Power Doppler** scan shows enhanced vascularity in lesion *(arrow)*. **G, Elastography** of same lesion *(arrow)* in **F** shows blue color in lesion, implying stiff tissue.

and has recommended that the examination be performed in the supine position.[25] Our experience is the opposite, with the upper side generally appearing more vascular. Also, we prefer to use the power Doppler mode, which is more sensitive to flow detection, gives a more uniform display of vascular density, and produces images that are more stable with different equipment settings (see Fig. 10-5).

There are pitfalls with Doppler imaging. Not all cancers are vascular. The absence of vascularity should not prevent biopsy of an otherwise suspicious nodule[139] (Fig. 10-15, *B*). The capsule of the prostate is very vascular, especially at the base and apex, and can mimic

neovascularity to the uninitiated operator. Prostate calcifications and corpora amylacea cause considerable Doppler artifact and may prevent diagnostic studies (see Fig. 10-6, *D*).

Contrast-Enhanced Ultrasound

Investigations are underway using microbubble contrast-enhanced ultrasound. Unlike conventional Doppler imaging, vascular contrast enhancement with microbubbles allows detection of microvessels.[135] Both **vascular density** and **time to peak enhancement** have been used. There are increases in tumor detection and possibly detection of tumors with a higher Gleason score, but false-positive results are also seen, especially with prostatitis. Premedication with dutasteride (Avodart), which decreases prostate size and suppresses normal vascularity, has been used with some success to increase the conspicuity of nonresponsive neovascularity. More work is being done with contrast enhancement and "targeted" bubbles that bind to specific tissues. At present, contrast enhancement remains investigational.[136,138-140,142]

When evaluating new approaches, the reader should remember to determine the *added value* of the new approaches compared with gray-scale TRUS and targeted biopsy, not only the isolated results of the new approaches.

Three-Dimensional Ultrasound Scans

Three-dimensional (3-D) scanning has been evaluated. Since 3-D depends on two-dimensional (2-D) scanning, generally there is no improvement in cancer detection, but there may be slight improvement in cancer staging.[138] There may be a role for 3-D imaging in accurate volume determinations when precise volumes are needed to monitor changes in gland size. Marketed 3-D approaches to biopsy include TargetScan and PercuNav. The **TargetScan** device is a dedicated ultrasound unit incorporating a biopsy channel on the probe and uses a unique flexible needle. It allows volumetric segmentation and computes biopsy sites to allow a more repeatable and uniform biopsy sampling pattern.[143] It may prove helpful in patients needing precise tumor mapping before focal therapy. The **PercuNav** device is used freehand, and probe motion is followed using electromagnetic methods. Such devices may facilitate accurate TRUS/MRI co-registration/fusion and help with biopsy guidance in men who have negative TRUS scan but an MRI detects a lesion needing biopsy or intervention. PercuNav can be used for any organ.

Elastography

Elastography is being evaluated. Elastography creates a color-coded map of tissue "stiffness" (elastic modulus). Some prostate tumors have increased cell density, leading to change of tissue elasticity and stiffness, which may be amenable to detection by "strain imaging." When the prostate is gently deformed by hand-controlled probe pressure, areas of different density/stiffness in the prostate are portrayed by different colors. Tumors tend to be stiffer than benign tissue. Areas containing cancer can be found, but currently the overall detection is similar or slightly better than systematic biopsy, and this technique cannot be used to avoid biopsy. False-positive results are seen with chronic inflammation and atrophy. Personal experience has shown that currently, elastography is subjective and has a long learning curve and that images are difficult to reproduce[10,136,144] (Fig. 10-15, *E-G*). New techniques that use sound waves to create tissue strain

are being developed to avoid variations seen with manual compression.

Summary

Careful TRUS to detect hypoechoic nodules and guidance of biopsy remains the cornerstone of cancer diagnosis with ultrasound.[1,84,145] Additional enhancements are being researched and show promise, but to date they significantly increase complexity and scan time and have provided only limited improvements in cancer detection over careful gray-scale examination.[84,145] At present in complex cases, such as those with multiple negative extensive biopsies but rising PSA, additional information may be more readily obtained using endorectal coil MRI and processing enhancements.[1] The only issue that generally remains is the use of TRUS to biopsy lesions found by MRI alone. These issues are being resolved by TRUS/MRI co-registration/fusion techniques and MRI-guided biopsy.

Staging to determine local extracapsular extension into periprostatic tissues or seminal vesicles remains imperfect with all modalities, including DRE, TRUS, CT, and MRI. Findings on TRUS that are suspicious for extracapsular extension include capsular bulging, distortion, angulated appearance of the lateral margin,[108,147] and also a hypoechoic nodule with length greater than 23 mm and base on the capsule[148] (see Figs. 10-7, *A,* and 10-12, *B*). Signs of seminal vesicle invasion are a posterior bulge at the base of the vesicle or asymmetry in seminal vesicle echogenicity, especially when associated with hypoechoic areas at the base. These findings are very subjective, and the positive predictive value is about 50% to 63%. In general, although extension can be suspected in some cases, the findings are not sufficiently reliable to consistently guide patient management. An advantage of TRUS is that staging biopsy can be performed to confirm extracapsular extension or seminal vesicle invasion. MRI also has variable accuracy, 54% to 93%. MRI seems to be most effective at excluding seminal vesicle invasion, with sensitivity of 23% to 80% but high specificity of 81% to 99%.[1] Again, because of wide variations in reported results, many clinicians, when staging prostate cancer, continue to rely on their clinical acumen or refer to nomograms (e.g., Partin, Kattan).[110,112]

ULTRASOUND-GUIDED BIOPSY

Prostate biopsy and cancer diagnosis has been revolutionized by TRUS guidance and the biopsy gun. This pairing allows effective, safe biopsy and likely is responsible for the increased interest in prostate cancer. The TRUS-guided approach has replaced the "blind" finger-guided transrectal, and earlier transperineal, approaches. Virtually all TRUS-guided biopsies are now done transrectally (Fig. 10-16, *A*). Many investigators have described their experiences.[1,21]

Preparation

Prostate biopsy is usually performed in an ambulatory setting and requires minimal patient preparation.[20,147] Experience has shown that it is best to schedule and prepare men for TRUS and biopsy at the same visit (vs. two visits). If TRUS shows a benign cause for the clinical findings, the biopsy can be deferred.

Informed consent is obtained. Some advocate the use of cleansing enemas before performing the biopsy. A rapidly absorbed, broad-spectrum antibiotic is administered, typically a quinolone such as ciprofloxacin, one dose an hour before and for several days after the biopsy.[21,150] However, antibiotic resistance is increasing, and about half the infectious complications are caused by *E. coli*, which have become ciprofloxacin resistant.[151]

Patients taking **anticoagulating agents** (e.g., aspirin, NSAIDs, clopidogrel [Plavix], warfarin)[149] should not undergo biopsy until these drugs have been discontinued for several days, depending on the agent. Aspirin is often taken by men in the prostate cancer age group. Even the 81-mg dose irreversibly blocks platelet function for 7 to 10 days. This area is controversial, and some suggest that aspirin-induced coagulation disturbance is not severe enough to prevent safe biopsy.[152-155] Because bleeding complications can occur after prostate biopsy, medical-legal defense may be difficult if an elective procedure was performed with the knowledge of anticoagulant ingestion. Acetaminophen (Tylenol) can be recommended to men who need analgesia for conditions such as arthritis because it is not an anticoagulant. Warfarin (Coumadin) needs to be discontinued. This is best arranged by the referring physician. Normal coagulation is confirmed with an international normalized ratio (INR) of less than 1.5 before biopsy. Patients with other coagulopathies should be seen by coagulation specialists.

Biopsy is avoided during urinary infections. The clinician should wait 4 to 6 weeks after symptoms have subsided and confirm antibiotic sensitivities to determine appropriate prophylaxis for biopsy. Endocarditis prophylaxis for genitourinary procedures such as prostate biopsy is no longer recommended in patients with valvular heart disease, although it is still recommended for dental procedures.[156]

Technique

The patient lies in the decubitus position. A DRE is performed before probe insertion to palpate the prostate and to confirm that probe insertion is safe. We insert the probe with needle guide attached at the outset to save time and examine the prostate. The decision to biopsy has already been made, so only target details need to be clarified.[3,21] A variety of probes and guides are available (Fig. 10-16; see also Fig. 10-7). Ching et al.[22] recently suggested that end-fire probes/guides provide better sampling than side-fire devices. Electronic guidelines direct the needle path (Fig. 10-16, D).

Local anesthesia lessens the discomfort of the biopsy. Typically, 5 to 10 mL of 1% lidocaine (Xylocaine) without epinephrine is injected either into the neurovascular bundles at the base of the prostate or, more easily, into the gland itself at the biopsy sites.[3,21] With direct injections into the gland, anesthesia is virtually instantaneous in most patients. Anesthetic gel has also been suggested. Some patients have some pain despite local anesthesia; acetaminophen should be available for their use after the biopsy.

The **automatic biopsy gun** with 18-gauge needles has remarkable patient acceptance and safety.[153] Biopsy is best done by a single operator who controls both the probe and the gun. With the gun cocked, the needle is "parked" in the guide, ensuring that the tip is safely inside the guide. The probe and contained needle are moved to the target using the targeting line (Fig. 10-16, D). A simple, swift motion advances the gun and needle tip to the surface of the lesion. Once in position, the device is triggered and the needle advances approximately 2 to 3 cm. Initially the inner stylet advances, and then the outer sheath advances to cut the tissue core and trap it in the beveled chamber of the inner needle (Fig. 10-16, C and D). We sample suspicious areas first, in case the patient cannot tolerate the entire procedure, and finish with systematic sampling. Biopsy through the urethra, internal urethral sphincter, and ejaculatory ducts is avoided because it can result in considerable urethral bleeding and potential injury to these structures. When the biopsy is finished and probe removed, the site is palpated for hematomas, and if present, finger pressure is applied for about a minute to help stop bleeding. After the biopsy, we keep the patient for an hour, the first 20 minutes lying down and the remainder seated. This helps prevent problems caused by late onset of vasovagal complications.

Cytology with and without TRUS guidance has been done in the past, but both false-positive and false-negative results can occur, and Gleason scoring is not possible.[65]

Side Effects and Complications

Minor side effects, including bleeding in the urine, stool, and sperm, are common and will be seen in most patients undergoing transrectal biopsy. This minor bleeding generally lasts only a few days but can continue for many weeks. The ejaculate may remain discolored for many months. Significant complications from prostate biopsy that require physician intervention have been relatively low, less than 1% to 2%, regardless of the mode of guidance, needle size, or approach.[21,153,155] These include sepsis, large hematoma, urinary retention, and significant rectal bleeding. With the use of prophylactic antibiotics, the incidence of septic complications requiring therapy is about 1%. Sepsis can rapidly increase in severity to septic shock. Patients should be advised to seek help promptly if they start feeling feverish or unwell.

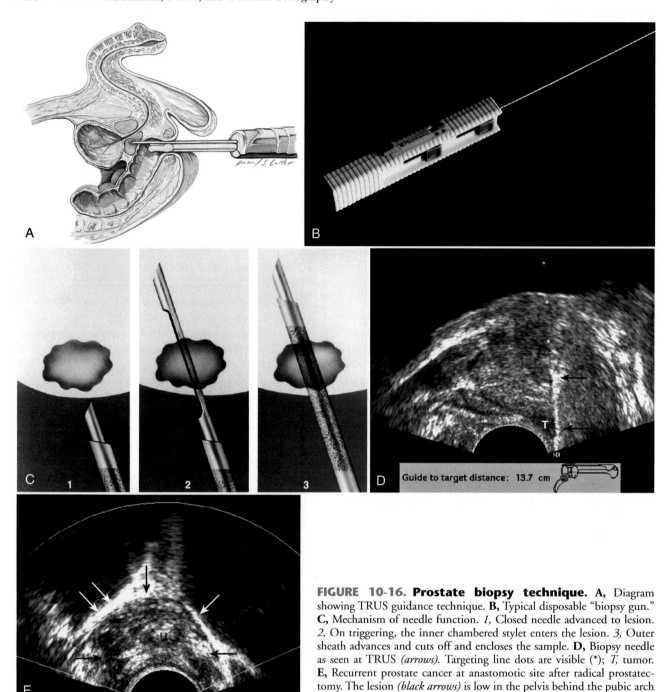

FIGURE 10-16. Prostate biopsy technique. A, Diagram showing TRUS guidance technique. **B,** Typical disposable "biopsy gun." **C,** Mechanism of needle function. *1,* Closed needle advanced to lesion. *2,* On triggering, the inner chambered stylet enters the lesion. *3,* Outer sheath advances and cuts off and encloses the sample. **D,** Biopsy needle as seen at TRUS *(arrows).* Targeting line dots are visible (*); *T,* tumor. **E,** Recurrent prostate cancer at anastomotic site after radical prostatectomy. The lesion *(black arrows)* is low in the pelvis behind the pubic arch bones *(white arrows)* and surrounds the urethra *(U).*

Infectious disease specialists can be consulted to help with antibiotic selection in men who need repeat biopsy but have had infections after prior biopsy. Tumor seeding is virtually unknown.

About 1% to 6% of patients have a hypotensive vasovagal-like reaction after the biopsy. This can occur even 30 to 60 minutes after the procedure.[153] It is characterized by pallor, sweating, nausea, and vomiting, often with bradycardia of 50 to 60 beats/min associated with significant hypotension. This usually occurs within 30 to 60 minutes after biopsy. Most men recover spontaneously and rapidly with rest, but rarely the patient may need intravenous atropine. We keep patients in the clinic for an hour after the biopsy to avoid problems with these delayed vasovagal hypotensive reactions.

Biopsy should never be taken lightly. Some patients have required prolonged hospitalization, and there are rare reports of patients dying from biopsy-related complications.[21]

Indications

Indications exist for both initial and repeat prostate biopsies to investigate cancer.

Initial Biopsy

Biopsy is performed in patients with a clinical suspicion of cancer in whom the results would alter clinical management. The **indications** include the following:

1. Abnormal DRE.
2. PSA of 10 ng/mL or greater. (Some advocate reducing the PSA criterion to 4 or even 2.5 ng/mL.)
3. Nodule visible at TRUS.
4. Excessive PSA velocity.
5. Positive chips at TURP.
6. Men with metastatic adenocarcinoma with undetermined primary.

The **number of samples and locations** used in prostate biopsy has been controversial. Initially it was thought that only suspicious areas should be sampled. It was quickly discovered, however, that only about 50% of hypoechoic areas contained cancer, and that cancer was present in normal-appearing areas of the prostate. This led to "targeted plus systematic" sextant (six-core) biopsy.[135,157] Subsequently, increased numbers of cores have been suggested because about 30% of cancers were being missed by the sextant biopsy. Ten to 12 cores is held to be appropriate on the initial visit.[3,21,158]

At the **first biopsy session,** suspicious hypoechoic or vascular areas are sampled first, followed by a systematic 10 to 12–core pattern. There is subtle variation between different operators[3,21] (Fig. 10-17). Typically, samples are obtained from the peripheral zone at the base, middle, and apex of the gland both medially and laterally from each lobe. Many emphasize obtaining lateral samples,

especially the "anterior horns" (part of peripheral zone that curves anteriorly around transition zone).[158,159] Others have found that both medial and lateral samples are equally important, and that it is important to search for hypoechoic nodules.[160] This approach should

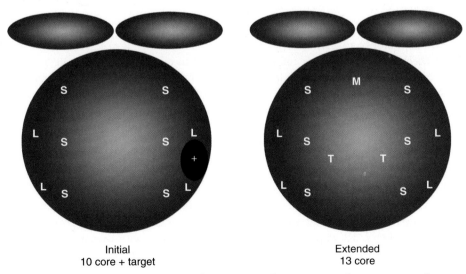

Initial
10 core + target

Extended
13 core

FIGURE 10-17. Biopsy sites as viewed en face from posterior aspect of prostate. Left image shows the standard 10 prostate biopsy sites; *S,* sextant; *L,* lateral or "anterior horn." Additional samples are taken of any lesion that is evident outside the systematic pattern (+). Right image shows a typical extended pattern of biopsies, in this case a 13-core pattern. In addition to the sextant sites *(S),* samples are taken from the lateral peripheral zones *(L),* deep in the anterior transition zone *(T),* and from the peripheral zone in the midline *(M)* at the base, cephalad to the verumontanum.

result in an overall 30% to 60% positive biopsy rate and about 60+% yield for lesions that are suspicious at ultrasound.[84]

Repeat Biopsy

Biopsy is repeated when needed, generally using a **more extensive sampling pattern,** in the following situations:
1. Initial biopsy is negative, but there is continued strong clinical suspicion of cancer (palpable nodule, PSA >10 or continuing to rise).
2. Initial biopsy shows suspicious histology that would not qualify for radical therapy (high-grade PIN, atypical cells, microscopic cancer).
3. Follow-up of men on active surveillance.

Because about 30% to 40% of cancers are not visible at TRUS, there is a chance that the initial samples missed the cancer and it is reasonable to repeat the biopsy. If the initial results are negative but PSA continues to rise, we generally repeat at about 1 year. If the initial histology is prostate intraepithelial neoplasia (PIN), atypical cells (atypical small acinar proliferation [ASAP]), or microscopic cancer, we generally repeat within 3 months because these lesions have a greater than 30% association with significant cancer.[21,158,161,162] In our hands in 2008, among 968 men undergoing their first biopsy we found cancer in 50%, microscopic cancer in 2%, PIN in 10%, and ASAP in 4%. Thus, about 16% of men would be asked to return promptly for follow-up biopsy (unpublished data).

Beyond three biopsy sessions, the yield becomes small, and most laboratories will revert to about 1 to 2–year follow-up. Cancer detection rates on repeat biopsies 1, 2, 3, and 4 are reported as 22% to 38%, 10%, 5%, and 4%.[21,163]

Repeat biopsies use a more extensive pattern of sampling[162,164] (Fig. 10-17). The sites of cancer missed by the initial sextant pattern have been evaluated[165] and several patterns for extended biopsy suggested.[3,21,158] We have found that a 13-core to 15-core pattern modeled after Babaian et al.[162] has been very effective. Samples are obtained for each lobe: lateral peripheral zone (2 cores), medial peripheral zone (3 cores = sextant sites), and transition zone (1 core), as well as one core from the midline at the base. Overall, 13 cores are obtained, and cancer yield at repeat biopsy can be as high as 40% in at-risk men. Most of the cancers will be found in the original systematic sites, with only a small contribution from the added transition zone and midline.[162] If repeated extensive biopsies are negative but indications keep increasing (rising PSA), we use MRI to help localize suspicious areas. At repeat biopsy, it is important to scrutinize the most anterior part of the gland in front of the internal urethral sphincter in the supposedly tumor-resistant anterior fibromuscular area. Often, large tumors "hide" there and are difficult to see, and this region is not well sampled at systematic biopsy.[137]

"Saturation" biopsy has been suggested using the transperineal approach and brachytherapy template to help systematically cover the entire prostate. Such biopsies are usually done under general anesthesia, and their added value beyond simple extensive 15-core biopsy is uncertain.[158,159] Color Doppler has slightly increased the sensitivity and specificity regardless of whether a gray-scale lesion is detected[139] (Fig. 10-14, C and D).

Biopsy after Radical Prostatectomy

Radical prostatectomy should reduce PSA to virtually undetectable levels. Recurrent disease is suspected if the PSA starts rising. In this situation, many urologists now just arrange for radiotherapy of the prostate bed and pelvis and do not rely on biopsy. If histologic proof is needed before therapy, TRUS with biopsy can be used to evaluate the anastomotic site to look for local lymphadenopathy and pelvic masses (Fig. 10-16, E). If requested, in such cases we obtain two samples from either side of the anastomosis and biopsy any other abnormal masses. Care must be taken not to mistake large pelvic vessels for masses; this can be avoided by using Doppler before biopsy.

Biopsy in Men with Absent Anus

Men who have had their anus closed by abdominoperineal resection present a difficult group to manage when their PSA becomes elevated. Prostate visibility is restricted through both the transabdominal and the transperineal approach. Transperineal ultrasound–guided biopsy with local anesthesia is moderately successful in obtaining prostate tissue. It is helpful to precede the biopsy with MRI, which may show suspicious areas that cannot be seen with ultrasound. We scan the patient in a lithotomy position and use the same transrectal probe because of its small size and just abut it firmly against the perineum and proceed as with a transrectal biopsy. About 20 mL of 1% lidocaine is needed for perineal anesthesia. Cancer yield in our hands is about 30%; others report it as high as 40% to 82%.[166,167] An alternative approach using MRI for initial lesion detection, followed by CT transsciatic biopsy, could be considered.

ULTRASOUND-GUIDED THERAPY

Transrectal ultrasound can be used to guide instrumentation into the prostate for therapy both transrectally and transperineally. This has become an increasingly important function with the advent of focal therapy. Need for guidance is seen with techniques such as radiotherapy (escalated-dose conformal radiotherapy; Fig. 10-18), brachytherapy (Fig. 10-19), and cryotherapy, as well as more contemporary treatments such as radiofrequency ablation therapy, HIFU, gene therapy with viral injection, and photodynamic therapy.[50,168] Many of these

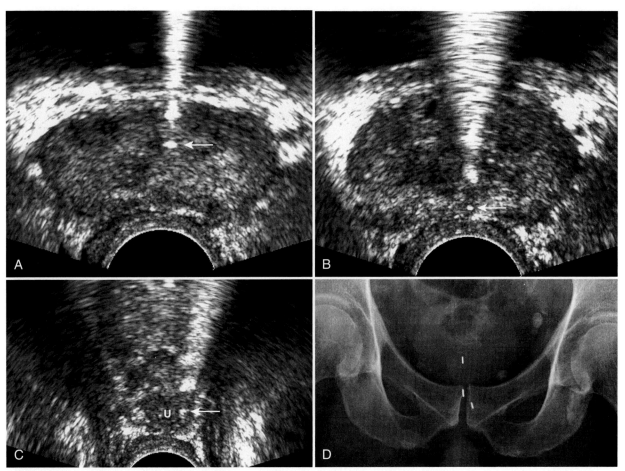

FIGURE 10-18. Ultrasound-guided radiotherapy. Fiducial marker seeds inserted with TRUS guidance and used to guide escalated-dose external beam radiotherapy. **A,** Transverse image shows basal seed *(arrow)* with characteristic comet-tail reverberation artifact. **B,** Rectal surface seed (arrow). **C,** Apical seed *(arrow)* just beside the urethra *(U).* **D,** Pelvic x-ray film shows the three marker seeds in place.

therapies can alter the texture of the prostate, making it impossible to detect recurrent cancer with TRUS. After such treatments we perform systematic 10-core biopsies of these patients when tissue is needed for patient management and often find solid, hard, almost woodlike tissues.

OTHER IMAGING TECHNIQUES

Magnetic resonance imaging is an increasingly useful technique to evaluate the prostate to detect and stage cancer. Its accuracy in tumor detection, sizing, and staging are improving with use of endorectal and pelvic coils, contrast agents, and specialized sequences. The main pitfalls to use of MRI are availability, cost, time, and intolerance of the endorectal coil. Biopsy equipment has been adapted for use with MRI.[1]

Computed tomography scan plays no role in primary tumor detection or local staging, but it helps with detection of lymphadenopathy and distant metastases. CT is of great value in radiotherapy planning and confirming seed placement with brachytherapy.[1]

Radionuclide bone scans play no role in primary tumor detection or local staging but they are the mainstay for detecting bone metastases in men with skeletal symptoms or PSA greater than 10 ng/mL.[1]

OTHER APPLICATIONS OF TRUS IN MEN AND WOMEN

In both men and women, the transrectal route is useful to evaluate and sample any pelvic mass that is within range of the probe and needle. TRUS also provides high-resolution pelvic access in girls and women when transvaginal ultrasound is not possible (Fig. 10-20).

A few caveats exist. Because of the large vessels in the pelvis, it is important to use Doppler ultrasound to interrogate any area where biopsy is contemplated. Remember that pelvic kidneys may mimic pathologic masses. Also, anterior meningoceles may mimic masses behind the rectum and should not be aspirated because of the risk of infection.

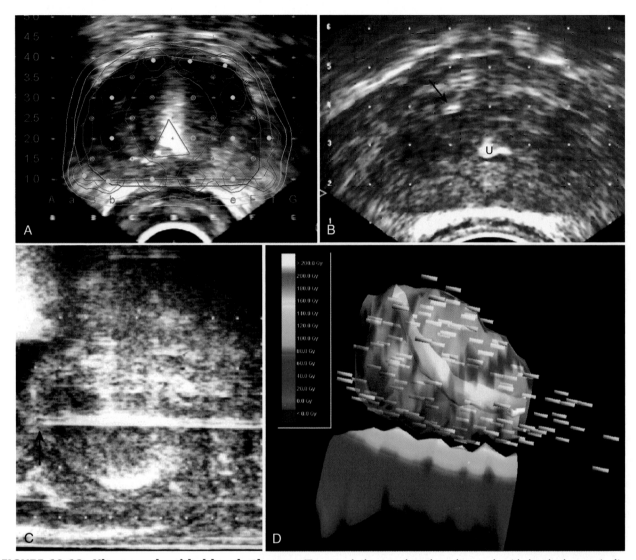

FIGURE 10-19. Ultrasound-guided brachytherapy. Transrectal ultrasound used to plane and guide brachytherapy (radioactive seed implantation) using a special stepping device and perineal needle template. **A,** One of multiple transverse prostate images used to plan seed sites *(dots)* and determine radiation isodose dose curves *(colored lines)*. Urethral dose is avoided *(white central area inside the green triangle)*. Note the grid markers at the bottom *(A, a, b . . . G)* and left side *(1.0, 1.5, 2.0 . . . 4.5)* and the grid dots superimposed on the field. **B,** TRUS-guided seed placement in the operating room; *U,* urethra. Transverse image shows the guiding grid dots and the tip of one inserting needle as a "hamburger-like" echo *(arrow)*. **C,** Sagittal images shows brachytherapy needle inserted to base of prostate *(arrow)* to insert a row of seeds. **D,** Postprocedural CT reconstruction shows the position of the seeds *(green)* and that the entire prostate is receiving a high *(white)* radiation dose. *(Images courtesy Dr. Juanita Crook, Radiation Oncology, Princess Margaret Hospital, Toronto.)*

FIGURE 10-20. Other TRUS application: pelvic mass. Woman with abnormal pelvic mass illustrates nonprostate uses of TRUS guidance and biopsy in men and women. This is a recurrent pelvic mass *(M)* following hysterectomy for uterine cancer. TRUS examination and biopsy provided the histologic proof needed before further therapy. The transrectal technique is useful to biopsy any pelvic mass that can be reached by the probe.

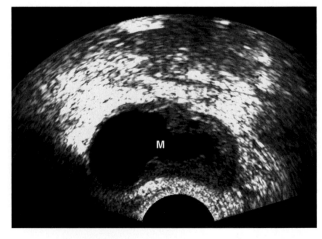

Nevertheless, we have performed abscess drainage and biopsies of numerous masses, including ovarian masses, recurrent masses after diverse primary tumor surgery, periureteric masses, bladder masses, and pericolonic masses in both men and women. All these procedures have the same preparation and protocol as the basic prostate biopsy.[169]

The distal ureters and ureterovesical junctions are readily accessible to evaluation for distal ureteric obstructing lesions, including calculi.

References

Background

1. Hricak H, Choyke PL, Eberhardt SC, et al. Imaging prostate cancer: a multidisciplinary perspective. Radiology 2007;243:28-53.
2. Fütterer JJ, Heijmink SW, Spermon JR. Imaging the male reproductive tract: current trends and future directions. Radiol Clin North Am 2008;46:133-147, vii.
3. Scherr DS, Eastham J, Ohori M, Scardino PT. Prostate biopsy techniques and indications: when, where, and how? Semin Urol Oncol 2002;20:18-31.
4. Meyer F, Fradet Y. Prostate cancer: 4. Screening. CMAJ 1998; 159:968-972.
5. Smith RA, Cokkinides V, Brawley OW. Cancer screening in the United States, 2009: a review of current American Cancer Society guidelines and issues in cancer screening. CA Cancer J Clin 2009; 59:27-41.
6. Watanabe H, Igari D, Tanahasi Y, et al. Development and application of new equipment for transrectal ultrasonography. J Clin Ultrasound 1974;2:91-98.
7. Watanabe H. History and applications of transrectal sonography of the prostate. Urol Clin North Am 1989;16:617-622.
8. Littrup PJ, Bailey SE. Prostate cancer: the role of transrectal ultrasound and its impact on cancer detection and management. Radiol Clin North Am 2000;38:87-113.
9. Mitterberger M, Pinggera GM, Pallwein L, et al. The value of three-dimensional transrectal ultrasonography in staging prostate cancer. BJU Int 2007;100:47-50.
10. Pallwein L, Mitterberger M, Pelzer A, et al. Ultrasound of prostate cancer: recent advances. Eur Radiol 2008;18:707-715.

Anatomy

11. Lee F, Torp-Pedersen ST, Siders DB, et al. Transrectal ultrasound in the diagnosis and staging of prostatic carcinoma. Radiology 1989;170:609-615.
12. Kutikov A, Guzzo TJ, Malkowicz SB. Clinical approach to the prostate: an update. Radiol Clin North Am 2006;44:649-663, vii.
13. McNeal JE. The zonal anatomy of the prostate. Prostate 1981; 2:35-49.
14. McNeal JE, Redwine EA, Freiha FS, Stamey TA. Zonal distribution of prostatic adenocarcinoma: correlation with histologic pattern and direction of spread. Am J Surg Pathol 1988;12:897-906.
15. Leventis AK, Shariat SF, Utsunomiya T, Slawin KM. Characteristics of normal prostate vascular anatomy as displayed by power Doppler. Prostate 2001;46:281-288.
16. Costello AJ, Brooks M, Cole OJ. Anatomical studies of the neurovascular bundle and cavernosal nerves. BJU Int 2004;94:1071-1076.
17. Lawrentschuk N, Lindner U, Fleshner N. Current textbooks and anatomy of the prostate: a case for an update. BJU Int 2009.
18. Walsh PC. The discovery of the cavernous nerves and development of nerve sparing radical retropubic prostatectomy. J Urol 2007; 177:1632-1635.

Sonographic Appearance

19. Ayala AG, Ro JY, Babaian R, et al. The prostatic capsule: does it exist? Its importance in the staging and treatment of prostatic carcinoma. Am J Surg Pathol 1989;13:21-27.

Equipment and Technique

20. Goldstein A. Pertinent physics of an optimal examination. Prog Clin Biol Res 1987;237:31-48.
21. Matlaga BR, Eskew LA, McCullough DL. Prostate biopsy: indications and technique. J Urol 2003;169:12-19.
22. Ching CB, Moussa AS, Li J, et al. Does transrectal ultrasound probe configuration really matter? End fire versus side fire probe prostate cancer detection rates. J Urol 2009;181:709.
23. Loeb S, Han M, Roehl KA, et al. Accuracy of prostate weight estimation by digital rectal examination versus transrectal ultrasonography. J Urol 2005;173:63-65.
24. Terris MK, Stamey TA. Determination of prostate volume by transrectal ultrasound. J Urol 1991;145:984-987.
25. Halpern EJ, Frauscher F, Forsberg F, et al. High-frequency Doppler ultrasound of the prostate: effect of patient position. Radiology 2002;222:634-639.

Benign Conditions

26. Barry MJ, Fowler Jr FJ, O'Leary MP, et al. The American Urological Association symptom index for benign prostatic hyperplasia. J Urol 1992;148:1549-1557; discussion 1564.
27. Lee F, Torp-Pedersen S, Littrup PJ, et al. Hypoechoic lesions of the prostate: clinical relevance of tumor size, digital rectal examination, and prostate-specific antigen. Radiology 1989;170:29-32.
28. Shinohara K, Scardino PT, Carter SS, Wheeler TM. Pathologic basis of the sonographic appearance of the normal and malignant prostate. Urol Clin North Am 1989;16:675-691.
29. Burks DD, Drolshagen LF, Fleischer AC, et al. Transrectal sonography of benign and malignant prostatic lesions. AJR Am J Roentgenol 1986;146:1187-1191.
30. Oyen RH, Van de Voorde WM, Van Poppel HP, et al. Benign hyperplastic nodules that originate in the peripheral zone of the prostate gland. Radiology 1993;189:707-711.
31. Pontari MA. Etiologic theories of chronic prostatitis/chronic pelvic pain syndrome. Curr Urol Rep 2007;8:307-312.
32. Rothman JR, Jaffe WI. Prostatitis: updates on diagnostic evaluation. Curr Urol Rep 2007;8:301-306.
33. Wasserman NF. Prostatitis: clinical presentations and transrectal ultrasound findings. Semin Roentgenol 1999;34:325-337.
34. Krieger JN, Nyberg Jr L, Nickel JC. NIH consensus definition and classification of prostatitis. JAMA 1999;282:236-237.
35. Nickel JC, Moon T. Chronic bacterial prostatitis: an evolving clinical enigma. Urology 2005;66:2-8.
36. Doble A, Carter SS. Ultrasonographic findings in prostatitis. Urol Clin North Am 1989;16:763-772.
37. Horcajada JP, Vilana R, Moreno-Martinez A, et al. Transrectal prostatic ultrasonography in acute bacterial prostatitis: findings and clinical implications. Scand J Infect Dis 2003;35:114-120.
38. Kravchick S, Cytron S, Agulansky L, Ben-Dor D. Acute prostatitis in middle-aged men: a prospective study. BJU Int 2004;93:93-96.
39. Varkarakis J, Sebe P, Pinggera GM, et al. Three-dimensional ultrasound guidance for percutaneous drainage of prostatic abscesses. Urology 2004;63:1017-1020; discussion 1020.
40. Lee HJ, Choe GY, Seong CG, Kim SH. Hypoechoic rim of chronically inflamed prostate, as seen at TRUS: histopathologic findings. Korean J Radiol 2001;2:159-163.
41. Dellabella M, Milanese G, Muzzonigro G. Correlation between ultrasound alterations of the preprostatic sphincter and symptoms in patients with chronic prostatitis/chronic pelvic pain syndrome. J Urol 2006;176:112-118.
42. Bude R, Bree RL, Adler RS, Jafri SZ. Transrectal ultrasound appearance of granulomatous prostatitis. J Ultrasound Med 1990;9:677-680.
43. Curran S, Akin O, Agildere AM, et al. Endorectal MRI of prostatic and periprostatic cystic lesions and their mimics. AJR Am J Roentgenol 2007;188:1373-1379.
44. Galosi AB, Montironi R, Fabiani A, et al. Cystic lesions of the prostate gland: an ultrasound classification with pathological correlation. J Urol 2009;181:647-657.
45. Nghiem HT, Kellman GM, Sandberg SA, Craig BM. Cystic lesions of the prostate. Radiographics 1990;10:635-650.
46. Parsons RB, Fisher AM, Bar-Chama N, Mitty HA. MR imaging in male infertility. Radiographics 1997;17:627-637.
47. Patel B, Gujral S, Jefferson K, et al. Seminal vesicle cysts and associated anomalies. BJU Int 2002;90:265-271.

48. Kim B, Kawashima A, Ryu JA, et al. Imaging of the seminal vesicle and vas deferens. Radiographics 2009;29:1105-1121.

49. Jarow JP, Sharlip ID, Belker AM, et al. Best practice policies for male infertility. J Urol 2002;167:2138-2144.

50. Campbell MF, Wein AJ, Kavoussi LR, et al, editors: Campbell-Walsh urology. 9th ed. Philadelphia: Saunders; 2007.

51. Fisch H, Lambert SM, Goluboff ET. Management of ejaculatory duct obstruction: etiology, diagnosis, and treatment. World J Urol 2006;24:604-610.

52. Smith JF, Walsh TJ, Turek PJ. Ejaculatory duct obstruction. Urol Clin North Am 2008;35:221-227, viii.

53. Fedder J, Cruger D, Oestergaard B, Petersen GB. Etiology of azoospermia in 100 consecutive nonvasectomized men. Fertil Steril 2004;82:1463-1465.

54. Kuligowska E, Fenlon HM. Transrectal ultrasound in male infertility: spectrum of findings and role in patient care. Radiology 1998;207:173-181.

55. Blau H, Freud E, Mussaffi H, et al. Urogenital abnormalities in male children with cystic fibrosis. Arch Dis Child 2002;87:135-138.

56. Jarvi K, McCallum S, Zielenski J, et al. Heterogeneity of reproductive tract abnormalities in men with absence of the vas deferens: role of cystic fibrosis transmembrane conductance regulator gene mutations. Fertil Steril 1998;70:724-728.

57. Schlegel PN, Shin D, Goldstein M. Urogenital anomalies in men with congenital absence of the vas deferens. J Urol 1996;155:1644-1648.

58. Ahmad I, Krishna NS. Hemospermia. J Urol 2007;177:1613-1618.

59. Torigian DA, Ramchandani P. Hematospermia: imaging findings. Abdom Imaging 2007;32:29-49.

60. Yagci C, Kupeli S, Tok C, et al. Efficacy of transrectal ultrasonography in the evaluation of hematospermia. Clin Imaging 2004;28:286-290.

61. Furuya S, Furuya R, Masumori N, et al. Magnetic resonance imaging is accurate to detect bleeding in the seminal vesicles in patients with hemospermia. Urology 2008;72:838-842.

Prostate Cancer

62. Sanda MG, Dunn RL, Michalski J, et al. Quality of life and satisfaction with outcome among prostate-cancer survivors. N Engl J Med 2008;358:1250-1261.

63. Sanda MG, Kaplan ID. A 64-year-old man with low-risk prostate cancer: review of prostate cancer treatment. JAMA 2009;301:2141-2151.

64. Iscoe NA. Prostate cancer screening: waiting for Godot. CMAJ 1998;159:1375-1377.

65. Nam RK, Jewett MA, Krahn MD. Prostate cancer. 2. Natural history. CMAJ 1998;159:685-691.

66. Thompson I, Thrasher JB, Aus G, et al. Guideline for the management of clinically localized prostate cancer: 2007 update. J Urol 2007;177:2106-2131.

67. Levy IG, Iscoe NA, Klotz LH. Prostate cancer. 1. The descriptive epidemiology in Canada. CMAJ 1998;159:509-513.

68. Neal DE, Leung HY, Powell PH, et al. Unanswered questions in screening for prostate cancer. Eur J Cancer 2000;36:1316-1321.

69. Rietbergen JB, Schroder FH. Screening for prostate cancer: more questions than answers. Acta Oncol 1998;37:515-532.

70. Bratt O. Hereditary prostate cancer: clinical aspects. J Urol 2002;168:906-913.

71. Eggener SE, Scardino PT, Carroll PR, et al. Focal therapy for localized prostate cancer: a critical appraisal of rationale and modalities. J Urol 2007;178:2260-2267.

72. Bostwick DG, Burke HB, Djakiew D, et al. Human prostate cancer risk factors. Cancer 2004;101:2371-2390.

73. Chang JJ, Shinohara K, Bhargava V, Presti Jr JC. Prospective evaluation of lateral biopsies of the peripheral zone for prostate cancer detection. J Urol 1998;160:2111-2114.

74. Carroll P, Albertsen P, Greene K, Babaian R. Prostate-specific antigen: best practice statement: 2009 update. American Urological Association.

75. Polascik TJ, Oesterling JE, Partin AW. Prostate-specific antigen: a decade of discovery—what we have learned and where we are going. J Urol 1999;162:293-306.

76. Thompson IM, Ankerst DP. Prostate-specific antigen in the early detection of prostate cancer. CMAJ 2007;176:1853-1858.

77. Thompson IM, Tangen CM, Kristal AR. Prostate-specific antigen: a misused and maligned prostate cancer biomarker. J Natl Cancer Inst 2008;100:1487-1488.

78. Bunting PS, DeBoer G, Choo R, et al. Intraindividual variation of PSA, free PSA and complexed PSA in a cohort of patients with prostate cancer managed with watchful observation. Clin Biochem 2002;35:471-475.

79. Alapont Alacreu JM, Navarro Rosales S, Budia Alba A, et al. [PSA and hK2 in the diagnosis of prostate cancer]. Actas Urol Esp 2008;32:575-588.

80. Jung K, Meyer A, Lein M, et al. Ratio of free-to-total prostate-specific antigen in serum cannot distinguish patients with prostate cancer from those with chronic inflammation of the prostate. J Urol 1998;159:1595-1598.

81. Loeb S, Catalona WJ. What to do with an abnormal PSA test. Oncologist 2008;13:299-305.

82. Price CP, Allard J, Davies G, et al. Pre- and post-analytical factors that may influence use of serum prostate-specific antigen and its isoforms in a screening programme for prostate cancer. Ann Clin Biochem 2001;38:188-216.

83. Bunting PS. A guide to the interpretation of serum prostate-specific antigen levels. Clin Biochem 1995;28:221-241.

84. Toi A, Neill MG, Lockwood GA, et al. The continuing importance of transrectal ultrasound identification of prostatic lesions. J Urol 2007;177:516-520.

85. Etzioni R, Penson DF, Legler JM, et al. Overdiagnosis due to prostate-specific antigen screening: lessons from U.S. prostate cancer incidence trends. J Natl Cancer Inst 2002;94:981-990.

86. Garnick MB. Prostate cancer: screening, diagnosis, and management. Ann Intern Med 1993;118:804-818.

87. Gonzalgo ML, Carter HB. Update on PSA testing. J Natl Compr Cancer Netw 2007;5:737-742.

88. Oesterling JE, Jacobsen SJ, Chute CG, et al. Serum prostate-specific antigen in a community-based population of healthy men: establishment of age-specific reference ranges. JAMA 1993;270:860-864.

89. Carter HB, Pearson JD, Metter EJ, et al. Longitudinal evaluation of prostate-specific antigen levels in men with and without prostate disease. JAMA 1992;267:2215-2220.

90. Moul JW, Mouraviev V, Sun L, et al. Prostate cancer: the new landscape. Curr Opin Urol 2009;19:154-160.

91. Catalona WJ, Smith DS, Ornstein DK. Prostate cancer detection in men with serum PSA concentrations of 2.6 to 4.0 ng/mL and benign prostate examination: enhancement of specificity with free PSA measurements. JAMA 1997;277:1452-1455.

92. Thompson IM, Pauler DK, Goodman PJ, et al. Prevalence of prostate cancer among men with a prostate-specific antigen level ≤4.0 ng per milliliter. N Engl J Med 2004;350:2239-2246.

93. Andriole G. Mortality results from a randomized prostate-cancer screening trial. N Engl J Med 2009;360:1310-1319.

94. Schröder F. Screening and prostate-cancer mortality in a randomized European study. N Engl J Med 2009;360:1320-1328.

95. Thompson IM, Ankerst DP, Chi C, et al. Operating characteristics of prostate-specific antigen in men with an initial PSA level of 3.0 ng/ml or lower. JAMA 2005;294:66-70.

96. Thompson IM, Ankerst DP, Etzioni R, Wang T. It's time to abandon an upper limit of normal for prostate-specific antigen: assessing the risk of prostate cancer. J Urol 2008;180:1219-1222.

97. Parekh DJ, Ankerst DP, Troyer D, et al. Biomarkers for prostate cancer detection. J Urol 2007;178:2252-2259.

98. Crawford ED, Thompson IM. Controversies regarding screening for prostate cancer. BJU Int 2007;100(Suppl 2):5-7.

99. Bartsch G, Horninger W, Klocker H, et al. Tyrol Prostate Cancer Demonstration Project: early detection, treatment, outcome, incidence and mortality. BJU Int 2008;101:809-816.

100. Nam RK, Toi A, Klotz LH, et al. Assessing individual risk for prostate cancer. J Clin Oncol 2007;25:3582-3588.

101. Barry M. Screening for prostate cancer: the controversy that refuses to die. N Engl J Med 2009;360:1351-1354.

102. Eng TY, Thomas CR, Herman TS. Primary radiation therapy for localized prostate cancer. Urol Oncol 2002;7:239-257.

103. Fuchsjager M, Shukla-Dave A, Akin O, et al. Prostate cancer imaging. Acta Radiol 2008;49:107-120.

104. Chang SS, Amin MB. Utilizing the tumor-node-metastasis staging for prostate cancer. CA Cancer J Clin 2008;58:54-59.

105. Greene FL, Page DL, Fleming ID. American Joint Committee on Cancer cancer staging manual. 7th ed. New York: Springer-Verlag; 2010.

106. Whitmore Jr WF. Natural history and staging of prostate cancer. Urol Clin North Am 1984;11:205-220.

107. Dugan JA, Bostwick DG, Myers RP, et al. The definition and preoperative prediction of clinically insignificant prostate cancer. JAMA 1996;275:288-294.

108. Engelbrecht MR, Jager GJ, Laheij RJ, et al. Local staging of prostate cancer using magnetic resonance imaging: a meta-analysis. Eur Radiol 2002;12:2294-2302.

109. Ross R, Harisinghani M. Prostate cancer imaging: what the urologic oncologist needs to know. Radiol Clin North Am 2006;44:711-722, viii.

110. Makarov DV, Trock BJ, Humphreys EB, et al. Updated nomogram to predict pathologic stage of prostate cancer given prostate-specific antigen level, clinical stage, and biopsy Gleason score (Partin tables) based on cases from 2000 to 2005. Urology 2007;69:1095-1101.

111. Ross PL, Scardino PT, Kattan MW. A catalog of prostate cancer nomograms. J Urol 2001;165:1562-1568.

112. Kattan MW, Cuzick J, Fisher G, et al. Nomogram incorporating PSA level to predict cancer-specific survival for men with clinically localized prostate cancer managed without curative intent. Cancer 2008;112:69-74.

113. Che M, Sakr W, Grignon D. Pathologic features the urologist should expect on a prostate biopsy. Urol Oncol 2003;21:153-161.

114. Gleason DF, Mellinger GT. Prediction of prognosis for prostatic adenocarcinoma by combined histological grading and clinical staging. J Urol 1974;111:58-64.

115. Epstein JI, Allsbrook Jr WC, Amin MB, Egevad LL. Update on the Gleason grading system for prostate cancer: results of an international consensus conference of urologic pathologists. Adv Anat Pathol 2006;13:57-59.

116. Wilt TJ, MacDonald R, Rutks I, et al. Systematic review: comparative effectiveness and harms of treatments for clinically localized prostate cancer. Ann Intern Med 2008;148:435-448.

117. Bill-Axelson A, Holmberg L, Ruutu M, et al. Radical prostatectomy versus watchful waiting in early prostate cancer. N Engl J Med 2005;352:1977-1984.

118. Thompson I, Leach RJ, Pollock BH, Naylor SL. Prostate cancer and prostate-specific antigen: the more we know, the less we understand. J Natl Cancer Inst 2003;95:1027-1028.

119. Epstein JI, Sanderson H, Carter HB, Scharfstein DO. Utility of saturation biopsy to predict insignificant cancer at radical prostatectomy. Urology 2005;66:356-360.

120. Klotz L. Active surveillance for favorable-risk prostate cancer: what are the results and how safe is it? Curr Urol Rep 2007;8:341-344.

121. Dall'Era MA, Cooperberg MR, Chan JM, et al. Active surveillance for early-stage prostate cancer: review of the current literature. Cancer 2008;112:1650-1659.

122. Allaf ME, Carter HB. Update on watchful waiting for prostate cancer. Curr Opin Urol 2004;14:171-175.

123. Engelbrecht MR, Barentsz JO, Jager GJ, et al. Prostate cancer staging using imaging. BJU Int 2000;86(Suppl 1):123-134.

124. Babaian RJ, Mettlin C, Kane R, et al. The relationship of prostate-specific antigen to digital rectal examination and transrectal ultrasonography. Findings of the American Cancer Society National Prostate Cancer Detection Project. Cancer 1992;69:1195-1200.

125. Eisenberg ML, Cowan JE, Davies BJ, et al. The importance of tumor palpability and transrectal ultrasonographic appearance in the contemporary clinical staging of prostate cancer. Urol Oncol Semin Orig Invest 2009.

126. Lee F, Gray JM, McLeary RD, et al. Transrectal ultrasound in the diagnosis of prostate cancer: location, echogenicity, histopathology, and staging. Prostate 1985;7:117-129.

127. Dahnert WF, Hamper UM, Eggleston JC, et al. Prostatic evaluation by transrectal sonography with histopathologic correlation: the echogenic appearance of early carcinoma. Radiology 1986;158:97-102.

128. Wink M, Frauscher F, Cosgrove D, et al. Contrast-enhanced ultrasound and prostate cancer; a multicentre European research coordination project. Eur Urol 2008;54:982-992.

129. Shinohara K, Wheeler TM, Scardino PT. The appearance of prostate cancer on transrectal ultrasonography: correlation of imaging and pathological examinations. J Urol 1989;142:76-82.

130. Hasegawa Y, Sakamoto N. Relationship of ultrasonographic findings to histology in prostate cancer. Eur Urol 1994;26:10-17.

131. Dahnert WF, Hamper UM, Walsh PC, et al. The echogenic focus in prostatic sonograms, with xeroradiographic and histopathologic correlation. Radiology 1986;159:95-100.

132. Rifkin MD, Dahnert W, Kurtz AB. State of the art: endorectal sonography of the prostate gland. AJR Am J Roentgenol 1990;154:691-700.

133. Hamper UM, Sheth S, Walsh PC, Epstein JI. Bright echogenic foci in early prostatic carcinoma: sonographic and pathologic correlation. Radiology 1990;176:339-343.

134. Dahnert W. Ultrasonography of the prostate: a critical review. Appl Radiol 1988;17:39-44.

135. Dyke CH, Toi A, Sweet JM. Value of random ultrasound-guided transrectal prostate biopsy. Radiology 1990;176:345-349.

136. Pallwein L, Aigner F, Faschingbauer R, et al. Prostate cancer diagnosis: value of real-time elastography. Abdom Imaging 2008;33:729-735.

137. Lawrentschuk N, Haider MA, Daljeet N, et al. "Prostatic evasive anterior tumours": the role of magnetic resonance imaging. BJU Int 2009 Oct 8. [Epub ahead of print.]

138. Amiel GE, Slawin KM. Newer modalities of ultrasound imaging and treatment of the prostate. Urol Clin North Am 2006;33:329-337.

139. Wijkstra H, Wink MH, de la Rosette JJ. Contrast-specific imaging in the detection and localization of prostate cancer. World J Urol 2004;22:346-350.

140. Frauscher F, Klauser A, Halpern EJ. Advances in ultrasound for the detection of prostate cancer. Ultrasound Q 2002;18:135-142.

141. Cornud F, Hamida K, Flam T, et al. Endorectal color Doppler sonography and endorectal MR imaging features of nonpalpable prostate cancer: correlation with radical prostatectomy findings. AJR Am J Roentgenol 2000;175:1161-1168.

142. Pepe P, Patane D, Panella P, Aragona F. Does the adjunct of echographic contrast medium Levovist improve the detection rate of prostate cancer? Prostate Cancer Prostatic Dis 2003;6:159-162.

143. Andriole GL, Bullock TL, Belani JS, et al. Is there a better way to biopsy the prostate? Prospects for a novel transrectal systematic biopsy approach. Urology 2007;70:22-26.

144. Pallwein L, Mitterberger M, Pinggera G, et al. Sonoelastography of the prostate: comparison with systematic biopsy findings in 492 patients. Eur J Radiol 2008;65:304-310.

145. Gosselaar C, Roobol MJ, Roemeling S, et al. The value of an additional hypoechoic lesion-directed biopsy core for detecting prostate cancer. BJU Int 2008;101:685-690.

146. Pallwein L, Mitterberger M, Gradl J, et al. Value of contrast-enhanced ultrasound and elastography in imaging of prostate cancer. Curr Opin Urol 2007;17:39-47.

147. Presti Jr JC, Hricak H, Narayan PA, et al. Local staging of prostatic carcinoma: comparison of transrectal sonography and endorectal MR imaging. AJR Am J Roentgenol 1996;166:103-108.

148. Ukimura O, Troncoso P, Ramirez EI, Babaian RJ. Prostate cancer staging: correlation between ultrasound determined tumor contact length and pathologically confirmed extraprostatic extension. J Urol 1998;159:1251-1259.

Ultrasound-Guided Biopsy

149. El-Hakim A, Moussa S. Guidelines on prostate biopsy methodology. Canadian Urological Association, 2009.

150. Carey JM, Korman HJ. Transrectal ultrasound guided biopsy of the prostate: do enemas decrease clinically significant complications? J Urol 2001;166:82-85.

151. Feliciano J, Teper E, Ferrandino M, et al. The incidence of fluoroquinolone-resistant infections after prostate biopsy: are fluoroquinolones still effective prophylaxis? J Urol 2008;179:952-925; discussion 925.

152. Somerville P, Seifert PJ, Destounis SV, et al. Anticoagulation and bleeding risk after core needle biopsy. AJR Am J Roentgenol 2008;191:1194-1197.

153. Rodriguez LV, Terris MK. Risks and complications of transrectal ultrasound guided prostate needle biopsy: a prospective study and review of the literature. J Urol 1998;160:2115-2120.

154. Herget EJ, Saliken JC, Donnelly BJ, et al. Transrectal ultrasound-guided biopsy of the prostate: relation between ASA use and bleeding complications. Can Assoc Radiol J 1999;50:173-176.

155. Ecke TH, Gunia S, Bartel P, et al. Complications and risk factors of transrectal ultrasound–guided needle biopsies of the prostate evaluated by questionnaire. Urol Oncol 2008;26:474-478.

156. Nishimura RA, Carabello BA, Faxon DP, et al. ACC/AHA 2008 Guideline Update on Valvular Heart Disease: focused update on infective endocarditis. A report of the American College of Cardiology/American Heart Association Task Force on Practice Guidelines endorsed by the Society of Cardiovascular Anesthesiologists, Society for Cardiovascular Angiography and Interventions, and Society of Thoracic Surgeons. J Am Coll Cardiol 2008;52:676-685.

157. Hodge KK, McNeal JE, Terris MK, Stamey TA. Random systematic versus directed ultrasound-guided transrectal core biopsies of the prostate. J Urol 1989;142:71-74; discussion 74-75.

158. Presti Jr JC. Prostate biopsy: how many cores are enough? Urol Oncol 2003;21:135-140.

159. Eichler K, Hempel S, Wilby J, et al. Diagnostic value of systematic biopsy methods in the investigation of prostate cancer: a systematic review. J Urol 2006;175:1605-1612.

160. Neill MG, Toi A, Lockwood GA, et al. Systematic lateral prostate biopsy: are the benefits worth the costs? J Urol 2008;179:1321-1326.

161. Borboroglu PG, Sur RL, Roberts JL, Amling CL. Repeat biopsy strategy in patients with atypical small acinar proliferation or high-grade prostatic intraepithelial neoplasia on initial prostate needle biopsy. J Urol 2001;166:866-870.

162. Babaian RJ, Toi A, Kamoi K, et al. A comparative analysis of sextant and an extended 11-core multisite directed biopsy strategy. J Urol 2000;163:152-157.

163. Djavan B, Remzi M, Schulman CC, et al. Repeat prostate biopsy: who, how and when? A review. Eur Urol 2002;42:93-103.

164. Chen ME, Troncoso P, Johnston DA, et al. Optimization of prostate biopsy strategy using computer-based analysis. J Urol 1997;158:2168-2175.

165. Chen ME, Johnston DA, Tang K, et al. Detailed mapping of prostate carcinoma foci: biopsy strategy implications. Cancer 2000;89:1800-1809.

166. Shinohara K, Gulati M, Koppie TM, Terris MK. Transperineal prostate biopsy after abdominoperineal resection. J Urol 2003;169:141-144.

167. Seaman EK, Sawczuk IS, Fatal M, et al. Transperineal prostate needle biopsy guided by transurethral ultrasound in patients without a rectum. Urology 1996;47:353-355.

Ultrasound-Guided Therapy
168. Mouraviev V, Madden JF. Focal therapy for prostate cancer: pathologic basis. Curr Opin Urol 2009;19:161-167.

Other Ultrasound Applications
169. Giede C, Toi A, Chapman W, Rosen B. The use of transrectal ultrasound to biopsy pelvic masses in women. Gynecol Oncol 2004;95:552-556.

CHAPTER 11

The Adrenal Glands

Amit R. Ahuja, Wendy Thurston, and Stephanie R. Wilson

Chapter Outline

The adrenal glands are the smallest paired organs in the abdomen, weighing approximately 4 g each in a nonstressed adult.[1] Despite their size, the adrenal glands are essential for maintaining homeostasis through hormone secretion. They also represent common sites for a wide range of disease. Numerous imaging techniques can be used to investigate a patient with suspected adrenal pathology. Computed tomography (CT) is widely regarded as the premier imaging modality, with recent advances in magnetic resonance imaging (MRI) and positron emission tomography (PET-CT) providing additional benefit. Sonography, however, remains a widely available, economical, and effective tool in the setting of adrenal disease. It is essential for the radiologist to understand not only the spectrum of adrenal pathology, but also the applications and limitations of all imaging techniques, to direct the most appropriate imaging strategy.

EMBRYOLOGY

The adrenal gland is composed of two parts, a **cortex** and a **medulla,** which have different embryologic origins. The cortex develops from the **mesoderm** and the medulla from the **neural crest.**

During the sixth week of fetal development, there is rapid proliferation of mesenchymal cells, originating from the posterior abdominal wall peritoneal epithelium near the cranial end of the mesonephros (primitive kidney). These cells penetrate the retroperitoneal mesenchyme to become the **primitive adrenal cortex.**[2] Further mesenchymal cell proliferation occurs, and these cells envelop the primitive cortex more compactly to become the **permanent adrenal cortex.** By the end of the eighth gestational week, the cortical mass separates from the posterior peritoneal surface and becomes surrounded by retroperitoneal connective tissue.

During the seventh week of development, cells originating from neuroectoderm migrate and invade the medial aspect of the developing primitive adrenal cortex. These cells differentiate into the chromaffin cells of the **adrenal medulla.**

At birth, the gland is composed predominantly of primitive fetal cortex and adrenal medulla. Immediately after birth, the primitive cortex begins to involute, disappearing by 1 year of age. Simultaneously, the thin, compact, **permanent adrenal cortex** further differentiates into the three zones (glomerulosa, fasciculata, and reticularis) of the adult gland[3] (Fig. 11-1).

ANATOMY AND PHYSIOLOGY

The adrenal glands are found at the level of the 11th or 12th thoracic rib, lateral to the first lumbar vertebra

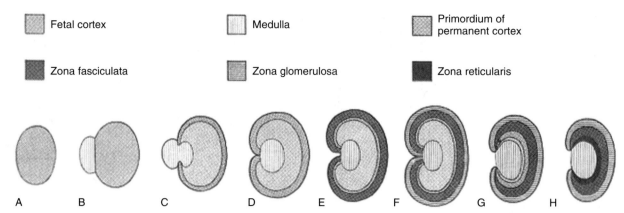

FIGURE 11-1. **Adrenal gland embryology. A,** Six weeks. **B,** Seven weeks. **C,** Eight weeks. **D** and **E,** Later stages of encapsulation of the medulla by the cortex. **F,** Newborn. **G,** One year, showing that fetal cortex has almost disappeared. **H,** Four years, showing the adult pattern of the cortical zones. *(Modified with permission from Moore KL, editor.* The developing human: clinically oriented embryology. *5th ed. Philadelphia, 1993, Saunders.)*

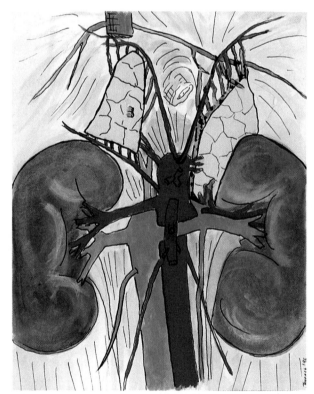

FIGURE 11-2. **Anatomy and blood supply of the adrenal glands.** *(Courtesy Jenny Tomash.)*

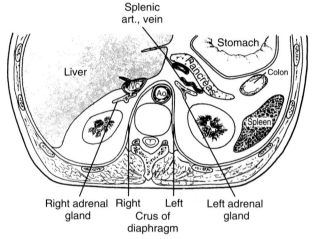

FIGURE 11-3. **Cross-sectional anatomy of the adrenal glands.** *(From Mitty HA, Yeh HC,* Radiology of the adrenals with sonography and CT. *Philadelphia, 1982, Saunders.)*

(Fig. 11-2). Each gland is composed of an **anteromedial ridge** and medial and lateral wings. This most often results in an inverted-V or inverted-Y appearance.

The glands are surrounded by fatty areolar tissue that has a thin, fibrous capsule and many fibrous extensions into the adrenal glands.[2] With their fascial support, the adrenals are relatively fixed, unlike the kidney, which is not anchored to the perinephric fascia. Thus the adrenal glands have a more constant relationship with the abdominal great vessels than they do with the kidneys

(Fig. 11-3). The adrenal gland and kidney will separate during deep inspiration or in the upright position. This may allow differentiation between renal and adrenal masses during sonographic examination.[4,5]

The **right adrenal gland** is located posterior to the inferior vena cava and cephalad to the upper pole of the right kidney (Fig. 11-4). Medially, the crus of the diaphragm runs parallel to the medial wing of the gland, whereas the lateral wing is adjacent to the posteromedial aspect of the liver (see Fig. 11-3). The medial wing may extend caudally along the medial aspect of the upper pole of the kidney. The tip of the gland always terminates cephalad to the renal vessels.[6]

The **left adrenal gland** is positioned anteromedially to the kidney (Fig. 11-5). It may extend from above the superior pole of the kidney to the level of the renal hilum in 10% of persons.[7,8] The aorta and crus of the diaphragm are on the medial aspect of the adrenal. The

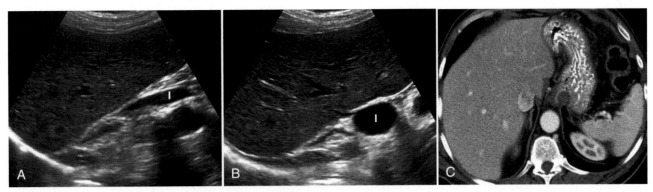

FIGURE 11-4. Normal adult right adrenal gland. A, Sagittal, and **B,** transverse, sonograms show the adrenal as a linear hypoechoic structure that lies deep to and slightly lateral to the inferior vena cava *(I)*. The kidney lies caudal to the right adrenal gland and therefore is not seen in the same plane. **C,** CT scan confirms the retrocaval position of the right adrenal gland. Only the tip of the upper pole of the right kidney is seen. The left adrenal gland, by comparison, is located anterior to the left kidney.

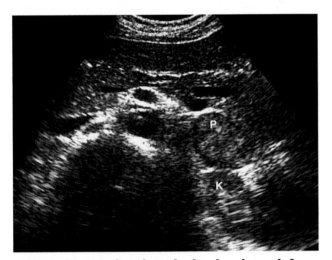

FIGURE 11-5. Left adrenal gland enlarged from pheochromocytoma. Visualization of this pheochromocytoma *(P)*, through a ventral epigastric approach. The adrenal is shown anterior to the upper pole of the left kidney (K).

cephalic two thirds of the gland is posterior to the stomach and therefore covered by peritoneum of the lesser sac. The caudal one third of the gland is related to the posterior aspect of the pancreatic body and splenic vasculature[9] (see Fig. 11-3).

The adrenal glands have a rich blood supply to facilitate their endocrine function. The superior, middle, and inferior suprarenal arteries arise off the inferior phrenic artery, aorta, and renal artery, respectively. Each gland drains through a main suprarenal vein, which on the right enters directly into the inferior vena cava (IVC) and on the left drains into the left renal vein.

On sonography, the adrenal cortex is less echogenic than the surrounding perirenal fat, whereas the medulla is evident as a highly echogenic, central linear structure. The echogenic linear medulla is most prominent in the fetus and newborn; however, it can also be identified in thin adults. Oppenheimer et al.[10] proposed that the increased medullary echogenicity in newborn infants is caused by increased collagen around the central vessels and haphazard orientation of its cell population, resulting in multiple reflective interfaces.

In their detailed assessment, Ma et al.[11] demonstrated that the average adrenal gland measures 3 to 4 cm length, 1 to 2 cm in width, and 2 to 3 mm in thickness. Although the shape of the adrenal glands can vary, the thickness of the limbs, particularly the lateral limbs, remain relatively constant and therefore are the most useful indicators of **gland hypertrophy.**

The **medial wing** of the adrenal gland is larger superiorly and smaller or absent inferiorly, whereas the **lateral wing** is larger inferiorly and smaller superiorly.[7] Complete visualization of the adrenal gland in a single sonographic plane is virtually impossible because of the complex shape of the organ.[12]

The adrenal gland performs a critical role in hormone secretion and maintenance of homeostasis. The cortex secretes steroid hormones and the medulla secretes catecholamines. The cortex is subdivided into three distinct zones. The **zona glomerulosa,** which is the outermost layer, produces and secretes the mineralocorticoid **aldosterone.** This hormone is part of a coordinated hormonal system (renin-angiotensin-aldosterone) involved in the homeostasis of fluid volume and blood pressure. The principal action of aldosterone is on the renal tubules, causing sodium retention. The **zona fasciculata** and **zona reticularis** act as a single unit and secrete **cortisol (glucocorticoid)** and **androgens.** The adrenal cortex in a nonstressed adult secretes about 20 mg of cortisol daily and with stressful stimuli may increase secretion up to 150 to 200 mg/day. The physiologic significance of the adrenal androgens is not known. In excess, androgens may cause hirsutism or virilization in females and precocious pseudopuberty in males.[13]

The adrenal medulla is responsible for the synthesis and secretion of the catecholamines **epinephrine** and **norepinephrine.** These hormones play an important role in the response to actual or anticipated stress but are not essential to life.[13]

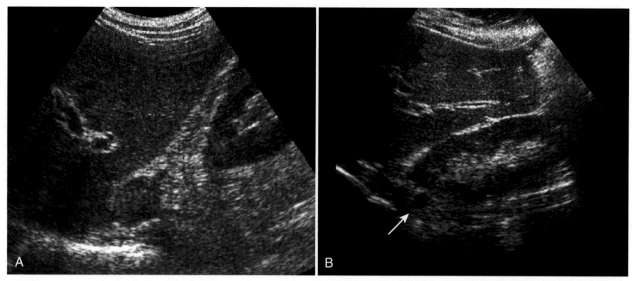

FIGURE 11-6. Importance of position in localization of pathology to the adrenal gland. A, Right adrenal mass. Sagittal sonogram shows a solid mass cephalad to upper pole of right kidney. **B,** Metastatic lymph node in a different patient. A sagittal sonogram shows a small, solid nodule *(arrow)* posterior to upper pole of right kidney. This location is not consistent with the adrenal gland.

ADRENAL SONOGRAPHY

Ability to visualize the adrenal glands sonographically is related to body habitus, operator experience, and type of equipment. With the introduction of high-resolution, real-time sector scanners, the adrenal glands have become easier to examine. Ideally, the patient should fast for 6 to 8 hours before the examination to reduce the amount of intervening bowel gas.

Marchal et al.[12] reported that the normal right and left adrenal glands were visualized by high-resolution real-time sonography in 92% and 71% of patients, respectively. Cortex and medulla were differentiated in 13% of patients. Alternatively, Günther et al.[14] studied 60 healthy subjects with high-resolution real-time sonography and identified adrenal glands in only one thin female. In newborn infants, real-time high-frequency scanning identified the right and left adrenal glands in 97% and 83% of patients, respectively.[10]

Multiplanar Scanning

Because of the complex shape of the adrenal gland, a comprehensive, systematic, multiplanar approach is necessary to evaluate it fully. The gland should be assessed in the transverse, coronal, and longitudinal planes, as well as in the supine, oblique, and lateral decubitus positions.

Right Adrenal Gland

The right adrenal gland is best evaluated intercostally at the midaxillary or anterior axillary line.[7,12,14] The key to the identification of the right adrenal is to remember its suprarenal location and its relationship to the IVC

(Fig. 11-6). The liver provides a good acoustic window. Alternatively, a subcostal oblique approach parallel to the rib cage at the midclavicular line can be used. Scanning from a direct anterior or posterior approach is typically poor because of overlying bowel gas or intervening muscle and fat interfaces (Fig. 11-7).

Left Adrenal Gland

The left adrenal gland is more difficult to visualize than the right and is best evaluated from the epigastrium or intercostally at the posterior axillary or midaxillary line through the spleen or kidney.[7,14] The key to the identification of the left adrenal is to remember it lies anterior to the upper pole of the left kidney (see Fig. 11-5). As with the right adrenal, a direct posterior approach is usually not helpful with the left adrenal gland.

Pitfalls

When the scan plane is parallel to the anterior surface of the lateral wing, false enlargement may be observed.[15] This could lead to erroneous diagnosis of hyperplasia or a small mass. Changing the angle of the insonating sound beam by altering the intercostal space should allow differentiation between real and false enlargement.

INFECTIOUS DISEASES

Tuberculosis (TB), histoplasmosis, blastomycosis, and meningococcal, echinococcal, cytomegalovirus (CMV), herpesvirus, and *Pneumocystis* infections are the most common infectious diseases of the adrenal gland.[16-18]

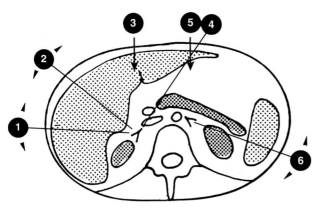

FIGURE 11-7. Scan planes for sonographic visualization of adrenal glands. *1, 2,* Lateral approach (right): *1,* midaxillary line; *2,* anterior axillary line. *3, 5,* Ventral approach (right and left): paramedian or midclavicular line. *4,* Ventral approach (right adrenal through left liver lobe): longitudinal oblique scan. *6,* Lateral approach (left): posterior axillary line. *(Modified from Günther RW, Kelbel C, Lenner V. Real-time ultrasound of normal adrenal glands and small tumors. J Clin Ultrasound 1984;12:211-217.)*

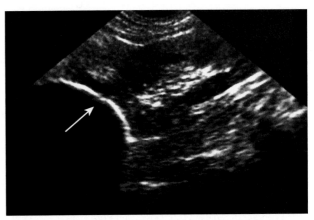

FIGURE 11-8. Adrenal gland calcification. Sagittal sonogram shows a large calcification of the adrenal gland with distal acoustic shadowing.

CAUSES OF ADRENAL CALCIFICATION

Infection
  Tuberculosis
  Histoplasmosis
  Echinococcus
Prior hemorrhage
Neoplasm
  Adrenocortical carcinoma
  Myelolipoma
  Pheochromocytoma
Hemangioma (rare)

ADRENAL PSEUDOMASSES

Thickened diaphragmatic crus
Accessory spleen
Gastric fundus
Gastric diverticulum
Renal vein
Retrocrural and retroperitoneal adenopathy
Upper-pole renal cysts and tumors
Pancreatic tumors
Hypertrophied caudate lobe of liver
Fluid-filled colon interposed between stomach and kidney

Tuberculosis has a variable appearance, depending on the stage of infection. Acutely, there is bilateral diffuse enlargement, often inhomogeneous, caused by caseous necrosis. Punctate calcification is a feature. Chronically, the adrenal glands become atrophic and more heavily calcified.[17,18] TB and **histoplasmosis** are the two most common causes of adrenal calcification in the adult population[19] (Fig. 11-8). Calcification in the absence of a soft tissue mass should suggest infection or prior hemorrhage rather than neoplasm. When TB infects the adrenal glands, chest radiographs and sputum cultures may be negative. Before antituberculous therapy, TB was the most common cause of Addison's disease (adrenal insufficiency). Currently, **autoimmune disorders** predominate as the most common etiology of adrenal insufficiency.

Echinococcal infection of the adrenal gland manifests similar to echinococcal disease seen elsewhere and is most often characterized by cysts with varying amounts of calcification.[20]

Immunosuppression resulting from acquired immunodeficiency syndrome (AIDS), transplantation, or other causes increases these patients' risk for infectious involvement of the adrenal gland. Common organisms include fungi (histoplasmosis), mycobacteria, CMV, herpesvirus, *Pneumocystis carinii (jiroveci),* human immunodeficiency virus (HIV), and toxoplasmosis.[17,18] Grizzle[18] described focal or diffuse damage of the glands by CMV in 70% of AIDS patients who died. Sonographically, these lesions are usually hypoechoic masses that may be heterogeneous and may contain gas if abscess formation occurs.

Bacterial adrenal abscesses are found more frequently in neonates and are relatively uncommon in adults.[21,22] In the neonate, hematogeneous seeding of normal glands or those affected by hemorrhage can result in abscess formation.[22] On sonography, adrenal abscesses typically appear as complex, avascular cystic masses.

BENIGN ADRENAL NEOPLASMS

Adenoma

Adenomas represent the most common adrenal tumor and have been found in as many as 9% of autopsy specimens.[23,24] Incidence increases with age, and adenomas are also reported more often in patients with hypertension, diabetes, hyperthyroidism, renal cell carcinoma,[25] or hereditary colorectal adenomatosis.[26] Bilateral adenomas are seen in 10% of cases.[27]

FEATURES OF ADRENAL ADENOMAS

- Most common adrenal tumor
- Most common cause of adrenal "incidentaloma"
- Nonhyperfunctioning > hyperfunctioning

DIAGNOSTIC FEATURES
- No specific ultrasound features
- Unenhanced CT adrenal mass <10 HU (lipid rich)
- Dynamic contrast-enhanced CT washout >60% (lipid poor)
- Loss of signal on chemical shift MRI (lipid rich)

Adenomas can be classified as either nonhyperfunctioning or hyperfunctioning. **Nonhyperfunctioning** adenomas are more common, typically asymptomatic, and most often discovered incidentally. **Hyperfunctioning** adenomas tend to present clinically with symptoms related to excess hormone production, most frequently manifesting as Cushing's syndrome or Conn's disease.

Cushing's Syndrome

Cushing's syndrome was described in 1932 by Harvey Cushing and is characterized by truncal obesity, hirsutism, amenorrhea, hypertension, weakness, and abdominal striae. This results from **excessive cortisol secretion,** which may occur with adrenal hyperplasia (70%), adenoma (20%), carcinoma (10%),[28] or from exogenous corticosteroid administration. **Cushing's disease** is caused by hyperplastic adrenal glands excreting excessive cortisol as a result of elevated adrenocorticotropic hormone (ACTH) production from a pituitary adenoma. A biochemical profile with high plasma cortisol and urinary 17-hydroxycorticoid levels and low serum ACTH suggests an autonomous adrenal tumor (adenoma/carcinoma) as the source of excessive hormone.

Conn's Disease

Conn's disease results from **excessive aldosterone secretion** and was first described in 1955.[29] Primary aldosteronism can result from adrenal adenoma (70%), adrenal hyperplasia (30%), and rarely adrenal carcinoma.[30] Clinically, **hyperaldosteronism** causes hypertension, muscular weakness, tetany, and electrocardiographic (ECG) abnormalities. Patients with unexplained hypertension and hypokalemia may have excess secretion of aldosterone. Patients with hyperaldosteronism from an adenoma typically are female,[31] whereas those with hyperaldosteronism from hyperplasia usually are male.[32] These tumors tend to be small (<2 cm). Biochemically, elevated urine

and serum aldosterone levels, hypokalemia, hypernatremia, and elevated bicarbonate and low plasma pH levels are found. A suppressed renin level indicates primary hyperaldosteronism.

Histologic Differentiation

Pathologically, it may be difficult to differentiate nodules of hyperplasia from adrenal adenomas. Nodules larger than 1 cm are likely to be adenomas.[1] Also, it may be impossible histologically to differentiate adenoma from adrenocortical carcinoma using only biologic indices. Histologically, nonhyperfunctioning adenomas are composed of lipid-filled cells indicative of their secretory inactivity.[1]

Management

Patients with an adrenal mass and evidence of excess hormone production typically require resection to alleviate their symptoms. When a nonhyperfunctioning adrenal mass is discovered, differentiation between benign and malignant etiologies will direct further management. Adrenal masses larger than 6 cm are considered suspicious for malignancy and typically are resected.[33-36] For lesions 4 to 6 cm, either close imaging follow-up or surgical excision is considered acceptable. Management of lesions less than 4 cm in size should be based on additional imaging findings, as described next.

Imaging Considerations

The number of incidentally discovered adrenal lesions has increased significantly over recent years as a result of increased utilization of cross-sectional imaging and improved imaging techniques. In patients with no known malignancy, these lesions are almost always benign. Even in patients with a known malignancy, an adrenal "incidentaloma" is still most likely to represent an adenoma.[37] However, distinguishing benign from malignant disease (i.e., metastases) is essential to the management of these patients. Accurate characterization of benign conditions based solely on imaging features can make biopsy unnecessary.

Two important features allow for accurate differentiation between adrenal adenomas and malignant disease: **intracytoplasmic lipid content** and **physiologic contrast washout.** Most adrenal adenomas contain sufficient intracytoplasmic lipid to produce characteristic low attenuation on unenhanced CT. Numerous studies to establish appropriate threshold criteria have concluded that an adrenal mass measuring less than 10 Hounsfield units (HU) on unenhanced CT can be classified as an adenoma with a sensitivity of 71% and specificity of 98%.[38] However, approximately 30% of adenomas are **lipid poor** and will demonstrate attenuation greater than 10 HU, thus overlapping with malignant disease. In this setting, multiphase contrast evaluation can be performed to distinguish these lesions as adrenal adenomas and will demonstrate more **rapid contrast washout** than malignant lesions. Caoili et al.[39] found that by applying a threshold level of >60% absolute washout or >40% relative washout at 15 minutes post-injection, adenomas could be differentiated from metastases with a 98% sensitivity and 97% specificity.

When a mass is still indeterminate on CT evaluation, chemical shift MRI can be performed to assess for the presence of microscopic fat. Reliable criteria for contrast washout evaluation using MRI have not yet been established.[40-42] PET-CT has also shown promise in differentiating benign from malignant disease.[43]

Given their prevalence, adrenal adenomas may be discovered on routine sonographic evaluations. They appear as small, round, well-defined solid masses (Fig. 11-9).

Unfortunately, these imaging features overlap considerably with malignant disease, and further imaging is required to establish a diagnosis.

When a very large abdominal mass is present, particularly in the right upper quadrant (RUQ), sonography can be superior to CT in determining the organ of origin. Gore et al.[44] demonstrated that the RUQ retroperitoneal fat reflection is displaced posteriorly by hepatic and subhepatic masses, whereas kidney and adrenal masses displace it anteriorly. This is best appreciated using a parasagittal plane (Fig. 11-10).

Myelolipoma

Adrenal myelolipomas are rare, benign, **nonhyperfunctioning** tumors composed of varying proportions of fat and bone marrow elements.[45] Their etiology and patho-

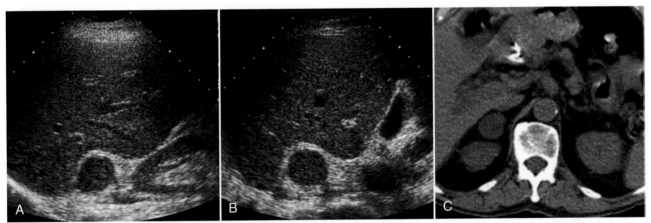

FIGURE 11-9. Adrenal adenoma. A, Sagittal, and **B,** transverse, sonograms show a small, solid right adrenal mass between the liver and upper pole of right kidney. Sonogram is indeterminate as to the significance. **C,** CT scan on a different patient with the same diagnosis demonstrates the classic and diagnostic low attenuation of the right adrenal gland, confirming the diagnosis of adenoma. *(A and B courtesy J William Charboneau.)*

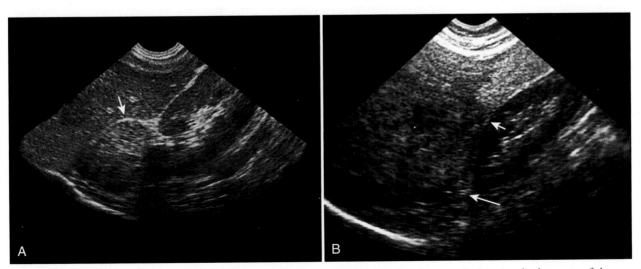

FIGURE 11-10. Retroperitoneal fat stripe displacement. Parasagittal sonograms. **A,** Anterior displacement of the retroperitoneal fat stripe *(arrow)* by a right adrenal cortical cancer. **B,** Posterior displacement of the retroperitoneal fat stripe *(arrows)* by a large hepatic adenoma.

genesis are unknown, although these lesions are thought to arise in the zona fasciculata of the adrenal cortex. Men and women are equally affected, with tumors most often occurring in the fifth or sixth decade of life. Myelolipomas are typically discovered incidentally in asymptomatic patients, with a 0.08% to 0.2% frequency at autopsy.[46] Although tumors can range in size from microscopic to 30 cm, most are less than 5 cm in diameter.[47] If these tumors undergo hemorrhage or necrosis or compress surrounding structures, symptoms may occur.

Imaging features of myelolipoma depend on the varying proportion of fat, myeloid element, hemorrhage, and calcification or ossification present. If a significant amount of fat is present, these tumors are typically seen sonographically as an echogenic mass in the adrenal bed (Fig. 11-11). When small, they may be difficult to differentiate from the adjacent echogenic retroperitoneal fat. **Propagation speed artifact** results from decreased sound velocity through fatty masses. **Apparent diaphragmatic disruption,** originally described by Richman et al.[48] with an adrenal myelolipoma, can result from this velocity change (Fig. 11-12). The presence of this artifact is good evidence as to the fatty nature of a mass. Musante et al.[46] found this artifact only when tumors were larger than 4 cm. The tumors may be homogeneous or heterogeneous and, if predominantly of myeloid component, will be isoechoic or hypoechoic. The heterogeneity may be caused by internal hemorrhage, which is common. Focal areas of calcification may be seen.

Computed tomography is very sensitive for the diagnosis of adrenal myelolipomas and should be performed to confirm the presence of macroscopic fat suspected sonographically (Fig. 11-12). Musante et al.[46] found that

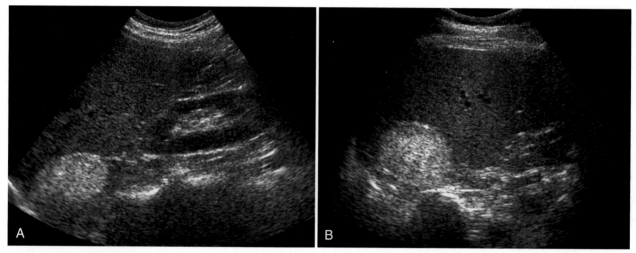

FIGURE 11-11. Myelolipoma. A, Sagittal, and **B,** transverse, sonograms show a homogeneous, highly echogenic, well-defined mass in the right adrenal gland.

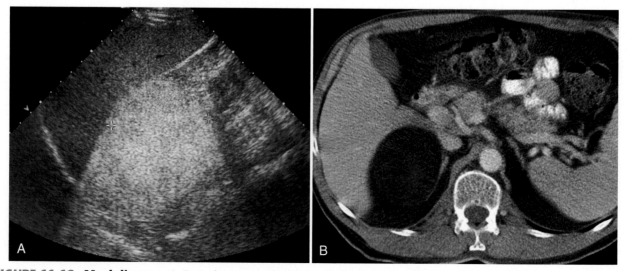

FIGURE 11-12. Myelolipoma. A, Sagittal sonogram shows a large, echogenic adrenal mass with apparent diaphragmatic disruption as a result of propagation speed artifact as the sound travels slower through the fatty mass than through the adjacent normal liver. **B,** Confirmatory CT demonstrates the presence of fat within the right adrenal mass. *(Courtesy J William Charboneau).*

unenhanced CT could explain confusing sonographic signs, including the demonstration of fat within isoechoic or hypoechoic, predominantly myeloid myelolipomas.

The differential diagnosis of a suprarenal fatty mass includes myelolipoma, renal angiomyolipoma, lipoma, retroperitoneal liposarcoma, lymphangioma, increased fat deposition, and teratoma.[49] If the adrenal origin of a fatty mass can be ascertained with imaging (US, CT, or MRI), the most likely diagnosis is adrenal myelolipoma. When large or atypical, fine-needle aspiration may be necessary to establish the diagnosis. The presence of mature fat cells and megakaryocytes is characteristic of adrenal myelolipoma.[49-51]

CAUSES OF FAT-CONTAINING SUPRARENAL MASS

Adrenal myelolipoma
Exophytic renal angiomyolipoma
Lipoma
Retroperitoneal liposarcoma
Retroperitoneal teratoma
Lymphangioma

Pheochromocytoma

Pheochromocytoma was first described by Frankel in 1886. Pheochromocytomas are usually **hyperfunctioning** tumors that secrete norepinephrine and epinephrine into the blood. The excess secretion of these catecholamines leads to the clinical manifestations of hypertension, pounding or severe headache, palpitations often with tachycardia, and excessive inappropriate perspiration.[52] These symptoms are often episodic.

Pheochromocytomas typically arise from the neuroectodermal tissue of the adrenal medulla. They are usually solitary, although 10% are bilateral. **Extraadrenal** pheochromocytomas occur in 10% of patients and have been described in the organ of Zuckerkandl, sympathetic nerve chains, aortic and carotid chemoreceptors, bladder, prostate, and chest. Multiple or extra-adrenal pheochromocytomas are more common in children.[53] From 10% to 13% of intra-adrenal pheochromocytomas and 40% of extra-adrenal pheochromocytomas are malignant.[16] Metastatic disease is the only reliable indicator of malignancy.

Pheochromocytomas are associated with many **neuroectodermal disorders,** including tuberous sclerosis, neurofibromatosis, von Hippel–Lindau disease, and multiple endocrine neoplasia IIa (50%) and IIb (90%).[16] Autopsy incidence of pheochromocytomas is about 0.1%, and the frequency in hypertensive patients is 0.4% to 2%.[54] This rare tumor occurs most frequently in adults between the fourth and sixth decades of life and is a curable cause of hypertension.

Biochemical screening is essential to confirm the diagnosis of pheochromocytoma, by measuring the level of **urinary catecholamines** and its metabolites **vanillylmandelic acid** (VMA) and **total metanephrines.**

Pathologically, pheochromocytomas are well encapsulated, weigh 90 to 100 g, and measure 5 to 6 cm in diameter.[54] The right gland is affected twice as frequently as the left gland. These tumors have a red-to-brown color on cut surface and microscopically demonstrate large pleomorphic cells with abundant cytoplasm and irregular nuclei. Calcification may be seen. Neurosecretory granules are seen ultrastructurally.[52]

Sonography has proved accurate in detecting adrenal pheochromocytomas, particularly because most are large and well marginated. In eight surgically confirmed cases of pheochromocytoma, Bowerman et al.[54] found that most were either heterogeneous or homogeneously solid. The heterogeneous tumors had areas of necrosis or hemorrhage (Fig. 11-13). Two tumors were predominantly cystic, which corresponded to old blood and necrotic debris, and one of these demonstrated a fluid-fluid level.

Extra-adrenal pheochromocytoma thought to lie in the retroperitoneum may be more difficult to localize with sonography because of body habitus and overlying bowel gas. In these patients, CT or MRI may be extremely useful for localization. For patients with suspected recurrent or metastatic disease, iodine-131 metaiodobenzylguanidine (^{131}I-MIBG) scintigraphy can play a significant role in screening.[55]

Multiple Endocrine Neoplasia

Multiple endocrine neoplasia (MEN) is a **familial** disease that is categorized into three types:
- **MEN I** affects pancreatic islets, the adrenal cortex, and pituitary and parathyroid glands.
- **MEN IIa** (Sipple's syndrome) includes medullary thyroid carcinoma, parathyroid hyperplasia, and pheochromocytoma.
- **MEN IIb** (III) includes all features of IIa, with marfanoid facies, mucosal neuromas, and gastrointestinal ganglioneuromatosis.

Inherited as an **autosomal dominant** trait, MEN II is believed to be caused by a genetic defect in the neural crest.[56] Pheochromocytomas in MEN syndromes are typically in the adrenal gland, usually bilateral (65%),[57] multicentric within the gland, more often malignant, and frequently asymptomatic. Patients diagnosed with MEN II should be screened biochemically and with imaging on a routine basis because they will eventually develop bilateral adrenal pheochromocytomas.

Rare Benign Tumors

Ganglioneuromas are benign tumors occurring most frequently in adults.[58] They are composed of ganglion and Schwann cells and arise most frequently in the sym-

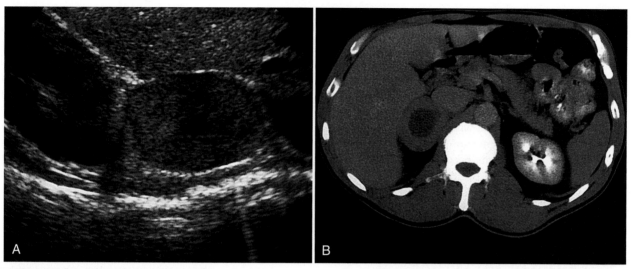

FIGURE 11-13. Pheochromocytoma. A, Transverse sonogram shows a solid right adrenal mass situated between the kidney and inferior vena cava. A central hypoechoic area corresponds to an area of necrosis. **B,** CT scan shows the large, partially necrotic tumor intimate to the posterior aspect of inferior vena cava.

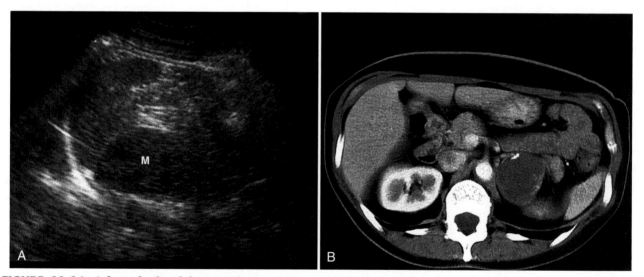

FIGURE 11-14. Adrenal gland hemangioma. A, Sagittal sonogram demonstrates a nonspecific solid mass *(M)* in the left adrenal gland. **B,** CT scan shows a nonspecific, enhancing, heterogeneous left adrenal mass with focal calcification.

pathetic chain, with 30% arising in the adrenal gland.[58] They are slow growing and usually clinically silent unless pressure phenomenon occurs. Rarely, ganglioneuromas increase urinary catecholamine levels, with symptoms of diarrhea, hypertension, and sweating.[58] Sonographically, they are solid and homogeneous and, because of their soft consistency, are pliable and change shape rather than displace organs.[59] The diagnosis can only be made histologically.

Hemangiomas of the adrenal gland are rare, benign, **nonhyperfunctioning** tumors. Most are small and discovered incidentally at autopsy. They may grow large and range from 2 to 15 cm in diameter.[60] Histologically, adrenal hemangiomas resemble hemangiomas elsewhere in the body and consist of **multiple dilated, endothelial-lined, blood-filled channels.**[61] Sonographically, they have a nonspecific structural pattern, with cystic, solid, and complex appearances. Calcification in the form of phleboliths may be seen[62] (Fig. 11-14). MRI has been useful in the differentiation of liver hemangiomas and may play a role in adrenal hemangiomas if the diagnosis is suspected. With time and growth, these lesions often hemorrhage; therefore surgical treatment is warranted.

Other rare benign adrenal tumors include **teratomas, lipomas, fibromas, leiomyomas, osteomas,** and **neurofibromas.** Radiologic findings are nonspecific. In most cases the diagnosis is made histologically.

MALIGNANT ADRENAL NEOPLASMS

Adrenocortical Cancer

Primary adrenal cortical (adrenocortical) cancer is a rare malignancy, with an incidence of 2 per million, and accounts for only 0.2% of all deaths from cancer.[63] It may arise from any of the layers in the adrenal cortex. Tumors may be **hyperfunctioning** (54%) or **nonhyperfunctioning** (46%).[63] Hyperfunctioning tumors are detected earlier because of the clinical manifestations of excess hormone production, including the following:

• Cushing's syndrome (most common)
• Adrenogenital syndrome (virilization or feminization)
• Precocious puberty
• Conn's syndrome (rare)

Hyperfunctioning tumors occur more often in females, whereas nonhyperfunctioning tumors are more common in males. Overall, adrenocortical cancer occurs more frequently in females. These tumors occur most often in the fourth decade, with equal frequency bilaterally. Tumors range in size from small to very large at presentation. On cut surface, they are predominantly yellow, with larger lesions exhibiting areas of hemorrhage and necrosis. Adrenocortical cancer is a highly malignant tumor and tends to invade the adrenal vein, IVC, and lymphatics[64] and to recur after surgery.

The sonographic appearance is variable, depending on the size of the mass. Hyperfunctioning tumors tend to be smaller when discovered and usually demonstrate a homogeneous echo pattern similar to renal cortex. The larger, nonhyperfunctioning lesions are more heterogeneous, with central areas of necrosis and hemorrhage. About 19% will demonstrate calcification. All lesions tend to be well defined with a lobulated border. Occasionally, a surrounding thin, echogenic, capsule-like rim is seen (27%).[63] Fishman et al.[65] suggested that this may represent a well-vascularized portion of the adrenocortical cancer and may be specific for this diagnosis.

Unfortunately, the sonographic appearance of adrenal masses does not allow differentiation between adenoma, carcinoma, pheochromocytoma, and metastases (Fig. 11-15). Smaller lesions are more likely benign, and larger masses with hemorrhage, necrosis, and calcification are more likely malignant (Fig. 11-16). If a large, necrotic, calcified adrenal mass is noted as an isolated finding, in the absence of a known primary tumor, adrenocortical cancer should be suspected. Sonography is an excellent screening method that allows rapid, noninvasive confirmation and localization of a lesion in patients clinically suspected of having an adrenal tumor. Duplex and color Doppler ultrasound are helpful to interrogate the veins for venous tumor extension, especially when other imaging modalities are equivocal. Ultrasound can be used to assess for metastatic spread and to guide fine-needle aspiration, which can be difficult when trying to differentiate adenoma from well-differentiated carcinoma.

Lymphoma

Primary lymphoma of the adrenal gland is rare but may arise from heterotrophic lymphoid elements occasionally found in normal adrenal glands.[66] More often, however, adrenal gland involvement is caused by **contiguous spread** from bulky retroperitoneal disease. **Non-Hodgkin's disease** is the most common cell type, with

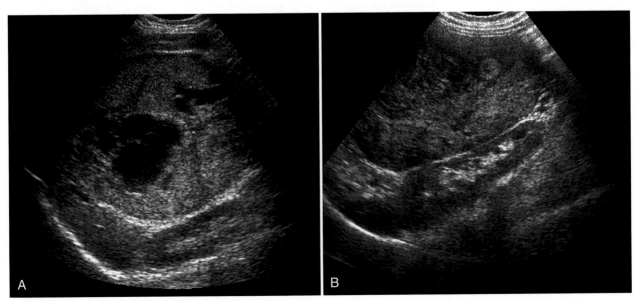

FIGURE 11-15. Large adrenal tumors. A, Adrenal pheochromocytoma. Sagittal sonogram of the left flank shows a large, complex mass with cystic components lying anterior to the left kidney. **B,** Adrenocortical carcinoma. Sagittal sonogram of the left flank shows an inhomogeneous solid mass anterior to the left kidney.

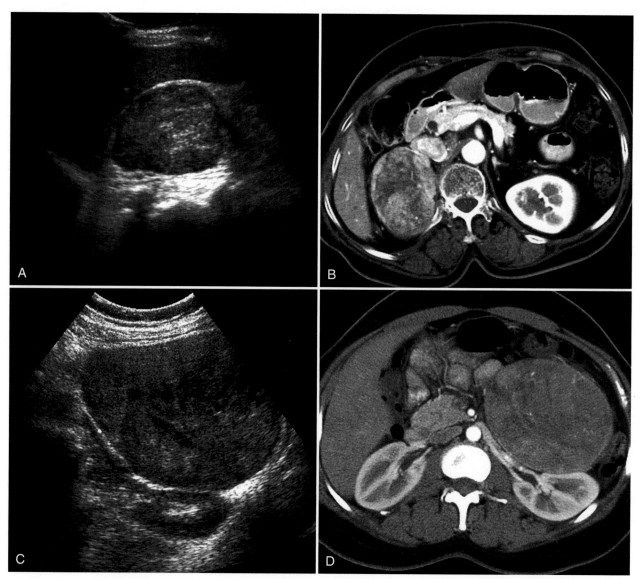

FIGURE 11-16. Adrenocortical carcinoma: value of localizing large flank mass to adrenal gland. A, Transverse sonogram, and **B,** corresponding CT scan, show a large, solid heterogeneous mass above the right kidney and impinging on posterior aspect of inferior vena cava. Right adrenal masses typically lie cephalad to the right kidney. **C,** Transverse sonogram, and **D,** corresponding CT scan, show a large, solid mass anterior to the left kidney. Left adrenal masses are often seen lying anterior to the left kidney.

4% of patients exhibiting discrete adrenal masses, often bilateral (46%).[67,68] Adrenal involvement is seen in 24% at autopsy.[67] After therapy, isolated adrenal gland recurrence may be seen. Necrosis and calcification within adrenal gland lymphoma are rare without prior treatment.[67]

On sonography, intranodal and extranodal lymphoma typically appears as a discrete or conglomerate hypoechoic mass (Fig. 11-17), likely related to the monotonous cell population within the tumor. Masses may be so hypoechoic as to simulate cysts; however, lack of appropriate through-transmission will indicate their solid nature.

Kaposi's Sarcoma

The adrenal glands of patients with AIDS demonstrate an increased incidence of both **opportunistic infection**

(CMV, histoplasmosis, *Candida, Cryptococcus,* herpesvirus, *Pneumocystis, Mycobacterium avium-intracellulare,* HIV, toxoplasmosis)[17,18,69,70] and **neoplasm** (Kaposi's sarcoma, lymphoma). If 90% or more of adrenal tissue is damaged by infection or tumor, frank adrenal insufficiency occurs.[71] This is often a late manifestation in AIDS patients.[69,70]

Sonographically, Kaposi's sarcoma of the adrenal gland is not well documented in the literature. A nonspecific solid mass with or without necrosis may be seen in the adrenal bed. Biopsy is necessary for confirmation (Fig. 11-18).

Metastases

The adrenal gland is the **fourth** most frequent site of metastatic disease after the lung, the liver, and bone. The

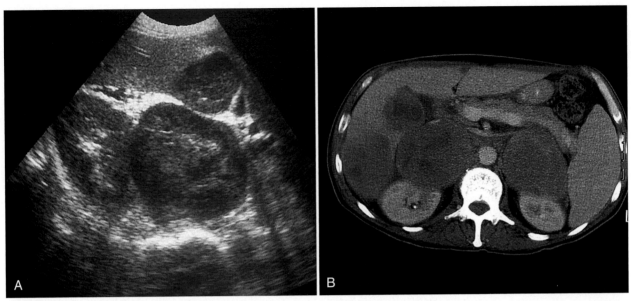

FIGURE 11-17. Adrenal lymphoma. A, Transverse sonogram shows a large, solid right adrenal mass as well as a large, solid hepatic mass in AIDS patient. **B,** CT scan shows bilateral solid adrenal masses, hepatic masses, and splenomegaly.

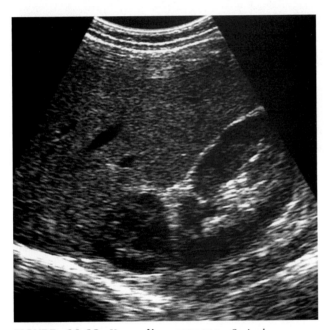

FIGURE 11-18. Kaposi's sarcoma. Sagittal sonogram shows a heterogeneous, predominantly solid right adrenal mass.

most common **primary tumors** giving rise to adrenal metastases include lung, breast, melanoma, kidney, thyroid, and colon cancer. Most are clinically silent. Although an adrenal mass found in a patient with a known primary malignancy is more likely to represent an adenoma than metastasis, accurate distinction between these two entities is necessary to guide patient management. The use of unenhanced CT, dynamic contrast analysis, and chemical shift MRI has significantly improved the ability to differentiate adrenal adenomas from metastatic lesions.[37] In some cases, PET-CT may play a complementary role.[43]

Adrenal metastases may be unilateral or bilateral and vary from microscopic deposits to enormous masses. Metastases are typically more heterogeneous, do not contain lipid, and demonstrate **delayed contrast washout** compared with adenomas. Central necrosis and hemorrhage may occur. Calcification in metastases is rare.[23]

Sonographically, the masses are solid and may demonstrate inhomogeneity because of necrosis or hemorrhage (Fig. 11-19). In some cases, percutaneous biopsy is necessary to confirm or exclude metastases. This may be performed with either ultrasound or CT guidance.

ADRENAL CYSTS

Adrenal cysts are rare benign lesions and are discovered most frequently as an incidental finding at autopsy, with a frequency of 0.06%.[72] Cysts are found with equal frequency on both sides and are typically unilateral, but may be bilateral in up to 15%.[73] Adrenal cysts can occur at any age but most often develop in the third through fifth decades. There is a 3 : 1 female preponderance.[74]

Most adrenal cysts are asymptomatic. With growth, however, cysts may cause symptoms related to displacement or compression of adjacent structures, including abdominal pain or discomfort, nausea, vomiting, and back pain. Adrenal cysts are classified into the following **four types** based on origin[61,75-77]:

- **Endothelial** (45%): angiomatous, lymphangiectatic, and hamartomatous
- **Pseudocysts** (39%): secondary to hemorrhage into normal adrenal gland or tumor
- **Epithelial** (9%)
- **Parasitic** (7%): most often, echinococcal infection

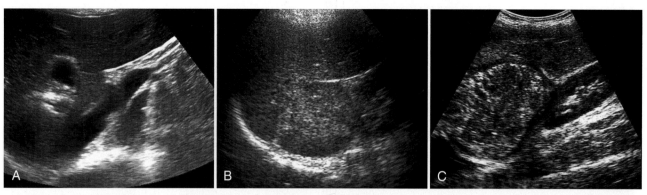

FIGURE 11-19. Right adrenal metastases in different patients. A, Sagittal sonogram shows a thickened adrenal that retains the shape of an adrenal limb. **B,** Sagittal sonogram shows a moderate-sized, solid mass superior to the kidney. **C,** Sagittal sonogram shows a large, inhomogeneous mass with a hypoechoic rim between the liver and upper pole of kidney.

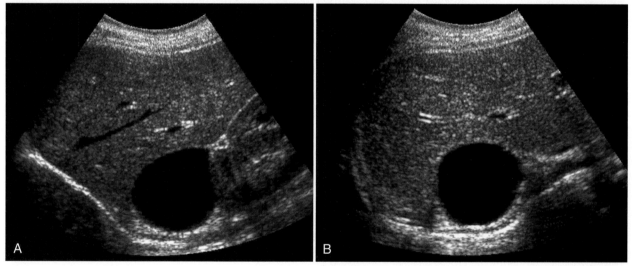

FIGURE 11-20. Adrenal cyst. A, Sagittal, and **B,** transverse, sonograms show a large, well-defined anechoic cyst with through-transmission.

Sonographically, adrenal cysts have the same characteristics as cysts elsewhere in the body (Fig. 11-20). They are usually round or oval with a thin, smooth wall. Good through-transmission is present, but internal debris is often noted. About 15% will display peripheral curvilinear wall calcification, usually in the pseudocysts and parasitic adrenal cysts (Fig. 11-21).

CYSTIC ADRENAL LESIONS

Pseudocyst
Endothelial cyst
Epithelial cyst
Infection (*Echinococcus,* abscess)
Necrotic neoplasm
Cystic pheochromocytoma
Lymphangioma

Percutaneous cyst aspiration showing **adrenal steroids** or **cholesterol** may be helpful to determine an adrenal origin if imaging techniques fail to do so.[74]

Adrenal cysts are benign and can be followed with serial imaging. If they are large and symptomatic, percutaneous aspiration, with or without sclerosis, or surgery may be necessary.

ADRENAL HEMORRHAGE

Spontaneous Hemorrhage

Spontaneous adrenal hemorrhage in the adult population is uncommon.[78] It is usually associated with **severe stress,** including septicemia, burns, trauma, and hypotension. It may also occur in patients with **hematologic abnormalities,** including thrombocytopenia and disseminated intravascular coagulation (DIC). Patients receiving **anticoagulation therapy** are also susceptible to adrenal hemorrhage, which usually occurs within the first 3 weeks after initiation of therapy.[61] Also, ligation and division of the right adrenal vein during **orthotopic liver transplantation** may cause venous congestion and hemorrhagic infarction or hematoma formation in

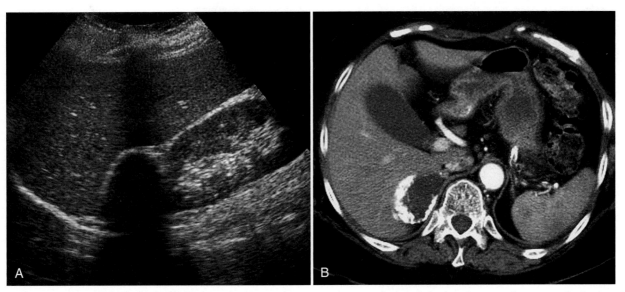

FIGURE 11-21. Adrenal pseudocyst. A, Sagittal sonogram shows a partially calcified adrenal mass with acoustic shadowing. **B,** CT scan shows a partially calcified cyst replacing the right adrenal gland. *(Courtesy Mitchell Tublin.)*

the right adrenal gland.[79] The resulting congested gland may rupture, causing excessive hemorrhage requiring reoperation.

Posttraumatic Hemorrhage

Posttraumatic adrenal hemorrhage may be present in up to 25% of severely injured patients.[80] Most patients will have ipsilateral thoracic, abdominal, or retroperitoneal injury.[81] The **right** adrenal gland is affected more often than the left. **Three mechanisms** have been proposed to explain traumatic adrenal hemorrhage, as follows[80,81]:

- Direct compression of the gland, with rupture of sinusoids and venules.
- Inferior vena cava compression, increasing right adrenal venous pressure as its vein drains directly into the IVC.
- Deceleration forces, causing shearing of small vessels and perforating the adrenal capsule.

Most often, the sonographic appearance of acute adrenal hemorrhage is a bright, echogenic mass in the adrenal bed, which becomes smaller and anechoic with time. Occasionally, an adrenal hemorrhage will initially appear as an anechoic mass, becoming more echoic with time (Fig. 11-22), likely because the initial hemorrhage consists of unclotted blood. With resolution of an adrenal hematoma, focal areas of calcification may develop. Most traumatic adrenal hematomas (83%) have a round or oval appearance and occur predominantly in the medulla.[81] The central hemorrhage may stretch or disrupt the cortex, resulting in periadrenal hemorrhage.

Unilateral adrenal hemorrhage has little clinical significance; however, patients with bilateral hemorrhage are at increased risk for development of **acute adrenal insufficiency.** It is crucial to exclude hemorrhage into a **preexisting underlying neoplasm;** therefore serial follow-up studies are necessary to document resolution of the adrenal hemorrhage, as done with sonography. Most hematomas will resolve with time, requiring no intervention.

DISORDERS OF METABOLISM

Hemochromatosis

Hemochromatosis may be primary (idiopathic) or secondary after repeated blood transfusions. Patients with **idiopathic hemochromatosis** have a defect in their intestinal mucosa that allows increased iron absorption and subsequent excess deposition in liver, pancreas, heart, spleen, kidneys, lymph nodes, endocrine glands, and skin. Clinically, they present with cirrhosis, diabetes mellitus, and hyperpigmentation.[82] Patients with **secondary hemochromatosis** have increased iron deposition in the reticuloendothelial cells of the spleen, liver, and bone marrow. Organ dysfunction does not usually occur.[82]

Excessive iron deposition in the adrenal glands often leads to **mild adrenocortical insufficiency,** but Addison's disease is rare.[83] The adrenal glands are usually small and may show increased attenuation on CT scan.

Wolman's Disease

Wolman's disease is a rare **autosomal recessive lipid storage disease** caused by a deficiency of liposomal acid lipase. Most patients die within 6 months of birth. The disease is characterized by marked hepatosplenomegaly

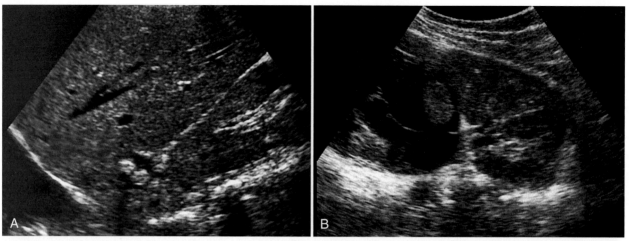

FIGURE 11-22. Spontaneous adrenal hemorrhage in two patients. A, Chronic hemorrhage. Sagittal sonogram shows two echogenic foci representing clotted blood in an enlarged right adrenal gland. **B, Acute hemorrhage.** Sagittal sonogram shows a large complex mass displacing the left kidney inferiorly and anteriorly.

and massive adrenal gland enlargement. The adrenal glands demonstrate diffuse punctate calcification.

ULTRASOUND-GUIDED INTERVENTION

Biopsy

Welch et al.[84] reviewed their 10-year experience with adrenal biopsy, which included 277 percutaneous biopsies in 270 patients. Sensitivity was 81%, specificity 99%, and accuracy 90%. Positive predictive value was 99%, and negative predictive value was 80%. Complication rate was 2.8%. Potential complications of percutaneous adrenal biopsy depend on the approach and include hematoma (0.05%-2.5%),[85] pneumothorax (most common),[85] pancreatitis (6%),[86] sepsis, and needle tract seeding. Needle biopsy of a pheochromocytoma may precipitate a hypertensive crisis and should be avoided.[87]

Most often, biopsies of the adrenal glands are performed with CT guidance. However, if the lesion is visible and readily accessible, ultrasound may be used to guide the procedure. Often, on the right, a transhepatic approach is chosen to avoid the pleural space (Fig. 11-23). On the left, a posterior, lateral, or anterior approach is chosen, depending on the lesion size and available safe access. A posterior approach is preferable to an anterior approach on the left in an attempt to avoid development of acute pancreatitis.

More recently, **endoscopic ultrasound** (EUS) has proved to be a safe, alternative method for adrenal gland sampling. Both left and right glands are readily accessible. In 24 patients with EUS-guided fine-needle aspiration of the adrenal glands, Jhala et al.[88] reported that adequate cellularity was obtained from all patients, with no significant complications.

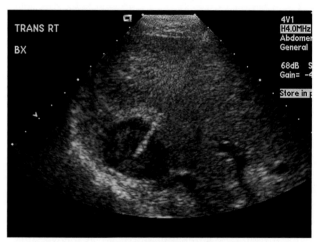

FIGURE 11-23. Percutaneous adrenal biopsy. Sagittal sonogram shows transhepatic placement of a needle (echogenic line) into a small right adrenal metastasis in a patient with lung cancer. (*Courtesy J. William Charboneau.*)

Drainage

Percutaneous drainage of an adrenal abscess or drainage and sclerosis of an adrenal cyst is possible provided safe access for catheter placement exists. Choice of catheter size depends on the viscosity of the material to be drained. Because of the deep location of the adrenal gland, these procedures are most frequently performed with CT guidance.

INTRAOPERATIVE ULTRASOUND

Intraoperative ultrasound with a 7.5-MHz transducer may be helpful when partial adrenalectomy is being performed. The exposed adrenal gland is scanned to allow precise localization of the pathology, which therefore allows the surgeon to obtain clear resection margins.

References

1. Cotran RS, Kumar V, Robbins SL, editors. Pathologic basis of disease. 5th ed. Philadelphia: Saunders; 1994. p. 1149-1165.

Embryology

2. Netter FH. The CIBA collection of medical illustrations. Vol. 4. Endocrine system and selected metabolic diseases. Summit, NJ: CIBA Pharmaceutical; 1981. p. 77-108.
3. Moore KL, editor. The developing human: clinically oriented embryology. 5th ed. Philadelphia: Saunders; 1993. p. 265-303.

Anatomy and Physiology

4. Mitty HA, Yeh HC. Radiology of the adrenals with sonography and CT. Philadelphia: Saunders; 1982.
5. Yeh HC, Mitty HA, Rose J, et al. Ultrasonography of adrenal masses: usual features. Radiology 1978;127:467-474.
6. Brownlie K, Kreel L. Computer assisted tomography of normal suprarenal glands. J Comput Assist Tomogr 1978;2:1-10.
7. Yeh HC. Ultrasonography of the adrenals. Semin Roentgenol 1988;23:250-258.
8. Yeh HC. Adrenal and retroperitoneal sonography. In: Leopold GR, editor. Ultrasound in breast and endocrine disorders. New York: Churchill Livingstone; 1984.
9. Mitty HA. Adrenal embryology, anatomy, and imaging techniques. In: Pollack HM, editor. Clinical urography: an atlas and textbook of urologic imaging. Philadelphia: Saunders; 1990. p. 2291-2305.
10. Oppenheimer DA, Carroll BA, Yousem S. Sonography of the normal neonatal adrenal gland. Radiology 1983;146:157-160.
11. Ma G, Liu SW, Zhao ZM, et al. Sectional anatomy of the adrenal gland in the coronal plane. Surg Radiol Anat 2008;30:271-280.
12. Marchal G, Gelin J, Verbeken E, et al. High-resolution real-time sonography of the adrenal glands: a routine examination? J Ultrasound Med 1986;5:65-68.
13. Lurie SN, Neelon FA. Physiology of the adrenal gland. In: Pollack HM, editor. Clinical urography: an atlas and textbook of urologic imaging. Philadelphia: Saunders; 1990. p. 2306-2312.

Adrenal sonography

14. Günther RW, Kelbel C, Lenner V. Real-time ultrasound of normal adrenal glands and small tumors. J Clin Ultrasound 1984;12:211-217.
15. Yeh HC. Sonography of the adrenal glands: normal glands and small masses. AJR Am J Roentgenol 1980;135:1167-1677.

Infectious Diseases

16. Shumam WP, Moss AA. The adrenal glands. In: Moss AA, Gamsu G, Genant H, editors. Computed tomography of the body with magnetic resonance imaging. Philadelphia: Saunders; 1992. p. 1021-1057.
17. Reznek RH, Armstrong P. The adrenal gland. Clin Endocrinol (Oxf) 1994;40:561-576.
18. Grizzle WE. Pathology of the adrenal gland. Semin Roentgenol 1988;23:323-331.
19. Dunnick NR. The adrenal gland. In: Taveras JM, Ferrucci T, editors. Radiology. Philadelphia: Lippincott; 1990.
20. Ilica AT, Kocaoglu M, Zeybek N, et al. Extrahepatic abdominal hydatid disease caused by *Echinococcus granulosus:* imaging findings. AJR Am J Roentgenol 2007;189:337-343.
21. O'Brien WM, Choyke PL, Copeland J, et al. Computed tomography of adrenal abscess. J Comput Assist Tomogr 1987;11:550-551.
22. Atkinson Jr GO, Kodroff MB, Gay Jr BB, Ricketts RR. Adrenal abscess in the neonate. Radiology 1985;155:101-104.

Benign Adrenal Neoplasms

23. Dunnick NR, Korobkin M, Francis I. Adrenal radiology: distinguishing benign from malignant adrenal masses. AJR Am J Roentgenol 1996;167:861-867.
24. Mayo-Smith WW, Boland GW, Noto RB, Lee MJ. State-of-the-art adrenal imaging. Radiographics 2001;21:995-1012.
25. Ambos MA, Bosniak MA, Lefleur RS, Mitty HA. Adrenal adenoma associated with renal cell carcinoma. AJR Am J Roentgenol 1981;136:81-84.
26. Painter TA, Jagelman DG. Adrenal adenomas and adrenal carcinomas in association with hereditary adenomatosis of the colon and rectum. Cancer 1985;55:2001-2004.
27. Commons RR, Callaway CP. Adenomas of the adrenal cortex. Arch Med Int 1948;81:37-41.
28. Dunnick NR. Hanson lecture. Adrenal imaging: current status. AJR Am J Roentgenol 1990;154:927-936.
29. Conn JW. Primary aldosteronism. J Lab Clin Med 1955;45:661-664.
30. Slee PH, Schaberg A, Van Brummelen P. Carcinoma of the adrenal cortex causing primary hyperaldosteronism: a case report and review of the literature. Cancer 1983;51:2341-2345.
31. Conn JW, Knopf RF, Nesbit RM. Clinical characteristics of primary aldosteronism from an analysis of 145 cases. Am J Surg 1964;107:159-172.
32. Grant CS, Carpenter P, van Heerden JA, Hamberger B. Primary aldosteronism: clinical management. Arch Surg 1984;119:585-590.
33. Hubbard MM, Husami TW, Abumrad NN. Nonfunctioning adrenal tumors: dilemmas in management. Am Surg 1989;55:516-522.
34. Bitter DA, Ross DS. Incidentally discovered adrenal masses. Am J Surg 1989;158:159-161.
35. Grumbach MM, Biller BM, Braunstein GD, et al. Management of the clinically inapparent adrenal mass ("incidentaloma"). Ann Intern Med 2003;138:424-429.
36. Mansmann G, Lau J, Balk E, et al. The clinically inapparent adrenal mass: update in diagnosis and management. Endocr Rev 2004;25:309-340.
37. Dunnick NR, Korobkin M. Imaging of adrenal incidentalomas: current status. AJR Am J Roentgenol 2002;179:559-568.
38. Boland GW, Lee MJ, Gazelle GS, et al. Characterization of adrenal masses using unenhanced CT: an analysis of the CT literature. AJR Am J Roentgenol 1998;171:201-204.
39. Caoili EM, Korobkin M, Francis IR, et al. Adrenal masses: characterization with combined unenhanced and delayed enhanced CT. Radiology 2002;222:629-633.
40. McNicholas MM, Lee MJ, Mayo-Smith WW, et al. An imaging algorithm for the differential diagnosis of adrenal adenomas and metastases. AJR Am J Roentgenol 1995;165:1453-1459.
41. Korobkin M, Giordano TJ, Brodeur FJ, et al. Adrenal adenomas: relationship between histologic lipid and CT and MR findings. Radiology 1996;200:743-747.
42. Outwater EK, Siegelman ES, Huang AB, Birnbaum BA. Adrenal masses: correlation between CT attenuation value and chemical shift ratio at MR imaging with in-phase and opposed-phase sequences. Radiology 1996;200:749-752.
43. Blake MA, Slattery JM, Kalra MK, et al. Adrenal lesions: characterization with fused PET/CT image in patients with proved or suspected malignancy: -initial experience. Radiology 2006;238:970-977.
44. Gore RM, Callen PW, Filly RA. Displaced retroperitoneal fat: sonographic guide to right upper quadrant mass localization. Radiology 1982;142:701-705.
45. Rao P, Kenney PJ, Wagner BJ, Davidson AJ. Imaging and pathologic features of myelolipoma. Radiographics 1997;17:1373-1385.
46. Musante F, Derchi LE, Zappasodi F, et al. Myelolipoma of the adrenal gland: sonographic and CT features. AJR Am J Roentgenol 1988;151:961-964.
47. Noble MJ, Montague DK, Levin HS. Myelolipoma: an unusual surgical lesion of the adrenal gland. Cancer 1982;49:952-958.
48. Richman TS, Taylor KJW, Kremkau FW. Propagation speed artifact in a fatty tumor (myelolipoma): significance for tissue differential diagnosis. J Ultrasound Med 1983;2:45-47.
49. Vick CW, Zeman RK, Mannes E, et al. Adrenal myelolipoma: CT and ultrasound findings. Urol Radiol 1984;6:7-13.
50. DeBlois GG, DeMay RM. Adrenal myelolipoma diagnosis by computed-tomography-guided fine-needle aspiration: a case report. Cancer 1985;55:848-850.
51. Galli L, Gaboardi F. Adrenal myelolipoma: report of diagnosis by fine needle aspiration. J Urol 1986;136:655-657.
52. Korobkin M. Pheochromocytoma. In: Pollack HM, editor. Clinical urography: an atlas and textbook of urologic imaging. Philadelphia: Saunders; 1990. p. 2347-2361.
53. Manger WM, Gifford Jr RW. Pheochromocytoma: diagnosis and management. NY State J Med 1980;80:216-226.
54. Bowerman RA, Silver TM, Jaffe MH, et al. Sonography of adrenal pheochromocytomas. AJR Am J Roentgenol 1981;137:1227-1231.
55. Quint LE, Glazer GM, Francis IR, et al. Pheochromocytoma and paraganglioma: comparison of MR imaging with CT and I-131 MIBG scintigraphy. Radiology 1987;165:89-93.

56. Cho KJ, Freier DT, McCormick TL, et al. Adrenal medullary disease in multiple endocrine neoplasia type II. AJR Am J Roentgenol 1980;134:23-29.

57. Brunt LM, Wells Jr SA. The multiple endocrine neoplasia syndromes. Invest Radiol 1985;20:916-927.

58. Silverman ML, Lee AK. Anatomy and pathology of the adrenal glands. Urol Clin North Am 1989;16:417-432.

59. Bosniak M. Neoplasms of the adrenal medulla. In: Pollack HM, editor. Clinical urography: an atlas and textbook of urologic imaging. Philadelphia: Saunders; 1990. p. 2344-2346.

60. Vargas AD. Adrenal hemangioma. Urology 1980;16:389-390.

61. Rumanick WM, Bosniak M. Miscellaneous conditions of the adrenals and adrenal pseudotumors. In: Pollack HM, editor. Clinical urography: an atlas and textbook of urologic imaging. Philadelphia: Saunders; 1990. p. 2399-2412.

62. Derchi LE, Rapaccini GL, Banderali A, et al. Ultrasound and CT findings in two cases of hemangioma of the adrenal gland. J Comput Assist Tomogr 1989;13:659-661.

Malignant Adrenal Neoplasms

63. Hamper UM, Fishman EK, Hartman DS, et al. Primary adrenocortical carcinoma: sonographic evaluation with clinical and pathologic correlation in 26 patients. AJR Am J Roentgenol 1987;148:915-919.

64. Ritchey ML, Kinard R, Novicki DE. Adrenal tumors: involvement of the inferior vena cava. J Urol 1987;138:1134-1136.

65. Fishman EK, Deutch BM, Hartman DS, et al. Primary adrenocortical carcinoma: CT evaluation with clinical correlation. AJR Am J Roentgenol 1987;148:531-535.

66. Glazer HS, Lee JK, Balfe DM, et al. Non-Hodgkin lymphoma: computed tomographic demonstration of unusual extranodal involvement. Radiology 1983;149:211-217.

67. Vicks BS, Perusek M, Johnson J, Tio F. Primary adrenal lymphoma: CT and sonographic appearances. J Clin Ultrasound 1987;15:135-139.

68. Feldberg MA, Hendriks MJ, Klinkhamer AC. Massive bilateral non-Hodgkin's lymphomas of the adrenals. Urol Radiol 1986;8:85-88.

69. Freda PU, Wardlaw SL, Brudney K, Goland RS. Primary adrenal insufficiency in patients with the acquired immunodeficiency syndrome: a report of five cases. J Clin Endocrinol Metab 1994;79:1540-1545.

70. Donovan DS, Dluhy RG. AIDS and its effect on the adrenal gland. Endocrinologist 1991;1:227-232.

71. Findling JW, Buggy BP, Gilson IH, et al. Longitudinal evaluation of adrenocortical function in patients infected with the human immunodeficiency virus. J Clin Endocrinol Metab 1994;79:1091-1096.

Adrenal Cysts

72. Wahl HR. Adrenal cysts. Am J Pathol 1951;27:758.

73. Scheible W, Coel M, Siemers PT, Siegel H. Percutaneous aspiration of adrenal cysts. AJR Am J Roentgenol 1977;128:1013-1016.

74. Tung GA, Pfister RC, Papanicolaou N, Yoder IC. Adrenal cysts: imaging and percutaneous aspiration. Radiology 1989;173:107-110.

75. Kearney GP, Mahoney EM. Adrenal cysts. Urol Clin North Am 1977;4:273-283.

76. Abeshouse GA, Goldstein RB, Abeshouse BS. Adrenal cysts: review of the literature and report of three cases. J Urol 1959;81:711-719.

77. Barron SH, Emanuel B. Adrenal cyst: a case report and a review ok the pediatric literature. J Pediatr 1961;59:592-599.

Adrenal Hemorrhage

78. Kawashima A, Sandler CM, Ernst RD, et al. Imaging of nontraumatic hemorrhage of the adrenal gland. Radiographics 1999;19:949-963.

79. Bowen AD, Keslar PJ, Newman B, Hashida Y. Adrenal hemorrhage after liver transplantation. Radiology 1990;176:85-88.

80. Murphy BJ, Casillas J, Yrizarry JM. Traumatic adrenal hemorrhage: radiologic findings. Radiology 1988;169:701-703.

81. Burks DW, Mirvis SE, Shanmuganathan K. Acute adrenal injury after blunt abdominal trauma: CT findings. AJR Am J Roentgenol 1992;158:503-507.

Disorders of Metabolism

82. Baron RL, Freeny PC, Moss AA. The liver. In: Moss AA, Gamsu G, Genant H, editors. CT of the body with magnetic resonance imaging. Philadelphia: Saunders: 1992. p. 735-821.

83. Doppman JL. Adrenal cortical hypofunction. In: Pollack HM, editor. Clinical urography: an atlas and textbook of urologic imaging. Philadelphia: Saunders; 1990. p. 2338-2343.

Ultrasound-Guided Intervention

84. Welch TJ, Sheedy 2nd PF, Stephens DH, et al. Percutaneous adrenal biopsy: review of a 10-year experience. Radiology 1994;193:341-344.

85. Zornoza J. Fine-needle biopsy of lymph nodes, adrenal glands and periureteral tissues. In: Pollack HM, editor. Clinical urography: an atlas and textbook of urologic imaging. Philadelphia: Saunders; 1990. p. 2854-2860.

86. Kane NM, Korobkin M, Francis IR, et al. Percutaneous biopsy of left adrenal masses: prevalence of pancreatitis after anterior approach. AJR Am J Roentgenol 1991;157:777-780.

87. Casola G, Nicolet V, van Sonnenberg E, et al. Unsuspected pheochromocytoma: risk of blood-pressure alterations during percutaneous adrenal biopsy. Radiology 1986;159:733-735.

88. Jhala NC, Jhala D, Eloubeidi MA, et al. Endoscopic ultrasound-guided fine-needle aspiration biopsy of the adrenal glands: analysis of 24 patients. Cancer 2004;102:308-314.

CHAPTER 12

The Retroperitoneum

Raymond E. Bertino, Nathan A. Saucier, and Daryl J. Barth

Chapter Outline

*O*ther than examination of the solid organs, ultrasound of the retroperitoneum is most often used in the diagnosis of **arterial vascular disease.**

ATHEROSCLEROSIS

The major cause of disease in human arteries is atherosclerosis.[1] It is the main cause of cardiovascular diseases, including heart disease, cerebrovascular accident (CVA, stroke), hypertension, and peripheral vascular disease. It is a primary contributor to several other conditions, such as heart failure, arrhythmias (including atrial fibrillation), and cardiomyopathy. **Cardiovascular disease (CVD)** has been the leading cause of death in the United States every year since 1900 except during the 1918 flu epidemic.[2]

However, there has been progress. Death rates from CVD dropped 27.0% between 1995 and 2005.[2] In 2005, CVD was listed as the underlying cause of death in 856,030 deaths. In 2005, **ischemic heart disease,** when considered separately from other cardiovascular diseases, was still by far the single leading cause of death (445,687 deaths) in the United States.[3] Stroke, when considered separately from other cardiovascular

diseases, was the third leading cause (143,579 deaths). According to the American Heart Association (AHA), if all major forms of heart and blood vessel disease were eliminated, U.S. life expectancy would rise by almost 7 years.[4]

Atherosclerosis is a complex process. It starts with injury to the endothelium, which results in increased permeability of the intima, allowing accumulation of low-density lipoprotein into the arterial wall.[5] Inflammation results and **plaque** is produced, consisting of lipids, smooth muscle cells, fibrous tissue, macrophages, and calcium within the arterial wall.[6,7] Hemorrhage may also be present within the plaque. Atherosclerotic plaque can cause decreased blood flow to target organs by narrowing the arterial lumen, which can result in ischemic signs and symptoms such as claudication and erectile dysfunction **(aortoiliac disease),** hypertension and renal insufficiency **(renal artery disease),** and mesenteric ischemia **(mesenteric artery disease).**

The processes inherent in atherosclerosis are also believed to contribute to aneurysm formation. Although there are other causes of aneurysms, including cystic medial necrosis, trauma, and infection, atherosclerosis is believed to account for approximately 90% of abdominal aortic aneurysms.

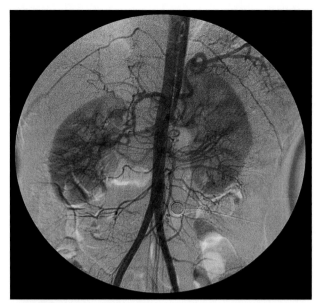

FIGURE 12-1. Abdominal aorta anatomy. The abdominal aorta tapers from the aortic hiatus to the aortic bifurcation. Much of the tapering occurs as it gives off its largest branch vessels: the celiac, superior mesenteric, and renal arteries.

ABDOMINAL AORTIC ANEURYSM

The abdominal aorta slowly tapers from the diaphragmatic hiatus to the aortic bifurcation (Fig. 12-1). Most of the tapering occurs in the proximal abdominal aorta as its largest branches (celiac, superior mesenteric, and renal arteries) arise. The normal size of the supraceliac abdominal aorta ranges from 2.5 to 2.7 cm in men and 2.1 to 2.3 cm in women. The normal diameter of the infrarenal aorta ranges from 2.0 to 2.4 cm in men and 1.7 to 2.2 cm in women.[8]

Mortality

Abdominal aortic aneurysm (AAA) is a common disease in the elderly population. Annually, 33,000 patients undergo elective repair in the United States.[9] AAA rupture is a catastrophic event accounting for 8500 in-hospital deaths per year.[10] Many patients with ruptured aneurysms die before reaching a hospital. Of those admitted with rupture, many do not survive to go to surgery. Of those who have surgery, the 30-day operative mortality is 50%. The overall mortality of a ruptured AAA is in the range of 80%.[10] Mortality for those undergoing elective repair is 3% to 5%.[11] These facts suggest that the majority of deaths from AAA ruptures are preventable (Fig. 12-2).

Much research has been conducted on reducing mortality from AAAs. Ultrasound screening has proved to be a cost-effective step. Medical therapies may reduce the rate of growth of AAAs once detected. For large aneurysms, surgical or endovascular repair is much safer when

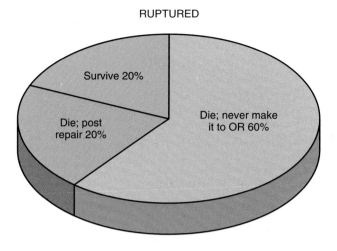

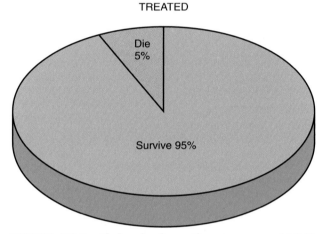

FIGURE 12-2. Abdominal aortic aneurysm (AAA) rupture: survival. Instead of the 20% of patients with a ruptured AAA who survive *(green wedge),* if AAA is treated before rupture, 95% survive.

done electively than emergently. With this knowledge, AAA mortality can be greatly reduced.

Definition

There are many definitions of an arterial aneurysm.[12] A general definition is an increase in the diameter of an artery of at least 50% compared to the normal diameter of that artery.[8] For example, if a patient has an aorta that measures 2.2 cm in diameter, the aorta would be classified as aneurysmal at 3.3 cm. This definition can be difficult to apply to an abdominal aorta because it may not be clear what constitutes the normal aortic diameter in a specific patient.

The majority of AAAs are infrarenal. The most practical and common definition of **infrarenal** AAA specifies that an aneurysm is present when the infrarenal aorta has a diameter of 3.0 cm or greater. This definition works well in most situations. However, the definition can be insufficient, particularly in small patients. It should be remembered that an aorta measuring 2.5 cm in diameter

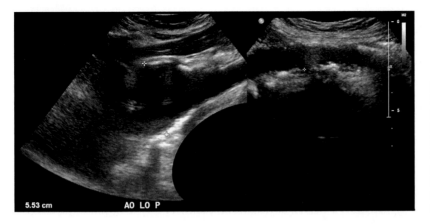

FIGURE 12-3. Isolated aneurysms of the suprarenal abdominal aorta are rare. Most suprarenal AAAs will extend also to involve the thoracic aorta above the diaphragm. Isolated suprarenal AAAs are included in the Crawford classification of thoracoabdominal aneurysms. Longitudinal ultrasound scan shows isolated suprarenal abdominal aortic aneurysm measuring 5.5 cm in a patient with an abdominal aortic diameter of 1.45 cm.

is properly called **aneurysmal** in a patient who has a more proximal aortic diameter measuring 1.6 cm.

Aneurysms that involve the renal arteries or the suprarenal aorta are less common and usually occur with an aneurysmal thoracic aorta. AAAs that occur at or above the renal arteries are included in the Crawford classification of thoracoabdominal aneurysms[13] (Fig. 12-3). The literature almost exclusively uses the term "abdominal aortic aneurysm" to refer to infrarenal aneurysms.

Pathophysiology

Arteries have three layers: intima, media, and adventitia. The **intima,** the inner layer, is composed of the endothelium and the internal elastic lamina, along with scant intervening tissue.[1] The **adventitia,** the outer layer, consists of connective tissue and carries nerves and the vaso vasorum.[5]

The **media** supplies much of the strength of the aorta and consists of elastin, collagen, smooth muscle cells, and extracellular matrix proteins. Elastin is only minimally produced in adult humans. With age there is a progressive loss of **elastin** in the body. Specifically, an aneurysmal aorta has a significant decrease in elastin content.[14] Destruction of elastin is mediated by enzymes such as matrix metalloproteinases (MMPs).[15] Medications may be able to reduce the rate of elastin destruction, either by suppression of the MMPs or inhibiting other biochemical pathways, and show promise in reducing the rate of AAA growth.[16] Statins and doxycycline are known inhibitors of MMP enzymes.

Natural History and Medical Therapy

Abdominal aortic aneurysm is a disease of elderly persons. AAAs are rare before age 50 and affect men four times more often than women. The risk of developing an AAA also increases with smoking and with a family history of AAA in a first-degree relative. Other factors that increase risk are a history of peripheral vascular disease, cardiovascular disease, and hypertension.[17] AAAs typically

increase in diameter at a rate of 1.7 to 2.6 mm per year. This rate of growth increases as the AAA becomes larger.[17] The rate of growth is faster in women.[18,19]

As the size of the AAA increases, the risk of rupture increases. Rupture is rare when the AAA is less than 4.0 cm in diameter, with a 0.3% risk per year. The rate of rupture increases to 1.9% when the AAA is 4 to 5 cm and to 6.5% for AAAs 5.0 to 6 cm in diameter. Although data for larger aneurysms are conflicting, when the diameter is greater than 6.0 cm, clearly the risk of rupture is significantly higher.[20,21] Other risk factors for rupture include current smoking and chronic obstructive pulmonary disease (COPD). In addition, the rupture rate for women is four times that of men.[22] Rupture in women occurs in smaller aneurysms, although the exact amount of increased risk is not well quantified. Because smaller AAAs in women have a risk similar to larger ones in men, the recommendation is that elective treatment in women should occur at a smaller aneurysm size than in men.[19] Recommendations about how much smaller vary from 3 mm to greater than 5 mm.

Current medical therapy is limited in its ability to prevent the growth of an AAA. Contradictory evidence surrounds whether smoking cessation[23] and control of hypertension is effective in decreasing the rate of AAA growth. Statins and doxycycline may reduce the rate of aneurysm growth.[24-26] Other promising medications in animal and in vitro studies include angiotensin II inhibitors and anti-inflammatory medications.

Screening

Recent Studies

The malady of AAA meets the 10 World Health Organization (WHO) criteria for the institution of screening programs.[27] Research has been extensive, particularly in Europe, on the effectiveness and cost-effectiveness of ultrasound screening for AAA. One large trial, the U.K. Multicentre Aneurysm Screening Study (MASS), documented a risk reduction of 42% in aneurysm-related deaths in a population of men age 65 to 74 years.[28] The study concluded that the cost per quality adjusted life year (QALY) was within the margin of acceptability for the British National Health Service.[29] A Danish trial had a reduction of in-hospital mortality of 68% for a group screened for AAA, concluding that AAA screening with ultrasound was cost-effective.[30] With few studies done, information on the utility of AAA screening in women remains inconclusive.[27]

A meta-analysis commissioned by the U.S. Preventive Services Task Force (USPSTF) combined analyses from a total of four studies, including the two European studies just mentioned. The study concluded that "for men age 65 to 75, an invitation to attend AAA screening reduces AAA-related mortality."[31] Based on these results, in 2005 the following recommendation was published[32]:

> The USPSTF recommends one-time screening for abdominal aortic aneurysm (AAA) by ultrasonography in men aged 65 to 75 who have ever smoked.
>
> Rationale: The USPSTF found good evidence that screening for AAA and surgical repair of large AAAs (5.5 cm or more) in men aged 65 to 75 who have ever smoked (current and former smokers) leads to decreased AAA-specific mortality. There is good evidence that abdominal ultrasonography, performed in a setting with adequate quality assurance (i.e., in an accredited facility with credentialed technologists), is an accurate screening test for AAA. There is also good evidence of important harms of screening and early treatment, including an increased number of surgeries with associated clinically significant morbidity and mortality, and short-term psychological harms. Based on the moderate magnitude of net benefit, the USPSTF concluded that the benefits of screening for AAA in men aged 65 to 75 who have ever smoked outweigh the harms.

The USPTF found that AAA mortality is also reduced by conducting screening for men with a negative smoking history. However, the magnitude of the mortality benefit was significantly smaller in nonsmokers, and the USPSTF concluded that the benefit did not clearly outweigh the negatives of screening (e.g., cost, anxiety of identified patients).[32]

Subsequently, the Screening Abdominal Aortic Aneurysms Very Efficiently (SAAAVE) Act was passed by the U.S. Congress and signed on February 8, 2006. Since January 1, 2007, Medicare has covered a one-time, ultrasound screening to check for AAA in qualified seniors. Qualified patients are men with a history of smoking (i.e., those who have smoked more than 100 cigarettes total during their lives) and men and women with a family history of AAA in a first-degree relative. To be covered, patients must undergo the AAA screening study as part of the Welcome to Medicare Physical Exam (WTMPE) and complete the screening within the first 6 months of Medicare eligibility.

Ultrasound Approach

Screening for AAA must have high sensitivity. It is mandatory that the entire infrarenal abdominal aorta be examined. The screening ultrasound has one of three results: positive, negative, or indeterminate. The number of expected indeterminate exams should be very low, much less than 5%.

There are currently two paradigms for ultrasound in the screening of AAAs. The first is embodied in the current guidelines issued by the American College of Radiology (ACR) and involves obtaining a full set of documentation images on every patient.[33] When the screening examination is positive for AAA, the recommended images are adequate to document aneurysm size accurately. The screening examination thus also serves as the first diagnostic exam. This type of screening exam is not very different from a full "diagnostic" examination and is probably the most common type in radiology departments performing high volumes of ultrasound.

The second paradigm has been used by several mobile companies offering aneurysm screening to the general population. These for-profit programs are prepaid by the individuals requesting screening; profit is based on doing a high volume of cases within a short time, keeping cost to a minimum. It is unclear whether adequate quality control mechanisms are in place for these exams, which often have only two possible results: positive and negative. Positive exams do not result in extension of the study to be diagnostic. Instead, a positive exam results in a recommendation to the patient to have a diagnostic evaluation. This allows the provider to save time and reduce cost.

The decreased cost of this type of examination offers a potential benefit. If the low cost of this type of service could be widely reproduced, and if the issue of quality control were addressed, screening that is both accurate and cost-effective could become available for a wider segment of the population.

Surveillance

Once an AAA is discovered, the patient moves from screening to a surveillance program, in which the aneurysm size is periodically checked. Because an AAA tends to grow more rapidly as its size increases, there is general agreement that a smaller aneurysm needs to be checked less frequently than a larger one. Otherwise, however, consensus is lacking on frequency of sonographic surveillance. Recommendations for assessing aneurysms less than 4.0 cm in diameter range from 1 to 3 years.[34] For the U.K. Small Aneurysm Trial, Brady et al.[35] concluded that surveillance could be performed at intervals of 36, 24, 12, and 3 months for aneurysms of 35, 40, 45, and 50 mm, respectively. Following this schedule, the risk of the AAA size on recheck being greater than 55 mm would be less than 1%. Achieving a 5% rate would require even less frequent surveillance.

Because of these results, our group's aneurysm clinic has moved to new guidelines for the surveillance of aneurysms. We now follow AAAs sonographically every 2 years when the aneurysm is less than 40 mm, every year for aneurysms 40 to 44 mm, and every 6 months once the aneurysm reaches 45 mm. As experience with surveillance programs progresses, we likely will follow AAAs even less frequently.

Surveillance of aneurysms lends itself well to being followed by a database. Our interventional radiology clinic started a database in 2003 to follow AAAs.[36] The service is offered to referring physicians of patients with known AAAs of any size, and patients are entered into the database as desired by the referrer. The clinic then orders all subsequent aortic ultrasounds and monitors all results. We found that primary care physicians are very receptive to the service. Patients are seen once in our interventional radiology clinic so that they can meet the physicians and advanced-practice nurses involved and can be informed about their disease, its treatment, and how their aneurysm is to be followed. After that first visit, all communication is by phone and by mail. The database is monitored periodically to make sure patients keep their appointments. When the aneurysm approaches treatment size, 4.5 cm in greatest diameter, patients again begin to be seen regularly in the clinic.

Sonographic Technique

Pertinent history should be obtained when doing surveillance on a known aneurysm. Questions of interest are whether the patient has back and/or abdominal pain or tenderness. These symptoms are considered an indication for aneurysm treatment.

The following principles apply both to screening examinations and studies for surveillance. Evaluation of the entire infrarenal aorta is necessary. Identifying the **aortic bifurcation** guarantees that one has seen far enough distally. By identifying the celiac, superior mesenteric, or renal arteries or the aortic hiatus of the diaphragm, one can guarantee that the proximal examination has been carried high enough. Images should be obtained in both transverse and longitudinal planes. The goal is to find the maximum diameter of the aorta, measured from outer edge of the wall to outer edge of the opposite wall. Measurements should be taken perpendicular to the axis of the lumen of the aorta. To guarantee that the measurement is perpendicular, longitudinal images are often best at obtaining the most accurate measurements (Fig. 12-4).

Most infrarenal aneurysms are **fusiform** in shape with a relatively circular cross section. With a fusiform aneurysm, measurement of its size taken from any longitudinal plane through the aorta will be the same (Fig. 12-5). The walls of the aorta are generally well seen with longitudinal imaging because they are parallel to the face of the transducer, resulting in a strong echo from the walls. Transverse imaging is particularly important to identify the smaller proportion of aneurysms that are eccentric. If the aneurysm is **eccentric,** the measurement must

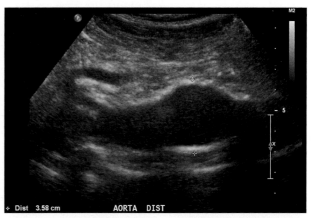

FIGURE 12-4. Measuring abdominal aorta. AAA measurements from longitudinal images are usually the most accurate, taken perpendicular to the lumen. The measurement includes both the front and the back walls, which generally are well seen.

be taken in the plane of the aneurysm's eccentricity to find the largest diameter of the aneurysm (Figs. 12-6 and 12-7).

We routinely image patients from two windows: the **anterior abdominal midline,** which allows imaging of the maximum length of the abdominal aorta, and the **left flank,** with the patient in the right lateral decubitus position. The middle and distal abdominal aorta is often better seen in this position, particularly with an obese patient. The proximal common iliac arteries may also be better seen in this position.

We obtain longitudinal and transverse cine loops from an anterior window and from a left lateral window. The **longitudinal cine loops** allow for easy remeasurement of the aorta. The **transverse cine loops** allow the reviewing physician to determine whether there is eccentricity of the aneurysm.

Computed Tomography

Computed tomography (CT) has a limited role in AAA screening and surveillance but should be used in any of the following situations:

1. The patient is so obese or otherwise difficult to image that whether the aneurysm may be eccentric cannot be determined with reasonable certainty on initial scanning. Once the aneurysm is shown to be fusiform, performing some or even most of the further surveillance with ultrasound is probably reasonable.
2. The aneurysm is known to be eccentric, and the area of eccentricity is not optimally seen with ultrasound.
3. The patient is acutely symptomatic (including emergency room patients).
4. Portions of the iliac arteries that are known to be aneurysmal are not well seen.

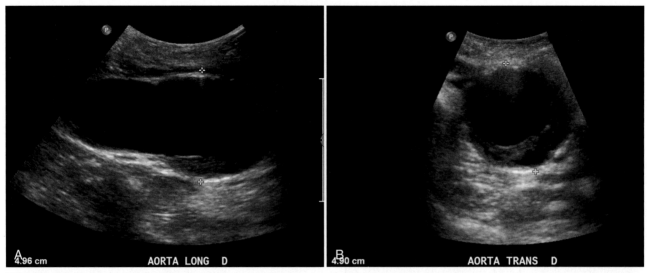

FIGURE 12-5. Most abdominal aortic aneurysms are fusiform. With this configuration, the AAA is circular in cross section. **A,** Longitudinal, and **B,** transverse, gray-scale sonograms show measurement of the AAA.

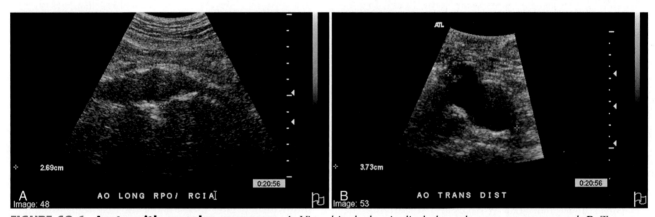

FIGURE 12-6. Aorta with saccular aneurysm. A, Viewed in the longitudinal plane, the aorta appears normal. **B,** Transverse imaging of the aorta is required to reliably detect this type of aneurysm. With a saccular aneurysm, unless a longitudinal image can be obtained in the plane of the greatest diameter of the aorta, transverse imaging must be used to measure the greatest diameter.

5. The AAA is suspected to be an inflammatory AAA (described later) and has not yet been imaged with CT.
6. The aneurysm is suspected of having reached a size at which treatment planning is needed.

False-Positive/False-Negative Results

Screening for aortic aneurysm should be highly accurate. Nonetheless, we have encountered two sets of circumstances where it is possible to have a **false-positive** study. The first can happen when the aorta at the diaphragmatic hiatus measures 3.0 cm or greater and is mistakenly called "aneurysmal." The normal size of the supraceliac aorta is 2.1 to 2.7 cm.[8] Using a definition of aneurysm that requires the diameter to be 1.5 times or more the normal diameter, a small aorta would not become aneurysmal until it reached approximately 3.2 cm in diameter, whereas the larger supraceliac aorta would not be aneurysmal even at 4.0 cm.

The second circumstance where we have seen several false-positive studies is when the spine is mistaken for the posterior wall of the aorta. This is particularly likely to occur when visualization is poor, as in a very obese patient. The true posterior wall of the aorta may then be difficult to determine. Usually, transverse imaging or imaging from the left flank will help define the true posterior wall to help determine if an aneurysm is present (Fig. 12-8).

False-negative studies may occur if visualization of the infrarenal aorta is incomplete. If the entire infrarenal aorta is well seen in longitudinal imaging, one can exclude the presence of a fusiform aneurysm, the most common type of AAA. However, if the entire infrarenal aorta is not well seen in the transverse plane, an eccentric aneurysm is not excluded (see Figs. 12-6 and 12-7).

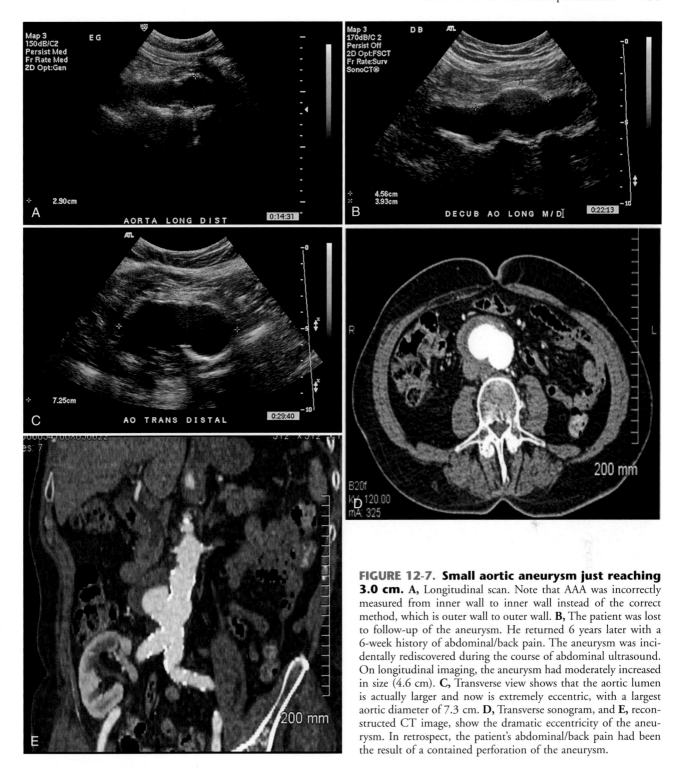

FIGURE 12-7. Small aortic aneurysm just reaching 3.0 cm. A, Longitudinal scan. Note that AAA was incorrectly measured from inner wall to inner wall instead of the correct method, which is outer wall to outer wall. **B,** The patient was lost to follow-up of the aneurysm. He returned 6 years later with a 6-week history of abdominal/back pain. The aneurysm was incidentally rediscovered during the course of abdominal ultrasound. On longitudinal imaging, the aneurysm had moderately increased in size (4.6 cm). **C,** Transverse view shows that the aortic lumen is actually larger and now is extremely eccentric, with a largest aortic diameter of 7.3 cm. **D,** Transverse sonogram, and **E,** reconstructed CT image, show the dramatic eccentricity of the aneurysm. In retrospect, the patient's abdominal/back pain had been the result of a contained perforation of the aneurysm.

Ultrasound versus CT for Evaluation of Rupture

As previously mentioned, rupture of aortic aneurysms is catastrophic, very often resulting in the patient's death. Although it played a role in the rapid diagnosis of ruptured AAAs in the emergency room 25 years ago,[37] ultra-

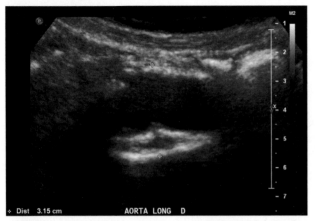

FIGURE 12-8. False-positive abdominal aortic aneurysm. The deep cursor has been placed on the echo caused by the lumbar spine, posterior to the aorta. This can easily cause a false-positive exam, most often when visualization is poor because of obesity. Transverse imaging can usually detect the error.

sound probably no longer has such a place at most institutions. The near ubiquitousness of high-speed multidetector CT scanners has made CT diagnosis extremely rapid. CT has a number of other advantages in comparison to ultrasound. CT is diagnostic of AAA in all cases, is highly diagnostic of retroperitoneal bleeding associated with aneurysm rupture, and is not operator dependent.

Because of these factors, obtaining a formal ultrasound in patients with an emergent need for diagnosis in most settings is probably unwise. If the patient has a ruptured AAA, time is of the essence, and the patient needs the most complete information possible obtained in a reliable way. Performing ultrasound risks wasting precious minutes that may be the difference between patient survival and death (Fig. 12-9).

Treatment Planning

Computed tomography angiography (CTA) is generally the most appropriate imaging method for AAA treatment planning. The distance of the renal arteries from the top of the aneurysm and the presence of accessory renal arteries and their location are important. If the patient is being considered for endoluminal grafting, knowledge of the three-dimensional (3-D) anatomy of the aneurysm and visualization of the iliac arteries are

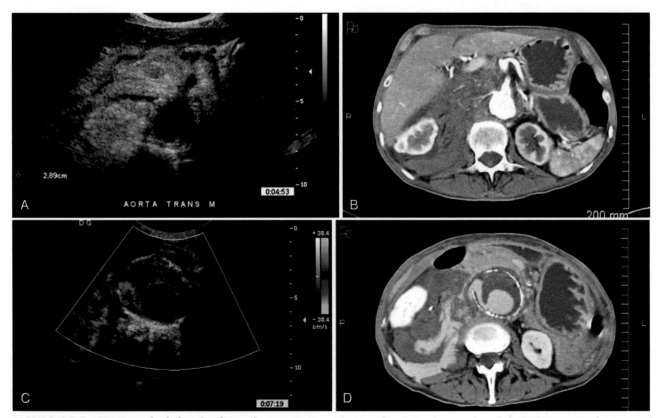

FIGURE 12-9. Ruptured abdominal aortic aneurysm. The use of both **A,** ultrasound, and **B,** CT, in suspected rupture of AAA should be avoided because of the addition of time for the workup, in this case 45 minutes *(white arrows).* CT is preferred in this setting because it can usually be done expeditiously and more reliably answers the pertinent questions. **C,** Transverse ultrasound, and **D,** contrast CT show the same AAA visualized at the site of rupture. The patient did not survive.

critical. In addition, evaluation of the mesenteric arteries is of value to determine whether reimplantation of the inferior mesenteric artery (IMA) is needed. All this information is most reliably obtained with CTA.

Postoperative Ultrasound Assessment

After open surgical repair of an aortic aneurysm, imaging surveillance generally is not performed. However, imaging is used to assess postoperative complications, including **thrombosis, infection, stenosis** (graft kink, neointimal hyperplasia, atherosclerosis), and **anastomotic pseudoaneurysm.** Ultrasound may play a role in the diagnosis of any of these complications. Another complication is **aortoenteric fistula**, generally to the third portion of the duodenum, which is potentially catastrophic and presents most often with upper gastrointestinal bleeding. Ultrasound does not play a role in the diagnosis of aortoenteric fistula.

Ultrasound has a larger, potentially much larger, role to play after repair of aortic aneurysms with endoluminal grafting. Current recommendations include lifelong imaging surveillance for endoleaks in patients who have undergone endoluminal grafting for AAA.[38] An **endoleak** is an area of the AAA that has been excluded by the **endoluminal graft** (ELG) that nonetheless continues to have blood flow. There are four types of endoleaks, categorized by four different sources of blood flowing into the aneurysmal sac (Fig. 12-10). Egress of blood from the sac is usually through patent aortic branches in all types of endoleak.

With a **type 1 leak**, one of the ends of the ELG is not tightly apposed to the arterial wall, allowing blood to enter the aneurysmal sac. A **type 2 leak** is caused by retrograde flow into the aneurysm sac through an aortic branch, usually the IMA or a lumbar artery. In a **type 3 leak**, there is disruption of the integrity of the ELG, caused by a fabric tear or a separation of component parts of the modular ELG. A **type 4 leak** is caused by

ENDOLEAKS

Type 1
Attachment leak

Type 2
Branch flow

A

B

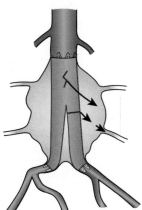

Type 3
Defect in graft or
modular disconnection

Type 4
Fabric porosity

C

D

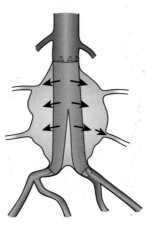

FIGURE 12-10. Endoleaks of abdominal aortic aneurysm after endoluminal graft (ELG) repair. A, Type 1 leak (attachment leak). Blood continues to enter the aneurysm sac at one of the three ends of the bifurcated ELG, the points where the ELG should be tightly affixed to the arterial wall. Egress, as with all endoleaks, is through branches of the aorta that remain patent. Treatment of type 1 leaks is indicated. **Type 2 leak (branch artery leak).** Blood enters the aneurysm sac through a patent branch artery. This type of leak can be self-limited and may be only observed. Treatment is indicated if the aneurysm enlarges. **B, Type 3 leak (loss of integrity of ELG).** Either the modules of the ELG have become separated or a rent has formed in the fabric of the ELG. Blood enters the sac from the ELG lumen through the site of loss of ELG integrity. Treatment is indicated. **Type 4 leak (fabric porosity).** Blood enters the sac from the ELG lumen through intact cloth of the ELG. This is self-limited and present only at surgery. The pores of the fabric quickly become occluded by blood products.

porosity of the ELG fabric with blood actually going through the pores in the fabric. This is seen only early after placement and is self-correcting. The term **endotension** refers to an aneurysm sac that stays pressurized in the presence of an ELG. This is sometimes referred to as a "type 5" endoleak. Its presence is inferred by continued growth in the aneurysm sac size in the absence of detecting another type of leak.[39,40]

With an endoleak, a treated aneurysm may continue to grow and eventually rupture. Endoleaks occur in approximately one third of AAAs treated with ELGs.[41] Types 1 and 3 endoleaks require immediate treatment when diagnosed. Type 4 endoleaks are generally seen only during placement of the graft and are self-limited, requiring no treatment. More judgment is involved in the care of type 2 leaks. Small leaks may be watched over time to see if they resolve and whether expansion of the aneurysm occurs.[41]

Because of the possibility of endoleaks, AAAs treated with ELGs undergo routine imaging surveillance. Imaging most often includes yearly, contrast-enhanced, multiphase CT examinations. This regular imaging greatly increases cost and exposes patients to contrast and significant radiation. Color duplex Doppler sonography alone can be used to visualize endoleaks (Fig. 12-11). Although clearly controversial, several studies suggest that standard color duplex Doppler ultrasound compares favorably with CT in the detection of leaks and may be the preferred method of surveillance.[42,43] Studies comparing contrast-enhanced duplex with standard color duplex have found the addition of contrast improves the quality of the study. Several studies suggest that contrast-enhanced ultrasound (CEUS) is at least as sensitive as CT for the detection of endoleaks[44,45] (Fig. 12-12). The issue is still a topic of research, although with more experience, duplex CEUS likely will play a significant role to play in AAA endoluminal graft surveillance.

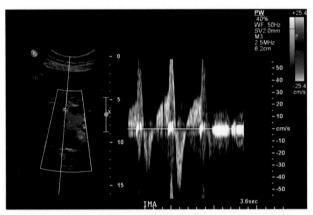

FIGURE 12-11. Inferior mesenteric artery (IMA) type 2 leak. Color duplex Doppler imaging from the left flank in this obese patient successfully decreased the distance to the IMA. Note the to-and-fro flow in the IMA.

OTHER ENTITIES CAUSING ABDOMINAL AORTIC DILATION

Inflammatory Abdominal Aortic Aneurysm

Inflammatory AAAs constitute approximately 5% of all AAAs.[46] According to some investigators, inflammatory AAA is likely related to retroperitoneal fibrosis (see later discussion), with both included as part of a classification referred to as **chronic periaortitis**.[47] Inflammatory AAAs are recognized by extremely thickened aortic wall and surrounding fibrosis that tends to spare the posterior wall. As in retroperitoneal fibrosis, the inflammation may involve the ureters, causing obstruction. Inflamma-

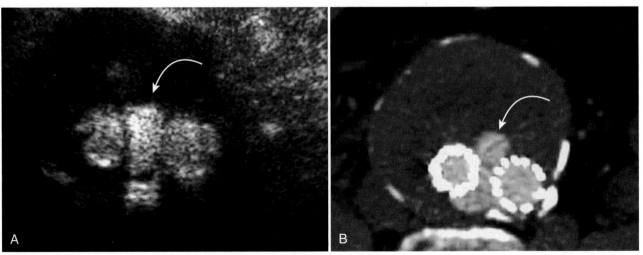

FIGURE 12-12. Endoleak after contrast injection. A, Ultrasound image, and **B,** comparison CT, correlate perfectly. (*Courtesy Stephanie Wilson, MD.*)

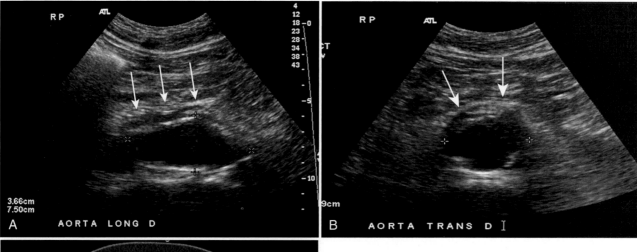

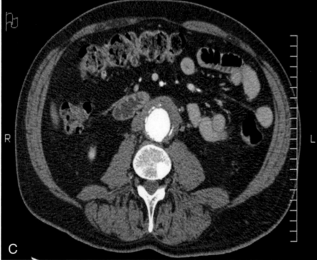

FIGURE 12-13. Inflammatory abdominal aortic aneurysm. Suspected inflammatory AAA with a rind of tissue approximately 7 mm in thickness projecting outside the anterior and lateral walls of the abdominal aorta *(arrows)*. **A,** Longitudinal, and **B,** transverse, sonograms. **C,** Diagnosis confirmed by CT, which shows a mildly enhancing rind of tissue outside the aorta. Note that the posterior wall is spared.

tory AAAs are less prone to rupture than other AAAs but are more prone to producing symptoms such as back pain. Anti-inflammatory drugs, including steroids and methotrexate, may be used to treat the inflammation.[47] With surgical or endovascular treatment, the inflammation surrounding many AAAs resolves. Sonographically, inflammatory AAAs may be recognized by a rind of tissue surrounding the aorta (Fig. 12-13).

Arteriomegaly and Aortic Ectasia

Arteriomegaly is diffuse arterial dilation involving several arteries, each with an increased diameter of at least 50% compared with the normal diameter. **Ectasia** refers to diffuse or focal dilation that is less than 50% increased in diameter.[8]

Pseudoaneurysm

A true aneurysm is a dilation of an artery that is contained by all three layers of the arterial wall. In contrast,

a **pseudoaneurysm** is a dilation that may be confined by only two layers, only one layer, or only adjacent soft tissue.[5] In the abdominal aorta, a pseudoaneurysm would be most likely to occur as a late surgical complication of aortic aneurysm repair or of other arterial surgery, almost always at sites of anastomosis. Sonographically, the appearance often is similar to a true aneurysm. With the proper findings, the diagnosis of pseudoaneurysm versus true aneurysm is largely made based on the clinical setting (e.g., previous trauma or aneurysm repair).

Penetrating Ulcer

Penetrating ulcer has been recognized for approximately 20 years. It is believed to result when an atherosclerotic ulceration penetrates the media, allowing an intramural hematoma to form.[48] This outpouching into the media can either develop or maintain flow, forming an aneurysmal-type structure. Penetrating ulcers occur more frequently in the thoracic aorta but are also seen in the abdominal aorta[49] (Fig. 12-14).

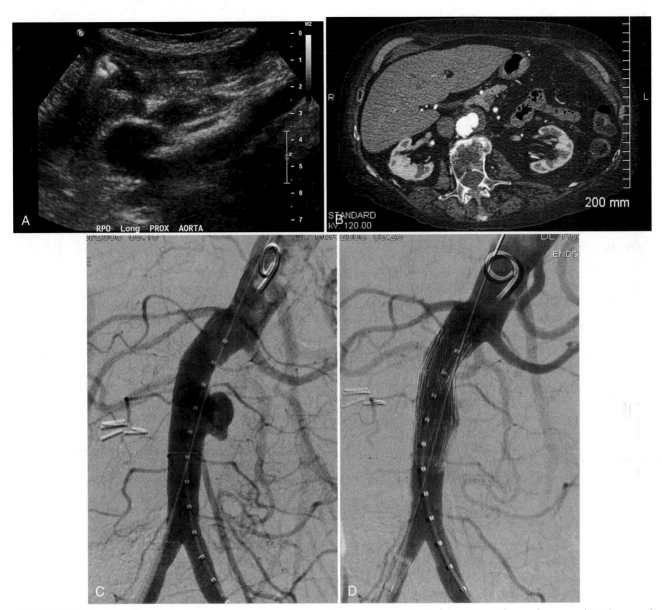

FIGURE 12-14. Penetrating ulcer. A, Longitudinal image shows an outpouching of the aorta with an otherwise relatively normal abdominal aorta. **B,** CT at level of outpouching. The rest of the aorta was not dilated and had no more than minimal atherosclerosis. **C** and **D,** Angiography images before and after placement of an endoluminal graft.

STENOTIC DISEASE OF THE ABDOMINAL AORTA

Stenosis or **occlusion** of the abdominal aorta can be congenital or may be caused by **atherosclerosis, vasculitis** (arteritis), **trauma,** or **embolus. Dissection** may also result in stenosis. **Midaortic syndrome** is a rare congenital stenosis that is also called **abdominal coarctation.**

Symptoms of aortic stenosis or occlusion may include intermittent claudication and impotence. These symptoms, along with the finding of decreased femoral pulses, are called **Leriche syndrome,** although the term is often is used more broadly to refer to all the signs and symptoms that may result from aortic occlusive disease or even the occlusion itself. In the great majority of patients with aortic stenosis or occlusion, the disease is caused by atherosclerosis. However, certain clinical settings suggest other causes.

With embolic disease, the dramatic abruptness of the onset of symptoms is the best historical evidence of the nature of the event. The patient can often relate exactly what he or she was doing when the symptoms started, even if the event was weeks in the past (e.g., "I had just gotten up from cutting roses . . ."). The rapidity with which the patient seeks treatment depends on the severity of the reduction in blood flow. Embolus to any artery must be viewed as a very serious and signal event. The majority of emboli to the abdominal aorta come from the heart. Having an arterial embolism of any type is similar to having a pulmonary embolism; having one means that the patient is at risk for having more. If the origin of the embolus was cardiac, the next one that forms may go to some less favorable place, such as the cerebral circulation, resulting in stroke, or to the mesenteric circulation, resulting in intestinal infarction. The workup of any patient identified as having an embolus should be expeditious, and anticoagulation is usually in order, at least until the source is determined and addressed.

Takayasu arteritis is a cause of aortic stenosis and is of particular note because it may occur in younger patients. It can affect the abdominal aorta or its branches.[50] Takayasu arteritis can present with symptoms resulting from aortic stenosis or branch vessel stenosis.

Posttraumatic aortic stenosis can occur in patients of any age, including younger patients. The initial aortic injury results from a forceful, nonpenetrating injury to the abdomen.[51] The resulting intimal injury can cause subintimal fibrosis, which can result in stenosis.

Isolated dissection of the abdominal aorta is rare. Involvement of the abdominal aorta more frequently results from extension of thoracic dissection, which can result in obstruction of the abdominal aorta or branch arteries.

In most cases of suspected aortic stenosis, we prefer to evaluate the aorta with CTA instead of duplex. Peripheral vascular disease is first confirmed in the patient by obtaining ankle brachial indices (ABIs) before and after exercise with or without arterial duplex sonography of the lower extremities. The next step in the workup is to obtain a map of the arteries supplying blood flow to the lower extremities to direct treatment. Maps of the arterial tree are more easily and reliably obtained either by CTA or by conventional catheter angiography than with duplex.

However, situations still arise in which aortic or iliac duplex Doppler sonography is indicated to assess for stenotic disease (Fig. 12-15). Several windows are necessary to complete an entire examination of the aorta and iliac arteries. Maintaining a proper Doppler angle of 60 degrees or less can be difficult.

DISEASES OF ABDOMINAL AORTA BRANCHES

Renal Arteries

Anatomy

The renal arteries arise distal to the **superior mesenteric artery** (SMA). Usually, they arise within 1-2 cm of the SMA but can originate as far distally as the common iliac

arteries. The main renal arteries are the only large lateral branches of the abdominal aorta.

When seen in cross section, viewing the aorta as if it were the face of a clock, the right renal artery arises from the aorta between the 9 and 11 o'clock positions. It then courses posterior to the inferior vena cava. The left renal artery most commonly arises between the 3 and 4 o'clock locations. The left renal artery typically arises directly posterior to the left renal vein.[52]

In most cases, a single renal artery supplies each kidney. In 30% of kidneys, however, one or both kidneys are supplied by two or more arteries.[53] When there are two renal arteries, the smaller artery is an **accessory artery.** Accessory arteries most often arise within 1 to 2 cm of the main renal artery. However, they may arise anywhere from the SMA to, in rare cases, as far distal as the common iliac arteries. Some accessory arteries do not enter the kidney at the hilum and instead enter the kidney at one of the poles. These accessory arteries are referred to as **polar arteries.**

Other arteries that can occasionally be confused for an accessory renal artery are the **lumbar arteries.** Occasionally seen near the abdominal aorta, lumbar arteries are small and arise more posteriorly than accessory renal arteries (Fig. 12-16). Lumbar arteries can be properly identified by their very-high-resistance waveform, similar to that in an extremity artery of a person at rest. Lumbar arteries can sometimes be identified by their course as they hug the vertebral body, coursing sharply posteriorly along the lateral vertebral bodies.

In renal anomalies such as crossed-fused ectopia or horseshoe kidney (see Chapter 9), the arterial supply is highly variable, making thorough duplex evaluation of the arteries challenging.[54,55]

Renal Artery Stenosis and Renovascular Hypertension

Recent data from the U.S. Department of Health and Human Services indicates that 31.3% of the population age 20 and older either have hypertension or are being treated for hypertension.[56] More than 90% of cases do not have a clear cause.[57] A minority of cases are caused by decreased arterial blood supply to the kidneys, activating the renin-angiotensin system that, through a complex series of events, results in elevated blood pressure. This mechanism causes only 1% to 5% of hypertension, but with the high prevalence of hypertension, the number of patients with renovascular hypertension is high.[58] Screening for renovascular hypertension is most appropriate in the presence of certain clinical features.

Treatment of renovascular hypertension caused by renal artery stenosis typically is endoluminal with percutaneous transluminal angioplasty or stent placement. The use of endovascular stenting has risen dramatically. Between 1996 and 2000, the volume of renal artery stent placement increased by 240%,[59,60] and it continues to

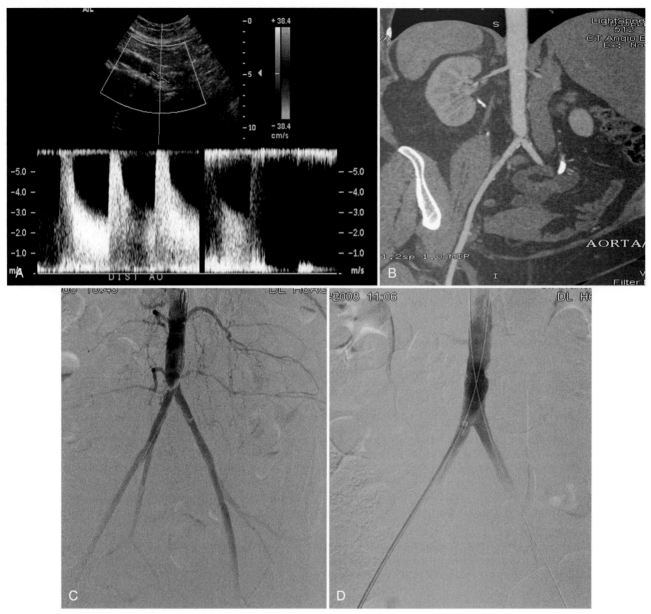

FIGURE 12-15. Stenotic aortic bifurcation. A, Duplex Doppler sonogram shows velocity of greater than 500 cm/sec at stenosis at the aortic bifurcation. Proximal to the stenosis, the aortic velocity varied from 35 to 50 cm/sec. **B,** CTA shows very focal stenosis of the abdominal aorta at its bifurcation. **C,** Angiography shows severe stenosis. **D,** Stenosis treated with "kissing" stents with good result.

increase. Many patients clearly benefit from endoluminal treatment of renal artery stenosis, but many others do not benefit, and a significant number even worsen when treated. Which patients should receive treatment still depends on clinical judgment.[60-62]

Many radiologic tests are available to assess for renal artery stenosis, including conventional angiography, CTA, magnetic resonance angiography (MRA), captopril scintigraphy, and renal artery duplex Doppler sonography. Opinions differ regarding the most advantageous strategy for using these tests.[58,63] The advantages of renal artery duplex Doppler sonography include low cost and the ability to achieve diagnostic information in almost all patients, regardless of the degree of renal function.

Many articles support the use of renal artery duplex Doppler in the diagnostic evaluation of renovascular hypertension.[64-66]

To be a good first-line test, renal artery duplex Doppler sonography must have high sensitivity and accuracy. Utility is greatest when there is proper clinical screening of patients for the test so that the pretest probability is higher than that of the hypertensive population as a whole. Performing the test must also be practical for ultrasound laboratories. A learning curve clearly exists, and while on the learning curve, the exam may suffer from inaccuracy or be unusually prolonged. The exam is probably best done in facilities capable of high volume, where it is practical to **periodically monitor** results

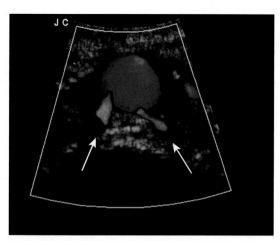

FIGURE 12-16. Lumbar arteries. Color Doppler sonogram of one set of the paired lumbar arteries shows their typical posterior origins *(arrows)*.

CLINICAL FINDINGS IN PATIENTS WITH HYPERTENSION THAT INCREASE PROBABILITY OF RENOVASCULAR CAUSE (RENAL ARTERY STENOSIS)

History of peripheral vascular disease, cerebrovascular disease, or coronary artery disease.

Recent onset of hypertension.

Refractory hypertension (not responsive with at least three medications).

Malignant hypertension (with papilledema) or accelerated (without papilledema but usually with fundus changes).

Abdominal or flank bruit.

Elevated creatinine and/or cholesterol levels (even higher suspicion if increased creatinine levels after treatment with angiotensin-converting enzyme [ACE] inhibitor).

Unexplained congestive heart failure or acute pulmonary edema.

Data from Safian RD, Textor SC. Renal-artery stenosis. N Engl J Med 2001;344:431-442; and Krijnen P, van Jaarsveld BC, Steyerberg EW, et al. A clinical prediction rule for renal artery stenosis. Ann Intern Med 1998;129:705-711.

---

versus the results of conventional angiography, CTA, or MRA. Such monitoring is invaluable for advancing on the learning curve and in raising the confidence in the examination. Once technologists are proficient in the examination, it can be performed fairly rapidly.

Feasibility of the examination in obese patients is also a concern. A few years after starting our duplex Doppler sonography program, we studied a total of 100 consecutive main renal arteries (50 patients), recording the **body mass index** (BMI) of each patient (unpublished data, 2002, Saint Francis Medical Center, Peoria, Ill). Of the 100 arteries, 20 were in obese patients (BMI ≥30) and four in extremely obese patients (BMI ≥40). 30 arteries were in overweight patients (BMI ≥25), and 46 were in patients of normal weight. We were able to complete a technically adequate examination in 96 of the 100 arteries. Of the four arteries with failed studies, three were in overweight patients, and one was in a patient of normal weight. All 24 arteries of the obese or morbidly obese patients were successfully studied.

Our technologists routinely score the quality of the duplex sonography of each renal artery on a 5-point scale. All examinations graded 2 or higher are considered diagnostically adequate; the entire extrarenal portion of the artery has been successfully interrogated. Table 12-1 lists quality score averages for the 100 arteries of our study. Our experience shows that renal duplex Doppler sonography can be completed successfully in most obese patients (Fig. 12-17).

Causes of Renal Artery Stenosis. The most common causes of renal artery stenosis in adults are atherosclerosis and fibromuscular dysplasia.[67] **Atherosclerotic disease** most often occurs in the proximal third of the artery, often at the origin of the artery[67] (Fig. 12-18). Percutaneous transluminal angioplasty alone has had mixed results in the treatment of atherosclerotic disease. In lesions that are at the origin of the artery, there tends to be a tremendous elastic recoil that allows the balloon to be inflated fully, but causes the artery to revert quickly to its stenotic state on deflation of the balloon. The development of stents has changed the situation by allowing the artery to be scaffolded. After stenting, there remains a risk of restenosis secondary to neointimal hyperplasia.[64,68] **Restenosis** is seen in 16% of patients between 6 and 12 months post-stenting[69] and is yet higher for patients followed for longer than one year. Because of the relatively low cost, lack of iodinated contrast, and high accuracy, renal artery duplex Doppler sonography is an ideal method to follow stented arteries.

Fibromuscular dysplasia (FMD) is the second most common cause of renovascular hypertension and typically occurs in women age 20 to 50 years. Multiple pathologic subtypes are seen; the most common FMD in the renal arteries is **medial fibroplasia.**[70,71] Histologically, these lesions are characterized by fibromuscular ridges.[72] The lesions most often occur in the distal two thirds of the renal artery and often have an angiographic appearance suggestive of a thin, fibrous web. The classic appearance on angiography is the "string of pearls," caused by multiple dysplastic regions in a row with short areas of post-stenotic dilation immediately distal to each stenosis (Fig. 12-19). FMD often responds well to simple percutaneous transluminal angioplasty. A single treatment often is effective in controlling blood pressure and is enduring.[73] Stent placement is rarely needed for FMD.

Another cause of impaired blood flow to the kidney that may result in renovascular hypertension is **dissection.** If the dissection extends to the renal artery, the

TABLE 12-1. SUCCESS OF RENAL ARTERY DUPLEX BY PATIENT BODY HABITUS

WEIGHT CATEGORY	NUMBER OF ARTERIES EXAMINED	NUMBER OF ARTERIES WITH FAILED EXAM	MEAN DUPLEX QUALITY SCORE
Extremely obese (BMI ≥40)	4	0	4.00
Obese (BMI ≥30 and <40)	20	0	4.30
Overweight (BMI ≥25 and <30)	30	3	4.00
Normal (BMI <25)	46	1	4.61

BMI, Body mass index.

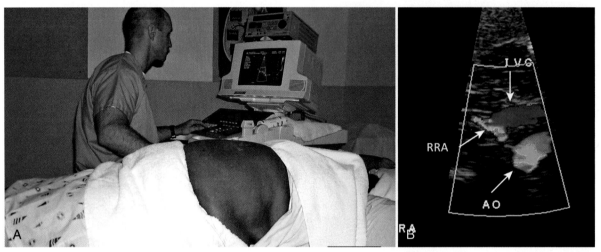

FIGURE 12-17. Renal artery duplex Doppler ultrasound in an obese patient. A, Photograph of patient (height, 5 ft 7 in; weight, 290 lb; BMI, 45.4). **B,** Image of right renal artery origin from the same patient. Imaging from the right flank, the origin of the artery is 13.5 cm from the transducer.

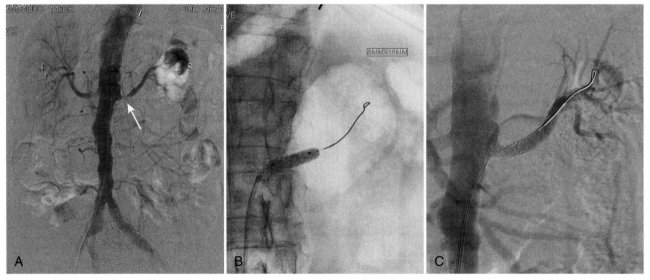

FIGURE 12-18. Atherosclerotic stenosis near origin of renal artery *(arrow)*. A, Angiogram. **B,** Single image during stent deployment. Because of elastic recoil, atherosclerotic lesions near the renal artery origins usually require stent placement. **C,** After stenting, the previously stenotic area is greatly improved.

raised intimal flap in the aorta may partially or completely occlude the renal artery orifice. Alternatively, if the dissection extends into the renal artery, the raised intima may cause stenosis or occlusion within the artery itself. Endovascular treatment is frequently successful either by stenting of the narrowed artery or by fenestration of the dissected intima[74] (Fig. 12-20).

Embolus can result in abruptly impaired blood flow to some or all of a kidney. The patient frequently complains of flank pain. Diagnosis often is delayed, resulting

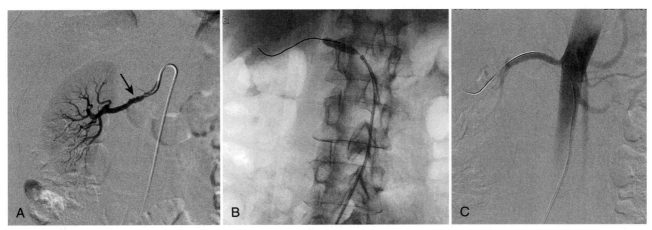

FIGURE 12-19. Fibromuscular dysplasia (FMD): angiography. A, Note the "string of beads" appearance, most often in the distal two thirds of the renal artery *(arrow)*. **B,** FMD generally responds well to balloon angioplasty. **C,** After balloon angioplasty, the appearance of the artery is improved.

in irreversible damage to the kidney involved. Revascularization of the kidney is unlikely to result in full return of function if delayed more than 90 minutes.[75]

Renal artery stenosis can also occur in children; FMD is the most common cause. **Neurofibromatosis** and **vasculitis** can also cause renal artery stenosis in children.[76] **Midaortic syndrome,** which is a hypoplasia of the abdominal aorta, can also result in reduced renal blood flow. Aortic coarctation most commonly is discovered in other ways but, if not recognized, also will cause renovascular hypertension (Fig. 12-21).

Renal Artery Duplex Doppler Sonography

When performing renal artery duplex Doppler sonography, it is critical to interrogate the **entire extrarenal portion** of the artery. The examination should not be considered adequate unless the entire extrarenal portion of the main renal artery is seen and interrogated by Doppler every 2 to 3 mm. Accessory arteries and large, early extrarenal branches of the main renal artery are also similarly assessed. Even then, stenoses in accessory arteries or branch renal arteries may be missed. Fortunately, nonvisualization of branch arteries or accessories is unlikely to affect patient management.[77,78]

Visualization of the renal artery is the key to successful ultrasound interrogation. At our institution, patients are prepared by eating a bland, low-fiber diet the day before and taking nothing by mouth (NPO) after 7 PM the night before. We ask them to avoid caffeine, smoking, and dairy products. The sonographic examination is significantly easier with a prepped patient.

Color Doppler sonography is usually necessary for visualization of the entire extrarenal portion of the artery. Rarely, however, the right renal artery can be seen better without color Doppler, using the liver as a window. Color Doppler sometimes makes the site of stenosis obvious because of a color bruit or increased diastolic velocity, causing a portion of the artery to remain filled with color throughout the cardiac cycle. At our facility, we do not screen by looking for **aliasing,** because we typically have the color scale set low to increase our ability to see the artery. This causes aliasing to occur in much of the artery, making it less useful as a screen but improving the ability to see the entire artery.

We set the **wall filter** low. **Color gain** is often set high. When necessary, power output is increased to aid visualization. On machines allowing control of the ensemble packet size, we set it to the highest size possible to increase sensitivity of flow detection. Maintaining an adequate **frame rate** (>10 frames/sec) is important. We keep the frame rate adequate by making the color window as narrow as reasonably possible. We also decrease the line density of the image and the sector width of the transducer. Our pictures of the renal artery often are not "pretty" because of the aliasing and the high color gain. Our goal, however, is to see the artery. With these settings, we can see the entire extrarenal portion of the artery in almost all patients, regardless of size.

We generally use a 5-2 or 5-1 curvilinear transducer (Phillips I-22 or HDI 5000). Some of our technologists prefer to use a phased array 4-1 or 5-1 transducer. With thin patients, interrogation from the anterior midline is likely to be successful. At our facility, however, the flank approach is most often used; it has a higher probability of seeing the entire renal artery in obese patients. Also, achieving an acceptable Doppler angle of less than 60 degrees is easier from the flank. Breath holding is often used, although it does not work well in many patients, either because the patient is dyspneic, or because of a slow but steady cephalad drift of the kidneys, which occurs in some patients despite breath holding. Even without breath holding, the examination often is successful.

When possible, we avoid examining patients who are in heart failure, who have acute dyspnea, who have

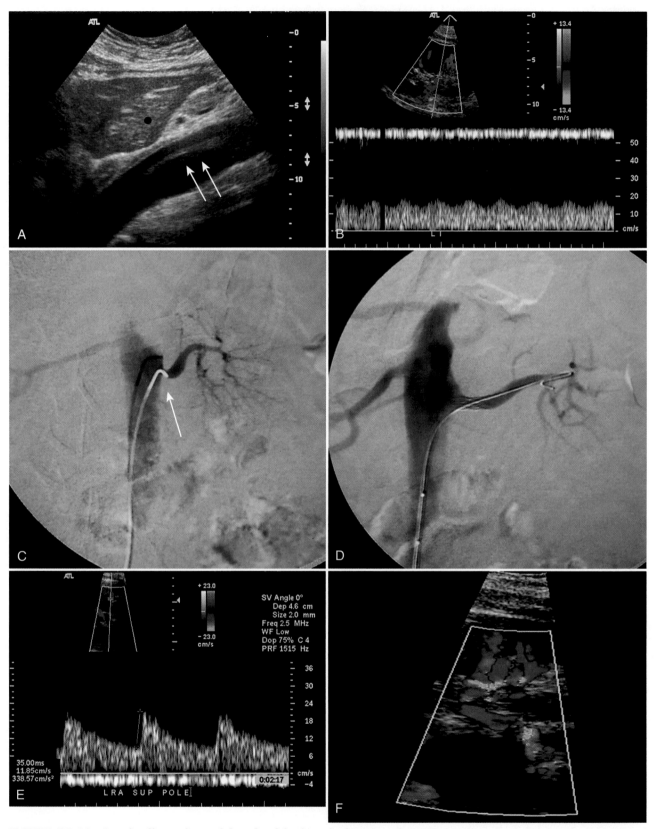

FIGURE 12-20. Aortic dissection with raised intima in lumen of aorta. A, Ultrasound of the proximal abdominal aorta in 30-year-old cocaine user. **B,** Duplex Doppler sonogram shows highly abnormal intrarenal waveforms from left kidney. Also, it is very difficult to see the main left renal artery with color Doppler. The systolic rise time is 190 msec and acceleration is 34 cm/sec². **C,** Selective injection of the left renal artery at angiography. Angiography shows moderate stenosis at origin of the left renal artery *(arrow).* **D,** After stenting of left renal artery, angiography shows origin is widely patent. **E,** Greatly improved intrarenal waveforms in left renal artery after stenting. Note that systolic rise time is 35 msec and acceleration is 339 cm/sec². **F,** Left renal artery is easy to see with color duplex after stenting because of increased flow.

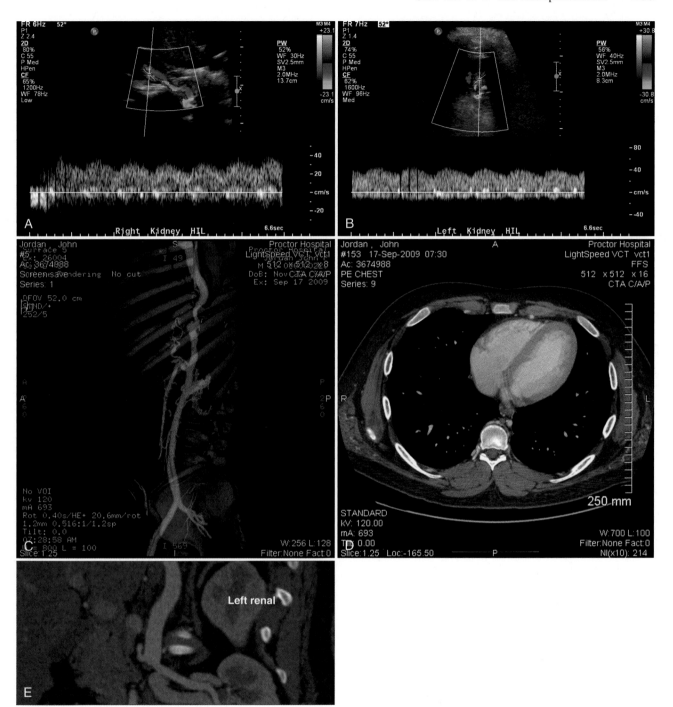

FIGURE 12-21 A and **B**, Renal duplex ultrasound of a 15-year-old football lineman presenting with hypertension. Waveforms from the right and left renal arteries. Waveforms bilaterally have low velocity, low resistance, and a rounded peak, all indications of a poststenotic waveform. No renal artery stenosis was seen. Waveforms suggested a more proximal aortic stenosis and are what might be expected with thoracic coarctation. **C**, 3D CT image of the thoracic aorta shows that severe narrowing was congenital. **D**, Axial CT shows a severely narrowed thoracic aorta. **E**, Curved reformatted CT image shows the widely patent left renal artery. There were two right renal arteries, which were also widely patent.

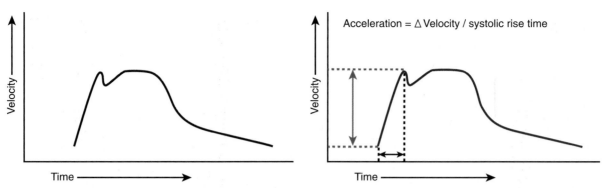

FIGURE 12-22. Renal artery systolic waveform. A, Normal waveform. **B,** Early systole. There is a rapid acceleration of blood in the renal artery. The systolic rise time *(purple arrow)* is the time expended during this rapid acceleration. The acceleration is the change in velocity during the systolic rise *(blue arrow)* divided by the systolic rise time.

acutely decreased mobility, or who are on ventilators. All these patients have a reduced ability to cooperate. Renal duplex Doppler sonograms generally are not emergent. The examination will likely become much easier, more successful, and more highly accurate once the patient's condition improves.

Performance of the renal artery duplex Doppler study mainly relies on obtaining accurate velocities throughout the main renal artery. However, measurement of the **resistive index** (RI) is also important. Treatment of renal artery stenosis is less likely to be effective in reducing blood pressure when the segmental artery RI is high (≥0.80), probably because of irreversible damage to the small blood vessels in kidneys with a high RI.[61]

Attention to **intrarenal waveforms** is also of some importance. A highly abnormal waveform can be a valuable indicator of stenosis. A delayed systolic peak (tardus, i.e., "tardy") and velocities that are greatly decreased (parvus, i.e., "puny") can be a strong sign of a more proximal stenosis. The intrarenal waveform can be analyzed quantitatively by calculating the systolic rise time and the acceleration (Fig. 12-22). Although we calculate these parameters, a qualitative assessment of the appearance of the waveform usually serves just as well. We only rely on a **tardus-parvus waveform** to make the diagnosis when the finding is pronounced (compare *B* and *E* of Fig. 12-20; see also *A* and *B* of Fig. 12-21).

Finally, because of the regular occurrence of renal lesions or abnormalities that affect patient care, we believe that ultrasound of the kidneys is indicated when renal artery duplex Doppler ultrasound is performed, unless the patient has had recent (<1 year) cross-sectional imaging. Incidental findings in our ultrasound department have included xanthogranulomatous pyelonephritis, adrenal tumors, hydronephrosis, and several renal cell carcinomas[79] (Fig. 12-23).

Doppler Interpretation. There are many proposed guidelines for Doppler interpretation. Proposed parameters to assess for stenosis include the **peak systolic velocity** (PSV), **renal aortic ratio** (RAR; defined as highest systolic velocity in renal artery divided by aortic systolic velocity, with aortic velocity measured at or above SMA origin), **acceleration time, acceleration index, renal interlobar ratio,**[80,81] and **renal-renal ratio.**[82-84] The Cleveland Clinic used a combination of RAR of 3.5 or greater *or* PSV of 200 or greater as the criterion for renal artery stenosis of more than 60%.[65] We use a variation of the Cleveland Clinic guidelines, using the same RAR as the study but a higher PSV. We have done internal validation of our guidelines but continue to look for ways to improve them.

False-Positive/False-Negative Results. To obtain the highest accuracy, it is important to avoid relying solely on the numerical data obtained. When a high velocity is seen or when the renal aortic ratio is high, the interpreting radiologist must also actively look for secondary signs of stenosis, such as a characteristic harsh audible signal at the site of stenosis, increased diastolic flow, color bruit, and post-stenotic turbulence (Fig. 12-24). Without ancillary findings, the interpreter must consider the possibility that the high velocity or high RAR represents a false-positive result.

False-negative findings are most a risk when visualization is marginal and the entire artery has not been adequately evaluated. In perhaps 5% to 10% of patients, accurate diagnosis cannot be made because of inadequate visualization of one or both arteries.

The examination is challenging to the uninitiated operator, but establishment of a renal artery duplex Doppler program can be rewarding. Because of the lower cost versus other diagnostic tests, Doppler ultrasound lowers the threshold for the diagnosis of renovascular hypertension. Hurdles mainly relate to the learning curve and the initial investment of time. Starting a program is more feasible in a large center where demand will likely be higher than in a smaller facility. Once the program is mature, the study is financially viable and can result in improved patient care.

Renal Artery Aneurysm

Renal artery aneurysms are uncommon and may be saccular or fusiform. They can be seen with atherosclerosis or FMD. Often, they are more reliably seen and followed with CT than with ultrasound. Most renal artery aneurysms do not result in significant morbidity or mortality.[85]

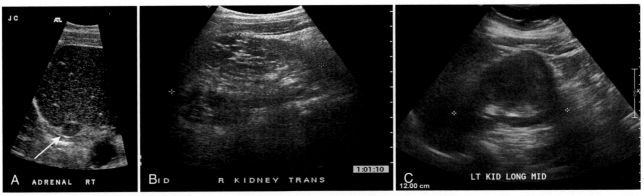

FIGURE 12-23. Gray-scale imaging of kidneys and surrounding structures. A, Small, aldosterone-secreting **right adrenal tumor** *(arrow)* is seen as part of the gray-scale examination. **B, Xanthogranulomatous pyelonephritis.** Gray-scale imaging of a Haitian teenager with hypertension shows renal distortion. The hypertension was cured by nephrectomy. **C,** Large left **renal cell carcinoma.** We have detected many renal cell tumors, of all sizes.

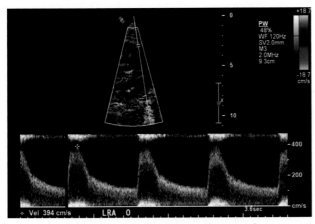

FIGURE 12-24. Secondary signs of stenosis. Increased diastolic flow, as seen here, can help confirm the presence of renal artery stenosis. Other secondary signs include a tardus-parvus waveform.

Treatment should be considered if (1) the aneurysm is greater than 2.0 cm, (2) it is believed to be causing symptoms (e.g., hematuria, pain, hypertension), or (3) the patient is a woman of childbearing age who anticipates becoming pregnant.[86,87] The patient and family must be made aware of a renal aneurysm to be alert to symptoms so that diagnosis and treatment can be expedited. Currently, no well-accepted guidelines address how often renal artery aneurysms should be imaged (Fig. 12-25).

Mesenteric Arteries

Anatomy

Three arteries constitute the main sources of arterial blood flow to the gastrointestinal tract: celiac, superior mesenteric, and inferior mesenteric. The **celiac artery** (CA) arises anteriorly from the abdominal aorta at the level of the aortic hiatus of the diaphragm. The CA supplies blood to the spleen, pancreas, and liver, along with the stomach and the proximal duodenum. The standard branching pattern of the CA is into the splenic and common hepatic arteries, which are easily identified. The third branch of the CA is the left gastric, which is much less frequently seen with sonography. The common hepatic artery branches into the proper hepatic artery and the gastroduodenal artery; the latter is important as a conduit for collateral blood flow to the celiac circulatory territory when the CA itself is highly stenosed or occluded.

The **superior mesenteric artery** typically arises from the anterior aorta 1 cm below the CA's origin. The SMA supplies blood to the pancreas, distal duodenum, jejunum, ileum, and proximal colon as far distal as the splenic flexure. In about 20% of people, the SMA supplies some of the hepatic blood flow through a replaced or accessory right hepatic artery. Other important branches of the SMA include the inferior pancreaticoduodenal artery (IPDA) and the middle colic artery. The IPDA and its branches form an arcade of blood vessels around the head of the pancreas with the gastroduodenal artery.[88,89] In celiac arterial occlusion, the IPDA-gastroduodenal arcade often becomes the primary route for blood to reach the celiac circulation (Fig. 12-26). In cases of SMA occlusion, blood flow often flows in the opposite direction through the arcade, supplying the occluded SMA with blood from the celiac artery.

The **inferior mesenteric artery** supplies the descending colon, sigmoid colon, and superior rectum. The IMA arises from the anterior aorta slightly to the left of midline, approximately two-thirds the distance between the renal artery origins and the aortic bifurcation. When the aorta is viewed transversely, the IMA arises at approximately the 1 o'clock position. Viewed longitudinally, the appearance is similar to that of the SMA, except the IMA is significantly smaller and always courses inferiorly to the left of the aorta. After 1 to 2 cm, the IMA bifurcates into a superior hemorrhoidal artery that runs caudally slightly to the left of midline and into a left colic artery that runs laterally to the descending colon. The

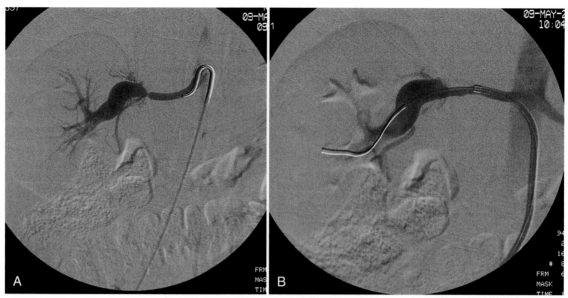

FIGURE 12-25. Most renal artery aneurysms are atherosclerotic or congenital. A, This 11-year-old boy with hypertension has severe renal artery stenosis, most likely caused by FMD. There is a post-stenotic aneurysm. **B,** Same artery immediately after balloon angioplasty. Two years later, the aneurysm had become much smaller.

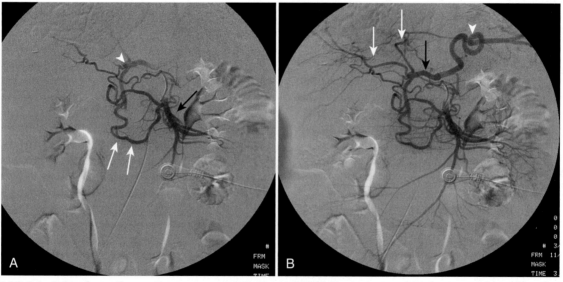

FIGURE 12-26. Injection of superior mesenteric artery (SMA) in patient with severe celiac artery stenosis. A, Early image from the angiographic run shows the SMA *(black arrow)* filling the inferior pancreaticoduodenal arcade *(white arrows)*. The gastroduodenal artery (GDA) is beginning to fill retrograde *(white arrowhead)*. **B,** Image from the same injection a few moments later. The retrograde flow in the GDA has filled the right and left hepatic arteries *(white arrows)*. In addition, there is retrograde flow in the short common hepatic artery *(black arrow)*, which then fills the splenic artery *(white arrowhead)*.

left colic artery immediately divides into ascending and descending branches. The superior hemorrhoidal artery gives off sigmoid branches as it courses inferiorly to the rectum (Fig. 12-27).

Connections between the SMA and IMA occur in the region of the splenic flexure. The IMA can supply blood to the SMA when the proximal SMA is occluded. Blood then flows from the IMA through the marginal artery of Drummond (Fig. 12-28) or through the sometimes present and more direct arch of Riolan to the middle colic artery and then into the SMA. The middle colic

artery is an anterior branch of the SMA and is generally identified sonographically only in cases of SMA occlusion (Fig. 12-29).

Mesenteric Ischemia

Acute Ischemia. Acute mesenteric ischemia occurs when there is an abrupt reduction of arterial flow to the intestines. The most common cause is cardiac embolus. Acute mesenteric ischemia also may be caused by aortic dissection. Less often, abrupt reduction of arterial flow

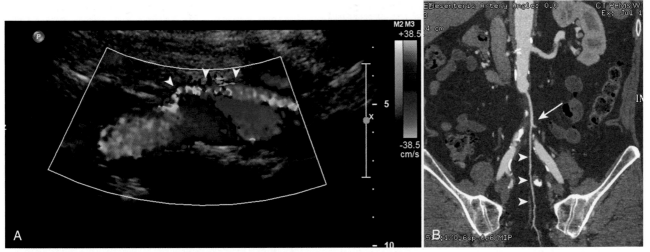

FIGURE 12-27. Inferior mesenteric artery (IMA) (arrowheads) has similar appearance to SMA when scanned longitudinally. A, Color Doppler longitudinal sonogram. **B,** Curved reformatted CT image of the IMA shows the early bifurcation into left colic (proximal section indicated by *arrow*) and superior hemorrhoidal arteries *(arrowheads).* The sigmoid branches of the superior hemorrhoidal artery are not visible on this image.

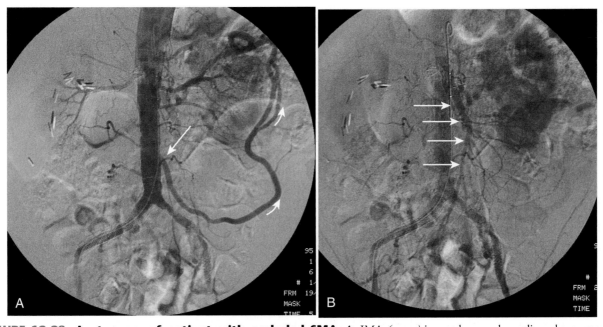

FIGURE 12-28. Aortogram of patient with occluded SMA. A, IMA *(arrow)* is very large and supplies a large artery of Drummond *(curved arrows).* **B,** A few moments later, flow through the artery of Drummond via the middle colic artery enters the SMA *(arrows).*

results from SMA thrombosis, decreased cardiac output without any obstruction of the arterial tree, or thrombosis of the superior mesenteric vein.[90] Only a single artery needs to be compromised acutely to cause mesenteric ischemia, most often the SMA. Patients present with an abrupt onset of severe abdominal pain, nausea and vomiting, and diarrhea. Later in the course, they may develop "currant jelly" stools from intestinal bleeding and mucosal sloughing.

Acute mesenteric ischemia is a medical emergency. Mortality is high, ranging from 30% to 95%.[91] The wide differences in reported mortality likely relate to the rapidity of diagnosis. Patient survival depends on quick and accurate diagnosis and treatment. In most cases, ultrasound has no role in the diagnosis of acute mesenteric ischemia.[92] These patients can be of any size and often have a large amount of gas in the bowel that compromises sonographic diagnosis. In most cases, the clinician simply cannot risk wasting time by initiating the diagnostic workup with mesenteric duplex Doppler sonography. CTA or angiography is the test of choice.[93]

Chronic Ischemia. Duplex Doppler sonography has a

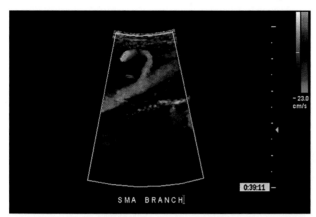

FIGURE 12-29. Major anterior branch of SMA. Middle colic artery is not usually seen sonographically, except when it is supplying collateral flow. Here, the middle colic artery is visible because of the thinness of the patient.

more central role in the diagnosis of chronic mesenteric ischemia. Chronic ischemia is usually the result of atherosclerosis slowly occluding the arteries that supply the intestines. Because the buildup of plaque is slow, collateral circulation has an opportunity to develop and supply some of the needed blood flow to the intestines. Mesenteric artery stenosis is relatively common, reported in 17.5% of the free-living elderly population. Most patients with severe narrowing of one or more of the arteries supplying the intestines have no symptoms and need no treatment.[93] These patients maintain adequate blood flow to the gut through collateral circulation. The collateral blood flow usually must itself be impaired before the patient becomes symptomatic. In most cases, two of the three arteries that supply mesenteric blood flow (CA, SMA, IMA) must be severely diseased before a patient experiences chronic mesenteric ischemia, but even many patients with multiple-artery disease are not symptomatic.[93] Again, the clinician must remember that, although uncommon, significant mesenteric ischemia can result from the narrowing of one artery, particularly the SMA.[94]

The onset of chronic ischemia is insidious, with the classic patient experiencing weight loss and postprandial pain. Atypical features in the history are common and often include complaints of "indigestion." Patients with chronic ischemia frequently are very thin, which facilitates ultrasound.

Vasculitis, most often Takayasu arteritis, can also lead to mesenteric ischemia. Although typically the symptoms are chronic, involvement of the mesenteric arteries can be rapidly progressive and result in bowel infarction.[95]

Median Arcuate Ligament Syndrome

Most commonly, patients with symptomatic mesenteric ischemia have at least two of the mesenteric arteries nar-rowed or completely occluded. Patients with the median arcuate ligament syndrome have narrowing only of the celiac artery.

The median arcuate ligament of the diaphragm is close to the CA. This ligament is a band of fibrous tissue that crosses the aorta, usually above the origin of the CA, although the crossing can be below. Deformity and narrowing of the CA caused by the median arcuate ligament are fairly common angiographic findings on lateral aortography. One study reported that 24% of aorto-grams performed for unrelated reasons showed CA stenosis of at least 50% caused by the median arcuate ligament.[96]

In median arcuate ligament syndrome, patients with only narrowing of the celiac artery experience significant postprandial pain that results in avoidance of eating and weight loss. The syndrome is poorly understood, but the pain is believed to be possibly related to ischemia.[97,98] Other investigators support a neurogenic cause.[99] Some patients respond dramatically to surgery and become symptom free.[97-100] Surgery consists of dividing the median arcuate ligament and may include CA revascularization.

Mesenteric Artery Duplex Doppler Sonography

Mesenteric artery duplex Doppler ultrasound is most often performed with the patient fasting. Most studies assessing the addition of a postprandial study conclude that it is not of value.[101-103]

Blood flow to the intestines in the fasting state is relatively low. Normal waveforms in the SMA and IMA are high resistance. When the patient eats, blood is shunted to the intestines, and the SMA has a lower-resistance waveform. The CA supplies the liver and spleen, which have a higher need for flow than the intestines when the patient is fasting. Accordingly, the CA has lower resistance than the SMA or IMA when interrogated with the patient fasting.

Because chronic mesenteric ischemia can be fatal, it is critical that the examination be performed and interpreted in a way that guarantees very high sensitivity. The majority of stenoses that result in chronic mesenteric ischemia are within the first 1 to 2 cm of the origin of the CA, SMA, and IMA. It is possible, although rare, to have a branch artery occlusion that results in chronic mesenteric ischemia. Ultrasound is not a reliable technique for screening for these more distal stenoses.

The evaluation of the CA starts at its origin and proceeds to its bifurcation into the splenic and common hepatic arteries. As with all duplex Doppler studies, the sample volume is advanced slowly through the CA with waveforms viewed every 2 to 3 mm and any abnormal sites documented with an image. A standard set of waveforms from the proximal, middle, and distal CA is also obtained.

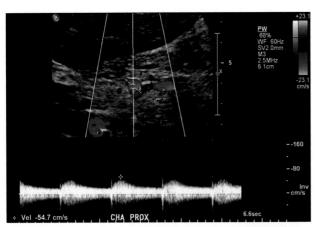

FIGURE 12-30. Patient with occluded celiac artery origin. Sample volume has been placed in the common hepatic artery *(CHA)* origin and shows a negative velocity (see velocity scale of spectral waveform) indicating retrograde flow (away from the transducer).

In patients with very severe celiac stenosis or occlusion, the CA often receives its blood supply from the SMA through the pancreaticoduodenal arcade. The blood flow in the gastroduodenal artery reverses, carrying the blood from the arcade back to the common hepatic artery. Blood flow then arrives at the liver through the proper hepatic artery. To arrive at the spleen, blood flow from the gastroduodenal artery flows retrograde in the common hepatic artery to reach the splenic artery. Assessment of blood flow direction in the common hepatic artery should be part of the sonographic examination of the celiac artery to detect cases in which this collateral flow is present (Fig. 12-30).

The evaluation of the SMA starts at the origin and is carried distally with viewing of waveforms every 2 to 3 mm, documenting waveforms in the proximal, middle, and distal artery. The examination can be performed with or without breath holding. However, without breath holding, motion of the sample volume with respect to the CA and SMA often occurs. With the patient breathing, the sonographer may believe a waveform is being obtained from the SMA when in fact the CA is being sampled or conversely in the CA when the SMA is being sampled. Great care should be exercised when not using breath holding to guarantee that the proper vessel is being evaluated.

The IMA has only a short trunk before it branches into the left colic, sigmoidal, and superior hemorrhoidal arteries. In most patients the IMA is readily found, being the only anterior branch of the abdominal aorta below the level of the renal arteries. The IMA requires Doppler interrogation only for 3 to 4 cm.

Finally, special maneuvers must be used when CA stenosis caused by the median arcuate ligament is suspected. The traditional test is to remeasure flow velocity in the artery when the patient takes a deep inspiration. We have found this test to be inconsistent. Reexamination of the artery with the patient standing may be superior in its ability to show normalization of velocities in the CA in the setting of compression by the median arcuate ligament.[104] Our experience indicates that examination with the patient standing is much superior to deep inspiration at normalizing waveforms (Fig. 12-31).

Mesenteric Duplex Interpretation. Probably the most widely accepted duplex criteria for mesenteric stenosis were some of the earliest to be developed. These state that PSVs greater than 275 cm/sec in the SMA and 200 cm/sec in the CA are indicative of stenosis of greater than 70% in these arteries.[105] Other investigators have found diastolic velocities to be a more accurate indicator. One group found an **end diastolic velocity** (EDV) greater than 45 cm/sec to be a highly accurate indicator of SMA stenosis greater than 50%.[86,106] Another group found EDV greater than 70 cm/sec to be highly accurate for diagnosing SMA stenosis of more than 50%, with an EDV greater than 100 cm/sec needed to diagnose CA stenosis of over 50%.[107]

In our laboratory, we have found the criteria using systolic velocities (but not diastolic) to be highly sensitive but to result in a significant number of false-positive studies. Because of the high sensitivity, we are confident that for a high-quality examination that does not show systolic velocities higher than those stated above, the diagnosis of chronic mesenteric ischemia is excluded. When velocities do reach the threshold given above, we look for secondary features that support the diagnosis of significant stenosis before we become confident that the stenosis is real. These secondary features include an increased diastolic velocity and the presence of significant post-stenotic turbulence. Color bruit is also supportive of severe stenosis (Fig. 12-32). In the absence of secondary findings, the radiologist must consider the possibility of a false-positive result. In this setting, we have a low threshold to recommend either CTA or MRA to assist in the diagnosis.

There have been no widely accepted duplex Doppler criteria for what constitutes significant stenosis of the IMA. Therefore, evaluation for severe stenosis must also be based on qualitative more than on quantitative data. High systolic velocity in the presence of high diastolic velocity and post-stenotic turbulence is indicative of severe stenosis. A PSV greater than 200 cm/sec in the IMA may be an accurate indicator of severe stenosis.[108] Stenosis of the IMA may be an important contributor to the development of mesenteric ischemia. We have seen and treated many patients with mesenteric ischemia in whom a stenotic IMA was the sole blood supply to the gut (Fig. 12-33).

Treatment of chronic mesenteric ischemia can be surgical or endoluminal. Rates of restenosis with endoluminal treatment are high, and thus, posttreatment surveillance is important. As with all arteries treated with

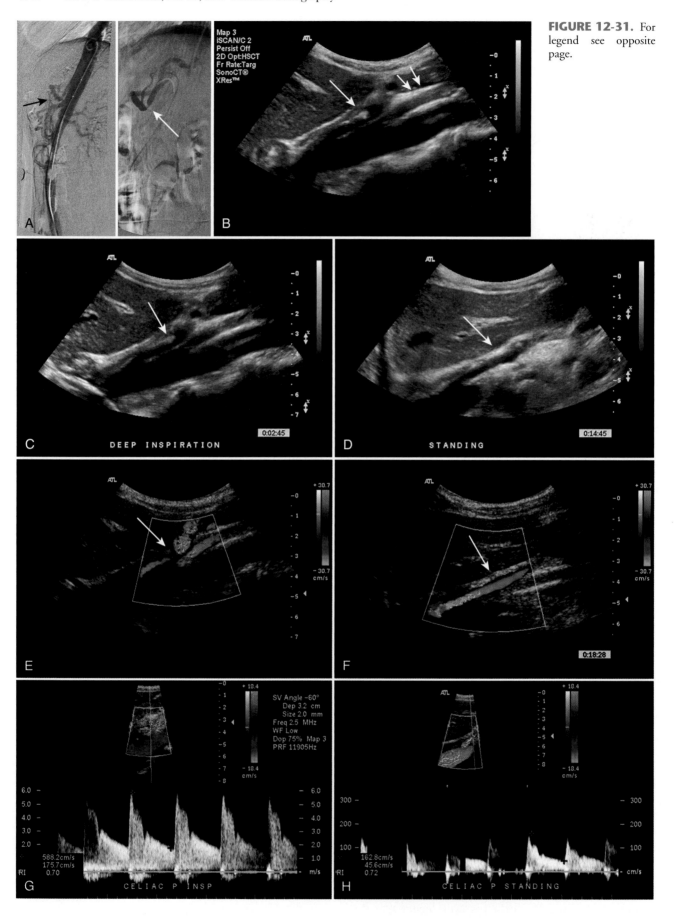

FIGURE 12-31. For legend see opposite page.

FIGURE 12-31. Kink in celiac artery caused by median arcuate ligament. Aortography shows typical appearance of kink in the celiac artery (CA) *(black arrow)* caused by the median arcuate ligament. **A,** Selective CA injection shows severe narrowing at site of the kink *(white arrow).* **B,** Gray-scale image with patient supine shows the kink in the celiac *(long arrow)* and its relation to the SMA *(short arrows).* **C,** Gray-scale image with patient supine in deep inspiration shows some improvement in the kink. **D,** Gray-scale image with patient standing shows resolution of kink. **E,** Color Doppler image with patient supine shows kink causing stenosis. **F,** With patient standing, the artery becomes straightened without narrowing. **G,** Spectral image shows high velocity of 588 cm/sec with the patient in deep inspiration. **H,** With patient standing the velocity is normal at 163 cm/sec.

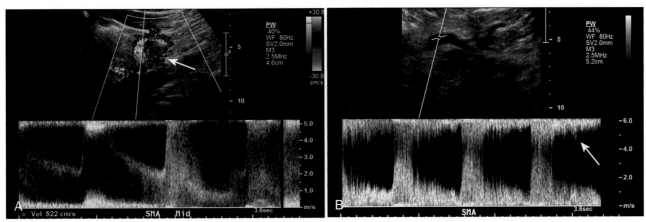

FIGURE 12-32. Post-stenotic turbulence. A, Spectral waveform at site of stenosis shows very high diastolic velocities of greater than 200 cm/sec. Color portion of the image shows color bruit *(arrow)* consisting of color outside the vessel near the stenosis site. thought to be caused by tissue vibration. **B,** Spectral waveform shows the typical "spike hairdo" waveform caused by post-stenotic turbulence. There is mirror-image artifact. Because of the very high velocities, the baseline of the waveform has been placed at the bottom, causing the mirror image to appear at the top of the tracing *(arrow).* Mirror-image artifact is also typical of turbulence.

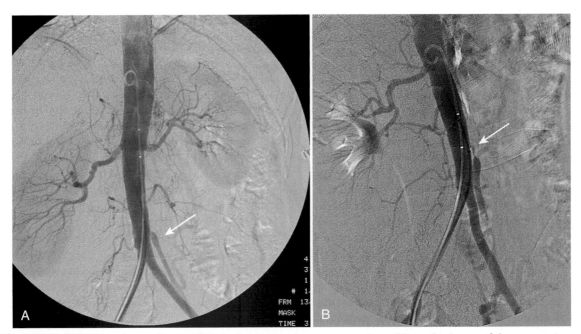

FIGURE 12-33. Mesenteric aortography. A, Anteroposterior aortogram shows filling of only one of the mesenteric arteries, a very large IMA *(arrow).* Also note incidental finding of FMD in the right renal artery. **B,** Oblique aortogram shows the severe stenosis at the IMA origin *(arrow).* The stenosis was successfully stented.

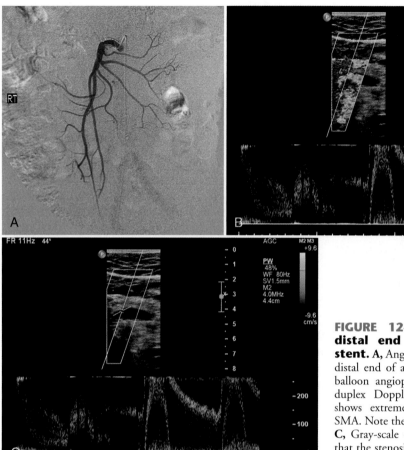

FIGURE 12-34. Stenotic SMA at distal end of previously placed stent. A, Angiogram showing stenosis at the distal end of a stent. This was treated with balloon angioplasty. **B,** Color and spectral duplex Doppler ultrasound 3 years later shows extremely elevated velocity in the SMA. Note the elevation in diastolic velocity. **C,** Gray-scale duplex Doppler image shows that the stenosis has recurred at distal end of the SMA stent.

stents, restenosis is usually caused by **intimal hyperplasia,** which is common within bare-metal stents but even more common at the end of the stent (Fig. 12-34).

However, posttreatment duplex surveillance is confounded by Doppler velocities often remaining high in stented SMAs.[109] Some speculate that this velocity elevation may be caused by a change in the elastic properties of the arterial wall induced by its incorporation of the stent. In addition, the goal of stenting often is not to restore normal flow, but only to restore enough flow to make the patient asymptomatic. Those arteries treated with stenting often supply collateral flow to any untreated arteries that remain stenotic or occluded. The stented arteries often have increased flow throughout their course. This results in velocities that are uniformly elevated throughout the artery. We have found this result not only in the SMA, but also in the other mesenteric arteries (Fig. 12-35). Treatment decisions after stenting must be made in the context of the entire clinical picture, not on the basis of velocities alone. If the patient is entirely asymptomatic, treatment will generally not be undertaken regardless of the results of mesenteric artery duplex.

Iliac Veins and Inferior Vena Cava

As with veins throughout the body, the range of pathology occurring in the iliac veins and inferior vena cava (IVC) is narrow. Thrombosis of the iliac veins and IVC is probably the most common pathology, but is much less common than lower extremity venous thrombosis.

Often, the iliac veins and the infrarenal IVC are not well evaluated directly with ultrasound. Therefore, ultrasound exams are infrequently done with the intent of doing a primary evaluation of the entire IVC and iliac veins. The main exception is infants, in whom IVC evaluation with ultrasound has a much better opportunity to provide good diagnostic information.

Anatomy

The IVC can be divided into several segments. The most proximal (i.e., central) segment is the **suprahepatic** (posthepatic), which is short and intrathoracic. In adults this segment is approximately 2.5 cm. in length and has the hepatic veins as tributaries. The next segment is **intrahepatic,** with accessory hepatic and caudate veins

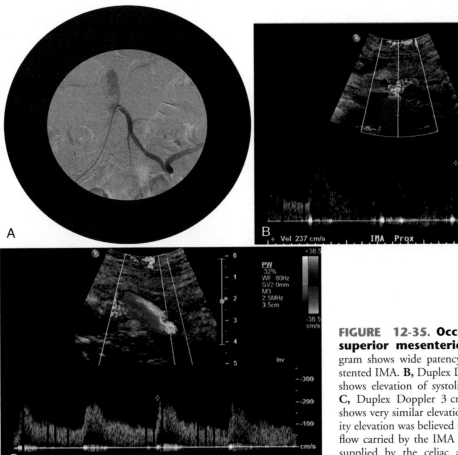

FIGURE 12-35. Occluded celiac and superior mesenteric arteries. A, Angiogram shows wide patency of origin of the large, stented IMA. **B,** Duplex Doppler at origin of IMA shows elevation of systolic and diastolic velocity. **C,** Duplex Doppler 3 cm distal to IMA origin shows very similar elevation of velocity. The velocity elevation was believed to be caused by increased flow carried by the IMA to supply organs usually supplied by the celiac and superior mesenteric arteries.

as tributaries. The next segment is the **infrahepatic/suprarenal,** which has the renal veins as tributaries. The last segment is **infrarenal,** which is the longest segment and has the right gonadal vein as a tributary. Proceeding distally, the IVC divides into the common iliac veins. The left common iliac vein passes between the right common iliac artery and the spine where it can become compressed producing **May-Thurner physiology** (called May-Thurner syndrome when it results in thrombosis) (Fig. 12-36). The common iliac veins have major tributaries of the internal and external iliac veins.

Anatomic Variants

There are three major variations of IVC anatomy, the most common a **duplicated** IVC. The duplication is of the infrarenal portion of the IVC, with incidence of approximately 2% (Fig. 12-37, *A*). Most often, the IVC's left channel enters the left renal vein. The suprarenal IVC has normal anatomy. The second most common anomaly is a **transposed** (left-sided) IVC (0.5%; Fig. 12-38, *B*), which also usually drains into the left renal vein. As with a duplicated IVC, anatomy above

the level of the renal veins is normal. With both these anomalies, the anomalous left-sided segment may cross the aorta below the level of the left renal vein. Also, the anomalous segment may cross either anterior or posterior to the aorta.[110]

The third major anomaly is **azygous continuation** of the IVC. The infrarenal IVC flows superiorly into the hemiazygous or azygous veins. The IVC does not course through the liver in this setting; there is no intrahepatic IVC. The hepatic veins drain normally into the short suprahepatic (posthepatic) IVC, which enters the right atrium. Incidence of azygous continuation is approximately 0.6%.[110]

Regarding IVC tributaries, there are variations in the anatomy of the hepatic veins, left renal vein, and gonadal veins. The hepatic veins have numerous variations important in preprocedural planning of liver resection or transplantation.[111] The most common variation is the presence of an **accessory right hepatic vein.**[112]

The **left renal vein** usually passes in front of the abdominal aorta to join the IVC. It also can be **circumaortic** (up to 8.7%),[110] where the left renal vein has two branches, one passing behind the aorta and the other anterior to the aorta. Less often, it can be **retroaortic**

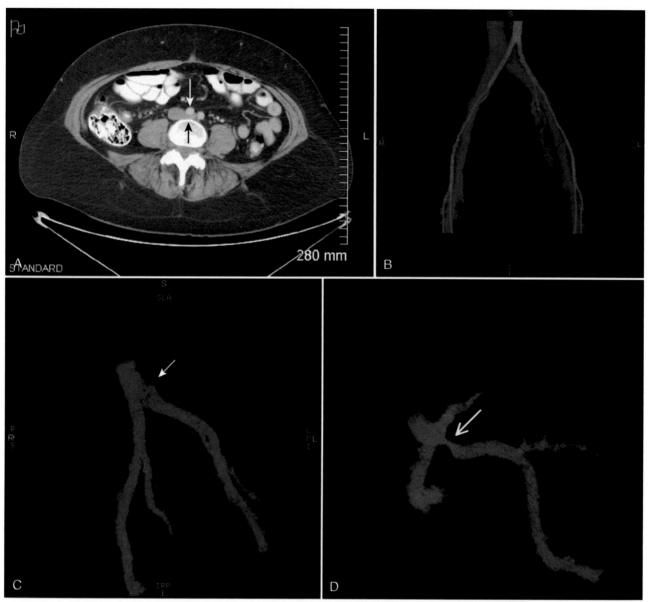

FIGURE 12-36. May-Thurner physiology. A, CT scan performed for a patient with greatly decreased phasicity in venous wave-forms of the left leg on duplex imaging. Left common iliac vein *(black arrow)* is compressed where it goes between the right common iliac artery *(white arrow)* and the spine. **B,** 3-D CT reconstruction showing the aorta and common iliac arteries *(light blue)* and the inferior vena cava (IVC) and common iliac veins *(purple)*. **C,** 3-D CT reconstruction of the IVC and iliac veins. Note the slight notch in the left common iliac vein at the point where it crosses behind the right common iliac artery. **D,** CT reconstruction of the IVC and iliac veins viewed to the left and superior to the pelvis. Right iliac veins and IVC overlap one another. The left external iliac (LEIV) and left common iliac (LCIV) veins are laid out well. The narrowing in the left common iliac vein *(yellow arrow)* is well seen in this projection.

(up to 2.4%), where a single left renal vein passes behind the aorta. In both cases, the portion of the left renal vein passing behind the aorta most frequently descends a short distance toward the pelvis as it passes behind the aorta.[110]

The **right gonadal vein** joins the IVC just below the level of the right renal vein or at the right renal vein in 90% of cases. In the remaining 10%, it joins the right renal vein. When IVC anatomy is standard, the **left gonadal vein** almost always drains into the left renal vein. In a duplicated or left IVC, the left gonadal vein most often drains into the left-sided IVC.[113]

Thrombosis

The iliac veins and IVC are large veins with high-volume flow. They are less prone to primary thrombosis than are deep veins of the extremities. Isolated iliac vein thrombosis is uncommon, occurring in 1.6% of cases of lower extremity deep venous thrombosis (DVT).[114]

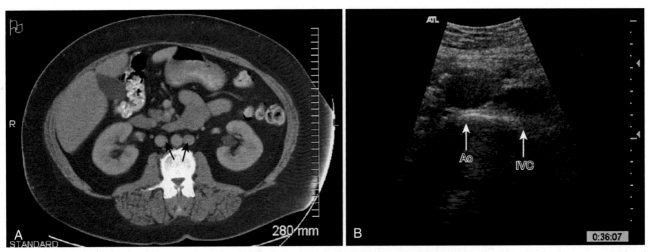

FIGURE 12-37. Inferior vena cava anomalies. A, CT image of duplicated IVC *(black arrows),* the most common anomaly of the IVC. The left IVC joined the left renal vein. The IVC above the level of the renal veins was in the normal location. **B,** Ultrasound of another IVC anomaly, a left IVC running to the left of the aorta. The left IVC joins the left renal vein.

In adults, thrombus in the iliac veins is more common than in the IVC. Thrombus most often results from extension of lower extremity venous thrombosis. Extrinsic compression of the IVC or iliac veins, as in May-Thurner physiology or a gravid uterus, may also result in thrombosis. Iliac vein thrombosis in adults is infrequently directly seen sonographically because of lack of an adequate window. Most often, the possibility of iliac thrombosis can only be inferred sonographically.

Sonographic clues to iliac vein thrombosis are found in the common femoral veins. When thrombus in the common femoral vein extends as far proximally as can be seen, it is easy to infer possible extension into the iliac veins. More subtle cases involve continuous, low, or absent flow in an open (nonthrombosed) common femoral vein. Common femoral vein waveforms generally show respiratory phasicity or cardiac phasicity, or both. When **phasicity** is not clearly seen, as in continuous, low, or absent flow, it suggests obstruction to flow more proximally (Fig. 12-38; see also Fig. 12-36). Before ordering other tests to look for more proximal obstruction, it is worthwhile to perform a few maneuvers to eliminate nonpathologic causes of lack of phasicity. First, remove underwear if it may be tight; this is a common cause of nonpathological obstruction. Second, sonographically check the fullness of the bladder. If moderately or greatly distended, the patient should be asked to empty the bladder. Third, if the patient is in the second or third trimester of pregnancy, check the waveforms in posterior oblique or decubitus positions. If the compression is caused by the gravid uterus compressing the veins, these maneuvers will often allow the waveform to return to normal, showing that there is no fixed blockage of the veins (Fig. 12-39).

If these maneuvers are not successful at restoring a normal waveform, there may be an obstruction proximal to the common femoral vein(s). If unilateral, there is likely to be iliac vein obstruction. If bilateral, the obstruction may be of the iliac veins bilaterally or of the IVC. In our experience the lack of common femoral vein phasicity is more likely to be a false-positive finding if it is bilateral rather than unilateral (Fig. 12-40).

In the setting of absent common femoral vein phasicity, more proximal obstruction may be caused by acute or chronic thrombosis, May-Thurner physiology, or extrinsic compression of the vein by a benign or malignant mass or fluid collection. When lack of phasicity is found, other imaging studies may be performed to evaluate possible etiologies. We typically use contrast-enhanced CT (Fig. 12-41) and, in pregnancy, MRI. Pelvic venography is another option.

In infants, particularly those with femoral venous catheters, scanning of the IVC can be valuable in assessing for thrombosis. The intrahepatic IVC is generally well seen. Thrombus can often be seen in gray scale and confirmed with color and spectral Doppler ultrasound. The infrahepatic IVC is more difficult to see but often can be adequately assessed using a far lateral approach obtaining coronal images using either kidney as a window.

Budd-Chiari Syndrome

Budd-Chiari syndrome is a rare condition caused by obstruction to outflow of the hepatic veins. In Caucasians the condition is often related to hypercoagulability. In Asians, membranous obstruction of the IVC is the most common cause.[115] When there is isolated stenosis of the IVC, percutaneous transluminal angioplasty with or without stent placement is often successful. Transjugular intrahepatic portosystemic shunt (TIPSS) placement is often effective for hepatic vein obstruction.[116]

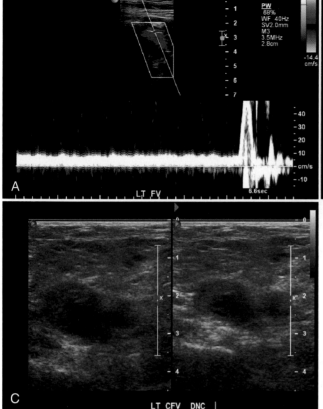

FIGURE 12-38. Venous duplex Doppler ultrasound for left leg swelling. A, Waveform in the left femoral vein lacks phasicity. All veins in the left thigh had similar waveforms. There was no thrombus found anywhere in the left leg. The examination was mistakenly read as normal. **B,** Normal waveform in the right common iliac vein. **C,** Left leg was reexamined the next day and now shows extensive thrombus. When the first exam was performed, there was likely iliac vein thrombus, which then had extended into the common femoral vein 24 hours later. Waveforms in the legs are often the only sonographic clue of iliac vein thrombosis.

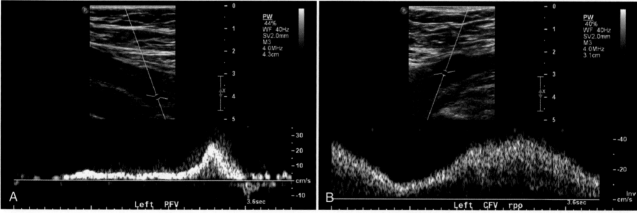

FIGURE 12-39. Patient in third trimester of pregnancy with leg swelling. A, Waveform in the left profunda femoral vein with patient supine shows decreased phasicity. All veins in the left thigh had a similar waveform. The only variation seen in flow is when an augmentation (calf or thigh squeeze) was performed, causing a brief increase in flow. **B,** Patient turned into right posterior oblique position. Turning has moved the gravid uterus off of the left iliac veins. Flow in the left common femoral vein shows normal respiratory phasicity.

Budd-Chiari syndrome has many intrahepatic manifestations.[117,118] IVC manifestations are visible sonographically and include an IVC web just above the hepatic veins,[115] narrowing of the intrahepatic IVC caused by swelling of the liver, and IVC thrombosis.[116]

Inferior Vena Cava Neoplasms

Neoplasm of the IVC is rare and most often occurs in the setting of extension of solid organ tumors extending through their venous drainage to enter the IVC. This

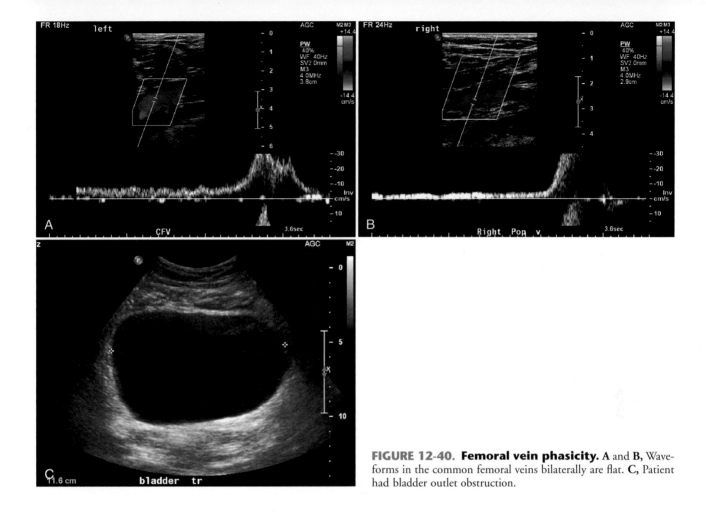

FIGURE 12-40. Femoral vein phasicity. A and **B,** Waveforms in the common femoral veins bilaterally are flat. **C,** Patient had bladder outlet obstruction.

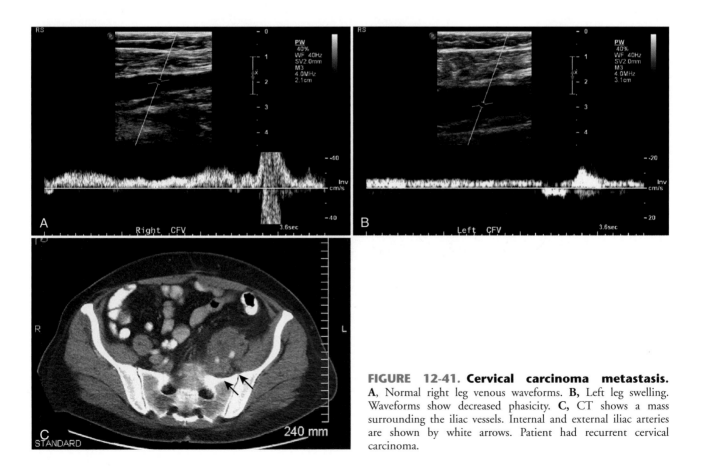

FIGURE 12-41. Cervical carcinoma metastasis. A, Normal right leg venous waveforms. **B,** Left leg swelling. Waveforms show decreased phasicity. **C,** CT shows a mass surrounding the iliac vessels. Internal and external iliac arteries are shown by white arrows. Patient had recurrent cervical carcinoma.

phenomenon is seen when **renal cell carcinoma** extends through the renal veins into the IVC. The same phenomenon can occur with **hepatocellular** and **adrenocortical carcinoma** extending through the hepatic and adrenal veins into the IVC.

Primary neoplasms of the IVC are even rarer. **Leiomyosarcoma** can occur at other sites in the systemic veins as well, but most often arises in the IVC.

Ultrasound is not the primary method of imaging these tumors. When findings of IVC tumor involvement are seen sonographically, cross-sectional imaging with CT or MRI should generally be recommended to determine the full extent of the abnormality.

Other Inferior Vena Cava Findings

Dilation of the IVC and hepatic vein orifices is seen in patients with congestive heart failure[119] (Fig. 12-42).

Placement of **IVC filters** has become more common. In our experience, they are inconsistently seen. When seen, filters appear as an echogenic foreign body in the IVC. It is rarely possible to determine more about the filter than its presence and approximate location (Fig. 12-43). The IVC may become sclerotic in patients with long-standing filters, in whom it may be possible to see an absence of the IVC along with retroperitoneal collateral veins. The legs of the filters can also penetrate the

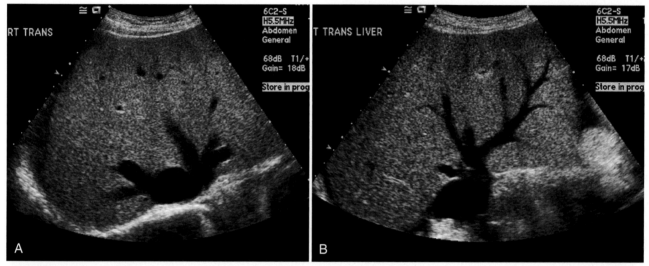

FIGURE 12-42. A and **B,** Two images show dilation of IVC and hepatic veins caused by congestive heart failure. *(Courtesy Carl Reading, MD.)*

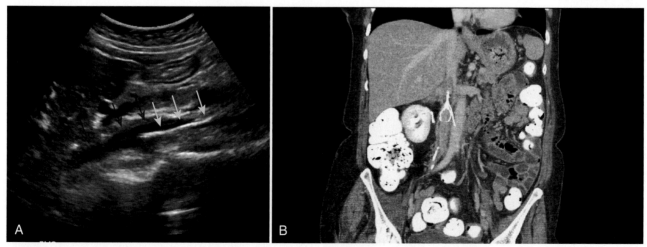

FIGURE 12-43. Inferior vena cava filters. A, IVC filters can be very difficult to see. Bright linear echoes *(yellow arrows)* indicate a tine of the filter within the IVC *(red arrows)*. This image represents an unusually good visualization of a filter. **B,** Coronal reconstruction of CT shows the location and form of the filter. *(Courtesy Anthony Hanbidge, MD.)*

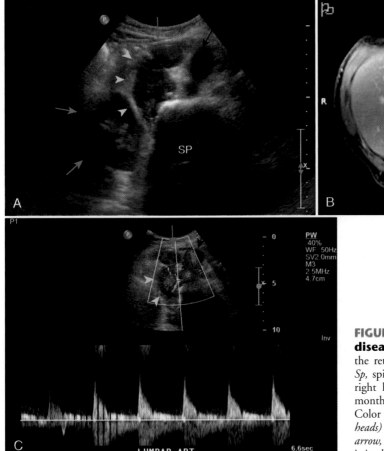

FIGURE 12-44. Metastatic retroperitoneal disease. A, Metastasis of esophageal adenocarcinoma to the retroperitoneum, probably nodal *(yellow arrowheads); Sp,* spine; *red arrow,* aorta; *blue arrow,* IVC; *green arrows,* right kidney. **B,** MR image of patient approximately 1 month later. Anatomy has only minimally changed. **C,** Color duplex Doppler shows that the lesion *(yellow arrowheads)* is vascular and is supplied by a lumbar artery; *red arrow,* aorta; *blue arrow,* IVC. The Doppler sample volume is in the enlarged lumbar artery that supplies the lesion.

wall of the IVC. This finding is fairly common on CT and most often is an incidental finding, although complications may result.[120] IVC penetration may be able to be observed sonographically as an echogenic foreign body extending outside of the IVC.

NONVASCULAR DISEASES OF THE RETROPERITONEUM

Ultrasound is not the primary modality used in defining nonvascular problems in the retroperitoneum. When the abnormalities described next are seen sonographically, in many cases further cross-sectional imaging with CT or MRI is needed to define the abnormality completely.

Solid Masses

Probably the most common solid mass is **lymphadenopathy** (enlarged lymph nodes). Causes of nodal enlargement can be benign or malignant (e.g., infection, lymphoma), but in all cases, malignancy must be excluded. Lymph nodes are most commonly hypoechoic. The iden-

tification of a structure as a probable lymph node is often by location in a para-aortic or paracaval region or in the mesentery.

Metastatic disease is another cause of solid masses in the retroperitoneum. Metastasis most frequently occurs to lymph nodes but can be seen in other sites. Often, it is impossible to tell with certainty whether the mass is nodal or is centered in some other type of tissue (Fig. 12-44).

Primary malignancies in the retroperitoneum are rare. The most common malignant retroperitoneal tumor is **lymphoma.**[121] The next most common are sarcomas: **liposarcoma, leiomyosarcoma,** and **fibrous histiocytoma.** These tumors generally undergo surgical resection and have a relatively high rate of recurrence.[122]

Benign masses also occur in the retroperitoneum, including **fibromas, schwannomas, neurofibromas,** and **lipomas.** Extra-adrenal **paragangliomas** (extra-adrenal **pheochromocytomas**) are usually benign but can be malignant.[123] The distinction between benign and malignant for retroperitoneal masses cannot generally be made sonographically, and the finding of an unexpected mass in the retroperitoneum should generally prompt further evaluation with CT or MRI.

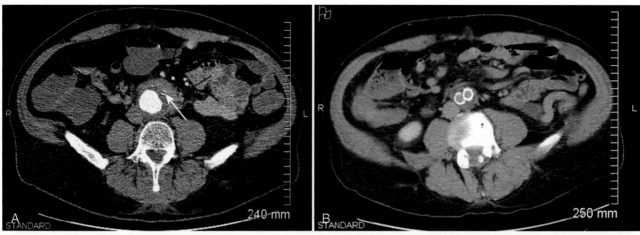

FIGURE 12-45. Chronic periaortitis. A, CT scan of chronic periaortitis with AAA (inflammatory AAA), which had maximal diameter of 4.9 cm. Patient was symptomatic and was treated with an endoluminal graft shortly after this scan. Note calcification *(white arrow)* indicating the aortic wall. Inflammatory tissue is present outside the aorta *(red arrows)*. **B,** CT scan 2 years later shows that aortic size is smaller. Inflammatory mass has disappeared.

Fluid collections may also be seen in the retroperitoneum, including hematoma, urinoma, lymphocele, abscess, and pancreatic pseudocyst. If well seen and when indicated, sonography in conjunction with fluoroscopy is often the best way to drain these collections.

Retroperitoneal Fibrosis

As mentioned previously, retroperitoneal fibrosis (RPF) is often grouped with inflammatory AAA in the disease process called **chronic periaortitis.** RPF can be seen as a mass usually surrounding the aorta and the common iliac arteries. It can involve adjacent structures, most often the ureters, resulting in displacement of the ureters and often in obstruction. When related to AAA, RPF usually regresses with repair of the AAA (Fig. 12-45).

In RPF, ultrasound shows a mass encasing the abdominal aorta (Fig. 12-46). The back wall of the aorta is usually spared. A periaortic mass seen to separate the aorta from the spine suggests that the cause is instead malignant.[124] Ultrasound is not sensitive for detection of RPF,[125] although it is sensitive for detection of AAA, which may be present. Sonography is also sensitive for the detection of ureteral obstruction and hydronephrosis, the most common complication.

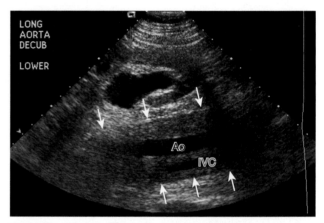

FIGURE 12-46. Chronic periaortitis. Coronal ultrasound image of chronic periaortitis with no AAA (retroperitoneal fibrosis) *(white arrows)* surrounding the aorta *(Ao).* Inferior vena cava *(IVC)* is also faintly visible, surrounded by the mass. Left kidney *(green arrows)* is hydronephrotic because of entrapment of the left ureter by the periaortic mass. *(Courtesy Carl Reading, MD.)*

CONCLUSION

Ultrasound often is used for targeted evaluation of solid organs and blood vessels in the retroperitoneum. Solid organ evaluation is covered in other chapters. For diseases of blood vessels of the retroperitoneum, ultrasound is generally an excellent diagnostic method and often the first modality used in diagnosis. For several reasons ultrasound is not a primary method for imaging the connective tissue regions of the retroperitoneum. To perform a thorough diagnostic examination when scanning the retroperitoneal organs and blood vessels, the clinician must have a clear concept of all retroperitoneal findings that may be encountered so that the best patient care can be provided.

References

Atherosclerosis

1. Stehbens WE. General features, structure, topography and adaptation of the circulatory system. In: Stehbens WE, Lie JT, editors. Vascular pathology. New York: Chapman & Hall; 1995.
2. American Heart Association. Heart disease and stroke statistics—2009 update. Dallas: AHA; 2009.
3. Kung HC, Hoyert DL, Xu J, Murphy SL. Deaths: final data for 2005. Natl Vital Stat Rep 2008;56:1-120.
4. American Heart Association. Heart disease and stroke statistics—2008 update. Dallas: AHA; 2008.

5. Schoen FJ, Cotran RS. Blood vessels. In: Cotran RS, Kumar V, Collins T, editors. Robbins pathologic basis of disease. 6th ed. Philadelphia: Saunders; 1999.

6. Schoen FJ. Blood vessels. In: Kumar V, Abbas A, Fausto N, editors. Robbins pathologic basis of disease. 7th ed. Philadelphia: Saunders-Elsevier; 2005.

7. Ross R. Atherosclerosis: an inflammatory disease. N Engl J Med 1999;340:115-126.

Abdominal Aortic Aneurysm

8. Johnston KW, Rutherford RB, Tilson MD, et al. Suggested standards for reporting on arterial aneurysms. Subcommittee on Reporting Standards for Arterial Aneurysms, Ad Hoc Committee on Reporting Standards, Society for Vascular Surgery, and North American Chapter, International Society for Cardiovascular Surgery. J Vasc Surg 1991;13:452-458.

9. Lederle FA, Wilson SE, Johnson GR, et al. Immediate repair compared with surveillance of small abdominal aortic aneurysms. N Engl J Med 2002;346:1437-1444.

10. Gillum RF. Epidemiology of aortic aneurysm in the United States. J Clin Epidemiol 1995;48:1289-1298.

11. Scott RA, Vardulaki KA, Walker NM, et al. The long-term benefits of a single scan for abdominal aortic aneurysm (AAA) at age 65. Eur J Vasc Endovasc Surg 2001;21:535-540.

12. Wanhainen A, Bjorck M, Boman K, et al. Influence of diagnostic criteria on the prevalence of abdominal aortic aneurysm. J Vasc Surg 2001;34:229-235.

13. Crawford ES, Snyder DM, Cho GC, Roehm Jr JO. Progress in treatment of thoracoabdominal and abdominal aortic aneurysms involving celiac, superior mesenteric, and renal arteries. Ann Surg 1978;188:404-422.

14. Wills A, Thompson MM, Crowther M, et al. Pathogenesis of abdominal aortic aneurysms: cellular and biochemical mechanisms. Eur J Vasc Endovasc Surg 1996;12:391-400.

15. Grange JJ, Davis V, Baxter BT. Pathogenesis of abdominal aortic aneurysm: an update and look toward the future. Cardiovasc Surg 1997;5:256-265.

16. Golledge J, Muller J, Daugherty A, Norman P. Abdominal aortic aneurysm: pathogenesis and implications for management. Arterioscler Thromb Vasc Biol 2006;26:2605-2613.

17. Wilmink AB, Quick CR. Epidemiology and potential for prevention of abdominal aortic aneurysm. Br J Surg 1998;85:155-162.

18. Solberg S, Singh K, Wilsgaard T, Jacobsen BK. Increased growth rate of abdominal aortic aneurysms in women. The Tromso Study. Eur J Vasc Endovasc Surg 2005;29:145-149.

19. Mofidi R, Goldie VJ, Kelman J, et al. Influence of sex on expansion rate of abdominal aortic aneurysms. Br J Surg 2007;94:310-314.

20. Schermerhorn ML, Cronenwett JL. Abdominal aortic and iliac aneurysms. In: Rutherford RB, Cronenwett JL, Gloviczki P, et al, editors. Vascular surgery. 6th ed. Philadelphia: Saunders-Elsevier; 2005.

21. Brown LC, Powell JT. Risk factors for aneurysm rupture in patients kept under ultrasound surveillance. UK Small Aneurysm Trial Participants. Ann Surg 1999;230:289-296; discussion 296-297.

22. Brown PM, Zelt DT, Sobolev B. The risk of rupture in untreated aneurysms: the impact of size, gender, and expansion rate. J Vasc Surg 2003;37:280-284.

23. MacSweeney ST, Ellis M, Worrell PC, et al. Smoking and growth rate of small abdominal aortic aneurysms. Lancet 1994;344:651-652.

24. Baxter BT, Pearce WH, Waltke EA, et al. Prolonged administration of doxycycline in patients with small asymptomatic abdominal aortic aneurysms: report of a prospective (Phase II) multicenter study. J Vasc Surg 2002;36:1-12.

25. Schlosser FJ, Tangelder MJ, Verhagen HJ, et al. Growth predictors and prognosis of small abdominal aortic aneurysms. J Vasc Surg 2008;47:1127-1133.

26. Mosorin M, Juvonen J, Biancari F, et al. Use of doxycycline to decrease the growth rate of abdominal aortic aneurysms: a randomized, double-blind, placebo-controlled pilot study. J Vasc Surg 2001;34:606-610.

27. Bergqvist D, Bjorck M, Wanhainen A. Abdominal aortic aneurysm—to screen or not to screen. Eur J Vasc Endovasc Surg 2008;35:13-18.

28. Ashton HA, Buxton MJ, Day NE, et al. The Multicentre Aneurysm Screening Study (MASS) into the effect of abdominal aortic aneurysm screening on mortality in men: a randomised controlled trial. Lancet 2002;360:1531-1539.

29. Multicentre Aneurysm Screening Study (MASS). cost effectiveness analysis of screening for abdominal aortic aneurysms based on four-year results from randomised controlled trial. BMJ 2002;325:1135.

30. Lindholt JS, Juul S, Fasting H, Henneberg EW. Hospital costs and benefits of screening for abdominal aortic aneurysms: results from a randomised population screening trial. Eur J Vasc Endovasc Surg 2002;23:55-60.

31. Fleming C, Whitlock EP, Beil TL, Lederle FA. Screening for abdominal aortic aneurysm: a best-evidence systematic review for the US Preventive Services Task Force. Ann Intern Med 2005;142:203-211.

32. US Preventive Services Task Force. Screening: abdominal aortic aneurysm. February 2005. http://www.ahrq.gov/clinic/uspstf/uspsaneu.htm. Accessed November 2008.

33. Bertino RE, Pellerito JS, Angtuaco TL, et al. ACR practice guideline for the performance of diagnostic and screening ultrasound of the abdominal aorta. American College of Radiology; 2005.

34. McCarthy RJ, Shaw E, Whyman MR, et al. Recommendations for screening intervals for small aortic aneurysms. Br J Surg 2003;90:821-826.

35. Brady AR, Thompson SG, Fowkes FG, et al. Abdominal aortic aneurysm expansion: risk factors and time intervals for surveillance. Circulation 2004;110:16-21.

36. Bertino R, Pai D, Beach D, et al. Establishment of an interventional radiology clinic to follow untreated abdominal aortic aneurysms. J Am Coll Radiol 2006;3:291-295.

37. Shuman WP, Hastrup Jr W, Kohler TR, et al. Suspected leaking abdominal aortic aneurysm: use of sonography in the emergency room. Radiology 1988;168:117-119.

38. Dill-Macky MJ. Aortic endografts: detecting endoleaks using contrast-enhanced ultrasound. Ultrasound Q 2006;22:49-52.

39. Bashir MR, Ferral H, Jacobs C, et al. Endoleaks after endovascular abdominal aortic aneurysm repair: management strategies according to CT findings. AJR Am J Roentgenol 2009;192:W178-W186.

40. Mennander A, Pimenoff G, Heikkinen M, et al. Nonoperative approach to endotension. J Vasc Surg 2005;42:194-199.

41. Baum RA, Stavropoulos SW, Fairman RM, Carpenter JP. Endoleaks after endovascular repair of abdominal aortic aneurysm. J Vasc Interv Radiol 2003;14:1111-1117.

42. Parent FN, Meier GH, Godziachvili V, et al. The incidence and natural history of type I and II endoleak: a 5-year follow-up assessment with color duplex ultrasound scan. J Vasc Surg 2002;35:474-481.

43. Manning BJ, O'Neill SM, Haider SN, et al. Duplex ultrasound in aneurysm surveillance following endovascular aneurysm repair: a comparison with computed tomography aortography. J Vasc Surg 2009;49:60-65.

44. Dill-Macky MJ, Wilson SR, Sternbach Y, et al. Detecting endoleaks in aortic endografts using contrast-enhanced sonography. AJR Am J Roentgenol 2007;188:W262-W268.

45. Giannoni MF, Palombo G, Sbarigia E, et al. Contrast-enhanced ultrasound imaging for aortic stent-graft surveillance. J Endovasc Ther 2003;10:208-217.

Other Entities Causing Abdominal Aortic Dilation

46. Lindblad B, Almgren B, Bergqvist D, et al. Abdominal aortic aneurysm with perianeurysmal fibrosis: experience from 11 Swedish vascular centers. J Vasc Surg 1991;13:231-237; discussion 237-239.

47. Hellmann DB, Grand DJ, Freischlag JA. Inflammatory abdominal aortic aneurysm. JAMA 2007;297:395-400.

48. Hayashi H, Matsuoka Y, Sakamoto I, et al. Penetrating atherosclerotic ulcer of the aorta: imaging features and disease concept. Radiographics 2000;20:995-1005.

49. Tsuji Y, Tanaka Y, Kitagawa A, et al. Endovascular stent-graft repair for penetrating atherosclerotic ulcer in the infrarenal abdominal aorta. J Vasc Surg 2003;38:383-388.

Stenotic Disease of the Abdominal Aorta

50. Chung JW, Kim HC, Choi YH, et al. Patterns of aortic involvement in Takayasu arteritis and its clinical implications: evaluation with spiral computed tomography angiography. J Vasc Surg 2007;45:906-914.

51. Diaz JA, Campbell BT, Moursi MM, et al. Delayed manifestation of abdominal aortic stenosis in a child presenting 10 years after blunt abdominal trauma. J Vasc Surg 2006;44:1104-1106.

Diseases of Abdominal Aorta Branches

52. Verschuyl EJ, Kaatee R, Beek FJ, et al. Renal artery origins: best angiographic projection angles. Radiology 1997;205:115-120.
53. Kadir S. Arterial and venous systems of the viscera: kidneys. In: Normal and variant angiographic anatomy. Philadelphia: Saunders; 1991.
54. Glodny B, Petersen J, Hofmann KJ, et al. Kidney fusion anomalies revisited: clinical and radiological analysis of 209 cases of crossed fused ectopia and horseshoe kidney. BJU Int 2009;103:224-225.
55. Boatman DL, Cornell SH, Kolln CP. The arterial supply of horseshoe kidneys. Am J Roentgenol Radium Ther Nucl Med 1971; 113:447-451.
56. US Department of Health and Human Services. DHHS Pub No 2009-1232. Health, United States, 2008. Centers for Disease Control and Prevention, National Center for Health Statistics, March 2009.
57. Oparil S, Zaman MA, Calhoun DA. Pathogenesis of hypertension. Ann Intern Med 2003;139:761-776.
58. Vasbinder GB, Nelemans PJ, Kessels AG, et al. Diagnostic tests for renal artery stenosis in patients suspected of having renovascular hypertension: a meta-analysis. Ann Intern Med 2001;135:401-411.
59. Murphy TP, Soares G, Kim M. Increase in utilization of percutaneous renal artery interventions by Medicare beneficiaries, 1996-2000. AJR Am J Roentgenol 2004;183:561-568.
60. Textor SC. Atherosclerotic renal artery stenosis: overtreated but underrated? J Am Soc Nephrol 2008;19:656-659.
61. Radermacher J, Chavan A, Bleck J, et al. Use of Doppler ultrasonography to predict the outcome of therapy for renal-artery stenosis. N Engl J Med 2001;344:410-417.
62. Beutler JJ, Van Ampting JM, Van De Ven PJ, et al. Long-term effects of arterial stenting on kidney function for patients with ostial atherosclerotic renal artery stenosis and renal insufficiency. J Am Soc Nephrol 2001;12:1475-1481.
63. Zucchelli PC. Hypertension and atherosclerotic renal artery stenosis: diagnostic approach. J Am Soc Nephrol 2002;13(Suppl 3):184-186.
64. White CJ. Catheter-based therapy for atherosclerotic renal artery stenosis. Circulation 2006;113:1464-1473.
65. Olin JW, Piedmonte MR, Young JR, et al. The utility of duplex ultrasound scanning of the renal arteries for diagnosing significant renal artery stenosis. Ann Intern Med 1995;122:833-838.
66. Labropoulos N, Ayuste B, Leon Jr LR. Renovascular disease among patients referred for renal duplex ultrasonography. J Vasc Surg 2007;46:731-737.
67. Safian RD, Textor SC. Renal artery stenosis. N Engl J Med 2001; 344:431-442.
68. Henry M, Amor M, Henry I, et al. Stents in the treatment of renal artery stenosis: long-term follow-up. J Endovasc Surg 1999;6:42-51.
69. Isles CG, Robertson S, Hill D. Management of renovascular disease: a review of renal artery stenting in ten studies. Q J Med 1999;92:159-167.
70. Plouin PF, Perdu J, La Batide-Alanore A, et al. Fibromuscular dysplasia. Orphanet J Rare Dis 2007;2:28.
71. Slovut DP, Olin JW. Fibromuscular dysplasia. N Engl J Med 2004;350:1862-1871.
72. Luscher TF, Noll G, Wenzel RR. Systemic hypertension and related vascular diseases. In: Stehbens WE, Lie JT, editors. Vascular pathology. New York: Chapman & Hall; 1995.
73. Sos TA, Pickering TG, Sniderman K, et al. Percutaneous transluminal renal angioplasty in renovascular hypertension due to atheroma or fibromuscular dysplasia. N Engl J Med 1983;309:274-279.
74. Williams DM, Lee DY, Hamilton BH, et al. The dissected aorta: percutaneous treatment of ischemic complications: principles and results. J Vasc Interv Radiol 1997;8:605-625.
75. Blum U, Billmann P, Krause T, et al. Effect of local low-dose thrombolysis on clinical outcome in acute embolic renal artery occlusion. Radiology 1993;189:549-554.
76. Courtel JV, Soto B, Niaudet P, et al. Percutaneous transluminal angioplasty of renal artery stenosis in children. Pediatr Radiol 1998;28:59-63.
77. Ritz E. Accessory renal arteries—mostly, but not always, innocuous. J Am Soc Nephrol 2006;17:3-4.

78. Bude RO, Forauer AR, Caoili EM, Nghiem HV. Is it necessary to study accessory arteries when screening the renal arteries for renovascular hypertension? Radiology 2003;226:411-416.
79. Bertino RE, Gooding GE, Ralls PW, et al. ACR practice guidelines for the performance of renal artery duplex sonography. American Collage of Radiology, 2008. Accessed at http://www.acr.org/SencondaryMainMenuCategories/quality_safety/guidelines/us/Renal_Artery_Sonography.aspx April 11, 2010.
80. Li JC, Wang L, Jiang YX, et al. Evaluation of renal artery stenosis with velocity parameters of Doppler sonography. J Ultrasound Med 2006;25:735-742; quiz 743-744.
81. Stavros AT, Parker SH, Yakes WF, et al. Segmental stenosis of the renal artery: pattern recognition of tardus and parvus abnormalities with duplex sonography. Radiology 1992;184:487-492.
82. Li JC, Jiang YX, Zhang SY, et al. Evaluation of renal artery stenosis with hemodynamic parameters of Doppler sonography. J Vasc Surg 2008;48:323-328.
83. Williams GJ, Macaskill P, Chan SF, et al. Comparative accuracy of renal duplex sonographic parameters in the diagnosis of renal artery stenosis: paired and unpaired analysis. AJR Am J Roentgenol 2007;188:798-811.
84. Taylor DC, Kettler MD, Moneta GL, et al. Duplex ultrasound scanning in the diagnosis of renal artery stenosis: a prospective evaluation. J Vasc Surg 1988;7:363-369.
85. Tham G, Ekelund L, Herrlin K, et al. Renal artery aneurysms: natural history and prognosis. Ann Surg 1983;197:348-352.
86. Nosher JL, Chung J, Brevetti LS, et al. Visceral and renal artery aneurysms: a pictorial essay on endovascular therapy. Radiographics 2006;26:1687-1704.
87. Bui BT, Oliva VL, Leclerc G, et al. Renal artery aneurysm: treatment with percutaneous placement of a stent-graft. Radiology 1995; 195:181-182.
88. Uflacker R. Abdominal aorta and branches. In: Atlas of vascular anatomy: an angiographic approach. 2nd ed. Philadelphia: Lippincott–Williams & Wilkins; 2007.
89. Kadir S, Lundell C, Saeed M. Celiac, superior and inferior mesenteric arteries. In: Atlas of normal and variant angiographic anatomy. Philadelphia: Saunders; 1991.
90. Oldenburg WA, Lau LL, Rodenberg TJ, et al. Acute mesenteric ischemia: a clinical review. Arch Intern Med 2004;164:1054-1062.
91. Moore EM, Endean ED. Treatment of acute intestinal ischemia caused by arterial occlusions. In: Rutherford RB, Johnston KW, editors. Vascular surgery. 6th ed. Philadelphia: Saunders-Elsevier; 2009.
92. Hirsch AT, Haskal ZJ, Hertzer NR, et al. ACC/AHA Guidelines for the Management of Patients with Peripheral Arterial Disease (lower extremity, renal, mesenteric, and abdominal aortic): a collaborative report from the American Associations for Vascular Surgery/Society for Vascular Surgery, Society for Cardiovascular Angiography and Interventions, Society for Vascular Medicine and Biology, Society of Interventional Radiology, and the ACC/AHA Task Force on Practice Guidelines (Writing Committee to Develop Guidelines for the Management of Patients with Peripheral Arterial Disease)—summary of recommendations. J Vasc Interv Radiol 2006;17:1383-1397; quiz 1398.
93. Wilson DB, Mostafavi K, Craven TE, et al. Clinical course of mesenteric artery stenosis in elderly Americans. Arch Intern Med 2006;166:2095-2100.
94. Huber TS, Lee WA, Seeger JM. Chronic mesenteric ischemia. In: Rutherford RB, Johnston KW, editors. Vascular surgery. 6th ed. Philadelphia: Saunders-Elsevier; 2009.
95. Simon S, Schittko G, Bosenberg H, et al. [Fulminant course of a Takayasu arteritis and rare mesenteric arterial maninfestation]. Z Rheumatol 2006;65:520-526.
96. Levin DC, Baltaxe HA. High incidence of celiac axis narrowing in asymptomatic individuals. Am J Roentgenol Radium Ther Nucl Med 1972;116:426-429.
97. Delis KT, Gloviczki P, Altuwaijri M, McKusick MA. Median arcuate ligament syndrome: open celiac artery reconstruction and ligament division after endovascular failure. J Vasc Surg 2007;46:799-802.
98. Mensink PB, van Petersen AS, Kolkman JJ, et al. Gastric exercise tonometry: the key investigation in patients with suspected celiac artery compression syndrome. J Vasc Surg 2006;44:277-281.
99. Balaban DH, Chen J, Lin Z, et al. Median arcuate ligament syndrome: a possible cause of idiopathic gastroparesis. Am J Gastroenterol 1997;92:519-523.

100. Loffeld RJ, Overtoom HA, Rauwerda JA. The celiac axis compression syndrome: report of 5 cases. Digestion 1995;56:534-537.

101. Volteas N, Labropoulos N, Leon M, et al. Detection of superior mesenteric and coeliac artery stenosis with colour flow Duplex imaging. Eur J Vasc Surg 1993;7:616-620.

102. Gentile AT, Moneta GL, Lee RW, et al. Usefulness of fasting and postprandial duplex ultrasound examinations for predicting high-grade superior mesenteric artery stenosis. Am J Surg 1995;169:476-479.

103. Muller AF. Role of duplex Doppler ultrasound in the assessment of patients with postprandial abdominal pain. Gut 1992;33:460-465.

104. Wolfman D, Bluth EI, Sossaman J. Median arcuate ligament syndrome. J Ultrasound Med 2003;22:1377-1380.

105. Moneta GL, Lee RW, Yeager RA, et al. Mesenteric duplex scanning: a blinded prospective study. J Vasc Surg 1993;17:79-84; discussion 55-86.

106. Bowersox JC, Zwolak RM, Walsh DB, et al. Duplex ultrasonography in the diagnosis of celiac and mesenteric artery occlusive disease. J Vasc Surg 1991;14:780-786; discussion 786-788.

107. Perko MJ, Just S, Schroeder TV. Importance of diastolic velocities in the detection of celiac and mesenteric artery disease by duplex ultrasound. J Vasc Surg 1997;26:288-293.

108. Pellerito JS, Revzin MV, Tsang JC, et al. Doppler sonographic criteria for the diagnosis of inferior mesenteric artery stenosis. J Ultrasound Med 2009;28:641-650.

109. Mitchell EL, Chang EY, Landry GJ, et al. Duplex criteria for native superior mesenteric artery stenosis overestimate stenosis in stented superior mesenteric arteries. J Vasc Surg 2009;50:335-340.

110. Kellman GM, Alpern MB, Sandler MA, Craig BM. Computed tomography of vena caval anomalies with embryologic correlation. Radiographics 1988;8:533-556.

111. Radtke A, Schroeder T, Sotiropoulos GC, et al. Anatomical and physiological classification of hepatic vein dominance applied to liver transplantation. Eur J Med Res 2005;10:187-194.

112. Xing X, Li H, Liu WG. Clinical studies on inferior right hepatic veins. Hepatobiliary Pancreat Dis Int 2007;6:579-584.

113. Kadir S. Gonadal vessels. In: Normal and variant angiographic anatomy. Philadelphia: Saunders; 1991.

114. Ouriel K, Green RM, Greenberg RK, Clair DG. The anatomy of deep venous thrombosis of the lower extremity. J Vasc Surg 2000;31:895-900.

115. Lee BB, Villavicencio L, Kim YW, et al. Primary Budd-Chiari syndrome: outcome of endovascular management for suprahepatic venous obstruction. J Vasc Surg 2006;43:101-108.

116. Cura M, Haskal Z, Lopera J. Diagnostic and interventional radiology for Budd-Chiari syndrome. Radiographics 2009;29:669-681.

117. Brancatelli G, Vilgrain V, Federle MP, et al. Budd-Chiari syndrome: spectrum of imaging findings. AJR Am J Roentgenol 2007;188:W168-W176.

118. Bargallo X, Gilabert R, Nicolau C, et al. Sonography of Budd-Chiari syndrome. AJR Am J Roentgenol 2006;187:W33-W41.

119. Gore RM, Mathieu DG, White EM, et al. Passive hepatic congestion: cross-sectional imaging features. AJR Am J Roentgenol 1994;162:71-75.

120. Kinney TB. Update on inferior vena cava filters. J Vasc Interv Radiol 2003;14:425-440.

Nonvascular Diseases of the Retroperitoneum

121. Sanyal R, Remer EM. Radiology of the retroperitoneum: case-based review. AJR Am J Roentgenol 2009;192:S112-S117; quiz S118-S121.

122. Gronchi A, Lo Vullo S, Fiore M, et al. Aggressive surgical policies in a retrospectively reviewed single-institution case series of retroperitoneal soft tissue sarcoma patients. J Clin Oncol 2009;27:24-30.

123. Nishino M, Hayakawa K, Minami M, et al. Primary retroperitoneal neoplasms: CT and MR imaging findings with anatomic and pathologic diagnostic clues. Radiographics 2003;23:45-57.

124. Cronin CG, Lohan DG, Blake MA, et al. Retroperitoneal fibrosis: a review of clinical features and imaging findings. AJR Am J Roentgenol 2008;191:423-431.

125. Moussavian B, Horrow MM. Retroperitoneal fibrosis. Ultrasound Q 2009;25:89-91.

CHAPTER 13

Dynamic Ultrasound of Hernias of the Groin and Anterior Abdominal Wall

A. Thomas Stavros and Cynthia T. Rapp

Chapter Outline

*P*atients with groin hernias typically present with an obvious lump or bulge and are often diagnosed clinically and infrequently require imaging (except to evaluate the contralateral side preoperatively). On the other hand, patients with hernias who present with pain but without a lump or bulge are more often referred for diagnostic imaging. In the past, "herniography" was the procedure of choice. More recently, CT and MRI have been used to identify and describe hernias (Fig. 13-1). However, real-time ultrasound has advantages over other imaging modalities: the ability to scan the patient in both upright and supine positions, to use **dynamic maneuvers** such as Valsalva and compression, and to document motion in real time (Fig. 13-2). Positioning and dynamic maneuvers affect the operator's ability to diagnose a hernia, alter its size and contents, and evaluate its reducibility. Sonography also enables the user to assess tenderness and clinical significance of a hernia.

There are various definitions of **the groin**. The most common definition is that the groin is represented by the ilioinguinal crease at the junction of the abdomen and the thigh and the adjacent areas immediately above and below. In the strictest sense, the only "groin hernias" are **inguinal.** However, **spigelian** and **femoral** hernias lie so close to the inguinal area that we consider them groin hernias as well. Sonographic evaluation of the groin should include assessment for spigelian, direct and indirect inguinal, and femoral hernias.

Hernias occur in areas of natural weakness—in areas where vessels penetrate the abdominal wall (femoral and spigelian), where fetal migration of testis, spermatic cord, or round ligament have occurred (**indirect** inguinal),

and through broad flat tendons called aponeuroses (**direct** inguinal). Hernias do not occur through the belly of abdominal wall muscles unless they have been surgically incised.

TECHNICAL REQUIREMENTS

A high-frequency ($\geq$12 MHz) 50-mm-long transducer should be used in the majority of patients. Only in very obese patients is a lower-frequency transducer necessary, usually a 7 to 9–MHz curved array. Using a 50-mm transducer is important because its larger field of view (FOV) allows better identification of landmarks, especially in patients who have diastasis of aponeuroses. In departments where the longest transducer available is 38 mm, using a trapezoidal or virtual convex display can be helpful. In some cases, extended-FOV modes can be helpful, particularly in indirect inguinal hernias that extend into the scrotum and long incisional hernias. It is important to be able to store and review video loops in order to capture dynamic events critical to diagnosis.

HERNIA CONTENTS

Most sonographically detected hernias do not contain bowel. In fact, most hernias contain only fat (Fig. 13-3). The fat may be **intraperitoneal** (mesenteric or omental) or **preperitoneal** in origin. Generally, it is not possible sonographically to distinguish whether the hernia contains intraperitoneal or preperitoneal fat. Only in rare cases of hernias that contain both intraperitoneal and preperitoneal fat can the distinction be made (**Video 13-1**). Hernias that contain intraperitoneal fat may contain bowel later and thus may be a greater risk than those that contain only preperitoneal fat. Some hernias contain free fluid of intraperitoneal origin (Fig. 13-4).

Hernias that contain bowel are considered higher risk because strangulation may lead to infarction of bowel (Fig. 13-5; **Video 13-2**). Large hernias that are the most likely to contain bowel are easier to detect clinically and less often require sonographic imaging for diagnosis. Hernias can contain small bowel, colon, or appendix. Other, much less common hernia contents include ovaries and "bladder ears."

DYNAMIC MANEUVERS

The dynamic maneuvers that are the key to ultrasound's advantage over computed tomography (CT) and magnetic resonance imaging (MRI) include the Valsalva maneuver, the compression maneuver, and upright positioning. Dynamic maneuvers are useful because many hernias spontaneously reduce when the patient is supine and breathing quietly, making the hernias undetectable. Hernias that contain only fat are almost isoechoic with surrounding tissues and therefore relatively inconspicuous. Dynamic maneuvers can cause the fat within a hernia to move, making the hernia contents more conspicuous. The direction of movement can be helpful, because movement of surrounding tissues is almost always in the anteroposterior (AP) direction, while hernia contents often move horizontally during compression maneuvers (**Video 13-3**). Hernia contents may change with dynamic maneuvers. Finally, reducibility and tenderness can be assessed.

The **Valsalva maneuver** is most useful when the patient is supine. It forces hernia contents anteriorly, and often horizontally in an inferomedial direction (Fig. 13-6; **Video 13-4**). Some hernias become visible only during the Valsalva maneuver (**Video 13-5**). In other cases, hernia sacs that can be seen in quiet respiration elongate and widen during the Valsalva maneuver. Hernias that appear to contain only fat during quiet respiration may be shown to contain bowel during the Valsalva maneuver (**Video 13-6**). In some patients the hernia becomes tender during the Valsalva maneuver.

The **compression maneuver** is essential to assess reducibility and tenderness in patients who have sono-

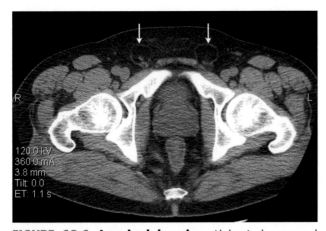

FIGURE 13-1. Inguinal hernias. Abdominal computed tomography (CT) scan shows moderate-sized, fat-containing, bilateral indirect inguinal hernias *(arrows)*.

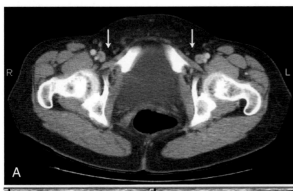

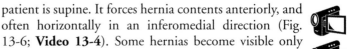

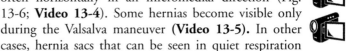

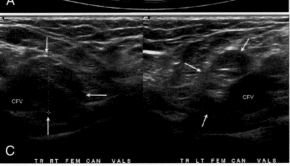

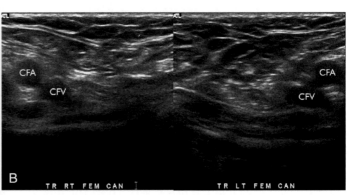

FIGURE 13-2. Femoral hernias. A, Abdominal CT image shows no evidence of femoral hernias. **B,** Transverse ultrasound image of the femoral canal during quite respiration appears normal. **C,** Transverse sonogram of the femoral canal during Valsalva maneuver, showing bilateral fat-containing hernias, with the right larger than the left *(arrows)*.

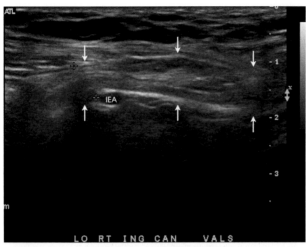

FIGURE 13-3. Indirect inguinal hernia. Long-axis ultrasound image of an indirect inguinal hernia *(arrows)* that contains only fat; *IEA,* inferior epigastric artery.

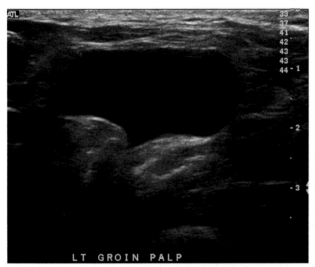

FIGURE 13-4. Femoral hernia. Long-axis image of a fluid-containing femoral hernia that presented with pain and swelling.

graphically detectable hernias, regardless of whether the patient is upright or supine. Compression maneuvers are also useful in supine patients in whom the Valsalva maneuver is ineffective. Compression helps assess **reducibility** of a hernia. Hernias may be completely reducible, partially reducible, or nonreducible (incarcerated) **(Videos 13-7, 13-8,** and **13-9).** The shape of hernias correlates with reducibility. A hernia with a broad fundus and narrow neck is likely to be nonreducible, whereas a hernia with a broad neck compared to the fundus is more likely to be reducible (Fig. 13-7). Assessing tenderness is very important because dynamic sonography is so sensitive that it detects many asymptomatic and clinically insignificant hernias. Furthermore, in some patients the pain is caused by other etiologies.

Upright positioning is essential in all patients being sonographically evaluated for groin hernia. Many patients

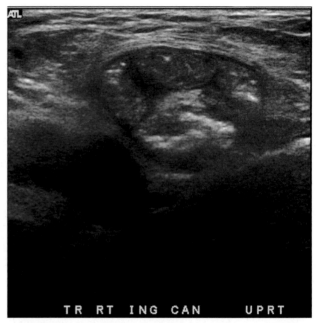

FIGURE 13-5. Indirect inguinal hernia. Short-axis view of the inguinal canal in the upright position shows an indirect inguinal hernia that contains bowel.

are symptomatic *only* in the upright position, or they are *more* symptomatic in the upright position. Fluid can best be demonstrated with the patient in the upright position, especially female patients. It may take minutes for the free fluid to "puddle" in the inferior end of the hernia sac once the patient has been placed in the upright position. Therefore, delayed imaging in the upright position may be helpful in demonstrating **peritoneal fluid** (Fig. 13-8). Other hernias contain bowel only in the upright position. Some hernias are either only present in the upright position or are much better demonstrated in the upright position (direct inguinal and femoral). The reducibility of a hernia may vary between supine and upright position, so it is important to assess reducibility in both positions **(Video 13-10).** In most patients, groin hernias are more reducible in the supine than in the upright position, whereas in others the opposite is true. Also, tenderness may vary between the supine and upright positions.

KEY SONOGRAPHIC LANDMARKS

Ultrasound shows characteristic features of groin hernias that lie above the inguinal ligament. Four types of hernias occur within the broader definition of the groin: indirect inguinal, direct inguinal, spigelian, and femoral. The key landmark in distinguishing between the first three types is the **inferior epigastric artery** (IEA). This artery arises from the external iliac artery and then courses superomedially, crossing the spigelian fascia and the semilunar line, eventually coursing along the midposterior aspect

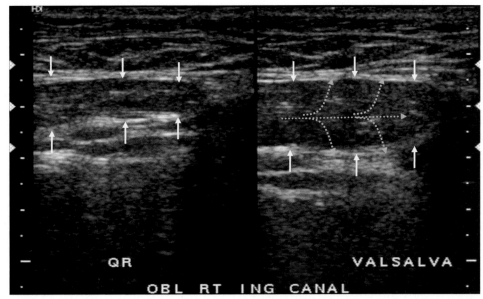

FIGURE 13-6. Indirect inguinal hernia. Split-screen long-axis views of a fat-containing indirect inguinal hernia during quiet respiration and Valsalva maneuvers. The left image shows the hernia during quiet respiration *(arrows)*. The right image, obtained during a Valsalva maneuver, shows the hernia contents being forced distally in a horizontal direction within the inguinal canal *(arrows and dotted arrows)*.

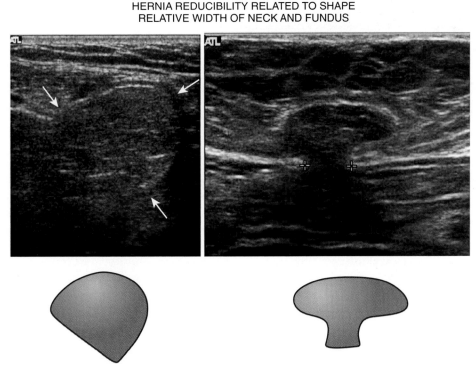

FIGURE 13-7. Typical hernia shapes. *Left,* Direct inguinal hernia shows a wide neck in comparison to the fundus. This hernia shape correlates with complete reducibility. *Right,* Linea alba hernia shows a very narrow neck in comparison to the fundal width. This hernia shape correlates with nonreducibility and increased risk of strangulation.

of the rectus abdominis muscle. The IEA can be identified sonographically in all patients along the midposterior surface of the rectus abdominis muscle at a level about halfway between the umbilicus and pubic symphysis while scanning in a transverse plane (Fig. 13-9). The

IEA lies anterior to the peritoneum and thus is never obscured by bowel gas. Once identified in the transverse plane, the IEA can be traced inferiorly and laterally to its origin from the external iliac artery. The **internal inguinal ring** (deep inguinal ring) lies in the crotch

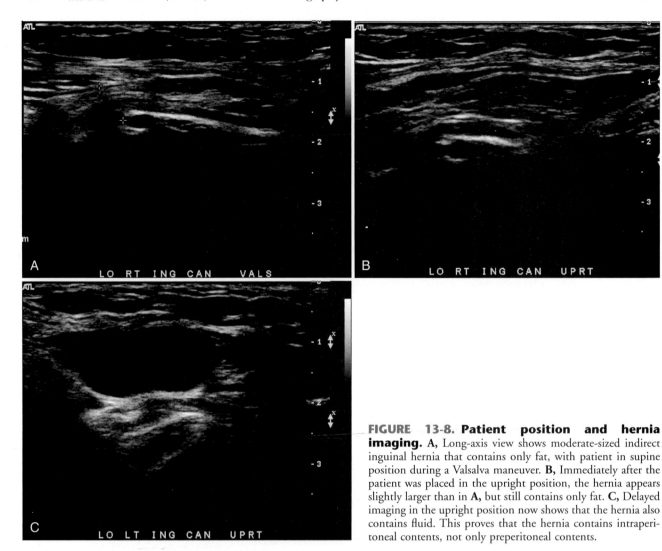

FIGURE 13-8. Patient position and hernia imaging. A, Long-axis view shows moderate-sized indirect inguinal hernia that contains only fat, with patient in supine position during a Valsalva maneuver. **B,** Immediately after the patient was placed in the upright position, the hernia appears slightly larger than in **A,** but still contains only fat. **C,** Delayed imaging in the upright position now shows that the hernia also contains fluid. This proves that the hernia contains intraperitoneal contents, not only preperitoneal contents.

between the external iliac artery and the proximal IEA. **Direct inguinal hernias** arise through the "conjoined tendon" inferior and medial to the IEA's origin. **Spigelian hernias** occur through the spigelian fascia just lateral to where it is penetrated by the IEA. **Femoral hernias** lie within the femoral canal inferior to the inguinal ligament (Fig. 13-10).

Once the origin of the inferior epigastric artery is identified, the transducer should be rotated into an axis that is parallel to the inguinal ligament, which courses obliquely from superolaterally to inferomedially. The patient should be scanned in long axis (LAX) parallel to the inguinal ligament and short axis (SAX) perpendicular to the inguinal ligament, rather than scanning transversely and longitudinally (see Fig. 13-9).

Inguinal Hernias

Inguinal hernias can be classified as direct or indirect. The terms **direct** and **indirect** refer to how hernias present during open surgical repairs. **Direct inguinal hernias** protrude into the surgically opened inguinal

canal "directly" from posteriorly. **Indirect inguinal hernias,** on the other hand, enter the surgically opened inguinal canal "indirectly" from a superolateral direction after passing through the internal inguinal ring (deep inguinal ring). From a sonographic point of view, "direct" and "indirect" are confusing. It would be less confusing to characterize them as internal inguinal ring (indirect) hernia and nonring (direct) hernia.

Indirect Inguinal Hernias

Indirect inguinal hernias are the most common type of groin hernia. They are congenital and represent a persistence of a patent process vaginalis. In males the testis descends from the abdominal cavity into the scrotum, which can result in delayed or incomplete closure of the inguinal canal. Thus, indirect inguinal hernias are more common in males. However, delayed or incomplete closure of the **canal of Nuck** can occur in females. The neck of an indirect inguinal hernia is the segment that lies within the internal inguinal ring, and the fundus lies within the inguinal canal (Fig. 13-11). The neck

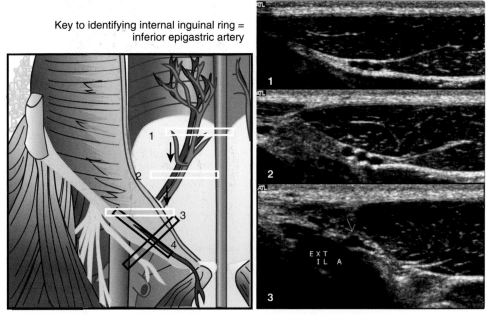

Key to identifying internal inguinal ring = inferior epigastric artery

Long axis and short axis —not longitudinal and transverse

FIGURE 13-9. Inferior epigastric vessels (IEVs) are main landmarks for evaluating inguinal area. Image 1 is obtained in a transverse plane about halfway between the umbilicus and the pubic symphysis. The inferior epigastric artery and its paired veins lie along the midlateral posterior surface of the rectus abdominis muscle. Image 2 is obtained several centimeters inferiorly, and the IEVs lie more laterally. Image 3 is obtained at a level where the IEVs *(arrow)* lie at the edge of the rectus muscle. This is the level at which most spigelian hernias occur. Image 4 shows that once the origin of the inferior epigastric artery is identified, the transducer should be rotated into planes that are parallel and perpendicular to the inguinal canal—long-axis and short-axis views.

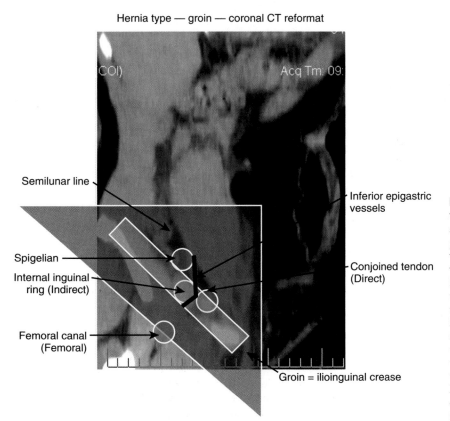

Hernia type — groin — coronal CT reformat

Semilunar line

Spigelian

Internal inguinal ring (Indirect)

Femoral canal (Femoral)

Inferior epigastric vessels

Conjoined tendon (Direct)

Groin = ilioinguinal crease

FIGURE 13-10. Locations of four types of "groin" hernias. Abdominal and pelvic CT image, reformatted in coronal plane. **Indirect inguinal hernias** arise within the internal or deep inguinal ring, which lies in the crotch between the external iliac artery and the proximal inferior epigastric artery. **Direct inguinal hernias** arise through the "conjoined tendon," which lies inferior and medial to the origin of the inferior epigastric artery. **Spigelian hernias** arise through the spigelian fascia just lateral to the inferior epigastric artery, where it reaches the lateral margin of the rectus muscle. **Femoral hernias** lie within the femoral canal, inferior to the inguinal canal and inguinal ligament.

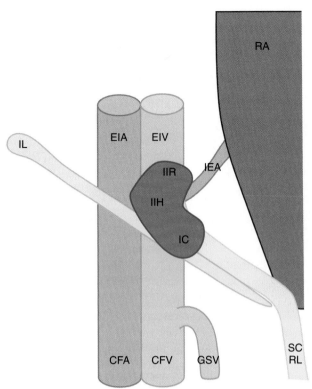

FIGURE 13-11. Relationship of indirect inguinal hernias (IIH) to inferior epigastric artery (IEA) origin from external iliac artery (EIA). The neck of the hernia arises in the internal inguinal ring (IIR), extends anteriorly, then extends inferomedially superficial to the proximal to the IEA and lies anterior to the spermatic cord (SC) in males or round ligament (RL) in females; RA, rectus abdominis; EIV, external iliac vein; CFA, common femoral artery; CFV, common femoral vein; GSV, greater saphenous vein; IL, inguinal ligament; IC, inguinal canal.

(internal inguinal ring) lies just superior and lateral to the IEA's origin and tends to be oriented in an AP direction, whereas the fundus (inguinal canal) is oriented horizontally and courses inferiorly and medially, passing superficial to the IEA's origin The fundus of an indirect inguinal hernia lies anterior and lateral to the **spermatic cord** in males and the **round ligament** in females (Fig. 13-12). In the short axis, the internal inguinal ring and the neck of the indirect inguinal hernia lie between the external iliac artery along its lateral side and the IEA along its medial side.

In the long axis, indirect inguinal hernias can have two appearances: sliding and nonsliding types. The **sliding type** of indirect inguinal hernia has a relatively wide neck compared with the fundus, with loss of the angle between the neck and fundus. It is usually reducible, at least in the supine position, and is more likely to contain bowel and other intraperitoneal contents. The **nonsliding type** has a relatively narrower neck compared with the fundus and maintains the almost 90-degree angle between the neck and fundus (Fig. 13-13). Nonsliding hernias usually contain only properitoneal fat and are nonreducible, frequently being misclassified as "spermatic cord lipoma"

or "inguinal canal lipoma" at surgery. True spermatic cord lipomas can occur, but are rare. Nonsliding indirect inguinal hernias are more difficult to diagnose sonographically than sliding types because (1) they tend to be smaller; (2) they contain only fat, which is almost isoechoic with surrounding tissues; and (3) their nonreducibility minimizes motion of contents during dynamic maneuvers. In the short axis, the sliding type of direct inguinal hernia can be diagnosed at either the level of the internal inguinal ring or the level of the inguinal canal. However, the nonsliding type can be diagnosed only at the level of the inguinal canal, where it is widest.

In some cases, it can be difficult to demonstrate the relationship of the hernia neck to the inferior epigastric vessels. In such cases, it is helpful to assess the relationship of the hernia sac to the spermatic cord. Indirect inguinal hernias tend to lie along the anterolateral aspect of the spermatic cord, while direct inguinal hernia sacs tend to lie posteromedial to the cord (Fig. 13-14; **Video 13-11**). In females, indirect inguinal hernias lie anterior to the round ligament (Fig. 13-15). Large indirect inguinal hernias can flatten and splay the spermatic cord (Figs. 13-16 and 13-17; **Video 13-12**), causing pain that radiates into the scrotum.

Indirect inguinal hernias are much more likely than direct inguinal hernias to extend into the scrotum or labium majorum (Fig. 13-18; **Video 13-13**).

Direct Inguinal Hernias

Direct inguinal hernias are the second most common type of groin hernia and are acquired. They arise in two ways, either a passing through a defect in the "conjoined tendon" (Fig. 13-19) or by greatly stretching the tendon into the inguinal canal (Fig. 13-20). During open hernia repair, direct inguinal hernias protrude "directly" into the opened inguinal canal from a posterior direction. Indirect inguinal hernias, on the other hand, extend into the opened inguinal canal "indirectly" from a superior and lateral direction. The conjoined tendon area, and thus the neck of a direct inguinal hernia, arises inferior and medial to the inferior epigastric vessels (Fig. 13-21).

The neck of direct inguinal hernias is typically wider than the fundus. This makes incarceration and strangulation of direct hernias rare. Most small to medium direct inguinal hernias are completely reducible, but large direct inguinal hernias may be incompletely reducible, especially in the upright position. Most direct inguinal hernias spontaneously reduce completely in the supine position during quiet respiration, and therefore they are visible only during Valsalva maneuvers or in the upright position.

The **conjoined tendon** consists of the aponeuroses of the internal oblique and transverse abdominis muscles and the underlying transversalis (transverse) fascia. It occurs inferior to the lower edge of the external oblique aponeurosis. In most patients the aponeuroses of the

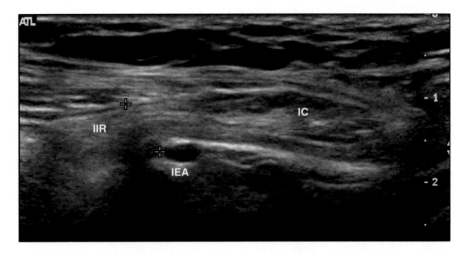

Long axis right internal
inguinal ring and inguinal canal

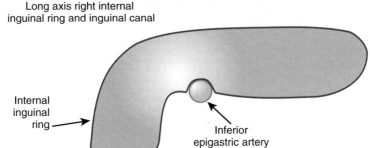

Internal
inguinal
ring

Inferior
epigastric artery

FIGURE 13-12. Indirect inguinal hernia. Long-axis view shows that neck of the hernia lies in the internal inguinal ring *(IIR)*, which lies superior and lateral to the proximal inferior epigastric artery *(IEA)*. Hernia sac then courses horizontally in an inferomedial direction within the inguinal canal *(IC)*. Indirect inguinal hernias always pass superficial to the IEA.

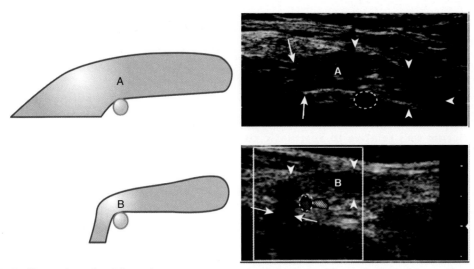

FIGURE 13-13. Indirect inguinal hernias: two types. A, Sliding type. The neck *(arrows)* is as wide as or wider than the fundus *(arrowheads)*, with loss of the angle between the internal inguinal ring and inguinal canal. Sliding hernias usually contain intraperitoneal contents and are reducible. **B, Nonsliding type.** The neck *(arrows)* is narrow in comparison to the fundus *(arrowheads)* and the nearly 90-degree angle between the internal inguinal ring and inguinal canal is preserved. Nonsliding hernias usually contain only properitoneal fat and are nonreducible. They have often been misclassified as "lipomas" of the inguinal canal or spermatic cord. *Circle,* Inferior epigastric artery.

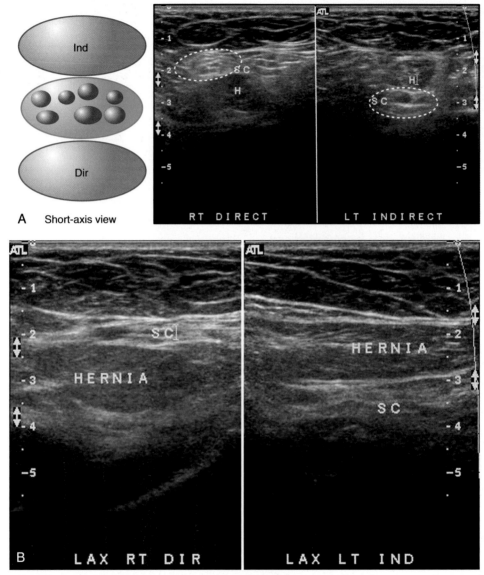

FIGURE 13-14. Hernia sacs relative to spermatic cord. A, Direct and indirect hernia sacs relative to the spermatic cord *(SC). Left,* Drawing shows that indirect inguinal hernia sac tends to lie anterior to spermatic cord, whereas direct inguinal hernia sac lies posterior to the cord. *Center,* Short-axis view shows fat-containing direct inguinal hernia *(H)* posterior and medial to the spermatic cord *(SC). Right,* Short-axis view shows fat-containing indirect inguinal hernia *(H)* lying anterior and lateral to the spermatic cord *(SC).* **B,** Long-axis views of right direct and left indirect inguinal hernias in the same patient. *Left,* Image shows the right direct inguinal hernia sac lying posterior to the spermatic cord *(SC). Right,* Image shows the left indirect inguinal hernia sac lying anterior to the spermatic cord *(SC).*

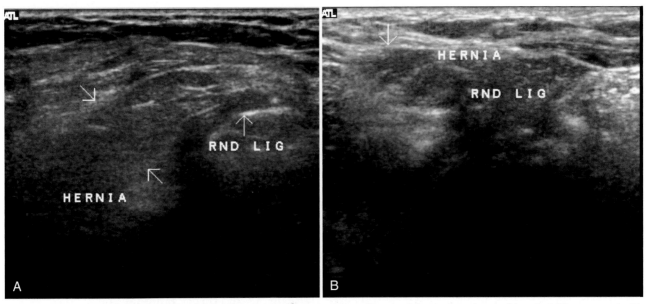

FIGURE 13-15. Indirect inguinal hernia. A, Long-axis view shows fat-containing indirect inguinal hernia *(oblique arrows)* with the sac anterior to the round ligament *(vertical arrow).* **B,** Short-axis view of hernia *(arrow)* in **A.**

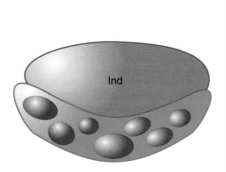

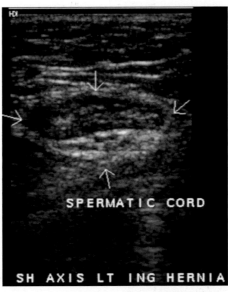

FIGURE 13-16. Indirect inguinal hernia. Short-axis view shows indirect inguinal hernia displacing and compressing the hyperechoic spermatic cord posteriorly.

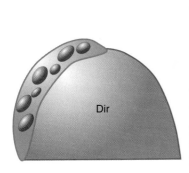

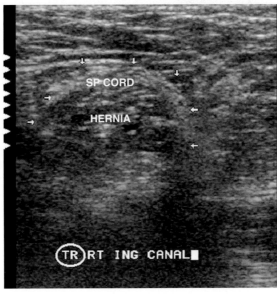

FIGURE 13-17. Direct inguinal hernia. Short-axis view shows direct inguinal hernia displacing and compressing the hyperechoic spermatic cord anteriorly and laterally.

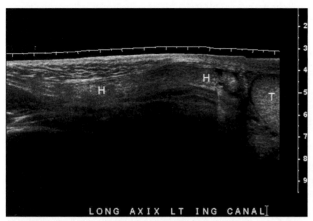

FIGURE 13-18. Indirect inguinal hernia. Long-axis extended–field of view (FOV) image shows extremely large, indirect inguinal hernia *(H)* extending down the entire length of the inguinal canal into the scrotum; *T,* testis.

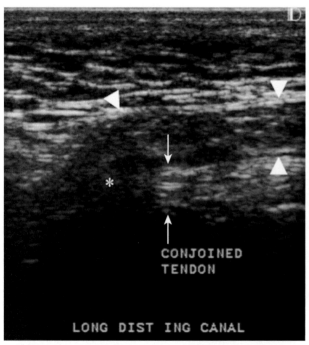

FIGURE 13-19. Direct inguinal hernia. Long-axis view shows fat-containing direct inguinal hernia passing through an acute tear (*) in the conjoined tendon *(arrows)* and extending down the inguinal canal *(arrowheads).*

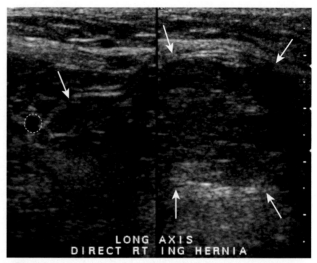

FIGURE 13-20. Direct inguinal hernia. Long-axis view of large, direct inguinal hernia shows the thinned and stretched conjoined tendon and underlying transversalis fascia and peritoneum *(arrows)* forming the hernia sac; *circle,* inferior epigastric artery. Note that the neck of direct inguinal hernias arised inferior and medial to the inferior epigastric artery *(circle).*

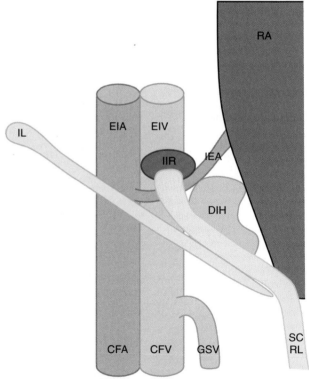

FIGURE 13-21. Direct inguinal hernia (DIH): relationship to surrounding anatomy. The neck of the hernia arises in the area of the conjoined tendon and lies inferior and medial to the proximal inferior epigastric artery *(IEA)*. The hernia sac does not pass superficial to the IEA and lies posterior and medial to the spermatic cord *(SC)* or round ligament *(RL)*. *RA,* Rectus abdominis muscle; *EIV,* external iliac vein; *EIA,* external iliac artery; *CFA,* common femoral artery; *CFV,* common femoral vein; *GSV,* greater saphenous vein; *SC/RL,* spermatic cord or round ligament; *IL,* inguinal ligament; *IIR,* internal inguinal ring.

internal oblique and transverse abdominis muscles are not closely adherent to each other; the aponeurosis of the transverse abdominis is separated from the underlying transversalis fascia and peritoneum by a variable layer of preperitoneal fat; and the conjoined tendon is not really a well-defined structure (Fig. 13-22).

Thinning and anterior bulging of the conjoined tendon ("conjoined tendon insufficiency") is a precursor to development of direct inguinal hernias. In males the anterior bulging displaces and rotates the spermatic cord laterally. The thinning and bulging of the conjoined tendon push the aponeuroses of the internal oblique and

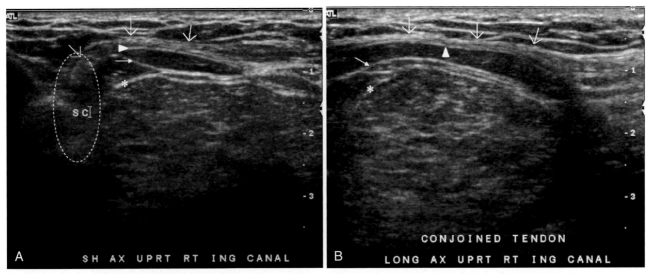

FIGURE 13-22. Direct inguinal hernia. A, Short-axis view of direct inguinal hernia shows a thinned and bulging conjoined tendon, consisting of the internal oblique aponeurosis *(superficial arrows)* and transverse abdominis aponeurosis *(arrowhead),* and underlying transversalis fascia *(horizontal arrow)* and peritoneum (*). **B,** Long-axis view shows the conjoined tendon *(between three vertical arrows and arrowhead),* underlying transversalis fascia *(oblique arrow),* and peritoneum (*).

transverse abdominis muscles closer together, making the conjoined tendon appear to be a more discrete structure than when the patient is in the supine position and in quiet respiration (Figs. 13-23 and 13-24). As the thinning and bulging progress, a **tear** can form within the tendon, leading to the formation of a direct inguinal hernia. Smaller direct inguinal hernias extend anteriorly into the floor of the inguinal canal, but larger hernias turn inferomedially, extending distally within the canal. Factors that can cause conjoined tendon insufficiency to progress to frank direct inguinal hernia over time include any cause of increased intra-abdominal pressure (obesity, pregnancy, ascites, coughing, straining) and generalized connective tissue weakness. Because these underlying causes affect both sides, direct inguinal hernias are frequently bilateral, although often asymmetrical (Fig. 13-25). It is difficult to explain why bilaterally symmetrical direct inguinal hernias can vary so much clinically. It is not unusual to find one direct inguinal hernia symptomatic and exquisitely tender, while the contralateral hernia is asymptomatic and nontender.

Direct inguinal hernias, and their precursors, posterior inguinal wall insufficiency, are common problems for athletes (see Sports Hernias).

Femoral Hernias

Femoral hernias reportedly are rare, because they are difficult to diagnose clinically unless strangulated, and in fact are much less common that inguinal hernias. However, sonographically detected femoral hernias are much more common than suggested. Unlike inguinal hernias, femoral hernias are more common in women than men. It is thought that the increased intrapelvic pressure that occurs during the third trimester of preg-

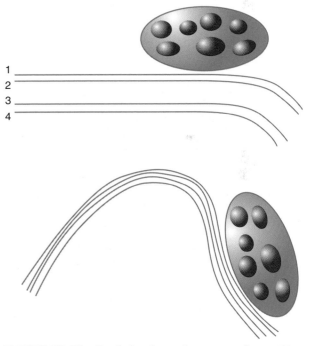

FIGURE 13-23. Conjoined tendon: two views. *Upper illustration,* Relationship of the conjoined tendon to the spermatic cord in quiet respiration in the supine position. The layers are separated by loose connective tissues or fat. *Lower illustration,* Bulging of the conjoined tendon during Valsalva maneuver or in the upright position. The layers tend to be pushed together and are more difficult to distinguish from each other. When the aponeuroses of the internal oblique *(1)* and transverse abdominis *(2)* muscles are pushed together, the conjoined tendon appears as a more discrete structure. *3,* Transversalis fascia; *4,* peritoneum. The anterior bulging of the conjoined tendon pushes the spermatic cord laterally and rotates it from a "wider-than-tall" orientation to a "taller-than-wider" orientation.

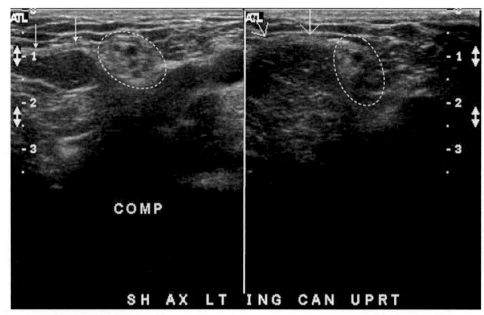

FIGURE 13-24. Conjoined tendon: two more views. *Left image,* Relationship of the conjoined tendon to the spermatic cord in quiet respiration in the supine position. The conjoined tendon lies posterior to the spermatic cord. *Right image,* Valsalva maneuver results in anterior bulging of the conjoined tendon, which now protrudes anterior to the spermatic cord and pushes and rotates the cord laterally.

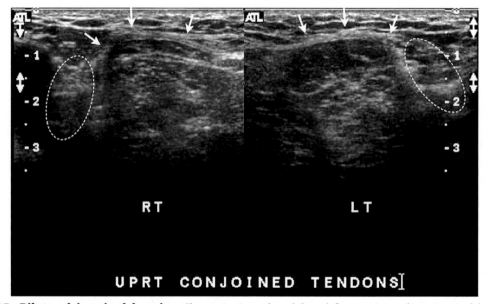

FIGURE 13-25. Bilateral inguinal hernias. Short-axis views show bilateral fat-containing direct inguinal hernias, which are common.

nancy, together with the hormone-induced softening of tissues, predisposes to the development of femoral hernias.

Femoral hernias arise within the femoral canal inferior to the inguinal canal and ilioinguinal crease. The **femoral canal** lies just medial to the **common femoral vein** (CFV) and just superior to the saphenofemoral junction (Fig. 13-26). The **saphenofemoral junction,** similar to the origin of the inferior epigastric artery for inguinal hernias, is the key landmark for identifying the femoral

canal **(Video 13-14).** The most common location for femoral hernias is medial to the CFV, but a few lie anterior to the common femoral vessels (Figs. 13-27 and 13-28). Most femoral hernias that lie anterior to the CFV arise medially and then extend anteriorly **(Video 13-15).** It is rare for a femoral hernia to actually arise anteriorly **(Teale's hernia)** (Fig. 13-29). Although femoral hernias reportedly can lie posterior or lateral to the CFV, we have never seen one in either of these locations. A femoral hernia tends to have a narrow neck in

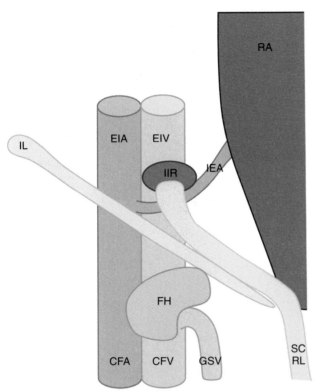

FIGURE 13-26. **Femoral hernia (FH): relationship to surrounding anatomy.** Femoral hernias arise within the femoral canal, which lies medial to the common femoral vein (CFV) just superior to the saphenofemoral junction and inferior to the inguinal ligament (IL). Small femoral hernias remain medial to the CFV, but larger hernias usually wrap around anterior to the CFV. RA, Rectus abdominis muscle; IEA, inferior epigastric artery; EIV, external iliac vein; EIA, external iliac artery; CFA, common femoral artery; GSV, greater saphenous vein; SC/RL, spermatic cord or round ligament; IIR, internal inguinal ring.

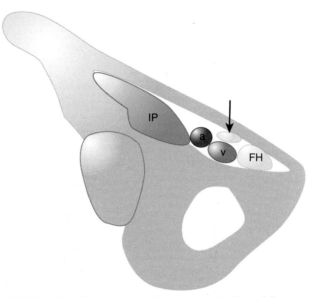

FIGURE 13-27. **Femoral hernia: relationship to femoral vessels.** Short-axis view shows that most femoral hernias arise medial to the common femoral vein (CFV) and can extend anterior to the CFV as they enlarge. A few small femoral hernias (Teale's hernia) may arise anterior to the CFV (arrows). IP, Iliopsoas muscle; a, common femoral artery; v, common femoral vein; FH and arrow, most common femoral hernia locations.

comparison to the width of its fundus, a shape that predisposes the femoral hernia to strangulation. In fact, femoral hernias are the most likely type of groin hernia to strangulate (Fig. 13-30). Femoral hernia contents vary, and most contain only fat. Femoral hernias that contain bowel are almost always nonreducible and frequently, strangulated as well.

The femoral canal lies deeper than the inguinal canal and may be more difficult to assess with a high-frequency linear array transducer. Small and even moderate-sized femoral hernias frequently reduce completely in the supine position during quiet respiration and are most readily demonstrated with the patient in the supine position during the Valsalva maneuver or in the upright position during compression maneuvers. Femoral hernias are often bilateral (see Fig. 13-2, C; **Video 13-16**).

Spigelian Hernias

Spigelian hernias that present clinically are rare. Sonographically detected spigelian hernias are more common than the literature would suggest. Spigelian hernias are usually considered anterior abdominal wall hernias rather than groin hernias. They can occur anywhere along the

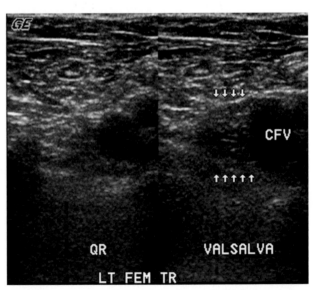

FIGURE 13-28. **Femoral hernia on Valsalva maneuver. A,** No evidence of a femoral hernia during quiet respiration. **B,** During a Valsalva maneuver, a fat-containing femoral hernia (arrows) appears medial to the common femoral vein (CFV).

course of the **spigelian fascia,** the complex aponeurotic tendon that lies between the oblique muscles laterally and the rectus muscles medially. However, almost all spigelian hernias occur at the inferior end of the **semicircular line,** inferior to the arcuate line, where the posterior rectus sheath is absent, and where the spigelian fascia is penetrated and weakened by the inferior epigastric vessels (Fig. 13-31). In many patients, this location is within 2 cm of the internal inguinal ring. Further-

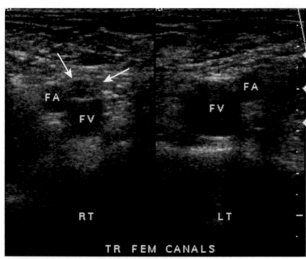

FIGURE 13-29. Teale's femoral hernia. Small, Teale's type of right femoral hernia lying anterior to the common femoral vein *(FV)*, but no femoral hernia on the left.

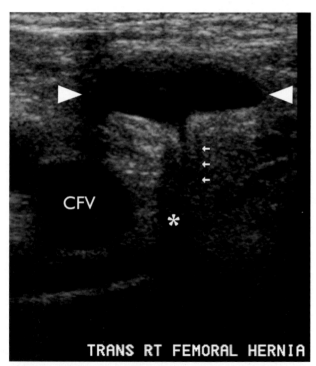

FIGURE 13-30. Nonreducible femoral hernia. Short-axis view shows large, nonreducible femoral hernia that arises within the femoral canal (*) medial to the common femoral vein *(CFV)*. The long, narrow neck *(arrows)* extends directly anteriorly, and the large fundus *(arrowheads)* filled with peritoneal fluid causes this hernia to be at extremely high risk for strangulation.

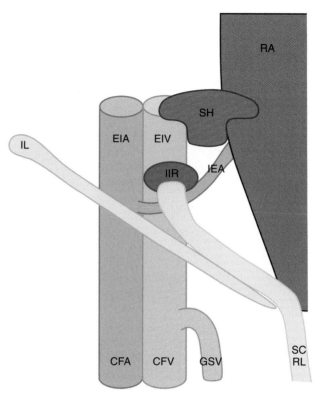

FIGURE 13-31. Spigelian hernia (SH): relationship to surrounding anatomy. Almost all spigelian hernias arise from the inferior end of the spigelian fascia just lateral to where it is penetrated by the inferior epigastric vessels, lateral to the lateral edge of the rectus abdominis muscle *(RA)*. Although these are usually considered **anterior abdominal wall** rather than "groin" hernias, the neck of spigelian hernias often lie within 2 cm of the internal inguinal ring *(IIR)*, where indirect inguinal hernias arise. *IEA,* Inferior epigastric artery; *EIV,* external iliac vein; *EIA,* external iliac artery; *CFA,* common femoral artery; *CFV,* common femoral vein; *GSV,* greater saphenous vein; *SC/RL,* spermatic cord or round ligament; *IL,* inguinal ligament.

more, when symptomatic, the pain caused by spigelian hernias can be difficult to distinguish from that caused by indirect inguinal hernias. Therefore, we are including spigelian hernias in our discussion of groin hernias.

The spigelian fascia is composed of several different layers of loosely apposed aponeurotic tendons. From external to internal lie the aponeuroses of the external oblique, internal oblique, and transverse abdominis muscles. Internal to the aponeuroses lie the transversalis fascia and peritoneum. In spigelian hernias the transverse abdominis tendon is always torn. In most cases the internal oblique aponeurosis is also torn (Fig. 13-32). The external oblique tendon is always intact and usually forces the hernia sac to extend either medially over the anterior aspect of the rectus abdominis muscle or laterally over the external oblique muscle, forcing it into the shape of an anvil or mushroom (Figs. 13-33 and 13-34). As with femoral hernias, spigelian hernias have narrow necks and broad fundi (**Videos 13-17** and **13-18**), making them at least partially nonreducible and predisposing them to strangulation (Fig. 13-35). Because spigelian hernias pass through multiple layers of tendons, projections of the hernia may also extend intraparietally between the multiple layers of lateral muscles (either between the transverse abdominis and internal oblique muscles or between the internal and external oblique muscles). In some cases the spigelian fascia, like the linea alba, can become diastatic and widen. Extended-FOV modes may be helpful in demonstrating the anatomy in such cases (see Figs. 13-32 and 13-33).

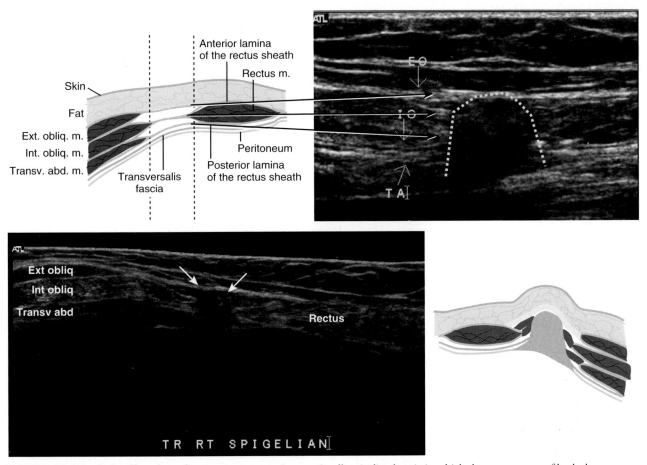

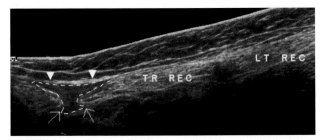

FIGURE 13-32. Spigelian hernia: torn aponeuroses. Small, spigelian hernia in which the aponeuroses of both the transverse abdominis *(TA)* and internal oblique *(IO)* muscles are torn, but in which the external oblique *(EO)* aponeurosis, as usual, is intact. This is the most common pattern of aponeurosis defects in spigelian hernias.

FIGURE 13-33. Spigelian hernia: "mushroom" shape. Transverse extended-FOV sonogram shows small, nonreducible, fat-containing right spigelian hernia. Because the external oblique aponeurosis is not torn, it forces the hernia sac to extend medially over the anterior surface of the right rectus muscle and laterally over the anterior aspect of the right external oblique muscle. This results in a mushroom or anvil shape, which correlates with nonreducibility and an increased risk of strangulation.

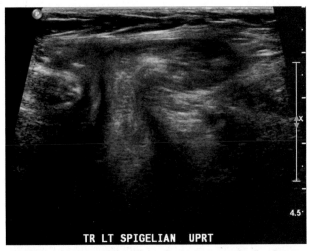

FIGURE 13-34. Spigelian hernia: typical shape. Nonreducible left spigelian hernia contains bowel and has a narrow neck and broad fundus, the typical shape for spigelian hernias.

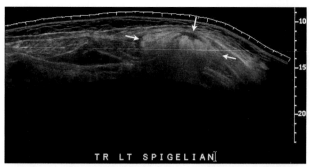

FIGURE 13-35. Strangulated spigelian hernia.
Transverse extended-FOV image shows strangulated left spigelian hernia containing large bowel and fat *(arrows)*. Note the hyperechoic texture of the edematous strangulated contents.

Sports Hernias

Sports hernia is a common cause of groin and pubic pain among elite and professional athletes. Sports hernia is a complex, confusing, and controversial subject. There is neither a universally accepted definition of sports hernia nor a uniform agreement on the best treatment. Sports hernia, also called "sportsman's hernia" and "athletic pubalgia," is complex because it occurs in an area where many tendons come together and are difficult to separate from each other, and where weakness in one tendon may lead to failure of another or to instability of the pubic symphysis. Also, multiple abnormalities often contribute to pain. Surgery may help some of the underlying causes, but not others.

Sports hernias most often occur in elite athletes who kick, bend over at the waist, and make sudden changes in direction. Soccer players, hockey players, and American and Australian-rules football players are most frequently affected. "Sports pubalgia" can be especially debilitating for elite and professional athletes, causing long periods of disability, and can be career threatening. Sports hernias are much more common in men than in women because of differences in the insertion of the rectus muscles into the pubis, but the incidence is increasing in women.

The type of hernia most often associated with groin pain in athletes is the **direct inguinal hernia** or its precursor, "posterior inguinal wall deficiency" (conjoined tendon insufficiency). In many athletes with groin pain, however, the hernia is not the only, or even the main, cause of pain.

Dynamic ultrasound is the best modality for demonstrating groin hernias associated with sports pubalgia, but MRI is generally better for demonstrating causes of pain other than hernia.

The underlying pathology is usually **tendinosis** (degenerative change in tendons without signs of inflammation) of either the adductor longus origin or the rectus abdominis insertion. The tendons of these two muscles interdigitate, making them inseparable from each other as they insert onto the pubis. Tendinosis of one tendon usually leads to tendinosis of the other, and eventually to instability of the pubic symphysis and osteitis pubis. Tendinosis of the rectus abdominis muscle can also lead to microtears in which the aponeuroses of the internal oblique and transverse abdominis muscles (components of conjoined tendon) insert onto the rectus sheath, causing them to bulge anteriorly into the inguinal canal (posterior inguinal wall insufficiency or conjoined tendon insufficiency) and also leading to dilation of the external (superficial) inguinal ring. The thinned and bulged conjoined tendon pushes the spermatic cord laterally, rotates it, and compresses it. Because of the effects on the spermatic cord, the resulting pain often radiates into the scrotum.

Posterior inguinal wall insufficiency is usually bilateral, even though symptoms may only be unilateral. In the short axis, posterior inguinal wall insufficiency appears indistinguishable from direct inguinal hernia (see Figs. 13-23 and 13-24). In the long axis, however, posterior inguinal wall insufficiency and direct inguinal hernia have different shapes. The posterior wall insufficiency is semicircular, whereas the direct inguinal hernia protrudes inferiorly within the inguinal canal in a finger-like projection (Fig. 13-36). At the level of the proximal inguinal canal, insufficiency and hernia can only be distinguished in the long axis, appearing identical in the short axis. More distally within the inguinal canal, however, the distinction can be made in the short axis. The direct inguinal hernia sac will be seen posterior to the spermatic cord (see Fig. 13-14 and **Video 13-11**), whereas in posterior inguinal wall insufficiency, the inguinal canal will appear normal.

Posterior inguinal wall insufficiency can progress to direct inguinal hernia in two ways: the conjoined tendon can tear completely, or the tendon can become so thinned and stretched that it is pushed inferomedially into the distal inguinal canal. Both complications arise inferior and medial to the origin of the inferior epigastric vessels. In patients with acute tendon tears, the neck is small, and the hernia sac appears thin (transversalis fascia and peritoneum) (Fig. 13-37). In severe stretching of the conjoined tendon, however, the neck is wide, and the hernia sac appears thicker (aponeuroses of internal oblique and transverse abdominis muscles as well as transversalis fascia and peritoneum) (see Figs. 13-20 and 13-36).

Because there is usually some degree of **tendinosis** or **osteitis pubis,** even when a direct inguinal hernia or posterior inguinal wall insufficiency is present, simply assessing sonographically for hernia is often insufficient for the workup of these patients. Ultrasound can show tendinosis in the rectus and adductor tendons in some cases (Fig. 13-38), but not as reliably as MRI, which can also demonstrate osteitis pubis and findings such as the secondary cleft. In a patient with other pathology, only repairing an inguinal hernia or posterior wall deficiency may not cure the patient's groin pain. Thus, optimal

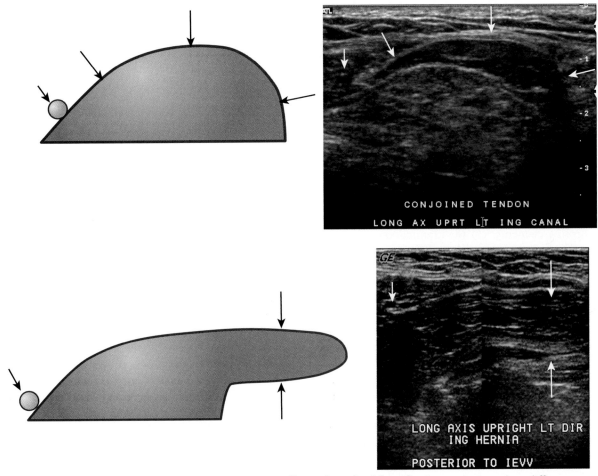

FIGURE 13-36. Inguinal wall insufficiency versus direct inguinal hernia. Long-axis views show different appearance of posterior inguinal wall insufficiency and direct inguinal hernia. **A,** Insufficiency of the posterior inguinal wall appears semicircular in shape. **B,** Frank direct inguinal hernia extends distally within the inguinal canal in a fingerlike projection posterior to the spermatic cord. At the level of the proximal inguinal canal, the distinction is possible only on long-axis views, because insufficiency and frank hernia appear identical on short-axis views obtained proximally.

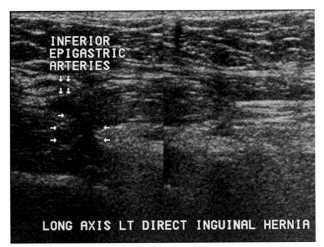

FIGURE 13-37. Acute tear of conjoined tendon (arrows). Note that the neck is small in comparison to the fundus in this long-axis view. This is an unusual configuration for a direct inguinal hernia.

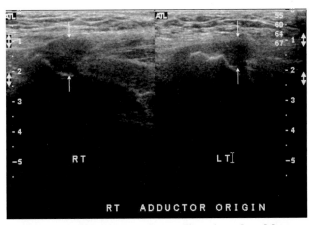

FIGURE 13-38. Bilateral tendinosis of adductor longus tendons. Note that the edema and thickening of the tendon *(arrows)* is greater on the symptomatic right side than on the contralateral left side. The tendinosis in patients with athletic pubalgia is usually bilateral, but asymmetrical.

imaging workup of athletes with groin pain usually requires both dynamic ultrasound of the groin and MRI. In patients with inguinal hernia or inguinal wall insufficiency, both surgical repair of the hernia and surgical or medical treatment of the associated tendinosis and pubic symphysis instability may be necessary.

THE REPORT FOR DYNAMIC ULTRASOUND OF GROIN HERNIAS

It is important to use correct terminology in reporting the results of a dynamic groin ultrasound examination. In addition to the indication, the report should contain the following elements: (1) the examination name; (2) the specific dynamic components of the examination; (3) the side examined; (4) presence or absence of a hernia; (5) hernia size; (6) hernia contents; (7) reducibility of the hernia; and (8) whether the hernia is tender or nontender. Surgeons who treat these patients expect to see all these elements in the report. If all these findings are not reported, the examination will be reviewed or repeated.

We generally do not measure hernias. We usually subjectively report size is **small, medium,** or **large.** A hernia may be **completely reducible, partially reducible,** or **nonreducible.** Nonreducibility may vary between **supine** and **upright** positions. Most hernias are more reducible in the supine than in the upright position, but in some the opposite is true. We report hernias as being either **nontender** or **mildly, moderately, or exquisitely tender** when compressed by the transducer. Tenderness is important in determining whether a hernia is more likely to be incidental or clinically significant.

When a hernia has been described in the report, we also report about our search for additional types of **ipsilateral** or **contralateral** groin hernias. A surgeon considering a laparoscopic hernia repair will want to know if additional ipsilateral and contralateral hernias are present. In a patient with an inguinal hernia, presence of an ipsilateral femoral or spigelian hernia may necessitate using a larger piece of mesh. Presence of a contralateral hernia may lead to bilateral rather than unilateral repair. If the contralateral side is not mentioned in the report, the surgeon may request that a repeat examination be performed at no cost to the patient to assess that side.

Linea Alba Hernias

Linea alba hernias are anterior abdominal wall hernias that protrude through the linea alba. Those that occur superior to the umbilicus are called **epigastric hernias,** and those that occur inferior to the umbilicus are called **hypogastric hernias.** Hypogastric hernias are much less common than epigastric hernias because the linea alba is much narrower and shorter inferior to the umbilicus than superior to the umbilicus.

DYNAMIC ULTRASOUND FOR GROIN HERNIA: NEGATIVE REPORT

Examination
Dynamic ultrasound of the right groin.

Indication
Right groin pain.

Procedure
The right groin was evaluated in both the supine and the upright position, with and without compression and Valsalva maneuvers, using a 12-MHz transducer.

Findings
There is no evidence of direct or indirect inguinal, femoral, or spigelian hernias.

Impression
There is no evidence of a right groin hernia.

DYNAMIC ULTRASOUND FOR GROIN HERNIA: POSITIVE UNILATERAL REPORT

Examination
Bilateral dynamic groin ultrasound.

Indication
Right groin pain.

Procedure
The right and left groin areas were evaluated in both supine and upright positions, with and without compression and Valsalva maneuvers, using a 12-MHz transducer.

Findings
Size: small
Contents: fat-containing
Reducibility: completely reducible
Tenderness: moderately tender
Side: right
Type: indirect inguinal hernia

Other Ipsilateral Hernias
There is no direct inguinal, femoral, or spigelian hernia on the right.

Contralateral Hernias
There are no contralateral left-sided groin hernias.

Impression
1. There is a small, fat-containing, completely reducible, but moderately tender, right indirect inguinal hernia that is the cause of the patient's pain.
2. There are no other ipsilateral groin hernias.
3. There are no contralateral groin hernias.

DYNAMIC ULTRASOUND FOR GROIN HERNIA: POSITIVE BILATERAL REPORT

Examination
Bilateral dynamic groin ultrasound.

Indication
Right groin pain.

Procedure
The right and left groin areas were evaluated in both supine and upright positions with and without compression and Valsalva maneuvers using a 12-MHz transducer.

Findings
Size: moderate sized
Contents: fat and bowel containing
Reducibility: reducible in the supine position, but nonreducible in the upright position
Tenderness: exquisitely tender
Side: right
Type: indirect inguinal hernia

Other Ipsilateral Hernias
There is no direct inguinal, femoral, or spigelian hernia on the right.

Contralateral Hernias
There is a small, fat-containing, completely reducible, nontender left indirect inguinal hernia.

Impression
1. There is a moderate-sized, fat-containing, exquisitely tender right indirect inguinal hernia that is completely reducible with transducer pressure when the patient is supine, but that is nonreducible in the upright position. This is the cause of the patient's right groin pain.
2. There are no other ipsilateral groin hernias.
3. There is also an incidental small, fat-containing, completely reducible, nontender left indirect inguinal hernia.

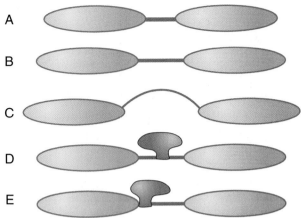

FIGURE 13-39. Linea alba between rectus abdominis muscles: spectrum of appearances. Transverse views. **A,** Normal, thick linea alba. **B,** Thinner but wider linea alba, possibly resulting from fewer decussations of rectus sheath fibers or representing diastasis recti when the patient is in the supine position in quiet respiration. **C,** Marked thinning and bulging of the linea alba that occurs in diastasis recti during a Valsalva maneuver or in the upright position. **D,** Typical small, epigastric linea alba hernia with its neck near the midline of the linea alba. **E,** Small linea alba hernia with neck occurring eccentrically near the right edge of the linea alba. Note that linea alba hernias typically have narrow necks and broad fundi in the transverse view, a shape that correlates with nonreducibility and increased risk of strangulation.

The **linea alba** is a thick layer of aponeurosis that separates the rectus abdominis muscles. It is formed by fusion and interlacing of fibers of the anterior and posterior sheaths of the right and left rectus muscles. Unlike the "conjoined tendon" and semilunar line, in which there are multiple thin layers of thin, loosely associated aponeuroses that do not form a discrete, well-defined structure, the linea alba is single, thick, well defined, extremely hyperechoic, and easily seen on ultrasound in most patients (Fig. 13-39, *A*). However, the degree of decussation of fibers from the right and left sides varies. Most patients have three layers of interlaced fibers, but a minority of patients may show only a single layer of interlaced fibers. In the latter group the linea alba is weaker and more predisposed to stretching (diastasis recti abdominis) and tearing (epigastric linea alba hernia).

Any cause of prolonged increased intra-abdominal pressure can predispose toward weakening of the linea alba, including pregnancy, morbid obesity, and ascites. The first step is often **diastasis recti abdominis,** thinning and stretching of the linea alba that is most apparent during straining or in the upright position. The stretching of the linea alba pulls the decussated fibers apart, decreasing their interlacing, weakening the tendon, and predisposing to **epigastric herniation.**

In patients with diastasis, the linea alba is thinner and wider than normal. When the patient is supine and in quiet respiration, the associated anterior bulging of the tendon is not evident (Fig. 13-39, *B*). However, having the patient perform a Valsalva maneuver or raise the head off the pillow while lying supine, or having the patient stand, will make the anterior bulging visible (Fig. 13-39, *C*; Fig. 13-40; **Video 13-19**). In patients with diastasis recti abdominis, the anterior bulging extends along the entire craniocaudal length of the epigastric segment of the linea alba. In patients with epigastric hernia, any bulging will be more localized along the craniocaudal axis. Although diastasis usually does not, epigastric hernias often do cause tenderness.

Epigastric linea alba hernias are easier to diagnose than are groin hernias as long as they are scanned with the proper transducer and the sonographer or physician is actually visually inspecting the linea alba. Epigastric hernias are usually superficial enough in location that

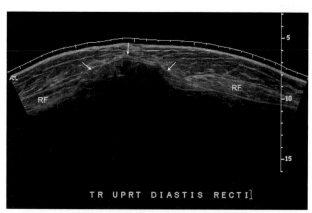

FIGURE 13-40. Linea alba–diastasis recti. Extended-FOV image obtained upright in the transverse plane shows marked widening, thinning, and bulging of the linea alba–diastasis recti abdominis.

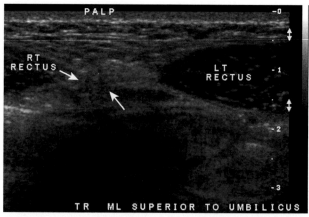

FIGURE 13-42. Epigastric linea alba hernia. Transverse view of small, fat-containing, nonreducible epigastric linea alba hernia arising from tear that is eccentrically located near the right edge of the linea alba (arrows).

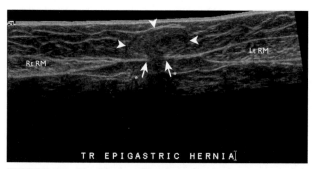

FIGURE 13-41. Linea alba hernia. Transverse extended-FOV image in upright position shows large, fat-containing, non-reducible epigastric linea alba hernia (arrowheads) demonstrating marked widening and thinning of the linea alba. Note that the neck, the defect in the linea alba (arrows) is narrow in comparison to the fundus (arrowheads). Note also that the fat within the hernia appears to be all preperitoneal, because the transversalis fascia deep to the neck is intact (asterisks). Linea alba hernias are more common in patients who have preexisting diastasis recti.

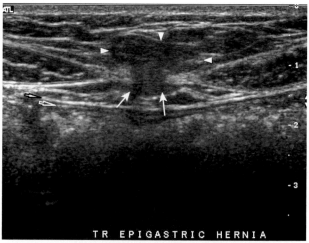

FIGURE 13-43. Epigastric linea alba hernia. Transverse view of small, mushroom-shaped, fat-containing, nonreducible epigastric linea alba hernia (arrowheads) shows a small tear of the linea alba. The fat within the hernia is preperitoneal fat. The underlying transversalis fascia (black open arrow) and peritoneal membrane (white open arrow) are intact and in the normal position.

they are best shown with 10- to 12-MHz linear array transducers. With these transducers, the defect through the linea alba is usually quite conspicuous because it is either isoechoic or hypoechoic compared with the extremely hyperechoic linea alba. The defect is usually very near the midline, but it may occur eccentrically toward the right or left side of the linea alba (Fig. 13-39, D and E; Figs. 13-41 and 13-42). The most frequent reason for missing an epigastric linea alba hernia is that the examination for abdominal pain was performed with the standard 3-MHz curved linear array transducer, focused too deep in the elevation axis to identify any structures except large hernias in obese patients. The clinician must have an index of suspicion to employ the appropriate transducer.

Although clinically detected epigastric hernias tend to be quite large and often contain bowel and other intra-peritoneal contents, sonographically detected epigastric

hernias are usually small to moderate-sized and contain only preperitoneal fat (Fig. 13-43). In hernias that contain only preperitoneal fat, the underlying peritoneal membrane and transversalis fascia are intact and the hernia cannot be seen or repaired laparoscopically. Epigastric hernias always have a very narrow neck in comparison to the size of the fundus and thus are usually not reducible (**Video 13-20**) and are at increased risk for strangulation, even when small. Some epigastric hernias that contain only preperitoneal fat are so small that it is difficult to believe that herniation is the cause of pain (Fig. 13-44). These hernias are not palpable, and patients typically present with pain, which more likely results

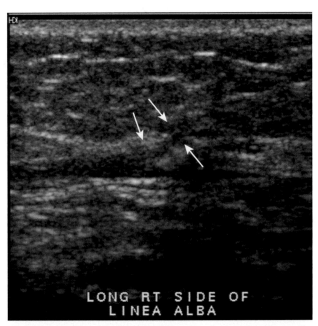

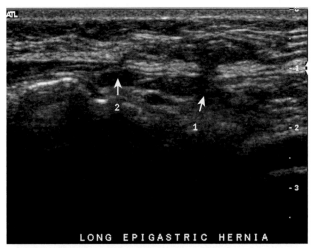

FIGURE 13-45. **Two epigastric hernias.** Longitudinal view shows a small, fat-containing, nonreducible, epigastric linea alba hernia inferiorly and a tiny tear superiorly. This patient had three other small hernias more superiorly. Multiple epigastric linea alba hernias are common enough that the entire length of the linea alba should be investigated in any patient with an identified epigastric hernia.

FIGURE 13-44. **Linea alba tear.** Tiny tear of the linea alba *(arrows)* caused pain but was not palpable. Such tears are relatively common in patients with preexisting diastasis recti abdominis.

from the tear or tendinosis of the linea alba than from herniation of a tiny amount of properitoneal fat.

Simply identifying diastasis in a patient who complains of epigastric midline pain is insufficient. The linea alba in the area of pain and along its entire epigastric segment must be examined for hernias, because patients with diastasis are at increased risk for multiple epigastric hernias. It is important to assess the entire length of the linea alba in any patient in whom one epigastric linea alba hernia is found. Most hernias contain only properitoneal fat, so they cannot be seen laparoscopically and must be repaired externally. If surgeons do not know that multiple hernias are present, they may use too small a piece of mesh to repair all the hernias. It is our experience that "recurrent" epigastric hernias are more likely to be secondary hernias that were not recognized and repaired, rather than true recurrences (Fig. 13-45; **Video 13-21**).

The much less common **hypogastric linea alba hernia** usually lies within a few centimeters of the umbilicus. Inferior to this area, the rectus muscles are more closely apposed or even fused. As with epigastric hernias, hypogastric linea alba hernias have narrow necks, usually are small to moderate-sized, contain only preperitoneal fat, are usually not reducible, and are prone to strangulation (Fig. 13-46).

Umbilical Hernias

Umbilical hernias occur through a widened **umbilical ring.** In newborns, they result from delayed return to the abdomen of bowel loops that lie in the base of the

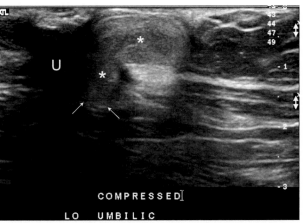

FIGURE 13-46. **Hypogastric linea alba hernia.** Longitudinal view shows a moderate-sized, fat-containing, periumbilical hypogastric linea alba hernia *(asterisk)* immediately inferior to the umbilicus *(U)*. Note that neck of the hernia *(arrows)* is very narrow and that the edematous strangulated fat is hyperechoic in comparison to the surrounding subcutaneous fat.

umbilical cord in the first trimester. In many cases, umbilical hernias in newborns will regress spontaneously by 3 or 4 years of age. Those that do not regress by age 4 are usually repaired.

Umbilical hernias can, however, develop at any time during life. Any cause of chronically increased intra-abdominal pressure or connective tissue weakness can lead to dilation of the umbilical ring and formation of an umbilical hernia. Umbilical hernias contain intraperitoneal contents, but smaller umbilical hernias usually contain only intraperitoneal fat (Fig. 13-47). We are asked to evaluate umbilical hernias sonographically

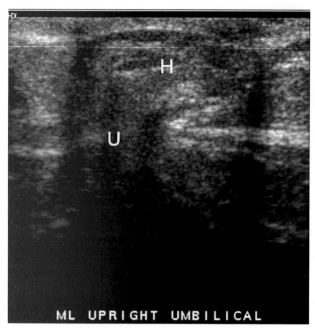

FIGURE 13-47. Umbilical hernia. Longitudinal view shows moderate-sized, fat and bowel–containing umbilical hernia *(H)*. Umbilical hernias pass through dilated umbilical rings *(U)*.

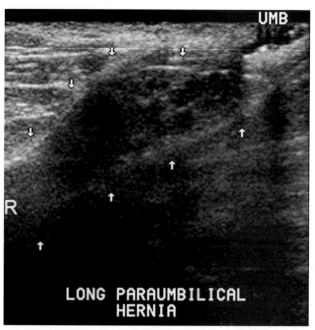

FIGURE 13-48. Umbilical hernia. Longitudinal view of moderate-sized, fat-containing umbilical hernia *(arrows)* in a morbidly obese patient who presented with umbilical pain. The hernia was not clinically apparent. In such obese patients the umbilicus lies several centimeters inferior to the umbilical ring. Thus, one must investigate superior to the umbilicus to identify small to moderate hernias.

much less frequently than we are asked to evaluate patients for groin pain, because the diagnosis of umbilical hernia is usually obvious clinically. The role of ultrasound is usually limited to evaluating for umbilical pain in patients who are so morbidly obese that an umbilical hernia cannot be detected clinically, or to assess for strangulation. In obese patients the umbilicus courses obliquely from deep superiorly to superficial inferiorly (Fig. 13-48). Thus the umbilical ring may be much more superiorly located that is suspected from the location of the umbilicus in obese patients. Untreated umbilical hernias tend to increase in size over time. They are usually reducible but may become nonreducible and can also become strangulated. Clinically, it may be difficult to distinguish between acute omphalitis and a strangulated small umbilical hernia. Both can present with pain and redness in the umbilical area. Sonography, however, can readily make the distinction (Figs. 13-49 and 13-50).

The sonographic evaluation of umbilical hernias is similar to that for any hernia. Dynamic maneuvers are used, with identification of type, size, contents, reducibility, and tenderness.

Paraumbilical or Periumbilical Hernias

A "paraumbilical" hernia is not really a distinct type of hernia. It is usually either an epigastric or a hypogastric **linea alba** hernia that lies very close to the umbilicus (Figs. 13-51 and 13-52). **Periumbilical** linea alba hernias, whether epigastric or hypogastric, are particularly likely to become strangulated (see Fig. 13-46).

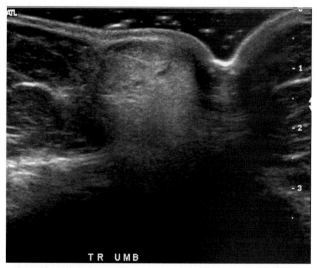

FIGURE 13-49. Small, nonreducible, strangulated umbilical hernia. Note in this transverse view that the edematous strangulated fat within the hernias is hyperechoic compared with the surrounding subcutaneous fat.

Incisional Hernias

Incisional hernias occur through surgical scars. Herniation can occur through any type of surgical scar, including laparoscopy ports and stomal sites. Incisional hernias can occur in any area along the anterior abdominal wall where an incision is made.

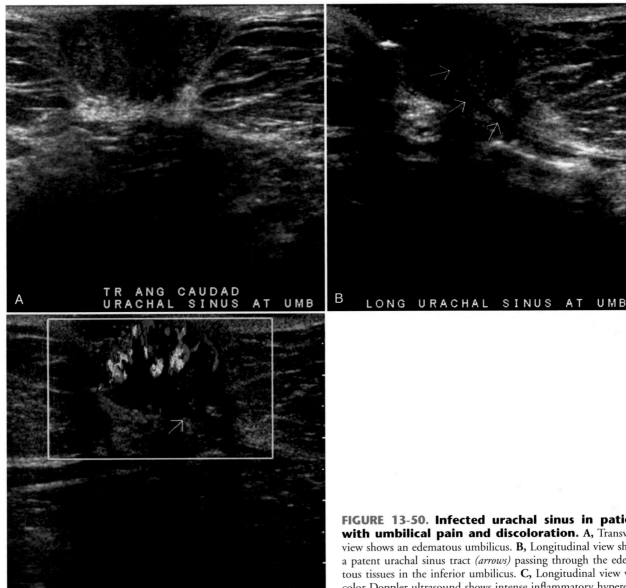

FIGURE 13-50. Infected urachal sinus in patient with umbilical pain and discoloration. A, Transverse view shows an edematous umbilicus. B, Longitudinal view shows a patent urachal sinus tract *(arrows)* passing through the edematous tissues in the inferior umbilicus. C, Longitudinal view with color Doppler ultrasound shows intense inflammatory hyperemia with the inflamed tissues that surround the infected patent urachal sinus tract *(arrow)*.

The herniation can result from thinning and stretching of the scar or from a tear in a segment of the scar. Whether the scar is stretched or torn affects the shape of the hernia, its reducibility, and its risk of strangulation. Incisional hernias resulting from **thinning and stretching** of the scar have wide necks and are reducible, whereas those resulting from **tears** in the scar are more likely to have narrow necks and to be nonreducible (Figs. 13-53 and 13-54). Incisional hernias can occur where natural hernias cannot, through the bellies of muscles that have been incised (Fig. 13-55). Incisional hernias can occur through very small scars (e.g., laparoscopy ports) **(Video 13-22).** Patients who have undergone transverse rectus abdominis myocutaneous (TRAM) flap breast reconstruction surgery are particularly likely to have one or more incisional hernias **(Video 13-23).**

Multiple Hernias

Patients who have one type of hernia are more likely to have additional hernias. These patients are more likely to have contralateral hernias of the same type, and they are more likely to have either ipsilateral or contralateral hernias of different types. There are several reasons for this. First, **bilateralism** may be caused by timing of closure of fetal canals, and delayed closure for any reason is likely to affect both sides simultaneously. Second, underlying factors that lead to formation of hernias can affect all sites simultaneously. Factors that increase the risk of hernias include any cause of chronically increased intra-abdominal pressure, as well as repetitive stress. Pregnancies, morbid obesity, and ascites can increase intra-abdominal pressure long enough to lead to development of hernias. Certain professions lead to repetitive

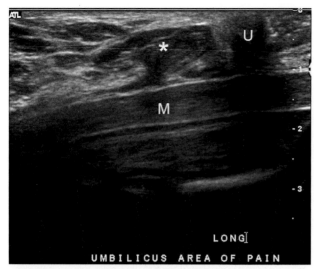

FIGURE 13-51. Small periumbilical hernia. Patient presented with periumbilical pain during the third trimester of pregnancy. Longitudinal view shows a fat-containing, nonreducible epigastric linea alba hernia (*asterisk*). The increased intra-abdominal pressure, together with the softening of ligaments that occurs in the late third trimester, predisposes to all types of hernias. *U,* Umbilicus; *M,* myometrium of gravid uterus.

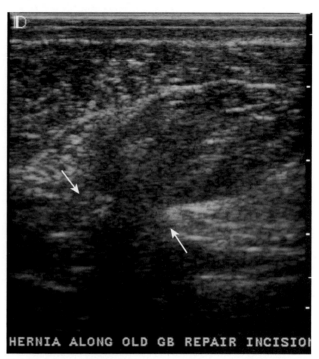

FIGURE 13-53. Incisional hernia. Fat-containing incisional hernia in the right upper quadrant (cholecystectomy scar) has a narrow neck *(arrows),* a broad fundus, and is nonreducible.

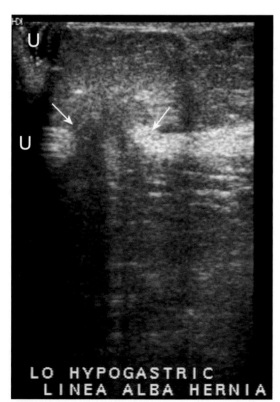

FIGURE 13-52. Periumbilical linea alba hernia. Longitudinal view shows a small, fat-containing, nonreducible periumbilical hypogastric linea alba hernia. Note that the defect is through the linea alba and lies inferior to the umbilicus and umbilical ring. *U,* Umbilicus.

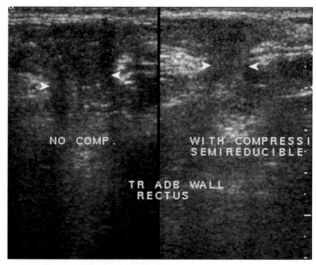

FIGURE 13-54. Incisional hernia. Narrow-necked, fat-containing ventral incisional hernia that is incompletely reducible, with no compression on the left, but with compression on the right.

stress injuries. Sedentary lifestyle, nutritional deficiencies, and hereditary factors can result in weak connective tissues. Evidence suggests that patients who have multiple hernias have increased levels of circulating metalloproteinases, which can weaken soft tissues.

In a patient with unilateral groin pain, but no demonstrable hernia on that side during dynamic ultrasound, the study can be stopped after examining the symptom-

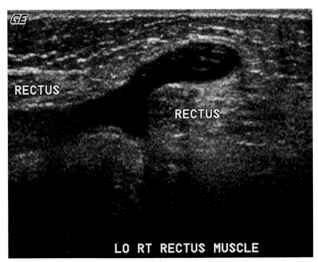

FIGURE 13-55. **Incisional hernia.** Longitudinal view shows moderate-sized, peritoneal fluid–containing incisional hernia through the belly of the rectus muscle, a site in which natural hernias do not occur.

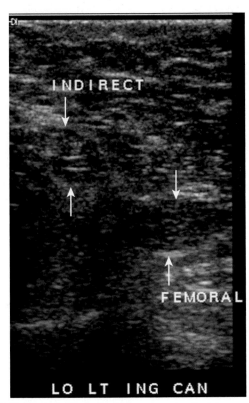

FIGURE 13-56. **Two hernias.** Longitudinal image of indirect inguinal and femoral hernias.

atic side. Again, however, in any patient in whom one type of groin hernia is found during the dynamic ultrasound examination, the clinician must look for the other three types of ipsilateral groin hernias. Femoral and indirect inguinal hernias can occur together (Fig. 13-56; **Video 13-24**). Additionally, direct and indirect inguinal hernias can occur on the same side. On long-axis views, the necks of the hernias resemble pant legs straddling the

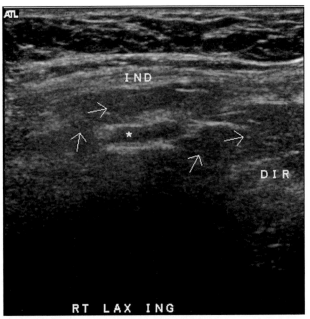

FIGURE 13-57. **"Pantaloon" hernia.** Long-axis view of right inguinal area shows both direct (*dir*) and indirect (*ind*) inguinal hernias with the inferior epigastric vessels (*) between them, a pantaloon hernia. The necks of the direct and indirect inguinal hernia resemble pant legs straddling the inferior epigastric vessels.

inferior epigastric vessels, explaining why the combination of the two hernias has been termed a **pantaloon hernia** (Fig. 13-57; **Video 13-25**). The contralateral groin is evaluated as well. This is especially important in patients who will undergo laparoscopic hernia repairs, because surgeons are more likely to perform bilateral repairs using a laparoscopic approach than when performing external herniorrhaphy. Direct inguinal hernias and femoral hernias are most likely to be bilateral. As many as four or five hernias may be found in a single patient (Fig. 13-58; **Videos 13-26**). Multiple linea alba and incisional hernias are also relatively common (see Videos 13-21 and 13-23).

Recurrent Groin Hernias

Hernia repair can be performed by direct anterior incision of the inguinal canal or laparoscopically. Hernia repairs performed decades ago were done without mesh. Originally, fascia was pulled up to reinforce the inguinal area, but this tended to widen the femoral canal and led to "recurrent" femoral hernias. "Tension free" external repairs using proline mesh were developed to prevent this. Recent data suggest that results of laparoscopic repairs equal those of external repairs. Laparoscopic repairs have the advantage of allowing bilateral repair, but require general anesthesia. External repairs are generally limited to one side, but can be done with regional anesthesia. Most hernia repairs now are "tension free" and employ mesh. Mesh can be used with both external

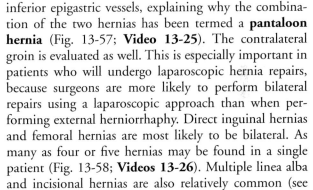

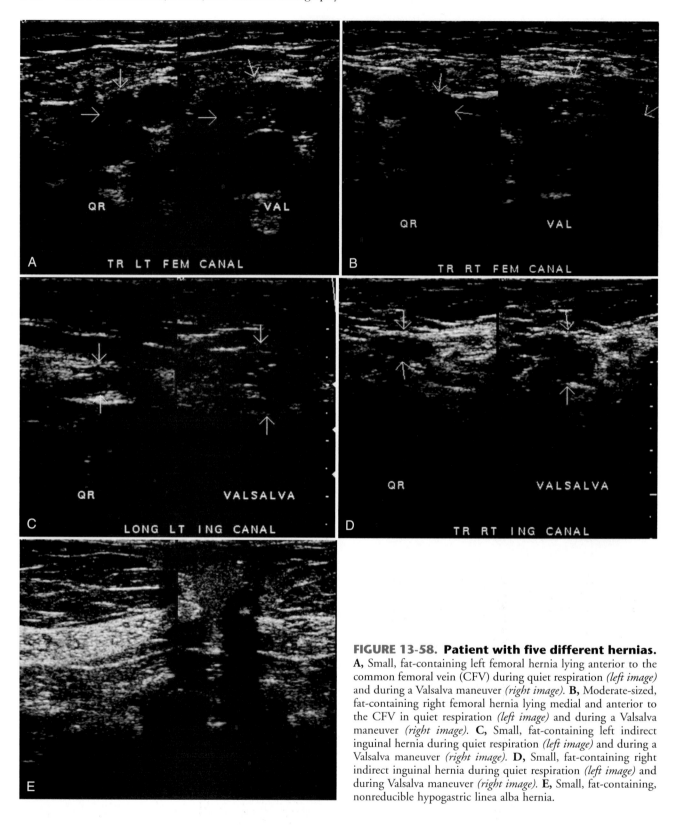

FIGURE 13-58. Patient with five different hernias. **A,** Small, fat-containing left femoral hernia lying anterior to the common femoral vein (CFV) during quiet respiration *(left image)* and during a Valsalva maneuver *(right image)*. **B,** Moderate-sized, fat-containing right femoral hernia lying medial and anterior to the CFV in quiet respiration *(left image)* and during a Valsalva maneuver *(right image)*. **C,** Small, fat-containing left indirect inguinal hernia during quiet respiration *(left image)* and during a Valsalva maneuver *(right image)*. **D,** Small, fat-containing right indirect inguinal hernia during quiet respiration *(left image)* and during Valsalva maneuver *(right image)*. **E,** Small, fat-containing, nonreducible hypogastric linea alba hernia.

and laparoscopic repairs. Several different types of mesh are used.

Unfortunately, recurrent or residual groin pain after herniorrhaphy is relatively common. Recurrent hernia is not the only cause of residual or recurrent groin pain after herniorrhaphy, and dynamic sonography is an inte-

gral part of the evaluation of other causes in patients with acute or chronic postherniorrhaphy pain.

In the acute phase, **residual pain** unchanged from preoperative pain is rare and usually the result of an unsuccessful hernia repair. The original hernia persists and can be demonstrated sonographically. More often, acute pain is caused by entities other than recurrent hernia, including incisional pain, pain caused by acute **hematomas** (Fig. 13-59) or **seromas** (Fig. 13-60), and sometimes pain radiating into the scrotum as the result of spermatic cord compression by a seroma, a hematoma, the mesh, or a repair that makes the internal inguinal ring too tight. In such cases, it is important to assess the ipsilateral scrotum and testis with gray-scale imaging and Doppler ultrasound, because cord compression of any etiology can lead to **testicular infarction** (Fig. 13-61, *A*). Doppler ultrasound evidence of testicular ischemia may indicate the need for emergency decompression by either evacuating an inguinal canal hematoma/seroma or

loosening the repaired internal inguinal ring (Fig. 13-61, *B*). Inguinal canal hematomas or seromas that do not compress the spermatic cord or cause testicular ischemia, on the other hand, can usually be managed conservatively. Postherniorrhaphy hematomas or seromas can become secondarily infected and evolve into abscesses. **Stitch granulomas** or **stitch abscesses** can cause pain (Fig. 13-62).

Late recurring pain also has a variety of causes, but recurrent hernia becomes a greater concern, particularly

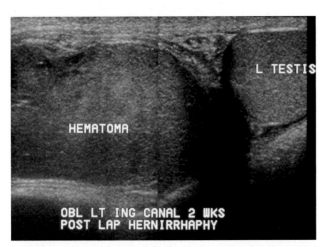

FIGURE 13-59. Hematoma. Severe pain, swelling, and ecchymosis 2 weeks after left inguinal herniorrhaphy, resulting from a huge hematoma filling the entire inguinal canal from the groin to the upper pole of the testis.

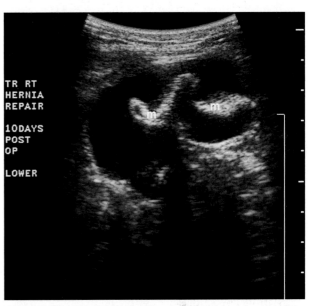

FIGURE 13-60. Seroma. Extremely large seroma around the mesh (*m*) caused severe right groin pain and swelling a few days after herniorrhaphy.

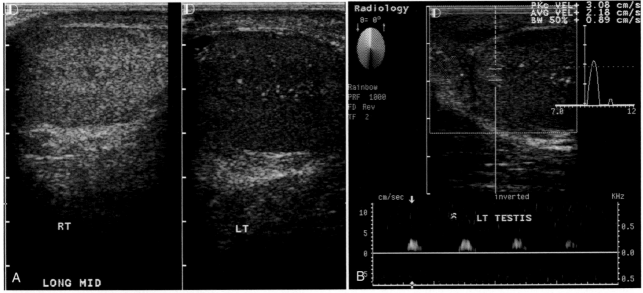

FIGURE 13-61. Testicular ischemia. Testicular ischemia caused by large, acute hematoma within the left inguinal canal after herniorrhaphy, with pain radiating into the scrotum. **A,** Left testis is swollen and edematous. **B,** Pulsed Doppler spectral analysis of the left testis shows decreased velocities and increased impedance from compression of the spermatic cord by the hematoma. Doppler ultrasound evidence of decreased flow to the ipsilateral testis in patients with postherniorrhaphy hematomas indicates the need to evacuate the hematoma.

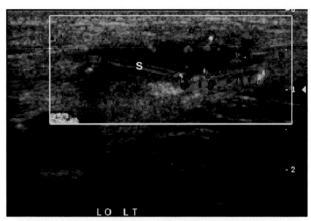

FIGURE 13-62. Subacute stitch abscess. This patient developed pain and redness in the left groin weeks after an otherwise successful herniorrhaphy. Sonography showed a stitch *(s)* within the center of a hyperemic complex fluid collection.

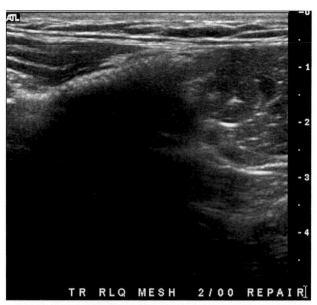

FIGURE 13-63. Normal mesh. The mesh used in this hernia repair is thick and echogenic, and individual fibers within the mesh are visible. It casts a strong acoustic shadow. The mesh can be well seen in only a small percentage of cases.

when the pain is similar in type to that present before surgery. Late pain etiologies include recurrent hernia, seroma, hematoma, abscess, traction on the edges of the mesh, immune reaction to the mesh, spiral clips, compression of the spermatic cord, and fibrosis and scarring of the ilioinguinal nerve. Again, dynamic sonography is essential in evaluating such patients, although it is more difficult than in patients not previously repaired.

In patients who had herniorrhaphy without mesh, the recurrent hernia is usually of the same type as the original. However, it is not unusual, even after tension-free repairs, to find a "recurrent" femoral hernia. In such cases, especially after external repair, the femoral hernia may have been present before the repair, but subclinical and unrecognized. This is a major reason why it is important to look for *all* types of groin hernias during dynamic sonography. In our experience, "recurrent" femoral hernias are less common after tension-free repairs that employ mesh, because they usually employ a piece of mesh large enough to cover the conjoined tendon, internal inguinal ring, femoral canal, and spigelian area.

In patients whose hernias were repaired with mesh, it is not possible to determine sonographically whether a recurrent inguinal hernia is direct or indirect. It is only possible to determine that it is a *recurrent* inguinal hernia. The key to finding recurrent hernias in patients who have mesh in place is to identify the mesh and then assess for herniations along the edges of the mesh with dynamic maneuvers. In patients being evaluated for recurrent hernia, the most useful dynamic maneuver is usually the compression maneuver with the patient in the upright position.

Because many types of mesh are available, the appearance varies greatly. In ideal cases, we can actually see the texture of the mesh (Fig. 13-63). In most cases, however, the mesh can be seen only as an echogenic line of variable thickness with variable shadowing or as an area of variable shadowing (Figs. 13-64 and 13-65). Some newer

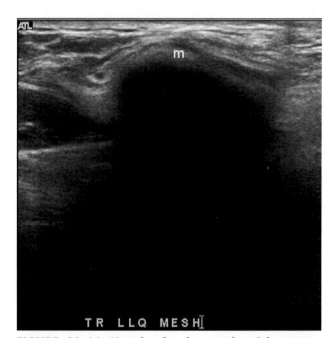

FIGURE 13-64. Herniorrhaphy mesh with strong shadow. Mesh typically appears thick and echogenic and casts a strong acoustic shadow, but individual fibers within the mesh are not visible sonographically.

types of mesh are thin and much more difficult to identify sonographically. Normal mesh can have folds and can be rolled at the edges, and it normally bulges mildly outward in the upright position and during Valsalva maneuvers (Fig. 13-66). Patient history is rarely helpful because patients are unaware of the type of mesh used.

However, every effort should be made to identify the mesh, because recurrent hernias do not occur though the

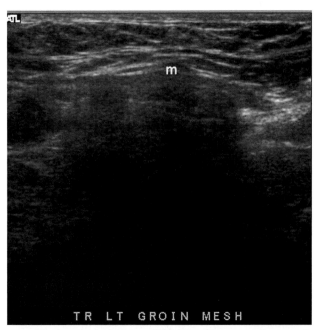

FIGURE 13-65. Herniorrhaphy mesh with weak shadow. Thin, poorly defined mesh casts only a weak acoustic shadow. Such mesh can only be identified with high-frequency transducers, optimal technique, and careful search.

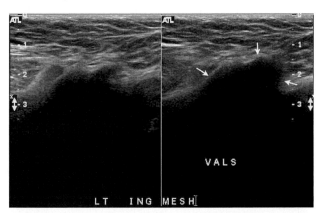

FIGURE 13-66. Wrinkled herniorrhaphy mesh. Mesh can bulge during the Valsalva maneuver or when the patient is scanned in the upright position; this may be normal. These split-screen images show wrinkled mesh in the supine position in quiet respiration *(left image)* and bulging with straightening of some of the wrinkles in the upright position *(right image).*

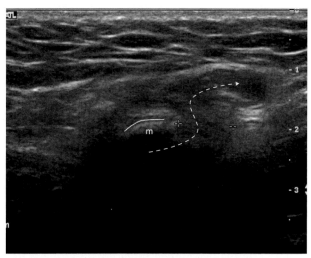

FIGURE 13-67. Recurrent inguinal hernia. Short-axis view shows small, fat-containing, reducible *(dotted line)* hernia arising from inferomedial edge of the mesh *(m)*, where recurrent inguinal hernias most often arise.

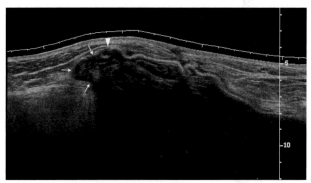

FIGURE 13-68. Detached mesh with hernia. Transverse extended-FOV image shows that a large piece of mesh used to repair a large ventral hernia has become detached along its right edge *(arrowhead)*, allowing a recurrent hernia to protrude from under the detached edge *(arrows)*.

center but rather at the *edges* of the mesh. Most recurrent hernias occur along the **inferomedial edge** of the mesh (Fig. 13-67; **Videos 13-27** and **13-28**), but it is still important to identify the mesh and then assess the entire periphery of the mesh, because hernias can occur along any edge of the mesh **(Video 13-29)**. Herniation from the edge of the mesh likely occurs because the affected edge has "pulled loose" (Fig. 13-68).

The edges of the mesh can be anchored to surrounding connective tissues with sutures, surgical clips, or special spiral clips. The sutures and clips hold the mesh in place for about the first 6 weeks after surgery. After

this, fibrosis forms and generally holds the mesh in place. It is during the first 6 postoperative weeks, before the mesh has fibrosed to the anterior abdominal wall, that mesh is most likely to pull loose from its anchors. In our experience, this is most likely to occur after laparoscopic repairs, not because the repair has been defective or because laparoscopic repair is less effective, but because the patient feels "too well, too soon" after the minimally invasive repair and resumes activities that put the repair at risk within the first 6 weeks. Some patients may complain of a tearing sensation during some movement, followed by the onset of recurrent inguinal pain, but in most patients the onset is more insidious.

A chronic hematoma/seroma can cause chronic pain, and its evacuation can relieve the pain. Therefore, searching for a hematoma or seroma is a standard part of the postherniorrhaphy sonogram. Some patients can develop an allergic or hypersensitivity reaction to the mesh, with a thin seroma localized to the mesh surface.

When sonography demonstrates no hernia, hematoma, or seroma, it is important to assess the mesh for tenderness. In many cases without sonographically demonstrable pathology, the mesh is tender, for a variety of reasons. First, the mesh may compress the spermatic cord; compressing the mesh will cause pain that radiates into the scrotum. Second, the mesh may be placing traction on the fibrosis that holds its edges in place; this is especially common in patients with significant weight gain since surgery. The mesh usually bulges anteriorly in such cases. In other cases, the fibrosis that holds the mesh in place has entrapped nerves, notably the **ilioinguinal nerve.** This has been a diagnosis of exclusion, confirmed by injecting the nerve, then surgically dissecting it free of the fibrosis. The normal ilioinguinal nerve can be identified sonographically superior to the inguinal canal. Ultrasound can be used to guide a block of the nerve, but we are unaware of sonography playing a role in diagnosing entrapment of the ilioinguinal nerve in patients who underwent herniorrhaphy.

The **spiral clips** used to anchor the mesh require special mention. Because these can become tender and a source of postherniorrhaphy pain, spiral clips are now seldom used. However, their past popularity means many patients have them. Spiral clips have a characteristic radiographic and sonographic appearance (Fig. 13-69). In some postherniorrhaphy patients with no other sonographically demonstrable pathology, the only finding is focal tenderness directly over the offending clip, which has a classic sonographic appearance (Fig. 13-70). Surgical removal of the clip will relieve the pain and tenderness and generally will not adversely affect the soundness of the repair, because the edge of the mesh will be held firmly in place by fibrosis, even after the clip is removed.

Hernia Complications

Hernia complications include incarceration, obstruction, and strangulation. **Incarcerated hernias** are simply hernias that are nonreducible. **Obstructed hernias** contain incarcerated bowel loops that have become mechanically obstructed. **Strangulated hernias** contain incarcerated contents with compromised vascularity. Not all strangulated hernias contain bowel loops; even preperitoneal fat can become strangulated. Most incarcerated hernias are neither obstructed nor strangulated, but all obstructed and strangulated hernias are also incarcerated. We prefer not to use the term "incarcerated" because many referring clinicians confuse incarceration with obstruction and strangulation, often believing that incarceration is a surgical emergency when it is not. Only incarcerated hernias that are also obstructed or strangulated are surgical emergencies. Even strangulated hernias that contain only preperitoneal fat may not be emergencies. It is the presence of bowel loops within strangulated hernias that makes them emergent. Instead of incarcerated, we use the term **nonreducible** because the referring clinician is less likely to confuse it with strangulation.

The **shape** of hernias affects their reducibility and their likelihood of becoming obstructed or strangulated in the future. The hernia type affects its shape. Hernias that have relatively **broad necks** in comparison to their fundi are usually completely reducible and rarely become obstructed or strangulated. Groin hernias that typically have broad necks and infrequently strangulate are direct inguinal hernias and some indirect inguinal hernias.

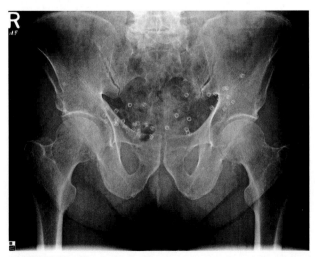

FIGURE 13-69. Spiral clips. Anteroposterior radiograph of the pelvis shows spiral clips in both inguinal areas from bilateral inguinal herniorrhaphies.

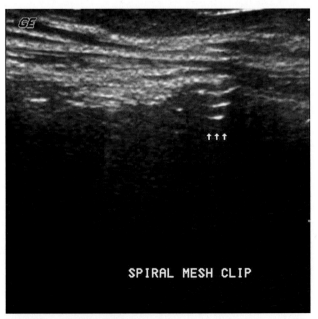

FIGURE 13-70. Spiral clip. Characteristic sonographic appearance of a spiral clip *(arrows)* used to anchor the edges of mesh in a repair of inguinal hernia and causing pain and tenderness.

Hernias that have relatively **narrow necks** in comparison to their fundi are more likely to be nonreducible, to become obstructed, and to strangulate. Hernia types that typically have narrow necks and are at high risk for strangulation include femoral **(Video 13-30)**, spigelian (see Fig. 13-35), linea alba (see Fig. 13-46), umbilical (see Fig. 13-47), and some indirect inguinal hernias.

Although **vascular compromise** is the hallmark of strangulation, Doppler ultrasound is not the most sensitive modality for demonstrating signs of strangulation. Gray-scale sonography, however, is sensitive. Doppler ultrasound shows arterial flow within hernias with some success, but generally is not sensitive enough to demonstrate venous flow and cannot show lymphatic flow at all. Lymphatic and venous vessel walls are very thin and easily compressed within by the tissues surrounding the neck of the hernia. Arteries, on the other hand, are relatively thick walled and incompressible and generally are not compressed by the surrounding tissues. Thus, in strangulated hernias, the lymphatics and veins become obstructed long before arterial flow decreases. Blood can still supply the strangulated hernia long after venous and lymphatic outflow stops. The continued inflow in the presence of obstructed outflow (1) increases intravascular pressure, (2) causes increased transudation and exudation of fluid into the extracellular spaces, and (3) changes the gray-scale appearance of the hernia even when Doppler ultrasound can still detect arterial inflow. The most sensitive findings of strangulation are the presence of the following:

- Hyperechoic fat (Fig. 13-71)
- Isoechoic thickening of the normally thin and echogenic hernia sac (Fig. 13-72)
- Fluid within the sac (Fig. 13-72; **Video 13-30**)
- Thickening of bowel wall in bowel-containing hernias (Fig. 13-73)

In most strangulated hernias, more than one of these gray-scale findings are present, even when Doppler ultra-sound demonstrates normal flow within the hernia contents (Fig. 13-74). Care should be taken in equating fluid within the hernia sac with strangulation; nonstrangulated hernias that contain intraperitoneal contents can contain peritoneal fluid, especially in female patients.

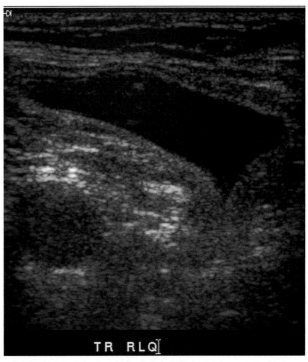

FIGURE 13-72. Femoral hernia. Short-axis view shows strangulated left femoral hernia that shows two additional gray-scale findings of strangulation: transudative or exudative fluid and isoechoic thickening of the hernia sac wall. The sac normally appears thin and echogenic.

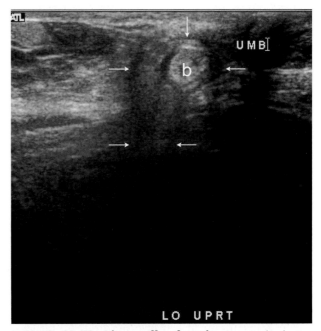

FIGURE 13-73. Linea alba hernia. Longitudinal view shows strangulated periumbilical epigastric linea alba hernia. The fat is hyperechoic, the sac wall is isoechoic and thickened, and a small bowel loop (b) has a thickened wall and is aperistaltic.

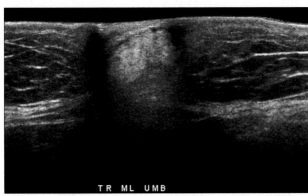

FIGURE 13-71. Linea alba hernia. Long-axis extended-FOV sonogram shows strangulated hypogastric linea alba hernia. The hallmark of strangulation is **hyperechogenicity** of the fat with the hernia.

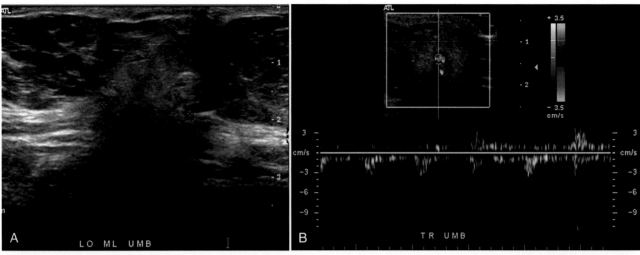

FIGURE 13-74. Strangulation. A, Abnormal hyperechogenicity of the fat within this umbilical hernia indicates that it is strangulated. **B,** Color Doppler and pulsed Doppler spectral ultrasound analysis shows normal flow within the hernia, despite it being strangulated. Gray-scale findings are more sensitive than Doppler ultrasound for detecting strangulation in a hernia.

Entities That Simulate Groin Hernias

A wide spectrum of space-occupying lesions in the groin can simulate hernias of the groin. Entities that can occur within the inguinal canal include lipomas; processus vaginalis cysts or hydroceles (hydroceles of canal of Nuck); round ligament cysts, leiomyomas, or varices; desmoids; endometriomas; sarcomas; hematomas; seromas; undescended testes; and metastatic peritoneal implants. Inguinal lymphadenopathy, common femoral or external iliac artery aneurysms and pseudoaneurysms, iliopsoas bursae, and sebaceous cysts can all occur within the groin, but *outside* the inguinal canal. Additionally, pain from intraabdominal inflammatory processes can simulate groin pain; acute appendicitis and acute diverticulitis can cause pain near the groin.

   Cysts or **hydroceles** of the inguinal canal can occur in both males and females. In males these localized fluid collections can occur when the segment of the processus vaginalis peritonei within the inguinal canal does not fuse while segments proximal and distal to it do fuse. This leads to accumulation of fluid within the unfused segment of processus vaginalis and forms a localized process hydrocele. In males these occur within the inguinal canal next to the spermatic cord and can compress the cord (Fig. 13-75). In females the unfused processus vaginalis is called the canal of Nuck, so this localized cyst or hydrocele is termed a **cyst** or **hydrocele of the canal of Nuck** (Fig. 13-76). Hydroceles are usually unilocular and fixed in position within the canal, but can become lobulated and septated as they enlarge.

   The round ligament can give rise to cysts and leiomyomas. Unlike inguinal canal hydroceles, which are fixed in position, **round ligament cysts** can be mobile and can move back and forth between the abdominal cavity and the inguinal canal **(Video 13-31).** The round

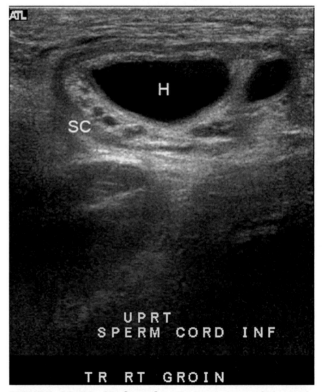

FIGURE 13-75. Hydrocele. Short-axis view of the mid–right inguinal canal shows a hydrocele *(H)* compressing the spermatic cord *(SC)* posteriorly and to the right.

ligament contains smooth muscle fibers from which **leiomyomas** can arise (Fig. 13-77).

   Round ligament varices develop as collateral pathways for uterine venous drainage during pregnancy. They are usually asymptomatic and incidental, but in some patients can cause a tender, palpable, inguinal or labial abnormality. They usually resolve spontaneously completely after delivery, but in a few patients can persist and cause inguinal pain and swelling months or years after the last pregnancy. They are relatively inapparent with the patient in the supine position, but become larger and have faster flow in the upright position (Fig. 13-78). Round ligament varices are typically more symptomatic and larger when the patient is upright and after exercise such as running, when varices become hyperemic. Occasionally, round ligament variceal **thrombosis** occurs spontaneously, most often in the postpartum period when collateral uterine flow through them regresses (Fig. 13-79).

Endometriomas can occur along the course of the round ligament within the inguinal canal (Fig. 13-80). They often have a history of cyclical variation in size and tenderness.

Most so-called inguinal canal lipomas are not true lipomas, but rather **nonsliding-type indirect inguinal hernias** that contain only properitoneal fat. However, true **lipomas** can occur anywhere along the length of the inguinal canal (Fig. 13-81) and into the scrotum or labium majorum (Fig. 13-82).

Entities that Simulate Anterior Abdominal Wall Hernias

Subcutaneous or intramuscular lipomas have a sonographic appearance identical to those of the inguinal canal or labium (Figs. 13-81 and 13-82).

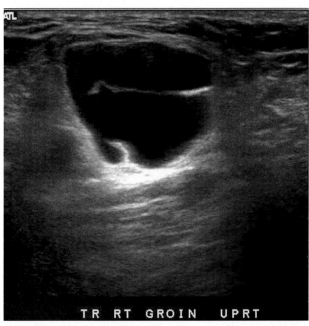

FIGURE 13-76. Hydrocele. Short-axis view in female patient shows a lobulated, thinly septated hydrocele of the canal of Nuck (inguinal canal).

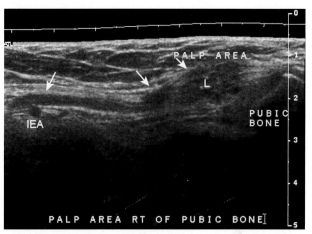

FIGURE 13-77. Leiomyoma. Long-axis view of the right inguinal canal in female patient shows a leiomyoma *(L)* arising from the round ligament *(arrows)* that presented as a palpable nodule; *IEA,* inferior epigastric artery.

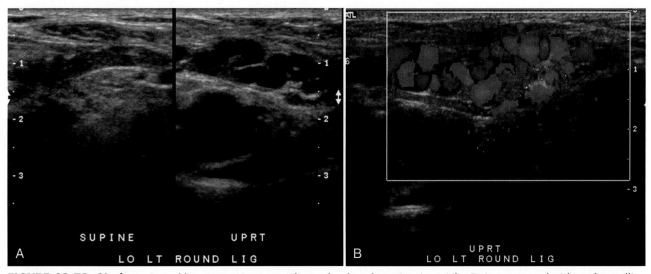

FIGURE 13-78. Varices. Round ligament varices are evident only when the patient is upright. Patient presented with tender swelling in the left labium majorum after running. **A,** Split-screen ultmage shows the round ligament during quiet respiration in the supine position *(left image)* and in the upright position *(right image).* **B,** Long-axis color Doppler ultrasound view shows abundant flow within the round ligament varices when the patient is upright.

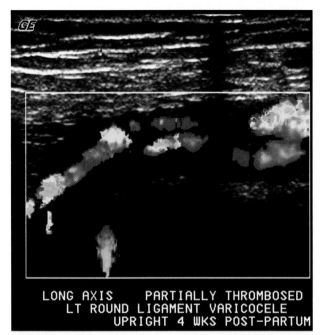

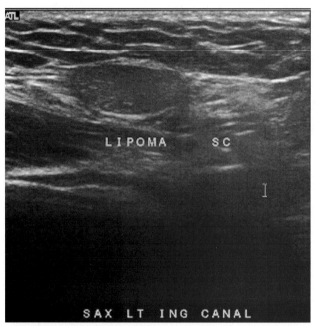

FIGURE 13-79. Varices. Long-axis view shows partially thrombosed left round ligament varices in a patient who presented with left groin pain 4 weeks postpartum. The decreasing uterine flow that occurs in the postpartum period can lead to thrombosis of round ligament varices that develop as collateral pathways during pregnancy.

FIGURE 13-81. Inguinal lipoma. Short-axis view of the right inguinal canal shows a true hyperechoic lipoma of the inguinal canal lying lateral to the spermatic cord (SC). Most "lipomas" of the inguinal canal are merely nonsliding-type inguinal hernias that contain only preperitoneal fat.

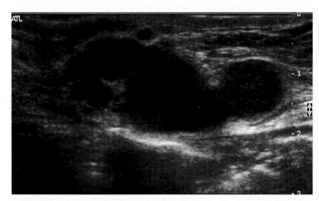

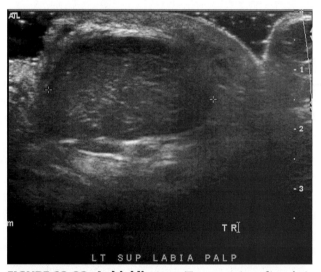

FIGURE 13-80. Endometrioma. Long-axis view of the left inguinal canal shows a multiloculated complex cyst, an endometrioma, in a patient who complained of intermittent inguinal pain and swelling.

FIGURE 13-82. Labial lipoma. Transverse view of isoechoic lipoma of the left labium majorum in patient who complained of painless swelling of the left labium.

In patients being evaluated for incisional hernias, **exuberant scars** (Fig. 13-83) and **fat necrosis** (Fig. 13-84) resulting from previous surgeries can clinically simulate an anterior abdominal wall incisional hernia.

Hematomas of the rectus abdominis (Fig. 13-85) or oblique muscles (Fig. 13-86) can cause pain and swelling that simulate anterior abdominal wall hernia. The patient usually (but not always) has a history of significant acute trauma. In patients without a classic history, sonography can be helpful.

Desmoid tumors (aggressive fibromatosis) are rare, except in patients with familial adenomatoid fibromatosis (FAP), whose tumors are usually intra-abdominal.

Anterior abdominal wall desmoids are usually sporadic. They arise from the fibrous elements of the anterior abdominal wall aponeuroses or muscle sheaths. Desmoids are locally invasive and tend to recur if not excised widely enough, but do not metastasize distantly. Sonographically, desmoids are solid nodules or masses that are irregular in shape and that have some internal vascularity (Figs. 13-87 and 13-88). Desmoids are difficult to distinguish from sarcomas, except for slightly less blood flow on color or power Doppler ultrasound. If not excised, desmoids grow progressively (Fig. 13-89).

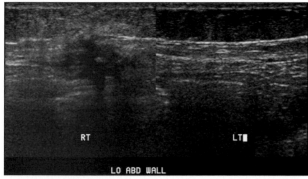

FIGURE 13-83. Incisional hernia. Exuberant scar tissue causes the palpable abnormality on the right side *(left image)* that was clinically suspicious for incisional hernia. The mirror-image location is normal on the left side *(right image)*. Patient presented with a painless lump in the area of a previous right lower quadrant surgical incision.

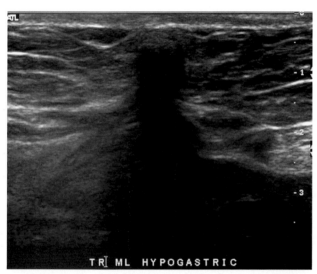

FIGURE 13-84. Calcified oil cyst. Transverse image shows mass that presented as a painless palpable lump in the vicinity of a previous hypogastric midline surgical incision, considered clinically suspicious for an incisional hernia.

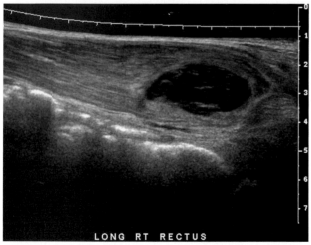

FIGURE 13-85. Tear and hematoma. Long-axis extended-FOV image shows an acute right rectus abdominis muscle tear and hematoma that presented with acute pain and swelling in the right groin and lower anterior abdominal wall. The referring physician was suspicious of an acute right sports hernia.

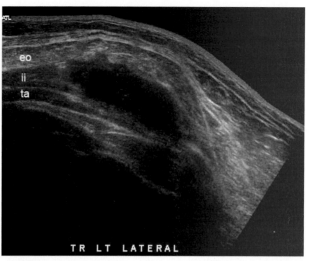

FIGURE 13-86. Tear and hematoma. Transverse extended-FOV image shows an acute tear and hematoma within the internal oblique muscle *(ii)* in a patient who presented with acute pain in the left lower quadrant; *eo,* external oblique muscle; *ta,* transverse abdominis muscle.

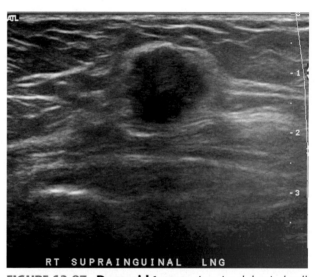

FIGURE 13-87. Desmoid tumor. Anterior abdominal wall desmoid tumor is highly hypoechoic, irregular in shape, and difficult to distinguish from a sarcoma. It presented as a painful and tender lump.

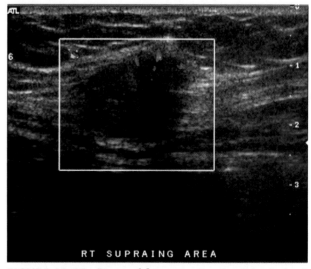

FIGURE 13-88. Desmoid tumor. Anterior abdominal wall desmoid tumor has a small amount of peripheral blood flow.

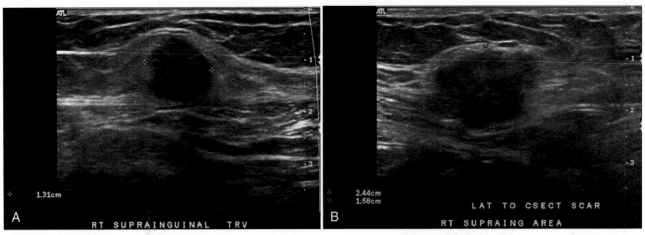

FIGURE 13-89. Desmoid tumor. Although desmoid tumors are considered histologically benign and do not metastasize, they are locally invasive and will enlarge if not excised. **A,** This desmoid tumor developed as a tender nodule a few months after pregnancy. The patient elected not to have it excised. **B,** In 23 months, desmoid tumor enlarged from 1.3 to 2.4 cm. The patient then elected to have it excised.

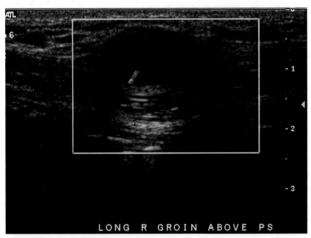

FIGURE 13-90. Fibroma. Long-axis view of a benign fibroma of the anterior rectus sheath of the inferior right rectus abdominis muscle that presented as a nontender swelling near the right groin. Note that there is minimal internal vascularity.

Benign and malignant connective tissue tumors of the anterior abdominal wall such as **fibromas** (Fig. 13-90) and **fibrosarcomas** (Fig. 13-91) can simulate anterior abdominal wall hernias.

SUMMARY

Dynamic ultrasound is the key examination for assessing groin or anterior abdominal wall pain. Dynamic components of the examination include Valsalva and compression maneuvers and scanning in both supine and upright positions. Dynamic sonography enables clinicians to determine hernia type, size, contents, reducibility, and tenderness. Each of these should be determined during the scan and specifically mentioned in the final report. We also venture an educated guess as to the clinical significance of the hernia based on type, size, contents, and

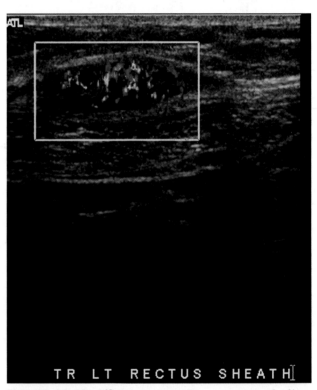

FIGURE 13-91. Fibrosarcoma. Transverse view of a fibrosarcoma of the anterior sheath of the left rectus abdominis muscle that presented as a painless lump. It is similar in appearance to the fibroma shown in Figure 13-90 but is much more vascular internally.

tenderness, because asymptomatic clinically insignificant groin hernias are frequently identified sonographically.

Evaluation of groin pain in athletes is frequently more complex than in nonathletes because of associated tendinosis and osteitis pubis. Adding MRI to dynamic ultrasound is usually necessary to identify underlying pathologic processes and decide the best combination of surgical and nonsurgical treatments.

Patients with one hernia frequently have multiple hernias, so in any patient in whom a hernia is sonographically demonstrable, the examination should be continued, looking for other types of ipsilateral and contralateral groin or anterior abdominal hernias. Even when no additional hernias are found, it is important to the surgeon to specifically mention in the report that a complete search of both groin areas was made and no additional hernias were found.

Strangulation is the most dreaded complication of groin hernias. Gray-scale findings of strangulation—hyperechoic fat, isoechoic thickening of the hernia sac, fluid within the sac, and thickening of the walls of bowel loops—are all more sensitive for strangulation than is Doppler ultrasound.

Recurrent pain after herniorrhaphy is a relatively common problem. Dynamic sonography can be helpful in assessing both acute and chronic recurrences of groin pain. Most hernia repairs now use mesh. The key to sonographic identification of recurrent hernias is to assess the edges of the mesh with dynamic maneuvers, because recurrent hernias arise from the edges of the mesh.

Many pathologic processes can simulate hernia, both rare and nonspecific, but cysts or hydroceles of the processus vaginalis (or canal of Nuck) and round ligament varices are relatively common and have virtually pathognomonic sonographic appearances.

Bibliography

Aguirre DA, Santosa AC, Casola G, Sirlin CB. Abdominal wall hernias: imaging features, complications, and diagnostic pitfalls at multi-detector row CT. Radiographics 2005;25:1501-1520.

Bradley M, Morgan D, Pentlow B, Roe A. The groin hernia: an ultrasound diagnosis? Ann R Coll Surg Engl 2003;85:178-180.

Brittenden J, Robinson P. Imaging of pelvic injuries in athletes. Br J Radiol 2005;78:457-468.

Caudill P, Nyland J, Smith C, et al. Sports hernias: a systematic literature review. Br J Sports Med 2008;42:954-964.

Courtney CA, Lee AC, Wilson C, O'Dwyer PJ. Ventral hernia repair: a study of current practice. Hernia 2003;7:44-46.

Emby DJ, Aoun G. CT technique for suspected anterior abdominal wall hernia. AJR Am J Roentgenol 2003;181:431-433.

Engel JM, Deitch EE. Sonography of the anterior abdominal wall. AJR Am J Roentgenol 1981;137:73-77.

Jaffe TA, O'Connell MJ, Harris JP, et al. MDCT of abdominal wall hernias: is there a role for Valsalva's maneuver? AJR Am J Roentgenol 2005;184:847-851.

Jamadar DA, Jacobson JA, Morag Y, et al. Sonography of inguinal region hernias. AJR Am J Roentgenol 2006;187:185-190.

Kervancioglu R, Bayram MM, Ertaskin I, Ozkur A. Ultrasonographic evaluation of bilateral groins in children with unilateral inguinal hernia. Acta Radiol 2000;41:653-657.

Miller PA, Mezwa DG, Feczko PJ, et al. Imaging of abdominal hernias. Radiographics 1995;15:333-347.

Mufid MM, Abu-Yousef MM, Kakish ME, et al. Spigelian hernia: diagnosis by high-resolution real-time sonography. J Ultrasound Med 1997;16:183-187.

Omar IM, Zoga AC, Kavanagh EC, et al. Athletic pubalgia and "sports hernia": optimal MR imaging technique and findings. Radiographics 2008;28:1415-1438.

Orchard JW, Read JW, Neophyton J, Garlick D. Groin pain associated with ultrasound finding of inguinal canal posterior wall deficiency in Australian Rules footballers. Br J Sports Med 1998;32:134-139.

Parra JA, Revuelta S, Gallego T, et al. Prosthetic mesh used for inguinal and ventral hernia repair: normal appearance and complications in ultrasound and CT. Br J Radiol 2004;77:261-265.

Rettenbacher T, Hollerweger A, Macheiner P, et al. Abdominal wall hernias: cross-sectional imaging signs of incarceration determined with sonography. AJR Am J Roentgenol 2001;177:1061-1066.

Robinson P, Hensor E, Lansdown MJ, et al. Inguinofemoral hernia: accuracy of sonography in patients with indeterminate clinical features. AJR Am J Roentgenol 2006;187:1168-1178.

Shadbolt CL, Heinze SB, Dietrich RB. Imaging of groin masses: inguinal anatomy and pathologic conditions revisited. Radiographics 2001;21 Spec No:261-271.

Wechsler RJ, Kurtz AB, Needleman L, et al. Cross-sectional imaging of abdominal wall hernias. AJR Am J Roentgenol 1989;153:517-521.

Yang DM, Kim HC, Lim JW, et al. Sonographic findings of groin masses. J Ultrasound Med 2007;26:605-614.

Zarvan NP, Lee Jr FT, Yandow DR, Unger JS. Abdominal hernias: CT findings. AJR Am J Roentgenol 1995;164:1391-1395.

CHAPTER 14

The Peritoneum

Anthony E. Hanbidge and Stephanie R. Wilson

Chapter Outline

$\mathcal{U}$ltrasound of the abdomen and pelvis has become an extension of the physical examination when evaluating patients with abdominal symptoms and signs. It is accurate, safe, readily available, and relatively inexpensive. Evaluations have traditionally focused on assessing the solid viscera, the gallbladder, and bile ducts. Frequently, images of only these organs are recorded, and the peritoneal cavity is often neglected or subjected to cursory evaluation. The general belief is that ultrasound is not particularly helpful at imaging the peritoneum because of technical limitations, such as poor visibility and interference from bowel gas. There is also unfamiliarity with the common sonographic features encountered with peritoneal disease, as reflected by extensive literature on ultrasound of the liver, gallbladder, bile ducts, pancreas, spleen, kidneys, bladder, and reproductive organs, but little on sonographic evaluation of the peritoneum and peritoneal cavity. As a result, teaching of optimal sonographic technique to evaluate these areas is minimal.

If peritoneal pathology is a clinical concern, computed tomography (CT)[1,2] or magnetic resonance imaging (MRI)[3-5] is generally used to investigate. We believe that ultrasound can also be sensitive and specific in this regard.[6] To be successful, however, two criteria must be met: (1) the operator must be aware of the potential involvement of the peritoneum and peritoneal cavity with a disease process, and (2) these areas must receive a thorough sonographic assessment.

PERITONEUM, OMENTUM, AND MESENTERY

The **peritoneum** is a serous membrane lined with epithelial cells. It is divided into the parietal and visceral peritoneum. The **parietal peritoneum** lines the anterior and posterior walls of the abdominal cavity and is visible with ultrasound as a thin, smooth, echogenic line in the deepest layer of the anterior abdominal wall. Bowel loops can usually be seen deep to the parietal peritoneum, moving independent of it with respiration. The **visceral peritoneum,** on the other hand, covers the intra-abdominal organs and is not visible with ultrasound in its normal state. The potential space between these two layers is known as the **peritoneal cavity**, which usually contains a small volume of fluid that acts as a lubricant.[7]

The **small bowel mesentery** is a specialized, fan-shaped, peritoneal fold extending from the second lumbar vertebra to the right iliac fossa. It connects the jejunum and ileum to the posterior abdominal wall. It is composed of a double layer of peritoneum, blood vessels, nerves, lacteals (lymphatic capillaries in villi), lymph nodes, and a variable amount of fat. Normal bowel mesentery is best assessed with ultrasound in the presence of **ascites;** it appears as freely floating, smooth leaves separated by fluid, directed toward the center of the abdomen, away from small bowel loops (Fig. 14-1). In the absence of ascites, the mesentery is more difficult

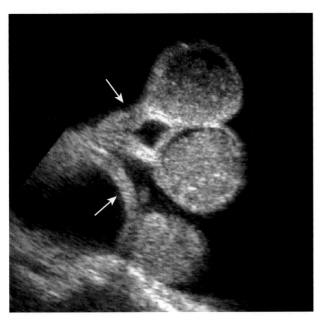

FIGURE 14-1. Normal mesentery with gross ascites. Oblique sagittal ultrasound image of the midabdomen shows the normal small bowel mesenteric leaves *(arrows)* outlined by fluid.

to appreciate but has been described as a series of elongated, aperistaltic structures separated from each other by specular echoes, best appreciated in the left lower quadrant.[8] It is frequently difficult to localize a disease process to the mesentery, and the relationship to other anatomic landmarks may be helpful. For example, lymphoma may be correctly localized to the mesentery if a mass is seen that encases the mesenteric vessels.

The **omenta** are also specialized peritoneal folds. They are composed of a double layer of peritoneum, blood vessels, lymphatics, and a variable amount of fat. The **lesser omentum** connects the lesser curvature of the stomach and proximal duodenum with the liver. The **greater omentum** descends from the greater curvature of the stomach, anterior to the abdominal contents, often as low as the pelvis, then reflects back on itself to form a four-layered structure that ascends and separates to enclose the transverse colon. A potential space exists between the two layers of the greater omentum, which is continuous with the lesser sac.

In the normal state, the omenta may be extremely difficult or impossible to distinguish with ultrasound. In the presence of ascites, the free inferior edge of the normal greater omentum may be visible floating in the fluid with variable thickness, depending on the fat content. In disease the greater omentum may become infiltrated, thickened, and nodular. Its superficial location allows for careful sonographic evaluation with high-frequency transducers, and disease processes may often be correctly identified and localized to the greater omentum even in the absence of ascites.

SONOGRAPHIC TECHNIQUE

Sonographic assessment of the peritoneum requires the motivation to evaluate, as far as possible, the parietal and visceral peritoneum, mesentery, omentum, and peritoneal cavity. The **initial survey** of the peritoneum and peritoneal cavity is performed with a standard-frequency, 3.5-MHz or 5-MHz, transducer (Fig. 14-2, *A*). The **field of view** (FOV) is set to include the full depth of the peritoneal cavity, but no more; this adds perspective to the image. The **focal zone** is continually adjusted to evaluate in detail different depths within the FOV. The **power** and **gain** settings are also adjusted using a high gain setting to characterize free fluid as anechoic or particulate and a low gain setting to visualize hypoechoic nodules or masses optimally. Once the initial survey is complete, higher-frequency transducers are used to more carefully evaluate and characterize abnormalities in the near field (Fig. 14-2, *B*).

When scanning transabdominally, graded compression is used to displace bowel gas. Determination of the site of origin of a peritoneal process may be aided by several techniques. Palpation of an abnormal mass, either with the transducer or with the free hand, will determine both the compliance and the mobility of a mass. Masses arising from the parietal peritoneum are often fixed, whereas masses arising from the visceral peritoneum may be mobile. This distinction may also be demonstrated by changing the patient's position or with changes in respiration. For example, in the right upper quadrant, a lesion in the near field is likely to be located on the parietal peritoneum if the liver moves independent of it with respiration.

A **transvaginal ultrasound examination** is critical for all female patients at risk for or with suspected peritoneal disease (Fig. 14-2, *C*). The pelvic pouch of Douglas is a common site of involvement, particularly in carcinomatosis and acute conditions. This technique allows exquisite assessment of both the parietal and the visceral pelvic peritoneum.[9,10] In addition to assessing the uterus and ovaries, the probe should be directed to the pouch of Douglas, by elevating the examining hand, and to both pelvic side-walls. The transvaginal scan may also facilitate improved visualization of pelvic bowel loops and the urinary bladder.

ASCITES

One of the earliest uses of sonography in the abdomen and pelvis involved the **detection** of ascites.[11] Normally, 50 to 75 mL of free fluid is present in the peritoneal cavity, acting as a lubricant. Ascites occurs with excess accumulation of peritoneal fluid. Ascites can be classified as **transudate** or **exudate** depending on the protein content. In North America, cirrhosis, peritoneal carcino-

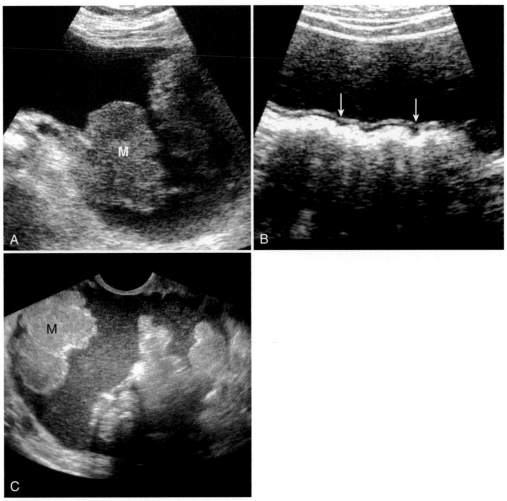

FIGURE 14-2. Optimization of technique. Stage 3 papillary serous adenocarcinoma of the ovary. A, Suprapubic sagittal image of the right adnexa using a 5.2-MHz curvilinear transducer, taken at the initial survey, shows ascites and a solid, lobulated, hypoechoic mass *(M)*. The field of view includes the full depth of the peritoneal cavity but no more. **B,** Transabdominal sagittal image of the left flank using a higher frequency, 7.4-MHz, curvilinear transducer shows ascites and hypoechoic seeding on the serosal surface of the descending colon *(arrows)*. A low gain setting is used to optimize visualization of the seeding, seen as a thin, continuous line on the serosal surface of the gut, which contains shadowing air. **C,** Transverse transvaginal image of the right adnexa using an 8.4-MHz transvaginal probe shows the right adnexal mass *(M)* and particulate ascites. A high gain setting is used to better characterize the particulate ascites.

matosis, congestive heart failure, and tuberculosis account for 90% of all cases. Accumulations of blood, urine, chyle, bile, or pancreatic juice are more unusual causes.

Ascites can be detected with physical examination when the volume reaches 500 mL. Transabdominal ultrasound can readily detect large volumes of ascites (Fig. 14-3). Transvaginal ultrasound is more sensitive in this regard, and volumes of free fluid as small as 0.8 mL can be demonstrated with the transvaginal probe[12] (Fig. 14-4). With the patient lying supine, free fluid tends to accumulate in the paracolic gutters and pelvis,[13] particularly the superior end of the right paracolic gutter and Morison's pouch. These areas should therefore be carefully assessed when ascites is suspected. Ultrasound is also accurate at **quantifying**[14] and **localizing** ascites and

may be used to guide both diagnostic and therapeutic paracentesis.

In addition to its excellent capability to quantify ascites, ultrasound can also **characterize** ascites as anechoic or particulate. This may be helpful at determining the source because **particulate** ascites suggests the presence of blood, pus, or neoplastic cells in the fluid. The observation of particulate ascites should prompt a more detailed assessment of the peritoneum with ultrasound,[15,16] further imaging with CT/MRI, and therapeutic paracentesis.

Hemoperitoneum has many causes, including trauma, ruptured aneurysm, ruptured ectopic pregnancy, ruptured liver mass (e.g., adenoma, hepatoma), and postsurgical bleeding. Spontaneous hemorrhage may occur in patients receiving anticoagulants. The appear-

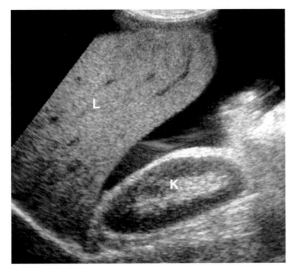

FIGURE 14-3. Cirrhosis of the liver with portal hypertension. Sagittal image of the right upper quadrant readily demonstrates a large amount of ascites surrounding an enlarged, bulbous, fatty liver *(L). K,* Right kidney.

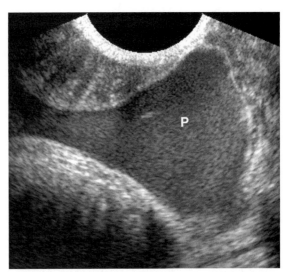

FIGURE 14-5. Hemoperitoneum in ruptured ectopic pregnancy. Oblique transverse transvaginal ultrasound image of the left adnexa shows particulate free fluid *(P).*

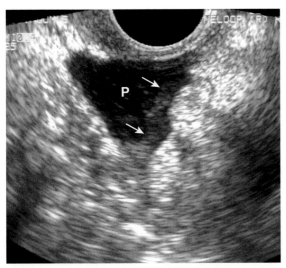

FIGURE 14-4. Grade 2/3 ovarian mucinous cystadenocarcinoma. Transverse transvaginal image of the right adnexa shows a small amount of particulate free fluid *(P)* and serosal seeding *(arrows)* on loops of bowel in the pelvis. This was visible only on the transvaginal scan.

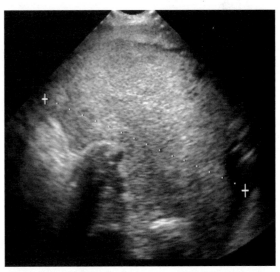

FIGURE 14-6. Blood clot. Acute blood clot secondary to rupture of a pseudoaneurysm at the hepatic artery anastomosis after liver transplantation. Sagittal ultrasound image of the left lower quadrant shows a solid, heterogeneous mass (calipers).

ance of acute blood is varied, including anechoic or particulate free fluid (Fig. 14-5). A fluid-debris level may develop if the patient has maintained a stable position for a time. Massive hemorrhage often results in a large, echogenic mass that may become more heterogeneous as lysis occurs over time (Figs. 14-6 and 14-7).

Focused abdominal sonography for trauma (FAST) has become an accepted screening modality for intra-abdominal injuries in the traumatized patient.[17-21] The primary focus of this limited study is to detect free intra-peritoneal fluid with ultrasound in the trauma center. Fluid detected in this setting strongly suggests significant intra-abdominal injury requiring urgent laparotomy. FAST has replaced peritoneal lavage in many centers.

Chylous ascites is an unusual condition in which lymph accumulates within the peritoneal cavity. The causes are varied, including **trauma, surgery, lymphangioma, lymphoma, intestinal lymphangiectasia,** and **cystic hygroma.** Sonography may show particulate ascites or a fluid-fluid level because of layering of the lymphatic fluid.[22,23]

It is sometimes difficult to decide if fluid visualized in the peritoneal cavity is free or loculated. Altering the patient's position may be helpful to establish if the fluid moves under the force of gravity. For example, free fluid in the right paracolic gutter with the patient lying supine may move from this location if the patient lies in a left lateral decubitus position. The morphology of the fluid collection may also be helpful. **Free fluid** tends to conform to the surrounding organs and will frequently exhibit acute angles when in contact with surrounding structures such as bowel loops. **Loculated fluid,** on the other hand, tends to have rounded margins and show

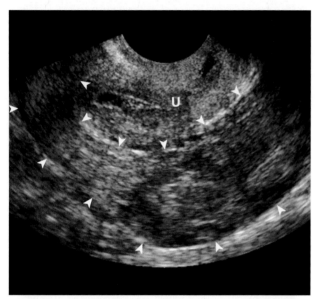

FIGURE 14-7. Pelvic hematoma 2 days after surgery in female patient taking anticoagulants. Midline sagittal transvaginal ultrasound image shows the uterus *(U),* with fluid in the endometrial canal, surrounded by a large, hypoechoic heterogeneous hematoma *(arrowheads).*

mass effect, frequently displacing surrounding structures from their usual location. Loculated fluid collections can occur anywhere in the abdomen and pelvis. Characterization of fluid and the demonstration of complexity of localized or generalized peritoneal fluid collections are strengths of ultrasound, and ultrasound is superior to CT scan in this regard (Fig. 14-8).

PERITONEAL INCLUSION CYSTS (BENIGN ENCYSTED FLUID)

The fluid produced by active ovaries in premenopausal patients is usually absorbed by the peritoneum. This balance can be upset by disease processes involving the pelvis, such as previous surgery, trauma, pelvic inflammatory disease (PID), inflammatory bowel disease (IBD), or endometriosis. In these patients the fluid produced by the ovaries may not be absorbed but may become trapped by adhesions. Over time, an inclusion cyst forms that frequently encases the ovary and may cause pelvic pain and pressure. Inclusion cysts vary in size and complexity and may be relatively simple or may contain internal echoes and septations.[24-26] They often cause confusion when imaging is performed and may be misinterpreted as representing ovarian cysts, parovarian cysts, hydrosalpinges, or even ovarian cancer. The key to the correct diagnosis is to suspect this condition based on the patient's profile, then demonstrate a normal ovary, either within or on the margin of the inclusion cyst, most often with the transvaginal scan (Fig. 14-9). Complex peritoneal inclusion cysts are also known as **multicystic mesotheliomas.**[27]

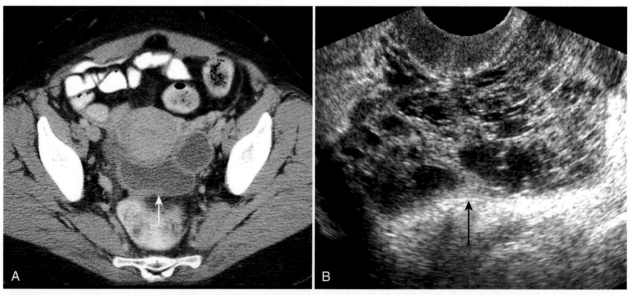

FIGURE 14-8. Fibrinous peritonitis. A, Axial, oral, and intravenously enhanced CT image through the midpelvis of female patient shows loculated fluid in the pouch of Douglas and left adnexa with an enhancing rim *(arrow).* **B,** Transverse transvaginal ultrasound image taken the same day shows the high degree of complexity of this fluid *(arrow)* to much better advantage.

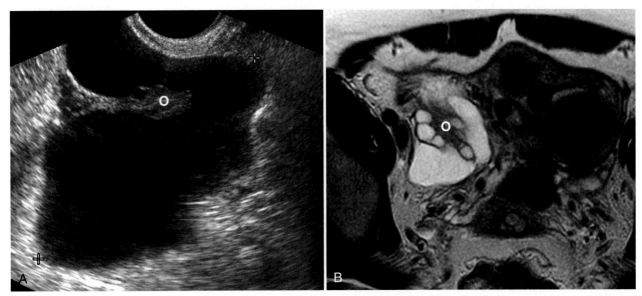

FIGURE 14-9. Peritoneal inclusion cyst. A, Transverse transvaginal ultrasound image of the right adnexa, and **B,** axial T2-weighted MR image through the midpelvis, show the normal right ovary *(O)* surrounded by encysted fluid, conforming to the contours of the peritoneal cavity. *(Reproduced from Wilson SR. Pseudomyxoma peritonei. In Cohen HL, editor. Gastrointestinal disease, test and syllabus. American College of Radiology 2004:73-84.)*

MESENTERIC CYSTS

Mesenteric cysts are rare intra-abdominal masses often discovered incidentally at imaging. However, they may present clinically with abdominal distention because of their size, or acutely with pain because of a complication such as hemorrhage, rupture, or torsion. Mesenteric cysts are most often of lymphatic (**lymphangioma**) or mesothelial origin but may also be of enteric (**enteric duplication cyst**) or urogenital origin. **Dermoid cysts** and **pseudocysts** (infectious, inflammatory, or traumatic) are seen as well.[28] Mesenteric cysts vary in size from less than 1 cm to greater than 25 cm, filling the entire peritoneal cavity. They may be entirely simple to highly complex with extensive internal septations, as sometimes seen with lymphangiomas[29,30] (Fig. 14-10). Smaller mesenteric cysts are frequently mobile, changing location with palpation or with changes in the patient's position. Asymptomatic cysts are frequently managed conservatively, particularly if simple or with the typical appearance of a lymphangioma. Surgery is usually reserved to alleviate pressure symptoms or to address acute complications.

PERITONEAL TUMORS

Tumors involving the peritoneum are often encountered with ultrasound and are generally malignant. **Metastatic tumors** are much more common than **primary peritoneal tumors.** The ovary is the primary site of disease in the vast majority of female patients. Other sites of primary disease with a propensity to spread to the peritoneum include the **stomach, colon, breast, pancreas, kidney, bladder, uterus,** and **skin** (melanoma).

Peritoneal Carcinomatosis

Peritoneal carcinomatosis is the term used to describe diffuse involvement of the peritoneum with metastatic disease. Carcinomatous seeding involving the parietal peritoneum (Fig. 14-11) or visceral peritoneum (Fig. 14-12) may produce discrete hypoechoic nodules, irregular masses, or hypoechoic rindlike thickening of the peritoneum.[16] Ascites is common and may be the only finding. The pouch of Douglas, greater omentum, Morison's pouch, and the right subphrenic space are common sites,[31] and therefore any sonographic evaluation of the peritoneum for metastatic disease should include careful and detailed assessment of these areas (Fig. 14-13). The **parietal peritoneal line** is often preserved on sonography with small seeds but is often lost as the lesion increases in size. Growth of a lesion is usually inward, toward the peritoneal cavity, but growth outward with invasion of the abdominal wall can occur (Fig. 14-14). If **psammomatous calcification** occurs within a peritoneal nodule, it appears echogenic with ultrasound, and if the calcification is dense, it may demonstrate posterior acoustic shadowing (Fig. 14-15).

Peritoneal carcinomatosis can be detected with ultrasound in the absence of ascites (Figs. 14-16 and 14-17), but its presence greatly enhances the detection of peritoneal lesions. Nodules as small as 2 to 3 mm may be seen on the parietal and visceral peritoneum with the transvaginal probe (Fig. 14-18). The detection of omental involvement is also enhanced by ascites. Infiltration of the omentum leads to an "omental cake,"[32] which may float freely in the ascitic fluid (Fig. 14-19). Alternatively, the omentum may be adherent to the parietal

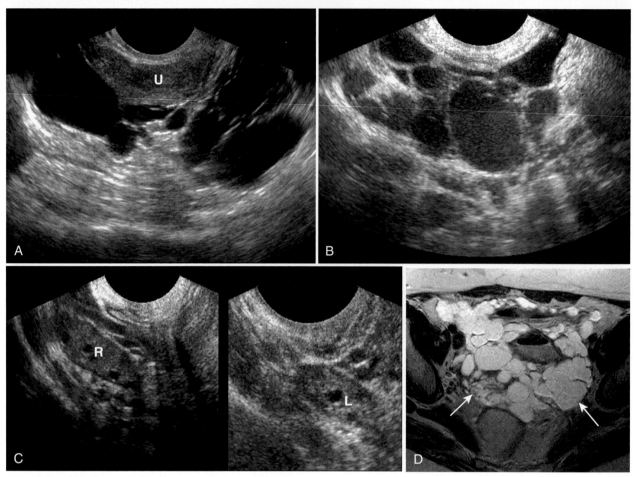

FIGURE 14-10. Pelvic lymphangioma in asymptomatic woman. A, Transverse transvaginal ultrasound image shows the normal uterus *(U)* in cross section, surrounded by innumerable cystic spaces with thin septations separating the fluid-filled components. There is no identified nodularity. Real-time examination suggested that these cysts were soft and compliant. **B,** Transvaginal image taken lateral to the uterus shows that the cystic changes are extensive. Their distribution and extent do not suggest an ovarian origin. **C,** Two transvaginal images shown side by side show a normal right *(R)* and a normal left *(L)* ovary. This excludes the ovaries as a source of the pathology. **D,** T2-weighted MR image confirms the extensive intraperitoneal cystic masses, which appear as areas of high signal intensity *(arrows).* The septations between the fluid components are thin. *(Reproduced from Wilson SR. Pseudomyxoma peritonei. In Cohen HL, editor. Gastrointestinal disease, test and syllabus. American College of Radiology 2004:73-84.)*

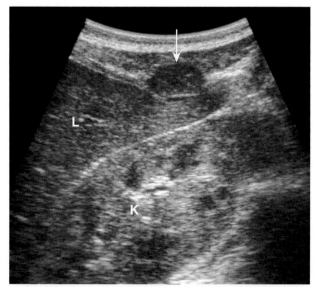

FIGURE 14-11. Parietal peritoneal metastasis from squamous cell carcinoma of the lung. Sagittal image of the right upper quadrant shows a hypoechoic nodule *(arrow)* anterior to the liver *(L).* With respiration, the liver moved freely and independent of the nodule, which stayed stationary, correctly suggesting its location on the parietal peritoneum. *K,* Kidney.

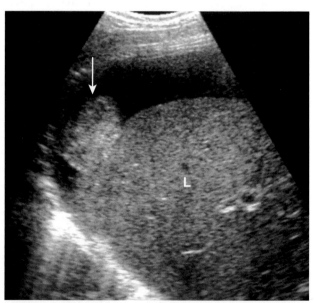

FIGURE 14-12. Visceral peritoneal metastasis from adenocarcinoma of the colon. Oblique sagittal image of the right upper quadrant shows an echogenic nodule *(arrow)* on the surface of the liver *(L),* surrounded by ascites. With respiration, the nodule moved in concert with the liver, correctly suggesting its location on the visceral peritoneum.

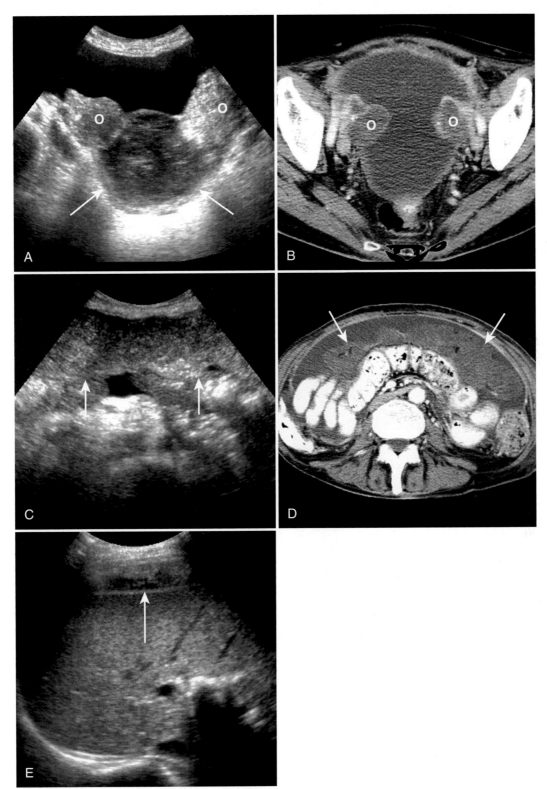

FIGURE 14-13. Peritoneal carcinomatosis from mucinous adenocarcinoma, presumably of gastrointestinal origin. A, Transverse ultrasound image in the pelvis, and **B,** CT scan at the same level, show ascites and bilateral ovarian solid masses *(O)* suggestive of Krukenberg tumors. The marked complexity of the fluid with particles and septations is better appreciated on the ultrasound scan *(arrows* in **A**). **C,** Transverse midabdominal ultrasound image, and **D,** corresponding CT scan, both show a thick "omental cake" *(arrows)* displacing bowel loops posteriorly in the peritoneal cavity. There is also a small volume of free fluid. **E,** Sagittal ultrasound image in the right upper quadrant shows a rim of complex, mixed-echogenic material overlying and indenting the convexity of the liver *(arrow).* There is echogenic nodularity on the parietal peritoneum of the diaphragm. This did not move with the liver on respiration, confirming its origin from the parietal peritoneum. *(Reproduced from Wilson SR. Pseudomyxoma peritonei. In Cohen HL, editor.* Gastrointestinal disease, test and syllabus. *American College of Radiology 2004:73-84.)*

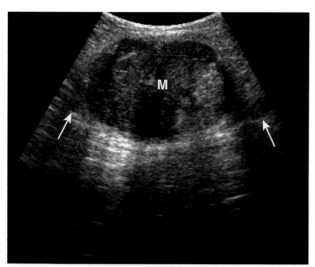

FIGURE 14-14. Abdominal wall seed in patient with known peritoneal carcinomatosis. Transverse ultrasound image of the midabdomen shows a hypoechoic solid mass *(M)* in the anterior abdominal wall, superficial to the parietal peritoneum *(arrows).*

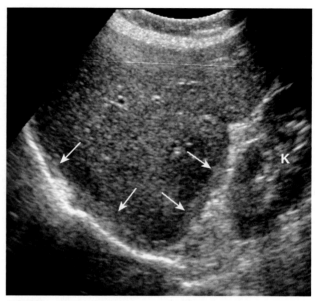

FIGURE 14-16. Stage 3 papillary serous ovarian cancer without ascites. Sagittal ultrasound image in the right upper quadrant shows a subtle, thin, echogenic "rind" of seeding *(arrows)* on the surface of the liver, extending into Morison's pouch. *K,* Kidney.

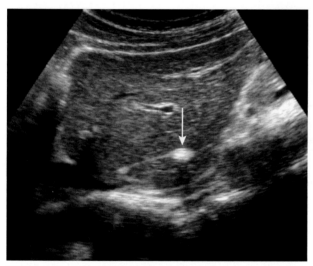

FIGURE 14-15. Well-differentiated stage 3 papillary serous ovarian cancer. Sagittal ultrasound image through the liver shows a calcified implant *(arrow)* in the ligamentum venosum, with posterior acoustic shadowing.

peritoneum in the near field (Fig. 14-20), or it may be deeper in the peritoneal cavity, adherent to the visceral peritoneum and surrounding small bowel loops (Fig. 14-21). **Thickening of the mesentery, mesenteric nodules,** and **lymphadenopathy** are other possible features of carcinomatosis.

After the full extent of peritoneal involvement has been documented with ultrasound, a careful search should be made for the primary lesion within the abdomen and pelvis, if not already identified. This search should not be limited to the solid organs, gallbladder, and bile ducts and should include the stomach and bowel.

Primary Tumors of Peritoneum

Primary tumors of the peritoneum are rare and include **primary peritoneal serous papillary carcinoma (PPSPC), malignant mesothelioma,** and **lymphoma.** PPSPC is a multicentric peritoneal tumor that is morphologically identical to **ovarian serous papillary carcinoma** (OSPC) of equivalent grade but that can spare or minimally invade the ovaries.[33] Women with PPSPC are more likely to present with ascites than women with OSPC and have a worse 3-year survival rate.[34] Imaging may demonstrate the typical features of peritoneal carcinomatosis, but no obvious primary site[35-39] (Fig. 14-22). The ovaries are generally normal in size but may be enlarged by surface involvement.

Primary peritoneal mesothelioma accounts for 10% to 30% of all cases of malignant mesothelioma[1,2,27,40] and is most common in middle-aged men. The tumor proves invariably fatal, and as with mesothelioma of the pleura, there is an association with asbestos exposure. Up to 65% of chest radiographs show evidence of asbestos exposure at diagnosis. In this condition the parietal and visceral peritoneums are diffusely thickened or are extensively involved by tumor plaques or nodules. These plaques and nodules may aggregate to form discrete masses. The viscera may be encased or invaded by tumor. Ascites is a common finding and is seen in up to 90% of cases.[41] As with peritoneal carcinomatosis, the nodules and plaques are often hypoechoic in peritoneal mesothelioma (Fig. 14-23). Pleural effusions and pleural plaques may also be appreciated with ultrasound. The solid organs should be evaluated for direct invasion or metas-

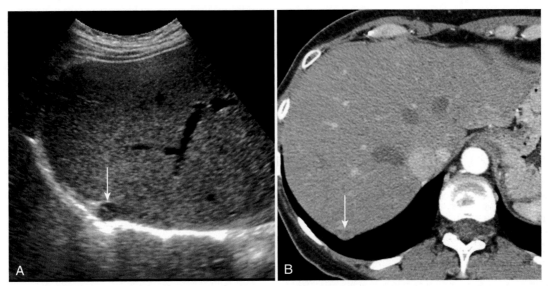

FIGURE 14-17. Peritoneal implant without ascites. A, Transverse ultrasound image, and **B,** axial CT image, of the right upper quadrant show a small peritoneal implant *(arrow)* overlying segment 7 of the liver. Note that the implant is better appreciated on the ultrasound image.

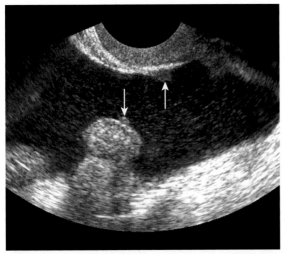

FIGURE 14-18. Peritoneal carcinomatosis from ovarian cancer. Oblique sagittal transvaginal ultrasound image shows small (<5 mm), parietal (near-field), and visceral (far-field) peritoneal implants *(arrows)*, surrounded by particulate ascites.

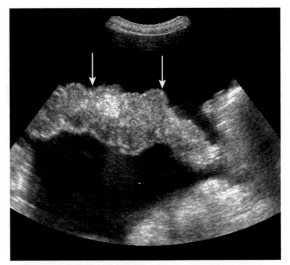

FIGURE 14-19. Free-floating "omental cake." Sagittal ultrasound image of the lower midline abdomen shows an omental cake *(arrows)* floating freely in the ascitic fluid. Note the free edge of the abnormal greater omentum inferiorly.

tases. Ultrasound-guided biopsy can be performed to confirm the diagnosis.[42] Generally, core biopsies from a number of locations are required because of difficulty sometimes encountered in establishing the diagnosis of peritoneal mesothelioma.

Primary lymphoma of the peritoneum is extremely rare and is the non-Hodgkin's variety.[2,43] There is an increased incidence in patients with acquired immunodeficiency syndrome (AIDS).[44] Again, features include diffuse peritoneal seeding, often with more focal masses. Lymphomatous masses may be extremely hypoechoic and can be mistaken for fluid collections with cursory assessment (Fig. 14-24).

Pseudomyxoma Peritonei

Pseudomyxoma peritonei (PP) is a rare, often fatal intraabdominal disease characterized by dissecting gelatinous ascites and multifocal peritoneal implants of columnar epithelium that secrete copious globules of extracellular mucin.[45] Controversy surrounds the origin of PP. Some studies suggest synchronous ovarian and appendiceal tumors in 90% of patients,[46] whereas most now believe that the condition almost always originates from a perforated appendiceal epithelial tumor.[47] The disease process tends to remain localized to the peritoneal cavity, and extraperitoneal spread is rare. PP encompasses

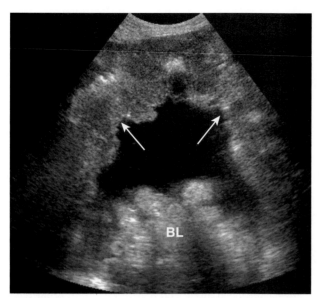

FIGURE 14-20. Omental cake adherent to parietal peritoneum. Transverse ultrasound image of the midabdomen shows an omental cake *(arrows)* in the near field, adherent to the parietal peritoneum. Small bowel loops *(BL)* are visible in the far field, outlined by ascites.

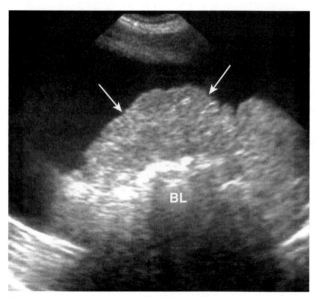

FIGURE 14-21. Omental cake adherent to visceral peritoneum. Transverse ultrasound image of the midabdomen shows a thick omental cake *(arrows)* adherent to the visceral peritoneum and encasing gas-filled small bowel loops *(BL).*

benign, borderline, and malignant mucinous neoplasms, resulting in a variable and poorly predictable prognosis. The overall 5-year survival is 40% to 50%, depending on cell type.[48]

Patients with PP present with abdominal pain and distention. Ultimately, the bowel becomes encased with mucinous material, and bowel obstruction may occur. Repeated surgical intervention to remove the accumulated mucinous material remains the treatment of choice.[49] Perioperative intraperitoneal chemotherapy

may add additional benefit.[50] Because patients present with abdominal symptoms, the diagnosis is frequently made preoperatively by ultrasound or CT.[51] Sonography frequently shows complex ascites reflecting the gelatinous nature of the fluid. The echogenic foci within the fluid are nonmobile, and the bowel loops, instead of floating freely, are displaced centrally and posteriorly by the surrounding mass, giving a characteristic "starburst" appearance (Fig. 14-25). **Scalloping** of the liver is another typical feature of PP.[52] Ultrasound may be helpful to guide paracentesis in these patients because less viscous areas may be identified, with a greater likelihood of successful aspiration.

INFLAMMATORY DISEASE OF PERITONEUM

Peritonitis is defined as diffuse inflammation of the parietal and visceral peritoneum, with both infectious and noninfectious causes.[3] Infectious causes include bacteria (including tuberculosis), viruses, fungi, and parasites. Noninfectious causes are less common and include **chemical peritonitis** (secondary to gastric or pancreatic juice or bile), **granulomatous peritonitis** (secondary to foreign bodies such as talc), and **sclerosing peritonitis** associated with **continuous ambulatory peritoneal dialysis** (CAPD).

Most cases of **infective peritonitis** are **bacterial, secondary to complications** of disease processes involving intra-abdominal organs. Common causes include bowel necrosis secondary to ischemia, perforated appendicitis, perforated diverticulitis, perforated duodenal ulcer, IBD, and postoperative leaks. Culture of the exudate generally reveals a mixed flora in this setting, with gram-negative bacilli and anaerobes predominating.

Primary or **spontaneous bacterial peritonitis** (SBP) occurs much less often, predominantly in association with cirrhosis and nephrotic syndrome. The clinical findings are often subtle, and correct diagnosis requires a high index of suspicion. SBP should be considered in any cirrhotic patient with ascites, fever, and an unexplained clinical deterioration. Culture of the ascitic fluid will characteristically reveal a single organism, usually *Escherichia coli.*

The sonographic appearance of infective peritonitis varies but may include particulate ascites (Fig. 14-26, *A*), loculated ascites, or ascitic fluid containing septations (Fig. 14-27), debris, or gas.[53] Diffuse thickening of the parietal and visceral peritoneum (Fig. 14-26, *B*), mesentery, and omentum may also be observed, and heterogeneous exudate may be seen interposed between bowel loops.

Peritonitis secondary to viruses, fungi, or parasites is rare and usually occurs in immunocompromised patients (Fig. 14-28) or CAPD patients. **Echinococcal disease** may involve the peritoneum.[54] A hepatic or splenic cyst

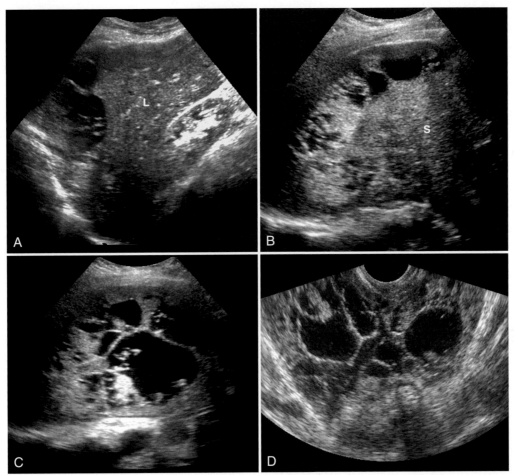

FIGURE 14-22. Primary peritoneal serous papillary carcinoma. A, Sagittal ultrasound image shows a highly complex peritoneal mass between the right hemidiaphragm and the liver *(L).* The liver border is scalloped. **B,** Sagittal ultrasound image in the left upper quadrant shows a similar complex peritoneal mass over the convexity of the spleen *(S).* **C,** Midabdominal image shows a complex peritoneal cystic and solid mass of enormous size. **D,** Transvaginal image taken in the pouch of Douglas shows no normal tissue. The entire pouch is filled with a complex cystic and solid tumor. *(Reproduced from Wilson SR. Pseudomyxoma peritonei. In Cohen HL, editor.* Gastrointestinal disease, test and syllabus. *American College of Radiology 2004:73-84.)*

may rupture, resulting in diffuse seeding of the peritoneal cavity. Ultrasound may reveal one or more of the typical appearances of hydatid cysts, including daughter cysts, the sonographic "water lily" sign, or multiple, closely folded echogenic membranes within the cyst cavity.

Abscess

Abscesses may occur at the site of a localized perforation or may result from delayed treatment of peritonitis, in which case they often develop in dependent areas of the abdomen and pelvis. The subphrenic or subhepatic spaces and the pouch of Douglas are common locations. Ultrasound is often limited in detecting intra-abdominal abscesses, particularly in postoperative patients. These patients are less mobile because of their recent surgery and frequently have open wounds and dressings, limiting access for the ultrasound probe. In addition, visibility is often limited by extensive bowel gas, a result of paralytic ileus. In this setting, it may prove extremely difficult to

distinguish between a dilated, aperistaltic, fluid-filled or gas-filled bowel loop and an extraluminal abscess collection.

Recognized features of intra-abdominal abscesses include round or oval fluid collections with well-defined and irregular walls. They usually contain internal debris and septations (Figs.14-29 and 14-30) and occasionally small pockets of gas that appear as echogenic foci with ultrasound, often with posterior reverberation artifact. The presence of gas within a collection is virtually diagnostic of infection.[55] Ultrasound-guided or CT-guided percutaneous drainage is generally the treatment of choice, and follow-up sonographic examinations are helpful at assessing response to therapeutic intervention.

Tuberculous Peritonitis

Tuberculosis (TB) is still prevalent in developing countries, with a recent resurgence in the developed world,

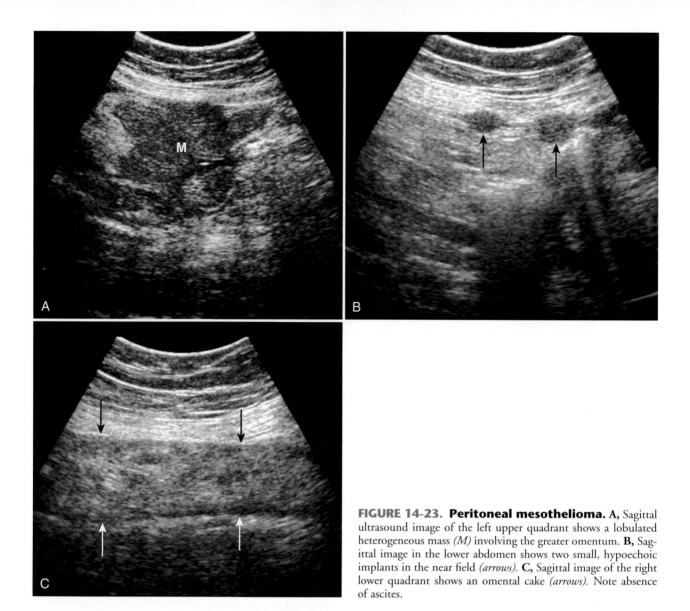

FIGURE 14-23. Peritoneal mesothelioma. A, Sagittal ultrasound image of the left upper quadrant shows a lobulated heterogeneous mass *(M)* involving the greater omentum. **B,** Sagittal image in the lower abdomen shows two small, hypoechoic implants in the near field *(arrows)*. **C,** Sagittal image of the right lower quadrant shows an omental cake *(arrows)*. Note absence of ascites.

FIGURE 14-24. Non-Hodgkin's lymphoma of the peritoneum. A, Transverse ultrasound image, and **B,** axial CT image, of the right lower quadrant show a mass *(M)* displacing bowel loops medially. Infiltrated fat *(arrows)* is seen lateral to the mass as echogenic mass effect on the sonogram.

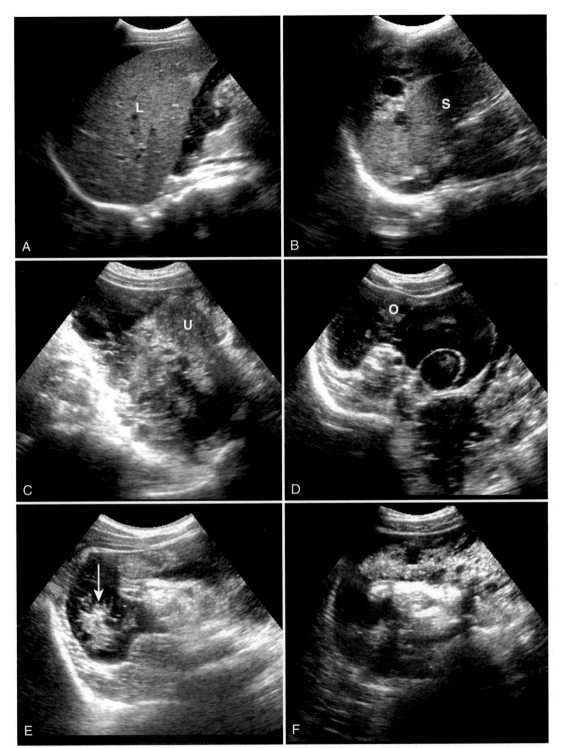

FIGURE 14-25. Pseudomyxoma peritonei. A, Sagittal ultrasound image of the right upper quadrant shows complex fluid surrounding the liver *(L)*. There is very mild and subtle scalloping of the deep border of the liver. **B,** Sagittal ultrasound image of the left upper quadrant shows the spleen *(S)* surrounded by highly complex and echogenic fluid. The echogenic components of the fluid do not move with gravity. There is an indentation on the convexity of the spleen where the peritoneal process appears to invaginate the splenic parenchyma. **C,** Sagittal ultrasound image of the midline pelvis shows a normal anteverted uterus *(U)*. The pouch of Douglas is filled with highly complex fluid. **D,** Oblique sagittal ultrasound image of the right abdomen at the pelvic brim shows a thin-walled intraperitoneal cyst with intracystic septations. This is not within the ovary. The normal right ovary *(O)* with small follicles is seen adjacent to the intraperitoneal cyst. The normal left ovary was seen elsewhere. **E,** Transverse image in the right paracolic gutter shows a "starburst" within the fluid *(arrow)*. This is associated, in our experience, with the presence of mucin in the peritoneal cavity. **F,** Highly echogenic plaquelike structure anteriorly represents a very thick and abnormal omentum, an "omental cake." There are hypoechoic nodules within the cake that are highly suggestive of tumor deposits.

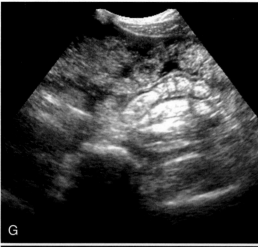

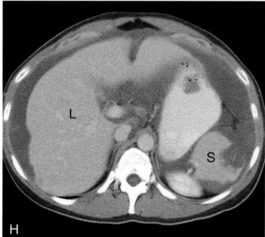

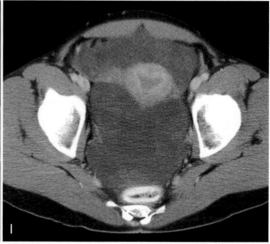

FIGURE 14-25, cont'd. G, Also taken in the peritoneal cavity, this image shows that the loops of bowel are compressed deep into the abdomen by the overlying abnormal and thick fluid and the omental cake. **H** and **I,** CT images taken in the upper abdomen and the pelvis, respectively (*L,* liver; *S,* spleen). They confirm the extensive peritoneal process, the organ scalloping, and the pouch of Douglas full of complex fluid. *(Reproduced from Wilson SR. Pseudomyxoma peritonei. In Cohen HL, editor.* Gastrointestinal disease, test and syllabus. *American College of Radiology 2004:73-84.)*

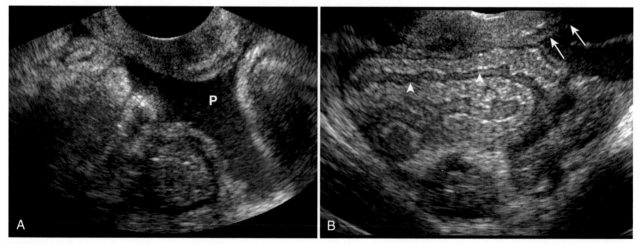

FIGURE 14-26. Suppurative peritonitis. A, Transverse transvaginal ultrasound image of the pouch of Douglas shows particulate free fluid (P). **B,** Transverse transvaginal ultrasound image more anteriorly in the pelvis shows diffuse thickening of both the parietal *(arrows)* and the visceral *(arrowheads)* peritoneum. An S-shaped small bowel loop is seen meandering through the thickened visceral peritoneum.

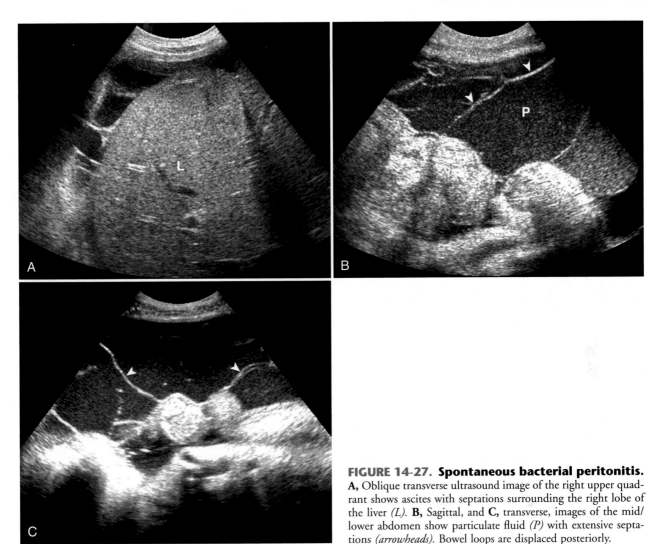

FIGURE 14-27. Spontaneous bacterial peritonitis.
A, Oblique transverse ultrasound image of the right upper quadrant shows ascites with septations surrounding the right lobe of the liver *(L)*. **B,** Sagittal, and **C,** transverse, images of the mid/lower abdomen show particulate fluid *(P)* with extensive septations *(arrowheads)*. Bowel loops are displaced posteriorly.

particularly among **AIDS patients** and **immigrant populations.**[56] Other groups at risk include patients with **alcoholism** and **cirrhosis.** Of all non-AIDS patients with TB, extrapulmonary disease occurs in only 10% to 15%; this increases to more than 50% in AIDS patients.[57] The peritoneum is a common site of extrapulmonary involvement,[58] but the chest radiograph will show evidence of pulmonary TB in only 14% of these patients. Therefore, a high index of suspicion, particularly in high-risk groups, and knowledge of the common sonographic features allow for earlier diagnosis of this potentially curable disease, thus reducing morbidity and mortality.

There are no pathognomonic sonographic features for **TB peritonitis** but, in the proper clinical setting, a diffuse peritoneal process may strongly suggest the diagnosis. Ascites is frequently present and may be free or loculated. It may be anechoic or more frequently particulate and may contain fine, mobile strands composed of fibrin (Fig. 14-31). These strands may produce a lattice-like pattern. Irregular and nodular hypoechoic thickening of the peritoneum, mesentery, and omentum is

another feature.[59] Associated **lymphadenopathy** in the mesentery and retroperitoneum is a common feature and is more common than in peritoneal carcinomatosis.[60,61] The nodes may be discrete or conglomerate because of periadenitis. Caseation may give rise to a hypoechoic center within the node, although a similar appearance can be seen with metastatic lymph nodes undergoing necrosis. Echogenic nodes caused by fat deposition may suggest the diagnosis of TB. Sonographic assessment of the solid viscera may show involvement, particularly hypoechoic masses in the spleen. Ultrasound helps guide diagnostic paracentesis in TB peritonitis and may also guide fine-needle aspiration of enlarged nodes.[62] Sonography can also readily document response to treatment.

Sclerosing Peritonitis

Sclerosing peritonitis is a major complication of CAPD and is characterized by the formation of a connective tissue membrane covering the peritoneum and eventually encasing and strangulating bowel loops.[63,64] Patients

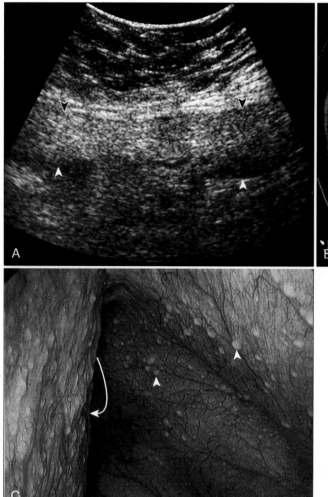

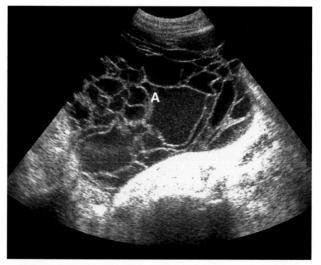

FIGURE 14-28. _Histoplasma_ peritonitis. A, Sagittal ultrasound image of the left upper quadrant shows omental infiltration _(arrowheads)_ in the absence of ascites. **B,** Axial CT image confirms omental infiltration _(arrowheads)._ **C,** Laparoscopic image shows the omentum dissected off the parietal peritoneum _(curved arrow)_ with multiple small granulomas on the parietal peritoneum _(arrowheads)._ Biopsy showed _Histoplasma_ peritonitis in this immunocompromised patient.

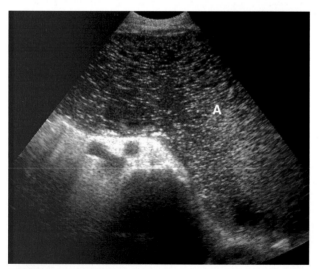

FIGURE 14-29. Abscess. Transverse ultrasound image of the midabdomen shows a large abscess collection _(A)._

FIGURE 14-30. Abscess. Sagittal ultrasound image of the right lower quadrant shows a large abscess collection with internal septations _(A)._

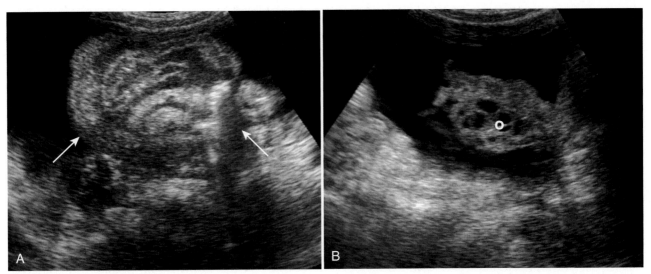

FIGURE 14-31. Tuberculous peritonitis. A, Midline transverse ultrasound image shows "matted" bowel loops *(arrows)* surrounded by ascites. Note thickening of the visceral peritoneum. **B,** Sagittal ultrasound image of the left adnexa shows the ovary *(O)* embedded in thickened visceral peritoneum and surrounded by ascites.

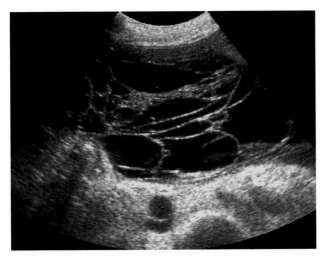

FIGURE 14-32. Sclerosing peritonitis. Transverse ultrasound image of the midabdomen shows extensive, complex, septated ascites.

initially complain of abdominal pain and loss of ultrafiltration. Ultimately, bowel obstruction occurs. Surgery is often difficult in these patients, and the prognosis is poor. Early diagnosis of sclerosing peritonitis may be important in reducing mortality.

Ultrasound is extremely helpful in the diagnosis.[65] Increased peristalsis in multiple bowel loops is one of the earliest findings in sclerosing peritonitis. Ascites, both free and loculated, is common. With time, the fluid becomes more complex with **stranding** (Fig. 14-32). Bowel loops become matted together and are tethered to the posterior abdominal wall by a characteristic enveloping membrane. This membrane can be seen with ultrasound as a uniformly echogenic layer measuring 1 to 4 mm in thickness.

LOCALIZED INFLAMMATORY PROCESS OF PERITONEAL CAVITY

The CT appearance and significance of inflamed peritoneal fat are familiar to sonographers. If ultrasound is to be successful at investigating patients with abdominal symptoms, the sonographic appearance of inflamed fat must become just as familiar.

Inflamed perienteric fat appears as an **echogenic** "mass effect," with ultrasound frequently displacing bowel loops out of the scanning plane. Compression sonography may greatly enhance the detection of focally inflamed fat, and gentle palpation with the transducer over this area will frequently show that it is the site of the patient's maximal tenderness. Frequently, an associated underlying abnormality, such as an abnormal bowel segment, can be identified with ultrasound[66] (Fig. 14-33). **Appendicitis** and **diverticulitis** are the most common acute processes giving rise to focally inflamed fat. Other possibilities include IBD, pancreatitis, and complicated acute cholecystitis. Progression to phlegmon typically shows development of a **hypoechoic** region within the echogenic fat without fluid content (Fig. 14-34). If untreated, this may progress to abscess formation. Color Doppler imaging frequently shows increased blood flow in the area of inflammation.[67]

RIGHT-SIDED SEGMENTAL OMENTAL INFARCTION

Right-sided segmental omental infarction is a rare clinical entity that usually presents with right-sided abdominal pain and is often mistaken for appendicitis. It is important to make the correct diagnosis because the

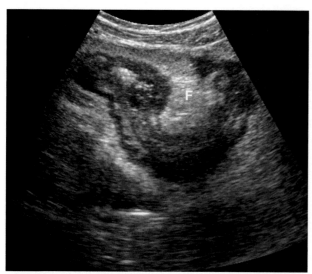

FIGURE 14-33. Inflamed fat. Transverse ultrasound image of the right lower quadrant shows echogenic inflamed fat *(F)* associated with a long segment of thickened terminal ileum in patient with Crohn's disease.

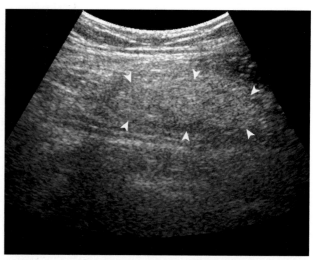

FIGURE 14-35. Right-sided segmental omental infarction. Sagittal image of the right midabdomen shows an ovoid echogenic mass *(arrowheads)*. This was the site of the patient's maximal tenderness.

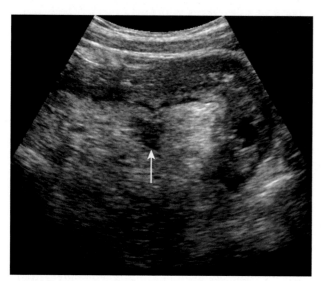

FIGURE 14-34. Inflamed fat with phlegmon. Oblique sagittal ultrasound image of the right lower quadrant shows the thickened terminal ileum with echogenic inflamed fat and hypoechoic perienteric phlegmon formation *(arrow).*

condition is self limiting and resolves spontaneously with supportive measures. Omental infarction occurs in all age groups and is thought to result from an embryologic variant in the blood supply to the right inferior portion of the omentum, leaving it prone to infarction. Precipitating factors include straining and eating a large meal.

Ultrasound reveals an **echogenic, ovoid,** or **cakelike mass** in the right midabdomen at the site of the patient's tenderness[68,69] (Fig. 14-35). Careful assessment will reveal no underlying bowel abnormality. The typical location of right-sided omental infarction is anterolateral to the hepatic flexure of the colon, and it corresponds to a circumscribed fatty mass on CT, with areas of strand-

ing. The mass often adheres to the parietal peritoneum, with bowel moving deep to it on respiration.

ENDOMETRIOSIS

Endometriosis is a common condition affecting predominantly premenopausal women and occurs when functional endometrium is located outside of the uterus. Patients may be asymptomatic but frequently present with pelvic pain, dyspareunia, or infertility. The ovaries and suspensory ligaments of the uterus are the sites most often affected, but endometriotic implants can involve the bowel, urinary bladder, peritoneum, chest, or soft tissues.[70]

Sonographic evaluation is often normal in patients with endometriosis. If **endometriomas** are present, transvaginal ultrasound is very sensitive at detecting and characterizing the masses, often showing the typical "chocolate" cysts with uniform, low-level internal echoes. There may be associated complex free fluid with stranding. Occasionally, **tiny echogenic foci** may be identified along the pelvic peritoneal surfaces. These foci are not specific for endometriosis and may also be seen with serous papillary ovarian neoplasms. Clinical correlation is essential, and occasionally, laparoscopic evaluation may be necessary, with biopsy of the peritoneum to rule out tumor.

Another possible sonographic finding in endometriosis is the presence of **hypoechoic endometrial plaques** on the serosal surface of pelvic bowel loops or urinary bladder. These plaques may tether the wall of the affected organ and show flow with color Doppler imaging. They are best demonstrated with the transvaginal probe (Fig. 14-36).

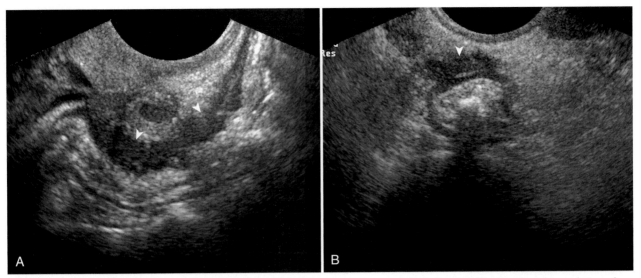

FIGURE 14-36. Endometriotic plaque. A, Sagittal, and **B,** transverse, transvaginal ultrasound images show hypoechoic endometriotic plaque *(arrowheads)* along one serosal surface of the sigmoid colon.

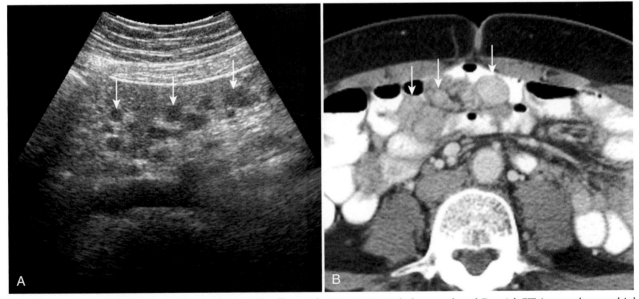

FIGURE 14-37. Leiomyomatosis peritonealis disseminata. A, Sagittal ultrasound, and **B,** axial CT, images show multiple small, hypoechoic, enhancing peritoneal nodules *(arrows).*

LEIOMYOMATOSIS PERITONEALIS DISSEMINATA

Leiomyomatosis peritonealis disseminata (LPD) is a relatively rare clinical entity characterized by multiple nodules, mainly the result of smooth muscle proliferation over the surface of the peritoneal cavity.[71] LPD often mimics a malignant process, but the diagnosis is easily made with biopsy.

Typically, LPD is an incidental finding at imaging or during procedures such as laparoscopy, cesarean section, laparotomy, and postpartum tubal ligation.[27] It occurs mainly in women, primarily during the reproductive period. Exposure to estrogen seems to play an etiologic role. Many patients have uterine leiomyomas as well. Conservative care is generally indicated. When LPD occurs during pregnancy or with the oral contraceptive (OC) use, it may regress spontaneously after delivery or with OC discontinuation. Malignant transformation of LPD remains uncertain. In a few isolated cases, malignant leiomyosarcomas have been described shortly after making the diagnosis of LPD. A clear association, however, has not been established. Sonographic evaluation may show multiple small, hypoechoic nodules throughout the peritoneal cavity (Fig. 14-37).

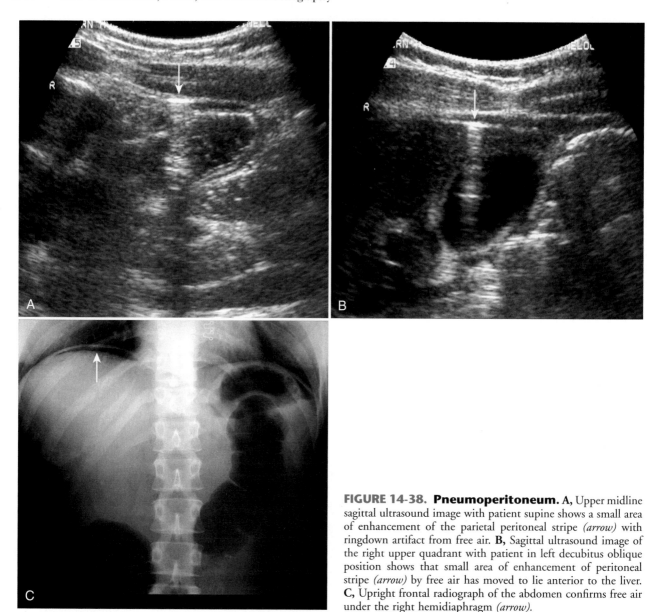

FIGURE 14-38. Pneumoperitoneum. A, Upper midline sagittal ultrasound image with patient supine shows a small area of enhancement of the parietal peritoneal stripe *(arrow)* with ringdown artifact from free air. **B,** Sagittal ultrasound image of the right upper quadrant with patient in left decubitus oblique position shows that small area of enhancement of peritoneal stripe *(arrow)* by free air has moved to lie anterior to the liver. **C,** Upright frontal radiograph of the abdomen confirms free air under the right hemidiaphragm *(arrow).*

PNEUMOPERITONEUM

Computed tomography is regarded as the standard for detecting, localizing, and quantifying free air.[72] Plain radiographs are also sensitive at detecting free air, with even 1 mL potentially visible on an erect chest radiograph. Ultrasound is often the initial imaging modality requested to assess abdominal pain, however, so the identification of free air is an extremely important finding.

Sonographic technique is critical when assessing for free air. The patient should be scanned in the supine and steep left posterior oblique positions, paying particular attention to the epigastrium and right upper quadrants, respectively.[73,74] **Free air in the epigastrium,** with the patient lying supine, will frequently shift to the right upper quadrant with the patient lying in a left posterior oblique position (Fig. 14-38). Free air is most often seen just deep to the parietal peritoneum, is best appreciated with a linear array transducer, and appears as **enhancement of the parietal peritoneal line,** often with posterior reverberation artifact.[75] Another sonographic sign of pneumoperitoneum in patients with ascites is gas bubbles in the ascitic fluid. Gas bubbles may appear as tiny, floating echogenic foci and have a high association with gut perforation and infection of the peritoneal fluid. When free air is detected, ultrasound will frequently reveal the underlying cause, so the remainder of the abdomen and pelvis should be carefully assessed for evidence of inflammation or tumor.[74]

CONCLUSION

Assessment of the peritoneum is easily performed with ultrasound in the majority of patients and should not add significantly to scanning time when the peritoneum is normal. There are limitations in extremely obese and postoperative patients, but in general, most peritoneal diseases can be readily detected and characterized with ultrasound. Many patterns of peritoneal disease are non-specific, however, and sonographic findings must be interpreted in light of the patient's clinical symptoms, physical findings, and laboratory investigations. When fluid or tissue is required to reach a specific diagnosis, ultrasound is an efficient, cost-effective modality for guidance.[76] It is also a safe, readily available, and relatively inexpensive modality for monitoring disease progression and response to treatment. In patients with ovarian cancer, ultrasound is invariably performed as part of the patient's initial clinical workup. Because peritoneal dissemination is the major determinant of both prognosis and treatment choices, we recommend including the peritoneal cavity in the sonographic assessment of this patient population.

References

1. Jeong YJ, Kim S, Kwak SW, et al. Neoplastic and nonneoplastic conditions of serosal membrane origin: CT findings. Radiographics 2008;28:801-817; discussion 817-818; quiz 912.
2. Pickhardt PJ, Bhalla S. Primary neoplasms of peritoneal and sub-peritoneal origin: CT findings. Radiographics 2005;25:983-995.
3. Elsayes KM, Staveteig PT, Narra VR, et al. MRI of the peritoneum: spectrum of abnormalities. AJR Am J Roentgenol 2006;186:1368-1379.
4. Low RN. Gadolinium-enhanced MR imaging of liver capsule and peritoneum. Magn Reson Imaging Clin North Am 2001;9:803-819, vii.
5. Low RN. MR imaging of the peritoneal spread of malignancy. Abdom Imaging 2007;32:267-283.
6. Hanbidge AE, Lynch D, Wilson SR. US of the peritoneum. Radiographics 2003;23:663-684; discussion 84-85.

Peritoneum, Omentum, and Mesentery
7. Healy JC, Reznek RH. The peritoneum, mesenteries and omenta: normal anatomy and pathological processes. Eur Radiol 1998;8:886-900.
8. Derchi LE, Solbiati L, Rizzatto G, De Pra L. Normal anatomy and pathologic changes of the small bowel mesentery: US appearance. Radiology 1987;164:649-652.

Sonographic Technique
9. Damani N, Wilson SR. Nongynecologic applications of transvaginal US. Radiographics 1999;19(Spec No):S179-S200; quiz S65-S66.
10. Serafini G, Gandolfo N, Gazzo P, et al. Transvaginal ultrasonography of nongynecologic pelvic lesions. Abdom Imaging 2001;26:540-549.

Ascites
11. Goldberg BB, Goodman GA, Clearfield HR. Evaluation of ascites by ultrasound. Radiology 1970;96:15-22.
12. Nichols JE, Steinkampf MP. Detection of free peritoneal fluid by transvaginal sonography. J Clin Ultrasound 1993;21:171-174.
13. Meyers MA. The spread and localization of acute intraperitoneal effusions. Radiology 1970;95:547-554.
14. Inadomi J, Cello JP, Koch J. Ultrasonographic determination of ascitic volume. Hepatology 1996;24:549-551.
15. Edell SL, Gefter WB. Ultrasonic differentiation of types of ascitic fluid. AJR Am J Roentgenol 1979;133:111-114.
16. Goerg C, Schwerk WB. Peritoneal carcinomatosis with ascites. AJR Am J Roentgenol 1991;156:1185-1187.
17. Chiu WC, Cushing BM, Rodriguez A, et al. Abdominal injuries without hemoperitoneum: a potential limitation of focused abdominal sonography for trauma (FAST). J Trauma 1997;42:617-623; discussion 23-25.
18. Kimura A, Otsuka T. Emergency center ultrasonography in the evaluation of hemoperitoneum: a prospective study. J Trauma 1991;31:20-23.
19. Rozycki GS, Ochsner MG, Schmidt JA, et al. A prospective study of surgeon-performed ultrasound as the primary adjuvant modality for injured patient assessment. J Trauma 1995;39:492-498; discussion 498-500.
20. Sirlin CB, Casola G, Brown MA, et al. Patterns of fluid accumulation on screening ultrasonography for blunt abdominal trauma: comparison with site of injury. J Ultrasound Med 2001;20:351-357.
21. Wherrett LJ, Boulanger BR, McLellan BA, et al. Hypotension after blunt abdominal trauma: the role of emergent abdominal sonography in surgical triage. J Trauma 1996;41:815-820.
22. Franklin JT, Azose AA. Sonographic appearance of chylous ascites. J Clin Ultrasound 1984;12:239-240.
23. Hibbeln JF, Wehmueller MD, Wilbur AC. Chylous ascites: CT and ultrasound appearance. Abdom Imaging 1995;20:138-140.

Peritoneal Inclusion Cysts (Benign Encysted Fluid)
24. Hoffer FA, Kozakewich H, Colodny A, Goldstein DP. Peritoneal inclusion cysts: ovarian fluid in peritoneal adhesions. Radiology 1988;169:189-191.
25. Kim JS, Lee HJ, Woo SK, Lee TS. Peritoneal inclusion cysts and their relationship to the ovaries: evaluation with sonography. Radiology 1997;204:481-484.
26. Sohaey R, Gardner TL, Woodward PJ, Peterson CM. Sonographic diagnosis of peritoneal inclusion cysts. J Ultrasound Med 1995;14:913-917.
27. Levy AD, Arnaiz J, Shaw JC, Sobin LH. From the archives of the AFIP: primary peritoneal tumors: imaging features with pathologic correlation. Radiographics 2008;28:583-607; quiz 621-622.

Mesenteric Cysts
28. De Perrot M, Brundler M, Totsch M, et al. Mesenteric cysts: toward less confusion? Dig Surg 2000;17:323-328.
29. Egozi EI, Ricketts RR. Mesenteric and omental cysts in children. Am Surg 1997;63:287-290.
30. Konen O, Rathaus V, Dlugy E, et al. Childhood abdominal cystic lymphangioma. Pediatr Radiol 2002;32:88-94.

Peritoneal Tumors
31. Meyers MA, Oliphant M, Berne AS, Feldberg MA. The peritoneal ligaments and mesenteries: pathways of intraabdominal spread of disease. Radiology 1987;163:593-604.
32. Rioux M, Michaud C. Sonographic detection of peritoneal carcinomatosis: a prospective study of 37 cases. Abdom Imaging 1995;20:47-51; discussion 56-57.
33. Koutselini HA, Lazaris AC, Thomopoulou G, et al. Papillary serous carcinoma of peritoneum: case study and review of the literature on the differential diagnosis of malignant peritoneal tumors. Adv Clin Pathol 2001;5:99-104.
34. Halperin R, Zehavi S, Langer R, et al. Primary peritoneal serous papillary carcinoma: a new epidemiologic trend? A matched-case comparison with ovarian serous papillary cancer. Int J Gynecol Cancer 2001;11:403-408.
35. Voultsinos V, Semelka RC, Elias Jr J, et al. Primary peritoneal carcinoma: computed tomography and magnetic resonance findings. J Comput Assist Tomogr 2008;32:541-547.
36. Morita H, Aoki J, Taketomi A, et al. Serous surface papillary carcinoma of the peritoneum: clinical, radiologic, and pathologic findings in 11 patients. AJR Am J Roentgenol 2004;183:923-928.
37. Zissin R, Hertz M, Shapiro-Feinberg M, et al. Primary serous papillary carcinoma of the peritoneum: CT findings. Clin Radiol 2001;56:740-745.
38. Chopra S, Laurie LR, Chintapalli KN, et al. Primary papillary serous carcinoma of the peritoneum: CT-pathologic correlation. J Comput Assist Tomogr 2000;24:395-399.

39. Furukawa T, Ueda J, Takahashi S, et al. Peritoneal serous papillary carcinoma: radiological appearance. Abdom Imaging 1999;24: 78-81.
40. Moertel CG. Peritoneal mesothelioma. Gastroenterology 1972;63: 346-350.
41. Guest PJ, Reznek RH, Selleslag D, et al. Peritoneal mesothelioma: the role of computed tomography in diagnosis and follow-up. Clin Radiol 1992;45:79-84.
42. Reuter K, Raptopoulos V, Reale F, et al. Diagnosis of peritoneal mesothelioma: computed tomography, sonography, and fine-needle aspiration biopsy. AJR Am J Roentgenol 1983;140:1189-1194.
43. Runyon BA, Hoefs JC. Peritoneal lymphomatosis with ascites: a characterization. Arch Intern Med 1986;146:887-888.
44. Lynch MA, Cho KC, Jeffrey Jr RB, et al. CT of peritoneal lymphomatosis. AJR Am J Roentgenol 1988;151:713-715.
45. O'Connell JT, Tomlinson JS, Roberts AA, et al. Pseudomyxoma peritonei is a disease of MUC2-expressing goblet cells. Am J Pathol 2002;161:551-564.
46. Hart WR. Ovarian epithelial tumors of borderline malignancy (carcinomas of low malignant potential). Hum Pathol 1977;8:541-549.
47. Yan H, Pestieau SR, Shmookler BM, Sugarbaker PH. Histopathologic analysis in 46 patients with pseudomyxoma peritonei syndrome: failure versus success with a second-look operation. Mod Pathol 2001;14:164-171.
48. Fox H. Pseudomyxoma peritonei. Br J Obstet Gynaecol 1996;103: 197-198.
49. Mann Jr WJ, Wagner J, Chumas J, Chalas E. The management of pseudomyxoma peritonei. Cancer 1990;66:1636-1640.
50. Sugarbaker PH. Cytoreductive surgery and perioperative intraperitoneal chemotherapy as a curative approach to pseudomyxoma peritonei syndrome. Tumori 2001;87:S3-S5.
51. Walensky RP, Venbrux AC, Prescott CA, Osterman Jr FA. Pseudomyxoma peritonei. AJR Am J Roentgenol 1996;167:471-474.
52. Seshul MB, Coulam CM. Pseudomyxoma peritonei: computed tomography and sonography. AJR Am J Roentgenol 1981;136: 803-806.

Inflammatory Disease of Peritoneum
53. Yeh HC, Wolf BS. Ultrasonography in ascites. Radiology 1977; 124:783-790.
54. Prousalidis J, Tzardinoglou K, Sgouradis L, et al. Uncommon sites of hydatid disease. World J Surg 1998;22:17-22.
55. Gazelle GS, Mueller PR. Abdominal abscess: imaging and intervention. Radiol Clin North Am 1994;32:913-932.
56. Snider Jr DE, Roper WL. The new tuberculosis. N Engl J Med 1992;326:703-705.
57. Marshall JB. Tuberculosis of the gastrointestinal tract and peritoneum. Am J Gastroenterol 1993;88:989-999.
58. Vanhoenacker FM, De Backer AI, Op de BB, et al. Imaging of gastrointestinal and abdominal tuberculosis. Eur Radiol 2004;14(Suppl 3):E103-115.
59. Akhan O, Pringot J. Imaging of abdominal tuberculosis. Eur Radiol 2002;12:312-323.
60. Kedar RP, Shah PP, Shivde RS, Malde HM. Sonographic findings in gastrointestinal and peritoneal tuberculosis. Clin Radiol 1994;49: 24-29.

61. Lee DH, Lim JH, Ko YT, Yoon Y. Sonographic findings in tuberculous peritonitis of wet-ascitic type. Clin Radiol 1991;44:306-310.
62. Malik A, Saxena NC. Ultrasound in abdominal tuberculosis. Abdom Imaging 2003;28:574-579.
63. Cohen O, Abrahamson J, Ben-Ari J, et al. Sclerosing encapsulating peritonitis. J Clin Gastroenterol 1996;22:54-57.
64. Hollman AS, McMillan MA, Briggs JD, et al. Ultrasound changes in sclerosing peritonitis following continuous ambulatory peritoneal dialysis. Clin Radiol 1991;43:176-179.
65. Krestin GP, Kacl G, Hauser M, et al. Imaging diagnosis of sclerosing peritonitis and relation of radiologic signs to the extent of the disease. Abdom Imaging 1995;20:414-420.

Localized Inflammatory Process of Peritoneal Cavity
66. Sarrazin J, Wilson SR. Manifestations of Crohn disease at US. Radiographics 1996;16:499-520; discussion 520-521.
67. McDonnell 3rd CH, Jeffrey Jr RB, Vierra MA. Inflamed pericholecystic fat: color Doppler flow imaging and clinical features. Radiology 1994;193:547-550.

Right-Sided Segmental Omental Infarction
68. McClure MJ, Khalili K, Sarrazin J, Hanbidge A. Radiological features of epiploic appendagitis and segmental omental infarction. Clin Radiol 2001;56:819-827.
69. Puylaert JB. Right-sided segmental infarction of the omentum: clinical, US, and CT findings. Radiology 1992;185:169-172.

Endometriosis
70. Woodward PJ, Sohaey R, Mezzetti Jr TP. Endometriosis: radiologic-pathologic correlation. Radiographics 2001;21:193-216; questionnaire 288-294.

Leiomyomatosis Peritonealis Disseminata
71. Bekkers RL, Willemsen WN, Schijf CP, et al. Leiomyomatosis peritonealis disseminata: does malignant transformation occur? A literature review. Gynecol Oncol 1999;75:158-163.

Pneumoperitoneum
72. Baker SR. Imaging of pneumoperitoneum. Abdom Imaging 1996; 21:413-414.
73. Braccini G, Lamacchia M, Boraschi P, et al. Ultrasound versus plain film in the detection of pneumoperitoneum. Abdom Imaging 1996;21:404-412.
74. Lee DH, Lim JH, Ko YT, Yoon Y. Sonographic detection of pneumoperitoneum in patients with acute abdomen. AJR Am J Roentgenol 1990;154:107-109.
75. Muradali D, Wilson S, Burns PN, et al. A specific sign of pneumoperitoneum on sonography: enhancement of the peritoneal stripe. AJR Am J Roentgenol 1999;173:1257-1262.

Conclusion
76. Gottlieb RH, Tan R, Widjaja J, et al. Extravisceral masses in the peritoneal cavity: sonographically guided biopsies in 52 patients. AJR Am J Roentgenol 1998;171:697-701.

Gynecology

Shia Salem

Chapter Outline

$\mathcal{S}$onography plays an integral role in the evaluation of gynecologic disease. It can determine the organ or site of abnormality and provide a diagnosis or short differential diagnosis in the vast majority of patients. Both transabdominal and transvaginal approaches are now well-established techniques for assessing the female pelvic organs. **Transvaginal** sonography is now considered an essential part of almost all pelvic ultrasound examinations. Color and spectral **Doppler** sonography helps assess normal and pathologic blood flow. Doppler ultrasound can also distinguish vascular structures from nonvascular structures, such as dilated fallopian tubes or fluid-filled bowel loops. **Sonohysterography** provides more detailed evaluation of the endometrium, allowing differentiation among intracavitary, endometrial, and submucosal lesions. More recently, **three-dimensional multiplanar sonography** has been shown to be an extremely useful addition, especially in evaluating the uterus and endometrium.[1] Sonography also plays an important role in guiding interventional procedures.

Magnetic resonance imaging has excellent tissue characterization and can be helpful when sonography is inconclusive and in the staging of pelvic malignancies. Computed tomography has a limited role but is also used for cancer staging.

NORMAL PELVIC ANATOMY

The **uterus** is a hollow, thick-walled muscular organ. Its internal structure consists of a muscular layer, or **myometrium,** which forms most of the substance of the uterus, and a mucous layer, the **endometrium,** which is firmly adherent to the myometrium. The uterus is located between the two layers of the broad ligament laterally, the bladder anteriorly, and the rectosigmoid colon posteriorly. The uterus is divided into two major portions, the body and the cervix, by a slight narrowing at the level of the internal os. The **fundus** is the superior area of the body above the entrance of the fallopian

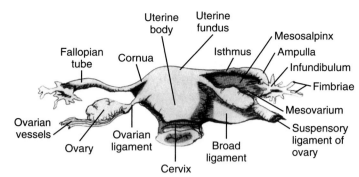

FIGURE 15-1. Normal gynecologic organs.
Diagram of uterus, ovaries, tubes, and related structures. On left side, broad ligament has been removed. (*Courtesy Jocelyne Salem.*)

tubes. The area of the body where the tubes enter the uterus is called the **cornua.** The anterior surface of the uterine fundus and body is covered by peritoneum. The peritoneal space anterior to the uterus is the **vesico-uterine pouch,** or **anterior cul-de-sac.** This space is usually empty, but it may contain small bowel loops. Posteriorly, the peritoneal reflection extends to the posterior fornix of the vagina, forming the **rectouterine recess,** or **posterior cul-de-sac.** Laterally, the peritoneal reflection forms the **broad ligaments,** which extend from the lateral aspect of the uterus to the lateral pelvic side walls (Fig. 15-1). The **round ligaments** arise from the uterine cornua anterior to the fallopian tubes in the broad ligaments, extend anterolaterally, and course through the inguinal canals to insert into the fascia of the labia majora.

The **cervix** is located posterior to the angle of the bladder and is anchored to the bladder angle by the parametrium. The cervix opens into the upper vagina through the external os. The **vagina** is a fibromuscular canal that lies in the midline and runs from the cervix to the vestibule of the external genitalia. The cervix projects into the proximal vagina, creating a space between the vaginal walls and the surface of the cervix called the **vaginal fornix.** Although the space is continuous, it is divided into anterior, posterior, and two lateral fornices.[2]

The two **fallopian tubes** run laterally from the uterus in the upper free margin of the broad ligament. Each tube varies from 7 to 12 cm in length and is divided into intramural, isthmic, ampullary, and infundibular portions.[2] The **intramural,** or interstitial, portion is approximately 1 cm long, is contained within the muscular wall of the uterus, and is the narrowest part of the tube. The **isthmus,** constituting the medial third, is slightly wider, round, cordlike, and continuous with the **ampulla,** which is tortuous and forms approximately one-half the length of the tube. The ampulla terminates in the most distal portion, the **infundibulum,** or fimbriated end, which is funnel shaped and opens into the peritoneal cavity (Fig. 15-1).

The **ovaries** are elliptical in shape, with the long axis usually oriented vertically. The surface of the ovary is not covered by peritoneum but by a single layer of cuboidal or columnar cells called the **germinal epithelium** that becomes continuous with the peritoneum at the hilum of the ovary. The internal structure of the ovary is divided into an outer cortex and inner medulla. The **cortex** consists of an interstitial framework, or **stroma,** which is composed of reticular fibers and spindle-shaped cells and which contains the ovarian follicles and corpus lutea. Beneath the germinal epithelium, the connective tissue of the cortex is condensed to form a fibrous capsule, the **tunica albuginea.** The **medulla,** which is smaller in volume than the cortex, is composed of fibrous tissue and blood vessels, especially veins. In the nulliparous female, the ovary is located in a depression on the lateral pelvic wall called the **ovarian fossa,** which is bounded anteriorly by the obliterated umbilical artery, posteriorly by the ureter and the internal iliac artery, and superiorly by the external iliac vein.[2] The fimbriae of the fallopian tube lie superior and lateral to the ovary. The anterior surface of the ovary is attached to the posterior surface of the broad ligament by a short mesovarium. The lower pole of the ovary is attached to the uterus by the **ovarian ligament,** whereas the upper pole is attached to the lateral wall of the pelvis by the lateral extension of the broad ligament known as the **suspensory** (infundibulopelvic) **ligament** of the ovary. The suspensory ligament contains the ovarian vessels and nerves. These ligaments are not rigid, and therefore the ovary can be quite mobile, especially in women who have had pregnancies.

The arterial blood supply to the uterus comes primarily from the **uterine artery,** a major branch of the anterior trunk of the internal iliac artery. The uterine artery ascends along the lateral margin of the uterus in the broad ligament and, at the level of the uterine cornua, runs laterally to anastomose with the ovarian artery. The uterine arteries anastomose extensively across the midline through the anterior and posterior arcuate arteries, which run within the broad ligament and then enter the myometrium.[2] The uterine plexus of veins accompanies the arteries.

The **ovarian arteries** arise from the aorta laterally, slightly inferior to the renal arteries. They cross the external iliac vessels at the pelvic brim and run medially within the suspensory ligament of the ovary. After giving off branches to the ovary, the ovarian arteries continue medially in the broad ligament to anastomose with the branches of the uterine artery. The **ovarian veins** leave the ovarian hilum and form a plexus of veins in the broad ligament that communicate with the uterine plexus of veins. The right ovarian vein drains into the inferior vena cava inferior to the right renal vein, whereas the left ovarian vein drains directly into the left renal vein.[2]

The **lymphatic drainage** of the pelvic organs is variable but tends to follow recognizable patterns. The lymph vessels of the ovary accompany the ovarian artery to the lateral aortic and periaortic lymph nodes. The lymphatics of the fundus and upper uterine body and fallopian tube accompany those of the ovary. The lymphatics of the lower uterine body course laterally to the external iliac lymph nodes, whereas those of the cervix course in three directions: laterally, to the external iliac lymph nodes; posterolaterally, to the internal iliac lymph nodes; and posteriorly, to the lateral sacral lymph nodes. The lymphatics of the upper vagina course laterally with the branches of the uterine artery to the external and internal iliac lymph nodes, whereas those of the middle vagina follow the vaginal artery branches to the internal iliac lymph nodes. The lymphatic vessels of the lower vagina near the orifice join those of the vulva and drain to the superficial inguinal lymph nodes.[2]

SONOGRAPHIC METHODS

Transabdominal versus Transvaginal Scanning

Transabdominal and transvaginal sonography are complementary techniques; both are used extensively in evaluation of the female pelvis. The **transabdominal** approach visualizes the entire pelvis and gives a global overview. Its main limitations involve the examination of patients unable to fill the bladder, obese patients, or patients with a retroverted uterus, in whom the fundus may be located beyond the focal zone of the transducer. The transabdominal technique also is less effective for characterization of adnexal masses.

Because of the proximity of the transducer to the uterus and adnexa, **transvaginal** sonography allows the use of higher-frequency transducers, producing much better resolution, which provides better image quality and anatomic detail. However, because of the higher frequencies, the field of view (FOV) is limited, which is the major disadvantage of the transvaginal technique. Large masses may fill or extend out of the FOV, making orientation difficult, and superiorly or laterally placed ovaries or masses may not be visualized. Transvaginal sonography better distinguishes adnexal masses from bowel loops and provides greater detail of the internal characteristics of a pelvic mass because of its improved resolution. Thus, transvaginal and transabdominal techniques complement each other.

ADVANTAGES OF TRANSVAGINAL SONOGRAPHY
Use of higher-frequency transducers with better resolution.
Examination of patients who are unable to fill their bladder.
Examination of obese patients.
Evaluation of a retroverted uterus.
Better distinction between adnexal masses and bowel loops.
Better characterization of the internal characteristics of a pelvic mass.
Better detail of a pelvic lesion.
Better detail of the endometrium.

Many women will require both transabdominal and transvaginal studies. If the initial study is completely normal; however, or if a well-defined abnormality is detected, no further study is usually necessary. The second study is added if the pelvic organs are not well visualized. At my laboratory, we begin with a transabdominal scan to look for large masses or any obvious abnormalities, but we do not ask the patient to fill her bladder. If the bladder is full, we will do a complete scan. If the bladder is empty, we will proceed directly with the transvaginal scan.

Transvaginal sonography should always be performed in women with suspected endometrial disorders, in patients who have a high risk of disease (e.g., strong family history of ovarian cancer), and to assess the internal characteristics of a pelvic mass. For follow-up examinations, only the more efficient diagnostic technique is needed.

Sonohysterography

Sonohysterography (SHG) involves the instillation of sterile saline into the endometrial cavity under ultrasound guidance. The saline distends the cavity, separating the walls of the endometrium. The most common indication for SHG is abnormal uterine bleeding in both premenopausal and postmenopausal women. Other indications include evaluation of endometrial or intracavitary abnormalities detected by transvaginal sonography or a suboptimally visualized endometrium by transvaginal sonography, infertile women, and suspected congenital uterine malformations.[3]

The procedure is explained to the patient and verbal consent obtained. A sterile speculum is inserted into the vagina and the cervix cleansed with an antiseptic solution. A special catheter, or a 5-F pediatric feeding tube, is inserted into the uterine cavity. The catheter should be prefilled with saline before insertion to minimize air artifact. A hysterosalpingography catheter with a balloon may be necessary in women with a patulous or incompetent cervix, to prevent retrograde leakage of saline into the vagina. The balloon should be placed as close to the internal os as possible and inflated with saline, not air.

The speculum is then removed and the transvaginal transducer inserted into the vagina. The catheter position in the endometrial cavity is identified and repositioned if necessary. Sterile saline is then injected slowly through the catheter under continuous sonographic control. The uterus is scanned systematically in sagittal and coronal planes to delineate the entire endometrial cavity, and appropriate images are recorded.

In premenopausal women with regular cycles, SHG is usually performed in the first 10 days of the menstrual cycle, preferably between days 4 and 7. This is when the endometrium is thinnest and avoids the possibility of disrupting an early pregnancy. For women with irregular cycles, the procedure is performed soon after the cessation of bleeding. In postmenopausal women receiving sequential **hormone replacement therapy** (HRT), SHG is performed shortly after the monthly bleeding period. In postmenopausal women not receiving HRT, the procedure can be performed at any time. SHG should not performed in women who are or could be pregnant or those with acute **pelvic inflammatory disease** (PID). In most cases, there is no special patient preparation. Prophylactic antibiotics may be given to women with chronic PID and those with cardiac disorders at risk for bacterial endocarditis.[4]

More recently, SHG has been combined with three-dimensional (3-D) multiplanar sonography, providing additional information to the standard SHG.[5,6] The 3-D volume data are analyzed after SHG is completed, decreasing the time that the endometrial cavity is distended.

UTERUS

Normal Sonographic Anatomy

The uterus lies in the true pelvis between the urinary bladder anteriorly and the rectosigmoid colon posteriorly (Fig. 15-2). Uterine position is variable and changes with varying degrees of bladder and rectal distention. The cervix is fixed in the midline, but the body is quite mobile and may lie obliquely on either side of the midline. **Flexion** refers to the axis of the uterine body relative to the cervix, whereas **version** refers to the axis of the cervix relative to the vagina. The uterus is usually anteverted and anteflexed, but it may appear straight or slightly retroflexed on transabdominal sonograms because of posterior displacement by the distended bladder. The uterus may also be retroflexed when the body is tilted posteriorly (relative to the cervix) or retroverted when the entire uterus is tilted backward (relative to the vagina) (Fig. 15-3). The fundus of a retroverted or retroflexed uterus is frequently difficult to assess by

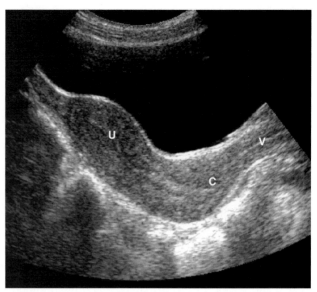

FIGURE 15-2. Normal uterus (U), cervix (C), and vagina (V). Sagittal ultrasound scan shows central linear echo representing apposed surfaces of vaginal mucosa (V).

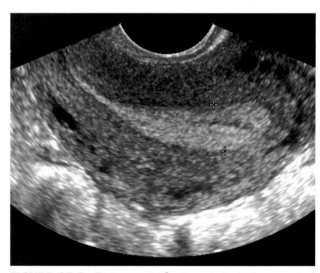

FIGURE 15-3. Retroverted uterus. Sagittal transvaginal sonogram shows retroverted uterus and secretory endometrium (cursors).

transabdominal sonography. Because this portion of the uterus is situated at a distance from the transducer, it may appear hypoechoic and simulate a fibroid. Transvaginal sonography has proved to be excellent for assessing the retroverted or retroflexed uterus because the transducer is close to the posteriorly located fundus.

The size and shape of the normal uterus vary throughout life and are related to age, hormonal status, and parity. The infantile or prepubertal uterus ranges from 2.0 to 3.3 cm (mean, 2.8 cm) in length, with the cervix accounting for two thirds of the total length, and 0.5 to 1.0 cm (mean, 0.8 cm) in anteroposterior (AP) diameter.[7] The prepubertal uterus has a tubular or inverse pear-shaped appearance, with the AP diameter of the cervix greater than that of the fundus.[8] In the immediate neonatal period, because of residual maternal hormone stimulation, the neonatal uterus is slightly larger, varying in length from 2.3 to 4.6 cm (mean, 3.4 cm) and AP diameter from 0.8 to 2.1 cm (mean, 1.2 cm).[9] Also, an echogenic endometrium is seen in the neonatal uterus in almost all babies (Fig. 15-4).

A small amount of endometrial fluid may be present in up to 25% of neonatal uteri.[10] Growth of the **prepubertal** uterus is minimal from infancy until approximately 8 years of age, when the uterus gradually increases in size until puberty.[11] At this time, there is a more dramatic increase in size with more pronounced growth in the body until it reaches the eventual adult, pear-shaped appearance, with the diameter and length of the body about double that of the cervix.[8] The normal **postpubertal,** or adult, uterus varies considerably in size. The maximal dimensions of the nulliparous uterus are approximately 8 cm in length, 5 cm in width, and 4 cm in AP diameter. **Parity** (pregnancy) increases the normal size by more than 1 cm in each dimension.[12-14] Merz et al.[13] also found a significant difference in uterine length between primiparas and multiparas, with an increase of approximately 1 cm in primiparas and 2 cm in multiparas. After menopause, the uterus atrophies, with the most rapid decrease in size occurring in the first 10 years after cessation of menstruation.[12] In patients over age 65 years, the uterus ranges from 3.5 to 6.5 cm in length and 1.2 to 1.8 cm in AP diameter.[14]

The normal **myometrium** consists of three layers that can be distinguished by sonography (Fig. 15-5). The **intermediate layer** is the thickest and has a uniformly homogeneous texture of low to moderate echogenicity. The **inner layer** of myometrium is thin, compact, and relatively hypovascular.[15,16] This inner layer, which is hypoechoic and surrounds the relatively echogenic endometrium, has also been referred to as the **subendometrial halo.** The thin **outer layer** is slightly less echogenic than the intermediate layer and is separated from it by the arcuate vessels.

The **arcuate arteries** lie between the outer and intermediate layers of the myometrium and branch into the **radial arteries,** which run in the intermediate layer to the level of the inner layer. The radial arteries then branch into the **spiral arteries,** which enter the endometrium and supply the functional layer. The **uterine veins** are larger than the accompanying arcuate arteries and are frequently identified as small, focal anechoic areas by both transabdominal and transvaginal sonography.[17] This vascular pattern can be confirmed by Doppler ultrasound (see Fig. 15-5).

Calcification may be seen in the arcuate arteries in postmenopausal women because of Mönckeberg's sclerosis.[18,19] On sonography, such calcification appears as peripheral linear echogenic areas with shadowing; they should be distinguished from calcified leiomyomas

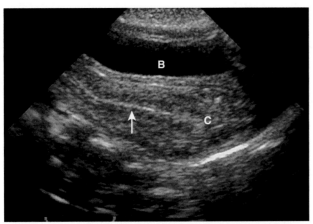

FIGURE 15-4. Normal neonatal uterus. Sagittal sonogram shows inverse pear shape with cervix *(C)* having greater anteroposterior diameter and length than uterine body; *B,* bladder. The echogenic endometrium *(arrow)* is thin and normal.

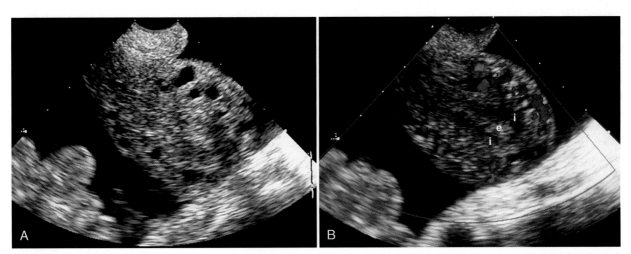

FIGURE 15-5. Uterine veins. A, Transvaginal sagittal scan of uterus surrounded by ascites shows multiple peripheral anechoic uterine veins. **B,** Confirmation by color Doppler ultrasound; *e,* endometrium; *i,* hypoechoic inner layer of myometrium. The outer layer of myometrium is separated from the intermediate layer by the arcuate uterine veins.

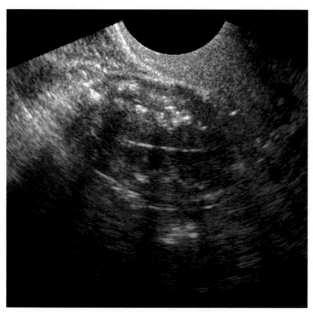

FIGURE 15-6. Arcuate artery calcification. Transvaginal sagittal scan shows multiple small, peripheral, linear hyperechoic calcific foci in the arcuate arteries.

(Fig. 15-6). This is a normal aging process that may be accelerated in diabetic patients.

Small, highly echogenic foci in the inner layer of myometrium may be seen in normal women. These foci, measuring only a few millimeters, may be single or multiple and are usually nonshadowing. They are thought to represent **dystrophic calcification** related to previous instrumentation, such as dilation and curettage (D&C) or endocervical biopsy.[20] Similar-appearing echogenic foci may be seen in the endometrium and endocervix and are most often caused by **microcalcification.**[21] These echogenic foci, whether within the endometrium or inner layer of myometrium, are thought to be incidental findings and of no clinical significance.

Uterine perfusion can be assessed by duplex Doppler ultrasound or color Doppler sonography of the uterine arteries. In normal women, the Doppler waveform usually shows a high-velocity, high-resistance pattern.

The normal **endometrial cavity** is seen as a thin echogenic line as a result of specular reflection from the interface between the opposing surfaces of the endometrium.[22] The sonographic appearance of the **endometrium** varies during the menstrual cycle (Fig. 15-7, A-D) and has been correlated with histology.[15,23,24] The endometrium is composed of a **superficial functional layer** and a **deep basal layer**. The functional layer thickens throughout the menstrual cycle and is shed with menses. The basal layer remains intact during the cycle and contains the spiral arteries, which become tortuous and elongated to supply the functional layer as it thickens. The **proliferative phase** of the cycle before ovulation is under the influence of estrogen, whereas progesterone is mainly responsible for maintenance of

PHASES OF PREMENOPAUSAL ENDOMETRIUM: SONOGRAPHIC APPEARANCE

Menstrual phase	Thin, broken echogenic line
Proliferative phase	Hypoechoic thickening (4-8 mm)
Periovulatory phase	Triple layer (6-10 mm)
Secretory phase	Hyperechoic thickening (7-14 mm)

the endometrium in the **secretory phase** following ovulation.

The **menstrual phase** endometrium consists of a thin echogenic line. During the **proliferative phase,** the endometrium thickens, reaching 4 to 8 mm. The endometrium is best measured on a midline sagittal scan of the uterus and should include both anterior and posterior portions of the endometrium. It is important not to include the thin hypoechoic inner layer of myometrium in this measurement. A relatively hypoechoic region that represents the functional layer can be seen around the central echogenic line. In the early proliferative phase, this hypoechoic area is thin, but it increases and becomes more clearly defined in the later proliferative phase **(periovulatory),** probably as a result of edema. The hypoechoic appearance of the proliferative endometrium has been related to the relatively homogeneous histologic structure because of the orderly arrangement of the glandular elements.

After **ovulation,** the functional layer of the endometrium changes from hypoechoic to hyperechoic as the endometrium progresses to the **secretory phase.**[23,24] The endometrium in this phase measures 7 to 14 mm in thickness. The hyperechoic texture in the secretory endometrium is related to increased mucus and glycogen within the glands, as well as to the increased number of interfaces caused by the tortuosity of the spiral arteries. Acoustic enhancement may be seen posterior to the secretory endometrium, but it is not specific because it has also been seen with the proliferative endometrium, although not as frequently.[24]

After **menopause,** the endometrium becomes atrophic because it is no longer under hormonal control. Sonographically, the endometrium is seen as a thin echogenic line measuring no more than 8 mm in the normal asymptomatic woman[25] (Fig. 15-7, E). The endometrial cavity is best seen with 3-D ultrasound using the rendered coronal image.

Congenital Abnormalities

The incidence of congenital uterine abnormalities is approximately 1%. They are associated with recurrent pregnancy loss and other obstetric complications, such

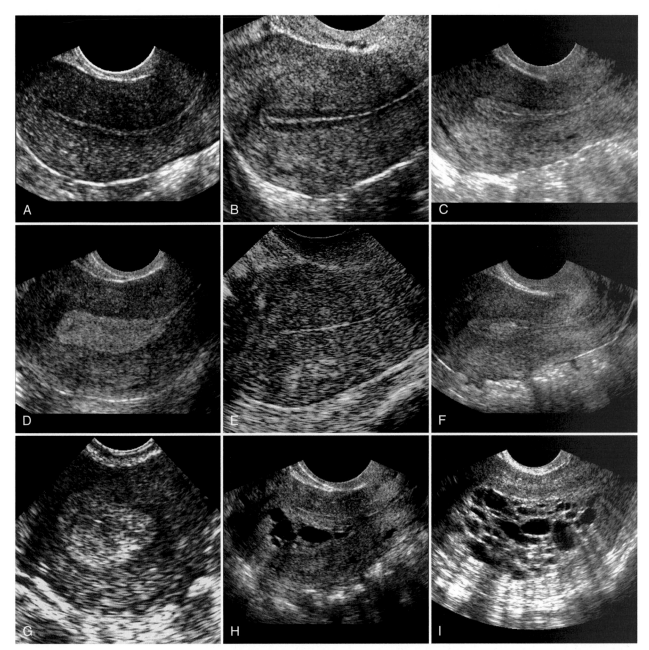

FIGURE 15-7. Endometrium: spectrum of appearances. Transvaginal scans. **A,** Normal, thin, early-proliferative endometrium. **B,** Normal, late-proliferative endometrium with triple-layer appearance. Central echogenic line is caused by opposed endometrial surfaces surrounded by a thicker hypoechoic functional layer, bounded by an outer echogenic basal layer. **C,** Normal, early-secretory phase endometrium. The functional layer surrounding the echogenic line has become hyperechoic. **D,** Normal, thick, hyperechoic late-secretory endometrium. **E,** Normal, thin, postmenopausal endometrium. **F,** Oval, well-defined polyp that is more hyperechoic than surrounding periovulatory endometrium. **G,** Thickened endometrium caused by multiple small **polyps** confirmed on sonohysterogram. **H,** Thick, cystic endometrium caused by **hyperplasia** in patient taking tamoxifen. **I,** Thick, cystic endometrium caused by large **polyp** in patient receiving tamoxifen.

as intrauterine growth restriction and preterm labor and birth. The fused caudal ends of the two müllerian (**paramesonephric**) ducts form the uterus, cervix, and upper two thirds of the vagina, whereas the unfused cranial ends form the paired fallopian tubes. It was previously believed that fusion occurs in a cephalad direction. However, descriptions of cases with cervical duplication and a fully fused uterine body and fundus have challenged this concept. A more recent hypothesis is that fusion occurs in the medial portion of the ducts and proceeds in either a cephalad or a caudal direction, or both.[26,27] The median septum formed by the medial walls of the müllerian ducts then resorbs, leaving a single uterine cavity. **Uterine malformations** may be caused by the following (Figs. 15-8 and 15-9):

• Arrested development of the müllerian ducts
• Failure of fusion of the müllerian ducts
• Failure of resorption of the median septum

Arrested development of the müllerian ducts may be either unilateral or bilateral. Arrested **bilateral** development is extremely rare and results in congenital absence of the uterus, or **uterine aplasia.** Arrested **unilateral** development results in a **uterus unicornis unicollis,** or one uterine horn and one cervix. Hypoplasia of one müllerian duct may result in a rudimentary uterine horn. Approximately 65% of unicornuate uteruses will have a rudimentary horn and about half of these will contain no endometrial cavity **(noncavitary).** The other half will have an endometrial cavity **(cavitary),** of which approximately 70% will not communicate with the other horn (noncommunicating) and approximately 30% will communicate with the other horn (communicating).[28,29]

Failure of fusion of the müllerian ducts may be **complete,** resulting in a **uterus didelphys,** or two cervices and two uterine horns, or **partial,** which may result in either a **uterus bicornis bicollis** (two cervices and two uterine horns) or a **uterus bicornis unicollis** (one cervix and two uterine horns). The didelphys uterus has an associated longitudinal vaginal septum in approximately 75% of cases, and there is complete separation of the uterine horns and cervices, whereas some communication exists between the uterine horns in a uterus bicornis bicollis.

Failure of resorption of the median septum results in a **septate uterus** or **subseptate uterus,** depending on whether the failure is **complete** (extending to the cervical os) in a septate or **partial** in a subseptate uterus. This septum results in complete or partial duplication of the uterine cavities without duplication of the uterine horns and is the most common müllerian duct anomaly (~55%).[29] The septate uterus is associated with some of the poorest reproductive outcomes, with a high rate of spontaneous abortion.[29] The septate or subseptate uterus can be distinguished from the bicornuate uterus by looking at the external contour of the uterus. The **arcuate uterus** is caused by almost complete resorption of the median septum, with only a mild indentation of the endometrium at the fundus. The external uterine contour is normal. There is still debate whether the arcuate uterus should be considered an anomaly or a normal variant.

Uterine abnormalities have also been seen in patients exposed in utero to **diethylstilbestrol** (DES), which was discontinued in 1971. DES given during the first trimester crosses the placenta and exerts a direct effect on the müllerian system of the fetus. Sonography may demonstrate a diffuse decrease in the size of the uterus and an irregular T-shaped uterine cavity.[30,31]

There is a high association between **uterine malformations** and **congenital renal abnormalities,** especially renal agenesis and ectopia.[32] In all patients with uterine malformations, the kidneys should be evaluated sonographically. In patients with an absent or ectopic kidney, the uterus should be scanned for malformations. Renal abnormalities are more common in patients with a unicornuate uterus (~40%) and are always on the same side as the uterine abnormality.

The most common classification system is that of the American Fertility Society (AFS), which is based on embryology (Table 15-1). However, this system is problematic because it does not consider more complicated uterine anomalies or vaginal anomalies, such as septa. It also does not provide measurements to help determine whether the uterus is arcuate, septate, or bicornuate. Salim et al.[33] modified the AFS system by

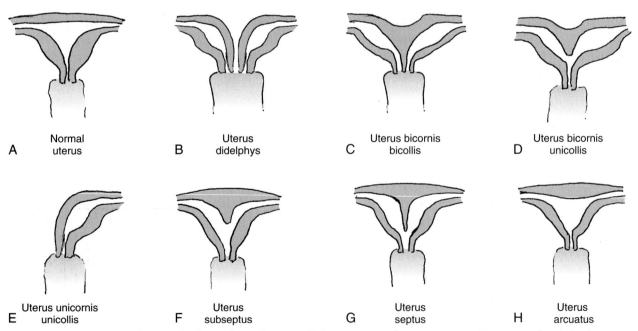

FIGURE 15-8. Congenital uterine abnormalities. Diagram of common types. *(Courtesy Jocelyne Salem.)*

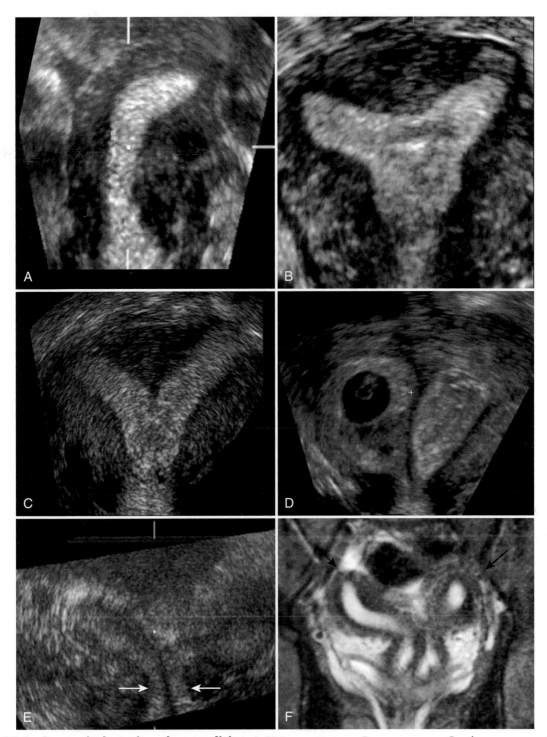

FIGURE 15-9. Congenital uterine abnormalities. A, Unicornuate uterus; **B,** arcuate uterus; **C,** subseptate uterus; **D,** septate uterus with pregnancy on right side; **E** and **F,** didelphys uterus with two separate uterine horns *(black arrows)* and cervices *(arrows).* **A** to **E,** 3-D coronal reconstructions; **F,** MR image. *(A, E, and F courtesy Anna Lev-Toaff, MD.)*

adding measurements obtained from the coronal view of the uterus.

Conventional two-dimensional (2-D) sonography is considered a good screening test because most uterine anomalies can be detected by this method.[34] The examination should be performed during the secretory phase of the menstrual cycle, when the endometrium is thick-

est. Two endometrial echo complexes may be seen in the bicornuate or septate uterus. Sonography can also outline the external contour of the uterus. In the **didelphys** and **bicornuate uterus** the endometrial cavities are widely separated, and there is a deep indentation on the fundal contour. The **septate uterus,** in contrast, has a relatively normal outline, and the two endometrial cavities are

TABLE 15-1. CLASSIFICATION OF MÜLLERIAN DUCT ANOMALIES

CLASS	ANOMALY
I	Partial or complete agenesis
II	Unicornuate uterus
III	Didelphys uterus
IV	Bicornuate uterus
V	Septate uterus
VI	Arcuate uterus
VII	DES-associated anomalies

From American Fertility Society.
DES, Diethylstilbestrol.

closer together and are separated by a septum. The septum has a poor blood supply and contains fibrous and/or myometrial tissue.[35,36] Sonography, combined with hysterosalpingography, has a high level of accuracy in distinguishing between the septate and the bicornuate uterus.[37] It is important to differentiate these two conditions because the septate uterus can be treated by outpatient hysteroscopic resection of the septum. Because the bicornuate uterus consists of two separate uterine horns, each containing a full complement of myometrium and endometrium, correction, if necessary, requires abdominal surgery.

The **unicornuate uterus** is difficult to differentiate from the normal uterus by conventional sonography. It may be suspected when the uterus appears small and laterally positioned. Hydrometra in the opposite rudimentary horn may be seen and mistaken for a uterine or adnexal mass. The **bicornuate uterus** may also be confused with a uterine or adnexal mass if the central endometrial echo complex is not seen in one horn. In many cases the bicornuate uterus is first diagnosed incidentally in early pregnancy when a gestational sac is present in one horn and there is decidual reaction in the other.

Three-dimensional ultrasound with multiplanar imaging has been shown to be more accurate in detecting and classifying uterine anomalies with high sensitivity and specificity[27,29,38,39] (see Fig. 15-9). The coronal view through the entire uterus, which cannot be obtained on routine 2-D ultrasound because of the limited mobility of the transducer in the vagina, is essential for accurate diagnosis. The coronal view provides more accurate visualization of the external uterine fundal contour and endometrium, which allows better differentiation among bicornuate, septate, and arcuate uterus. The normal, septate and arcuate uterus usually have a normal convex or flat external fundal contour but may have a shallow fundal indentation measuring less than 1 cm in depth, whereas the bicornuate uterus has an external fundal cleft of at least 1 cm dividing the two cornua.[33,39] The unicornuate uterus is small, with only one cornual angle

laterally positioned with a curved banana-like shape. The arcuate uterus has a normal external fundal contour with a broad smooth indentation on the fundal endometrium forming an obtuse angle at its central point and measuring less than 1 cm when measured from the cornual angle.[39] Magnetic resonance imaging (MRI) is also highly accurate in demonstrating uterine anomalies.[29,35] Because of its relatively high cost, however, MRI is usually reserved for the more complicated anomalies.

Abnormalities of the Myometrium

Leiomyoma

Leiomyomas **(fibroids)** are the most common neoplasms of the uterus. They occur in 20% to 30% of females over age 30 years[40] and are more common in black women. Fibroids are usually multiple and are the most common cause of enlargement of the nonpregnant uterus. Although frequently asymptomatic, women with leiomyomas can experience pain and uterine bleeding. Leiomyomas may be classified as **intramural**, confined to the myometrium; **submucosal**, projecting into the uterine cavity and displacing or distorting the endometrium; or **subserosal**, projecting from the peritoneal surface of the uterus.

LEIOMYOMA CLASSIFICATION

Intramural	Confined to the myometrium
Submucosal	Projecting into the uterine cavity
Subserosal	Projecting from the peritoneal surface

Intramural fibroids are the most common. Submucosal fibroids, although less common, produce symptoms most frequently and may also be associated with infertility. Subserosal fibroids may be pedunculated and may present as an adnexal mass. They may also project between the leaves of the broad ligament, where they are referred to as "intraligamentous." Cervical fibroids account for approximately 8% of all fibroids.

Fibroids are **estrogen dependent** and may increase in size during anovulatory cycles, as a result of unopposed estrogen stimulation,[41] and during pregnancy, although about one half of all fibroids show little significant change during pregnancy.[42] Fibroids identified in the first trimester are associated with increased risk of pregnancy loss, which is higher in patients with multiple fibroids than in those with a single fibroid.[43] Large fibroids do not interfere with pregnancy or normal vaginal delivery except when located in the lower uterine segment or the cervix. Leiomyomas rarely develop in postmenopausal women, and most stabilize or decrease in size after menopause. They may increase in size in postmenopausal patients who are undergoing HRT. Tamoxifen has also been reported to cause growth in leiomyomas.[44] A rapid increase in fibroid size, especially in a postmenopausal patient, should raise the possibility of sarcomatous change.

Pathologically, leiomyomas are composed of spindle-shaped, smooth muscle cells arranged in whorl-like patterns separated by variable amounts of fibrous connective tissue. The surrounding myometrium may become compressed to form a pseudocapsule. As they enlarge, leio-myomas may outgrow their blood supply, resulting in ischemia and cystic degeneration.

Sonographically, leiomyomas have variable appearances (Fig. 15-10, *A-H*). Leiomyomas are most often hypoechoic (Fig. 15-10, *A* and *B*) or heterogeneous in echotexture. They frequently distort the external contour of the uterus. Many leiomyomas demonstrate areas of **acoustic attenuation** or **shadowing** without a discrete

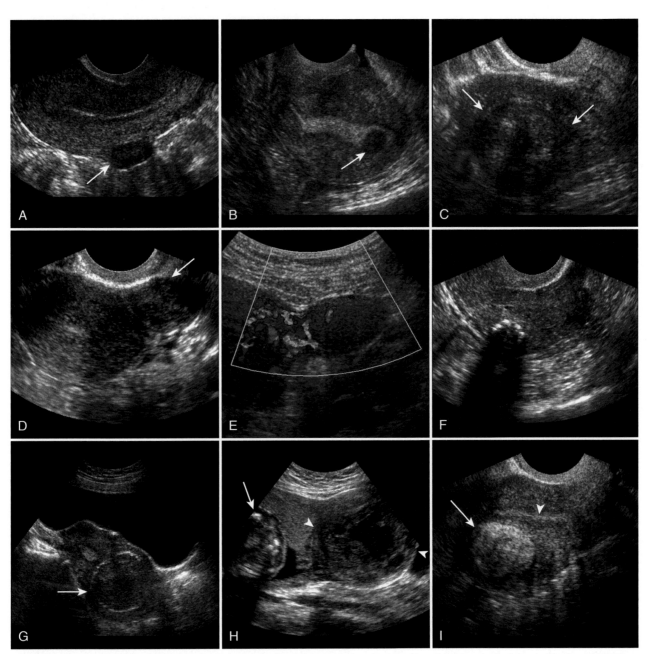

FIGURE 15-10. Uterine fibroids: spectrum of appearances. A to **D, F,** and **I,** Transvaginal scans. **E, G,** and **H,** Transabdominal scans. **A,** Localized hypoechoic **subserosal fibroid** *(arrow).* **B,** Hypoechoic **submucosal fibroid** *(arrow).* **C,** Marked attenuation of sound beam by fibroid *(arrows).* **D, Pedunculated subserosal fibroid** *(arrow)* presenting as solid left adnexal mass. **E,** Color Doppler sonogram of **pedunculated subserosal fibroid** shows blood supply arising from uterus. **F, Fibroid with calcification** causing posterior shadowing. **G, Calcified fibroid** with curvilinear peripheral calcification *(arrow)* mimicking a fetal head. **H, Fibroid with cystic degeneration** *(arrowheads)* in pregnancy. Patient presented with pain and tenderness over degenerating fibroid *(arrow,* fetus). **I, Lipoleiomyoma.** Highly echogenic mass within myometrium *(arrow)* with posterior attenuation *(arrowhead,* endometrium).

LEIOMYOMAS: SONOGRAPHIC FEATURES

Variable appearance
Hypoechoic or heterogeneous mass
Distortion of external uterine contour
Attenuation or shadowing without discrete mass
Calcification
Degeneration or necrosis

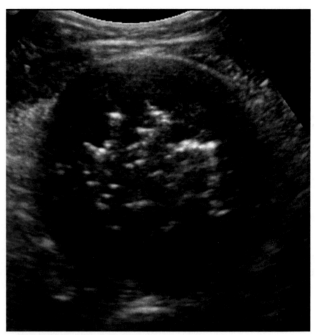

FIGURE 15-11. Fibroid containing extensive air after uterine artery embolization.

mass, making it impossible to estimate size (Fig. 15-10, C). The attenuation is thought to be caused by dense fibrosis within the substance of the tumor. Kliewer et al.[45] suggest that posterior shadowing arising from within the substance of a leiomyoma (but not from echogenic foci) originates from transitional zones between apposed tissues. Histologically, the transitional zone includes the margins of the leiomyoma with adjacent normal myometrium, the borders between fibrous tissue and smooth muscle, and the edges of whorls and bundles of smooth muscle. This type of shadowing is a very useful diagnostic feature in distinguishing a **pedunculated** or **exophytic** leiomyoma from other types of adnexal masses.[46]

Calcification may occur in fibroids of older females, frequently appearing as focal areas of increased echogenicity with shadowing (Fig. 15-10, F) or as a curvilinear echogenic rim, which may simulate the outline of a fetal head[47] (Fig. 15-10, G). When fibroids undergo rapid growth, they tend to outgrow their blood supply, leading to **degeneration** and **necrosis** and producing areas of decreased echogenicity or cystic spaces within the fibroid (Fig. 15-10, H). This tends to occur more often during pregnancy, affecting about 7% to 8% of pregnant patients with fibroids, who may present with pain over this area.[40] Although uncommon, pedunculated fibroids may undergo torsion. Giant leiomyomas with multiple cystic spaces resulting from edema have been described.[48]

Submucosal fibroids may impinge on the endometrium, distorting the cavity with varying degrees of intracavitary extension. Transvaginal sonography allows better differentiation between a submucosal and an intramural lesion and its relationship to the endometrial cavity.[49]

Sonohysterography and more recently 3-D ultrasound is very helpful to determine the exact location and relationship of the fibroid to the endometrium, the amount of intracavitary extension, and its potential resectability.[50] Fibroids with at least 50% of the mass projecting into the endometrial cavity can be resected hysteroscopically.[51,52] In many cases, SHG and 3-D sonography may also be necessary to distinguish a submucosal leiomyoma from an endometrial lesion. Submucosal fibroids are usually broad-based solid hypoechoic masses with an overlying layer of echogenic endometrium.

Transvaginal sonography can detect very small leiomyomas and may be diagnostic in showing the uterine origin of large, pedunculated, subserosal leiomyomas that simulate adnexal masses. Color Doppler ultrasound is valuable in showing uterine vessels supplying the fibroid (Fig. 15-10, D and E). Large fibroids are usually better assessed transabdominally, and subserosal or pedunculated fibroids may be missed if the transvaginal approach alone is used, because of the limited FOV.[53] Leiomyomas in the fundus of a retroverted uterus are much better delineated by transvaginal sonography.

Uterine artery embolization (UAE) is now an accepted alternative to surgical and medical treatment of symptomatic fibroids. Air may be seen within the fibroid as early as 1 month after UAE (Fig. 15-11). This is thought to be caused by air filling potential spaces left by tissue infarction and is rarely from infection.[54] There are no reliable imaging findings to diagnose an infected fibroid after UAE, and correlation with clinical and laboratory findings is essential to exclude an infected fibroid. Endometritis is uncommon and can occur days to weeks after UAE. Transcervical expulsion of a fibroid may occur in up to 3% of patients after UAE. This occurs in fibroids that are in contact with the endometrial surface (i.e., submucosal) or intramural fibroids with a submucosal component.[54,55] Most are expelled spontaneously.

Lipomatous Uterine Tumors

Lipomatous uterine tumors (**lipoleiomyomas**) are uncommon, benign neoplasms consisting of variable portions of mature lipocytes, smooth muscle, or fibrous tissue. Histologically, these tumors comprise a spectrum that includes pure lipomas, lipoleiomyomas, and fibrolipomyomas. Sonographically, the finding of a highly echogenic, attenuating mass within the myometrium is virtually diagnostic of this condition[56] (Fig. 15-10, *I*). Color Doppler sonography shows complete absence of flow within the mass.[57] It is important to identify the lesion within the uterus so as not to confuse it with the more common, similar-appearing, fat-containing ovarian dermoid.[58] Because lipomatous uterine tumors are usually asymptomatic, they do not require surgery.

Leiomyosarcoma

Leiomyosarcoma is rare, accounting for 1.3% of uterine malignancies, and may arise from a preexisting uterine leiomyoma.[40] Frequently, patients are asymptomatic, although uterine bleeding may occur. This condition is rarely diagnosed preoperatively. Sonographically, the appearance is similar to that of a rapidly growing or degenerating leiomyoma, except when there is evidence of local invasion or distant metastases (Fig. 15-12).

Adenomyosis

Adenomyosis is a common condition characterized pathologically by the presence of endometrial glands and stroma within the myometrium, associated with adjacent smooth muscle hyperplasia. It is usually more extensive in the posterior wall.[40] The endometrial glands arise from the basal layer and are typically resistant to hormonal stimulation. Adenomyosis can occur in both diffuse and nodular forms. The more common **diffuse** adenomyosis is composed of widely scattered adenomyosis foci within the myometrium, whereas **nodular** adenomyosis consists of circumscribed nodules called **adenomyomas**. The clinical presentation is usually nonspecific: uterine enlargement, pelvic pain, dysmenorrhea, and menorrhagia. Adenomyosis is more often seen in women who have had children and much less often in nulliparous or postmenopausal women.

Before the advent of transvaginal sonography, the diagnosis was rarely made by transabdominal sonography. Transvaginal sonography has made the diagnosis of adenomyosis easier and more accurate, and this condition is now being detected with increasing frequency[59-62] (Fig. 15-13). The uterus may be enlarged, having a globular configuration with a diffusely heterogeneous-appearing myometrium without a discrete mass or contour deformity. The myometrium may be asymmetrically thickened. The endometrial-myometrial border may be poorly defined. Small **myometrial cysts,** frequently subendometrial, may also be present within the myometrium and histologically represent dilated glands in ectopic endometrial tissue.[60] Subendometrial echogenic linear **striations** and subendometrial echogenic **nodules** *(D)* have been described, as well as inhomogeneous hypoechoic areas with indistinct margins in the myometrium.[63] Focal uterine tenderness may be elicited by the transvaginal transducer. Subendometrial echogenic linear striations/nodules and asymmetrical thickening have been reported to improve the specificity and positive predictive value in diagnosing adenomyosis.[63] The variable sonographic appearance is related to the distribution of the heterotopic endometrial tissue, the degree of associated muscle hypertrophy, and the presence and size of the cysts within the heterotopic endometrial tissue.[63] Adenomyosis and leiomyomas frequently occur together in the same uterus.[61] The presence of fibroids has been

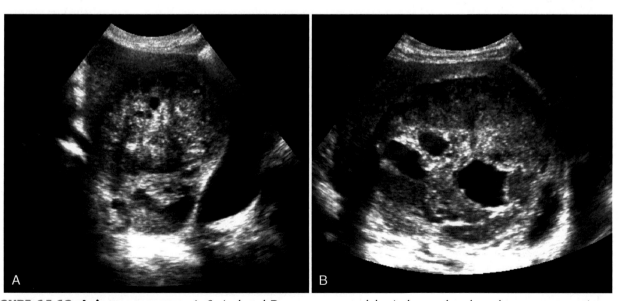

FIGURE 15-12. Leiomyosarcoma. A, Sagittal, and **B,** transverse, transabdominal scans show large, heterogeneous uterine mass with cystic areas. There is a rim of remaining normal myometrium.

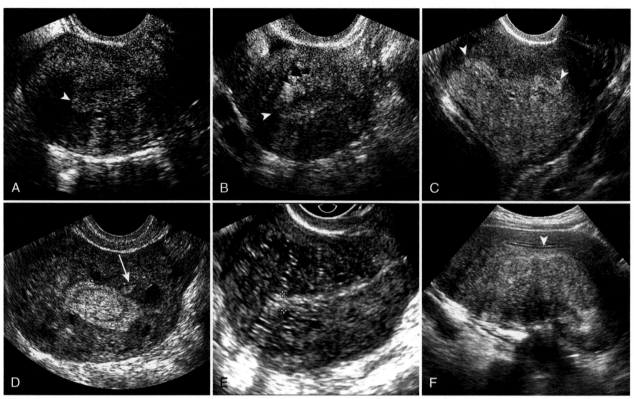

FIGURE 15-13. Adenomyosis on transvaginal scans: spectrum of appearances. A, Subendometrial cyst *(arrowhead, endometrium).* **B,** Cysts and heterogeneity in anterior myometrium with poorly defined anterior endometrial border *(arrowhead).* **C,** Myometrial heterogeneity with poorly defined endometrial borders *(arrowheads).* **D,** Multiple subendometrial cysts and echogenic nodules *(arrow).* **E,** Diffuse heterogeneous myometrium with multiple cysts and poorly defined endometrial borders *(cursors).* **F,** Large area of myometrial heterogeneity producing a focal mass effect and displacing endometrium *(arrowhead).* This may mimic a fibroid.

ADENOMYOSIS: SONOGRAPHIC FEATURES

Diffuse uterine enlargement
Diffusely heterogeneous myometrium
Asymmetrical thickening of myometrium
Inhomogeneous hypoechoic areas
Myometrial cysts
Poor definition of endometrial-myometrial border
Focal tenderness elicited by vaginal transducer
Subendometrial echogenic linear striations
Subendometrial echogenic nodules

shown to limit the ability to diagnose the severity of adenomyosis.[62]

Localized adenomyomas may be seen by transvaginal sonography as inhomogeneous, circumscribed areas in the myometrium with indistinct margins and containing cysts.[59,64,65] However, these adenomyomas are usually difficult to distinguish from leiomyomas. The borders of the mass and the Doppler sonographic vascular pattern may help to differentiate these two conditions. Usually, leiomyomas have well-defined borders and adenomyo-

mas have poorly defined borders. In adenomyomas, Doppler ultrasound shows internal vascularity, whereas fibroids frequently have a peripheral pattern.[66,67] MRI is highly accurate in demonstrating adenomyosis, which appears as poorly defined areas of decreased signal within the myometrium or diffuse or focal thickening of the junctional zone (>12 mm) on T2-weighted images.[68-70] Reinhold et al.[69] found MRI and sonography to be of comparable accuracy in the diagnosis of adenomyosis.

Arteriovenous Malformations

Uterine arteriovenous malformations (AVMs) consist of a vascular plexus of arteries and veins without an intervening capillary network. These rare lesions usually involve the myometrium and at times the endometrium. Most cases are acquired from pelvic trauma, surgery, and gestational trophoblastic neoplasia (GTN). Uterine AVMs are more often diagnosed in the postabortion and postpartum periods and often present with severe vaginal bleeding with hemoglobin-decreasing blood loss. Diagnosis is critical because D&C will likely worsen the bleeding and may lead to catastrophic hemorrhage.

On sonography, uterine AVMs may be nonspecific, with minimal findings (Fig. 15-14, *A*). They may be seen

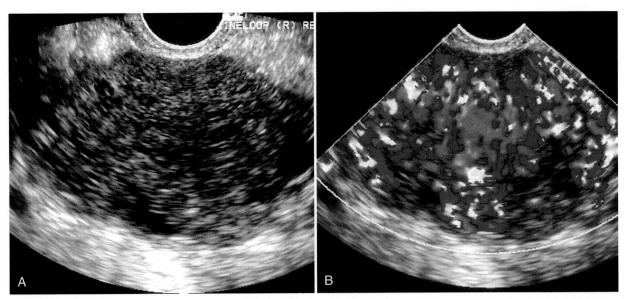

FIGURE 15-14. Uterine arteriovenous malformation. A, Transverse transvaginal sonogram shows a textural inhomogeneity in the uterine fundus. **B,** Color Doppler ultrasound image shows a floridly colored mosaic pattern with apparent flow reversals and areas of color aliasing. *(From Huang M, Muradali D, Thurston WA, et al: Uterine arteriovenous malformations: Gray-scale ultrasound and Doppler US features with MR imaging correlation. Radiology 1998;206;115-123.)*

as multiple serpiginous anechoic structures within the myometrium, as subtle myometrial heterogeneity, or as a myometrial or endometrial mass. Color Doppler ultrasound is more specific, showing abundant blood flow within the anechoic structures[71,72] (Fig. 15-14, *B*). There is a florid color mosaic, which is more extensive than the gray-scale abnormality. Spectral Doppler sonography shows high-velocity, low-resistance arterial flow, with high-velocity venous flow often indistinguishable from the arterial signal.[72] The diagnosis is confirmed by angiography, which shows early venous filling. AVMs can be treated by uterine artery embolization.

Uterine AVMs may be overdiagnosed in the early postabortion or postpartum period.[73] Many sonographically diagnosed AVMs have resolved on follow-up sonography. Focal high-resistance flow can also occur with **retained products of conception** and GTN or as a normal finding caused by **subinvolution of the placental bed.**[73] A negative serum human chorionic gonadotropin (hCG) level is helpful in distinguishing an AVM from GTN and many cases of retained products. If the patient is stable, conservative management should be considered with follow-up sonography to see if the lesion resolves.[73,74] Despite considerable overlap, peak systolic velocity (PSV) is useful in differentiating low-risk and high-risk patients. Timmerman et al.[74] reviewed 30 patients with sonographically diagnosed uterine AVMs, defined as an abnormal hypervascular area in the myometrium with turbulent flow. Lesions with PSV greater than 83 cm/sec had higher probability of further treatment such as embolization, whereas no lesion with PSV less than 39 cm/sec required embolization.[74] However, severe bleeding is an indication for immediate treatment (e.g., embolization).

CAUSES OF ENDOMETRIAL THICKENING

Early intrauterine pregnancy
Incomplete abortion
Ectopic pregnancy
Retained products of conception
Trophoblastic disease
Endometritis
Adhesions
Hyperplasia
Polyps
Carcinoma

Abnormalities of the Endometrium

Because of its improved resolution, transvaginal sonography is better able to image and depict subtle abnormalities within the endometrium and clearly define the endometrial-myometrial border.[75] Knowledge of the normal sonographic appearance of the endometrium allows for earlier recognition of pathologic conditions manifested by endometrial thickening with well-defined or poorly defined or irregular margins. Many endometrial pathologies, such as **hyperplasia, polyps,** and **carcinoma,** can cause abnormal bleeding, especially in the postmenopausal patient. All these conditions can have a similar sonographic appearance. A hyperechoic line partially or completely surrounding the endometrium has been described as a sign of a focal intracavitary process, likely caused by the interface between the intraluminal mass and the surrounding endometrium or the endometrium itself.[76]

Sonohysterography has been shown to be of great value in further evaluating the abnormally thickened endometrium.[51,52,77-80] SHG can distinguish between focal and diffuse endometrial abnormalities and help determine further management. If the abnormality is diffuse, a blind, nondirected biopsy can be done, but a focal process requires hysteroscopy with directed biopsy or excision.[52,80] SHG may also be able to distinguish benign from malignant endometrial processes.[81,82] Patients with endometrial cancer may have poorly distensible endometrial cavities, despite successful cervical os cannulation.[82]

With the reconstructed coronal view, 3-D sonography also has been a valuable addition to standard transvaginal ultrasound in patients with suspected endometrial abnormalities and in those with an endometrium greater than 6 mm.[1]

Postmenopausal Endometrium

Postmenopausal bleeding is considered to be any vaginal bleeding that occurs in a postmenopausal woman other than the expected cyclic bleeding with sequential HRT. Because the prevalence of endometrial cancer is low, the negative predictive value of a thin endometrium is high; therefore a thin endometrium can be reliably used to exclude cancer. Several studies have shown that in patients with postmenopausal bleeding who have had endometrial sampling, an endometrial measurement of **4 mm or less**[83-85] or **5 mm or less**[86-88] can be considered **normal.** The bleeding in these patients is usually caused by an **atrophic endometrium.** In 1168 women with postmenopausal bleeding, in whom 114 endometrial cancers were found, no women with endometrial cancer had an endometrium measuring less than 5 mm.[84]

A meta-analysis of 35 published studies that included 5892 women showed that an endometrial thickness greater than 5 mm detected 96% of endometrial cancer and 92% of any endometrial disease.[89] Using this meta-analysis, a multispecialty consensus conference sponsored by the Society of Radiologists in Ultrasound to discuss the role of sonography in women with postmenopausal bleeding concluded that an **endometrial thickness of greater than 5 mm is abnormal.**[90]

Transvaginal assessment of endometrial thickness has been shown to be highly reproducible, with excellent intraobserver and good interobserver agreement.[91] If the endometrium cannot be visualized in its entirety or its margins are indistinct, the examination should be considered "nondiagnostic" and lead to further investigation (e.g., SHG, hysteroscopy).[90] The consensus conference also addressed when SHG or hysteroscopy should be used in the evaluation of postmenopausal bleeding, agreeing that either is appropriate if a focal abnormality is suspected on transvaginal sonography, and that sonohysterography is more sensitive than transvaginal sonography alone in detecting focal abnormalities in women with postmenopausal bleeding. Some recommend that all women with postmenopausal bleeding should undergo SHG, even if the transvaginal sonogram is normal.[92,93] Neele et al.[94] found 30% of 111 healthy asymptomatic postmenopausal women with a normal transvaginal sonogram had SHG-detected endometrial abnormalities. The important question is whether finding and treating these benign conditions improves the patient's quality of life, morbidity, and survival; further investigation is warranted.[90]

Other studies have assessed the endometrium in **asymptomatic postmenopausal patients** and concluded that an **endometrium of 8 mm or less** can be considered **normal.**[25,95-97] Most of these reports have included a mixed group of patients, with some undergoing HRT and some not undergoing HRT. In a theoretical cohort of postmenopausal women age 50 years or older who were not bleeding or receiving HRT, Smith-Bindman et al.[98] recommended that biopsy should be considered if the endometrium measures greater than 11 mm, because the risk of cancer is 6.7% (similar to that of a postmenopausal woman with bleeding and endometrial thickness >5 mm). **If the endometrium measures 11 mm or less, biopsy is not needed because the risk of cancer is extremely low.**[98] Using this cutoff provides an acceptable trade-off between cancer detection and unnecessary biopsies prompted by an incidental finding.

Postmenopausal patients may be receiving HRT, because estrogen replacement decreases the risk of osteoporosis and relieves menopausal symptoms. However, unopposed estrogen replacement is associated with an increased risk of endometrial hyperplasia and carcinoma. Therefore, estrogen therapy is frequently combined with progesterone in **continuous combined** or in **sequential** regimens. Patients receiving sequential HRT have a changing endometrial appearance on sonography similar to the premenopausal endometrium. If noncyclic bleeding occurs, endometrial hyperplasia, polyps, and malignancy must be considered. In these patients, sonography should be done 4 to 5 days after completion of the cyclic bleeding, when the endometrium is thinnest.[90,99]

A small amount of fluid within the endometrial canal, detected by transvaginal sonography, may be a normal finding in asymptomatic patients[100] (Fig. 15-15). Larger amounts of fluid may be associated with benign conditions, most often related to cervical stenosis, or with malignancy.[101,102] The fluid should be excluded when measuring the endometrium. Because the fluid allows better detail of the endometrium, it is extremely important to assess the endometrium carefully for irregularities and polypoid masses.[103]

Hydrometrocolpos and Hematometrocolpos

Obstruction of the genital tract results in the accumulation of secretions and blood in the uterus (metro)

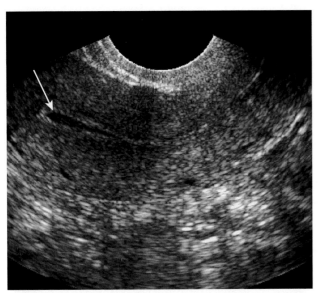

FIGURE 15-15. Normal postmenopausal endometrium on transvaginal scan. Small amount of fluid *(arrow)* is seen in postmenopausal endometrial canal.

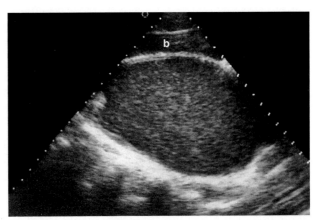

FIGURE 15-16. Hematocolpos in young patient with imperforate hymen. Sagittal transabdominal scan shows distended vagina filled with echogenic material and compressing the bladder *(b)* anteriorly.

and/or vagina *(colpos),* with the location depending on the amount of obstruction. Before menstruation, the accumulation of secretions in the vagina and uterus is referred to as **hydrometrocolpos.** After menstruation, **hematometrocolpos** results from the presence of retained menstrual blood. The obstruction may be congenital and is usually caused by an **imperforate hymen.** Other congenital causes include a **vaginal septum, vaginal atresia,** or a **rudimentary uterine horn.**[104] Hydrometra and hematometra may also be acquired as a result of cervical stenosis from endometrial or cervical **tumors** or from postirradiation **fibrosis.**[101,105]

Sonographically, if the obstruction is at the vaginal level, there is marked distention of the vagina and endometrial cavity with fluid. If seen before puberty, the accumulation of secretions is anechoic. After menstruation, the presence of old blood results in echogenic material in the fluid (Fig. 15-16). There may also be layering of the echogenic material, resulting in a fluid-fluid level.

Acquired hydrometra or hematometra usually shows a distended, fluid-filled endometrial cavity that may contain echogenic material (Fig. 15-17). Superimposed infection **(pyometra)** is difficult to distinguish from hydrometra on sonography, and this diagnosis is usually made clinically in the presence of hydrometra.[105]

Endometrial Hyperplasia

Hyperplasia of the endometrium is defined as a proliferation of glands of irregular size and shape, with an increase in the gland/stroma ratio compared with the normal proliferative endometrium.[40] The process is diffuse but may not involve the entire endometrium. Histologically,

endometrial hyperplasia can be divided into hyperplasia without cellular atypia and hyperplasia with cellular atypia **(atypical hyperplasia).** Long-term follow-up studies have shown that about 25% of atypical hyperplasia will progress to carcinoma, versus less than 2% of hyperplasia without cellular atypia.[40] Each of these types may be further subdivided into **simple** or **complex** hyperplasia, depending on the amount of glandular complexity and crowding. In simple **(cystic)** hyperplasia, the glands are cystically dilated and surrounded by abundant cellular stroma, whereas in complex **(adenomatous)** hyperplasia, the glands are crowded together with little intervening stroma.

Endometrial hyperplasia is a common cause of abnormal uterine bleeding. Hyperplasia develops from unopposed estrogen stimulation; in postmenopausal and perimenopausal women, it is usually caused by unopposed estrogen HRT. Hyperplasia is less often seen during the reproductive years, but it may occur in women with persistent anovulatory cycles, polycystic ovarian disease, and in obese women with increased production of endogenous estrogens. Hyperplasia may also be seen in women with estrogen-producing tumors, such as ovarian granulosa cell tumors and thecomas.

Sonographically, the endometrium is usually diffusely thick and echogenic, with well-defined margins (Fig. 15-18). Focal or asymmetrical thickening can also occur. Small cysts may be seen within the endometrium in **cystic hyperplasia;** however, a similar appearance may be seen in **cystic atrophy,** and cystic changes can also be seen in endometrial **polyps.** These cystic areas represent the dilated cystic glands seen at histology.[106,107] Although cystic changes within a thickened endometrium are more frequently seen in benign conditions, they can also be seen in endometrial **carcinoma.**[108] Because hyperplasia has a nonspecific sonographic appearance, biopsy is necessary for diagnosis.

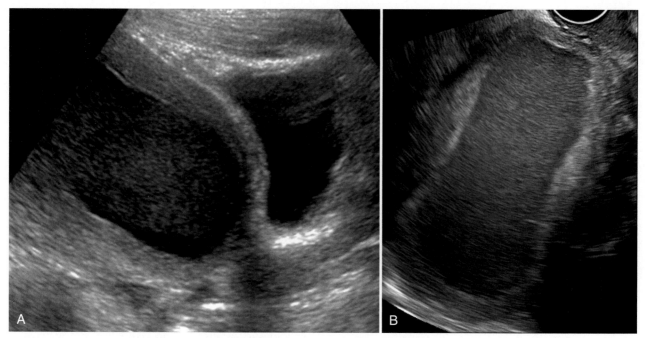

FIGURE 15-17. Hematometra in patient with cervical stenosis secondary to cervical carcinoma. A, Transabdominal, and **B,** transvaginal, scans show greatly distended endometrial canal filled with particulate echogenic material, a result of blood and debris.

Endometrial Atrophy

The majority of women with postmenopausal uterine bleeding have endometrial atrophy.[84-88,109] On transvaginal sonography, an atrophic endometrium is usually thin, measuring less than 5 mm, and in these patients, no further investigation or therapy is necessary. Histologically, the endometrial glands may be dilated, but the cells are cuboidal or flat, and the stroma is fibrotic. A thin endometrium with cystic changes on transvaginal sonography is consistent with a diagnosis of cystic atrophy, but when the endometrium is thick, the appearance is indistinguishable from that of cystic hyperplasia.[108]

Endometrial Polyps

Endometrial polyps are common benign lesions more frequently seen in perimenopausal and postmenopausal women. Polyps may cause uterine bleeding, although most are asymptomatic. In the menstruating woman, endometrial polyps may be associated with intermenstrual bleeding or menometrorrhagia and may be a cause of infertility. Histologically, polyps are localized overgrowths of endometrial tissue covered by epithelium and projecting above the adjacent surface epithelium.[40] They may be pedunculated or broad based, or may have a thin stalk. Approximately 20% of endometrial polyps are multiple. Malignant degeneration is uncommon. Occasionally, a polyp will have a long stalk, allowing it to protrude into the cervix or even into the vagina.

On sonography, polyps may appear as nonspecific echogenic endometrial thickening, which may be diffuse or focal (see Fig. 15-7, *G*). However, they may also appear as a focal, round, echogenic mass within the endometrial cavity[110] (see Figs. 15-7, *F,* and 15-18). This appearance is much more easily identified when there is fluid within the endometrial cavity outlining the mass. Because fluid is instilled into the endometrial cavity during SHG, this technique is ideal for demonstrating polyps (Fig. 15-19, *A-F*). SHG is also a valuable technique when transvaginal sonography is unable to differentiate an **endometrial polyp** from a **submucosal leiomyoma** (Figs. 15-19, *G* and *H*). The polyp can be seen arising from the endometrium, whereas a normal layer of endometrium is seen overlying the submucosal fibroid. Cystic areas may be seen within a polyp (see Fig. 15-7, *I*), representing the histologically dilated glands.[106,107] A feeding artery in the pedicle can frequently be seen with color Doppler ultrasound (pedicle artery sign) and negate the need for sonohysterography[111,112] (see Fig. 15-18, *B*).

Endometrial polyps may not be diagnosed on D&C because a polyp on a pliable stalk may be missed by the curette. If abnormal bleeding persists after a nondiagnostic D&C in a postmenopausal woman with an endometrial thickness greater than 8 mm, hysteroscopy with direct visualization of the endometrial cavity is recommended.[113]

Endometrial Carcinoma

Endometrial carcinoma is the most common gynecologic malignancy in North America. The American Cancer Society (ACS) estimated 40,100 new cases of

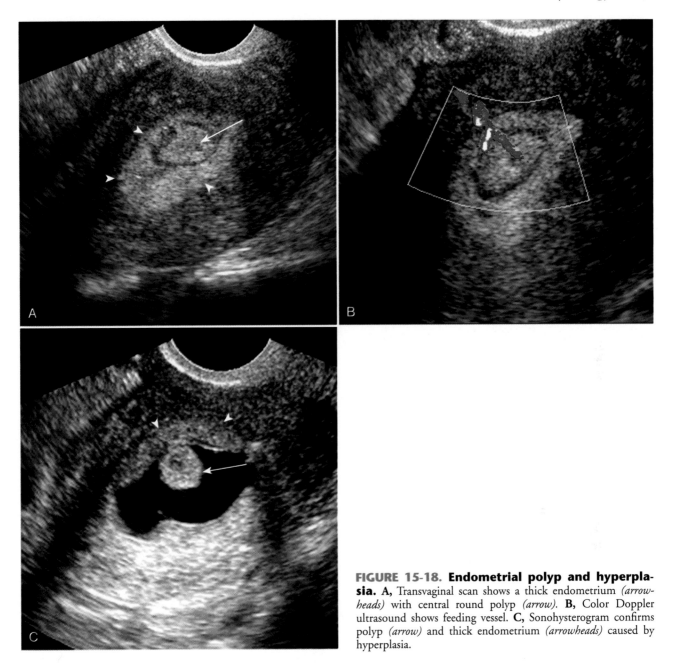

FIGURE 15-18. Endometrial polyp and hyperplasia. A, Transvaginal scan shows a thick endometrium *(arrowheads)* with central round polyp *(arrow).* **B,** Color Doppler ultrasound shows feeding vessel. **C,** Sonohysterogram confirms polyp *(arrow)* and thick endometrium *(arrowheads)* caused by hyperplasia.

endometrial cancer in the United States in 2008, with about 7470 deaths. Since 1998, the incidence has been decreasing by about 0.8% a year after a period of increase during the previous decade. Mortality rates have been stable since 1992.[114] Endometrial carcinoma is highly curable because more than 75% are confined to the uterus at clinical presentation. Most endometrial carcinomas (75%-80%) occur in postmenopausal women. The most common clinical presentation is uterine bleeding, although only about **10% of women with postmenopausal bleeding will have endometrial carcinoma.** There is a strong association with estrogen replacement therapy in postmenopausal women and anovulatory cycles in premenopausal women. Other risk factors include obesity, diabetes, hypertension, and low

parity. Approximately 25% of patients with atypical endometrial hyperplasia will progress to well-differentiated endometrial carcinoma.[40]

Sonographically, **a thickened endometrium must be considered cancer until proven otherwise.** The thickened endometrium may be well defined, uniformly echogenic, and indistinguishable from hyperplasia and polyps. Cancer is more likely when the endometrium has a heterogeneous echotexture with irregular or poorly defined margins (Fig. 15-20). Cystic changes within the endometrium are more frequently seen in endometrial atrophy, hyperplasia, and polyps but can also be seen with carcinoma. Endometrial carcinoma may also obstruct the endometrial canal, resulting in hydrometra or hematometra. Although certain sonographic appear-

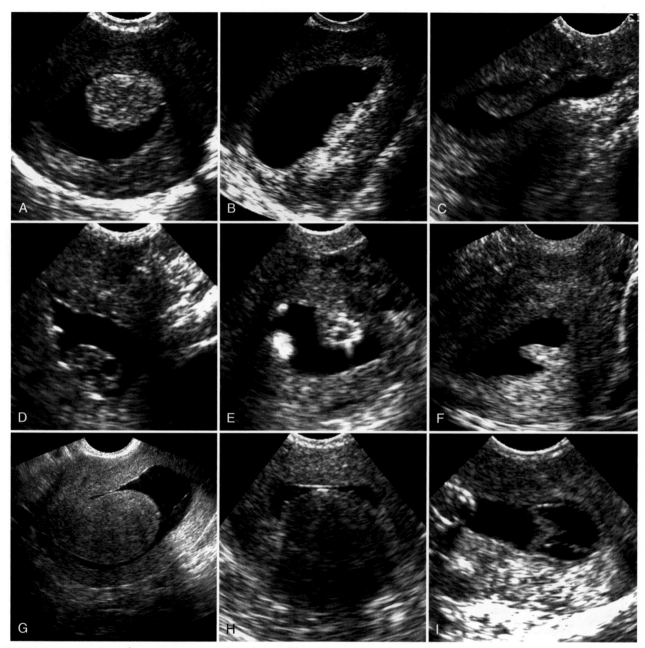

FIGURE 15-19. Sonohysterograms of polyps, fibroids, and adhesions. A, Well-defined, round echogenic polyp. **B,** Carpet of small polyps. **C,** Polyp on a stalk. **D,** Polyp with cystic areas. **E,** Small polyp. **F,** Small polyp. **G,** Hypoechoic submucosal fibroid. **H,** Hypoechoic attenuating submucosal fibroid. **I,** Endometrial adhesions. Note bridging bands of tissue within fluid-filled endometrial canal.

ances tend to favor a benign or malignant etiology, there are overlapping features, and endometrial biopsy is usually required for a definitive diagnosis.

The role of color and spectral Doppler ultrasound in the diagnosis of endometrial carcinoma is still controversial. Blood flow is difficult to detect in the normal endometrium. Initial studies using transvaginal color and spectral Doppler ultrasound suggested that endometrial carcinoma could be differentiated from a normal or benign postmenopausal endometrium by the presence of low-resistance flow in the uterine arteries in women with endometrial cancer, compared with high-resistance flow

in women with normal or benign endometria.[115,116] Subsequent reports, however, have shown no significant difference in uterine blood flow between benign and malignant endometrial processes.[117-119] Low-resistance flow in the uterine artery has also been reported in association with uterine fibroids.[116] Some reports have shown low-resistance flow in the subendometrial and endometrial arteries in malignant endometrial lesions,[97,120] whereas others have found no statistically significant difference.[118,119,121] Sladkevicius et al.[119] found that endometrial thickness is a better method for discriminating between normal and pathologic or benign and malignant

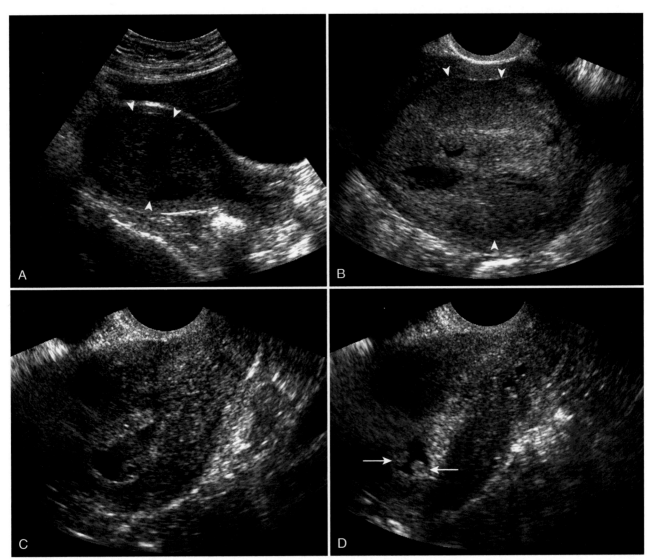

FIGURE 15-20. Endometrial carcinoma: varying appearance in two patients. A, Transabdominal scan, and **B,** transvaginal scan, show a large, heterogeneous endometrial mass *(arrowheads)* compressing the surrounding myometrium. **C** and **D,** Transvaginal scans show localized irregular endometrial thickening with echogenic polypoid projections *(arrows)* into the fluid-filled endometrial canal.

endometrium than Doppler ultrasound of the uterine, subendometrial, or intraendometrial arteries.[119]

Sonography may be used in the preoperative evaluation of a patient with endometrial carcinoma by determining myometrial invasion.[122-124] An intact **subendometrial halo** (inner layer of myometrium) usually indicates superficial invasion, whereas obliteration of the halo indicates deep invasion.[124] Transvaginal sonography and unenhanced T2-weighted MRI have been reported to have similar accuracy,[125] but contrast-enhanced MRI has been shown to be superior to both in demonstrating myometrial invasion.[126-128] MRI can also assess cervical extension (stage II) and extrauterine extension (stages III and IV).

Tamoxifen, a nonsteroidal antiestrogen compound, is widely used for adjuvant therapy in premenopausal and postmenopausal women with breast cancer. Tamoxifen acts by competing with estrogen for estrogen receptors.

In premenopausal women, tamoxifen has an antiestrogenic effect, but in postmenopausal women it may have estrogenic effects. An **increased risk of endometrial carcinoma** has been reported in patients receiving tamoxifen therapy,[129] as well as an **increased risk of endometrial hyperplasia and polyps**.[130,131] On sonography, tamoxifen-related endometrial changes are nonspecific and similar to those described in hyperplasia, polyps, and carcinoma.[131-133] Cystic changes within the thickened endometrium are frequently seen (see Fig. 15-7, *H* and *I*). Polyps are frequently seen and have a higher incidence in women receiving tamoxifen than in untreated women, and these polyps can be quite large.[134,135] A correlation exists between increased endometrial thickness and duration of tamoxifen therapy longer than 5 years.[134] In some patients taking tamoxifen, the cystic changes actually have been shown to be subendometrial in location and represent abnormal

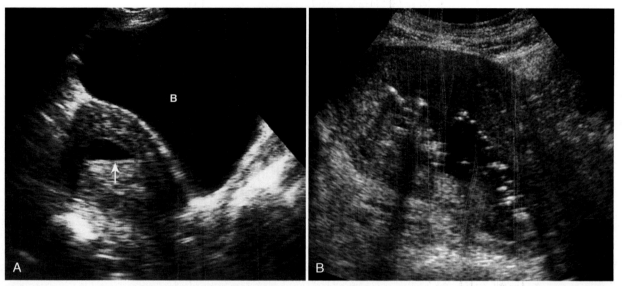

FIGURE 15-21. Endometritis: varying appearance in two patients. Transabdominal sagittal scans. **A,** Fluid-fluid level *(arrow)* within endometrial canal in patient with pelvic inflammatory disease; *B,* bladder. This resolved after antibiotic therapy. **B,** Multiple linear hyperechogenic foci with shadowing caused by gas are seen within a distended endometrial canal in a febrile postpartum patient.

adenomyosis-like changes in the inner layer of myometrium.[136] Because it may be difficult to distinguish the endometrial-myometrial border in many of these patients, sonohysterography is valuable in determining whether an abnormality is endometrial or subendometrial.[137,138] Routine ultrasound screening of asymptomatic women receiving tamoxifen has not been effective in increasing the early detection of endometrial cancer and is therefore not recommended.[139]

Endometritis

Endometritis may occur postpartum, after D&C, or in association with PID. Sonographically, the endometrium may appear thick and/or irregular, and the cavity may or may not contain fluid (Fig. 15-21). Gas with distal acoustic shadowing may be seen within the endometrial canal. However, gas can also be seen in up to 21% of clinically normal women, after uncomplicated vaginal delivery in the first 3 weeks postpartum.[140] Clinical correlation is necessary when endometrial gas is seen in the postpartum patient.

Endometrial Adhesions

Endometrial adhesions (synechiae, Asherman's syndrome) are posttraumatic or postsurgical in nature and may be a cause of infertility or recurrent pregnancy loss. The sonographic diagnosis is difficult unless fluid is distending the endometrial cavity. The endometrium usually appears normal on transabdominal and transvaginal sonograms, although adhesions may be seen transvaginally as irregularities or a hypoechoic bridgelike band within the endometrium.[141] This is best seen during the secretory phase, when the endometrium is more

hyperechoic. SHG is an excellent technique for demonstrating adhesions and should be performed in all cases of suspected adhesions.[142] Adhesions appear as bridging bands of tissue that distort the cavity (see Fig. 15-19, *I*) or as thin, undulating membranes best seen on real-time sonography.[4] Thick, broad-based adhesions may prevent distention of the uterine cavity.[77] The adhesions can be divided under hysteroscopy.

Intrauterine Contraceptive Devices

Sonography has an important role in evaluating the location of intrauterine contraceptive devices (IUCDs). IUCDs are readily demonstrated on both transabdominal and transvaginal sonography (Fig. 15-22). They appear as highly echogenic linear structures in the endometrial cavity in the body of the uterus. Several types of IUCDs demonstrate a characteristic appearance on sonography, reflecting their gross appearance. Acoustic shadowing from the IUCD is usually demonstrated, and two parallel echoes (entrance-exit reflections), representing the anterior and posterior surfaces of the IUCD, may also be observed[143] (Fig. 15-22, *A*). Newer hormone-containing IUCDs (e.g., Mirena) may be difficult to visualize sonographically.[144] 3DUS has been extremely useful in providing a more complete assessment of IUCD location by imaging the entire IUCD simultaneously in the coronal plane[144,145] (Fig. 15-22, *D*). Sonography can demonstrate malposition, perforation, and incomplete removal (Fig. 15-22, *E-H*). Eccentric position of an IUCD suggests myometrial penetration. If the IUCD is not seen on sonography, a radiograph should be taken to assess whether it is lying free in the peritoneal cavity or is not present, having been previously expelled. The IUCD may be hidden by coexisting intrauterine

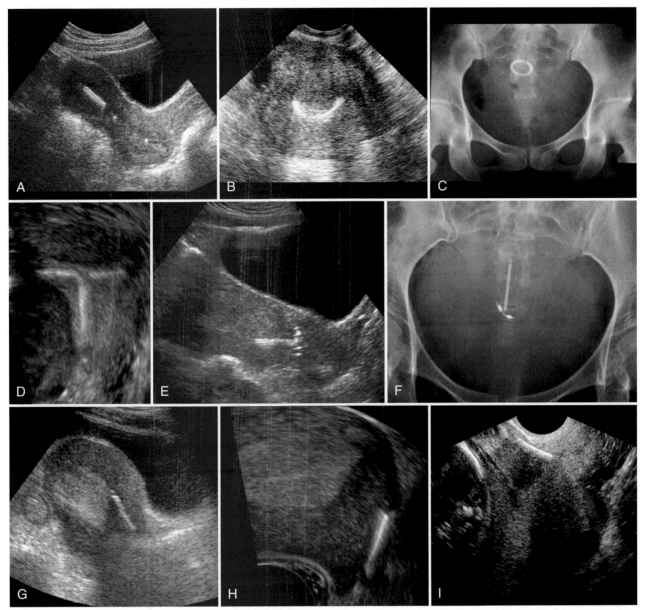

FIGURE 15-22. Intrauterine contraceptive devices (IUCDs). A, B, E, and **G,** Transabdominal scans; **H** and **I,** transvaginal scans. **A,** Highly echogenic linear structure in normal location within endometrial canal in body of uterus. **B,** Unusual Chinese ring IUCD, **C,** Radiograph of **B. D,** 3-D coronal reconstruction shows entire IUCD in normal location. **E,** IUCD in upside-down position with limbs positioned inferiorly. **F,** Radiograph of **E. G,** IUCD abnormally positioned in lower uterine segment. **H,** IUCD located in outer myometrium. **I,** IUCD in a 30-week gravid uterus.

abnormalities, such as blood clots or an incomplete abortion. When an IUCD is present in the uterus in association with an intrauterine pregnancy (Fig. 15-22, *I*), it can be seen reliably early in the first trimester, but it is rarely identified thereafter. In the first trimester the device can usually be removed safely under ultrasound guidance.

Abnormalities of the Cervix

The cervix may be difficult to assess adequately by transabdominal sonography because it lies low in the pelvis,

posterior to the bladder. Better visualization is obtained by transvaginal sonography, which can reliably diagnose normal and benign cervical conditions.[146]

Nabothian (inclusion) cysts of the cervix are often seen during routine sonography (Fig. 15-23). They may vary in size from a few millimeters to 4 cm, may be single or multiple, and are usually diagnosed incidentally, although they may be associated with healing chronic cervicitis. Occasionally, nabothian cysts have internal echoes, possibly caused by hemorrhage or infection. Multiple cysts may be a cause of benign enlargement of the cervix.[147]

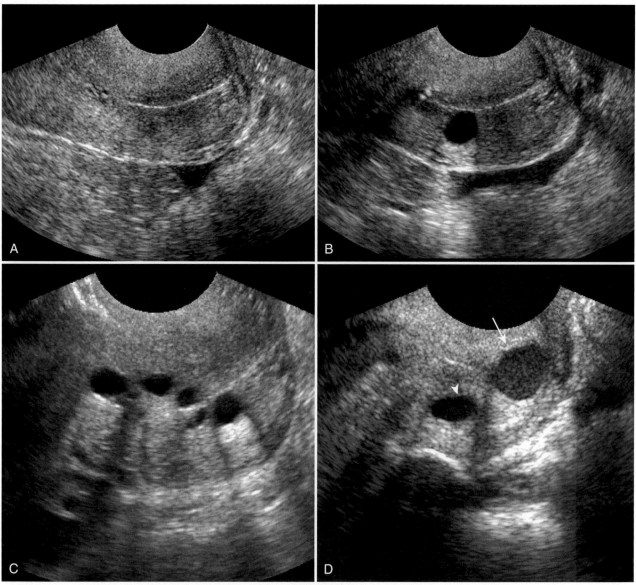

FIGURE 15-23. Nabothian cysts on transvaginal scans. A, Normal cervix. **B,** Single nabothian cyst in cervix. **C,** Multiple nabothian cysts. **D,** Hemorrhagic nabothian cyst *(arrow)* and simple nabothian cyst *(arrowhead)*.

Cervical polyps are a frequent cause of vaginal bleeding and may be seen on sonography, although the diagnosis is usually made clinically. Approximately 8% of **leiomyomas** arise in the cervix. They may be pedunculated and may prolapse into the vagina. In patients who underwent supracervical hysterectomy, the **cervical remnant** occasionally simulates a mass. Transvaginal sonography is usually diagnostic; it can demonstrate a normal cervix. The cervical remnant may measure up to 4.4 cm in AP diameter and 4.3 cm in length.[148] **Cervical stenosis** may be secondary to previous radiation therapy, previous cone biopsy, postmenopausal cervical atrophy, or cervical carcinoma.

Cervical carcinoma is usually diagnosed clinically, and patients are rarely referred for sonographic evaluation. Sonography may demonstrate a solid retrovesical mass, which may be indistinguishable from a cervical fibroid (Fig. 15-24). MRI is used for staging cervical carcinoma.

Adenoma malignum, also termed "minimal deviation adenocarcinoma," is a rare cervical neoplasm arising from the endocervical glands and often associated with Peutz-Jeghers syndrome.[149] Multiple cystic areas are seen within a solid cervical mass[149,150] (Fig. 15-25). This condition should be easily differentiated from deep nabothian cysts because nabothian cysts do not have an associated mass.

VAGINA

The vagina runs anteriorly and caudally from the cervix between the bladder and rectum. It is best seen on midline sagittal sonograms with a slight caudal angula-

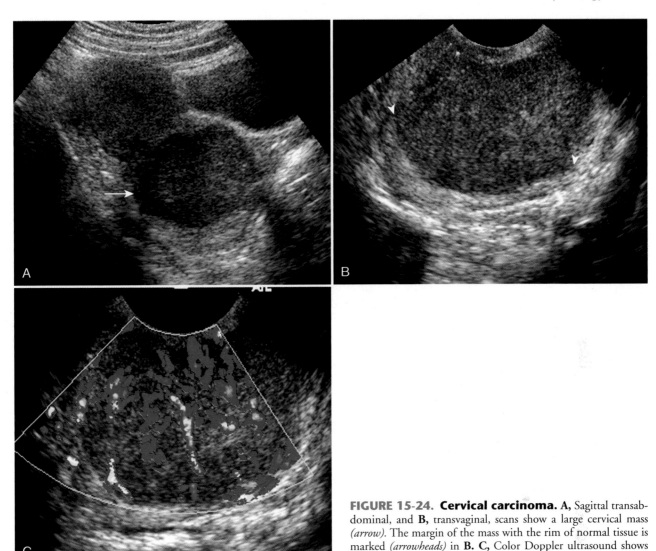

FIGURE 15-24. Cervical carcinoma. A, Sagittal transabdominal, and **B,** transvaginal, scans show a large cervical mass *(arrow).* The margin of the mass with the rim of normal tissue is marked *(arrowheads)* in **B. C,** Color Doppler ultrasound shows hypervascularity of the mass.

tion of the transducer. It appears as a collapsed hypoechoic tubular structure with a central, high-amplitude, linear echo representing the apposed surfaces of the vaginal mucosa (see Fig. 15-2). The most common congenital abnormality of the female genital tract is an **imperforate hymen** resulting in **hematocolpos.** Occasionally, sonography is used to characterize a vaginal mass. **Gartner's duct cysts** are remnants of the caudal end of the mesonephric duct that form single or multiple masses along the lateral or anterolateral wall of the vagina. These are the most common cystic lesions of the vagina and are usually found incidentally during sonographic examination. They are usually small and asymptomatic and may be associated with renal and ureteral abnormalities.[151] Solid masses of the vagina are rare. Two cases of **neurofibroma** of the vagina that appear as solid masses have been described.[152] As in carcinoma of the cervix, sonography is not used for diagnosis of carcinoma of the vagina, although it may play a role in staging.

In patients with hysterectomy, a **vaginal cuff** should not be mistaken for a mass. Stein et al.[148] found the upper limit of normal for the vaginal cuff to be 2.2 cm in women who had had a transvaginal hysterectomy and 2.4 cm in those that had had a transabdominal hysterectomy. Also, the AP diameter decreased significantly with advancing age, and color Doppler ultrasound typically showed flow within the cuff. A cuff larger than 2.2 cm or containing a definite mass suggests malignancy. Nodular areas may be caused by postradiation fibrosis.[153]

RECTOUTERINE RECESS

The rectouterine recess **(posterior cul-de-sac)** is the most posterior and inferior reflection of the peritoneal cavity. It is located between the rectum and vagina and is also known as the **pouch of Douglas.** The posterior fornix of the vagina is closely related to the posterior cul-de-sac and is separated by the thickness of the vaginal wall and the peritoneal membrane. The cul-de-sac is a potential space, and because of its location, it is fre-

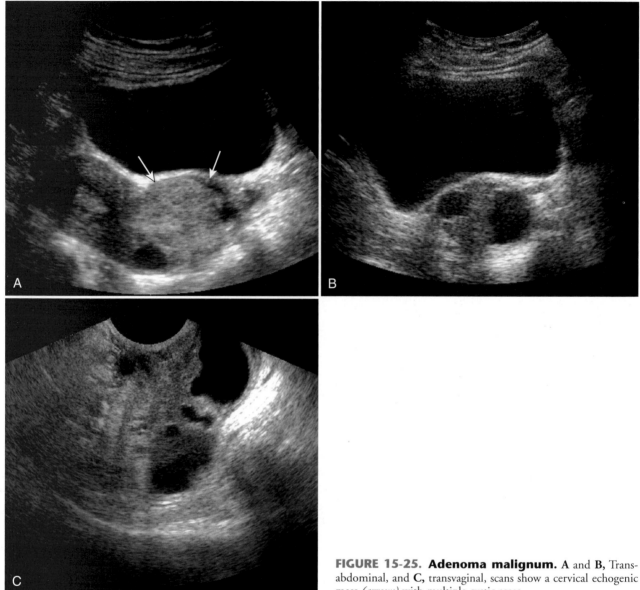

FIGURE 15-25. Adenoma malignum. A and B, Trans-abdominal, and C, transvaginal, scans show a cervical echogenic mass *(arrows)* with multiple cystic areas.

quently the initial site for intraperitoneal fluid collection. As little as 5 mL of fluid has been detected by transvaginal sonography.[154]

Fluid in the cul-de-sac is a normal finding in asymptomatic women and can be seen during all phases of the menstrual cycle. Possible sources include blood or fluid caused by follicular rupture, blood from retrograde menstruation, and increased capillary permeability of the ovarian surface caused by the influence of estrogen.[155,156] Pathologic fluid collections in the pouch of Douglas may be seen in association with generalized **ascites**, **blood** resulting from a ruptured ectopic pregnancy or hemorrhagic cyst, or **pus** from infection. Sonography may aid in differentiating the type of fluid, because blood, pus, mucin, and malignant exudates usually contain echoes within the fluid, whereas serous fluid (either physiologic or pathologic) is usually anechoic. Clotted blood may be

very echogenic.[157] Transvaginal sonography can demonstrate echoes within the fluid more frequently because of its improved resolution (Fig. 15-26). Pelvic abscesses and hematomas can also occur in the cul-de-sac.

OVARY

Normal Sonographic Anatomy

Uterine location influences the position of the ovaries. The normal ovaries are usually identified laterally or posterolaterally to the anteflexed midline uterus. When the uterus lies to one side of the midline (a normal variant), the ipsilateral ovary often lies superior to the uterine fundus. In a retroverted uterus, the ovaries tend to be located laterally and superiorly, near the uterine

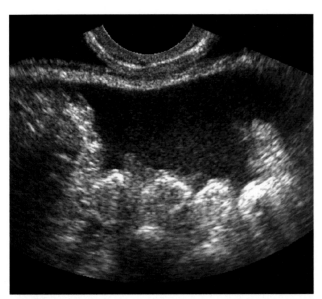

FIGURE 15-26. **Echogenic fluid** in cul-de-sac caused by blood on transvaginal scan.

fundus. When the uterus is enlarged, the ovaries tend to be displaced more superiorly and laterally. After hysterectomy, the ovaries tend to be located more medially and directly superior to the vaginal cuff.

Because of the laxity of the ligamentous attachments, the ovary can be quite variable in position and may be located high in the pelvis or in the cul-de-sac. Because of their **variable position,** superiorly or extremely laterally placed ovaries may not be visualized by the transvaginal approach because they are out of the FOV. The ovaries are ellipsoid in shape, with their craniocaudad axes paralleling the internal iliac vessels, which lie posteriorly and serve as a helpful reference (Fig. 15-27).

On sonography, the normal ovary has a relatively homogeneous echotexture with a central, more echogenic medulla. Small, well-defined anechoic or cystic follicles may be seen peripherally in the cortex. The appearance of the ovary changes with age and phase of the menstrual cycle. During the early **proliferative phase,** many follicles that are stimulated by both follicle-stimulating hormone (FSH) and luteinizing hormone (LH) develop and increase in size until about day 8 or 9 of the menstrual cycle. At that time, one follicle becomes dominant, destined for ovulation, and increases in size, reaching up to 2.0 to 2.5 cm at ovulation. The other follicles become atretic. A **follicular cyst** develops if the fluid in one of these nondominant follicles is not resorbed. After ovulation, the **corpus luteum** develops and may be identified sonographically as a small, hypoechoic or isoechoic structure peripherally within the ovary. The corpus luteum involutes before menstruation.

Because of the variability in shape, **ovarian volume** has been considered the best method for determining ovarian size. The volume measurement is based on the formula for a prolate ellipse (0.523 × length × width ×

height). Studies have shown that ovarian volumes are larger than previously thought. In the first 2 years of life, the mean ovarian volume is slightly greater than 1 cubic centimeters (cc) in the first year and 0.7 cc in the second year.[158] The upper limit of normal has been reported as 3.6 cc in the first 3 months, 2.7 cc from 4 to 12 months, and 1.7 cc in the second year.[158] Ovarian volume remains relatively stable up to 5 years of age and then gradually increases up to menarche, when the mean volume is 4.2 ± 2.3 cc, with an upper limit of 8.0 cc.[8] Small follicles or cysts are frequently seen in neonatal and premenarchal ovaries. One study showed follicle activity in 87% of prepubertal girls.[11] These follicles usually measure less than 9 mm but may be as large as 17 mm.[159]

In the menstruating adult female, a normal ovary may have a volume as large as 22 cc. Cohen et al.[160] assessed 866 normal ovaries by transabdominal sonography and reported a mean ovarian volume of 9.8 ± 5.8 cc, with an upper limit of 21.9 cc.[160] Another study of 406 patients with normal ovaries used transvaginal sonography and reported a mean ovarian volume of 6.8 cc, with an upper limit of 18.0 cc.[161] There is no significant parity-related change in ovarian volume in premenopausal women.[13]

Echogenic ovarian foci are commonly seen in an otherwise normal-appearing ovary (Fig. 15-28). These are tiny (1-3 mm) nonshadowing foci, usually multiple and peripherally located, although they can be diffuse. They were thought to represent inclusion cysts and associated psammomatous calcifications.[162] In a study with histopathologic correlation in seven normal ovaries with echogenic foci, Muradali et al.[163] showed that these foci are caused by a specular reflection from the walls of **tiny unresolved cysts** below the spatial resolution of ultrasound rather than calcification. These echogenic foci do not indicate significant underlying disease, so no further investigation or follow-up is necessary.

Focal calcification may occasionally be seen in an otherwise normal-appearing ovary and is thought to represent stromal reaction to previous hemorrhage or infection.[164] However, the calcification may be the initial or early manifestation of a neoplasm, so follow-up sonography is recommended.

Postmenopausal Ovary

After menopause, the ovary atrophies and the follicles disappear over the subsequent few years, with the ovary decreasing in size with increasing age.[13,165-167] Because of its smaller size and lack of follicles, the postmenopausal ovary may be difficult to visualize sonographically (Fig. 15-29). A stationary loop of bowel may be mistaken for a normal ovary; therefore, scanning must be done slowly to look for peristalsis. Sonographic visualization of normal postmenopausal ovaries varies greatly in the literature, from a low of 20% to a high of 99%, using either the transabdominal or the transvaginal approach.[161,165-170] The variation is likely caused by differences in technique

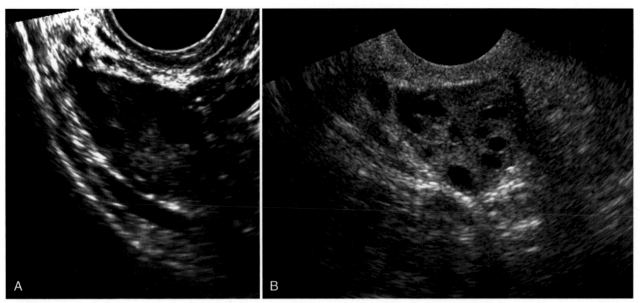

FIGURE 15-27. Normal ovary. A and **B,** Transvaginal scans show normal ovaries with a few follicles in two patients. Internal iliac vein is posterior to ovary.

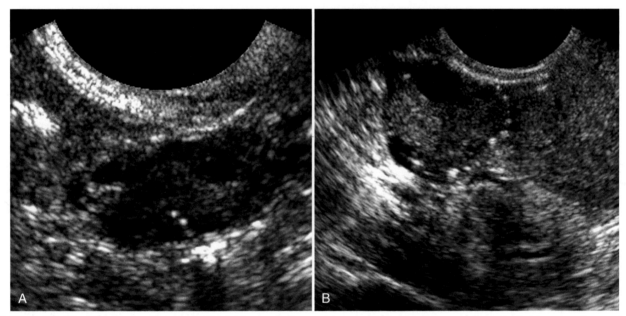

FIGURE 15-28. Ovarian echogenic foci. Transvaginal scans in two patients. **A,** Two tiny echogenic foci in normal-appearing ovary. **B,** Multiple peripheral tiny echogenic foci (tiny unresolved cysts).

and length of time since menopause. The ovary decreases in size with increasing age, and therefore the ability to see the ovaries decreases with lengthening time since menopause.[171]

Also, the absence of the uterus may play a role because the ovaries are less likely to be seen after hysterectomy because of the loss of normal anatomic landmarks. In 290 postmenopausal ovaries known to be present, Wolf et al.[171] visualized only 41% of ovaries transvaginally and 58% transabdominally. Using both transabdominal and transvaginal techniques resulted in their visualizing more ovaries (68%) than when they used either approach

alone. Highly placed ovaries may be out of the FOV of transvaginal transducers, and transabdominal sonography may not image very small or deeply placed ovaries. Nonvisualization of an ovary does not exclude an ovarian lesion.

Mean ovarian volume ranges are reported from 1.2 to 5.8 cc.[160,161,165-169] The mean values in these studies may be somewhat high because nonvisualized ovaries were not included. One study assessing 563 patients with normal postmenopausal ovaries by transvaginal sonography reported a mean ovarian volume of 2.0 cc with an upper limit of normal of 8.0 cc.[161] An **ovarian volume**

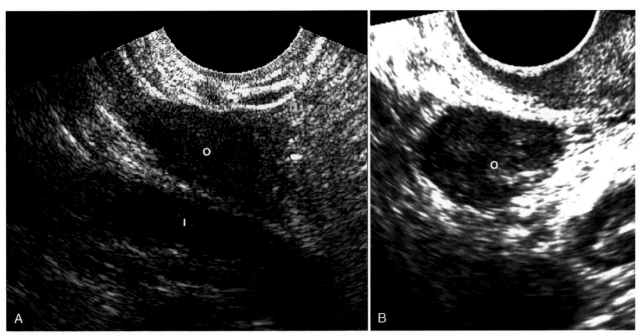

FIGURE 15-29. Normal postmenopausal ovary. A and **B,** Transvaginal scans in two patients show a normal postmenopausal ovary *(O)*; *I,* internal iliac vein. Note small size and lack of follicles.

of more than 8.0 cc is definitely considered abnormal. Some authors suggest that an ovarian volume more than twice that of the opposite side should also be considered abnormal, regardless of the actual size.[166,168]

Postmenopausal Cysts

Simple cysts may be seen in up to 15% of postmenopausal ovaries and are not related to age, length of time since menopause, or hormone use.[171] These cysts are more frequently seen by transvaginal sonography with its improved resolution, but in some women, especially those with hysterectomy or highly placed ovaries, the cysts may be seen only by transabdominal sonography. Most of these cysts either disappear or decrease in size over time[172-174] (Fig. 15-30).

Several studies have shown a very low incidence of malignancy in unilocular postmenopausal cysts less than 5 cm in diameter and without septation or solid components.[173-178] Ekerhovd et al.[178] found four borderline or malignant tumors in 247 postmenopausal women (1.6%) who underwent surgery for simple ovarian cysts detected by transvaginal sonography. These four tumors were all greater than 7.5 cm in diameter. It is generally recommended that postmenopausal women with simple ovarian cysts less than 5 cm in diameter be followed by serial sonographic examinations without surgical intervention unless there is an increase in size or change in the characteristics of the lesion. Surgery is generally recommended for postmenopausal cysts greater than 5 cm and for those containing internal septations or solid nodules.

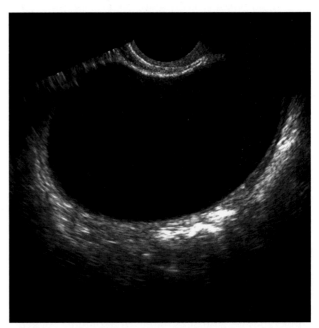

FIGURE 15-30. Postmenopausal large ovarian cyst. Transvaginal scan shows a 7-cm ovarian cyst that contains no internal echoes or septations and that had not changed in size over 4 years.

Nonneoplastic Lesions

Functional Cysts

Functional cysts of the ovary include follicular, corpus luteum, and theca lutein cysts. A **follicular cyst** occurs when a mature follicle fails to ovulate or to involute.

Because normal follicles can vary from a few millimeters up to 2.5 cm, a follicular cyst cannot be diagnosed with certainty until it is greater than 2.5 cm. Therefore, a simple cyst less than 2.5 cm in a premenopausal woman should be referred to as a **follicle** and considered to be **normal.** Follicles and follicular cysts are usually unilateral, asymptomatic, and frequently detected incidentally on sonographic examination. Follicular cysts usually regress spontaneously.

After ovulation, the **corpus luteum** develops and may be identified sonographically as a small, hypoechoic or isoechoic structure within the ovary. The corpus luteum usually contains low-level internal echoes, frequently with a thicker wall than a follicle and a crenulated appearance. It typically has a peripheral rim of color around the wall on color Doppler ultrasound (ring of fire; see Fig. 15-31, C). The corpus luteum usually involutes before menstruation but may persist because of failure of absorption or excess bleeding into the corpus luteum. Timor-Tritsch and Goldstein[179] recommend using the term "corpus luteum" rather than "corpus luteal cyst" unless it is greater than 4 to 5 cm. **Corpus luteal cysts** are less common than follicular cysts but tend to be larger and more symptomatic. Pain is the major symptom. These cysts are usually unilateral and more prone to hemorrhage and rupture. If the ovum is fertilized, the corpus luteum continues as the corpus luteum of pregnancy, which may become enlarged and cystic. Maximum size is reached at 8 to 10 weeks, and by 16 weeks the cyst has usually resolved.[180]

Hemorrhagic Cysts

Internal hemorrhage may occur in both types of functional cysts, although it is much more frequently seen in corpus luteal cysts. Women with hemorrhagic cysts frequently present with acute onset of pelvic pain. Hemorrhagic cysts show a spectrum of findings because of the variable sonographic appearance of blood (Fig. 15-31). The appearance depends on the amount of hemorrhage and the time of the hemorrhage relative to the time of the sonographic examination.[181-183] The internal characteristics are much better appreciated on transvaginal sonography because of its improved resolution. An **acute hemorrhagic cyst** is usually hyperechoic and may mimic a solid mass (Fig. 15-31, A-C). However, it usually has a smooth posterior wall and shows posterior acoustic enhancement, indicating the cystic nature of the lesion. Diffuse low-level internal echoes may be seen (Fig. 15-31, D), but this appearance is more frequently seen in endometriomas. As the clot hemolyzes, the internal pattern becomes more complex, with a reticular-type pattern containing internal echoes and interdigitating lines believed to result from fibrin strands[184] (Fig. 15-31, E and F). These should not be confused with septations, which are thicker. As the clot retracts (Fig. 15-31, G-I),

it will have a concave outer margin with angularity rather than a solid mural nodule, which will have a convex outer margin. Color Doppler ultrasound will show no flow within the clot. Patel et al.[184] found that a specific diagnosis could be made in approximately 90% of hemorrhagic cysts by demonstrating the presence of a reticular pattern or a retractile clot. The presence of echogenic, free intraperitoneal fluid in the cul-de-sac helps confirm the diagnosis of a leaking or ruptured hemorrhagic cyst. Rupture of a hemorrhagic cyst may mimic a ruptured ectopic pregnancy, both clinically and sonographically.

Functional cysts are the **most common cause of ovarian enlargement** in young women. Because functional cysts typically resolve within one to two menstrual cycles, follow-up is usually not required for small, simple cysts or typical hemorrhagic cysts. However, follow-up of larger cysts can be performed at a different time of the menstrual cycle, usually in 6 weeks, to show a changing appearance or resolution.

Surface epithelial inclusion cysts are nonfunctional cysts usually seen in postmenopausal women, although they may be seen at any age, and usually located peripherally in the cortex. They arise from cortical invaginations of the ovarian surface epithelium.[40] Although usually tiny, unilocular, and thin walled, these cysts can measure up to several centimeters in diameter. Occasionally, surface epithelial inclusion cysts may be hemorrhagic, particularly if torsion has occurred.

Pregnancy-Associated Ovarian Lesions

Ovarian lesions unique to pregnancy include hyperstimulated ovaries, ovarian hyperstimulation syndrome, theca lutein cysts, hyperreactio luteinalis, and the rare luteoma of pregnancy.[180] **Hyperstimulated ovaries** are a normal response to elevated circulating levels of hCG. It is usually diagnosed in women who have undergone ovulation induction. Sonographically, the ovaries are enlarged with multiple cysts, some of which may be hemorrhagic. The enlarged ovaries may undergo torsion.[185] They usually regress spontaneously during the pregnancy.

Ovarian hyperstimulation syndrome (OHS) is used when the hyperstimulation is accompanied by fluid shifts[186] (Fig. 15-32). Clinically, three degrees of OHS are described: mild, moderate, and severe. The **mild** form is associated with lower abdominal discomfort, but no significant weight gain. The ovaries are enlarged, but less than 5 cm in average diameter. **Moderate** OHS presents with weight gain of 5 to 10 lb and ovarian enlargement between 5 and 12 cm. The patient may have nausea and vomiting. With **severe** OHS, there is weight gain greater than 10 lb and the patient complains of severe abdominal pain and distention. The ovaries are greatly enlarged (>12 cm in diameter) and contain numerous large, thin-walled cysts, which may replace most of the ovary. The associated ascites and pleural

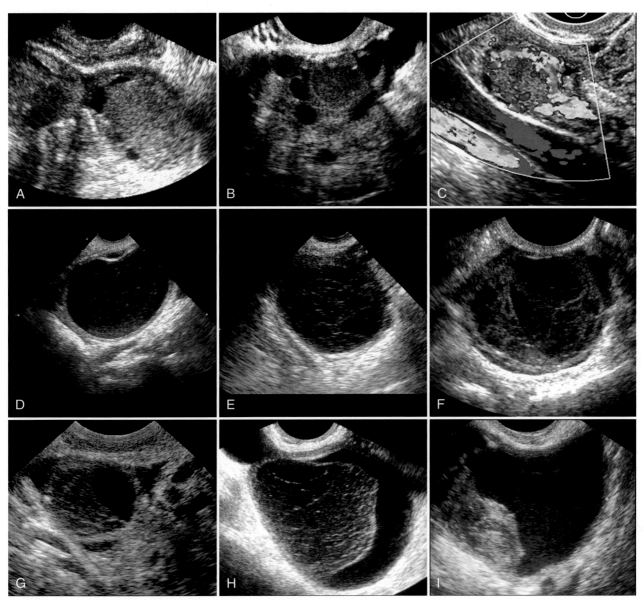

FIGURE 15-31. Hemorrhagic cysts on transvaginal scans: spectrum of appearances. A, Acute hyperechoic hemorrhagic cyst. **B,** Acute hemorrhagic cyst mimicking a solid lesion. **C,** Color Doppler ultrasound shows peripheral ring of vascularity (**ring of fire**), typical of a corpus luteum, but no vascularity within the cyst. **D,** Large cyst containing multiple internal low-level echoes. **E,** Reticular pattern of internal echoes and septations within cyst. **F,** Reticular pattern. **G, H,** and **I,** Variations in clot retraction. The clot in **I** suggests a solid mass. Lack of color Doppler ultrasound signal supports its benign nature.

effusions may lead to depletion of intravascular fluids and electrolytes, resulting in hemoconcentration with hypotension, oliguria, and electrolyte imbalance.[187] Severe OHS is usually treated conservatively to correct the depleted intravascular volume and electrolyte imbalance and usually resolves within 2 to 3 weeks.

Theca luteal cysts are the largest of the functional ovarian cysts and are associated with high hCG levels. These cysts typically occur in patients with gestational trophoblastic disease but can also be seen in OHS as a complication of drug therapy for infertility. Sonographically, theca luteal cysts are usually bilateral, multilocular, and very large. They may undergo hemorrhage, rupture, and torsion.

Hyperreactio luteinalis (HL) is caused by an abnormal response to circulating hCG in the absence of ovulation induction therapy. Approximately 60% of HL cases occur in singleton pregnancies with normal circulating levels of hCG. HL usually occurs in the third trimester or less often in the puerperium. Patients are usually asymptomatic, although maternal virilization may be seen in up to 25% of patients. Incidence of HL increases in patients with polycystic ovarian disease.[188] In contrast to OHS, body fluid shifts are rare. Sonographically, there are bilaterally enlarged ovaries with multiple cysts similar to OHS, although the ovaries tend to be not as large and the condition occurs later in pregnancy. HL is a self-limited condition that resolves spontaneously.

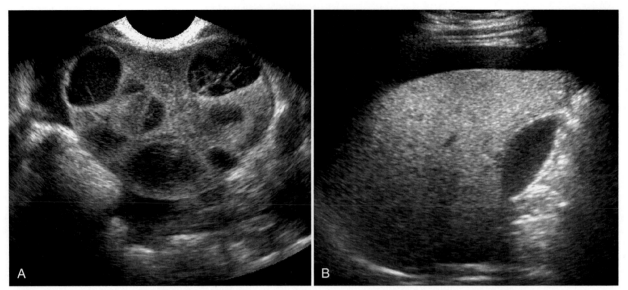

FIGURE 15-32. Ovarian hyperstimulation. A, Transvaginal sonogram shows a round, greatly enlarged ovary with multiple complicated cysts. **B,** Sagittal sonogram in right upper quadrant shows large volume of free intraperitoneal fluid.

Luteoma of pregnancy is a rare benign process unique to pregnancy that resolves spontaneously. Luteinized stromal cells may become hormonally active, producing androgens and replacing the normal ovarian parenchyma. Most patients are asymptomatic, although maternal virilization may occur in up to 30%. These patients have a 50% risk of virilization of the female fetus.[189] The male fetus is unaffected. Sonographically, luteomas usually present as a nonspecific, heterogeneous, predominantly hypoechoic mass that may be highly vascular. An ovarian mass in a pregnant patient with signs of virilization should suggest this diagnosis, because luteoma is the most common cause of maternal virilization during pregnancy.

Ovarian Remnant Syndrome

Infrequently, a cystic mass may be encountered in a patient who has undergone bilateral oophorectomy; a small amount of residual ovarian tissue has been unintentionally left behind. The surgery has usually been technically difficult because of adhesions from endometriosis, PID, or tumor.[190] The residual ovarian tissue can become functional and produce pelvic pain or extrinsic compression of the distal ureter, or both. Sonographically, the cysts vary from small to relatively large, completely cystic or complex masses.[191,192] A thin rim of ovarian tissue is usually present in the wall of the cyst.[192]

Parovarian Cysts

Parovarian (paratubal) cysts account for about 10% to 20% of all adnexal masses. They are found in the broad ligament and are usually of mesothelial or parameso-

nephric origin, or rarely, of mesonephric origin.[193] They may occur at any age but are most common in the third and fourth decades. These cysts are typically small but vary in size, and on sonography they have the typical appearance of cysts. Parovarian cysts show no cyclic changes and are frequently located superior to the uterine fundus;[193] they may contain internal echoes as a result of hemorrhage.[194] Larger cysts may undergo torsion and rupture similar to other cystic masses. Benign neoplasms such as cystadenomas and cystadenofibromas of parovarian origin are uncommon. On sonography, parovarian cysts may appear as simple cysts or may contain small nodular areas and occasionally have septations.[195] Malignancy has been reported in 2% to 3% of parovarian cystic masses on histopathology;[196,197] it occurs even less often in masses less than 5 cm.[198,199] A specific diagnosis of a parovarian cyst is possible only by demonstrating a normal ipsilateral ovary close to, but separate from, the cyst.[199,200]

Peritoneal Inclusion Cysts

Peritoneal inclusion cysts occur predominantly in premenopausal women with a history of previous abdominal surgery, but they may also be seen in patients with a history of trauma, PID, or endometriosis. The ovaries are the main producers of peritoneal fluid in women.[156] In patients with peritoneal adhesions, fluid may accumulate within the adhesions and entrap the ovaries, resulting in a large, adnexal mass.[201-204] Peritoneal inclusion cysts are lined with mesothelial cells; this condition has also been referred to as **benign cystic mesothelioma** or **benign encysted fluid.** Clinically, most patients present with pain and/or a pelvic mass.

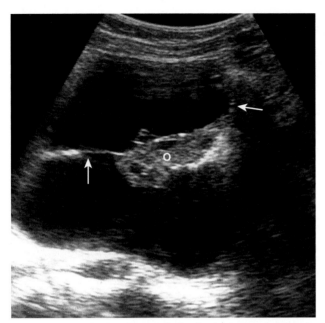

FIGURE 15-33. Peritoneal inclusion cyst. Transabdominal scan shows multiple fluid-filled cystic areas with linear septations *(arrows)* representing adhesions attached to normal ovary *(O)*.

On sonography, peritoneal inclusion cysts are multiloculated cystic adnexal masses, often with a bizarre shape[205] (Fig. 15-33). The diagnostic finding is the presence of an intact ovary amid septations and fluid.[202-204] This indicates the extraovarian origin of the mass. The ovary may be located centrally or displaced peripherally, and although it may appear distorted, it is easily identified. The septations represent the mesothelial and fibrous strands seen pathologically. The fluid is usually anechoic but may contain echoes in some compartments as a result of hemorrhage or proteinaceous fluid. Peritoneal inclusion cysts must be differentiated from parovarian cysts and hydrosalpinx. All these conditions are extraovarian, but parovarian cysts are separate from the ovary, whereas the ovary lies inside or in the wall of a peritoneal inclusion cyst. **Parovarian cysts** are usually round or ovoid and not associated with a history of pelvic surgery, trauma, or inflammation. **Hydrosalpinx** appears as a tubular or ovoid cystic structure with often visible folds, and the ovary is shown to be outside the cystic structure. Accurate diagnosis of peritoneal inclusion cysts is important because the risk of recurrence after surgical resection is 30% to 50%.[206] Conservative therapy, such as ovarian suppression with oral contraceptives or fluid aspiration, is recommended.[204] Peritoneal inclusion cysts have no malignant potential.

Endometriosis

Endometriosis is defined as the presence of functioning endometrial tissue outside the uterus. Endometriosis most often occurs in the ovary, fallopian tube, broad ligament, and posterior cul-de-sac, but it can occur almost anywhere in the body, including the bladder and bowel. Two forms have been described: **diffuse** and **localized** (endometrioma) (Fig. 15-34). The diffuse form, which is more common, consists of minute endometrial implants involving the pelvic viscera and their ligamentous attachments. The ectopic endometrium is hormonally responsive and undergoes bleeding during the menses, resulting in a local inflammatory reaction with adhesions. This diffuse form of endometriosis is rarely diagnosed by sonography because the implants are too small to be imaged. However, they may occasionally be seen as nodular or plaquelike deposits in the pelvis associated with particulate ascites and endometriomas in the ovary. They may be difficult to distinguish from peritoneal metastases (Fig. 15-34, *E* and *F*). Endometriosis commonly affects women during the reproductive years, and clinical symptoms include dysmenorrhea, dyspareunia, and infertility.

The localized form of endometriosis consists of a discrete mass referred to as an **endometrioma,** or **chocolate cyst.** Although endometriosis is frequently associated with infertility, an endometrioma may be seen in a pregnant patient. Endometriomas are usually asymptomatic and are frequently multiple, with a variety of appearances, from an anechoic cyst to a solid-appearing mass caused by the degradation of blood products over time.[207] The characteristic sonographic appearance is that of a well-defined, unilocular or multilocular, predominantly cystic mass containing diffuse, homogeneous, low-level internal echoes (Fig. 15-34, *A-D*). This is much better appreciated on transvaginal sonography.[208] The low-level internal echoes may be seen diffusely throughout the mass or in the dependent portion. Occasionally, a fluid-fluid level may be seen.

Small, linear, hyperechoic foci may be present in the wall of the cyst (Fig. 15-34, *A*), likely caused by cholesterol deposits accumulating in the cyst wall.[209] In a retrospective study, Patel et al.[209] found diffuse, low-level internal echoes in 95% of endometriomas. They concluded that this finding in the absence of neoplastic features is highly likely to be an endometrioma, especially if multilocularity or hyperechoic wall foci are present, whereas an endometrioma is highly unlikely when no component of the mass contains low-level echoes. A prospective study by Dogan et al.[210] found a positive predictive value of 97% for typically appearing endometriomas with low-level internal echoes, regular margins, round shape, and thick walls. Calcification is occasionally present in an endometrioma and misdiagnosed as a dermoid.[211] Rarely, in pregnancy, decidualization of the wall of an endometrioma may occur, resulting in a solid vascular mural mass that cannot be differentiated from malignancy[212,213] (Fig. 15-35, *A-D*). Endometrioid and clear cell carcinomas can also occur within endometriomas[40] (Fig. 15-35, *D*).

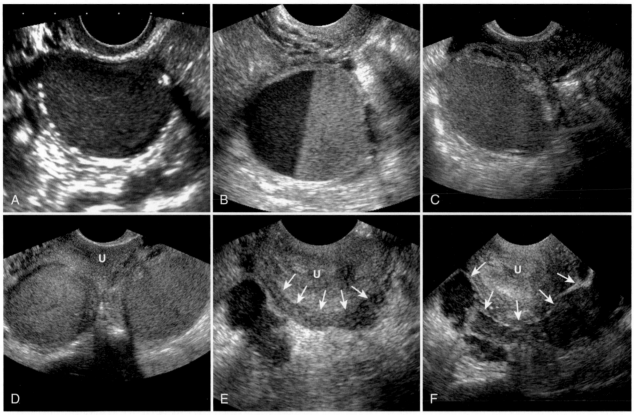

FIGURE 15-34. Endometriosis: spectrum of appearances. Transvaginal scans. **A** to **D,** Uniform low-level echoes within a cystic ovarian mass. **A,** Typical peripheral echogenic foci. **B,** Fluid-fluid level. **C,** Avascular marginal echogenic nodules. **D,** Bilateral disease. **E,** Endometriotic plaque on posterior surface of uterus *(arrows).* **F,** Filling the pouch of Douglas *(arrows). U,* Uterus.

The appearance of an endometrioma may be similar to a **hemorrhagic ovarian cyst** because both are cystic masses that contain blood of variable age. However, a hemorrhagic cyst more frequently demonstrates a reticular internal pattern and is more frequently associated with free fluid in the cul-de-sac. A hemorrhagic cyst will resolve or show a significant decrease in size over the next few menstrual cycles, whereas endometriomas tend to show little change in size and internal echo pattern. Clinically, most women with an acute hemorrhagic cyst present with acute pelvic pain, whereas women with an endometrioma are asymptomatic or have more chronic discomfort associated with their menses.

Polycystic Ovarian Syndrome

Polycystic ovarian syndrome (PCOS) is a complex endocrinologic disorder of abnormal estrogen and androgen production resulting in chronic anovulation. The serum LH level is elevated and the FSH level is depressed; an elevated LH/FSH ratio is a characteristic finding. Pathologically, the ovaries contain an increased number of follicles in various stages of maturation and atresia, and increased local concentration of androgens produces stromal abnormality. PCOS is a common cause of infertility and a higher-than-usual rate of early pregnancy loss.[214,215] Clinical manifestations of PCOS range from mild signs of hyperandrogenism in thin, normally menstruating women to the classic Stein-Leventhal syndrome (oligomenorrhea or amenorrhea, hirsutism, and obesity).

The typical sonographic findings of polycystic ovaries are those of bilaterally enlarged ovaries containing multiple small follicles and increased stromal echogenicity (Fig. 15-36). The ovaries have a more rounded shape, with the follicles usually located peripherally ("string of pearls"), although they can also occur randomly throughout the ovarian parenchyma. Transvaginal sonography, because of its superior resolution, is more sensitive in detecting the small follicles. However, many women with PCOS will not have these typical sonographic findings. Ovarian volume may be normal in 30% of patients.[216,217]

Using transvaginal sonography, increased stromal echogenicity is believed to be the most sensitive and specific sign of polycystic ovaries.[218,219] In a small number of patients, the sonographic findings may be unilateral.[215,220] A 2003 consensus meeting of the American Society for Reproductive Medicine and European Society of Human Reproduction and Embryology defined PCOS as requiring two of three criteria: (1) oligo-ovulation and/or anovulation, (2) hyperandrogenism (clinical and/or biochemical), and (3) polycystic ovaries.[221]

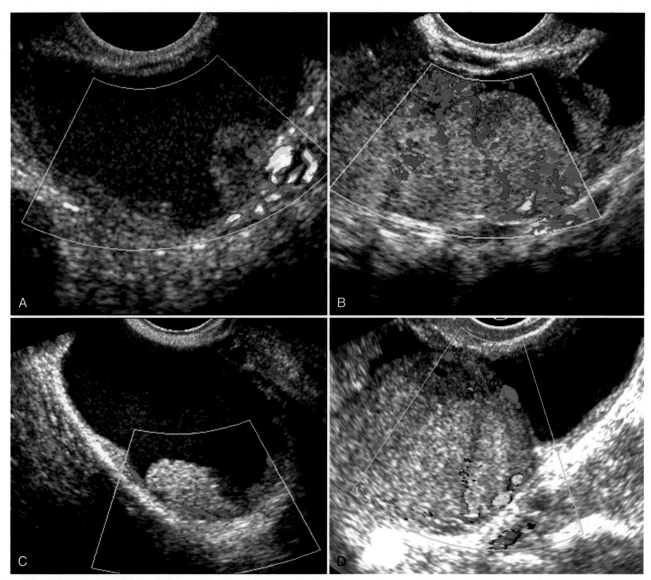

FIGURE 15-35. Ovarian masses in four pregnant patients. Transvaginal color Doppler ultrasound images. **A** and **B,** **Decidualization of endometrioma** in two patients. **A,** Ovarian mass filled with low-level internal echoes typical of endometrioma, with solid vascular mural nodule, at 23 weeks' gestation. Nodule disappeared and mass became smaller after delivery. **B,** Another patient, at 24 weeks' gestation, shows a large, predominantly solid vascular ovarian mass with a small cystic component. The mass had continued to increase during the pregnancy and was confirmed at surgery. **C, Ovarian cystadenocarcinoma of low malignant potential.** Ovarian mass filled with low-level internal echoes with solid vascular mural nodule at 11 weeks' gestation; surgery at 16 weeks. **D, Clear cell carcinoma in an endometrioma.** Ovarian mass with low-level internal echoes and large solid vascular component, which had been growing; 26 weeks' gestation; confirmed at surgery.

Also, the diagnosis of polycystic ovaries should have either 12 or more follicles measuring 2 to 9 mm in diameter *or* increased ovarian volume greater than 10 cc. Although increased stromal echogenicity was considered specific for polycystic ovaries, because of its subjective nature, it was not included in the criteria. The consensus thought that measurement of ovarian volume worked as well as stromal evaluation in clinical practice. Jonard et al.[222] reported that more than 12 follicles was the best diagnostic criterion.[222] These criteria are not considered valid if the patient is taking oral contraceptives or there is a dominant follicle greater than 10 mm.

Because ovulation does not occur, the follicles will persist on serial studies. Long-term follow-up is recommended in patients with PCOS because the unopposed high estrogen levels appear to be associated with an increased risk of endometrial and breast carcinoma.

Ovarian Torsion

Torsion of the ovary is an acute abdominal condition requiring prompt surgical intervention (Fig. 15-37). It is caused by partial or complete rotation of the ovarian pedicle on its axis. This results in compromise of the

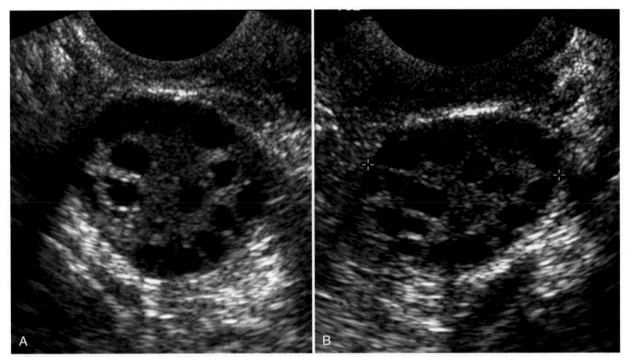

FIGURE 15-36. Polycystic ovaries: typical appearance on transvaginal scans. A and **B,** Enlarged round ovaries *(outlined by cursors)* with mildly increased stromal echogenicity and multiple peripheral follicles, "string of pearls" sign, and central follicles.

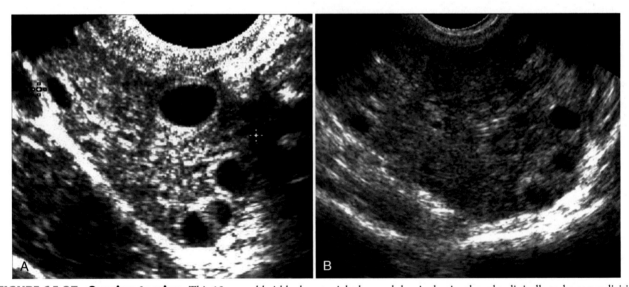

FIGURE 15-37. Ovarian torsion. This 18-year-old girl had acute right lower abdominal pain, thought clinically to be appendicitis. **A,** Enlarged right ovary with enlarged peripheral follicles. Color Doppler ultrasound evaluation shows minimal flow, much less than on the normal side. **B,** One day later, the ovary had quadrupled in size, with no flow demonstrated on Doppler ultrasound.

lymphatic and venous drainage, causing congestion and edema of the ovarian parenchyma and leading to eventual loss of arterial perfusion and resultant infarction. Torsion usually occurs in childhood and during the reproductive years and is uncommon after menopause. There is an increased risk during pregnancy, especially if the patient has hyperstimulated ovaries.[223] Clinically, there is severe pelvic pain, nausea, and vomiting. A palpable mass may be present. Torsion occurs more fre-

quently on the right side, and the pain may clinically mimic acute appendicitis. This may be caused by the decreased space on the left side, which is occupied by the sigmoid colon and protects the left ovary.[224]

Torsion may occur in normal ovaries or in association with a preexisting ovarian cyst or mass, which is usually benign.[225] In postmenopausal women, however, the mass has a higher frequency of being malignant, with a higher frequency of ovarian necrosis resulting from delayed

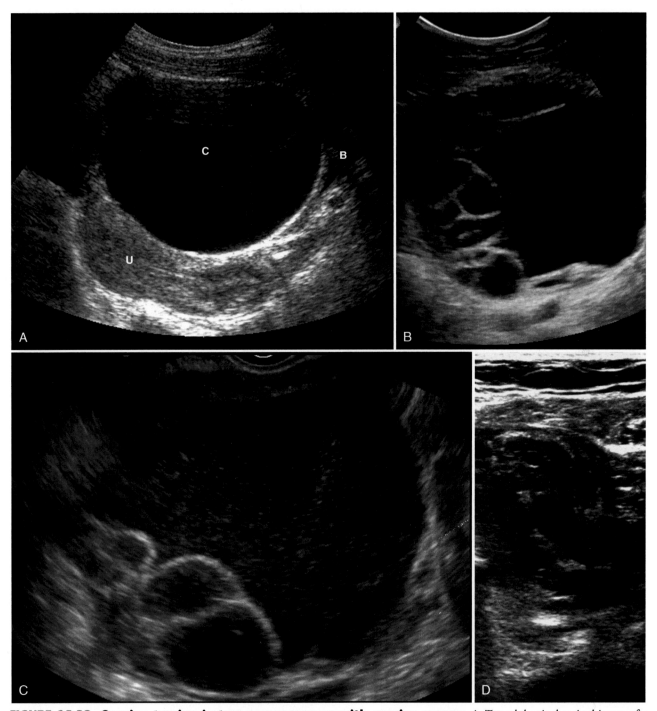

FIGURE 15-38. Ovarian torsion in two young women with ovarian masses. A, Transabdominal sagittal image of a young woman with acute pain shows a large, simple cyst *(C)* that lies anterior to the uterus *(U)* and cephalad to the bladder *(B)*. This unusual position should raise the suspicion of torsion. No blood flow could be detected in the ovary on color Doppler ultrasound. **B, C,** and **D,** Another young woman with acute pain. **B,** Transabdominal image shows a large, multiloculated midline cystic mass. Neither ovary could be definitely identified. **C,** Transvaginal image shows echogenic fluid within the cystic component. **D,** Transabdominal image to right of mass shows tortuous tubular structures, which showed no flow on Doppler, suggesting a twisted ovarian pedicle. A torsed, nonviable right ovary was confirmed at surgery, and pathology showed a large, mucinous cystadenoma.

diagnosis.[226,227] Torsion of a normal ovary usually occurs in children and younger women with especially mobile adnexa, allowing torsion at the mesosalpinx.[228]

The sonographic findings are variable, depending on the duration and degree of vascular compromise and

whether an adnexal mass is present (Fig. 15-38). The ovary is enlarged. Multiple cortical follicles in an enlarged ovary are considered a specific sign, although they are not always present.[228] The multifollicular enlargement is the result of transudation of fluid into the follicles from the circulatory impairment. Free fluid in the cul-de-sac is often seen.[229] Color and spectral Doppler ultrasound examination may show absent flow in the affected ovary. However, Doppler findings may vary depending on the degree and chronicity of the torsion and whether there is an associated adnexal mass.[230] The presence of arterial or venous flow or both does not exclude the diagnosis of torsion. Doppler arterial waveforms and color flow have been reported in surgically proven cases of torsion.[231,232] The possible explanations proposed are that venous thrombosis leads to symptoms before arterial occlusion occurs and that persistent adnexal arterial flow is related to the dual-ovarian arterial blood supply (ovarian artery and ovarian branches of uterine artery).[232] A twisted vascular pedicle (consisting of broad ligament, fallopian tube, and adnexal and ovarian branches of uterine artery and vein) may be demonstrated as a round hyperechoic structure with multiple concentric hypoechoic stripes (target appearance) or as an ellipsoid or tubular structure with internal heterogeneous echoes.[233] On color Doppler ultrasound, the presence of circular or coiled twisted vessels within the vascular pedicle (whirlpool sign) is helpful in diagnosing torsion.[233] Absence of blood flow within the vascular pedicle suggests a nonviable ovary.[233,234] Comparison with the morphologic appearance and flow patterns of the contralateral ovary should always be done and can be helpful because decreased flow may be present in the torsed ovary.[229,235] The most constant finding in ovarian torsion is a unilateral enlarged ovary. In the appropriate clinical setting, an enlarged ovary should suggest torsion even in the presence of ovarian Doppler ultrasound flow.[235,236] Torsion is extremely unlikely if the ovary is morphologically normal, regardless of Doppler findings.

Massive Edema of the Ovary

Massive edema is a rare condition resulting from partial or intermittent torsion of the ovary, causing venous and lymphatic obstruction but not arterial occlusion. This results in ovarian enlargement caused by marked stromal edema. The few cases described on sonography show a large, predominantly multicystic adnexal mass.[237-239]

Neoplasms

Ovarian Cancer

Ovarian cancer is the fifth leading cause of cancer death among U.S. women. The ACS estimated 21,650 new cases of ovarian cancer in the United States in 2008, with about 15,520 deaths. Between 1987 and 2004, the incidence has decreased at a rate of 0.9% a year.[114] Ovarian cancer represents 25% of all gynecologic malignancies, with peak incidence in the sixth decade of life. Although only the third most common gynecologic malignancy, it has the highest mortality rate as a result of late

diagnosis. Because there are few clinical symptoms, 60% to 70% of women have advanced disease (stages III or IV) at diagnosis. The overall 5-year survival rate is 20% to 30%, but with early detection in stage I, the rate rises to 80% to 90%. Therefore, efforts have been directed at developing methods of early diagnosis of ovarian cancer.

Increasing age, nulliparity, a family history of ovarian cancer, and a patient history of breast, endometrial, or colon cancer have been associated with increased risk of ovarian cancer. Family history is considered to be the most important risk factor. The lifetime risk of a woman developing ovarian cancer is 1 in 70 (1.4%). However, if a woman has a first-degree relative (mother, daughter, sister) or second-degree relative (aunt or grandmother) who has had ovarian cancer, the risk is 5%. With two or more relatives, the lifetime risk increases to 7%.[240] About 3% to 5% of women with a family history of ovarian cancer will have a hereditary ovarian cancer syndrome. The three main hereditary syndromes associated with ovarian cancer are the breast-ovarian cancer syndrome, the most common, caused by mutations in the suppressor genes BRCA1 and BRCA2, with a high frequency of both cancers; the hereditary nonpolyposis colorectal cancer syndrome (Lynch II) in which ovarian cancer occurs in association with nonpolyposis colorectal cancer or endometrial cancer, or both; and site-specific ovarian cancer syndrome, the least common, without an excess of breast or colorectal cancer.[241] Hereditary ovarian cancer syndromes are thought to have an autosomal dominant inheritance, and the lifetime risk of ovarian cancer in these patients is 40% to 50%. They have an earlier age of onset (10-15 years) than do other ovarian cancers.[241]

A number of clinical screening trials of asymptomatic women have been reported using transvaginal sonography either alone or in combination with Doppler sonography and/or biologic markers such as cancer antigen (CA) 125.[242-247] CA 125 is a high-molecular-weight glycoprotein recognized by the OC 125 monoclonal antibody. It has proved extremely useful in following the clinical course of patients undergoing chemotherapy and in detecting recurrent subclinical disease.[248,249] Although serum CA 125 is elevated in approximately 80% of women with epithelial ovarian cancer, it detects less than 50% of stage I disease and is insensitive to mucinous and germ cell tumors.[249] Other malignancies, as well as several benign conditions, may be associated with elevated serum CA 125. The use of serum CA 125 and/or sonography as a screening test for ovarian cancer is not recommended for routine clinical use.[250] Routine screening has resulted in unnecessary surgery with its attendant potential risks.[250]

Histologically, epithelial neoplasms represent 65% to 75% of ovarian tumors and 90% of ovarian malignancies[40] (Table 15-2). The remaining neoplasms consist of germ cell tumors (15%-20%), sex cord–

TABLE 15-2. OVARIAN NEOPLASMS: HISTOLOGIC OUTLINE

TYPE	ANOMALY	INCIDENCE	EXAMPLES
I	Surface epithelial–stromal tumors	65%-75%	Serous cystadenoma (carcinoma) Mucinous cystadenoma (carcinoma) Endometrioid carcinoma Clear cell carcinoma Transitional cell tumor
II	Germ cell tumors	15%-20%	Teratoma 　Dermoid 　Immature Dysgerminoma Yolk sac tumor
III	Sex cord–stromal tumors	5%-10%	Granulosa cell tumor Sertoli-Leydig cell tumor Thecoma and fibroma
IV	Metastatic tumors	5%-10%	Genital primary 　Uterus Extragenital primary 　Stomach 　Colon 　Breast Lymphoma

stromal tumors (5%-10%), and **metastatic tumors** (5%-10%).

Sonographically, ovarian cancer usually presents as an adnexal mass (Fig. 15-39). Well-defined anechoic lesions are more likely to be benign, whereas lesions with irregular walls, thick irregular septations, mural nodules, and solid echogenic elements favor malignancy.[251,252] Many scoring systems and mathematical models based on the morphologic characteristics have been proposed for distinguishing between benign and malignant masses. However, **subjective evaluation** of the ultrasound morphologic features (**pattern recognition**) by an experienced interpreting physician has been shown to be the superior method.[253,254] Using this method, a physician should be able to distinguish benign from malignant masses in approximately 90% of cases.[255] Van Calster et al.[256] found pattern recognition by an experienced sonologist to be superior to CA 125 for discrimination between benign and malignant masses.

Color and pulsed Doppler sonography have been advocated for distinguishing benign from malignant ovarian masses. Support is based on the premise that malignant masses, because of internal neovascularization, will have high diastolic flow that can be detected on spectral Doppler ultrasound waveforms. Malignant tumor growth depends on angiogenesis, with the development of abnormal tumor vessels.[257] These abnormal vessels lack smooth muscle within their walls, which, along with arteriovenous shunting, leads to decreased vascular resistance and thus higher diastolic flow velocity. Therefore, the pulsatility index (PI) and resistive index (RI) should be lower in malignant lesions. Although many reports have found a tendency for both PI and RI to be lower in malignant lesions, there has been too much overlap to differentiate reliably between benign

and malignant lesions in the individual patient.[258-263] Other parameters such as vessel location have been suggested to improve the specificity of Doppler ultrasound assessment of ovarian masses.[264] Malignant lesions tend to have more central flow, whereas benign lesions tend to have more peripheral flow. However, Stein et al.[259] found considerable overlap, with 21% of malignant lesions having only peripheral flow and 31% of benign lesions having central flow. Guerriero et al.[265] found a higher accuracy in predicting malignancy when color Doppler US demonstrated arterial flow within the solid portions of the mass.

Studies comparing the morphologic features on sonography with the Doppler findings found that Doppler ultrasound showed no more diagnostic information than morphologic assessment alone.[253,260,261,266] Valentin[253] concluded that, in experienced hands, morphologic assessment is the best method for discriminating between benign and malignant masses—with the main advantage of adding Doppler ultrasound being to increase the confidence with which a correct diagnosis is made. Others have found that Doppler ultrasound, when added to sonographic morphologic assessment, improves specificity and positive predictive value.[263,267-269] Brown et al.[270] found that a nonhyperechoic solid component was the most statistically significant predictor of malignancy. Schelling et al.[271] also found that a solid component in an adnexal mass with central vascularity achieved high accuracy, sensitivity, and specificity in predicting malignancy. A meta-analysis of 46 published studies concluded that ultrasound techniques that combine morphologic assessment with color Doppler flow imaging (CDFI) is significantly better in characterizing ovarian masses than morphologic assessment, CDFI, or Doppler indices alone.[272] Doppler ultra-

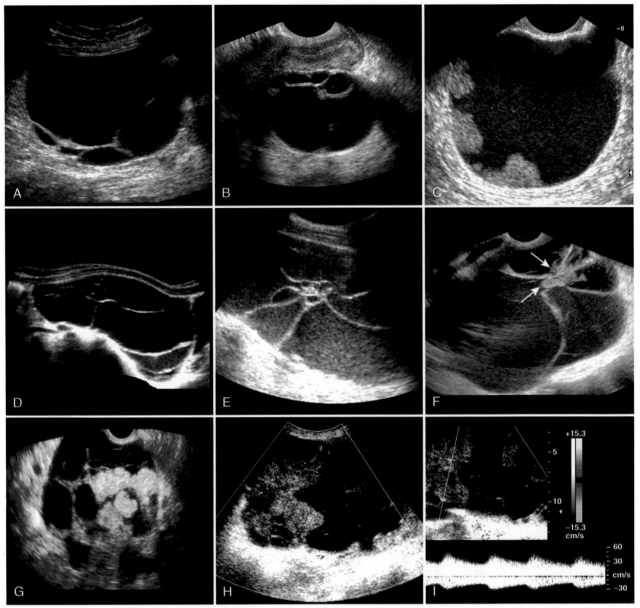

FIGURE 15-39. Epithelial ovarian neoplasms: spectrum of appearances. A and B, Serous cystadenomas. A, Septations within a cystic mass are fairly thin. **B,** Septations are thicker. **C, Serous cystadenoma of low malignant potential.** Low-level echogenic particles and mural nodules. **D and E, Mucinous cystadenomas. F, Mucinous cystadenocarcinoma.** Large size and septations are characteristic; septal nodularity is marked *(arrows)*. **G, H,** and **I,** Patient with **serous cystadenocarcinoma.** Extensive nodularity shows vascularity, confirming the morphologic suspicion of a malignant mass. There is high diastolic flow resulting in a low resistive index.

sound is probably not needed if the mass has a characteristic benign morphology, because morphologic assessment is highly accurate in this group of lesions.[259,262] Doppler ultrasound is likely valuable in assessing the mass that is morphologically indeterminant or suggestive of malignancy. Doppler findings should be combined with morphologic assessment, clinical findings, patient age, and phase of menstrual cycle for optimal evaluation of an adnexal mass.[273]

Surface Epithelial–Stromal Tumors

Surface epithelial–stromal tumors are generally considered to arise from the surface epithelium that covers

the ovary and the underlying ovarian stroma (Fig. 15-39). These tumors can be divided into five broad categories based on epithelial differentiation: **serous, mucinous, endometrioid, clear cell,** and **transitional cell (Brenner).**[40] This group of tumors accounts for 65% to 75% of all ovarian neoplasms and 80% to 90% of all ovarian malignancies. The mode of spread of the malignant tumors is primarily intraperitoneal, although direct extension to contiguous structures and lymphatic spread can occur. Lymphatic spread is predominantly to the paraortic nodes. Hematogeneous spread usually occurs late in the course of the disease.

Serous Cystadenoma and Cystadenocarcinoma.
Serous tumors are the most common surface epithelial–

stromal tumors, representing 30% of all ovarian neoplasms. Approximately 50% to 70% of serous tumors are benign. Serous **cystadenomas** account for about 25% of all benign ovarian neoplasms, and serous **cystadenocarcinomas** account for about 50% of all malignant ovarian neoplasms.[40] The peak incidence of serous cystadenomas is in the fourth and fifth decades, whereas serous cystadenocarcinomas most frequently occur in perimenopausal and postmenopausal women. Approximately 20% of benign serous tumors and 50% of malignant serous tumors are bilateral. Their sizes vary greatly, but in general they are smaller than mucinous tumors.

Sonographically, **serous cystadenomas** are usually large, thin-walled, unilocular cystic masses that may contain thin septations (Fig. 15-39, *A* and *B*). Papillary projections are occasionally seen. **Serous cystadenocarcinomas** may be quite large and usually present as multilocular cystic masses containing multiple papillary projections arising from the cyst walls and septa (Fig. 15-39, *G-I*). The septa and walls may be thick. Echogenic solid material may be seen within the loculations. Papillary projections may form on the surface of the cyst and surrounding organs, resulting in fixation of the mass. Ascites is frequently seen.

Mucinous Cystadenoma and Cystadenocarcinoma. Mucinous tumors are the second most common ovarian epithelial tumor, accounting for 20% to 25% of ovarian neoplasms. Mucinous **cystadenomas** constitute 20% to 25% of all benign ovarian neoplasms, and mucinous **cystadenocarcinomas** make up 5% to 10% of all primary malignant ovarian neoplasms.[40] Mucinous cystadenomas occur most often in the third to sixth decades, but may be seen in very young women, whereas mucinous cystadenocarcinomas most frequently occur in the fourth to seventh decades. Mucinous tumors are less frequently bilateral than their serous counterparts, with only 5% of the benign and 15% to 20% of the malignant lesions occurring on both sides; 80% to 85% of mucinous tumors are benign.[274]

On sonographic examination, **mucinous cystadenomas** can be huge cystic masses, measuring up to 15 to 30 cm and filling the entire pelvis and abdomen (Figs. 15-39, *D*, and 15-40). Multiple thin septa are present, and low-level echoes caused by the mucoid material may be seen in the dependent portions of the mass (Fig. 15-39, *D* and *E*). Papillary projections are less frequently seen than in the serous counterpart. **Mucinous cystadenocarcinomas** are usually large, multiloculated cystic masses containing papillary projections and echogenic material; they generally have a sonographic appearance similar to that of serous cystadenocarcinomas (Fig. 15-39, *F*).

Penetration of the tumor capsule or rupture may lead to intraperitoneal spread of mucin-secreting cells that fill the peritoneal cavity with a gelatinous material. This condition, known as **pseudomyxoma peritonei,** may be similar sonographically to ascites or may contain multiple septations in the fluid that fills much of the pelvis and abdomen. Low-level echogenic material may be seen

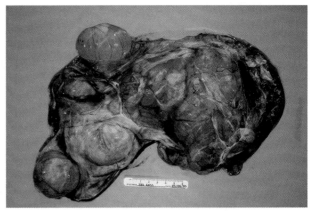

FIGURE 15-40. Mucinous cystadenoma. Gross pathologic specimen shows multiple cystic loculations.

within the fluid. This condition may occur in mucinous cystadenomas and in mucinous cystadenocarcinomas. A ruptured mucocele of the appendix and mucinous tumors of the appendix and colon can also lead to pseudomyxoma peritonei.

Borderline Ovarian Tumors or Tumors of Low Malignant Potential. There is an intermediate group of epithelial tumors that are histologically categorized as "borderline" or of "low malignant potential" (LMP). They are much more common in the serous and mucinous tumors, occurring in 10% to 15% of each. These tumors have cytologic features of malignancy but do not invade the stroma and, although malignant, have a much better prognosis. They present at an earlier age than cystadenocarcinomas and have a 5-year and 20-year survival of 95% and 80%, respectively. They may be treated by ovary-sparing surgery to preserve fertility.

Sonographic features suggestive of LMP tumors are a small to medium-sized cyst containing low-level echoes (similar to an endometrioma) with vascular mural nodules (Figs. 15-35, *C*, and 15-39, *C*) or a cystic mass with a well-defined multilocular (honeycomb) nodule.[275,276] Normal ovarian tissue may be seen adjacent to the lesion and may be helpful in excluding invasive ovarian cancer.[275,277] This has been referred to as the **ovarian crescent sign.**[277]

Endometrioid Tumor. Almost all endometrioid tumors are malignant. They are the second most common epithelial malignancy, representing 20% to 25% of ovarian malignancies; 25% to 30% are bilateral, and they occur most frequently in the fifth and sixth decades. Their histologic characteristics are identical to those of endometrial adenocarcinoma, and approximately 30% of patients have associated endometrial adenocarcinoma, which is thought to represent an independent primary tumor. Approximately 15% to 20% of endometrioid cancer is associated with endometriosis, which may occur within the endometriosis, the ipsilateral or contralateral ovary.[40] The endometrioid tumor has a better prognosis than other epithelial malignancies, probably related to diagnosis at an earlier stage. Sonographically, it usually presents as a cystic mass containing papillary projections, although some endometrioid tumors are predominantly a solid mass that may contain areas of hemorrhage or necrosis.[274]

Clear Cell Tumor. This tumor is considered to be of müllerian duct origin and a variant of endometrioid carcinoma. Clear cell tumor is almost always malignant and constitutes 5% to 10% of primary ovarian carcinomas. It occurs most frequently in the fifth to seventh decades and is bilateral in about 20% of patients. Associated pelvic endometriosis is present in 50% to 70% of clear cell carcinomas, and approximately one third arise within the lining of endometriomas[40] (see Fig. 15-35, C and D). Sonographically, it usually presents as a nonspecific, complex, predominantly cystic mass.[274]

Transitional Cell Tumor. Also known as **Brenner tumor**, transitional cell tumor is derived from the surface epithelium that undergoes metaplasia to form typical uroepithelial-like components.[274] It is uncommon, accounting for 2% to 3% of all ovarian neoplasms, and is almost always benign; 6% to 7% are bilateral. Most patients are asymptomatic, and the tumor is discovered incidentally on sonographic examination or at surgery. About 30% are associated with cystic neoplasms, usually serous or mucinous cystadenomas or cystic teratomas, frequently in the ipsilateral ovary[278] (Fig. 15-41). Sonographically, Brenner tumors are hypoechoic solid masses. Calcification may occur in the outer wall. A cystic component is uncommon, but when present, usually results from a coexistent cystadenoma.[274,279] Pathologically, transitional cell masses are solid tumors composed of

dense fibrous stroma. They appear similar to ovarian fibromas and thecomas and to uterine leiomyomas, both sonographically and pathologically.

Germ Cell Tumors

Germ cell tumors are derived from the primitive germ cells of the embryonic gonad. They account for 15% to 20% of ovarian neoplasms, with 95% **benign cystic teratomas.** The others, including **dysgerminomas** and **endodermal sinus** (yolk sac) **tumors,** occur mainly in children and young adults and are almost always malignant. Germ cell tumors are the most common ovarian malignancies in children and young adults. When a large, predominantly solid ovarian mass is present in a girl or young woman, the diagnosis of a malignant germ cell tumor should be strongly considered.[280]

Cystic Teratoma. Cystic teratomas make up approximately 15% to 25% of ovarian neoplasms; 10% to 15% are bilateral. They are composed of well-differentiated derivatives of the **three germ layers:** ectoderm, mesoderm, and endoderm. Because **ectodermal elements** generally predominate, cystic teratomas are virtually always benign and are also called **dermoid cysts.** Cystic teratomas and serous cystadenomas are the two most common ovarian neoplasms. In contrast to surface epithelial–stromal tumors, cystic teratomas are more frequently seen in the active reproductive years, but can occur at any age and can be seen in postmenopausal women. These tumors may present as a clinically palpable mass. Cystic teratomas are usually asymptomatic and often are discovered incidentally during sonography. In approximately 10% of cases, the tumor is diagnosed during pregnancy.[40] Torsion is the most common complication, whereas rupture is uncommon, occurring in 1% of patients and causing a secondary chemical peritonitis. Malignant transformation is also uncommon, occurring in 2% of patients, usually older women.[40]

Sonographically, cystic teratomas have a variable appearance ranging from completely anechoic to completely hyperechoic. However, certain features are considered specific (Figs. 15-42 and 15-43). These include a predominantly cystic mass with an echogenic mural nodule, the **dermoid plug.**[281] The dermoid plug usually

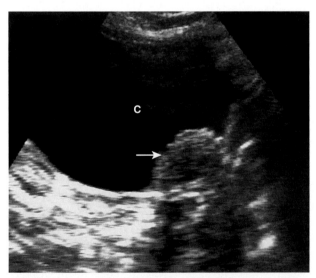

FIGURE 15-41. Transitional cell (Brenner) tumor in wall of mucinous cystadenoma. Transabdominal scan shows a large, well-defined cystic mass *(C)* with a solid hypoechoic mural nodule *(arrow)*. Pathology showed a Brenner tumor within the wall of a large, mucinous cystadenoma.

CYSTIC TERATOMAS: SONOGRAPHIC FEATURES

Dermoid plug
"Tip of the iceberg" sign
Dermoid mesh
Mobile spherules (rare)
Fat-fluid level with echogenic nondependent layer

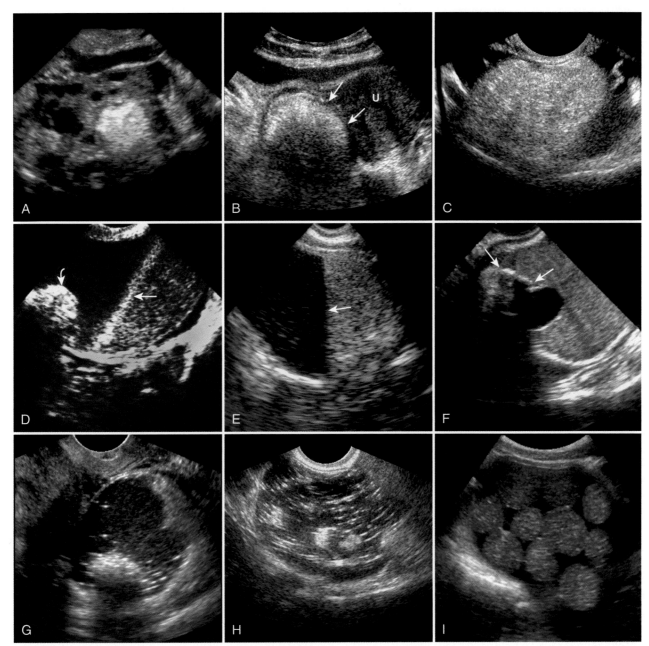

FIGURE 15-42. Dermoid cysts: spectrum of appearances. A, Small, highly echogenic mass in an otherwise normal ovary. **B,** Transverse transabdominal scan shows the uterus *(U)*. In the right adnexal region, there is a highly echogenic and attenuating mass *(arrows)*, the "tip of the iceberg" sign. **C,** Highly echogenic intraovarian mass with no normal ovarian tissue. **D,** Mass of varying echogenicity with **hair-fluid level** *(straight arrow)* and highly echogenic, fat-containing **dermoid plug** *(curved arrow)* with shadowing. **E,** Mass with fat-fluid level *(arrow)*, with dependent layer more echogenic. **F,** Mass containing uniform echoes, small cystic area, and calcification *(arrows)* with shadowing. **G,** Combination of **dermoid mesh** and **dermoid plug** appearances. **H, Dermoid mesh,** multiple linear hyperechogenic interfaces floating within cystic mass. **I,** Multiple mobile spherical echogenic structures floating in a large, cystic pelvic mass.

contains hair, teeth, or fat and frequently casts an acoustic shadow. Correlation with computed tomography (CT) images has shown that in many cases the cystic component is pure **sebum** (which is liquid at body temperature) rather than fluid.[282]

A mixture of matted hair and sebum is highly echogenic because of multiple tissue interfaces, and it produces poorly defined acoustic shadowing that obscures

the posterior wall of the lesion. This has been termed the **"tip of the iceberg"** sign[283] (Fig. 15-42, *B*). Highly echogenic foci with well-defined acoustic shadowing may arise from other elements, including teeth and bone. Multiple linear hyperechogenic interfaces may be seen floating within the cyst and have been shown to be hair fibers.[284] This is also considered a specific sign and has been referred to as the **dermoid mesh**[285] (Fig. 15-42, *D*).

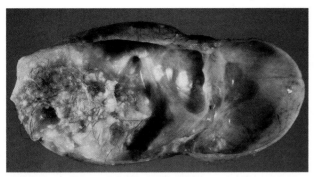

FIGURE 15-43. Cystic teratoma. Pathologic specimen shows large ovarian mass containing fluid, fat, hair, and teeth.

A **fat-fluid** or **hair-fluid level** may also be seen (Fig. 15-42, *D* and *E*). In most cases, as in other lesions such as endometriomas and hemorrhagic cysts, the dependent layer will be more echogenic. However, in approximately 30% of dermoids, the nondependent layer will be more echogenic.[286] Another rare but characteristic feature is multiple mobile spherical echogenic structures floating in a large, cystic pelvic mass[287] (Fig. 15-42, *I*). Microscopically, these structures were composed of desquamative keratin-containing fibrin, hemosiderin, and hair.

Patel et al.[288] found that an adnexal mass showing two or more characteristic sonographic dermoid features had a positive predictive value of 100%. Pitfalls in the diagnosis of cystic teratomas have been described.[289] Acute hemorrhage into an ovarian cyst or an endometrioma may be so echogenic that it resembles a dermoid plug. However, posterior sound enhancement is usually seen with acute hemorrhage, whereas the dermoid plug tends to attenuate sound. Other pitfalls include pedunculated fibroids, especially lipoleiomyomas, and perforated appendicitis with an appendicolith. An echogenic dermoid may appear similar to bowel gas and may be overlooked. If a definite pelvic mass is clinically palpable and the sonogram appears normal, the patient should be reexamined, to look carefully for a dermoid.

Struma ovarii is a teratoma composed entirely or predominantly of thyroid tissue. It occurs in 2% to 3% of teratomas. Color Doppler sonography detected central blood flow in solid tissue in four reported cases of struma ovarii, compared with absent central blood flow in benign cystic teratomas.[290] This is likely caused by the highly vascularized thyroid tissue in struma ovarii, versus the avascular fat and hair found in benign cystic teratomas. Although associated hormonal effects are rare, sonography may be valuable in identifying a pelvic lesion in a hyperthyroid patient when there is no evidence of a thyroid lesion in the neck.[291]

Immature teratoma is uncommon, representing less than 1% of all teratomas, and contains immature tissue from all three germ-cell layers. It is a rapidly growing malignant tumor that most often occurs in the first two decades of life. Sonographically, the tumor usually presents as a solid mass, but cystic structures of varying size may also be seen.[280] Calcifications are typically seen in immature teratoma.

Dysgerminoma. Dysgerminomas are malignant germ cell tumors that constitute approximately 1% to 2% of primary ovarian neoplasms and 3% to 5% of ovarian malignancies.[40] They are composed of undifferentiated germ cells and are morphologically identical to the male testicular **seminoma.** Dysgerminomas are highly radiosensitive and have a 5-year survival of 75% to 90%. This tumor occurs predominantly in women under age 30 and is bilateral in approximately 15% of cases.

The **dysgerminoma, cystic teratoma,** and **serous cystadenoma** are the most common ovarian neoplasms seen in pregnancy.[40] Sonographically, they are solid masses that are predominantly echogenic but that may contain small anechoic areas caused by hemorrhage or necrosis[280] (Fig. 15-44). CT and MRI have shown these solid masses to be lobulated with fibrovascular septa between the lobules.[292] A report using color Doppler ultrasound in three dysgerminomas showed prominent arterial flow within the fibrovascular septa of a multilobulated, solid, echogenic mass.[293]

Yolk Sac Tumor. This rare, rapidly growing tumor, also called **endodermal sinus tumor**, is the second most common malignant ovarian germ cell neoplasm after dysgerminoma. Yolk sac tumor has a poor prognosis. It is thought to arise from the undifferentiated, multipotential embryonal carcinoma by selective differentiation toward yolk sac or vitelline structures.[40] It usually occurs in females under 20 years of age and is almost always unilateral. Increased levels of serum alpha-fetoprotein (AFP) may be seen in association with endodermal sinus tumor. The sonographic appearance is similar to that of the dysgerminoma.[280]

Sex Cord–Stromal Tumors

Sex cord–stromal tumors arise from the sex cords of the embryonic gonad and from the ovarian stroma. The main tumors in this group include the **granulosa cell tumor, Sertoli-Leydig cell tumor** (androblastoma), **thecoma,** and **fibroma.** This group accounts for 5% to 10% of all ovarian neoplasms and 2% of all ovarian malignancies.

Granulosa Cell Tumor. Representing 1% to 2% of ovarian neoplasms, granulosa cell tumor has a low malignancy potential. About 95% are of the **adult type** and occur predominantly in postmenopausal women; almost all are unilateral. Granulosa cell tumors are the most common estrogenically active ovarian tumor,[40] and clinical signs of estrogen production can occur. Approximately 10% to 15% of patients eventually develop endometrial carcinoma. The **juvenile type** makes up 5% of granulosa cell tumors, occurring mainly in patients younger than 30 years and in children. In premenarchal girls, these tumors usually produce sexual precocity as a

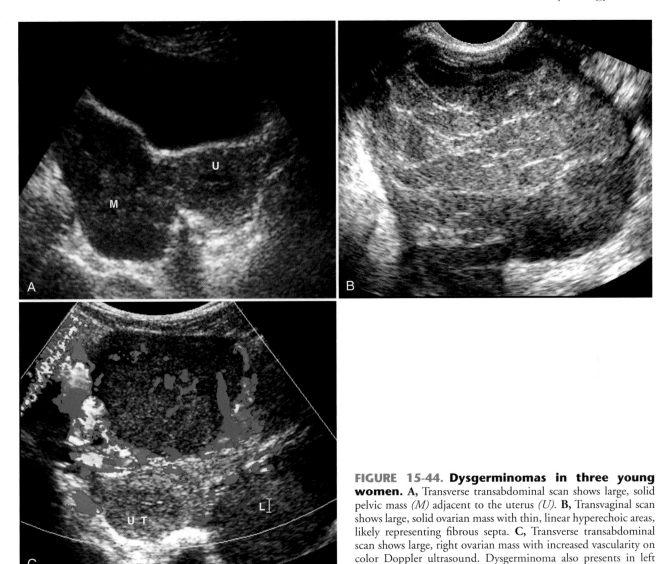

FIGURE 15-44. Dysgerminomas in three young women. A, Transverse transabdominal scan shows large, solid pelvic mass *(M)* adjacent to the uterus *(U).* **B,** Transvaginal scan shows large, solid ovarian mass with thin, linear hyperechoic areas, likely representing fibrous septa. **C,** Transverse transabdominal scan shows large, right ovarian mass with increased vascularity on color Doppler ultrasound. Dysgerminoma also presents in left ovary *(L); UT,* uterus.

result of estrogen secretion. Sonographically, adult granulosa cell tumors have a variable appearance, ranging from small solid masses to tumors with variable degrees of hemorrhage or fibrotic changes, to multilocular cystic lesions.[294] Metastases, although uncommon, appear as peritoneal-based masses, similar to epithelial neoplasms, or as cystic liver masses.[295]

Sertoli-Leydig Cell Tumor. This rare tumor, also called **androblastoma,** constitutes less than 0.5% of ovarian neoplasms. It generally occurs in women under 30 years of age; almost all are unilateral. Malignancy occurs in 10% to 20% of these tumors. The malignant tumors tend to recur relatively soon after initial diagnosis, with few recurrences after 5 years.[296] Clinically, signs and symptoms of virilization occur in about 30% of patients, although about half will have no endocrine manifestations.[40] Occasionally, these tumors may be associated with estrogen production. Sonographically, Sertoli-Leydig cell tumors usually appear as solid

hypoechoic masses or may be similar in appearance to granulosa cell tumors.[296]

Thecoma and Fibroma. Both these tumors arise from the ovarian stroma and may be difficult to distinguish from each other pathologically. Tumors with an abundance of thecal cells are classified as **thecomas,** whereas those with fewer thecal cells and abundant fibrous tissue are classified as **thecofibromas** and **fibromas. Thecomas** constitute approximately 1% of all ovarian neoplasms, and 70% occur in postmenopausal females. They are unilateral, almost always benign, and frequently show clinical signs of estrogen production. **Fibromas** represent about 4% of ovarian neoplasms, are benign, usually unilateral, and occur most often in menopausal and postmenopausal women. Unlike thecomas, fibromas are rarely associated with estrogen production and therefore are frequently asymptomatic, despite reaching a large size. Ascites has been reported to be present in up to 50% of patients with fibromas larger than 5 cm in diameter.[297]

Meigs syndrome (associated ascites and pleural effusion) occurs in 1% to 3% of patients with ovarian fibromas but is not specific, having been reported in association with other ovarian neoplasms as well. Fibromas also occur in approximately 17% of patients with the **basal cell nevus (Gorlin) syndrome.** In this condition the fibromas are usually bilateral, calcified, and occur in younger women (mean age, 30 years).[296]

Sonographically, these tumors have a characteristic appearance (Fig. 15-45). A hypoechoic mass with marked posterior attenuation of the sound beam is seen as a result of the homogeneous fibrous tissue in these tumors.[297] The main differential diagnosis is a Brenner tumor or pedunculated uterine fibroid. Not all fibromas and thecomas show this characteristic appearance, and a variety of sonographic appearances have been noted, probably because edema and cystic degeneration tend to occur within these tumors.[298]

Metastatic Tumors

About 5% to 10% of ovarian neoplasms are metastatic in origin. The most common primary sites of ovarian metastases are tumors of the breast and gastrointestinal tract. The term **Krukenberg tumor** should be reserved for those tumors containing the typical mucin-secreting "signet ring" cells, usually of gastric or colonic origin. Endometrial carcinoma frequently metastasizes to the ovary, but it may be difficult to distinguish from primary endometrioid carcinoma, as discussed earlier. Sonographically, **ovarian metastases** are usually bilateral solid masses, but they may become necrotic and may have a complex, predominantly cystic appearance that simulates primary cystadenocarcinoma[299,300] (Fig. 15-46). Testa et al.[301] found that almost all ovarian metastases from primary tumors of the breast, stomach, and uterus were solid, whereas those from the colon and rectum were

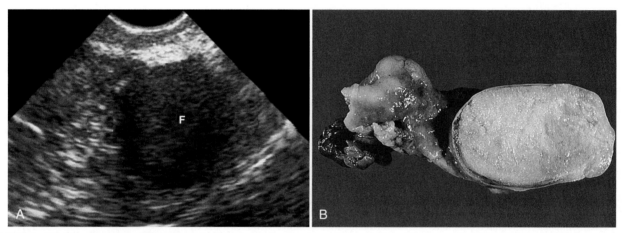

FIGURE 15-45. Ovarian fibroma. A, Transvaginal scan shows hypoechoic solid mass *(F)* with some posterior attenuation. **B,** Pathologic specimen shows homogeneous, solid nature of fibroma.

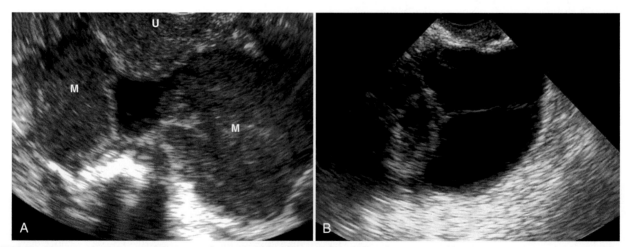

FIGURE 15-46. Ovarian metastases from carcinoma of the colon in two patients. A, Bilateral solid ovarian masses *(M)* or Krukenberg tumors in young woman; *U,* uterus. **B,** Complex, predominantly cystic mass with septations and nodules mimicking a primary ovarian cystadenocarcinoma in postmenopausal woman.

more heterogeneous, most being multicystic with irregular borders. Ascites may be seen in either primary or metastatic tumors. **Lymphoma** may involve the ovary, usually in a diffuse, disseminated form that is frequently bilateral. The sonographic appearance is that of a solid hypoechoic mass similar to lymphoma elsewhere in the body.

FALLOPIAN TUBE

The normal fallopian tube is difficult to identify by transabdominal or transvaginal sonography unless it is dilated or surrounded by fluid. The normal fallopian tube is an undulating echogenic structure approximately 8 to 10 mm in width, running posterolaterally from the uterus to lie within the posterior cul-de-sac near the ovary. The lumen is not seen unless it is fluid filled.[302] Developmental abnormalities of the fallopian tube are rare. Abnormalities of the tube include pregnancy, infection, and neoplasm.

Pelvic Inflammatory Disease

Pelvic inflammatory disease is a common condition that is increasing in frequency. PID is usually caused by sexually transmitted diseases (STDs), most often associated with gonorrhea and chlamydia. The infection typically spreads by ascent from the cervix and endometrium. Less common causes include direct extension from appendiceal, diverticular, or postsurgical abscesses that have ruptured into the pelvis, as well as puerperal and postabortion complications. Hematogenous spread is rare but can occur from tuberculosis. PID is usually bilateral, except when caused by direct extension of an adjacent inflammatory process, when it is most often unilateral. The presence of an IUCD increases the risk of PID. Long-term sequelae include chronic pelvic pain, infertility, and increased risk of ectopic pregnancy.

Sexually transmitted PID spreads along the mucosa of the pelvic organs, initially infecting the cervix and uterine endometrium (endometritis), the fallopian tubes (acute salpingitis), and finally the region of both ovaries and the peritoneum. A pyosalpinx develops as a result of occlusion of the tube. The patients usually present clinically with pain, fever, pelvic tenderness, and vaginal discharge. A pelvic mass may be palpated.

The sonographic findings may be normal early in the course of PID.[303] As the disease progresses or becomes chronic, a spectrum of findings may occur (Figs. 15-47 and 15-48). Endometrial thickening or fluid may indicate **endometritis.** Pus may be demonstrated in the cul-de-sac and contains echogenic particles, which distinguish pus from serous fluid in this region. Enlarged ovaries with multiple cysts and indistinct margins may be seen as a result of periovarian inflammation.[303] On transabdominal sonography, dilated tubes appear as complex,

predominantly cystic masses that are often indistinguishable from other adnexal masses. However, transvaginal sonography recognizes the fluid-filled tube by its tubular shape, somewhat folded configuration, and well-defined echogenic walls.[304] The dilated tube can be distinguished from a fluid-filled bowel loop by the lack of peristalsis. Low-level internal echoes may be seen within the fluid-filled tube as a result of pus (**pyosalpinx**), and a fluid-pus level may occasionally be seen. Anechoic fluid within the tube indicates **hydrosalpinx.** A thickened tubal wall (≥5 mm) is indicative of acute disease.[305,306] In assessing 14 acute and 60 chronic cases of PID, Timor-Tritsch et al.[306] described three appearances of tubal wall structure: (1) **cogwheel sign,** an anechoic "cogwheel-shaped" structure visible in the cross section of the tube with thick walls, seen mainly in acute disease; (2) **"beads on a string" sign,** hyperechoic mural nodules measuring 2 to 3 mm on cross section of the fluid-filled distended tube, caused by degenerated and flattened endosalpingeal fold remnants and seen only in chronic disease; and (3) **incomplete septa,** hyperechoic septa that originate as a triangular protrusion from one of the walls, but do not reach the opposite wall, seen frequently in both acute and chronic disease and not discriminatory. Patel et al.[307] found that the presence of a tubular fluid-filled mass with diametrically opposed indentations in the wall (**"waist sign"**) had the highest likelihood ratio in discriminating hydrosalpinx from other adnexal masses.[307]

As the infection worsens, periovarian adhesions may form, with fusion of the inflamed dilated tube and ovary, which is called the **tubo-ovarian complex** (Fig. 15-48, *B*). The ovary is still recognizable but cannot be separated from the tube by pushing with the vaginal transducer.[306] Further progression leads to complete breakdown, and a separate tube and ovary are no longer identified, resulting in a **tubo-ovarian abscess.** Sono-

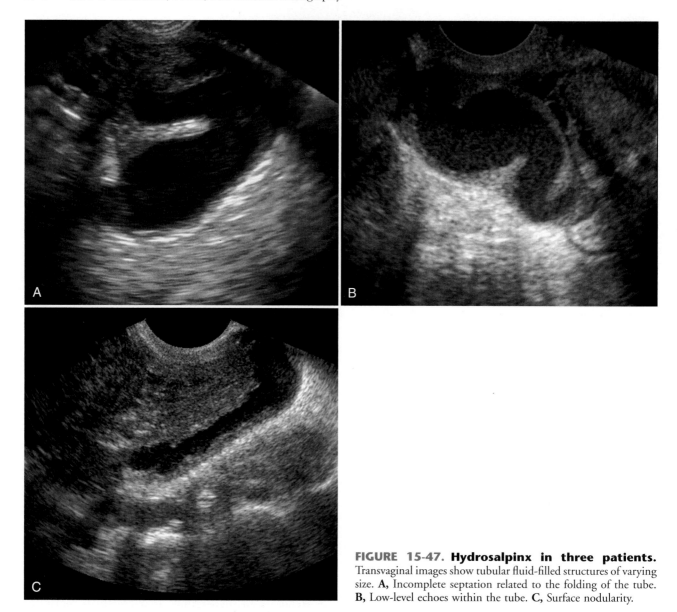

FIGURE 15-47. Hydrosalpinx in three patients.
Transvaginal images show tubular fluid-filled structures of varying size. **A,** Incomplete septation related to the folding of the tube. **B,** Low-level echoes within the tube. **C,** Surface nodularity.

graphically, this appears as a complex multiloculated mass with variable septations, irregular margins, and scattered internal echoes. There is usually posterior acoustic enhancement, and a fluid-debris level or gas may occasionally be seen within the mass. The sonographic appearance may be indistinguishable from other benign and malignant adnexal masses, and clinical correlation is necessary for suggesting the correct diagnosis. Because the ovaries are relatively resistant to infection, areas of recognizable ovarian tissue may be seen within the inflammatory mass by transvaginal sonography.[154]

Both transabdominal and transvaginal sonography are useful in assessing patients with PID. The transabdominal approach is helpful in assessing the extent of the disease, whereas the transvaginal approach is sensitive to detecting dilated tubes, periovarian inflammatory change, and the internal characteristics of tubo-ovarian abscesses.[303,308] Sonography is also useful in following the

response to antibiotic therapy. Tubo-ovarian abscesses may be treated by sonographically guided transvaginal aspiration and drainage.

In **chronic PID**, extensive fibrosis and adhesions may obscure the margins of the pelvic organs, which blend into a large, poorly defined mass. Isolated torsion of the fallopian tube is uncommon, but it occurs in association with chronic hydrosalpinx.[309] The patient presents with abrupt onset of severe pelvic pain. Hydrosalpinx and tubal torsion have also been reported as late complications in patients undergoing tubal ligation.[310]

Carcinoma

Carcinoma of the fallopian tube is the least common (0.3%) of all gynecologic malignancies, with adenocarcinoma being the most common histologic type. It occurs most frequently in postmenopausal women in

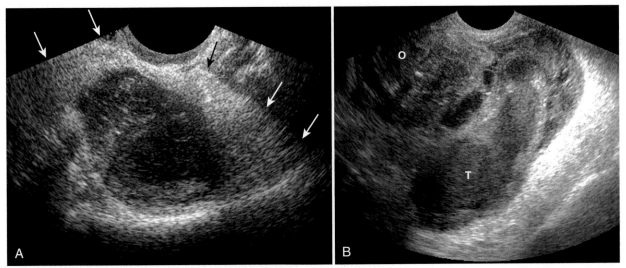

FIGURE 15-48. Pelvic inflammatory disease in two patients. A, Transvaginal image shows a very large ovary surrounded by a rim of highly echogenic and inflamed fat *(arrows)*. There are complex fluid collections within the ovary. There is no normal architecture. **B,** The tube *(T)* is distended and elongated and filled with debris representing pus. The ovary *(O)* is similarly filled with pus, with indistinct borders, showing a tubo-ovarian complex.

their sixth decade, who present clinically with pain, vaginal bleeding, and a pelvic mass. A minority of patients will have a profuse watery discharge, known as **hydrops tubae profluens.** The tumor usually involves the distal end, but it may involve the entire length of the tube. The clinical and sonographic findings are quite similar to those of ovarian carcinoma. Sonographically, carcinoma of the fallopian tube has been described as a sausage-shaped, solid, or cystic mass with papillary projections.[311-314] Patlas et al.[315] stated that this diagnosis should be considered when a solid vascular mass corresponding to the expected location of the fallopian tube is seen in association with normal ovaries, especially if the mass is mobile.[315]

SONOGRAPHIC EVALUATION OF A PELVIC MASS IN ADULT WOMEN

Sonography is often used to evaluate a pelvic mass (Table 15-3). Clinical features such as patient age, symptoms, menstrual status, and family history should also be considered when evaluating the mass. Comparison with previous examinations, if available, should be done to determine if the mass was previously present and if there has been any change in size or internal characteristics.

When a mass is found on sonography, it should be characterized by the following:

- Location (uterine or extrauterine)
- Size
- External contour (well-defined, poorly defined, or irregular borders)
- Internal consistency (cystic, complex predominantly cystic, complex predominantly solid, or solid)

Generally, uterine masses are mainly solid, as opposed to ovarian masses, which are mainly cystic. If the mass can be shown to arise from the uterus, it is usually a benign leiomyoma. Leiomyomas are common causes of solid adnexal masses, in which case showing their origin from the uterus is diagnostic. Occasionally, it may be impossible to determine the exact origin of the mass by sonography, and MRI may be helpful.

The vast majority of ovarian masses are functional in nature. Ovarian masses that are purely cystic and have well-defined borders are almost always benign. The size of the mass is important. In premenopausal women, simple cysts or typical hemorrhagic cysts less than 3 cm can be considered functional, and no follow-up is required. Simple cysts greater than 3 cm are also likely functional, but resolution should be confirmed with a follow-up examination. In postmenopausal women, cysts less than 5 cm are usually benign. Larger masses, especially those greater than 10 cm, have a higher incidence of malignancy. Solid ovarian masses are usually malignant, except for teratomas, fibromas, and transitional cell (Brenner) tumors, which frequently have a specific sonographic appearance. Complex masses may be either benign or malignant and should be further assessed for wall contour, septations, and mural nodules. Irregular borders, thick irregular septations, papillary projections, and echogenic solid nodules favor malignancy. Color and spectral Doppler ultrasound may demonstrate vascularity within the septae or nodules. High-resistance flow strongly suggests benign disease, whereas low-resistance flow suggests malignancy, although it can also be seen with benign disease. Although ascites may be associated with benign masses, it is much more frequently seen with malignant disease. Malignant ascites often contains echogenic particulate matter.

TABLE 15-3. OVARIAN MASSES: SONOGRAPHIC FEATURES SUGGESTIVE OF DISEASE

SONOGRAPHIC CHARACTERISTIC	SUGGESTIVE OF BENIGN DISEASE	SUGGESTIVE OF MALIGNANT DISEASE
Size	Small (<5 cm)	Large (>10 cm)
External contour	Thin wall	Thick wall
	Well-defined borders	Poorly defined or irregular borders
Internal consistency	Purely cystic	Solid or complex
	Thin septations	Thick or irregular septations
		Echogenic solid nodules
		Papillary projections
Doppler findings	High-resistance or no flow	Low-resistance flow
	Avascular nodules	Vascular nodules
Associated findings		Ascites; peritoneal implants

If a pelvic mass is suspected of being malignant, the abdomen should also be evaluated for evidence of ascites and peritoneal implants, obstructive uropathy, lymphadenopathy, and hepatic and splenic metastases. Hepatic and splenic metastases are uncommon in ovarian carcinoma, but when they occur, they are usually peripheral on the surface of the liver or spleen as a result of peritoneal implantation. Hematogenous metastases within the liver or splenic parenchyma may occur late in the course of the disease.

NONGYNECOLOGIC PELVIC MASSES

Pelvic masses and pseudomasses may not be of gynecologic origin. To make this diagnosis, it is important to visualize the uterus and ovaries separately from the mass (Fig. 15-49). This is frequently not possible because of displacement of the normal pelvic structures by the mass. Nongynecologic pelvic masses most frequently originate from the gastrointestinal or urinary tract or may develop after surgery.

Postoperative Pelvic Masses

Postoperative masses may be abscesses, hematomas, lymphoceles, urinomas, or seromas. Sonographically, **abscesses** are ovoid-shaped, anechoic masses with thick, irregular walls and posterior acoustic enhancement. Variable internal echogenicity may be seen, and high-intensity echoes with shadowing caused by gas may be demonstrated. **Hematomas** show a spectrum of sonographic findings, varying with time.[316] During the initial acute phase, hematomas are anechoic. After organization and clot formation, they become highly echogenic. With lysis of the clot, hematomas become more complex, until finally, with complete lysis, they are again anechoic. It is frequently not possible to distinguish an abscess from a hematoma sonographically, and clinical correlation is usually necessary.

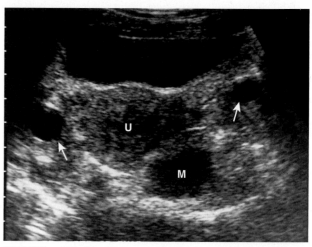

FIGURE 15-49. Extramedullary hematopoiesis. Transverse scan in 44-year-old asymptomatic woman with thalassemia shows anechoic mass *(M)* to left and separate from uterus *(U)* and both ovaries, which contain cysts *(arrows)*. Diagnosis was made by percutaneous biopsy under CT guidance.

Pelvic **lymphoceles** occur after surgical disruption of lymphatic channels, usually after pelvic lymph node dissection or renal transplantation. Sonographically, lymphoceles are cystic, having an appearance similar to that of **urinomas**, which are localized collections of urine, or **seromas**, which are collections of serum. Sonography-guided aspiration may be necessary to differentiate these conditions.

Gastrointestinal Tract Masses

The most frequent pelvic pseudomasses are fecal material in the rectum simulating a complex mass in the cul-de-sac and a fluid-filled rectosigmoid colon presenting as a cystic adnexal mass. Transvaginal sonography can usually distinguish the pseudomass from a true mass, but when it cannot, a repeat examination or MRI may be necessary. **Bowel neoplasms,** especially those involving the rectosigmoid, cecum, and ileum, may simulate an adnexal mass. These tumors frequently show the characteristic target sign of a gastrointestinal mass, consisting of a central echogenic focus caused by air within the lumen, surrounded by a thickened hypoechoic wall.[317] **Abscesses** related to inflammatory disease of the gastrointestinal tract may also present as an adnexal mass. On the right side, this is most frequently caused by appendicitis or Crohn's disease, whereas abscesses on the left side are usually caused by diverticular disease and are seen in an older age group.

Urinary Tract Masses

Patients with a **pelvic kidney** may present with a clinically palpable mass. This is readily recognized sonographically by the typical reniform appearance and the absence of a kidney in the normal location. Occasionally, a greatly distended bladder may be mistaken for an ovarian cyst. When a cystic pelvic mass is identified, it is imperative that the bladder be seen separately from the mass. **Bladder diverticula** may also simulate a cystic adnexal mass. The diagnosis can be confirmed by demonstrating communication with the bladder and a changing appearance after voiding. **Dilated distal ureters** may simulate adnexal cysts on transverse scans; however, sagittal scans show their tubular appearance and continuity with the bladder.

POSTPARTUM PELVIC PATHOLOGIC CONDITIONS

The uterus is enlarged during the postpartum period and gradually returns to a nongravid size within 6 to 8 weeks. The endometrium returns to its nongravid state by 3 to 6 weeks.[318] Small amounts of fluid and echogenic material (likely blood) can be seen normally within the endometrial canal.[319,320] Gas can also be seen normally for up to 3 weeks after uncomplicated vaginal delivery.[140] Pathologic states in the postpartum period are usually the result of infection and hemorrhage. Specific pathologic conditions occurring in the postpartum period include endometritis, retained products of conception, and ovarian vein thrombophlebitis. **Endometritis** is more frequent after cesarean than vaginal delivery. It usually occurs in patients who have had prolonged labor or premature rupture of membranes or who have retained products of conception. The most common source of organisms is the normal vaginal flora. Clinically, there is pelvic pain or unexplained fever.

Retained Products of Conception

Retained products of conception after an abortion or delivery may cause secondary hemorrhage or may serve as a nidus for infection. Sonographically, an **echogenic mass** in the endometrial cavity suggests this diagnosis (Fig. 15-50), although blood clot may also present as a mass.[321] Calcifications may be seen within the mass and strongly suggests retained placental tissue. The calcification is caused by retained mature placenta or the chronicity of the process.[322] Endometrial thickness is variable, however, when the endometrial thickness is less than 10 mm and there is no endometrial mass, either in the postabortion or postpartum state, the likelihood of clinically significant retained products is low.[318,323] **Vascularity** within the mass or thickened endometrium suggests retained products (Fig. 15-50, *A*), whereas absent vascularity favors blood clot. However, absent vascularity does not exclude retained products.

Ovarian Vein Thrombophlebitis

Puerperal ovarian vein thrombosis or thrombophlebitis is an uncommon but potentially life-threatening condition (Fig. 15-51). Patients present with fever, lower abdominal pain, and a palpable mass, usually 48 to 96 hours postpartum. The underlying cause is venous stasis and spread of bacterial infection from endometritis. The right ovarian vein is involved in 90% of cases. Retrograde venous flow occurs in the left ovarian vein during the puerperium, which protects this side from bacterial spread from the uterus.[40] This condition may be diagnosed by sonography, CT, or MRI.[324,325] Sonography may demonstrate an inflammatory mass lateral to the uterus and anterior to the psoas muscle. The ovarian vein may be seen as a tubular, anechoic structure directed cephalad from the mass and containing echogenic thrombus. The thrombus usually affects the most cephalic portion of the right ovarian vein and can be demonstrated sonographically at the junction of the right ovarian vein with the inferior vena cava, sometimes extending into the inferior vena cava.[326] Thrombus in the inferior vena cava may also be seen. Doppler ultrasound may demonstrate absence of flow in these veins.[327] Most patients respond to anticoagulant and antibiotic therapy, and follow-up sonography may show resolution of the thrombus and normal flow on duplex Doppler imaging.

Cesarean Section Complications

A lower uterine transverse incision site is typically used for cesarean section. On sonographic examination, the **incision site** can be identified as an oval, symmetrical region of hypoechogenicity relative to the myometrium, located between the posterior wall of the bladder and the lower uterine segment.[328] **Sutures** within the incision site may be recognized as small, punctate, high-amplitude echoes (Fig. 15-52).

Hematomas may develop from hemorrhage at the incision site (bladder flap hematomas) or within the prevesical space (subfascial hematomas). **Bladder flap hematomas** can be diagnosed sonographically when a complex or anechoic mass greater than 2 cm in diameter is located adjacent to the scar and between the

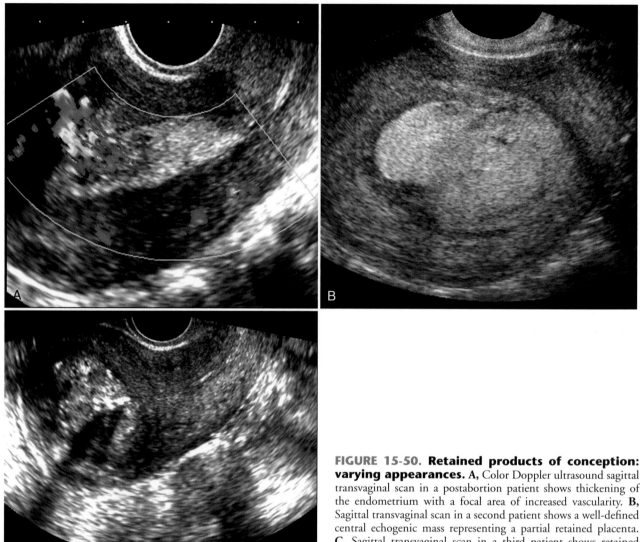

FIGURE 15-50. Retained products of conception: varying appearances. A, Color Doppler ultrasound sagittal transvaginal scan in a postabortion patient shows thickening of the endometrium with a focal area of increased vascularity. **B,** Sagittal transvaginal scan in a second patient shows a well-defined central echogenic mass representing a partial retained placenta. **C,** Sagittal transvaginal scan in a third patient shows retained placental tissue containing calcification in the fundus, extending into the myometrium—retained placenta increta.

lower uterine segment and the posterior bladder wall (Fig. 15-53). The echogenicity varies depending on the amount of organization within the hematoma.[316] The presence of air within the mass is highly suggestive of an infected hematoma.[329] **Subfascial hematomas** are extraperitoneal in location, contained within the prevesical space, and caused by disruption of the inferior epigastric vessels or their branches during cesarean section[330] or traumatic vaginal delivery.[331] Sonographically, a complex or cystic mass is seen anterior to the bladder. High-frequency, short-focus transducers are often necessary to recognize the superficial mass. It is important to identify the rectus muscle in order to distinguish the **superficial wound hematoma,** which is located anterior to the rectus muscle, from the subfascial hematoma, located posterior to it.[330] Bladder flap and subfascial hematomas may be seen together in the same patient; however, they have different sources of bleeding and should be treated as separate conditions.

GESTATIONAL TROPHOBLASTIC NEOPLASIA

Gestational trophoblastic neoplasia (GTN) represents a spectrum of conditions, including hydatidiform molar pregnancy, invasive mole, choriocarcinoma, and placental-site trophoblastic tumor. The latter three conditions are referred to as **persistent trophoblastic neoplasia** (PTN). All these conditions show abnormal trophoblastic proliferation histologically.

Hydatidiform Molar Pregnancy

Hydatidiform molar pregnancy is the most common and benign form of GTN, with an incidence of 1 in 1000 pregnancies in North America.[332] The incidence is much higher in the Asian population. There is an increased risk in teenagers, in women over 35 years of age, and in

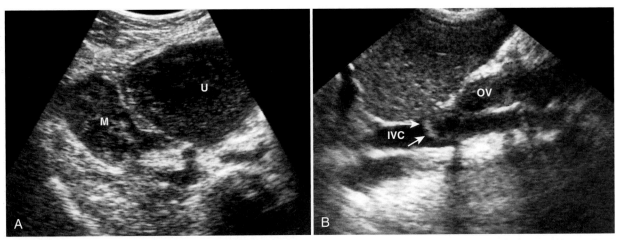

FIGURE 15-51. Ovarian vein thrombophlebitis. A, Transverse scan in patient with fever and right lower abdominal pain 4 days after cesarean section shows mass *(M)* to right of postpartum uterus *(U)*. **B,** Sagittal scan of abdomen shows echogenic thrombus in distended right ovarian vein *(OV)*. Thrombus *(arrows)* is seen extending into inferior vena cava *(IVC)*.

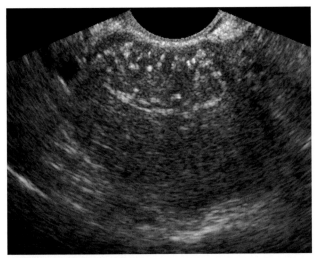

FIGURE 15-52. Cesarean section sutures. Transverse transvaginal image shows multiple bright, echogenic foci in the surgical site.

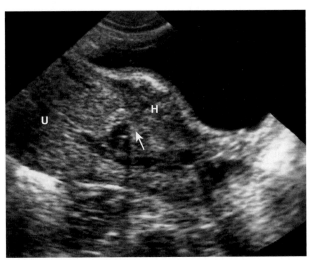

FIGURE 15-53. Bladder-flap hematoma. Sagittal scan in patient with fever and lower abdominal pain 8 days after cesarean section shows hematoma *(H)* between bladder and cesarean section scar *(arrow); U,* uterus.

women with a previous molar pregnancy. The risk also increases with the number of previous spontaneous abortions.[333] Molar pregnancy is characterized histologically by cystic (hydatidiform) degeneration of chorionic villi, with absent or inadequate vascularization and abnormal trophoblastic proliferation.

The most frequent presenting symptom is **vaginal bleeding,** which occurs in more than 90% of cases. Passage of vesicles (hydropic villi) through the vagina occurs frequently and is considered specific for the diagnosis of molar pregnancy.[334] The uterus may be enlarged for dates, and there may also be rapid uterine enlargement. Medical complications include pregnancy-induced hypertension, hyperemesis gravidarum, preeclampsia, and hyperthyroidism. The routine use of ultrasound for any woman with bleeding in pregnancy now allows for early diagnosis, and few women show the classic features of hyperemesis and preeclampsia.[335]

Serum hCG levels in molar pregnancy are abnormally elevated, usually greater than 100,000 mIU/mL. Theca lutein cysts of the ovaries occur in approximately 15% to 30% of cases and reflect the abnormally high hCG levels.

Molar pregnancy is treated by uterine evacuation, which is adequate in most patients. Approximately 80% of complete moles and 95% of partial moles will subsequently follow a benign course.[334,336] However, accurate diagnosis and classification of molar pregnancy are important because of the risk of PTN. For this reason, all patients with molar pregnancy are monitored with weekly serum hCG determinations and are counseled to avoid pregnancy for at least 1 year.

Hydatidiform molar pregnancy is classified as either complete molar pregnancy or partial molar pregnancy on the basis of cytogenetic and pathologic features.

Complete Molar Pregnancy

Complete molar pregnancy is characterized by a **diploid karyotype** of 46,XX in approximately 80% to 90% of cases, with the chromosomal DNA being exclusively paternal in origin.[337] This occurs when an ovum with absent or inactive maternal chromosomes is fertilized by a normal haploid sperm. Occasionally, fertilization of an empty ovum by two haploid sperm results in a 46,XY pattern.[333] As the embryo dies at an early stage, **no fetal parts** are seen.[337] The placenta is entirely replaced by abnormal, hydropic chorionic villi with excessive trophoblastic proliferation.

The classic sonographic features of complete molar pregnancy include an enlarged uterus with a central heterogeneous echogenic mass that expands the endometrial canal. The mass contains multiple cystic spaces of varying size, representing the hydropic villi (Fig. 15-54). These cystic spaces may vary in size from a few millimeters to 2 to 3 cm. In the second trimester, transabdominal sonographic diagnosis is highly accurate. In the first trimester, however, molar tissue may appear as a predominantly solid, echogenic mass on transabdominal sonography because tiny hydropic villi may not be adequately resolved. With its better resolution, transvaginal sonography may depict the hydropic villi earlier and to better advantage. In complete moles, a fetus is absent except in the rare event of a coexistent twin pregnancy; in such cases, sonography is accurate in establishing the diagnosis.

The ovaries may be greatly enlarged in complete molar pregnancy by multiple, bilateral theca lutein cysts. These are large, usually multilocular, and may undergo hemorrhage or torsion and can be a source of pelvic pain. Theca lutein cysts are most marked when trophoblastic proliferation is severe. They are seen much less often in the first trimester.[338,339]

Partial Molar Pregnancy

Partial molar pregnancy has a **triploid karyotype** of 69,XXX, 69,XXY, or 69,XYY. Most partial moles have one set of maternal chromosomes and two sets of paternal chromosomes, resulting from fertilization of a normal ovum by two haploid sperm. Triploidy of maternal origin is not associated with GTN.[340] Pathologically, partial molar pregnancy has well-developed but generally **anomalous (triploid) fetal tissues.** Hydropic degeneration of placental villi is focal, interspersed with normal placental villi. Trophoblastic proliferation is mild. Symptoms and signs are less frequent and less severe because of the mild trophoblastic proliferation. The diagnosis of partial molar pregnancy is rarely made prospectively,

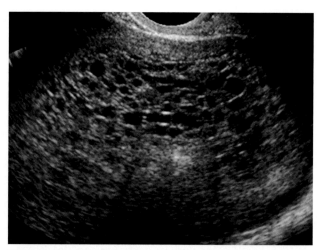

FIGURE 15-54. Complete molar pregnancy: classic appearance. Transabdominal scan shows a vesicular echogenic mass distending the endometrium. The mass is filled with innumerable uniformly distributed cystic spaces that corresponded to hydropic chorionic villi at pathology.

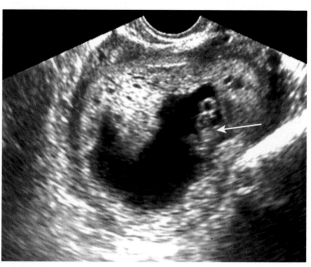

FIGURE 15-55. Partial molar pregnancy at 8 weeks' gestation. Transvaginal scan shows a gravid uterus with a yolk sac and live 8-week embryo *(arrow)*. On the right is a large placenta with multiple small cystic spaces consistent with hydropic villi. Pathology confirmed partial mole.

with most cases diagnosed clinically as an incomplete abortion.[334,336]

The sonographic features of partial molar pregnancy are less frequently described and overlap with other conditions, such as an anembryonic pregnancy or an incomplete abortion.[335] In partial molar pregnancy, the placenta is excessive in size and contains numerous cystic spaces distributed in a nonuniform manner (Fig. 15-55). Fine et al.[341] found that a ratio of transverse to anteroposterior dimension of the gestational sac of greater than 1.5, as well as cystic changes, irregularity, or increased echogenicity in the decidual reaction/placenta or myometrium, was significantly associated with this diagnosis. A growth-impaired fetus is present and may show multiple anomalies.

Placental **hydropic degeneration** (unrelated to trophoblastic neoplasia) may also show similar sonographic features. Hydropic degeneration occurs frequently in first-trimester abortion of any cause. The associated cystic spaces may be difficult or impossible to differentiate from an early mole. Therefore, in cases with equivocal ultrasound features, the products of conception should be carefully evaluated to avoid missing a hydatidiform mole.

Recent studies have shown that **sonography is much more accurate in diagnosing complete molar pregnancy than partial molar pregnancy.** Kirk et al.[342] evaluated sonography in the first trimester and found an accuracy of 95% for the diagnosis of complete mole and 20% for partial mole, with an overall accuracy for hydatidiform mole of 44%. In 859 pathologically diagnosed hydatidiform moles, Fowler et al.[343] found that sonography performed in the first and early second trimester had a similar 44% overall accuracy and an accuracy of 79% and 29% for complete and partial moles, respectively. Also, the sonographic detection rate improved after 14 weeks' gestation.

Coexistent Hydatidiform Mole and Normal Fetus

Twin pregnancies with an apparently normal fetus and a hydatidiform mole are uncommon, with an estimated incidence of 1 in 20,000 to 100,000 pregnancies.[344,345] It is differentiated from a partial molar pregnancy by identifying a normal-appearing fetus with a corresponding normal placenta adjacent to a mass of placental tissue that demonstrates molar changes (Fig. 15-56). Initial studies suggested that these patients were at high risk for developing PTN.[344] However, a larger study of 77 cases showed that the risk of PTN was similar to that after a singleton complete mole and was not increased by continuing the pregnancy.[345] The 53 women who decided to continue the pregnancy had an increased risk of pregnancy complications, but 20 (38%) delivered a live baby, usually after 32 weeks.

Persistent Trophoblastic Neoplasia

Persistent trophoblastic neoplasia is a life-threatening complication of pregnancy that includes invasive mole, choriocarcinoma, and the extremely rare placental-site trophoblastic tumor. PTN occurs most often after molar pregnancy; up to 20% of complete moles develop persistent disease requiring additional therapy.[332,334] Complete moles with severe degrees of trophoblastic proliferation are at the highest risk, with persistent disease developing in 50% or more of these patients.[336] The risk is also increased in patients over 40 years of age and in women who have had multiple molar pregnancies.[337] The risk of persistent disease after partial molar pregnancy is much lower, occurring in approximately 5% of cases.[334,337] Less often, PTN develops after a normal term delivery, spontaneous abortion, or rarely an ectopic pregnancy.[332]

Invasive Mole

Invasive mole is the **most common form of PTN,** accounting for 80% to 95% of cases.[346] Patients usually present with vaginal bleeding and persistent elevation of serum hCG within 1 to 3 months after molar evacuation.[347] Histologically, invasive mole is characterized by the presence of formed chorionic villi and trophoblastic proliferation deep in the myometrium (Fig. 15-57). It is

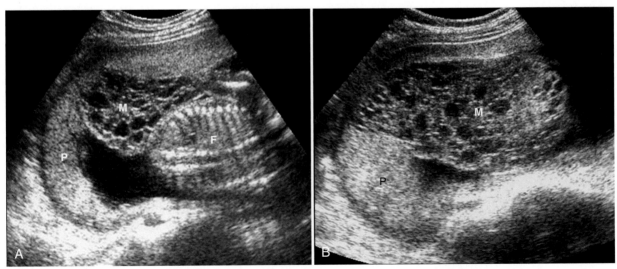

FIGURE 15-56. Complete mole with a coexistent fetus at 16 weeks' gestation. A and **B,** Large echogenic mass with innumerable tiny cystic spaces, the classic morphology for a complete mole *(M),* with a normal fetus *(F)* and a normal anterior placenta *(P).*

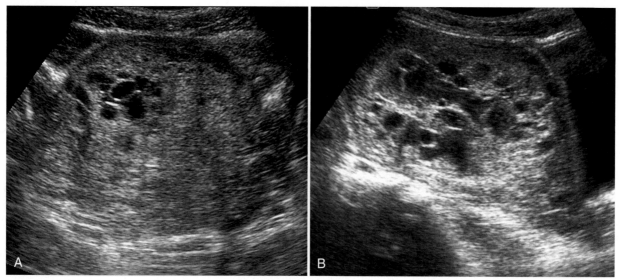

FIGURE 15-57. Invasive mole 6 weeks after evacuation of complete mole. A, Transverse, and **B,** sagittal, transabdominal scans show large mass filled with multiple cystic spaces extending deep into the myometrium on the right side.

considered biologically benign and is usually confined to the uterus; rarely, molar tissue can penetrate the whole thickness of the myometrium, leading to uterine perforation, which may cause severe hemorrhage.[348] Lesions can invade beyond the uterus to parametrial tissues, adjacent organs, and blood vessels. Rarely, invasive molar villi may embolize to distant sites, including the lungs and brain.

Choriocarcinoma

Choriocarcinoma is an extremely rare malignancy with an incidence of 1 in 30,000 pregnancies. As with other forms of PTN, the most important risk factor for choriocarcinoma is molar pregnancy. Molar gestations precede 50% to 80% of cases, and 1 in 40 molar pregnancies gives rise to choriocarcinoma. Choriocarcinoma is a purely cellular lesion characterized histologically by the invasion of the myometrium by abnormal, proliferating trophoblast and the absence of formed villi. Hemorrhage and necrosis are prominent features.[333] Early vascular invasion is common, resulting in distant metastases, most frequently affecting the lungs, followed by the liver, brain, gastrointestinal tract, and kidney. Respiratory compromise may be the initial presentation.[349] Venous invasion and retrograde metastases to the vagina and pelvic structures are also common.[349]

Placental-Site Trophoblastic Tumor

Placental-site trophoblastic tumor (PSTT) is the **rarest and most fatal form of PTN**.[350] As with choriocarcinoma and invasive mole, PSTT can follow any type of gestation, but in more than 90% of cases it develops after a normal term delivery.[348] The tumor may occur from as early as 1 week to many years after pregnancy. Vaginal bleeding is the most common symptom, although some

women may present with amenorrhea. Histologically, PSTT is distinct from other forms of trophoblastic neoplasia. It arises from nonvillous, "intermediate" trophoblast that infiltrates the decidua, spiral arteries, and myometrium at the placental bed. PSTT may be confined to the uterus, may be locally invasive in the pelvis, or may metastasize to the lungs, lymph nodes, peritoneum, liver, pancreas, or brain. Serum hCG is not a reliable marker for PSTT; it is usually negative or only mildly elevated. Histochemical staining of intermediate trophoblast for hCG is weak or absent, whereas staining for human placental lactogen (hPL) is strongly positive. Unfortunately, serum hPL is not a reliable predictor of tumor behavior.[350] Surgical therapy is recommended because these lesions tend to resist chemotherapy and have a high risk of metastasis.

Sonographic Features of PTN

Sonography plays an important role in detecting and staging PTN and in monitoring response to therapy. The sonographic features of PTN are less familiar than those of primary molar pregnancy. Whereas transvaginal sonography is frequently unnecessary for the diagnosis of primary molar pregnancy, it is essential for the diagnosis of PTN. The small, myometrial lesions typical of this condition may not be apparent on transabdominal scanning.[351] Invasive mole, choriocarcinoma, and PSTT may appear similar sonographically.[352,353] The most frequently described sonographic abnormality in PTN is a **focal, echogenic myometrial nodule**[349,351-353] (Fig. 15-58). The lesion usually lies close to the endometrial canal, but it may be found deep in the myometrium. Lesions may appear solid and uniformly echogenic, hypoechoic, or complex and multicystic, similar to molar tissue. Thick-walled, irregular anechoic areas may be seen, resulting

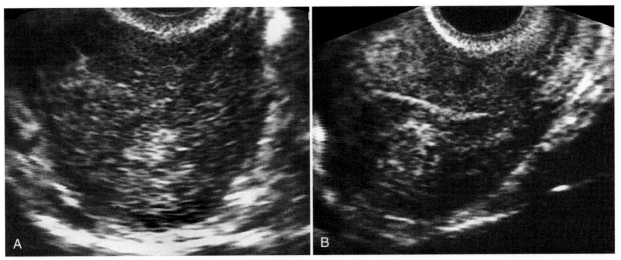

FIGURE 15-58. Focal echogenic myometrial nodule of persistent trophoblastic neoplasia (PTN). A, Transverse transvaginal sonogram shows central focal uterine echogenicity that could be mistaken for a thick endometrium. **B,** Sagittal image shows that the echogenic area lies within the myometrium posterior to a normal endometrial canal. *(Courtesy Drs. Margaret Fraser-Hill, Peter Burns, and Stephanie Wilson.)*

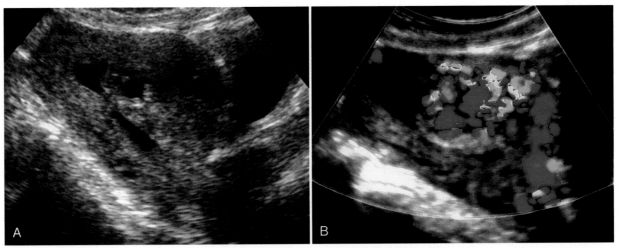

FIGURE 15-59. Cystic spaces representing vessels and hemorrhage in PTN. A, Sagittal sonogram shows a mildly enlarged uterus with a complex anterior myometrial mass and blood in the endometrial cavity. **B,** Color Doppler ultrasound shows a florid-color mosaic pattern in the anterior myometrial tumor and blood in the endometrial cavity. *(Courtesy of Drs. Margaret Fraser-Hill, Peter Burns and Stephanie Wilson.)*

from tissue necrosis and hemorrhage[351-353] (Fig. 15-59). In other cases, anechoic areas within lesions represent vascular spaces. When tumor replaces the entire myometrium, the uterus is enlarged, with the myometrium appearing heterogeneous and lobulated. The tumor may extend beyond the uterus to the parametrium, pelvic side wall, and adjacent organs. In extreme cases, PTN appears as a large, undifferentiated pelvic mass (Fig. 15-60). Sonography can be diagnostic in the correct setting (e.g., recent molar pregnancy, rising serum hCG, previously documented normal sonogram).

After effective therapy, sonographic lesions become progressively more hypoechoic and smaller in size. Even-tually, no residual abnormality is apparent in many cases. However, up to 50% of patients will have persistent abnormalities after therapy that may be difficult to distinguish from active lesions sonographically.

Duplex and color Doppler ultrasound features of PTN reflect the marked hypervascularity of invasive trophoblast.[354,355] Uterine spiral arteries feed directly into prominent vascular spaces, which then communicate with draining veins. These **functional arteriovenous shunts** produce abnormal uterine hypervascularity and high-velocity, low-impedance blood flow on duplex interrogation.[354] **Trophoblastic blood flow** has characteristic, high PSV and low RI. PSV is usually greater than

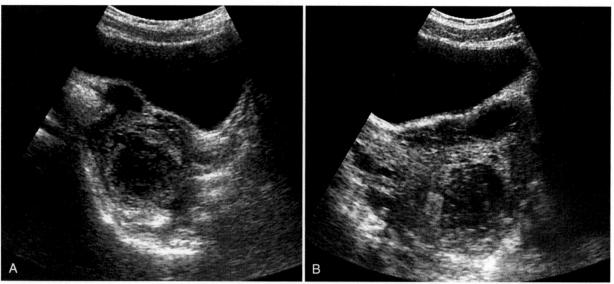

FIGURE 15-60. Choriocarcinoma after normal pregnancy producing pelvic mass in PTN. A, Sagittal, and **B,** transverse, sonograms show a large, poorly defined, complex pelvic mass with both cystic and solid components. The uterus could not be identified. Doppler ultrasound *(not shown)* showed trophoblastic signals everywhere within this mass. Choriocarcinoma in PTN was not suspected clinically or on sonography until Doppler ultrasound was performed. *(Courtesy Drs. Margaret Fraser-Hill, Peter Burns, and Stephanie Wilson.)*

50 cm/sec and is often over 100 cm/sec. RI is usually less than 0.5 and is often well below 0.4. In contrast, normal myometrial blood flow usually has a PSV of less than 50 cm/sec and an RI in the range of 0.7. Color Doppler sonographic features typical of PTN include extensive color aliasing, admixture of color signals, loss of discreteness of vessels, and chaotic vascular arrangement. Regions of abnormal color Doppler ultrasound frequently appear larger than corresponding sonographic abnormalities.

Duplex and color Doppler ultrasound studies are noninvasive and are reliable alternatives to conventional angiography for detecting and staging pelvic PTN.[355,356] Doppler is also helpful in detecting disease recurrence and following response to therapy.[357] **Abnormal vascularity** may be difficult or impossible to detect in primary molar pregnancy but is a major feature of PTN. Qualitative assessments of vascularity on color Doppler ultrasound are not diagnostic of PTN. However, the marked color Doppler hypervascularity in PTN is seen in a few other conditions, such as the extremely rare uterine AVMs, a potential pitfall.[72]

Trophoblastic signals on spectral Doppler ultrasound are not unique to PTN. They are seen in all conditions with functioning trophoblast, including failed pregnancy, retained products of conception, and ectopic pregnancy. These potential pitfalls are distinguished from PTN by clinical findings, sonographic morphology, and pathology. However, PSTT should remain a consideration even with a normal hCG level (see Fig. 15-61). In most patients the diagnosis of PTN is fairly straightforward, and additional information provided by Doppler ultrasound is supportive but not critical.

However, when PTN is not suspected clinically, duplex and color Doppler sonography may provide the first indication of trophoblastic disease by showing marked hypervascularity and typical trophoblastic blood flow within lesions. Doppler ultrasound also improves diagnostic specificity by showing normal uterine waveforms when PTN is absent and sonography is abnormal, as when other uterine lesions mimic the appearance of PTN, or persistent nonspecific abnormalities remain after effective therapy.[355]

Diagnosis and Treatment

Because PTN arises most often after a molar pregnancy, the diagnosis is usually based on abnormal regression of hCG after uterine evacuation. A histologic diagnosis is not considered mandatory because curettage risks uterine perforation and does not significantly alter management or outcome.[349,358] Patients are treated on the basis of clinical staging that includes CT of the brain, chest, abdomen, and pelvis. Again, although the diagnosis of PTN is usually straightforward, PTN may go unrecognized in some patients, as when inadequate pathologic examination fails to detect hydatidiform mole in a first-trimester abortion. PTN developing in such cases or after nonmolar gestations will be mistaken for a failed pregnancy or retained products of conception. Recognition of PSTT is further complicated by negative or low hCG levels. In addition, patients with PTN may present with a confusing variety of nongynecologic problems, including respiratory compromise and cerebral, gastrointestinal, or urologic hemorrhage.[346,349] In difficult cases, imaging may be the first study to suggest the diagnosis (Fig. 15-61).

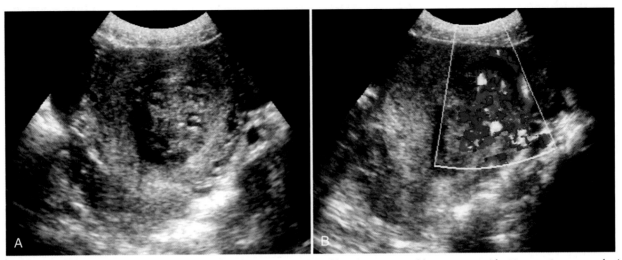

FIGURE 15-61. Placental-site trophoblastic tumor (PSTT). This 28-year-old woman, gravida 10, para 2, presented with heavy bleeding requiring transfusion (hCG negative). **A,** Transverse transvaginal sonogram shows a central, complex, 3-cm-diameter uterine mass involving both the endometrial canal and the myometrium. **B,** Color Doppler ultrasound shows extensive color, more extensive than the gray-scale abnormality. *(Courtesy Drs. Margaret Fraser-Hill, Peter Burns, and Stephanie Wilson.)*

With the exception of PSTT, hCG level is a sensitive and specific marker for detecting and monitoring PTN. Normal mean disappearance time of hCG in benign moles ranges from 7 to 14 weeks (median, 11 weeks), but can be as long as a year.

Persistent trophoblastic neoplasia is broadly classified as **nonmetastatic** or **metastatic** on the basis of staging computed tomography of the brain, chest, abdomen, and pelvis.[349,358] Nonmetastatic PTN has an excellent prognosis. Single-agent therapy with methotrexate achieves sustained remission in virtually 100% of cases.[358] Metastatic PTN is subdivided into **low-risk** and **high-risk** groups. Virtually all patients with low-risk metastatic disease are cured with simple chemotherapy.[349] In contrast, patients with high-risk disease have a significantly worse prognosis and a high likelihood of failure with single-agent therapy. High-risk, poor-prognosis disease is indicated by duration of disease for more than 4 months, pretreatment hCG levels greater than 40,000 mIU/mL, presence of brain or liver metastases, antecedent term pregnancy, and prior history of failed chemotherapy. These patients are treated aggressively with appropriate combinations of intense multiagent chemotherapy, adjuvant radiotherapy, and surgery. By tailoring therapy in this way, even high-risk patients have cure rates of 80% to 90%.[349,359]

References

1. Benacerraf BR, Shipp TD, Bromley B, et al. Which patients benefit from a 3D-reconstructed coronal view of the uterus added to standard routine 2D pelvic sonography? AJR Am J Roentgenol 2008; 190:626-629.

Normal Pelvic Anatomy
2. Williams PL, Warwick R, editors. Gray's anatomy, 37th ed. Edinburgh: Churchill Livingstone; 1989.

Sonographic Methods
3. American Institute of Ultrasound in Medicine. AIUM practice guidelines for the performance of sonohysterography. AUIM; 2007.
4. Cullinan JA, Fleischer AC, Kepple DM, Arnold AL. Sonohysterography: a technique for endometrial evaluation. Radiographics 1995;15:501-514; discussion 515-516.
5. Lev-Toaff AS, Pinheiro LW, Bega G, et al. Three-dimensional multiplanar sonohysterography: comparison with conventional two-dimensional sonohysterography and x-ray hysterosalpingography. J Ultrasound Med 2001;20:295-306.
6. De Kroon CD, Louwe LA, Trimbos JB, et al. The clinical value of 3-dimensional saline infusion sonography in addition to 2-dimensional saline infusion sonography in women with abnormal uterine bleeding: work in progress. J Ultrasound Med 2004;23:1433-1440.

Uterus
7. Sample WF, Lippe BM, Gyepes MT. Gray-scale ultrasonography of the normal female pelvis. Radiology 1977;125:477-483.
8. Orsini LF, Salardi S, Pilu G, et al. Pelvic organs in premenarcheal girls: real-time ultrasonography. Radiology 1984;153:113-116.
9. Nussbaum AR, Sanders RC, Jones MD. Neonatal uterine morphology as seen on real-time ultrasound. Radiology 1986;160:641-643.
10. Siegel MJ. Pediatric gynecologic sonography. Radiology 1991; 179:593-600.
11. Holm K, Laursen EM, Brocks V, Muller J. Pubertal maturation of the internal genitalia: an ultrasound evaluation of 166 healthy girls [see comment]. Ultrasound Obstet Gynecol 1995;6:175-181.
12. Platt JF, Bree RL, Davidson D. Ultrasound of the normal nongravid uterus: correlation with gross and histopathology. J Clin Ultrasound 1990;18:15-19.
13. Merz E, Miric-Tesanic D, Bahlmann F, et al. Sonographic size of uterus and ovaries in pre- and postmenopausal women. Ultrasound Obstet Gynecol 1996;7:38-42.
14. Miller EI, Thomas RH, Lines P. The atrophic postmenopausal uterus. J Clin Ultrasound 1977;5:261-263.
15. Fleischer AC, Kalemeris GC, Machin JE, et al. Sonographic depiction of normal and abnormal endometrium with histopathologic correlation. J Ultrasound Med 1986;5:445-452.
16. Farrer-Brown G, Beilby JO, Tarbit MH. The blood supply of the uterus. 2. Venous pattern. J Obstet Gynaecol 1970;77:682-689.
17. DuBose TJ, Hill LW, Hennigan Jr HW, et al. Sonography of arcuate uterine blood vessels. J Ultrasound Med 1985;4:229-233.
18. Occhipinti K, Kutcher R, Rosenblatt R. Sonographic appearance and significance of arcuate artery calcification. J Ultrasound Med 1991;10:97-100.

19. Atri M, de Stempel J, Senterman MK, Bret PM. Diffuse peripheral uterine calcification (manifestation of Monckeberg's arteriosclerosis) detected by ultrasonography. J Clin Ultrasound 1992;20:211-216.

20. Burks DD, Stainken BF, Burkhard TK, Balsara ZN. Uterine inner myometrial echogenic foci: relationship to prior dilatation and curettage and endocervical biopsy. J Ultrasound Med 1991;10:487-492.

21. Duffield C, Gerscovich EO, Gillen MA, et al. Endometrial and endocervical micro echogenic foci: sonographic appearance with clinical and histologic correlation. J Ultrasound Med 2005;24:583-590.

22. Callen PW, DeMartini WJ, Filly RA. The central uterine cavity echo: a useful anatomic sign in the ultrasonographic evaluation of the female pelvis. Radiology 1979;131:187-190.

23. Fleischer AC, Kalemeris GC, Entman SS. Sonographic depiction of the endometrium during normal cycles. Ultrasound Med Biol 1986;12:271-277.

24. Forrest TS, Elyaderani MK, Muilenburg MI, et al. Cyclic endometrial changes: ultrasound assessment with histologic correlation. Radiology 1988;167:233-237.

25. Lin MC, Gosink BB, Wolf SI, et al. Endometrial thickness after menopause: effect of hormone replacement [see comment]. Radiology 1991;180:427-432.

26. Ergun A, Pabuccu R, Atay V, et al. Three sisters with septate uteri: another reference to bidirectional theory. Hum Reprod 1997;12:140-142.

27. Deutch TD, Abuhamad AZ, Deutch TD, Abuhamad AZ. The role of 3-dimensional ultrasonography and magnetic resonance imaging in the diagnosis of müllerian duct anomalies: a review of the literature. J Ultrasound Med 2008;27:413-423.

28. Brody JM, Koelliker SL, Frishman GN. Unicornuate uterus: imaging appearance, associated anomalies, and clinical implications. AJR Am J Roentgenol 1998;171:1341-1347.

29. Troiano RN, McCarthy SM, Troiano RN, McCarthy SM. Müllerian duct anomalies: imaging and clinical issues. Radiology 2004;233:19-34.

30. Viscomi GN, Gonzalez R, Taylor KJ. Ultrasound detection of uterine abnormalities after diethylstilbestrol (DES) exposure. Radiology 1980;136:733-735.

31. Lev-Toaff AS, Toaff ME, Friedman AC. Endovaginal sonographic appearance of a DES uterus. J Ultrasound Med 1990;9:661-664.

32. Fedele L, Bianchi S, Agnoli B, et al. Urinary tract anomalies associated with unicornuate uterus. J Urol 1996;155:847-848.

33. Salim R, Woelfer B, Backos M, et al. Reproducibility of three-dimensional ultrasound diagnosis of congenital uterine anomalies. Ultrasound Obstet Gynecol 2003;21:578-582.

34. Nicolini U, Bellotti M, Bonazzi B, et al. Can ultrasound be used to screen uterine malformations? Fertil Steril 1987;47:89-93.

35. Pellerito JS, McCarthy SM, Doyle MB, et al. Diagnosis of uterine anomalies: relative accuracy of MR imaging, endovaginal sonography, and hysterosalpingography. Radiology 1992;183:795-800.

36. Zreik TG, Troiano RN, Ghoussoub RA, et al. Myometrial tissue in uterine septa. J Am Assoc Gynecol Laparosc 1998;5:155-160.

37. Reuter KL, Daly DC, Cohen SM. Septate versus bicornuate uteri: errors in imaging diagnosis. Radiology 1989;172:749-752.

38. Jurkovic D, Geipel A, Gruboeck K, et al. Three-dimensional ultrasound for the assessment of uterine anatomy and detection of congenital anomalies: a comparison with hysterosalpingography and two-dimensional sonography [see comment]. Ultrasound Obstet Gynecol 1995;5:233-237.

39. Bega G, Lev-Toaff AS, O'Kane P, et al. Three-dimensional ultrasonography in gynecology: technical aspects and clinical applications. J Ultrasound Med 2003;22:1249-1269.

40. Kurman RJ, editor. Blaustein's pathology of the female genital tract, 5th ed. New York: Springer-Verlag; 2002.

41. Smith JP, Weiser EB, Karnei Jr RF, Hoskins WJ. Ultrasonography of rapidly growing uterine leiomyomata associated with anovulatory cycles. Radiology 1980;134:713-716.

42. Lev-Toaff AS, Coleman BG, Arger PH, et al. Leiomyomas in pregnancy: sonographic study. Radiology 1987;164:375-380.

43. Benson CB, Chow JS, Chang-Lee W, et al. Outcome of pregnancies in women with uterine leiomyomas identified by sonography in the first trimester. J Clin Ultrasound 2001;29:261-264.

44. Dilts Jr PV, Hopkins MP, Chang AE, Cody RL. Rapid growth of leiomyoma in patient receiving tamoxifen. Am J Obstet Gynecol 1992;166:167-168.

45. Kliewer MA, Hertzberg BS, George PY, et al. Acoustic shadowing from uterine leiomyomas: sonographic-pathologic correlation. Radiology 1995;196:99-102.

46. Caoili EM, Hertzberg BS, Kliewer MA, et al. Refractory shadowing from pelvic masses on sonography: a useful diagnostic sign for uterine leiomyomas. AJR Am J Roentgenol 2000;174:97-101.

47. Baltarowich OH, Kurtz AB, Pennell RG, et al. Pitfalls in the sonographic diagnosis of uterine fibroids. AJR Am J Roentgenol 1988;151:725-728.

48. Moore L, Wilson S, Rosen B. Giant hydropic uterine leiomyoma in pregnancy: unusual sonographic and Doppler appearance. J Ultrasound Med 1994;13:416-418.

49. Fedele L, Bianchi S, Dorta M, et al. Transvaginal ultrasonography versus hysteroscopy in the diagnosis of uterine submucous myomas. Obstet Gynecol 1991;77:745-748.

50. Becker Jr E, Lev-Toaff AS, Kaufman EP, et al. The added value of transvaginal sonohysterography over transvaginal sonography alone in women with known or suspected leiomyoma. J Ultrasound Med 2002;21:237-247.

51. Lev-Toaff AS, Toaff ME, Liu JB, et al. Value of sonohysterography in the diagnosis and management of abnormal uterine bleeding. Radiology 1996;201:179-184.

52. Davis PC, O'Neill MJ, Yoder IC, et al. Sonohysterographic findings of endometrial and subendometrial conditions. Radiographics 2002;22:803-816.

53. Karasick S, Lev-Toaff AS, Toaff ME. Imaging of uterine leiomyomas [see comment]. AJR Am J Roentgenol 1992;158:799-805.

54. Ghai S, Rajan DK, Benjamin MS, et al. Uterine artery embolization for leiomyomas: pre- and postprocedural evaluation with ultrasound. Radiographics 2005;25:1159-1172; discussion 1173-1176.

55. Spies JB, Spector A, Roth AR, et al. Complications after uterine artery embolization for leiomyomas. Obstet Gynecol 2002;100:873-880.

56. Dodd 3rd GD, Budzik Jr RF. Lipomatous uterine tumors: diagnosis by ultrasound, CT, and MR. J Comput Assist Tomogr 1990;14:629-632.

57. Serafini G, Martinoli C, Quadri P, et al. Lipomatous tumors of the uterus: ultrasonographic findings in 11 cases. J Ultrasound Med 1996;15:195-199; quiz 201-202.

58. Hertzberg BS, Kliewer MA, George P, et al. Lipomatous uterine masses: potential to mimic ovarian dermoids on endovaginal sonography. J Ultrasound Med 1995;14:689-692; quiz 693-694.

59. Fedele L, Bianchi S, Dorta M, et al. Transvaginal ultrasonography in the diagnosis of diffuse adenomyosis [see comment]. Fertil Steril 1992;58:94-97.

60. Reinhold C, Atri M, Mehio A, et al. Diffuse uterine adenomyosis: morphologic criteria and diagnostic accuracy of endovaginal sonography. Radiology 1995;197:609-614.

61. Bromley B, Shipp TD, Benacerraf B. Adenomyosis: sonographic findings and diagnostic accuracy. J Ultrasound Med 2000;19:529-534; quiz 535-536.

62. Hulka CA, Hall DA, McCarthy K, et al. Sonographic findings in patients with adenomyosis: can sonography assist in predicting extent of disease? AJR Am J Roentgenol 2002;179:379-383.

63. Atri M, Reinhold C, Mehio AR, et al. Adenomyosis: ultrasound features with histologic correlation in an in vitro study. Radiology 2000;215:783-790.

64. Botsis D, Kassanos D, Antoniou G, et al. Adenomyoma and leiomyoma: differential diagnosis with transvaginal sonography. J Clin Ultrasound 1998;26:21-25.

65. Fedele L, Bianchi S, Dorta M, et al. Transvaginal ultrasonography in the differential diagnosis of adenomyoma versus leiomyoma. Am J Obstet Gynecol 1992;167:603-606.

66. Kuligowska E, Deeds 3rd L, Lu 3rd K, et al. Pelvic pain: overlooked and underdiagnosed gynecologic conditions. Radiographics 2005;25:3-20.

67. Chopra S, Lev-Toaff AS, Ors F, et al. Adenomyosis: common and uncommon manifestations on sonography and magnetic resonance imaging. J Ultrasound Med 2006;25:617-627; quiz 629.

68. Andreotti RF, Fleischer AC, Andreotti RF, Fleischer AC. The sonographic diagnosis of adenomyosis. Ultrasound Q 2005;21:167-170.

69. Reinhold C, McCarthy S, Bret PM, et al. Diffuse adenomyosis: comparison of endovaginal ultrasound and MR imaging with histopathologic correlation. Radiology 1996;199:151-158.

70. Togashi K, Ozasa H, Konishi I, et al. Enlarged uterus: differentiation between adenomyosis and leiomyoma with MR imaging. Radiology 1989;171:531-534.

71. Abu Musa A, Hata T, Hata K, Kitao M. Pelvic arteriovenous malformation diagnosed by color flow Doppler imaging. AJR Am J Roentgenol 1989;152:1311-1312.

72. Huang MW, Muradali D, Thurston WA, et al. Uterine arteriovenous malformations: gray-scale and Doppler ultrasound features with MR imaging correlation [see comment]. Radiology 1998;206:115-123.

73. Mungen E. Vascular abnormalities of the uterus: have we recently over-diagnosed them? Ultrasound Obstet Gynecol 2003;21:529-531.

74. Timmerman D, Wauters J, Van Calenbergh S, et al. Color Doppler imaging is a valuable tool for the diagnosis and management of uterine vascular malformations [see comment]. Ultrasound Obstet Gynecol 2003;21:570-577.

75. Mendelson EB, Bohm-Velez M, Joseph N, Neiman HL. Endometrial abnormalities: evaluation with transvaginal sonography. AJR Am J Roentgenol 1988;150:139-142.

76. Baldwin MT, Dudiak KM, Gorman B, Marks CA. Focal intracavitary masses recognized with the hyperechoic line sign at endovaginal ultrasound and characterized with hysterosonography. Radiographics 1999;19:927-935.

77. Parsons AK, Lense JJ. Sonohysterography for endometrial abnormalities: preliminary results. J Clin Ultrasound 1993;21:87-95.

78. Gaucherand P, Piacenza JM, Salle B, Rudigoz RC. Sonohysterography of the uterine cavity: preliminary investigations. J Clin Ultrasound 1995;23:339-348.

79. Dubinsky TJ, Parvey HR, Gormaz G, Makland N. Transvaginal hysterosonography in the evaluation of small endoluminal masses. J Ultrasound Med 1995;14:1-6.

80. Jorizzo JR, Riccio GJ, Chen MY, Carr JJ. Sonohysterography: the next step in the evaluation of the abnormal endometrium. Radiographics 1999;19(Spec No):117-130.

81. Dubinsky TJ, Stroehlein K, Abu-Ghazzeh Y, et al. Prediction of benign and malignant endometrial disease: hysterosonographic-pathologic correlation. Radiology 1999;210:393-397.

82. Laifer-Narin SL, Ragavendra N, Lu DS, et al. Transvaginal saline hysterosonography: characteristics distinguishing malignant and various benign conditions. AJR Am J Roentgenol 1999;172:1513-1520.

83. Varner RE, Sparks JM, Cameron CD, et al. Transvaginal sonography of the endometrium in postmenopausal women. Obstet Gynecol 1991;78:195-199.

84. Karlsson B, Granberg S, Wikland M, et al. Transvaginal ultrasonography of the endometrium in women with postmenopausal bleeding: a Nordic multicenter study [see comment]. Am J Obstet Gynecol 1995;172:1488-1494.

85. Ferrazzi E, Torri V, Trio D, et al. Sonographic endometrial thickness: a useful test to predict atrophy in patients with postmenopausal bleeding: an Italian multicenter study. Ultrasound Obstet Gynecol 1996;7:315-321.

86. Granberg S, Wikland M, Karlsson B, et al. Endometrial thickness as measured by endovaginal ultrasonography for identifying endometrial abnormality. Am J Obstet Gynecol 1991;164:47-52.

87. Nasri MN, Shepherd JH, Setchell ME, et al. The role of vaginal scan in measurement of endometrial thickness in postmenopausal women. Br J Obstet Gynaecol 1991;98:470-475.

88. Goldstein SR, Nachtigall M, Snyder JR, Nachtigall L. Endometrial assessment by vaginal ultrasonography before endometrial sampling in patients with postmenopausal bleeding. Am J Obstet Gynecol 1990;163:119-123.

89. Smith-Bindman R, Kerlikowske K, Feldstein VA, et al. Endovaginal ultrasound to exclude endometrial cancer and other endometrial abnormalities [see comment]. JAMA 1998;280:1510-1517.

90. Goldstein RB, Bree RL, Benson CB, et al. Evaluation of the woman with postmenopausal bleeding: Society of Radiologists in Ultrasound–Sponsored Consensus Conference statement. J Ultrasound Med 2001;20:1025-1036.

91. Delisle MF, Villeneuve M, Boulvain M. Measurement of endometrial thickness with transvaginal ultrasonography: is it reproducible? J Ultrasound Med 1998;17:481-484; quiz 485-486.

92. Bree RL, Bowerman RA, Bohm-Velez M, et al. Ultrasound evaluation of the uterus in patients with postmenopausal bleeding: a posi-tive effect on diagnostic decision making. Radiology 2000;216:260-264.

93. Laifer-Narin S, Ragavendra N, Parmenter EK, et al. False-normal appearance of the endometrium on conventional transvaginal sonography: comparison with saline hysterosonography. AJR Am J Roentgenol 2002;178:129-133.

94. Neele SJ, Marchien van Baal W, van der Mooren MJ, et al. Ultrasound assessment of the endometrium in healthy, asymptomatic early post-menopausal women: saline infusion sonohysterography versus transvaginal ultrasound. Ultrasound Obstet Gynecol 2000;16:254-259.

95. Osmers R, Volksen M, Schauer A. Vaginosonography for early detection of endometrial carcinoma? Lancet 1990;335:1569-1571.

96. Shipley 3rd CF, Simmons CL, Nelson GH. Comparison of transvaginal sonography with endometrial biopsy in asymptomatic postmenopausal women. J Ultrasound Med 1994;13:99-104.

97. Aleem F, Predanic M, Calame R, et al. Transvaginal color and pulsed Doppler sonography of the endometrium: a possible role in reducing the number of dilatation and curettage procedures. J Ultrasound Med 1995;14:139-145; quiz 147-148.

98. Smith-Bindman R, Weiss E, Feldstein V. How thick is too thick? When endometrial thickness should prompt biopsy in postmenopausal women without vaginal bleeding. Ultrasound Obstet Gynecol 2004;24:558-565.

99. Levine D, Gosink BB, Johnson LA. Change in endometrial thickness in postmenopausal women undergoing hormone replacement therapy. Radiology 1995;197:603-608.

100. Lewit N, Thaler I, Rottem S. The uterus: a new look with transvaginal sonography. J Clin Ultrasound 1990;18:331-336.

101. Breckenridge JW, Kurtz AB, Ritchie WG, Macht Jr EL. Postmenopausal uterine fluid collection: indicator of carcinoma. AJR Am J Roentgenol 1982;139:529-534.

102. McCarthy KA, Hall DA, Kopans DB, Swann CA. Postmenopausal endometrial fluid collections: always an indicator of malignancy? J Ultrasound Med 1986;5:647-649.

103. Goldstein SR. Postmenopausal endometrial fluid collections revisited: look at the doughnut rather than the hole. Obstet Gynecol 1994;83:738-740.

104. Wilson DA, Stacy TM, Smith EI. Ultrasound diagnosis of hydrocolpos and hydrometrocolpos. Radiology 1978;128:451-454.

105. Scott Jr WW, Rosenshein NB, Siegelman SS, Sanders RC. The obstructed uterus. Radiology 1981;141:767-770.

106. Sheth S, Hamper UM, Kurman RJ. Thickened endometrium in the postmenopausal woman: sonographic-pathologic correlation. Radiology 1993;187:135-139.

107. Hulka CA, Hall DA, McCarthy K, Simeone JF. Endometrial polyps, hyperplasia, and carcinoma in postmenopausal women: differentiation with endovaginal sonography. Radiology 1994;191:755-758.

108. Atri M, Nazarnia S, Aldis AE, et al. Transvaginal ultrasound appearance of endometrial abnormalities. Radiographics 1994;14:483-492.

109. Choo YC, Mak KC, Hsu C, et al. Postmenopausal uterine bleeding of nonorganic cause. Obstet Gynecol 1985;66:225-228.

110. Kupfer MC, Schiller VL, Hansen GC, Tessler FN. Transvaginal sonographic evaluation of endometrial polyps. J Ultrasound Med 1994;13:535-539.

111. Timmerman D, Verguts J, Konstantinovic ML, et al. The pedicle artery sign based on sonography with color Doppler imaging can replace second-stage tests in women with abnormal vaginal bleeding. Ultrasound Obstet Gynecol 2003;22:166-171.

112. Alcazar JL, Galan MJ, Minguez JA, et al. Transvaginal color Doppler sonography versus sonohysterography in the diagnosis of endometrial polyps. J Ultrasound Med 2004;23:743-748.

113. Karlsson B, Granberg S, Hellberg P, Wikland M. Comparative study of transvaginal sonography and hysteroscopy for the detection of pathologic endometrial lesions in women with postmenopausal bleeding. J Ultrasound Med 1994;13:757-762.

114. American Cancer Society. Cancer facts and figures 2008.

115. Bourne TH, Campbell S, Steer CV, et al. Detection of endometrial cancer by transvaginal ultrasonography with color flow imaging and blood flow analysis: a preliminary report. Gynecol Oncol 1991;40:253-259.

116. Weiner Z, Beck D, Rottem S, et al. Uterine artery flow velocity waveforms and color flow imaging in women with perimenopausal and postmenopausal bleeding: correlation to endometrial histopathology. Acta Obstet Gynecol Scand 1993;72:162-166.

117. Chan FY, Chau MT, Pun TC, et al. Limitations of transvaginal sonography and color Doppler imaging in the differentiation of endometrial carcinoma from benign lesions. J Ultrasound Med 1994;13:623-628.

118. Carter JR, Lau M, Saltzman AK, et al. Gray scale and color flow Doppler characterization of uterine tumors. J Ultrasound Med 1994;13:835-840.

119. Sladkevicius P, Valentin L, Marsal K. Endometrial thickness and Doppler velocimetry of the uterine arteries as discriminators of endometrial status in women with postmenopausal bleeding: a comparative study [see comment]. Am J Obstet Gynecol 1994;171:722-728.

120. Kurjak A, Shalan H, Sosic A, et al. Endometrial carcinoma in postmenopausal women: evaluation by transvaginal color Doppler ultrasonography. Am J Obstet Gynecol 1993;169:1597-1603.

121. Sheth S, Hamper UM, McCollum ME, et al. Endometrial blood flow analysis in postmenopausal women: can it help differentiate benign from malignant causes of endometrial thickening? Radiology 1995;195:661-665.

122. Cacciatore B, Lehtovirta P, Wahlstrom T, Ylostalo P. Preoperative sonographic evaluation of endometrial cancer. Am J Obstet Gynecol 1989;160:133-137.

123. Gordon AN, Fleischer AC, Reed GW. Depth of myometrial invasion in endometrial cancer: preoperative assessment by transvaginal ultrasonography. Gynecol Oncol 1990;39:321-327.

124. Fleischer AC, Dudley BS, Entman SS, et al. Myometrial invasion by endometrial carcinoma: sonographic assessment. Radiology 1987;162:307-310.

125. DelMaschio A, Vanzulli A, Sironi S, et al. Estimating the depth of myometrial involvement by endometrial carcinoma: efficacy of transvaginal sonography vs MR imaging. AJR Am J Roentgenol 1993;160:533-538.

126. Yamashita Y, Mizutani H, Torashima M, et al. Assessment of myometrial invasion by endometrial carcinoma: transvaginal sonography vs contrast-enhanced MR imaging. AJR Am J Roentgenol 1993; 161:595-599.

127. Kinkel K, Kaji Y, Yu KK, et al. Radiologic staging in patients with endometrial cancer: a meta-analysis. Radiology 1999;212:711-718.

128. Frei KA, Kinkel K, Bonel HM, et al. Prediction of deep myometrial invasion in patients with endometrial cancer: clinical utility of contrast-enhanced MR imaging: a meta-analysis and bayesian analysis. Radiology 2000;216:444-449.

129. Malfetano JH. Tamoxifen-associated endometrial carcinoma in postmenopausal breast cancer patients [see comment]. Gynecol Oncol 1990;39:82-84.

130. Kedar RP, Bourne TH, Powles TJ, et al. Effects of tamoxifen on uterus and ovaries of postmenopausal women in a randomised breast cancer prevention trial [see comment]. Lancet 1994;343:1318-1321.

131. Lahti E, Blanco G, Kauppila A, et al. Endometrial changes in postmenopausal breast cancer patients receiving tamoxifen. Obstet Gynecol 1993;81:660-664.

132. Cohen I, Rosen DJ, Tepper R, et al. Ultrasonographic evaluation of the endometrium and correlation with endometrial sampling in postmenopausal patients treated with tamoxifen. J Ultrasound Med 1993;12:275-280.

133. Hulka CA, Hall DA. Endometrial abnormalities associated with tamoxifen therapy for breast cancer: sonographic and pathologic correlation. AJR Am J Roentgenol 1993;160:809-812.

134. Hann LE, Giess CS, Bach AM, et al. Endometrial thickness in tamoxifen-treated patients: correlation with clinical and pathologic findings. AJR Am J Roentgenol 1997;168:657-661.

135. Ascher SM, Imaoka I, Lage JM. Tamoxifen-induced uterine abnormalities: the role of imaging [see comment]. Radiology 2000; 214:29-38.

136. Goldstein SR. Unusual ultrasonographic appearance of the uterus in patients receiving tamoxifen [see comment]. Am J Obstet Gynecol 1994;170:447-451.

137. Hann LE, Gretz EM, Bach AM, Francis SM. Sonohysterography for evaluation of the endometrium in women treated with tamoxifen. AJR Am J Roentgenol 2001;177:337-342.

138. Fong K, Kung R, Lytwyn A, et al. Endometrial evaluation with transvaginal ultrasound and hysterosonography in asymptomatic postmenopausal women with breast cancer receiving tamoxifen. Radiology 2001;220:765-773.

139. American College of Obstetricians and Gynecologists. Committee Opinion 336. Tamoxifen and uterine cancer. Obstet Gynecol 2006;107:1475-1478.

140. Wachsberg RH, Kurtz AB. Gas within the endometrial cavity at postpartum ultrasound: a normal finding after spontaneous vaginal delivery. Radiology 1992;183:431-433.

141. Fedele L, Bianchi S, Dorta M, Vignali M. Intrauterine adhesions: detection with transvaginal ultrasound. Radiology 1996;199:757-759.

142. Salle B, Gaucherand P, de Saint Hilaire P, Rudigoz RC. Transvaginal sonohysterographic evaluation of intrauterine adhesions. J Clin Ultrasound 1999;27:131-134.

143. Callen PW, Filly RA, Munyer TP. Intrauterine contraceptive devices: evaluation by sonography. AJR Am J Roentgenol 1980; 135:797-800.

144. Peri N, Graham D, Levine D, et al. Imaging of intrauterine contraceptive devices. J Ultrasound Med 2007;26:1389-1401.

145. Lee A, Eppel W, Sam C, et al. Intrauterine device localization by three-dimensional transvaginal sonography. Ultrasound Obstet Gynecol 1997;10:289-292.

146. Bajo J, Moreno-Calvo FJ, Uguet-de-Resayre C, et al. Contribution of transvaginal sonography to the evaluation of benign cervical conditions. J Clin Ultrasound 1999;27:61-64.

147. Fogel SR, Slasky BS. Sonography of nabothian cysts. AJR Am J Roentgenol 1982;138:927-930.

148. Stein MW, Grishina A, Shaw RJ, et al. Gray-scale and color Doppler sonographic features of the vaginal cuff and cervical remnant after hysterectomy. AJR Am J Roentgenol 2006;187:1372-1376.

149. Choi CG, Kim SH, Kim JS, et al. Adenoma malignum of uterine cervix in Peutz-Jeghers syndrome: CT and ultrasound features. J Comput Assist Tomogr 1993;17:819-821.

150. Yamashita Y, Takahashi M, Katabuchi H, et al. Adenoma malignum: MR appearances mimicking nabothian cysts. AJR Am J Roentgenol 1994;162:649-650.

Vagina

151. Sherer DM, Abulafia O. Transvaginal ultrasonographic depiction of a Gartner duct cyst. J Ultrasound Med 2001;20:1253-1255.

152. McCarthy S, Taylor KJ. Sonography of vaginal masses. AJR Am J Roentgenol 1983;140:1005-1008.

153. Schoenfeld A, Levavi H, Hirsch M, et al. Transvaginal sonography in postmenopausal women. J Clin Ultrasound 1990;18:350-358.

Rectouterine Recess

154. Mendelson EB, Bohm-Velez M, Neiman HL, Russo J. Transvaginal sonography in gynecologic imaging. Semin Ultrasound CT MR 1988;9:102-121.

155. Davis JA, Gosink BB. Fluid in the female pelvis: cyclic patterns. J Ultrasound Med 1986;5:75-79.

156. Koninckx PR, Renaer M, Brosens IA. Origin of peritoneal fluid in women: an ovarian exudation product. Br J Obstet Gynaecol 1980;87:177-183.

157. Jeffrey RB, Laing FC. Echogenic clot: a useful sign of pelvic hemoperitoneum. Radiology 1982;145:139-141.

Ovary

158. Cohen HL, Shapiro MA, Mandel FS, Shapiro ML. Normal ovaries in neonates and infants: a sonographic study of 77 patients 1 day to 24 months old. AJR Am J Roentgenol 1993;160:583-586.

159. Cohen HL, Eisenberg P, Mandel F, Haller JO. Ovarian cysts are common in premenarchal girls: a sonographic study of 101 children 2-12 years old. AJR Am J Roentgenol 1992;159:89-91.

160. Cohen HL, Tice HM, Mandel FS. Ovarian volumes measured by ultrasound: bigger than we think. Radiology 1990;177:189-192.

161. Van Nagell Jr JR, Higgins RV, Donaldson ES, et al. Transvaginal sonography as a screening method for ovarian cancer: a report of the first 1000 cases screened. Cancer 1990;65:573-577.

162. Kupfer MC, Ralls PW, Fu YS. Transvaginal sonographic evaluation of multiple peripherally distributed echogenic foci of the ovary: prevalence and histologic correlation. AJR Am J Roentgenol 1998; 171:483-486.

163. Muradali D, Colgan T, Hayeems E, et al. Echogenic ovarian foci without shadowing: are they caused by psammomatous calcifications? Radiology 2002;224:429-435.

164. Brandt KR, Thurmond AS, McCarthy JL. Focal calcifications in otherwise ultrasonographically normal ovaries. Radiology 1996; 198:415-417.

165. Goswamy RK, Campbell S, Royston JP, et al. Ovarian size in post-menopausal women. Br J Obstet Gynaecol 1988;95:795-801.

166. Granberg S, Wikland M. A comparison between ultrasound and gynecologic examination for detection of enlarged ovaries in a group of women at risk for ovarian carcinoma. J Ultrasound Med 1988; 7:59-64.

167. Andolf E, Jorgensen C, Svalenius E, Sunden B. Ultrasound measurement of the ovarian volume. Acta Obstet Gynecol Scand 1987;66:387-389.

168. Hall DA, McCarthy KA, Kopans DB. Sonographic visualization of the normal postmenopausal ovary. J Ultrasound Med 1986;5:9-11.

169. Fleischer AC, McKee MS, Gordon AN, et al. Transvaginal sonography of postmenopausal ovaries with pathologic correlation. J Ultrasound Med 1990;9:637-644.

170. DiSantis DJ, Scatarige JC, Kemp G, et al. A prospective evaluation of transvaginal sonography for detection of ovarian disease [see comment]. AJR Am J Roentgenol 1993;161:91-94.

171. Wolf SI, Gosink BB, Feldesman MR, et al. Prevalence of simple adnexal cysts in postmenopausal women. Radiology 1991;180:65-71.

172. Levine D, Gosink BB, Wolf SI, et al. Simple adnexal cysts: the natural history in postmenopausal women [see comment]. Radiology 1992;184:653-659.

173. Goldstein SR, Subramanyam B, Snyder JR, et al. The postmenopausal cystic adnexal mass: the potential role of ultrasound in conservative management. Obstet Gynecol 1989;73:8-10.

174. Conway C, Zalud I, Dilena M, et al. Simple cyst in the postmenopausal patient: detection and management. J Ultrasound Med 1998;17:369-372; quiz 373-374.

175. Bailey CL, Ueland FR, Land GL, et al. The malignant potential of small cystic ovarian tumors in women over 50 years of age [see comment]. Gynecol Oncol 1998;69:3-7.

176. Modesitt SC, Pavlik EJ, Ueland FR, et al. Risk of malignancy in unilocular ovarian cystic tumors less than 10 cm in diameter. Obstet Gynecol 2003;102:594-599.

177. Nardo LG, Kroon ND, Reginald PW, et al. Persistent unilocular ovarian cysts in a general population of postmenopausal women: is there a place for expectant management? Obstet Gynecol 2003;102: 589-593.

178. Ekerhovd E, Wienerroith H, Staudach A, Granberg S. Preoperative assessment of unilocular adnexal cysts by transvaginal ultrasonography: a comparison between ultrasonographic morphologic imaging and histopathologic diagnosis. Am J Obstet Gynecol 2001;184: 48-54.

179. Timor-Tritsch IE, Goldstein SR. The complexity of a "complex mass" and the simplicity of a "simple cyst." J Ultrasound Med 2005;24:255-258.

180. Glanc P, Salem S, Farine D, et al. Adnexal masses in the pregnant patient: a diagnostic and management challenge. Ultrasound Q 2008;24:225-240.

181. Baltarowich OH, Kurtz AB, Pasto ME, et al. The spectrum of sonographic findings in hemorrhagic ovarian cysts. AJR Am J Roentgenol 1987;148:901-905.

182. Yoffe N, Bronshtein M, Brandes J, Blumenfeld Z. Hemorrhagic ovarian cyst detection by transvaginal sonography: the great imitator. Gynecol Endocrinol 1991;5:123-129.

183. Jain KA, Jain KA. Sonographic spectrum of hemorrhagic ovarian cysts. J Ultrasound Med 2002;21:879-886.

184. Patel MD, Feldstein VA, Filly RA. The likelihood ratio of sonographic findings for the diagnosis of hemorrhagic ovarian cysts. J Ultrasound Med 2005;24:607-614; quiz 615.

185. Wiser A, Levron J, Kreizer D, et al. Outcome of pregnancies complicated by severe ovarian hyperstimulation syndrome (OHSS): a follow-up beyond the second trimester. Hum Reprod 2005;20:910-914.

186. Foulk RA, Martin MC, Jerkins GL, Laros RK. Hyperreactio luteinalis differentiated from severe ovarian hyperstimulation syndrome in a spontaneously conceived pregnancy. Am J Obstet Gynecol 1997;176:1300-1302; discussion 1302-1304.

187. Golan A, Ron-el R, Herman A, et al. Ovarian hyperstimulation syndrome: an update review. Obstet Gynecol Surv 1989;44:430-440.

188. Manganiello PD, Adams LV, Harris RD, Ornvold K. Virilization during pregnancy with spontaneous resolution postpartum: a case report and review of the English literature. Obstet Gynecol Surv 1995;50:404-410.

189. Choi JR, Levine D, Finberg H. Luteoma of pregnancy: sonographic findings in two cases. J Ultrasound Med 2000;19:877-881.

190. Price FV, Edwards R, Buchsbaum HJ. Ovarian remnant syndrome: difficulties in diagnosis and management. Obstetr Gynecol Surv 1990;45:151-156.

191. Phillips HE, McGahan JP. Ovarian remnant syndrome. Radiology 1982;142:487-488.

192. Fleischer AC, Tait D, Mayo J, et al. Sonographic features of ovarian remnants. J Ultrasound Med 1998;17:551-555.

193. Athey PA, Cooper NB. Sonographic features of parovarian cysts. AJR Am J Roentgenol 1985;144:83-86.

194. Alpern MB, Sandler MA, Madrazo BL. Sonographic features of parovarian cysts and their complications. AJR Am J Roentgenol 1984;143:157-160.

195. Korbin CD, Brown DL, Welch WR. Paraovarian cystadenomas and cystadenofibromas: sonographic characteristics in 14 cases. Radiology 1998;208:459-462.

196. Honore LH, O'Hara KE. Serous papillary neoplasms arising in paramesonephric parovarian cysts: a report of eight cases. Acta Obstet Gynecol Scand 1980;59:525-528.

197. Genadry R, Parmley T, Woodruff JD. The origin and clinical behavior of the parovarian tumor. Am J Obstet Gynecol 1977;129:873-880.

198. Savelli L, Ghi T, De Iaco P, et al. Paraovarian/paratubal cysts: comparison of transvaginal sonographic and pathological findings to establish diagnostic criteria. Ultrasound Obstet Gynecol 2006; 28:330-334.

199. Stein AL, Koonings PP, Schlaerth JB, et al. Relative frequency of malignant paraovarian tumors: should parovarian tumors be aspirated? Obstet Gynecol 1990;75:1029-1031.

200. Kim JS, Woo SK, Suh SJ, Morettin LB. Sonographic diagnosis of paraovarian cysts: value of detecting a separate ipsilateral ovary. AJR Am J Roentgenol 1995;164:1441-1444.

201. Hoffer FA, Kozakewich H, Colodny A, Goldstein DP. Peritoneal inclusion cysts: ovarian fluid in peritoneal adhesions. Radiology 1988;169:189-191.

202. Sohaey R, Gardner TL, Woodward PJ, Peterson CM. Sonographic diagnosis of peritoneal inclusion cysts. J Ultrasound Med 1995; 14:913-917.

203. Kim JS, Lee HJ, Woo SK, Lee TS. Peritoneal inclusion cysts and their relationship to the ovaries: evaluation with sonography. Radiology 1997;204:481-484.

204. Jain KA. Imaging of peritoneal inclusion cysts. AJR Am J Roentgenol 2000;174:1559-1563.

205. Savelli L, de Iaco P, Ghi T, et al. Transvaginal sonographic appearance of peritoneal pseudocysts. Ultrasound Obstet Gynecol 2004; 23:284-288.

206. Ross MJ, Welch WR, Scully RE. Multilocular peritoneal inclusion cysts (so-called cystic mesotheliomas). Cancer 1989;64:1336-1346.

207. Asch E, Levine D, Asch E, Levine D. Variations in appearance of endometriomas. J Ultrasound Med 2007;26:993-1002.

208. Kupfer MC, Schwimer SR, Lebovic J. Transvaginal sonographic appearance of endometriomata: spectrum of findings. J Ultrasound Med 1992;11:129-133.

209. Patel MD, Feldstein VA, Chen DC, et al. Endometriomas: diagnostic performance of ultrasound [see comment]. Radiology 1999;210: 739-745; erratum 1999;213:930.

210. Dogan MM, Ugur M, Soysal SK, et al. Transvaginal sonographic diagnosis of ovarian endometrioma. Int J Gynaecol Obstet 1996;52: 145-149.

211. Jain KA, Jain KA. Endometrioma with calcification simulating a dermoid on sonography. J Ultrasound Med 2006;25:1237-1241.

212. Sammour RN, Leibovitz Z, Shapiro I, et al. Decidualization of ovarian endometriosis during pregnancy mimicking malignancy. J Ultrasound Med 2005;24:1289-1294.

213. Fruscella E, Testa AC, Ferrandina G, et al. Sonographic features of decidualized ovarian endometriosis suspicious for malignancy [see comment]. Ultrasound Obstet Gynecol 2004;24:578-580.

214. Balen AH, Tan SL, Jacobs HS. Hypersecretion of luteinising hormone: a significant cause of infertility and miscarriage [see comment]. Br J Obstet Gynaecol 1993;100:1082-1089.

215. Eden JA, Warren P. A review of 1019 consecutive cases of polycystic ovary syndrome demonstrated by ultrasound. Australas Radiol 1999;43:41-46.

216. Yeh HC, Futterweit W, Thornton JC. Polycystic ovarian disease: ultrasound features in 104 patients. Radiology 1987;163:111-116.

217. Hann LE, Hall DA, McArdle CR, Seibel M. Polycystic ovarian disease: sonographic spectrum. Radiology 1984;150:531-534.

218. Pache TD, Wladimiroff JW, Hop WC, Fauser BC. How to discriminate between normal and polycystic ovaries: transvaginal ultrasound study. Radiology 1992;183:421-423.

219. Ardaens Y, Robert Y, Lemaitre L, et al. Polycystic ovarian disease: contribution of vaginal endosonography and reassessment of ultrasonic diagnosis. Fertil Steril 1991;55:1062-1068.

220. Battaglia C, Regnani G, Petraglia F, et al. Polycystic ovary syndrome: it is always bilateral? Ultrasound Obstet Gynecol 1999;14:183-187.

221. Balen AH, Laven JS, Tan SL, et al. Ultrasound assessment of the polycystic ovary: international consensus definitions. Hum Reprod Update 2003;9:505-514.

222. Jonard S, Robert Y, Dewailly D, et al. Revisiting the ovarian volume as a diagnostic criterion for polycystic ovaries. Hum Reprod 2005; 20:2893-2898.

223. Mashiach S, Bider D, Moran O, et al. Adnexal torsion of hyperstimulated ovaries in pregnancies after gonadotropin therapy. Fertil Steril 1990;53:76-80.

224. Warner MA, Fleischer AC, Edell SL, et al. Uterine adnexal torsion: sonographic findings. Radiology 1985;154:773-775.

225. Sommerville M, Grimes DA, Koonings PP, Campbell K. Ovarian neoplasms and the risk of adnexal torsion. Am J Obstet Gynecol 1991;164:577-578.

226. Chiou SY, Lev-Toaff AS, Masuda E, et al. Adnexal torsion: new clinical and imaging observations by sonography, computed tomography, and magnetic resonance imaging. J Ultrasound Med 2007;26:1289-1301.

227. Eitan R, Galoyan N, Zuckerman B, et al. The risk of malignancy in post-menopausal women presenting with adnexal torsion. Gynecologic Oncology 2007;106:211-214.

228. Graif M, Itzchak Y. Sonographic evaluation of ovarian torsion in childhood and adolescence. AJR Am J Roentgenol 1988;150:647-649.

229. Albayram F, Hamper UM. Ovarian and adnexal torsion: spectrum of sonographic findings with pathologic correlation. J Ultrasound Med 2001;20:1083-1089.

230. Fleischer AC, Stein SM, Cullinan JA, Warner MA. Color Doppler sonography of adnexal torsion. J Ultrasound Med 1995;14:523-528.

231. Stark JE, Siegel MJ. Ovarian torsion in prepubertal and pubertal girls: sonographic findings. AJR Am J Roentgenol 1994;163: 1479-1482.

232. Rosado Jr WM, Trambert MA, Gosink BB, Pretorius DH. Adnexal torsion: diagnosis by using Doppler sonography. AJR Am J Roentgenol 1992;159:1251-1253.

233. Lee EJ, Kwon HC, Joo HJ, et al. Diagnosis of ovarian torsion with color Doppler sonography: depiction of twisted vascular pedicle. J Ultrasound Med 1998;17:83-89.

234. Vijayaraghavan SB, Vijayaraghavan SB. Sonographic whirlpool sign in ovarian torsion. J Ultrasound Med 2004;23:1643-1649; quiz 1650-1651.

235. Chang HC, Bhatt S, Dogra VS, et al. Pearls and pitfalls in diagnosis of ovarian torsion. Radiographics 2008;28:1355-1368.

236. Shadinger LL, Andreotti RF, Kurian RL, et al. Preoperative sonographic and clinical characteristics as predictors of ovarian torsion. J Ultrasound Med 2008;27:7-13.

237. Kapadia R, Sternhill V, Schwartz E. Massive edema of the ovary. J Clin Ultrasound 1982;10:469-471.

238. Lee AR, Kim KH, Lee BH, Chin SY. Massive edema of the ovary: imaging findings. AJR Am J Roentgenol 1993;161:343-344.

239. Hill LM, Pelekanos M, Kanbour A. Massive edema of an ovary previously fixed to the pelvic side wall. J Ultrasound Med 1993; 12:629-632.

240. Kerlikowske K, Brown JS, Grady DG. Should women with familial ovarian cancer undergo prophylactic oophorectomy? Obstet Gynecol 1992;80:700-707.

241. Lynch HT, Watson P, Lynch JF, et al. Hereditary ovarian cancer: heterogeneity in age at onset. Cancer 1993;71:573-581.

242. Jacobs I, Davies AP, Bridges J, et al. Prevalence screening for ovarian cancer in postmenopausal women by CA 125 measurement and ultrasonography [see comment]. BMJ 1993;306:1030-1034.

243. DePriest PD, Gallion HH, Pavlik EJ, et al. Transvaginal sonography as a screening method for the detection of early ovarian cancer. Gynecol Oncol 1997;65:408-414.

244. Kurjak A, Shalan H, Kupesic S, et al. An attempt to screen asymptomatic women for ovarian and endometrial cancer with transvaginal color and pulsed Doppler sonography. J Ultrasound Med 1994; 13:295-301.

245. Bourne TH, Campbell S, Reynolds KM, et al. Screening for early familial ovarian cancer with transvaginal ultrasonography and colour blood flow imaging [see comment]. BMJ 1993;306:1025-1029.

246. Karlan BY, Raffel LJ, Crvenkovic G, et al. A multidisciplinary approach to the early detection of ovarian carcinoma: rationale, protocol design, and early results. Am J Obstet Gynecol 1993; 169:494-501.

247. Weiner Z, Beck D, Shteiner M, et al. Screening for ovarian cancer in women with breast cancer with transvaginal sonography and color flow imaging. J Ultrasound Med 1993;12:387-393.

248. Bast Jr RC, Klug TL, St John E, et al. A radioimmunoassay using a monoclonal antibody to monitor the course of epithelial ovarian cancer. N Engl J Med 1983;309:883-887.

249. Jacobs I, Bast Jr RC. The CA 125 tumour–associated antigen: a review of the literature. Hum Reprod 1989;4:1-12.

250. National Institute of Health. Ovarian cancer: screening, treatment, and follow-up. NIH Consensus Development Panel on Ovarian Cancer [see comment]. JAMA 1995;273:491-497.

251. Moyle JW, Rochester D, Sider L, et al. Sonography of ovarian tumors: predictability of tumor type. AJR Am J Roentgenol 1983;141:985-991.

252. Granberg S, Wikland M, Jansson I. Macroscopic characterization of ovarian tumors and the relation to the histological diagnosis: criteria to be used for ultrasound evaluation. Gynecol Oncol 1989; 35:139-144.

253. Valentin L. Prospective cross-validation of Doppler ultrasound examination and gray-scale ultrasound imaging for discrimination of benign and malignant pelvic masses. Ultrasound Obstet Gynecol 1999;14:273-283.

254. Timmerman D, Schwarzler P, Collins WP, et al. Subjective assessment of adnexal masses with the use of ultrasonography: an analysis of interobserver variability and experience [see comment]. Ultrasound Obstet Gynecol 1999;13:11-16.

255. Valentin L, Ameye L, Jurkovic D, et al. Which extrauterine pelvic masses are difficult to correctly classify as benign or malignant on the basis of ultrasound findings and is there a way of making a correct diagnosis? Ultrasound Obstet Gynecol 2006;27:438-444.

256. Van Calster B, Timmerman D, Bourne T, et al. Discrimination between benign and malignant adnexal masses by specialist ultrasound examination versus serum CA-125. J Natl Cancer Inst 2007; 99:1706-1714.

257. Folkman J, Watson K, Ingber D, Hanahan D. Induction of angiogenesis during the transition from hyperplasia to neoplasia. Nature 1989;339:58-61.

258. Brown DL, Frates MC, Laing FC, et al. Ovarian masses: can benign and malignant lesions be differentiated with color and pulsed Doppler ultrasound? Radiology 1994;190:333-336.

259. Stein SM, Laifer-Narin S, Johnson MB, et al. Differentiation of benign and malignant adnexal masses: relative value of gray-scale, color Doppler, and spectral Doppler sonography. AJR Am J Roentgenol 1995;164:381-386.

260. Jain KA. Prospective evaluation of adnexal masses with endovaginal gray-scale and duplex and color Doppler ultrasound: correlation with pathologic findings [see comment]. Radiology 1994;191: 63-67.

261. Levine D, Feldstein VA, Babcook CJ, Filly RA. Sonography of ovarian masses: poor sensitivity of resistive index for identifying malignant lesions. AJR Am J Roentgenol 1994;162:1355-1359.

262. Salem S, White LM, Lai J. Doppler sonography of adnexal masses: the predictive value of the pulsatility index in benign and malignant disease. AJR Am J Roentgenol 1994;163:1147-1150.

263. Buy JN, Ghossain MA, Hugol D, et al. Characterization of adnexal masses: combination of color Doppler and conventional sonography compared with spectral Doppler analysis alone and conventional sonography alone. AJR Am J Roentgenol 1996;166:385-393.

264. Fleischer AC, Jones 3rd HW. Color Doppler sonography of ovarian masses: the importance of a multiparameter approach. Gynecologic Oncology 1993;50:1-2.
265. Guerriero S, Alcazar JL, Coccia ME, et al. Complex pelvic mass as a target of evaluation of vessel distribution by color Doppler sonography for the diagnosis of adnexal malignancies: results of a multicenter European study. J Ultrasound Med 2002;21:1105-1111.
266. Bromley B, Goodman H, Benacerraf BR. Comparison between sonographic morphology and Doppler waveform for the diagnosis of ovarian malignancy. Obstet Gynecol 1994;83:434-437.
267. Carter J, Saltzman A, Hartenbach E, et al. Flow characteristics in benign and malignant gynecologic tumors using transvaginal color flow Doppler. Obstet Gynecol 1994;83:125-130.
268. Reles A, Wein U, Lichtenegger W. Transvaginal color Doppler sonography and conventional sonography in the preoperative assessment of adnexal masses. J Clin Ultrasound 1997;25:217-225.
269. Fleischer AC, Cullinan JA, Kepple DM, Williams LL. Conventional and color Doppler transvaginal sonography of pelvic masses: a comparison of relative histologic specificities. J Ultrasound Med 1993;12:705-712.
270. Brown DL, Doubilet PM, Miller FH, et al. Benign and malignant ovarian masses: selection of the most discriminating gray-scale and Doppler sonographic features. Radiology 1998;208:103-110.
271. Schelling M, Braun M, Kuhn W, et al. Combined transvaginal B-mode and color Doppler sonography for differential diagnosis of ovarian tumors: results of a multivariate logistic regression analysis. Gynecol Oncol 2000;77:78-86.
272. Kinkel K, Hricak H, Lu Y, et al. Ultrasound characterization of ovarian masses: a meta-analysis. Radiology 2000;217:803-811.
273. Laing FC. Ultrasound analysis of adnexal masses: the art of making the correct diagnosis [see comment]. Radiology 1994;191:21-22.
274. Wagner BJ, Buck JL, Seidman JD, McCabe KM. From the archives of the AFIP. Ovarian epithelial neoplasms: radiologic-pathologic correlation. Radiographics 1994;14:1351-1374; quiz 1375-1376.
275. Alfuhaid TR, Rosen BP, Wilson SR. Low-malignant-potential tumor of the ovary: sonographic features with clinicopathologic correlation in 41 patients. Ultrasound Q 2003;19:13-26.
276. Yazbek J, Raju KS, Ben-Nagi J, et al. Accuracy of ultrasound subjective "pattern recognition" for the diagnosis of borderline ovarian tumors. Ultrasound Obstet Gynecol 2007;29:489-495.
277. Yazbek J, Aslam N, Tailor A, et al. A comparative study of the risk of malignancy index and the ovarian crescent sign for the diagnosis of invasive ovarian cancer. Ultrasound Obstet Gynecol 2006;28:320-324.
278. Athey PA, Siegel MF. Sonographic features of Brenner tumor of the ovary. J Ultrasound Med 1987;6:367-372.
279. Green GE, Mortele KJ, Glickman JN, et al. Brenner tumors of the ovary: sonographic and computed tomographic imaging features. J Ultrasound Med 2006;25:1245-1251; quiz 1252-1254.
280. Brammer 3rd HM, Buck JL, Hayes WS, et al. From the archives of the AFIP. Malignant germ cell tumors of the ovary: radiologic-pathologic correlation. Radiographics 1990;10:715-724.
281. Quinn SF, Erickson S, Black WC. Cystic ovarian teratomas: the sonographic appearance of the dermoid plug. Radiology 1985;155:477-478.
282. Sheth S, Fishman EK, Buck JL, et al. The variable sonographic appearances of ovarian teratomas: correlation with CT. AJR Am J Roentgenol 1988;151:331-334.
283. Guttman Jr PH. In search of the elusive benign cystic ovarian teratoma: application of the ultrasound "tip of the iceberg" sign. J Clin Ultrasound 1977;5:403-406.
284. Bronshtein M, Yoffe N, Brandes JM, Blumenfeld Z. Hair as a sonographic marker of ovarian teratomas: improved identification using transvaginal sonography and simulation model. J Clin Ultrasound 1991;19:351-355.
285. Malde HM, Kedar RP, Chadha D, Nayak S. Dermoid mesh: a sonographic sign of ovarian teratoma. AJR Am J Roentgenol 1992;159:1349-1350.
286. Kim HC, Kim SH, Lee HJ, et al. Fluid-fluid levels in ovarian teratomas. Abdom Imaging 2002;27:100-105.
287. Kawamoto S, Sato K, Matsumoto H, et al. Multiple mobile spherules in mature cystic teratoma of the ovary. AJR Am J Roentgenol 2001;176:1455-1457.
288. Patel MD, Feldstein VA, Lipson SD, et al. Cystic teratomas of the ovary: diagnostic value of sonography. AJR Am J Roentgenol 1998;171:1061-1065.
289. Hertzberg BS, Kliewer MA. Sonography of benign cystic teratoma of the ovary: pitfalls in diagnosis. AJR Am J Roentgenol 1996;167:1127-1133.
290. Zalel Y, Caspi B, Tepper R. Doppler flow characteristics of dermoid cysts: unique appearance of struma ovarii. J Ultrasound Med 1997;16:355-358.
291. O'Malley BP, Richmond H. Struma ovarii. J Ultrasound Med 1982;1:177-178.
292. Tanaka YO, Kurosaki Y, Nishida M, et al. Ovarian dysgerminoma: MR and CT appearance. J Comput Assist Tomogr 1994;18:443-448.
293. Kim SH, Kang SB. Ovarian dysgerminoma: color Doppler ultrasonographic findings and comparison with CT and MR imaging findings. J Ultrasound Med 1995;14:843-848.
294. Ko SF, Wan YL, Ng SH, et al. Adult ovarian granulosa cell tumors: spectrum of sonographic and CT findings with pathologic correlation. AJR Am J Roentgenol 1999;172:1227-1233.
295. Neste MG, Francis IR, Bude RO. Hepatic metastases from granulosa cell tumor of the ovary: CT and sonographic findings. AJR Am J Roentgenol 1996;166:1122-1124.
296. Outwater EK, Wagner BJ, Mannion C, et al. Sex cord–stromal and steroid cell tumors of the ovary. Radiographics 1998;18:1523-1546.
297. Stephenson WM, Laing FC. Sonography of ovarian fibromas. AJR Am J Roentgenol 1985;144:1239-1240.
298. Athey PA, Malone RS. Sonography of ovarian fibromas/thecomas. J Ultrasound Med 1987;6:431-436.
299. Athey PA, Butters HE. Sonographic and CT appearance of Krukenberg tumors. J Clin Ultrasound 1984;12:205-210.
300. Shimizu H, Yamasaki M, Ohama K, et al. Characteristic ultrasonographic appearance of the Krukenberg tumor. J Clin Ultrasound 1990;18:697-703.
301. Testa AC, Ferrandina G, Timmerman D, et al. Imaging in gynecological disease (1): ultrasound features of metastases in the ovaries differ depending on the origin of the primary tumor. Ultrasound Obstet Gynecol 2007;29:505-511.

Fallopian Tube
302. Timor-Tritsch IE, Rottem S. Transvaginal ultrasonographic study of the fallopian tube. Obstet Gynecol 1987;70:424-428.
303. Patten RM, Vincent LM, Wolner-Hanssen P, Thorpe Jr E. Pelvic inflammatory disease: endovaginal sonography with laparoscopic correlation. J Ultrasound Med 1990;9:681-689.
304. Tessler FN, Perrella RR, Fleischer AC, Grant EG. Endovaginal sonographic diagnosis of dilated fallopian tubes. AJR Am J Roentgenol 1989;153:523-525.
305. Taipale P, Tarjanne H, Ylostalo P. Transvaginal sonography in suspected pelvic inflammatory disease. Ultrasound Obstet Gynecol 1995;6:430-434.
306. Timor-Tritsch IE, Lerner JP, Monteagudo A, et al. Transvaginal sonographic markers of tubal inflammatory disease. Ultrasound Obstet Gynecol 1998;12:56-66.
307. Patel MD, Acord DL, Young SW. Likelihood ratio of sonographic findings in discriminating hydrosalpinx from other adnexal masses. AJR Am J Roentgenol 2006;186:1033-1038.
308. Bulas DI, Ahlstrom PA, Sivit CJ, et al. Pelvic inflammatory disease in the adolescent: comparison of transabdominal and transvaginal sonographic evaluation. Radiology 1992;183:435-439.
309. Sherer DM, Liberto L, Abramowicz JS, Woods Jr JR. Endovaginal sonographic features associated with isolated torsion of the fallopian tube. J Ultrasound Med 1991;10:107-109.
310. Russin LD. Hydrosalpinx and tubal torsion: a late complication of tubal ligation. Radiology 1986;159:115-116.
311. Subramanyam BR, Raghavendra BN, Whalen CA, Yee J. Ultrasonic features of fallopian tube carcinoma. J Ultrasound Med 1984;3:391-393.
312. Ajjimakorn S, Bhamarapravati Y. Transvaginal ultrasound and the diagnosis of fallopian tubal carcinoma. J Clin Ultrasound 1991;19:116-119.
313. Slanetz PJ, Whitman GJ, Halpern EF, et al. Imaging of fallopian tube tumors. AJR Am J Roentgenol 1997;169:1321-1324.
314. Kurjak A, Kupesic S, Ilijas M, et al. Preoperative diagnosis of primary fallopian tube carcinoma. Gynecologic Oncology 1998;68:29-34.
315. Patlas M, Rosen B, Chapman W, et al. Sonographic diagnosis of primary malignant tumors of the fallopian tube. Ultrasound Q 2004;20:59-64.

Nongynecologic Pelvic Masses

316. Wicks JD, Silver TM, Bree RL. Gray-scale features of hematomas: an ultrasonic spectrum. AJR Am J Roentgenol 1978;131:977-980.
317. Salem S, O'Malley BP, Hiltz CW. Ultrasonographic appearance of gastrointestinal masses. J Can Assoc Radiol 1980;31:163-167.

Postpartum Pelvic Pathologic Conditions

318. Brown DL, Brown DL. Pelvic ultrasound in the postabortion and postpartum patient. Ultrasound Q 2005;21:27-37.
319. Edwards A, Ellwood DA. Ultrasonographic evaluation of the postpartum uterus. Ultrasound Obstet Gynecol 2000;16:640-643.
320. Mulic-Lutvica A, Bekuretsion M, Bakos O, Axelsson O. Ultrasonic evaluation of the uterus and uterine cavity after normal, vaginal delivery. Ultrasound Obstet Gynecol 2001;18:491-498.
321. Hertzberg BS, Bowie JD. Ultrasound of the postpartum uterus: prediction of retained placental tissue. J Ultrasound Med 1991;10:451-456.
322. Zuckerman J, Levine D, McNicholas MM, et al. Imaging of pelvic postpartum complications [see comment]. AJR Am J Roentgenol 1997;168:663-668.
323. Durfee SM, Frates MC, Luong A, et al. The sonographic and color Doppler features of retained products of conception. J Ultrasound Med 2005;24:1181-1186; quiz 1188-1189.
324. Wilson PC, Lerner RM. Diagnosis of ovarian vein thrombophlebitis by ultrasonography. J Ultrasound Med 1983;2:187-190.
325. Savader SJ, Otero RR, Savader BL. Puerperal ovarian vein thrombosis: evaluation with CT, ultrasound, and MR imaging. Radiology 1988;167:637-639.
326. Grant TH, Schoettle BW, Buchsbaum MS. Postpartum ovarian vein thrombosis: diagnosis by clot protrusion into the inferior vena cava at sonography. AJR Am J Roentgenol 1993;160:551-552.
327. Baran GW, Frisch KM. Duplex Doppler evaluation of puerperal ovarian vein thrombosis. AJR Am J Roentgenol 1987;149:321-322.
328. Baker ME, Kay H, Mahony BS, et al. Sonography of the low transverse incision, cesarean section: a prospective study. J Ultrasound Med 1988;7:389-393.
329. Baker ME, Bowie JD, Killam AP. Sonography of post-cesarean-section bladder-flap hematoma. AJR Am J Roentgenol 1985;144:757-759.
330. Wiener MD, Bowie JD, Baker ME, Kay HH. Sonography of subfascial hematoma after cesarean delivery. AJR Am J Roentgenol 1987;148:907-910.
331. Al-Naib S. Sonographic appearance of postpartum retropubic hematoma. J Clin Ultrasound 1990;18:520-521.

Gestational Trophoblastic Neoplasia

332. Semer DA, Macfee MS. Gestational trophoblastic disease: epidemiology. Semin Oncol 1995;22:109-112.
333. Wagner BJ, Woodward PJ, Dickey GE. From the archives of the AFIP. Gestational trophoblastic disease: radiologic-pathologic correlation. Radiographics 1996;16:131-148.
334. Rose PG. Hydatidiform mole: diagnosis and management. Semin Oncol 1995;22:149-156.
335. Sebire NJ, Rees H, Paradinas F, et al. The diagnostic implications of routine ultrasound examination in histologically confirmed early molar pregnancies. Ultrasound Obstet Gynecol 2001;18:662-665.
336. Goldstein DP, Berkowitz RS. Current management of complete and partial molar pregnancy. J Reprod Med 1994;39:139-146.
337. Berkowitz RS, Goldstein DP. Chorionic tumors. N Engl J Med 1996;335:1740-1748.
338. Lazarus E, Hulka C, Siewert B, Levine D. Sonographic appearance of early complete molar pregnancies. J Ultrasound Med 1999;18:589-594; quiz 595-596.
339. Benson CB, Genest DR, Bernstein MR, et al. Sonographic appearance of first trimester complete hydatidiform moles. Ultrasound Obstet Gynecol 2000;16:188-191.
340. Green CL, Angtuaco TL, Shah HR, Parmley TH. Gestational trophoblastic disease: a spectrum of radiologic diagnosis. Radiographics 1996;16:1371-1384.
341. Fine C, Bundy AL, Berkowitz RS, et al. Sonographic diagnosis of partial hydatidiform mole. Obstet Gynecol 1989;73:414-418.
342. Kirk E, Papageorghiou AT, Condous G, et al. The accuracy of first trimester ultrasound in the diagnosis of hydatidiform mole. Ultrasound Obstet Gynecol 2007;29:70-75.
343. Fowler DJ, Lindsay I, Seckl MJ, Sebire NJ. Routine pre-evacuation ultrasound diagnosis of hydatidiform mole: experience of more than 1000 cases from a regional referral center. Ultrasound Obstet Gynecol 2006;27:56-60.
344. Steller MA, Genest DR, Bernstein MR, et al. Natural history of twin pregnancy with complete hydatidiform mole and coexisting fetus. Obstet Gynecol 1994;83:35-42.
345. Sebire NJ, Foskett M, Paradinas FJ, et al. Outcome of twin pregnancies with complete hydatidiform mole and healthy co-twin. Lancet 2002;359:2165-2166.
346. Greenfield AW. Gestational trophoblastic disease: prognostic variables and staging. Semin Oncol 1995;22:142-148.
347. Jain KA, Jain KA. Gestational trophoblastic disease: pictorial review. Ultrasound Q 2005;21:245-253.
348. Jauniaux E. Ultrasound diagnosis and follow-up of gestational trophoblastic disease. Ultrasound Obstet Gynecol 1998;11:367-377.
349. Soper JT. Identification and management of high-risk gestational trophoblastic disease. Semin Oncol 1995;22:172-184.
350. Finkler NJ. Placental site trophoblastic tumor: diagnosis, clinical behavior and treatment. J Reprod Med 1991;36:27-30.
351. Mangili G, Spagnolo D, Valsecchi L, Maggi R. Transvaginal ultrasonography in persistent trophoblastic tumor [see comment]. Am J Obstet Gynecol 1993;169:1218-1223.
352. Caspi B, Elchalal U, Dgani R, et al. Invasive mole and placental site trophoblastic tumor: two entities of gestational trophoblastic disease with a common ultrasonographic appearance. J Ultrasound Med 1991;10:517-519.
353. Sakamoto C, Oikawa K, Kashimura M, Egashira K. Sonographic appearance of placental site trophoblastic tumor. J Ultrasound Med 1990;9:533-535.
354. Desai RK, Desberg AL. Diagnosis of gestational trophoblastic disease: value of endovaginal color flow Doppler sonography. AJR Am J Roentgenol 1991;157:787-788.
355. Chan FY, Chau MT, Pun TC, et al. A comparison of colour Doppler sonography and the pelvic arteriogram in assessment of patients with gestational trophoblastic disease. Br J Obstet Gynaecol 1995;102:720-725.
356. Yalcin OT, Ozalp SS, Tanir HM. Assessment of gestational trophoblastic disease by Doppler ultrasonography. Eur J Obstet Gynecol Reprod Biol 2002;103:83-87.
357. Zhou Q, Lei XY, Xie Q, et al. Sonographic and Doppler imaging in the diagnosis and treatment of gestational trophoblastic disease: a 12-year experience. J Ultrasound Med 2005;24:15-24.
358. Kennedy AW. Persistent nonmetastatic gestational trophoblastic disease. Semin Oncol 1995;22:161-165.
359. Lurain JR. High-risk metastatic gestational trophoblastic tumors: current management. J Reprod Med 1994;39:217-222.

CHAPTER 16

Ultrasound-Guided Biopsy of Abdomen and Pelvis

Thomas Atwell, J. William Charboneau, John McGahan, and Carl C. Reading

Chapter Outline

*U*ltrasound-guided percutaneous biopsy and abscess drainage are invaluable diagnostic and therapeutic procedures for the management of patients. Growing experience with ultrasound and technical advances have significantly broadened the applications of ultrasound as a guidance method for interventional techniques. An approach to this topic requires knowledge of the current fundamental methods and applications of these procedures in general and in terms of specific anatomic locations.

PERCUTANEOUS NEEDLE BIOPSY

Because of its relatively low cost and wide availability, ultrasound-guided biopsy has become one of the most important methods of tissue diagnosis in radiology practices worldwide. Ultrasound-guided biopsy is a safe and accurate technique for confirmation of suspected malignant masses and characterization of benign lesions in locations throughout the body.[1,2] Secondarily, minimally invasive tissue confirmation decreases patient costs by obviating the need for a surgical diagnosis and decreasing duration of hospital stay and number of ancillary diagnostic tests. In addition, lack of ionizing radiation and real-time imaging during the procedure both make these procedures safer.

Indications and Contraindications

In most cases a biopsy is performed in the setting of possible malignancy, for either initial diagnosis of cancer or confirmation of metastatic disease. In many patients, biopsy is performed to gauge the presence of parenchymal disease in a native organ or rejection in a transplanted organ. Occasionally, biopsy is indicated simply to determine the nature of an incidentally discovered mass.

Relative contraindications to percutaneous needle biopsy include uncorrectable coagulopathy, lack of a safe biopsy route, and an uncooperative patient. To assess for inherent **coagulopathy,** the most valuable information comes from the patient history,[3] including bleeding tendency or need for transfusion or a family history of bleeding diathesis. Patient medications should also be reviewed for recent use of blood-thinning agents such as warfarin, heparin, or adenosine diphosphate (ADP) inhibitors (e.g., clopidogrel), which are relative contraindications to biopsy. If this initial screening is unremarkable, most superficial biopsies can be performed without additional laboratory testing. However, if the history suggests a bleeding disorder, prothrombin time (PT), activated partial thromboplastin time (aPTT), and platelet count should be obtained.[4] The role of bleeding time measurement is of uncertain value in determining bleeding risk; in most cases, no good evidence supports the value of the bleeding time to predict bleeding.[3,5]

Mild coagulopathies may result from the use of aspirin and some antibiotics. In this setting, the procedure may be postponed and the drug discontinued until the medication effect resolves. Some coagulopathies can be corrected with the transfusion of appropriate blood products. Desmopressin (DDAVP) can be given to a uremic patient or a patient with a history of recent aspirin therapy to improve functioning platelet activity.[6] Postbiopsy embolization of the needle track has been reported to control hemorrhage in patients at high risk for bleeding and in whom the need for biopsy outweighs any risk.[7,8]

The second relative contraindication is the **lack of a safe biopsy route**. A biopsy path extending through large vessels such as the splenic or extrahepatic portal vein may increase the risk of hemorrhage. A biopsy path free of overlying stomach or bowel is also a preferable route, although such biopsies have been safely performed using smaller (21 gauge) needles.[9] Biopsies performed through ascites have also proved to be safe.[10,11]

The third relative contraindication to needle biopsy is an **uncooperative patient** in whom uncontrolled motion during needle placement increases the risk of unanticipated injury and hemorrhage. This is a particularly common problem in pediatric patients, and sedation may be required.

Imaging Methods

Both ultrasound and computed tomography (CT) can be used to guide percutaneous needle intervention. The choice of method depends on multiple factors, including lesion size and location, relative lesion conspicuity on the two modalities, and equipment availability. Most masses can be successfully biopsied using either ultrasound or CT, with the choice depending on personal preference.

Ultrasound

Ultrasound has several strengths as a means of guiding percutaneous intervention. It is readily available, relatively inexpensive, and portable. Ultrasound uses no ionizing radiation and can provide guidance in almost any anatomic plane. The greatest advantage, however, is that sonography allows the real-time visualization of the needle tip as it passes through tissue into the target. This allows precise and confident needle placement and avoidance of important intervening structures. In addition, **color Doppler flow imaging** (CDFI) may help prevent complications of needle placement by identifying the vascular nature of a mass and by allowing the clinician to avoid vascular structures lying within the needle path.

Ultrasound guidance can be used for the biopsy of many organs and regions of the body. The technique is optimal for lesions located superficially or at moderate depth in a thin to average-sized person, as well as for lesions within organs prone to respiratory motion (e.g., liver, kidney). In the latter scenario, the advantage of real-time ultrasound-guidance allows continuous visualization of the target during the biopsy. Lesions located within or behind bone or gas-filled bowel cannot be visualized because of near-complete reflection of sound from the bone or air interface.

Theoretically, any mass that is well visualized with ultrasound is amenable to ultrasound-guided needle biopsy. In our practice, most liver and kidney biopsies are performed with ultrasound guidance, as are biopsies of the thyroid and parathyroid glands. Superficial lymph nodes are also particularly well suited to real-time ultrasound-guided biopsy. Occasionally, the pancreas (particularly pancreas transplants) and other sites in the abdomen and pelvis undergo biopsy with ultrasound guidance if lesion visualization is adequate.

Compared with CT, ultrasound-guided procedures require less time to perform and can be more cost-effective.[12-14] Ultrasound-guided biopsy has been shown to be more accurate than CT, with a lower false-negative rate.[13,15]

Computed Tomography

Computed tomography is well established as an accurate guidance method for percutaneous biopsy of most regions in the body. It provides excellent spatial resolution of structures between the skin surface and targeted lesion, and it provides an accurate image of the needle tip. In addition, lesions located deep in the abdomen or within bone are better seen with CT than with ultrasound. In our practice, many pelvic, adrenal, pancreatic, retroperitoneal, and bone biopsies are performed with CT guidance because these structures are often best seen with this imaging method.

Historically, CT was limited by its lack of continuous visualization of the needle during insertion and biopsy. In the past decade, CT **fluoroscopy** has allowed real-time visualization of needle positioning. This has reduced the time required for interventional procedures at the cost of increased radiation dosage.[16]

Needle Selection

A variety of needles with a spectrum of calibers (shaft diameter), lengths, and tip designs are commercially available for use in percutaneous biopsy. Needle caliber is based on outer diameter, with larger-caliber needles having a lower gauge number. Conceptually, needles can be grouped into small-caliber (20 gauge or smaller) or large-caliber (19 gauge or larger) sizes. **Small-caliber needles** are traditionally used to obtain cells for cytologic analysis by using a procedure commonly referred to as **fine-needle aspiration** (FNA). However, small pieces of tissue may be obtained for histologic examination as well. With these small-caliber needles, masses behind loops of bowel can be punctured with minimal likelihood of infection.[9] The smaller samples yielded by small-caliber needles are appropriate to confirm tumor recurrence or metastasis in a patient known to have a previous primary malignancy. Even if the sample is small, the pathologist is usually able to make an accurate diagnosis by comparing the biopsy specimen with the original tissue.

Large-caliber needles can be used to obtain greater amounts of tissue for more thorough histologic and cytologic analysis. Larger needles may be necessary to obtain sufficient tissue to diagnose and subtype some types of malignancies (e.g., lymphoma), many benign lesions, and most chronic diffuse parenchymal diseases (e.g., hepatic cirrhosis, renal glomerulonephritis, renal allograft rejection).[17] The large-caliber tissue sample can also be used to generate an additional "touch prep" specimen, whereby the tissue is manually swiped across a glass pathology slide, leaving a cellular sample on the slide for cytologic analysis.[18]

The preference and level of expertise of the pathologist involved in the interpretation of biopsy specimens are considerations in the selection of needle size and type. **Cytopathologists** specialize in the interpretation of cellular samples, rendering a diagnosis based on the cells provided. Unfortunately, some clinical facilities do not offer cytopathologic interpretation. **Histopathologists,** in contrast, often prefer a large biopsy specimen for interpretation. For example, a large biopsy specimen from a metastatic lesion often allows a more reliable prediction of the primary site of the malignancy than a tiny sample or a cytologic aspirate. Determination of the primary site allows the oncologist to tailor subsequent treatment.

Biopsy Procedure

Before any invasive procedure is performed, the procedure, risks, alternatives, and benefits should be explained in terms that the patient can understand so that informed consent can be obtained. The performing physician must address patient apprehension about potential pain during the procedure and possible complications of the biopsy. After discussing the procedure, any patient questions should be answered fully.

Biopsies are frequently performed on an outpatient basis. Discomfort from the procedure is rarely severe and is usually controlled by appropriate administration of local anesthetic after the skin is cleaned and draped. An intravenous (IV) access may be established before the biopsy in the event that fluid or medications are necessary during the procedure. Premedication is usually not necessary. Sedatives and analgesics such as midazolam or fentanyl can be administered intravenously after consent has been obtained.[19] If the patient's history suggests a bleeding disorder, coagulation studies should be reviewed before biopsy. In patients with an increased risk of bleeding, a larger or second IV access site may be prudent.

There are two options to **sterilize the transducer**. The transducer may be covered with a sterile plastic sheath, although this may degrade image quality and make the transducer more difficult to handle. Alternatively, the transducer itself may be directly sterilized with povidone-iodine (Betadine) and placed directly on the skin. Sterile gel is used as an acoustic coupling agent. After the biopsy, the transducer is soaked for 10 minutes in a bactericidal dialdehyde solution.

Most ultrasound-guided biopsies are performed under continuous real-time visualization. **Needle guidance systems** designed to facilitate proper needle placement are commercially available. These guides direct the needle to various depths from the transducer surface, depending on the preselected angle of the guide relative to the transducer (Fig. 16-1). Many radiologists prefer the **"freehand" technique** in which the needle is inserted through the skin directly into the view of the transducer without the use of a guide. The needle is then independently directed to the target lesion by the operator under real-time ultrasound visualization.

In contrasting these two biopsy techniques, one can appreciate the technical ease provided by the needle guidance method. This can decrease the time to perform a biopsy, particularly in the hands of a novice operator.[20] However, the freehand technique allows greater flexibility to the operator in performing subtle adjustments to the needle path in the event of patient movement, particularly with respiration.

Fine-needle aspiration biopsies are performed by placing the tip of the needle into the target lesion and rapidly "bobbing" the needle within the mass, collecting cellular samples within the lumen of the small needle. Some biopsy devices include a syringe on the end to provide negative pressure within the lumen, increasing the cellular yield.

Large-caliber needles are used to obtain cores of tissue. With the typical spring-loaded core biopsy device (biopsy "gun"), the needle tip is advanced to the margin of the target lesion. Careful attention is made to the anticipated excursion of the device to prevent injury to deeper structures. Some biopsy devices allow initial manual advancement of the stylet through the target lesion to the desired depth. When the spring-loaded cutting sheath is activated, the sheath advances over the stylet, but there is no additional forward motion of the needle (Fig. 16-2).

Most biopsies are performed by making one or more passes into a mass with a single needle. Occasionally, two needles are used in a **coaxial** manner, whereby a larger introducer needle is first placed into the mass. The inner stylet of this needle is then removed, and a longer, smaller-caliber needle is placed through its lumen. Multiple samples can then be obtained with the smaller needle without the need to reposition the larger intro-

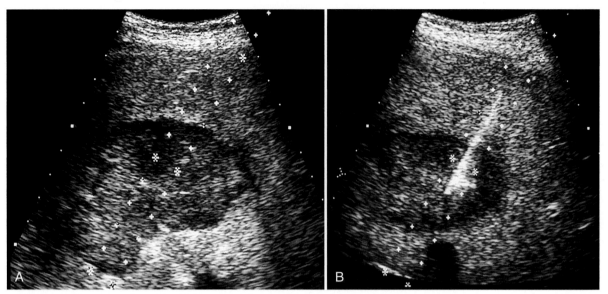

FIGURE 16-1. Ultrasound-guided biopsy with needle guide. A, Ultrasound image shows a mass in the right lobe of the liver. **B,** The needle is seen within the preselected angle boundaries, with the tip in the mass.

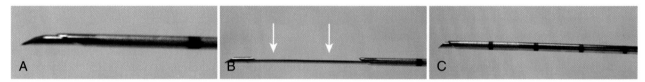

FIGURE 16-2. Biopsy needle with central stylet. A, Biopsy needle tip before stylet deployment. **B,** Stylet is deployed, with the biopsy trough *(arrows)* evident on the exposed stylet. **C,** Outer cannula is fired over the stylet, allowing tissue to be obtained in the trough.

ducer needle. This technique allows a large amount of tissue to be obtained with only one puncture of the organ capsule. While intuitively this should decrease bleeding complications, this has not been conclusively demonstrated in real practice.[21] This may be related to the large caliber of the introducer needle or the extended time during which the introducer needle lies within the organ, potentially tearing the capsule.

After the biopsy is performed, the patient is typically observed in the radiology department for 1 to 2 hours. Longer observation may be appropriate after kidney biopsy or if there is clinical concern about a potential complication. In many medical centers, initial cytologic results are available within this time. If the results of the initial cytologic analysis are not conclusive, a **repeat biopsy** is usually performed while the patient is in the department. When core biopsy tissue samples are obtained, frozen-section analysis may be performed for diagnosis if the touch-prep cytology specimen is inconclusive. In this case, additional samples may be necessary if permanent fixation or special staining is required.

Needle Visualization

Continuous real-time visualization of needle tip advancement is one of ultrasound's greatest strengths as a biopsy guidance method. Unfortunately, this is frequently the most technically difficult aspect of ultrasound-guided biopsy for many radiologists. Beginners may choose to practice on a homemade ultrasound biopsy phantom to develop the coordination necessary for ultrasound-guided procedures.[22,23]

The most common reason for nonvisualization of the needle tip is **improper alignment** of the needle tip and transducer. To visualize the entire needle, the needle and central ultrasound beam of the transducer must be in the same plane. This allows the entire shaft of the needle to be visualized. Although this rarely occurs with the use of a mechanical needle guide, such parallel placement can be challenging using the freehand technique, particularly when the radiologist is focused on the ultrasound image. In many cases the radiologist can simply look at the alignment of the needle with the transducer to allow gross correction of path deviation (Fig. 16-3), then fine-tune the needle alignment with ultrasound imaging.

A **bobbing** or in-and-out jiggling movement of the biopsy needle during insertion improves needle visualization. This bobbing motion causes deflection of the soft tissues adjacent to the needle and makes the trajectory of the needle much more discernible within the otherwise stationary field. Alternatively, if using a coaxial

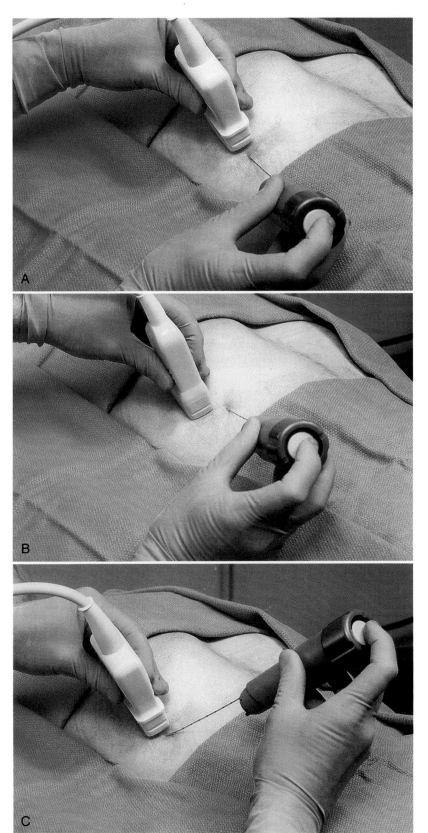

FIGURE 16-3. Freehand alignment of biopsy needle with ultrasound transducer. A, Correct alignment for optimal sonographic visualization. Biopsy needle is aligned precisely within the central plane of the transducer. **B** and **C,** Incorrect alignment. **B,** Biopsy needle is aligned off-center relative to the transducer. **C,** Biopsy needle is aligned correctly with the center of the transducer but is angled away from the central plane.

system, the inner, smaller needle can be "pumped" or moved in and out within the larger cannula.

Needle visualization can also be improved by **increasing the reflectivity** of the biopsy needle. Large-caliber needles are more readily visualized than small-caliber needles. Keeping the bevel of the needle directed toward the transducer may also increase the conspicuity of the needle tip. Some authors have found CDFI helpful to visualize needle motion,[24] although we have not routinely incorporated Doppler ultrasound into our practice. Modifications in needle tip design to enhance needle visualization include scoring the needle tip and using a screw stylet. Extrareflective needles specifically designed for ultrasound guidance are commercially available. Most needles, however, are sufficiently visible sonographically as long as the needle and transducer are aligned.

The **echogenicity** of the parenchyma of the organ undergoing biopsy also affects the visibility of the biopsy needle. If the parenchyma is relatively hypoechoic, such as liver, kidney, or spleen, the echogenic needle can usually be identified easily. Conversely, if the organ or soft tissues are relatively hyperechoic, it is usually difficult to visualize the echogenic needle tip in this background. This is particularly relevant in the biopsy of masses in obese patients or masses surrounded by complex fat, as in the retroperitoneum.

Linear or curved array transducers are frequently used for guiding procedures because of their good near-field resolution, which allows visualization of the needle after relatively little tissue penetration. The **focal zone of the ultrasound beam should also be placed in the near field** for better needle visualization. Sector transducers are often used if there is a small acoustic window or if there is a deep lesion situated at steep angles.

Clear visualization of the biopsy needle is an important element in the success of ultrasound-guided needle biopsies. The various techniques described here can be used to enhance needle visualization. However, considerable real-time scanning **experience** remains the key factor to the successful performance of ultrasound-guided biopsies.

Specific Anatomic Applications

Liver

The liver is the abdominal organ in which percutaneous biopsy is most frequently performed. Common indications for biopsy include nonsurgical confirmation of metastatic disease, characterization of focal liver mass(es) with inconclusive imaging, and diagnosis of parenchymal disease. Biopsy of large or superficial lesions is most easily done. With experience, deep lesions and lesions smaller than 1cm can undergo accurate biopsy[25,26] (Fig. 16-4).

In our practice, liver biopsy is almost universally performed under ultrasound guidance because of the real-time visualization of the needle. This advantage becomes particularly obvious when there is significant movement of the liver caused by respiration and diaphragm excursion.

Lesions in the left lobe of the liver and in the inferior portion of the right lobe can usually undergo biopsy through a subcostal approach. Lesions located superiorly in the dome of the liver present a technical challenge for traditional CT-guided biopsy, but real-time, off-axial imaging with ultrasound allows for accurate needle targeting of such tumors, often through an intercostal approach. Although the intercostal approach may violate the pleural space, aerated lung is rarely punctured because it is well visualized sonographically and can be avoided. We usually place the patient in the **left posterior oblique** (LPO) rather than the supine position when an intercostal approach is used to improve visibility of the liver through the intercostal spaces. If working along the right side of the patient, such a position also prevents the patient from watching needle manipulation. As feasible, **orienting the transducer along the longitudinal axis** of the patient is preferable. Such orientation minimizes the interference of respiration, because the tumor and needle remain in the field of view throughout the procedure.

Benign hepatic lesions such as focal fatty infiltration, focal areas of normal liver within a fatty infiltrated liver, and atypical hemangiomas can occasionally mimic the appearance of malignancy on imaging studies. Biopsy of these processes can be done with ultrasound guidance to exclude malignancy and to confirm their benign nature (Fig. 16-5). Although **cavernous hemangiomas** are vascular lesions, these masses have undergone successful percutaneous biopsy without significant complications.[27-29] Particular care must be taken to avoid direct puncture of a cavernous hemangiomas without intervening liver parenchyma because this may result in catastrophic bleeding.[30] Normal overlying liver may tamponade potential bleeding from the hemangioma.

Percutaneous ultrasound-guided biopsy of **portal vein thrombus** has proved to be a safe and accurate diagnostic procedure for staging of hepatocellular carcinoma.[31] The implication of tumor thrombus has important implications for specific treatment options.

Liver biopsies are relatively safe, with an overall significant complication rate of less than 1%.[32-36] Hemorrhage is most common. Such significant bleeding complications are more likely to occur in the biopsy of patients with malignancy and those with acute liver failure, chronic active hepatitis, or cirrhosis.[35,37,38] Most complications occur soon after the biopsy procedure, with about 60% occurring within 2 hours and 80% within 10 hours.[35] Several large series report mortality of percutaneous liver biopsy as 0.1% or less.[35-37]

Pancreas

Despite the growing use of **endoscopic ultrasound** (EUS) and EUS-guided FNA, percutaneous biopsy of

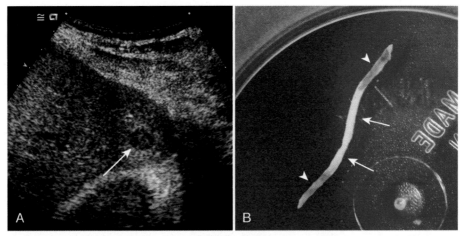

FIGURE 16-4. Ultrasound-guided biopsy of small hepatic metastasis. A, Longitudinal ultrasound image of inferior right lobe of the liver shows a 1-cm mass *(arrow)*. **B,** Gross photograph of the core biopsy sample shows the typical white core of pathologic tissue *(arrows)* bordered by typical-appearing normal liver parenchyma *(arrowheads).*

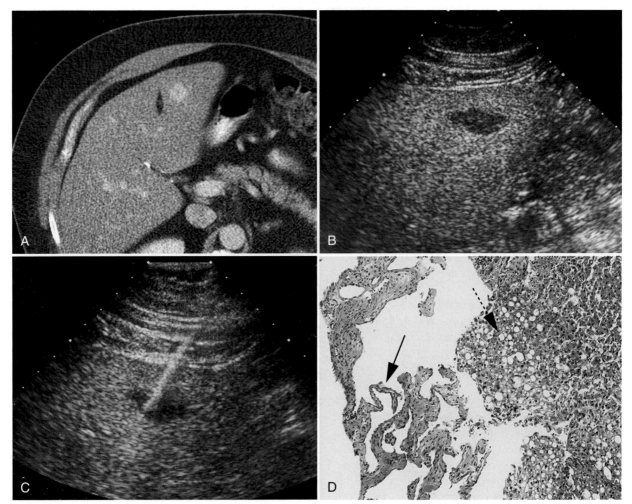

FIGURE 16-5. Biopsy of cavernous hemangioma. A, Contrast-enhanced computed tomography (CT) scan shows a 1.5-cm vascular mass in left lobe of the liver. **B,** Transverse ultrasound demonstrates a hypoechoic ellipsoid mass in a fatty infiltrated liver. **C,** Ultrasound-guided biopsy using an 18-gauge needle. **D,** Histologic specimen shows endothelial-lined vascular spaces *(arrow)* diagnostic of cavernous hemangioma, as well as small, round, fat globules *(dashed arrow)* within hematoxylin and eosin–stained hepatocytes.

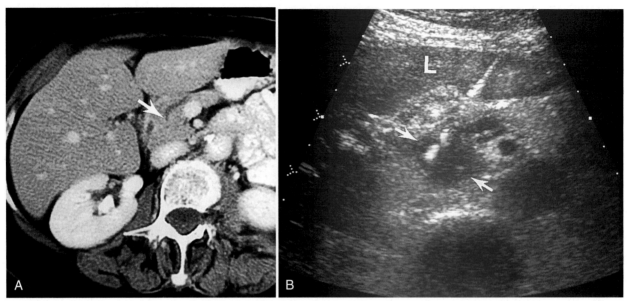

FIGURE 16-6. Ultrasound-guided pancreatic biopsy. A, Contrast-enhanced CT scan shows a mildly dilated pancreatic duct with abrupt termination in the head of the pancreas *(arrow)*. No definite mass is identified on CT scan. **B,** Ultrasound for guided biopsy shows a 19-gauge needle passing through left lobe of the liver *(L)*, with needle tip within a 2-cm hypoechoic mass in the head of the pancreas *(arrows)*. The biopsy was positive for adenocarcinoma.

pancreatic tumors frequently remains necessary when the tumor is in the tail of the pancreas or when EUS is unavailable. Biopsy is often required to document malignancy or differentiate malignancy from a benign condition, such as focal pancreatitis.

At our institution, most pancreatic biopsies are done with CT guidance because depth of the pancreas and presence of overlying bowel gas and hyperechoic abdominal fat can make visualization of the needle difficult. Nevertheless, biopsy of pancreatic masses in normal-size and slender patients can be done accurately under ultrasound guidance (Fig. 16-6).

The **gastrointestinal (GI) tract** may be traversed when biopsying the pancreas. With ultrasound, the stomach or bowel is either displaced or compressed. Brandt et al.[9] demonstrated the safety of traversing the GI tract (stomach, small bowel, colon) in performing percutaneous biopsies in 66 procedures. Most of these biopsies were performed using a 21-gauge needle, with no complications related to the biopsy route in these patients.

A particular advantage of ultrasound over CT is the ability to biopsy pancreatic masses in an off-axis plane, which is very useful if overlying vessels are present on CT. Ultrasound-guided biopsy has 93% to 95% accuracy, compared with 86% to 100% accuracy for CT guidance.[9,39,40]

In some series, the biopsy success rate for the diagnosis of pancreatic carcinoma has been lower than the success rate for the diagnosis of malignant lesions in other organs of the abdomen.[9,41,42] This may be related to sampling error, because significant desmoplastic reaction often accompanies pancreatic adenocarcinoma. By **targeting**

the central hypoechoic portion of the pancreatic mass, the clinician can improve their diagnostic yield. In addition, core biopsy, either alone or in addition to FNA, results in improved diagnostic performance compared with FNA alone.[40]

The differentiation between **benign serous** and potentially **malignant mucinous** pancreatic tumors can be difficult with imaging alone. Unfortunately, cystic pancreatic malignancies are difficult to accurately diagnose with percutaneous biopsy; a definitive diagnosis was achieved in only 60% of patients in one study.[43] In biopsy of a cystic pancreatic lesion, it is critical to obtain **epithelial cells,** either in the wall of the lesion or within the cyst fluid. Analysis of **percutaneous fluid aspirates** from a cystic lesion has also been proposed as an aid to distinguish cystic neoplasms from pseudocysts.[43-45] A high amylase level is consistent with a pseudocyst. The presence of tumor markers with the cyst fluid may also be helpful in suggesting a cystic neoplasm.

The safety of percutaneous biopsy of the pancreas has been well established, with a complication rate of 1% to 2%.[9,39] An historic review reported six deaths related to pancreas biopsy.[46] Five of these deaths were attributed to pancreatitis and one to sepsis. No pancreatic cancer was found in either the biopsy specimen or the postmortem examination of these patients, suggesting an increased risk for developing pancreatitis after biopsy of normal pancreas. In this same large review of percutaneous biopsies, 10 of 23 cases of needle track seeding occurred after the biopsy of pancreatic malignancies. For this reason, biopsy may not be indicated in patients who are surgical candidates.

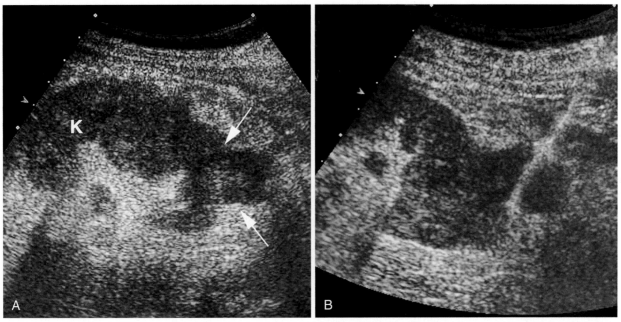

FIGURE 16-7. Ultrasound-guided biopsy of renal mass. A, Longitudinal image shows a 2-cm solid mass extending from lower pole of the left kidney *(K)*. **B,** Mass was biopsied using an 18-gauge biopsy device, confirming renal cell carcinoma.

Kidney

Biopsy of the kidney is performed to assess intrinsic parenchymal disease or to characterize a renal mass. The latter situation is controversial, with respect to the indication for biopsy, as well as the accuracy of biopsy in characterizing a renal mass (Fig. 16-7).

Cross-sectional imaging has allowed accurate characterization of many benign renal masses, notably benign **cysts** and fat-containing **angiomyolipomas.** The problem is with the indeterminate, enhancing renal mass, specifically the **oncocytoma** and **renal cell carcinoma,** which cannot be differentiated by imaging.[47] As such and as outlined by Silverman et al.,[48] currently accepted indications for biopsy of a renal mass include the following:

1. Renal mass and known extrarenal primary malignancy.
2. Renal mass and imaging findings that suggest unresectable renal cancer.
3. Patients with a renal mass and surgical comorbidity.
4. Renal mass that may have been caused by infection.

When performed in the appropriate circumstances, biopsy may affect a change in clinical management in approximately 40% of patients.[49] Although these indications are generally accepted in the radiology community, controversy exists over the routine biopsy of tumors before definitive surgical resection.

Such a biopsy approach is based on the growing incidence of incidentally detected, small (<3 cm) tumors, particularly in older persons, of which 25% will be benign.[50] Percutaneous renal mass biopsy has exceptional results,[49,51,52] but these studies are frequently limited by the mode of determining true-negative results, which is based on stability on imaging follow-up. However, we know that the lack of growth in a renal mass does not imply a true-negative result, because 25% of renal tumors will not grow.[53]

The best measure to determine the true value of renal mass biopsy is comparison with the **explanted** (surgically resected) specimen. Studies show mixed results, however, including nondiagnostic rates up to 30% and accuracy of 72% to 97%.[47,54-58] Unfortunately, a negative result often remains a clinical concern because of the imaging findings. Wunderlich et al.[56] summarized the role of percutaneous biopsy as follows: "a negative result with sufficiently suspicious imaging findings should be interpreted as suspicious for malignancy and, therefore, should be an indication for surgical exploration."

Sonographic-guidance can be used in the biopsy of kidneys with **diffuse parenchymal disease.** Insertion of the needle into the cortex of the lower-pole renal parenchyma under continuous real-time guidance results in few complications and produces a tissue sample of excellent quality for analysis. An **18-gauge biopsy needle** provides a biopsy specimen that is equivalent in diagnostic quality to the biopsy specimen obtained by the traditional 14-gauge cutting needle.[59] In fact, Hergesell et al.[60] found a 99% success rate in obtaining diagnostic tissue using an 18-gauge needle, with only 0.36% of patients experiencing a significant bleeding complication. In this series, postbiopsy ultrasound revealed a clinically occult hematoma greater than 2 cm in 2% of patients. Similarly, asymptomatic hemorrhage may be detected by CT in up to 90% of patients after uncomplicated kidney biopsy.[61] **Arteriovenous (AV) fistulas**

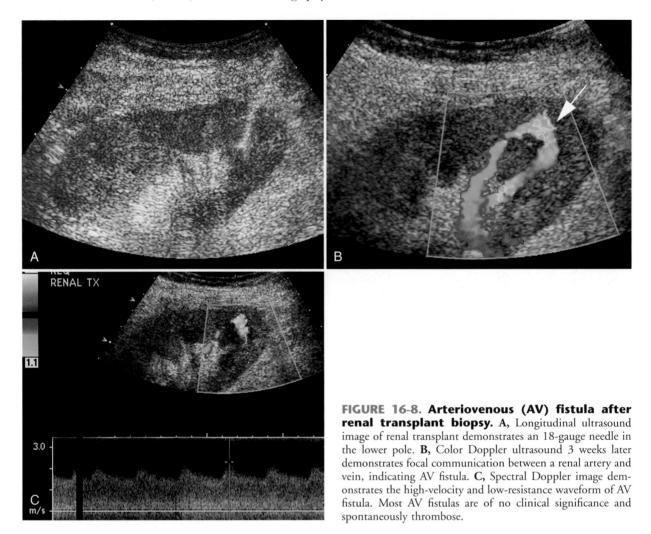

FIGURE 16-8. Arteriovenous (AV) fistula after renal transplant biopsy. A, Longitudinal ultrasound image of renal transplant demonstrates an 18-gauge needle in the lower pole. **B,** Color Doppler ultrasound 3 weeks later demonstrates focal communication between a renal artery and vein, indicating AV fistula. **C,** Spectral Doppler image demonstrates the high-velocity and low-resistance waveform of AV fistula. Most AV fistulas are of no clinical significance and spontaneously thrombose.

may be seen in about 10% of patients immediately after kidney biopsy and usually resolve spontaneously (Fig. 16-8).

Clinically important bleeding is the most serious complication after kidney biopsy, occurring in 0.3% to 6.3% of patients.[60,62-65] Gross hematuria may occur in 5% to 7% and usually stops within 6 to 12 hours.[66] Microscopic hematuria can occur in up to 100% of patients and should not be regarded as a complication.

Adrenal Gland

The most common indication for adrenal biopsy is to **confirm metastatic disease** in a patient with an adrenal mass and a known primary malignancy elsewhere. Currently, CT and magnetic resonance imaging (MRI) characterization of adrenal masses has supplanted biopsy in many cases in establishing benignity of an adrenal mass. Nevertheless, occasional histologic diagnosis is required. In this case, CT-guidance is generally the preferred adrenal biopsy technique because of the deep location of the adrenal glands in the retroperitoneum. Percutaneous

biopsy can yield a diagnosis in more than 93% to 96% of patients.[67,68]

The right adrenal gland is more accessible to ultrasound-guided biopsy than the left adrenal gland because the right lobe of the liver provides a sonographic window to optimize imaging (Fig. 16-9). Bright, echogenic, fat-containing adrenal masses and homogeneous, thin-walled, fluid-filled adrenal masses may not require biopsy because these should represent benign adrenal **myelolipomas** and **cysts**, respectively. CT or MRI can be performed to confirm this before considering biopsy.

Although **benign adenomas** can be larger than 3 cm, the likelihood of silent adrenal carcinoma increases significantly if an incidentally discovered adrenal mass is larger than 4 cm.[69] In this setting, surgical excision is recommended because biopsy will yield insufficient tissue to differentiate a benign adenoma from adrenocortical carcinoma.

Radiologists performing adrenal biopsies should be familiar with the management of a hypertensive crisis after inadvertent biopsy of a **pheochromocytoma.**[70] Although adrenal pheochromocytomas have been safely

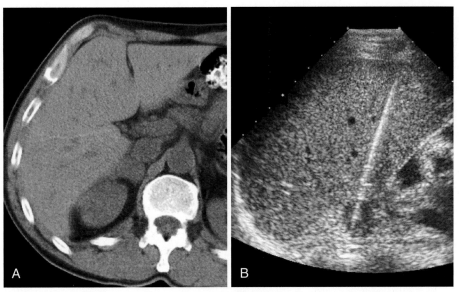

FIGURE 16-9. Ultrasound-guided biopsy of adrenal mass. A, CT scan without contrast demonstrates a 2-cm mass *(arrow)* in the right adrenal gland. **B,** Longitudinal ultrasound image shows value of the liver as a biopsy path to the right adrenal gland.

biopsied without premedication,[67] if the clinical history suggests pheochromocytoma, further laboratory tests should establish the diagnosis rather than biopsy. If biopsy is necessary, consultation with an endocrine specialist and pretreatment with alpha-adrenergic blockers and metyrosine should be considered.[71]

Spleen

The spleen is the abdominal organ that undergoes biopsy **least** often. First, isolated metastases to the spleen are exceptionally rare. In most cases, when the splenic tumor is visualized, there is concomitant disease in other abdominal organs, such as the liver or lymph nodes, in which a biopsy can be performed. Second, the spleen is a highly vascular organ, and the risk of needle biopsy would seem to be high. The reported rate of significant hemorrhage from needle biopsy varies from 0% to 8%.[72-79] In some cases, splenectomy is required.[73,75] Pneumothorax may also occur as a complication after spleen biopsy.[79]

At this time, the main clinical reason for performing percutaneous biopsy of the spleen is to differentiate recurrent **lymphoma, metastasis,** and **infection** in a patient who has a new splenic lesion but no disease elsewhere in the abdomen (Fig. 16-10). In the immunocompromised patient, differentiation between **malignancy** and **fungal infection** can be critical in patient management. Percutaneous biopsy can yield a specific diagnosis in approximately 90% of patients.[72,73,80]

Lung

Percutaneous biopsy of the lung is typically performed with CT guidance. However, ultrasound has proved to

be effective in the biopsy of masses that abut the chest wall, without the imaging interference of aerated lung parenchyma[81,82] (Fig. 16-11). Such lesions include **pulmonary, pleural,** and **mediastinal** masses. Notable advantages of ultrasound in the lung include (1) real-time guidance during patient respiration, (2) ability to biopsy efficiently in the off-axial plane, (3) ability to biopsy lesions in patients who would otherwise have difficulty cooperating, and (4) absence of ionizing radiation.[83] Ultrasound biopsy of mediastinal masses can be performed if the mass is visible. Mediastinal vessels in the path of the needle may be avoided with the use of color Doppler ultrasound before needle placement.

Complications

Image-guided percutaneous needle biopsy is a widely accepted mode of obtaining tissue for diagnosis, in part because of its well-documented safety. Several large reviews using multi-institutional questionnaires have reported major complication rates of 0.05% to 0.19% and mortality rates of 0.008% to 0.038%.[46,84-86]

Although rare, **hemorrhage** is the most common major complication of solid-organ biopsy and accounts for most biopsy-associated deaths. If hemorrhage is suspected after biopsy and the patient is hemodynamically stable, CT should be obtained. CT is more accurate than ultrasound to evaluate for hemorrhage.[61] On ultrasound, fresh blood has an echogenicity similar to that of surrounding tissues and can be overlooked (Fig. 16-12).

The difference in the complication rates associated with the use of larger-caliber core biopsy needles and small-caliber needles is not as great as might be expected. An early comparative study found complication rates of 0.8% with fine needle (22 gauge) and 1.4% with

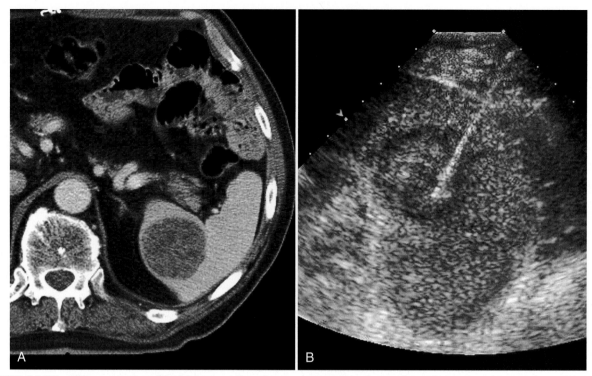

FIGURE 16-10. Ultrasound-guided biopsy of melanoma metastasis to the spleen. A, Contrast-enhanced CT shows a 4-cm mass in the spleen. **B,** Transverse ultrasound demonstrates the 18-gauge biopsy needle within the mass.

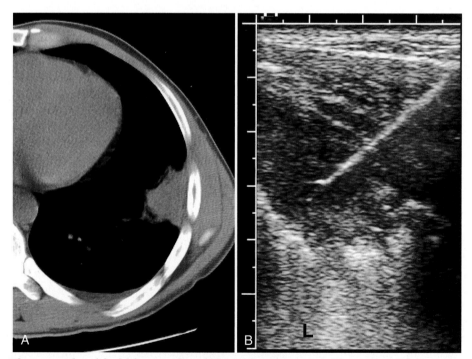

FIGURE 16-11. Ultrasound-guided biopsy of peripheral lung mass. A, Noncontrast CT demonstrates an indeterminate peripheral left lung mass. **B,** Oblique ultrasound image shows a 20-gauge biopsy needle isolated within the hypoechoic mass, which is surrounded by aerated lung *(L).* Biopsy confirmed histoplasmosis.

large-caliber needles (14 and 18 gauge); this difference was not statistically significant.[87] In addition, the larger needles provided a diagnostic tissue in 90% of biopsies, versus 65% in fine-needle biopsies. Welch et al.[88] found equal rates of complications from the use of 18-gauge and 21-gauge biopsy needles (0.3%).

Other major complications secondary to biopsy include **pneumothorax, pancreatitis, bile leakage, peritonitis, infection** (Fig. 16-13), and **needle track seeding.** An exceedingly rare complication (0.003%),[46] needle track seeding has been reported after biopsy of various malignancies, including those arising from the pancreas, prostate, liver, kidney, lung, neck, pleura, breast, eye, and retroperitoneum.[46,89-100] Because seeding is so rare, in most cases it should not affect the decision to perform percutaneous biopsy.

Minor complications more often encountered include **vasovagal reactions** and **pain.**

ULTRASOUND-GUIDED DRAINAGE

As with needle biopsy, percutaneous aspiration and drainage procedures have gained wide acceptance in clinical practice because of their safety, simplicity, and effectiveness. Ultrasound provides precise needle guidance to allow for needle aspiration or catheter drainage of superficial and deep fluid collections throughout the body.

Indications and Contraindications

Original criteria for percutaneous drainage specified that the fluid collection be unilocular with no communications, and surgical backup was considered essential.[101,102] Currently, percutaneous abscess drainage is performed safely for solitary, multilocular, and multifocal fluid collections with or without communication to the GI tract.[102,103] Such collections include complex solid-organ abscesses, enteric-related abdominal abscesses (e.g., caused by appendicitis and diverticulitis), tubo-ovarian abscesses, and percutaneous cholecystostomy for an inflamed gallbladder. Percutaneous drainage is more likely to be successful in abscesses with air-fluid levels or superficial gas collections, whereas abscesses with deep, trapped gas bubbles are less likely to be successfully managed with percutaneous drainage.[104] Poorly defined fluid in the peritoneum with an underlying surgically correctable abnormality (e.g., perforated bowel) is better treated with surgery.

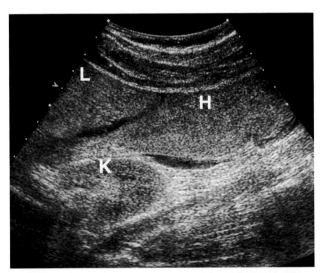

FIGURE 16-12. Isoechoic hematoma after biopsy of pancreas transplant. Large, fresh, postbiopsy intraperitoneal hematoma *(H)* is isoechoic with the adjacent liver *(L)* and right kidney *(K)*. Newly evolving clot (<30 min) can be echogenic and therefore overlooked.

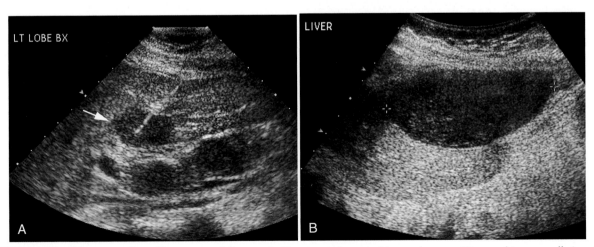

FIGURE 16-13. Abscess after liver mass biopsy. A, Transverse ultrasound image shows an 18-gauge biopsy needle in a 3-cm metastasis *(arrow)*. **B,** Longitudinal image obtained 2 weeks later demonstrates a 6-cm debris-containing fluid collection, anterior to left lobe of the liver, at biopsy site. Subsequent aspiration and drain placement confirmed abscess.

Most percutaneous abscess drainage is performed to achieve a cure without the need for surgery. In other patients, it is a temporizing procedure that either postpones definitive surgery until the patient is stable (e.g., periappendiceal abscess drainage) or permits a single-stage rather than a multistage surgery (e.g., peridiverticular abscess drainage). This is particularly desirable in high-risk, medically complicated patients who present with sepsis.

Contraindications to image-guided percutaneous catheter drainage are all relative and are similar to those for percutaneous biopsy. Although uncommon, lack of a safe route for percutaneous drainage precludes the procedure. Unlike percutaneous biopsy, in which bowel may be traversed without complication, fluid aspiration and percutaneous abscess drainage through bowel should be avoided. Initial advancement of the drain through normally contaminated bowel may seed a sterile fluid collection, resulting in iatrogenic infection. In addition, drain placement through bowel may result in not only significant perforation, but also enteric fistula.

Bleeding diathesis should be maximally corrected before drain placement, and appropriate sedation (local and systemic) should be given, as appropriate.

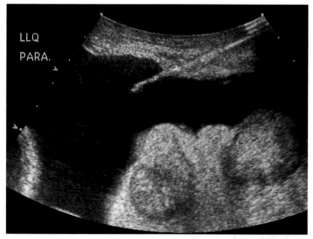

FIGURE 16-14. Ultrasound-guided paracentesis. Longitudinal image shows a 5-French angiocatheter with side holes in the left lower peritoneal cavity during a paracentesis.

Imaging Methods

Selection of ultrasound or CT for guidance of aspiration and drainage is influenced by several factors, including the location of the fluid collection and the strengths and weaknesses of each imaging modality, as discussed earlier. For example, a **simple paracentesis** is best performed under ultrasound guidance (Fig. 16-14). More complicated drainage procedures in the retroperitoneum or pelvis are best performed with CT guidance. More **superficial abdominal fluid collections** may be aspirated or drained easily with ultrasound guidance. Obtaining a CT scan before the procedure often provides a more detailed view of potentially deeper components to the collection and an anatomic map for planning a safe access route.

In certain anatomic areas, such as the gallbladder, biliary tract, and kidneys, combined ultrasound and **fluoroscopic guidance** of catheter placement may be preferred. The combined use of ultrasound for initial needle placement and fluoroscopy for catheter placement, using the **guidewire exchange technique** (Seldinger), optimizes the strengths of both guidance modalities. Fluoroscopy can then be used to opacify the area drained and confirm final catheter placement and adequacy of drainage.

No single method of guidance for percutaneous drainage is appropriate for all abdominal fluid collections or abscesses. The approach to any fluid collection or potential abscess must be tailored to the patient, procedure, and specific circumstances.

Catheter Selection

Various catheters and introducing systems are available for percutaneous abscess drainage; choice depends mainly on operator preference. As with most interventional procedures, the clinician or radiologist must be familiar and comfortable with the system chosen. In general, thicker fluid is best drained with larger-caliber catheters. A 10- to 14-French catheter provides adequate drainage for most abscesses. Smaller (6-8 French) catheters are adequate for less viscous collections. Catheters with retention devices, such as a locking loop, are frequently used to prevent catheter dislodgement (Fig. 16-15).

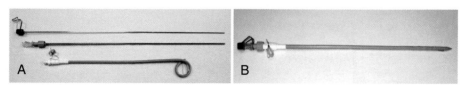

FIGURE 16-15. Locking-loop drainage catheter. A, Three components of the locking-loop catheter are sharpened inner stylet *(top),* stiffener *(middle),* and catheter with distal locking loop *(bottom).* **B,** Assembled catheter is ready for placement using trocar technique.

Patient Preparation

The procedure and risks should be explained to the patient and informed consent obtained. The patient's hemostatic status should be assessed through clinical history, and recent coagulation studies should be available. We routinely require platelets and PT for drainage procedures. IV access is obtained in all patients for administration of medications and for emergency access, in the event of a complication, such as hemorrhage, sepsis, or hypotension. Patients often receive broad-spectrum antibiotics intravenously to decrease the risk of sepsis. Satisfactory analgesia is necessary throughout the procedure to provide optimal patient comfort and cooperation. Local anesthesia is usually sufficient for needle aspiration; however, IV sedatives and analgesics such as midazolam (Versed) or fentanyl (Sublimaze) are beneficial for percutaneous catheter insertion; dilation of the drain tract can be extremely painful to the patient.

Diagnostic Aspiration

Because fluid collections often have a nonspecific appearance, diagnostic aspiration is the first step. A fine needle is guided into the fluid collection by the selected imaging modality. This needle insertion defines a precise and safe route to the fluid collection. A small amount of fluid is aspirated and sent for appropriate microbiologic evaluation. The resulting culture and sensitivity data are used to direct the antibiotic therapy. If the fluid does not appear infected (i.e., clear, colorless, and odorless), the radiologist may elect to aspirate the cavity completely and not perform the drainage procedure. This is important, because a catheter placed in a sterile fluid collection will eventually serve as a nidus of infection, with subsequent infection of the collection. If pus is aspirated, care should be taken to aspirate only a small amount of fluid, because any decrease in the cavity size may make subsequent catheter placement more difficult.

Catheter Placement

Catheter insertion can be performed using the trocar or the Seldinger technique; the choice usually depends on operator preference. In the **trocar technique** the catheter fits over a stiffening cannula, and a sharp inner stylet is placed within the cannula for insertion (see Fig. 16-15). The catheter assembly is advanced into the fluid collection. The catheter is then pushed from the cannula, and the distal loop is formed and tightened to secure the catheter within the fluid collection. This method works best for large and superficial fluid collections.

With the **Seldinger technique** (guidewire exchange technique), a guidewire is advanced through the aspiration needle and coiled within the fluid collection. The needle is then removed, and the guidewire is used as an anchor for passage of a dilator to widen the catheter

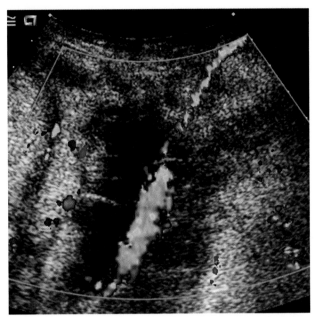

FIGURE 16-16. Drain within deep pelvic abscess. With aspiration of the abscess and subsequent fluid motion within the drain, longitudinal transperineal Doppler ultrasound image shows a color shift, allowing good visualization of the catheter.

track. The catheter-cannula assembly is placed over the guidewire into the fluid collection. The guidewire and inner cannula are removed as the catheter is simultaneously advanced. The distal locking loop of the catheter is re-formed to prevent catheter dislodgement. If the catheter is difficult to see with ultrasound, the use of CDFI may improve conspicuity. During aspiration or irrigation, Doppler shifts improve catheter visualization (Fig. 16-16).

Final positioning of the catheter is important in maximizing the effectiveness of drainage. For this purpose, ultrasound and CT are complementary and should be used together. CT provides an anatomic road map for ideal catheter placement. Because this ideal position seldom lies in the true axial plane, ultrasound can be used to direct the needle, guidewire, and catheter into the ideal position. Final placement can then be verified with CT.

Drainage Procedure

After the drainage catheter is placed, the cavity is completely aspirated and gently irrigated. Care should be taken not to distend the cavity during the irrigation because this may increase the risk of bacteremia. Repeat images are obtained to determine the size of the residual cavity, the position of the drainage tube, and whether the entire abscess communicates with the drainage tube. If the abscess cavity has not completely resolved, the drainage catheter may need to be repositioned, or a second drain may need to be placed. Such manipulations are often performed under fluoroscopy the day after initial drain placement. Correct catheter position and adequate catheter size are the most important factors for successful drainage.

Follow-up Care

All drains must be **irrigated regularly.** Injection and aspiration of 10 mL of isotonic saline three or four times daily is usually sufficient. If drainage is especially tenacious or the abscess is large, more frequent irrigations with greater volumes of saline may be necessary. The fluid collection can be drained dependently or by low, intermittent suction. The character and volume of the output should be recorded each nursing shift and checked daily on rounds by the radiology service. If the drainage changes significantly in volume or character or if fever recurs, the patient should be reexamined to check for fistulas, catheter blockage, reaccumulation of the abscess, or a previously undiagnosed collection.

From 24 to 48 hours after tube placement, a sinogram should be performed to look at the abscess cavity size, completeness of drainage, and catheter position and to look for fistulas. Simple abscess cavities may drain for 5 to 10 days. Abscesses secondary to fistulas from bowel, biliary, or urinary tracts may drain for 6 weeks or longer. As long as drainage persists, sinograms are performed every 3 to 4 days, and the drains are left in place. Outpatient care is possible for selected patients.

Catheter Removal

The three criteria for catheter removal are as follows:
1. Negligible drainage over 24 hours
2. Afebrile patient
3. Minimal residual cavity

Drains in small, superficial abscess cavities can be pulled all at once, whereas drains in large, deeper cavities may be gradually removed over a few days, which promotes healing by secondary intention.

Abdominal and Pelvic Abscesses: General

Most abdominal and pelvic abscesses are secondary to underlying bowel pathology or seen after surgery. Percutaneous abscess drainage for postoperative abdominal abscesses has become the accepted primary treatment of choice, with cure being the expected goal. Percutaneous drainage has also played a principal role in the treatment of **diverticular, appendiceal,** and Crohn's disease–related abscesses.[105,106] Drainage of abscesses in these acutely ill patients can help alleviate sepsis and allow the necessary curative surgery to be performed on an elective basis.

Drainage of **abdominal abscesses** is often best performed with CT guidance, which allows the best visualization and avoids adjacent bowel loops. CT also provides an overview of the entire abdomen, to ensure all collec-

tions are drained. Ultrasound can provide excellent guidance for percutaneous abscess drainage; however, careful review of CT imaging assists in planning an optimal approach free of intervening bowel. Unlike CT, ultrasound is especially valuable in the treatment of critically ill patients who cannot be transported to the radiology department.

Pelvic abscesses are of variable origin and have been notoriously difficult to access because of their deep location, overlying bowel, blood vessels, and urinary bladder. Traditional approaches include an **anterior transperitoneal** approach or a **posterior transgluteal** approach. The transgluteal approach is relatively painful, and care must be taken to avoid the sciatic nerve. Small, deep pelvic abscesses may be difficult to access safely using traditional approaches.

Ultrasound-guided **transvaginal drainage** has been established as a viable alternative to these traditional approaches[107,108] (Fig. 16-17). Needle guides are available for endovaginal probes that help guide the needle into the fluid collection. This transvaginal approach can be used to drain tubo-ovarian abscesses unresponsive to medical treatment. The trocar technique may also be used successfully for transvaginal drain placement. **Transrectal** ultrasound-guided drainage has also been described in the drainage of pelvic fluid collections,[109] but such an approach is infrequently used.

For **nonpurulent pelvic collections,** immediate catheter drainage is not necessarily indicated. Many of these patients respond to a one-step aspiration, lavage, and antibiotic therapy based on results of cultures of the aspirates.[110,111]

Enteric abscesses often have **communication with the GI tract.** For these abscesses to be drained successfully, the GI communication first must be recognized, then allowed to heal and close before removal of the catheter. Fistulas will not close if there is distal obstruction, tumor, or persistent infection. Even with the most aggressive techniques, however, success in treating abscesses with enteric communication is lower than for noncommunicating abscesses.[112,113] A particular challenge exists in the percutaneous treatment of **Crohn's-related abscesses.** Obviating surgery in the short term can only be achieved in about 50% of patients, with a much lower success rate in patients with preexisting bowel fistulas.[106,114] **Enterocutaneous fistulas** may develop along the drain tract in these patients.

Specific Anatomic Applications

Liver

In addition to antibiotics, percutaneous aspiration or drainage should be considered as a primary treatment for most **pyogenic liver abscesses** (Fig. 16-18). Pyogenic liver abscesses are most often caused by (1) hematogenous seeding from intestinal sources, such as appendicitis

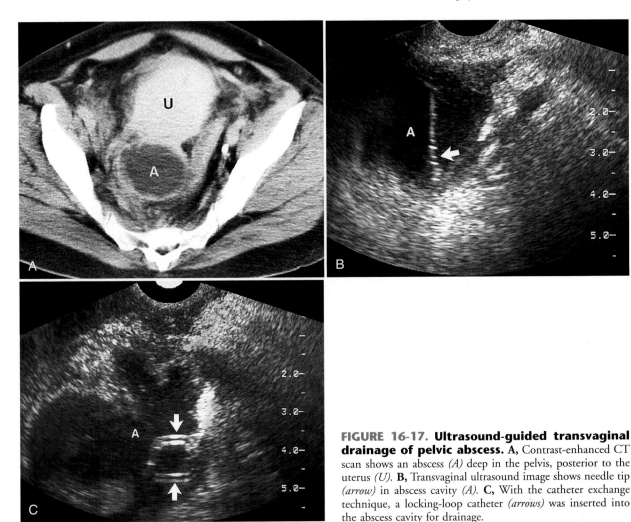

FIGURE 16-17. Ultrasound-guided transvaginal drainage of pelvic abscess. A, Contrast-enhanced CT scan shows an abscess *(A)* deep in the pelvis, posterior to the uterus *(U)*. **B,** Transvaginal ultrasound image shows needle tip *(arrow)* in abscess cavity *(A)*. **C,** With the catheter exchange technique, a locking-loop catheter *(arrows)* was inserted into the abscess cavity for drainage.

or diverticulitis; (2) direct extension from cholecystitis or cholangitis (Fig. 16-19); or (3) surgery or trauma. As with abscesses elsewhere in the body, the sonographic appearance of hepatic abscess is usually a complex fluid collection, although it can also appear as a solid mass. Both ultrasound and CT provide excellent guidance for percutaneous aspiration or drainage of hepatic abscesses, with a 67% to 94% cure rate.[112,115-117]

Some suggest treating pyogenic liver abscesses with antibiotics and percutaneous needle aspiration alone, without catheter drainage, although multiple aspiration procedures may be required.[118] Such an approach is particularly reasonable in smaller abscesses, less than 5 cm.[119,120] Multiple small (<1 cm) **microabscesses** are typically treated with antibiotics alone after diagnostic aspiration.[121] Final cure often depends on identification and appropriate treatment of the infectious source.

Amebic liver abscesses are caused by *Entamoeba histolytica*. Most amebic liver abscesses are effectively treated with metronidazole alone with 85% to 95% success.[122,123] However, percutaneous abscess drainage of amebic abscesses is indicated if the diagnosis is uncertain, the cavity is large (>5 cm) or enlarging, pyogenic superinfec-

tion is a concern, or there are signs of abscess cavity rupture.[123,124] Catheter drainage in these situations is safe and generally provides a rapid cure.

Historically, liver **hydatid abscesses** caused by *Echinococcus granulosus* were considered a contraindication to percutaneous abscess drainage because of the concern of **anaphylactic reaction** to cyst contents. More recently, these abscesses have been successfully treated with percutaneous aspiration combined with appropriate anthelmintic therapy.[125] The procedure is typically divided into three steps: (1) partial aspiration of the cyst contents; (2) instillation of a scolicidal agent, such as silver nitrate, hypertonic saline, or albendazole; and (3) complete aspiration of the cyst. This technique has been shown to be more than 98% successful.[125-127] Appropriate precautions must be taken before treatment because anaphylactic reactions may be seen in 2% to 4% of patients.[126-128]

Complications of percutaneous hepatic abscess drainage include sepsis, hemorrhage, and catheter transgression of the pleura. Sepsis may occur in up to 25% of patients, even with antibiotic therapy.[120] Intercostal placement of a drain should be avoided; such a path could introduce bacteria into the pleural space.

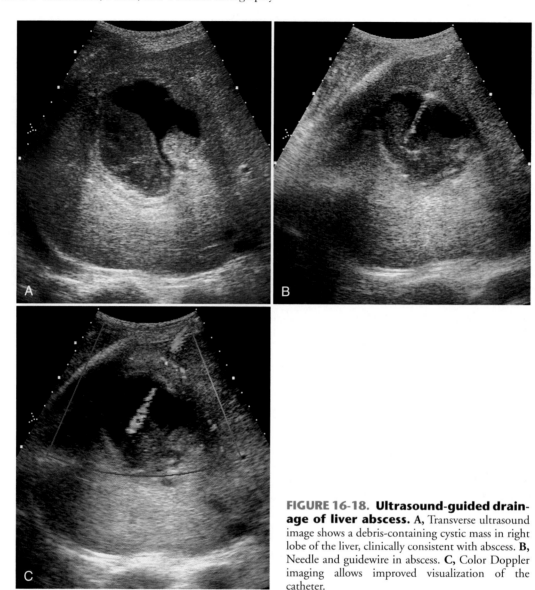

FIGURE 16-18. Ultrasound-guided drainage of liver abscess. A, Transverse ultrasound image shows a debris-containing cystic mass in right lobe of the liver, clinically consistent with abscess. **B,** Needle and guidewire in abscess. **C,** Color Doppler imaging allows improved visualization of the catheter.

Biliary Tract

Gallbladder. Percutaneous **cholecystostomy** has evolved into a favorable alternative to surgery in critically ill patients with acute calculous and acalculous **cholecystitis.** In contrast to surgical cholecystostomy, a major advantage of ultrasound-guided cholecystostomy is that the procedure may be performed at the patient's bedside. Thus, critically ill patients need not be moved to surgery or the radiology department. Similar to other drainage catheters, the cholecystostomy is easily placed with ultrasound guidance using a transhepatic route and either the trocar method or guidewire exchange (Seldinger) technique (Fig. 16-20).

Cholecystostomy placement can be successfully performed in up to 100% of cases, with rapid clinical improvement in 56% to 95% of patients.[129-131] Because of the severe comorbidities of these patients, mortality rates of 36% to 59% have been reported in hospitalized patients after cholecystostomy tube placement.[129,132]

Gallbladder aspiration alone may also be considered in treating the noncritically ill patient with acute cholecystitis who is a high surgical risk (Fig. 16-21). Given that positive blood cultures are present in less than 50% of patients with acute cholecystitis, continuous drainage may not be as critical in the management of this condition. One study showed a 77% clinical response in high-risk surgical patients using aspiration alone, compared with a 90% response in those treated with percutaneous cholecystostomy.[133] Care must be taken to avoid direct puncture of the gallbladder wall in patients with biliary obstruction because of the risk of significant bile leakage.[134]

Bile Ducts. Percutaneous **transhepatic cholangiography** and drainage is traditionally performed using "blind" cholangiography with fluoroscopy for initial needle placement. However, the combined use of ultrasound

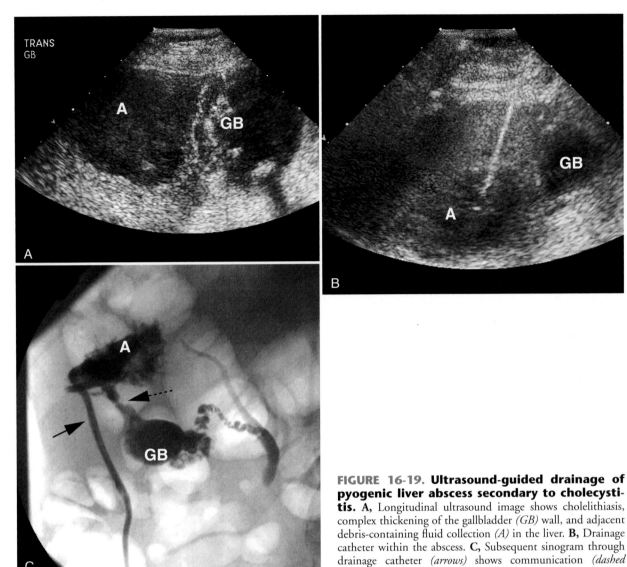

FIGURE 16-19. Ultrasound-guided drainage of pyogenic liver abscess secondary to cholecystitis. A, Longitudinal ultrasound image shows cholelithiasis, complex thickening of the gallbladder *(GB)* wall, and adjacent debris-containing fluid collection *(A)* in the liver. **B,** Drainage catheter within the abscess. **C,** Subsequent sinogram through drainage catheter *(arrows)* shows communication *(dashed arrow)* between the gallbladder *(GB)* and abscess *(A).*

for the initial needle puncture and fluoroscopy for final catheter placement using the guidewire exchange technique optimizes the advantages of both guidance systems for transhepatic cholangiography, biliary drainage, and other invasive procedures. Select ducts may be punctured under ultrasound guidance for transhepatic cholangiography or as the site of definitive catheter placement. In patients with segmental biliary obstruction, a blind technique allows initial opacification of the biliary system only by "chance," whereas ultrasound allows guided, direct puncture of the appropriate bile duct.

Pancreas

Percutaneous aspiration or drainage of pancreatic fluid collections typically arises in the setting of pancreatitis. In the absence of infection or obstruction of an adjacent hollow viscus, acute pancreatis-related peripancreatic fluid collections require no therapy.[135] Similarly, sterile pancreatic necrosis does not usually require treatment.

Infected **pancreatic necrosis** and some **pseudocysts** eventually require percutaneous intervention. Although CT is superior to ultrasound in evaluation of pancreatitis, ultrasound provides easy guidance for percutaneous interventional procedures (e.g., fluid aspiration) in these patients. Standard management of infected pancreatic necrosis is surgical debridement.[136] However, percutaneous drainage may provide short-term control of sepsis in almost 75% and cure in 50% of patients. Such a procedure typically involves very-large-bore catheters with frequent, vigorous irrigation, essentially resulting in a "percutaneous necrosectomy."[137]

The definition of **pancreatic abscess** is controversial. In general, a pancreatic abscess is a loculated collection of pus adjacent to the pancreas containing little or no pancreatic necrosis and resulting from pancreatitis or pancreatic trauma.[138] Percutaneous drainage of these abscesses is effective and can result in cure in about 90% of patients.[139,140] Key in the management of these often

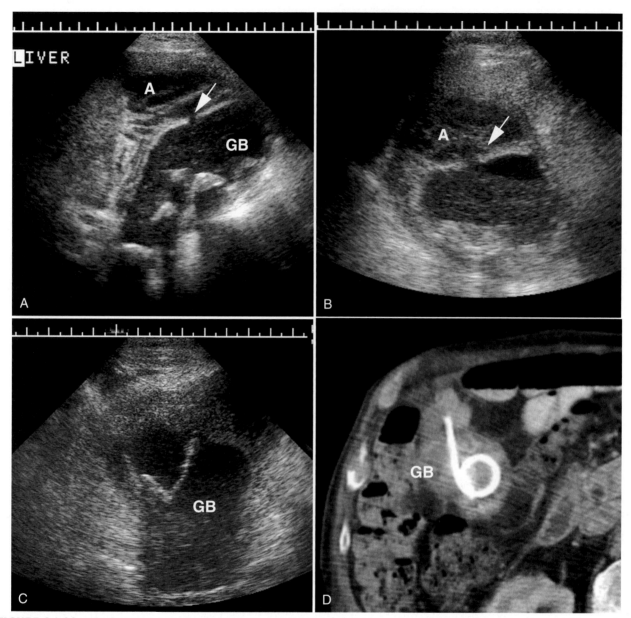

FIGURE 16-20. Cholecystostomy using ultrasound guidance. A, Longitudinal, and **B,** transverse, ultrasound images show stones within the gallbladder *(GB)* and adjacent debris-containing fluid collection representing abscess *(A)*. Perforation of gallbladder wall is identified *(arrow)*. **C,** Drainage catheter was placed using ultrasound guidance. **D,** Subsequent CT confirms catheter placement within gallbladder lumen.

complex collections is optimized placement of the drain within the infected cavity and frequent monitoring of drain function and cavity size. Frequent drain manipulations are often necessary, with drains varying in size from 8 to 30 French.[140] Drainage catheters may be in place for several weeks to several months.

Pancreatic pseudocysts arise in about 6% of patients following an episode of acute pancreatitis.[139] About half of pseudocysts will resolve spontaneously (but only a third of those >6 cm).[141,142] Simple aspiration of pancreatic pseudocysts is associated with a high rate of recurrence; therefore percutaneous catheter drainage is preferred in select cases[141-144] (Fig. 16-22). Indications for pancreatic pseudocyst drainage include the following[145]:

- Symptoms related to pseudocyst
- Complication of infection or bleeding
- Increase in size during the observation period
- A diameter of 6 cm or more
- No decrease in size during last 6 weeks of observation

Success of percutaneous pseudocyst drainage ranges from 70% to 100%.[143] Ultimate success may be related to the integrity of the pancreatic duct.[146]

Spleen

Splenic abscesses are uncommon, and in the past were often managed surgically. However, with increasing

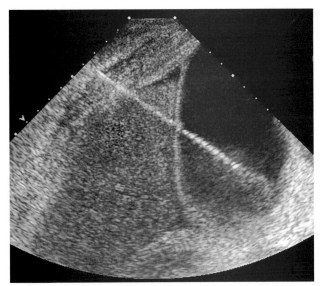

FIGURE 16-21. Ultrasound-guided gallbladder aspiration. Using freehand technique, a needle is advanced transhepatically into the lumen of a sludge-filled gallbladder.

experience in percutaneous abscess management, image-guided drain placement into select splenic abscesses has been successfully performed in up to 100% of patients.[147-149] With smaller (≤3 cm) infected splenic fluid collections, a trial of aspiration may be reasonable, with drain placement if reaccumulation of fluid occurs. More complex, multiloculated abscesses or deep-seated collections should be managed surgically. The primary risk of spleen drainage is bleeding.[75]

Kidney

Most **renal abscesses** can be successfully managed with percutaneous drainage combined with systemic antibiotics (Fig. 16-23). The size of the abscess should be considered when determining the type of treatment. For abscesses smaller than 3 cm, antibiotics alone are typically sufficient for treatment.[150] Success in the percutaneous drainage of larger abscesses ranges from 70% to 90%, with better results in treating smaller abscesses.[150]

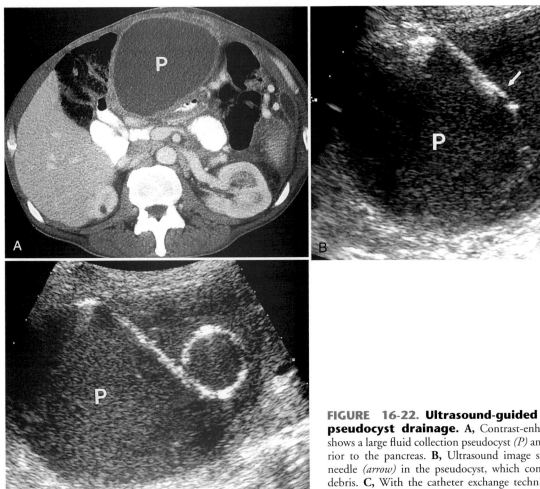

FIGURE 16-22. Ultrasound-guided pancreatic pseudocyst drainage. A, Contrast-enhanced CT scan shows a large fluid collection pseudocyst *(P)* anterior and superior to the pancreas. **B,** Ultrasound image shows aspiration needle *(arrow)* in the pseudocyst, which contains echogenic debris. **C,** With the catheter exchange technique, a locking-loop catheter was placed into pancreatic pseudocyst for drainage.

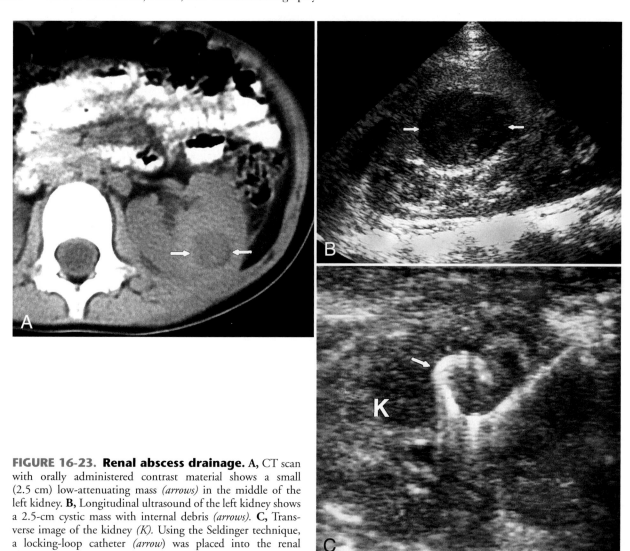

FIGURE 16-23. Renal abscess drainage. A, CT scan with orally administered contrast material shows a small (2.5 cm) low-attenuating mass *(arrows)* in the middle of the left kidney. **B,** Longitudinal ultrasound of the left kidney shows a 2.5-cm cystic mass with internal debris *(arrows)*. **C,** Transverse image of the kidney *(K)*. Using the Seldinger technique, a locking-loop catheter *(arrow)* was placed into the renal abscess.

PERCUTANEOUS CYST MANAGEMENT

Renal Cyst

Simple aspiration of large, symptomatic or obstructing renal cysts is ineffective in the long-term management of renal cysts because of rapid reaccumulation of cyst fluid within the cavity.[151] This has led to interest in **aspiration combined with sclerosis** to provide more permanent ablation of the cyst (Fig. 16-24).

The procedure involves placing a 6- to 8-French drain into the cyst with aspiration of the cyst fluid. If the cyst's true benign nature is in doubt, the fluid may be sent for cytology and other chemical markers to confirm a serous nature of the fluid. If there is no evidence of malignancy, the cyst is then injected with contrast material under fluoroscopy to exclude a communication with the urinary collecting system; sclerosis should not be performed if such a communication exists. The cyst is then injected with 95% alcohol at half the cyst volume, not to exceed 100 mL.[152] Injection of lidocaine with the alcohol minimizes the burning pain that often accompanies alcohol injection. The patient is turned in various positions over a 20-minute period to facilitate exposure of the cyst wall to the sclerosing agent. The alcohol is aspirated and the drain removed or placed to continuous suction. Repeat injections may be performed over the subsequent 2 to 3 days to maximize sclerosis. This technique is successful in more than 95% of patients.[151,153] Although alcohol is the sclerosing agent typically used, other agents include tetracycline, doxycycline, talc, and iodine.

Liver Cyst

Similar to renal cysts, hepatic cysts can be effectively sclerosed to provide long-term relief of symptoms. A communication to the biliary tract is usually excluded by injecting the cyst with contrast under fluoroscopy.

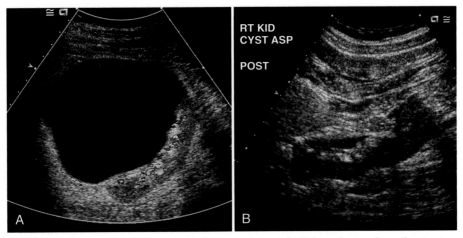

FIGURE 16-24. Renal cyst sclerosis. A, Longitudinal image of the right kidney shows a large, benign cyst. **B,** After aspiration and sclerosis, the cyst is completely decompressed.

A smaller amount of alcohol (25% cyst volume) has been proposed.[154] In one study, investigators used alcohol and/or tetracycline or doxycycline in successfully treating 85% of symptomatic hepatic cysts.[155]

Ovarian Cyst

Historically, surgical extirpation of symptomatic ovarian cysts has been the standard of care. Percutaneous management has been discouraged because of the concern about seeding malignant cells in the inadvertent aspiration of a low-grade neoplasm and the poor sensitivity in characterizing aspirated cyst fluid.[156,157] However, given the well-recognized sonographic criteria of benign ovarian cysts, the confidence level in percutaneous aspiration of such symptomatic simple cysts has improved.

Ultrasound-guided aspiration of symptomatic, benign ovarian cysts is highly effective in alleviating patient symptoms.[158] A thorough ultrasound examination should be performed initially to fully characterize the symptomatic cyst. If the cyst can be confidently characterized as benign with no worrisome features, aspiration can be performed. Some recommend obtaining preprocedural serum tumor markers to help exclude malignancy.[159] Using either a transabdominal or an endovaginal approach, a 20-gauge or 22-gauge needle can be used to aspirate the cyst completely, with 100% relief in one series.[158] Fluid should be sent for appropriate studies, including cytology. Recurrence of the cyst may be seen in 11% to 26% of patients.[160,161]

References

Percutaneous Needle Biopsy

1. Ojalehto M, Tikkakoski T, Rissanen T, Apaja-Sarkkinen M. Ultrasound-guided percutaneous thoracoabdominal biopsy. Acta Radiol 2002;43:152-158.
2. Winter TC, Lee Jr FT, Hinshaw JL. Ultrasound-guided biopsies in the abdomen and pelvis. Ultrasound Q 2008;24:45-68.
3. Peterson P, Hayes TE, Arkin CF, et al. The preoperative bleeding time test lacks clinical benefit. College of American Pathologists' and American Society of Clinical Pathologists' position article. Arch Surg 1998;133:134-139.
4. Silverman S, Mueller P, Pfister R. Hemostatic evaluation before abdominal interventions: an overview and proposal. AJR Am J Roentgenol 1990;154:233-238.
5. Channing Rodgers R, Levin J. A critical appraisal of the bleeding time. Semin Thromb Hemostasis 1990;16:1-20.
6. Peter FW, Benkovic C, Muehlberger T, et al. Effects of desmopressin on thrombogenesis in aspirin-induced platelet dysfunction. Br J Haematol 2002;117:658-663.
7. Smith TP, McDermott VG, Ayoub DM, et al. Percutaneous transhepatic liver biopsy with tract embolization. Radiology 1996;198:769-774.
8. Zines M, Vilgrain V, Gayno S, et al. Ultrasound-guided percutaneous liver biopsy with plugging of the needle track: a prospective study in 72 high-risk patients. Radiology 1992;184:841-843.
9. Brandt KR, Charboneau JW, Stephens DH, et al. CT- and ultrasound-guided biopsy of the pancreas. Radiology 1993;187:99-104.
10. Little AF, Ferris JV, Dodd 3rd GD, Baron RL. Image-guided percutaneous hepatic biopsy: effect of ascites on the complication rate. Radiology 1996;199:79-83.
11. Murphy F, Barefield K, Steinberg H, et al. CT- or sonography-guided biopsy of the liver in the presence of ascites: frequency of complications. AJR Am J Roentgenol 1988;151:485-486.
12. Sheafor D, Paulson E, Kleiwer M, et al. Comparison of sonographic and CT guidance techniques: does CT fluoroscopy decrease procedure time? AJR Am J Roentgenol 2000;2000:939-942.
13. Sheafor DH, Paulson EK, Simmons CM, et al. Abdominal percutaneous interventional procedures: comparison of CT and ultrasound guidance. Radiology 1998;207:705-710.
14. Kleiwer M, Sheafor D, Paulson E. Percutaneous liver biopsy: a cost-benefit analysis comparing sonographic and CT guidance. AJR Am J Roentgenol 1999;173:1199-1202.
15. Dameron R, Paulson E, Fisher A, et al. Indeterminate findings on imaging-guided biopsy. AJR Am J Roentgenol 1999;173:461-464.
16. Kirchner J, Kickuth R, Laufer U, et al. CT fluoroscopically assisted puncture of thoracic and abdominal masses: a randomized trial. Clin Radiol 2002;57:188-192.
17. Erwin BC, Brynes RK, Chan WC, et al. Percutaneous needle biopsy in the diagnosis and classification of lymphoma. Cancer 1986;57:1074-1078.
18. Hahn PF, Eisenberg PJ, Pitman MB, et al. Cytopathologic touch preparations (imprints) from core needle biopsies: accuracy compared with that of fine-needle aspirates. AJR Am J Roentgenol 1995;165:1277-1279.
19. Miller DL, Wall RT. Fentanyl and diazepam for analgesia and sedation during radiologic special procedures. Radiology 1987;162:195-198.
20. Phal PM, Brooks DM, Wolfe R. Sonographically guided biopsy of focal lesions: a comparison of freehand and probe-guided techniques using a phantom. AJR Am J Roentgenol 2005;184:1652-1656.

21. Hatfield MK, Beres RA, Sane SS, Zaleski GX. Percutaneous imaging-guided solid organ core needle biopsy: coaxial versus noncoaxial method. AJR Am J Roentgenol 2008;190:413-417.

22. Fornage BD. A simple phantom for training in ultrasound-guided needle biopsy using the freehand technique. J Ultrasound Med 1989;8:701-703.

23. McNamara Jr MP, McNamara ME. Preparation of a homemade ultrasound biopsy phantom. J Clin Ultrasound 1989;17:456-458.

24. Hamper UM, Savader BL, Sheth S. Improved needle-tip visualization by color Doppler sonography. AJR Am J Roentgenol 1991;156:401-402.

25. Yu SC, Liew CT, Lau WY, et al. Ultrasound-guided percutaneous biopsy of small (≤1-cm) hepatic lesions. Radiology 2001;218:195-199.

26. Buscarini L, Fornari F, Bolondi L, et al. Ultrasound-guided fine-needle biopsy of focal liver lesions: techniques, diagnostic accuracy and complications—a retrospective study on 2091 biopsies. J Hepatol 1990;11:344-348.

27. Caturelli E, Rapaccini GL, Sabelli C, et al. Ultrasound-guided fine-needle aspiration biopsy in the diagnosis of hepatic hemangioma. Liver 1986;6:326-330.

28. Cronan JJ, Esparza AR, Dorfman GS, et al. Cavernous hemangioma of the liver: role of percutaneous biopsy. Radiology 1988;166:135-138.

29. Tung GA, Cronan JJ. Percutaneous needle biopsy of hepatic cavernous hemangioma. J Clin Gastroenterol 1993;16:117-122.

30. Terriff BA, Gibney RG, Scudamore CH. Fatality from fine-needle aspiration biopsy of a hepatic hemangioma. AJR Am J Roentgenol 1990;154:203-204.

31. Dodd 3rd GD, Carr BI. Percutaneous biopsy of portal vein thrombus: a new staging technique for hepatocellular carcinoma. AJR Am J Roentgenol 1993;161:229-233.

32. Van der Poorten D, Kwok A, Lam T, et al. Twenty-year audit of percutaneous liver biopsy in a major Australian teaching hospital. Intern Med J 2006;36:692-699.

33. Firpi RJ, Soldevila-Pico C, Abdelmalek MF, et al. Short recovery time after percutaneous liver biopsy: should we change our current practices? Clin Gastroenterol Hepatol 2005;3:926-929.

34. Garcia-Tsao G, Boyer JL. Outpatient liver biopsy: how safe is it? Ann Intern Med 1993;118:150-153.

35. Piccinino F, Sagnelli E, Pasquale G, Giusti G. Complications following percutaneous liver biopsy: a multicentre retrospective study on 68,276 biopsies. J Hepatol 1986;2:165-173.

36. Van Thiel DH, Gavaler JS, Wright H, Tzakis A. Liver biopsy: its safety and complications as seen at a liver transplant center. Transplantation 1993;55:1087-1090.

37. McGill DB, Rakela J, Zinsmeister AR, Ott BJ. A 21-year experience with major hemorrhage after percutaneous liver biopsy. Gastroenterology 1990;99:1396-1400.

38. Terjung B, Lemnitzer I, Dumoulin FL, et al. Bleeding complications after percutaneous liver biopsy: an analysis of risk factors. Digestion 2003;67:138-145.

39. Paulsen SD, Nghiem HV, Negussie E, et al. Evaluation of imaging-guided core biopsy of pancreatic masses. AJR Am J Roentgenol 2006;187:769-772.

40. Matsubara J, Okusaka T, Morizane C, et al. Ultrasound-guided percutaneous pancreatic tumor biopsy in pancreatic cancer: a comparison with metastatic liver tumor biopsy, including sensitivity, specificity, and complications. J Gastroenterol 2008;43:225-232.

41. Hall-Craggs MA, Lees WR. Fine-needle aspiration biopsy: pancreatic and biliary tumors. AJR Am J Roentgenol 1986;147:399-403.

42. Lees WR, Hall-Craggs MA, Manhire A. Five years' experience of fine-needle aspiration biopsy: 454 consecutive cases. Clin Radiol 1985;36:517-520.

43. Carlson SK, Johnson CD, Brandt KR, et al. Pancreatic cystic neoplasms: the role and sensitivity of needle aspiration and biopsy. Abdom Imaging 1998;23:387-393.

44. Lewandrowski K, Lee J, Southern J, et al. Cyst fluid analysis in the differential diagnosis of pancreatic cysts: a new approach to the preoperative assessment of pancreatic cystic lesions. AJR Am J Roentgenol 1995;164:815-819.

45. Yong WH, Southern JF, Pins MR, et al. Cyst fluid NB/70K concentration and leukocyte esterase: two new markers for differentiating pancreatic serous tumors from pseudocysts. Pancreas 1995;10:342-346.

46. Smith EH. Complications of percutaneous abdominal fine-needle biopsy: review. Radiology 1991;178:253-258.

47. Dechet CB, Zincke H, Sebo TJ, et al. Prospective analysis of computerized tomography and needle biopsy with permanent sectioning to determine the nature of solid renal masses in adults. J Urol 2003;169:71-74.

48. Silverman SG, Gan YU, Mortele KJ, et al. Renal masses in the adult patient: the role of percutaneous biopsy. Radiology 2006;240:6-22.

49. Wood BJ, Khan MA, McGovern F, et al. Imaging-guided biopsy of renal masses: indications, accuracy and impact on clinical management. J Urol 1999;161:1470-1474.

50. Frank I, Blute ML, Cheville JC, et al. Solid renal tumors: an analysis of pathological features related to tumor size. J Urol 2003;170:2217-2220.

51. Caoili EM, Bude RO, Higgins EJ, et al. Evaluation of sonographically guided percutaneous core biopsy of renal masses. AJR Am J Roentgenol 2002;179:373-378.

52. Richter F, Kasabian NG, Irwin Jr RJ, et al. Accuracy of diagnosis by guided biopsy of renal mass lesions classified indeterminate by imaging studies. Urology 2000;55:348-352.

53. Kunkle DA, Crispen PL, Chen DY, et al. Enhancing renal masses with zero net growth during active surveillance. J Urol 2007;177:849-853; discussion 853-854.

54. Barocas DA, Rohan SM, Kao J, et al. Diagnosis of renal tumors on needle biopsy specimens by histological and molecular analysis. J Urol 2006;176:1957-1962.

55. Dechet CB, Sebo T, Farrow G, et al. Prospective analysis of intraoperative frozen needle biopsy of solid renal masses in adults. J Urol 1999;162:1282-1284; discussion 1284-1285.

56. Wunderlich H, Hindermann W, Al Mustafa AM, et al. The accuracy of 250 fine-needle biopsies of renal tumors. J Urol 2005;174:44-46.

57. Mondal A, Ghosh E. Fine-needle aspiration cytology (FNAC) in the diagnosis of solid renal masses: a study of 92 cases. Indian J Pathol Microbiol 1992;35:333-339.

58. Schmidbauer J, Remzi M, Memarsadeghi M, et al. Diagnostic accuracy of computed tomography–guided percutaneous biopsy of renal masses. Eur Urol 2008;53:1003-1011.

59. Bogan ML, Kopecky KK, Kraft JL, et al. Needle biopsy of renal allografts: comparison of two techniques. Radiology 1990;174:273-277.

60. Hergesell O, Felten H, Andrassy K, et al. Safety of ultrasound-guided percutaneous renal biopsy: retrospective analysis of 1090 consecutive cases. Nephrol Dial Transplant 1998;13:975-977.

61. Ralls PW, Barakos JA, Kaptein EM, et al. Renal biopsy–related hemorrhage: frequency and comparison of CT and sonography. J Comput Assist Tomogr 1987;11:1031-1034.

62. Shidham GB, Siddiqi N, Beres JA, et al. Clinical risk factors associated with bleeding after native kidney biopsy. Nephrology (Carlton) 2005;10:305-310.

63. Whittier WL, Korbet SM. Timing of complications in percutaneous renal biopsy. J Am Soc Nephrol 2004;15:142-147.

64. Meola M, Barsotti G, Cupisti A, et al. Free-hand ultrasound-guided renal biopsy: report of 650 consecutive cases. Nephron 1994;67:425-430.

65. Parrish AE. Complications of percutaneous renal biopsy: a review of 37 years' experience. Clin Nephrol 1992;38:135-141.

66. Wickre CG, Golper TA. Complications of percutaneous needle biopsy of the kidney. Am J Nephrol 1982;2:173-178.

67. Paulsen SD, Nghiem HV, Korobkin M, et al. Changing role of imaging-guided percutaneous biopsy of adrenal masses: evaluation of 50 adrenal biopsies. AJR Am J Roentgenol 2004;182:1033-1037.

68. Welch TJ, Sheedy 2nd PF, Stephens DH, et al. Percutaneous adrenal biopsy: review of a 10-year experience. Radiology 1994;193:341-344.

69. Mantero F, Terzolo M, Arnaldi G, et al. A survey on adrenal incidentaloma in Italy. Study Group on Adrenal Tumors of the Italian Society of Endocrinology. J Clin Endocrinol Metab 2000;85:637-644.

70. Casola G, Nicolet V, vanSonnenberg E, et al. Unsuspected pheochromocytoma: risk of blood pressure alterations during percutaneous adrenal biopsy. Radiology 1986;159:733-735.

71. Steinsapir J, Carr AA, Prisant LM, Bransome Jr ED. Metyrosine and pheochromocytoma. Arch Intern Med 1997;157:901-906.

72. Lieberman S, Libson E, Maly B, et al. Imaging-guided percutaneous splenic biopsy using a 20- or 22-gauge cutting-edge core biopsy needle for the diagnosis of malignant lymphoma. AJR Am J Roentgenol 2003;181:1025-1027.

73. Tam A, Krishnamurthy S, Pillsbury EP, et al. Percutaneous image-guided splenic biopsy in the oncology patient: an audit of 156 consecutive cases. J Vasc Interv Radiol 2008;19:80-87.

74. Keogan MT, Freed KS, Paulson EK, et al. Imaging-guided percutaneous biopsy of focal splenic lesions: update on safety and effectiveness. AJR Am J Roentgenol 1999;172:933-937.

75. Lucey BC, Boland GW, Maher MM, et al. Percutaneous nonvascular splenic intervention: a 10-year review. AJR Am J Roentgenol 2002;179:1591-1596.

76. Jansson SE, Bondestam S, Heinonen E, et al. Value of liver and spleen aspiration biopsy in malignant diseases when these organs show no signs of involvement in sonography. Acta Med Scand 1983;213:279-281.

77. Solbiati L, Bossi MC, Bellotti E, et al. Focal lesions in the spleen: sonographic patterns and guided biopsy. AJR Am J Roentgenol 1983;140:59-65.

78. Soderstrom N. How to use cytodiagnostic spleen puncture. Acta Med Scand 1976;199:1-5.

79. Caraway NP, Fanning CV. Use of fine-needle aspiration biopsy in the evaluation of splenic lesions in a cancer center. Diagn Cytopathol 1997;16:312-316.

80. Civardi G, Vallisa D, Berte R, et al. Ultrasound-guided fine-needle biopsy of the spleen: high clinical efficacy and low risk in a multicenter Italian study. Am J Hematol 2001;67:93-99.

81. Liao WY, Chen MZ, Chang YL, et al. Ultrasound-guided transthoracic cutting biopsy for peripheral thoracic lesions less than 3 cm in diameter. Radiology 2000;217:685-691.

82. Sheth S, Hamper UM, Stanley DB, et al. Ultrasound guidance for thoracic biopsy: a valuable alternative to CT. Radiology 1999;210:721-726.

83. Douglas BR, Charboneau JW, Reading CC. Ultrasound-guided intervention: expanding horizons. Radiol Clin North Am 2001;39:415-428.

84. Nolsoe C, Nielsen L, Torp-Pedersen S, Holm HH. Major complications and deaths due to interventional ultrasonography: a review of 8000 cases. J Clin Ultrasound 1990;18:179-184.

85. Livraghi T, Damascelli B, Lombardi C, Spagnoli I. Risk in fine-needle abdominal biopsy. J Clin Ultrasound 1983;11:77-81.

86. Fornari F, Civardi G, Cavanna L, et al. Complications of ultrasonically guided fine-needle abdominal biopsy: results of a multicenter Italian study and review of the literature. The Cooperative Italian Study Group. Scand J Gastroenterol 1989;24:949-955.

87. Martino CR, Haaga JR, Bryan PJ, et al. CT-guided liver biopsies: eight years' experience—work in progress. Radiology 1984;152:755-757.

88. Welch T, Sheedy PI, Johnson C, et al. CT-guided biopsy: prospective analysis of 1,000 procedures. Radiology 1989;171:493-496.

89. Bergenfeldt M, Genell S, Lindholm K, et al. Needle track seeding after percutaneous fine-needle biopsy of pancreatic carcinoma: case report. Acta Chir Scand 1988;154:77-79.

90. Caturelli E, Rapaccini GL, Anti M, et al. Malignant seeding after fine-needle aspiration biopsy of the pancreas. Diagn Imaging Clin Med 1985;54:88-91.

91. Haddad FS, Somsin AA. Seeding and perineal implantation of prostatic cancer in the track of the biopsy needle: three case reports and a review of the literature. J Surg Oncol 1987;35:184-191.

92. Greenstein A, Merimsky E, Baratz M, Braf Z. Late appearance of perineal implantation of prostatic carcinoma after perineal needle biopsy. Urology 1989;33:59-60.

93. Onodera H, Oikawa M, Abe M, et al. Cutaneous seeding of hepatocellular carcinoma after fine-needle aspiration biopsy. J Ultrasound Med 1987;6:273-275.

94. Kiser GC, Totonchy M, Barry JM. Needle track seeding after percutaneous renal adenocarcinoma aspiration. J Urol 1986;136:1292-1293.

95. Muller NL, Bergin CJ, Miller RR, Ostrow DN. Seeding of malignant cells into the needle track after lung and pleural biopsy. Can Assoc Radiol J 1986;37:192-194.

96. Fajardo LL. Breast tumor seeding along localization guide wire tracks. Radiology 1988;169:580-581.

97. Glasgow BJ, Brown HH, Zargoza AM, Foos RY. Quantitation of tumor seeding from fine-needle aspiration of ocular melanomas. Am J Ophthalmol 1988;105:538-546.

98. Hidai H, Sakuramoto T, Miura T, et al. Needle track seeding following puncture of retroperitoneal liposarcoma. Eur Urol 1983;9:368-369.

99. Raftopoulos Y, Furey WW, Kacey DJ, Podbielski FJ. Tumor implantation after computed tomography–guided biopsy of lung cancer. J Thorac Cardiovasc Surg 2000;119:1288-1289.

100. Shinohara S, Yamamoto E, Tanabe M, et al. Implantation metastasis of head and neck cancer after fine-needle aspiration biopsy. Auris Nasus Larynx 2001;28:377-380.

Ultrasound-Guided Drainage

101. Haaga JR, Alfidi RJ, Havrilla TR, et al. CT detection and aspiration of abdominal abscesses. AJR Am J Roentgenol 1977;128:465-474.

102. VanSonnenberg E, D'Agostino HB, Casola G, et al. Percutaneous abscess drainage: current concepts. Radiology 1991;181:617-626.

103. Gazelle GS, Mueller PR. Abdominal abscess: imaging and intervention. Radiol Clin North Am 1994;32:913-932.

104. Hui GC, Amaral J, Stephens D, et al. Gas distribution in intraabdominal and pelvic abscesses on CT is associated with drainability. AJR Am J Roentgenol 2005;184:915-919.

105. Sahai A, Belair M, Gianfelice D, et al. Percutaneous drainage of intra-abdominal abscess in Crohn's disease: short- and long-term outcome. Am J Gastroenterol 1997;92:275-278.

106. Men S, Akhan O, Koroglu M. Percutaneous drainage of abdominal abscess. Eur J Radiol 2002;43:204-218.

107. Saokar A, Arellano RS, Gervais DA, et al. Transvaginal drainage of pelvic fluid collections: results, expectations, and experience. AJR Am J Roentgenol 2008;191:1352-1358.

108. McGahan JP, Wu C. Sonographically guided transvaginal or transrectal pelvic abscess drainage using the trocar method with a new drainage guide attachment. AJR Am J Roentgenol 2008;191:1540-1544.

109. Nosher JL, Needell GS, Amorosa JK, Krasna IH. Transrectal pelvic abscess drainage with sonographic guidance. AJR Am J Roentgenol 1986;146:1047-1048.

110. Kuligowska E, Keller E, Ferrucci JT. Treatment of pelvic abscesses: value of one-step sonographically guided transrectal needle aspiration and lavage. AJR Am J Roentgenol 1995;164:201-206.

111. Feld R, Eschelman DJ, Sagerman JE, et al. Treatment of pelvic abscesses and other fluid collections: efficacy of transvaginal sonographically guided aspiration and drainage. AJR Am J Roentgenol 1994;163:1141-1145.

112. Lambiase RE, Deyoe L, Cronan JJ, Dorfman GS. Percutaneous drainage of 335 consecutive abscesses: results of primary drainage with 1-year follow-up. Radiology 1992;184:167-179.

113. Schuster MR, Crummy AB, Wojtowycz MM, McDermott JC. Abdominal abscesses associated with enteric fistulas: percutaneous management. J Vasc Interv Radiol 1992;3:359-363.

114. Gervais DA, Hahn PF, O'Neill MJ, Mueller PR. Percutaneous abscess drainage in Crohn disease: technical success and short- and long-term outcomes during 14 years. Radiology 2002;222:645-651.

115. Johnson RD, Mueller PR, Ferrucci Jr JT, et al. Percutaneous drainage of pyogenic liver abscesses. AJR Am J Roentgenol 1985;144:463-467.

116. VanSonnenberg E, Mueller PR, Ferrucci Jr JT. Percutaneous drainage of 250 abdominal abscesses and fluid collections. Part I. Results, failures, and complications. Radiology 1984;151:337-341.

117. Wong WM, Wong BC, Hui CK, et al. Pyogenic liver abscess: retrospective analysis of 80 cases over a 10- year period. J Gastroenterol Hepatol 2002;17:1001-1007.

118. Giorgio A, Tarantino L, Mariniello N, et al. Pyogenic liver abscesses: 13 years of experience in percutaneous needle aspiration with ultrasound guidance. Radiology 1995;195:122-124.

119. Zerem E, Hadzic A. Sonographically guided percutaneous catheter drainage versus needle aspiration in the management of pyogenic liver abscess. AJR Am J Roentgenol 2007;189:W138-W142.

120. Thomas J, Turner SR, Nelson RC, Paulson EK. Postprocedure sepsis in imaging-guided percutaneous hepatic abscess drainage: how often does it occur? AJR Am J Roentgenol 2006;186:1419-1422.

121. Shankar S, vanSonnenberg E, Silverman SG, Tuncali K. Interventional radiology procedures in the liver: biopsy, drainage, and ablation. Clin Liver Dis 2002;6:91-118.

122. Krige JE, Beckingham IJ. ABC of diseases of liver, pancreas, and biliary system. BMJ 2001;322:537-540.

123. VanSonnenberg E, Mueller PR, Schiffman HR, et al. Intrahepatic amebic abscesses: indications for and results of percutaneous catheter drainage. Radiology 1985;156:631-635.

124. Gervais DA, Brown SD, Connolly SA, et al. Percutaneous imaging-guided abdominal and pelvic abscess drainage in children. Radiographics 2004;24:737-754.

125. Paksoy Y, Odev K, Sahin M, et al. Percutaneous treatment of liver hydatid cysts: comparison of direct injection of albendazole and hypertonic saline solution. AJR Am J Roentgenol 2005;185:727-734.

126. Khuroo MS, Wani NA, Javid G, et al. Percutaneous drainage compared with surgery for hepatic hydatid cysts. N Engl J Med 1997;337:881-887.

127. Aygun E, Sahin M, Odev K, et al. The management of liver hydatid cysts by percutaneous drainage. Can J Surg 2001;44:203-209.

128. Odev K, Paksoy Y, Arslan A, et al. Sonographically guided percutaneous treatment of hepatic hydatid cysts: long-term results. J Clin Ultrasound 2000;28:469-478.

129. Davis CA, Landercasper J, Gundersen LH, Lambert PJ. Effective use of percutaneous cholecystostomy in high-risk surgical patients: techniques, tube management, and results. Arch Surg 1999;134:727-731; discussion 731-732.

130. Granlund A, Karlson BM, Elvin A, Rasmussen I. Ultrasound-guided percutaneous cholecystostomy in high-risk surgical patients. Langenbecks Arch Surg 2001;386:212-217.

131. Sugiyama M, Tokuhara M, Atomi Y. Is percutaneous cholecystostomy the optimal treatment for acute cholecystitis in the very elderly? World J Surg 1998;22:459-463.

132. McGahan JP, Lindfors KK. Percutaneous cholecystostomy: an alternative to surgical cholecystostomy for acute cholecystitis? Radiology 1989;173:481-485.

133. Chopra S, Dodd 3rd GD, Mumbower AL, et al. Treatment of acute cholecystitis in non-critically ill patients at high surgical risk: comparison of clinical outcomes after gallbladder aspiration and after percutaneous cholecystostomy. AJR Am J Roentgenol 2001;176:1025-1031.

134. Phillips G, Bank S, Kumari-Subaiya S, Kurtz LM. Percutaneous ultrasound-guided puncture of the gallbladder (PUPG). Radiology 1982;145:769-772.

135. AGA Institute. Medical position statement on acute pancreatitis. Gastroenterology 2007;132:2019-2021.

136. Forsmark CE, Baillie J. AGA Institute technical review on acute pancreatitis. Gastroenterology 2007;132:2022-2044.

137. Freeny PC, Hauptmann E, Althaus SJ, et al. Percutaneous CT-guided catheter drainage of infected acute necrotizing pancreatitis: techniques and results. AJR Am J Roentgenol 1998;170:969-975.

138. Bollen TL, van Santvoort HC, Besselink MG, et al. The Atlanta Classification of acute pancreatitis revisited. Br J Surg 2008;95:6-21.

139. Beger HG, Rau B, Mayer J, Pralle U. Natural course of acute pancreatitis. World J Surg 1997;21:130-135.

140. VanSonnenberg E, Wittich GR, Chon KS, et al. Percutaneous radiologic drainage of pancreatic abscesses. AJR Am J Roentgenol 1997;168:979-984.

141. Pitchumoni CS, Agarwal N. Pancreatic pseudocysts: when and how should drainage be performed? Gastroenterol Clin North Am 1999;28:615-639.

142. Yeo CJ, Bastidas JA, Lynch-Nyhan A, et al. The natural history of pancreatic pseudocysts documented by computed tomography. Surg Gynecol Obstet 1990;170:411-417.

143. Neff R. Pancreatic pseudocysts and fluid collections: percutaneous approaches. Surg Clin North Am 2001;81:399-403, xii.

144. Grosso M, Gandini G, Cassinis MC, et al. Percutaneous treatment (including pseudocystogastrostomy) of 74 pancreatic pseudocysts. Radiology 1989;173:493-497.

145. Isaji S, Takada T, Kawarada Y, et al. JPN Guidelines for the management of acute pancreatitis: surgical management. J Hepatobiliary Pancreat Surg 2006;13:48-55.

146. Nealon WH, Walser E. Main pancreatic ductal anatomy can direct choice of modality for treating pancreatic pseudocysts (surgery versus percutaneous drainage). Ann Surg 2002;235:751-758.

147. Kang M, Kalra N, Gulati M, et al. Image-guided percutaneous splenic interventions. Eur J Radiol 2007;64:140-146.

148. Chou YH, Tiu CM, Chiou HJ, et al. Ultrasound-guided interventional procedures in splenic abscesses. Eur J Radiol 1998;28:167-170.

149. Thanos L, Dailiana T, Papaioannou G, et al. Percutaneous CT-guided drainage of splenic abscess. AJR Am J Roentgenol 2002;179:629-632.

150. Siegel JF, Smith A, Moldwin R. Minimally invasive treatment of renal abscess. J Urol 1996;155:52-55.

Percutaneous Cyst Management

151. Fontana D, Porpiglia F, Morra I, Destefanis P. Treatment of simple renal cysts by percutaneous drainage with three repeated alcohol injection. Urology 1999;53:904-907.

152. Lohela P. Ultrasound-guided drainages and sclerotherapy. Eur Radiol 2002;12:288-295.

153. Mohsen T, Gomha MA. Treatment of symptomatic simple renal cysts by percutaneous aspiration and ethanol sclerotherapy. BJU Int 2005;96:1369-1372.

154. Moorthy K, Mihssin N, Houghton PW. The management of simple hepatic cysts: sclerotherapy or laparoscopic fenestration. Ann R Coll Surg Engl 2001;83:409-414.

155. VanSonnenberg E, Wroblicka JT, D'Agostino HB, et al. Symptomatic hepatic cysts: percutaneous drainage and sclerosis. Radiology 1994;190:387-392.

156. Higgins RV, Matkins JF, Marroum MC. Comparison of fine-needle aspiration cytologic findings of ovarian cysts with ovarian histologic findings. Am J Obstet Gynecol 1999;180:550-553.

157. Martinez-Onsurbe P, Ruiz Villaespesa A, Sanz Anquela JM, Valenzuela Ruiz PL. Aspiration cytology of 147 adnexal cysts with histologic correlation. Acta Cytol 2001;45:941-947.

158. Troiano RN, Taylor KJ. Sonographically guided therapeutic aspiration of benign-appearing ovarian cysts and endometriomas. AJR Am J Roentgenol 1998;171:1601-1605.

159. Mathevet P, Dargent D. [Role of ultrasound guided puncture in the management of ovarian cysts]. J Gynecol Obstet Biol Reprod (Paris) 2001;30(Suppl 1):53-58.

160. Lee CL, Lai YM, Chang SY, et al. The management of ovarian cysts by sono-guided transvaginal cyst aspiration. J Clin Ultrasound 1993;21:511-514.

161. Balat O, Sarac K, Sonmez S. Ultrasound guided aspiration of benign ovarian cysts: an alternative to surgery? Eur J Radiol 1996;22:136-137.

CHAPTER 17

Organ Transplantation

Derek Muradali and Tanya Chawla

Chapter Outline

Organ transplantation is the preferred treatment for patients with end-stage liver, renal, and pancreatic disease. Patients with fulminant liver failure have no other treatment option apart from orthotopic liver transplantation. Although patients with renal or pancreatic failure may be treated with dialysis or medical therapy, their long-term survival and quality of life are far superior with organ transplantation. Recent improvements in graft survival have been attributed to a combination of better donor-recipient matching,[1] more effective immunosuppressive therapy, improvements in surgical technique, and early recognition of transplant-related complications. These improvements have resulted in a 1-year patient survival rate of over 80% for each of these organ transplants.[2,3]

Because the clinical presentation of posttransplant complications varies widely and is often nonspecific, imaging studies are essential for monitoring the status of the allograft. If diagnosis is delayed, the function of the allograft may be permanently compromised, and in severe cases with complete loss of function, retransplantation may be warranted. However, the chronic shortage of suitable donor organs may delay or preclude immediate retransplantation, with devastating clinical consequences. Therefore, preservation of the allograft function and early detection of complications, with institution of appropriate treatment, is essential in the clinical management of these patients.

Ultrasound has revolutionized the practice of organ transplantation because gray-scale sonography permits optimal assessment of the textural and morphologic changes of the parenchyma, and color and spectral Doppler ultrasound permits evaluation of both parenchymal perfusion and the status of the major transplanted artery and vein. During routine transplant sonography, however, multiple artifacts are encountered that may be related to the intrinsic property of the structure or the scanning technique. Differentiation of these pseudolesions from true pathology depends on an understanding of the physical basis of the artifact; awareness of the spectrum of ultrasound appearances of common transplant-related complications is requisite knowledge. This chapter focuses on the ultrasound appearances of the normal organ transplant, acute and chronic transplant-related complications, and potential errors of interpretation that can lead to misdiagnoses.

LIVER TRANSPLANTATION

From 1988 to 2008 in the United States, 91,861 patients underwent liver transplantation.[4] One-year survival in liver transplant patients is approximately 87%, with 1-year graft survival of 80.3%. Patients are selected for transplantation when their life expectancy without transplantation is less than their life expectancy after the procedure. **Hepatitis C** is the most common disease requiring transplantation, followed by **alcoholic liver disease** and **cryptogenic cirrhosis.** Other end-stage liver disorders treated by transplantation include **chronic cholestatic diseases,** such as primary biliary cirrhosis and primary sclerosing cholangitis; **metabolic diseases,** including hemochromatosis and Wilson's disease; and **other hepatitides,** such as autoimmune hepatitis, chronic hepatitis B, and acute liver failure. Patients with end-stage hepatitis B cirrhosis were initially regarded as poor transplant candidates because of the high recurrence of infection in the implant, associated with rapid progression to cirrhosis. The use of hyperimmunoglobulins and nucleoside analogs has changed these expectations to a more favorable outcome.[5]

Most centers consider transplantation only in patients with **early-stage hepatocellular carcinoma** (HCC) or rarely **neuroendocrine metastasis.** The generally accepted guidelines for transplantation in patients with HCC are the Milan criteria of (1) no lesion greater than 5 cm in diameter or (2) no more than three lesions greater than 3 cm in diameter.[5,6]

Contraindications for liver transplantation include compensated cirrhosis without complications, extrahepatic malignancy, cholangiocarcinoma, active untreated sepsis, advanced cardiopulmonary disease, active alcoholism or substance abuse, or an anatomic abnormality precluding the surgical procedure. Although portal vein thrombosis is not an absolute contraindication to liver transplantation, its presence makes the surgery more complex, and posttransplantation patients show higher morbidity and mortality rates.[5]

Surgical Technique

Traditionally, most adult liver transplants involve explantation of the recipient liver and replacement with a cadaveric allograft. The surgery requires four **vascular anastomoses** (suprahepatic/infrahepatic vena cava, hepatic artery, portal vein) as well as a **biliary anastomosis** (Fig. 17-1).

The **hepatic artery** is reconstructed with a "fish-mouth" anastomosis between the donor celiac artery and either the bifurcation of the right and left hepatic arteries or the branch point of the gastroduodenal and proper hepatic arteries of the recipient. When the native hepatic artery is small in diameter or shows

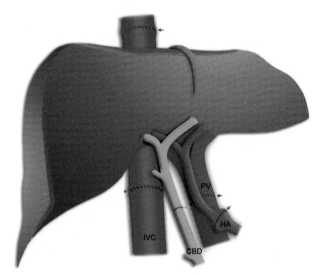

FIGURE 17-1. Normal liver transplant: surgical approach. The transplanted liver shows four vascular anastomoses and a biliary anastomosis. The inferior vena cava (*IVC,* blue) is transplanted with a suprahepatic and infrahepatic anastomosis. An end-to-end anastomosis is often used for the common bile duct (*CBD,* green) and portal vein (*PV,* purple), whereas the hepatic artery (*HA,* red) is reconstructed with a fish-mouth anastomosis.

minimal flow, a donor iliac artery interposition graft may be anastomosed directly to the supraceliac or infrarenal aorta.[7]

The **portal vein anastomosis** is usually end to end between the donor and recipient portal veins. In cases of extensive recipient portal vein thrombosis, a venous jump graft from the donor portal vein or the iliac vein may be used, or as a last resort, an anastomosis between both the portal vein and the hepatic artery of the donor and the arterial vessels of the recipient.[7,8]

During hepatectomy, the **inferior vena cava** (IVC) of the recipient usually is transected above and below the intrahepatic portion. The donor IVC is then anastomosed with two end-to-end suprahepatic and infrahepatic anastomoses. In an attempt to preserve the recipient retrohepatic IVC, some techniques advocate creation of an anastomosis between the donor and recipient IVC in an end-to-side or side-to-side configuration ("piggyback" anastomosis) or an end-to-end anastomosis between the donor IVC and a common stump of the three hepatic veins.[7]

The donor and recipient **common bile duct** are usually anastomosed end to end, after cholecystectomy. With this technique the sphincter of Oddi is preserved and acts as a barrier to the spread of infection. A T-tube is typically left in situ for about 3 months and permits access for cholangiography or other biliary procedures.

When the recipient common hepatic duct is diseased (e.g., sclerosing cholangitis), too short, or too narrow in diameter, a **choledochojejunostomy** is performed.[7]

This procedure involves an end-to-side anastomosis between the donor bile duct and a 40-cm recipient jejunal loop. It is associated with a higher risk of bile leaks, bleeding, and recurrent cholangitis compared with an end-to-end anastomosis.

The growing discrepancy between the number of patients awaiting transplantation and the lack of available cadaveric donor organs has led to a progressive increase in the number of **living related donor transplantations**. The recipient liver is replaced with the right lobe of a living donor. In the pediatric population, the lateral segment of the left lobe or the entire left lobe has been used successfully; the relative small size of the left lobe is not sufficient, however, to sustain adequate liver function in an adult. Another advantage of using a right lobe (vs. left lobe) as the donor portion for transplantation is the relative ease of positioning the right lobe in the right subphrenic space, allowing a technically less challenging hepatic venous anastomosis, with a decrease in the incidence of torsion, compared with left lobe grafts.[9]

For living related transplants, **donor** surgery consists of cholecystectomy followed by right hepatectomy, removing segments V, VI, VII, and VIII as well as the right hepatic vein. Occasionally an extended right hepatectomy may be done to include a portion of segment IV and the middle hepatic vein. However, most surgeons prefer not to remove the middle hepatic vein, but to leave it intact in the donor because of the intimate relationship of the middle and left hepatic veins near their drainage into the IVC.[9]

Regardless of the type of liver transplantation, routine imaging evaluation of each anastomosis must be assessed with gray-scale ultrasound, color Doppler, and spectral Doppler interrogation. To interpret the gray-scale appearance and Doppler features of these anastomotic regions, the sonographer should be aware of the surgical techniques used in liver transplantation.

Normal Liver Transplant Ultrasound

The normal liver transplant has a homogeneous or slightly heterogeneous echotexture on gray-scale ultrasound, appearing identical to a normal, nontransplanted liver. In the early postoperative period, there is usually a small amount of free intraperitoneal fluid or small, perihepatic seromas or hematomas, which tend to resolve within 7 to 10 days.

The **biliary tree** should have a normal appearance, with an anechoic lumen and thin, imperceptible walls. If a T-tube is in situ, the adjacent duct wall may appear mildly prominent secondary to irritation and edema. Ideally, the biliary anastomosis (end to end or biliary enteric) should be visualized and inspected for changes in caliber or wall thickness.

Pneumobilia is often observed in patients with choledochojejunostomy and appears as bright, echogenic foci with or without posterior acoustic shadowing in the bile duct lumen. The disappearance of previously documented pneumobilia should alert the sonographer to possible interval development of a biliary stricture at the biliary-enteric anastomosis. In addition, the sonographer should be aware that **intraductal biliary air** may be confused with tiny biliary stones or adjacent hepatic arterial calcifications because these structures can appear identical on gray-scale imaging (Fig. 17-2).

Vascular patency of the transplanted vessels (hepatic artery, portal vein, hepatic veins, IVC) is assessed by (1) direct inspection for narrowing of the diameter, (2) presence of thrombus within the vessel lumen, and (3) documentation of normal spectral waveforms with appropriate directional flow. Particular attention should be paid to the anastomotic regions because these areas have a higher propensity to develop a hemodynamically significant stenosis compared with the remaining vessel. Because intrahepatic segmental stenoses or occlusions can develop, the hepatic artery and main portal vein, as well as their major

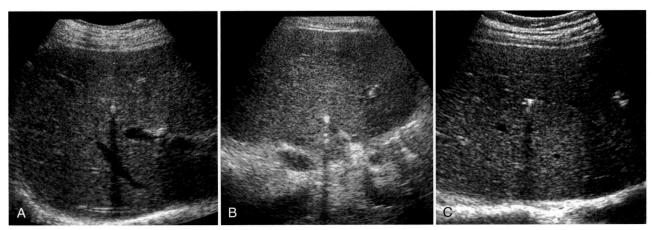

FIGURE 17-2. Echogenic foci in liver transplant. Transverse sonograms show similar bright echogenic foci with posterior acoustic shadowing secondary to **A,** intrahepatic calcification; **B,** hepatic arterial calcifications; and **C,** pneumobilia.

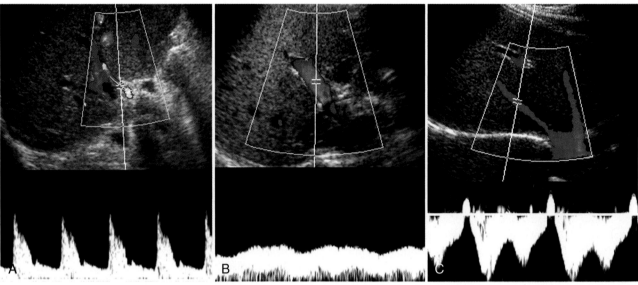

FIGURE 17-3. Normal liver transplant: color and spectral Doppler. Color and spectral Doppler images of normal **A,** hepatic artery; **B,** main portal vein; and **C,** right hepatic vein. *(From Crossin J, Muradali D, Wilson SR. Ultrasound of liver transplants: normal and abnormal. Radiographics 2003;23:1093-1114.)*

right and left branches, should be interrogated with color and spectral Doppler.

The **normal hepatic artery** shows a rapid systolic upstroke, with an acceleration time (AT; time from end diastole to first systolic peak) of less than 100 cm/sec, and continuous flow throughout diastole, with a resistive index (RI) of 0.5 to 0.7 (Fig. 17-3, *A*). A **normal portal vein** is typically smooth in contour, has an anechoic lumen, and may show a subtle change in caliber at the surgical anastomosis. The portal veins show continuous, monophasic, hepatopetal flow with mild velocity variations caused by respiration (Fig. 17-3, *B*). The Doppler appearance of the **hepatic veins** shows a phasic waveform, reflecting physiologic changes in blood flow during the cardiac cycle (Fig. 17-3, *C*).

Biliary Complications

Biliary tract complications are a significant cause of morbidity and mortality in 15% to 30% of patients with orthotopic liver transplantation and may be seen in up to 25% of all transplant patients.[10-12] Complications related to biliary-enteric anastomoses usually present within the first month of surgery and include anastomotic breakdown, bleeding, and an increased risk of ascending cholangitis from bacterial overgrowth. Choledochocholedochostomy-related complications most frequently present after the first posttransplantation month and are often managed by endoscopic retrograde cholangiopancreatography (ERCP).[11] Regardless of the type of anastomoses used, biliary tract complications can be broadly classified as those related to leaks, strictures, intraluminal sludge or stones, dysfunction of the sphincter of Oddi, and recurrent disease.

Biliary Strictures

Early diagnosis of biliary tree complications may be difficult because transplant recipients do not typically experience colic; the transplanted liver has a poor supply of nerves.[13] Therefore, patients with biliary strictures may be asymptomatic or may present with painless obstructive jaundice or abnormalities in liver function tests (LFTs).[11] These strictures can be categorized based on location and pathophysiology as anastomotic (extrahepatic) and intrahepatic strictures (Fig. 17-4).

Anastomotic strictures are the most common cause of biliary obstruction after transplantation[14,15] and arise from postsurgical scarring, resulting in retraction of the duct wall and narrowing of the luminal diameter.[16] These strictures are more common in patients with a Roux-en-Y choledochojejunostomy than in patients with an end-to-end biliary anastomosis. On ultrasound, a focal narrowing can sometimes be observed at the anastomoses, associated with dilation of the intrahepatic bile ducts, with a normal-sized or near-normal-sized distal common bile duct (CBD).

Intrahepatic strictures occur proximal to the anastomosis and may be unifocal or multifocal. The arterial supply of the distal CBD (recipient duct) is rich because of prominent collateral flow, whereas the reconstructed hepatic artery is the only blood supply to the proximal CBD and intrahepatic bile ducts (donor ducts).[11,17] Therefore, most intrahepatic duct strictures result from ischemia caused by **hepatic artery occlusion** (thrombosis or significant stenosis). In rare cases, biliary ischemia may also be caused by **prolonged cold preservation time** of the donor organ.[16,18] Other causes of intrahepatic strictures include immunogenic injury pro-

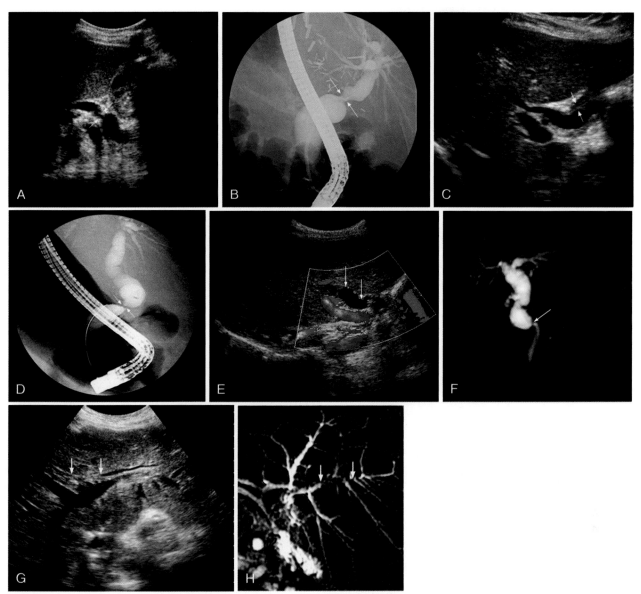

FIGURE 17-4. Bile duct: strictures in four patients. *Patient 1:* **A,** Gray-scale sonogram of common bile duct (CBD) shows anastomotic stricture *(arrows),* which is confirmed on **B,** endoscopic retrograde cholangiopancreatography (ERCP; *arrows*). *Patient 2:* **C,** Gray-scale sonogram shows grossly thickened CBD walls *(arrows),* secondary to ascending cholangitis, a consequence of an anastomotic stricture; **D,** correlative ERCP shows anastomotic stricture *(arrows).* In both ERCP images the CBD distal to the stricture appears dilated because of the pressure of contrast injection during the procedure. *Patient 3:* **E,** Transverse sonogram shows central biliary dilation *(arrows).* **F,** Magnetic resonance cholangiopancreatography (MRCP) radial image shows anastomotic stricture *(arrow). Patient 4:* **G,** Transverse sonogram, and **H,** radial T2-weighted MRCP image, show left intrahepatic bile duct stricture *(between arrows),* secondary to ischemia from hepatic artery stenosis. (*A and B from Crossin J, Muradali D, Wilson SR. Ultrasound of liver transplants: normal and abnormal. Radiographics 2003;23:1093-1114.)*

duced by chronic rejection, recurrent sclerosing cholangitis, ascending cholangitis, and cytomegalovirus (CMV) infections.

Ultrasound findings include focal areas of narrowing in the intrahepatic or proximal CBD and segmental dilation of the intrahepatic bile ducts, without evidence of an obstructing mass. The presence of echogenic intraluminal material within a dilated biliary tree is an ominous sign, sometimes caused by severe biliary ischemia, resulting in sloughing of the entire biliary epithelium. In this scenario the **intraluminal echogenic material** represents a combination of biliary sludge or stones, sloughed biliary epithelium, and intraluminal hemorrhage[16] (Fig. 17-5).

Bile Leaks

The incidence of bile leaks in patients with cadaveric liver transplants is 5.3% to 23%. The biliary complication rate may be significantly higher in living related

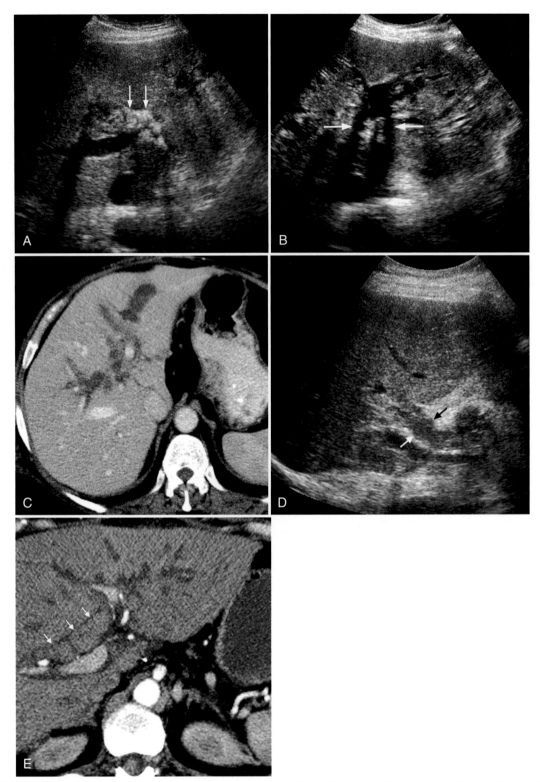

FIGURE 17-5. Bile duct: ischemia secondary to hepatic artery thrombosis in two patients. *Patient 1:* Transverse sonograms of **A,** right, and **B,** left, hepatic lobes show dilated intrahepatic bile ducts *(arrows)* with intraluminal echogenic material secondary to sloughed mucosa. **C,** Correlative contrast-enhanced computed tomography (CT) scan shows high-density material within the dilated intrahepatic bile ducts. *Patient 2:* **D,** Transverse sonogram of ischemic common bile duct *(arrows)* shows intraluminal echogenic material secondary to blood and sloughed mucosa. **E,** Corresponding CT scan shows intraluminal debris extending into the central intrahepatic bile ducts *(arrows).*

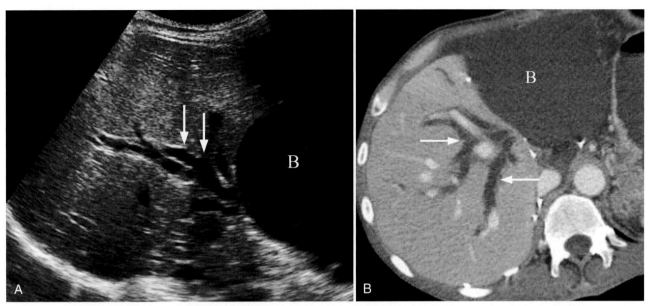

FIGURE 17-6. Bile duct: anastomotic leak. A, Transverse sonogram, and **B,** correlative CT scan, show large biloma *(B)* abutting the surgical margin of a living related donor transplant, secondary to anastomotic leak. The biloma exerts mass effect on the anastomosis, producing intrahepatic bile duct dilation *(arrows).*

transplant recipients, possibly because of (1) leaks caused by division of the liver at retrieval, (2) variant biliary anatomy resulting in more than one bile duct orifice at the resection margin, and (3) ischemia of the right biliary tree.[19] Overall, biliary leaks can be categorized as occurring (1) at the anastomotic site, (2) at the T-tube exit site, (3) as a result of bile duct necrosis, and (4) secondary to percutaneous liver biopsies[20] (Fig. 17-6).

Most anastomotic leaks and T-tube exit site leaks occur within the *first postsurgical month.* **Anastomotic leaks** may be related to surgical technique or may result from ischemia caused by hepatic artery compromise. Clinically, anastomotic leaks are associated with bile peritonitis or intra-abdominal sepsis and may present on ultrasound as a large periportal collection, a subhepatic collection, or ascites. **T-tube exit leaks** are related to technical errors when placing the T-tube and are usually detected incidentally at cholangiography. The resulting biloma is usually small, and patients with these types of bile leaks are usually asymptomatic.[20]

Leaks from **bile duct necrosis** usually occur *after the first postsurgical month* and are a result of severe hepatic artery stenosis or hepatic artery thrombosis. This condition is often associated with progressive hepatic dysfunction, and a poor clinical course, eventually requiring retransplantation. On ultrasound, the biliary tree may be dilated, thick walled, and may communicate with multiple surrounding bilomas.[20]

In rare cases, bile leaks can occur as a result of bile duct injury from **percutaneous liver biopsies.** Bile may leak from the needle track into the peritoneal cavity. These leaks can resolve without treatment or may persist and become clinically noticeable if distal biliary obstruction is present.[20]

Recurrent Sclerosing Cholangitis

Recurrent sclerosing cholangitis occurs in up to 20% of recipients undergoing orthotopic transplantation for sclerosing cholangitis, with a mean interval of 350 days.[5,8,21] Ultrasound findings include diffuse mural thickening of the intrahepatic and common bile duct and diverticulum-like outpouchings of the CBD[16,22] (Fig. 17-7). Recurrent disease should be suspected in patients transplanted for end-stage primary sclerosing cholangitis presenting with biliary dilation and mural thickening in the presence of a normal hepatic arterial waveform.

Occasionally, patients with ascending cholangitis may present with an identical ultrasound appearance. Infectious etiologies include both enteric flora and opportunistic infections (e.g., CMV, *Cryptosporidium*).[16]

Biliary Sludge and Stones

Biliary sludge can be detected within the hepatobiliary tree in up to 10% to 29% of liver transplant patients, as early as 6 days or as late as $8\frac{1}{2}$ years after surgery. The pathogenesis of biliary sludge in these patients is uncertain, although it has been related to ischemia, infection, rejection, mechanical obstruction, biliary leaks, and presence of stents or T-tubes and is more common in patients with hepaticojejunostomy.[13] Once in the donor or recipient biliary tree, sludge can cause biliary obstruction and life-threatening **ascending cholangitis** (Fig. 17-8). The detection of biliary sludge is an ominous sign that should prompt meticulous evaluation of the CBD to rule out an obstructing lesion or leak, evaluation of the hepatic artery to ensure an optimal

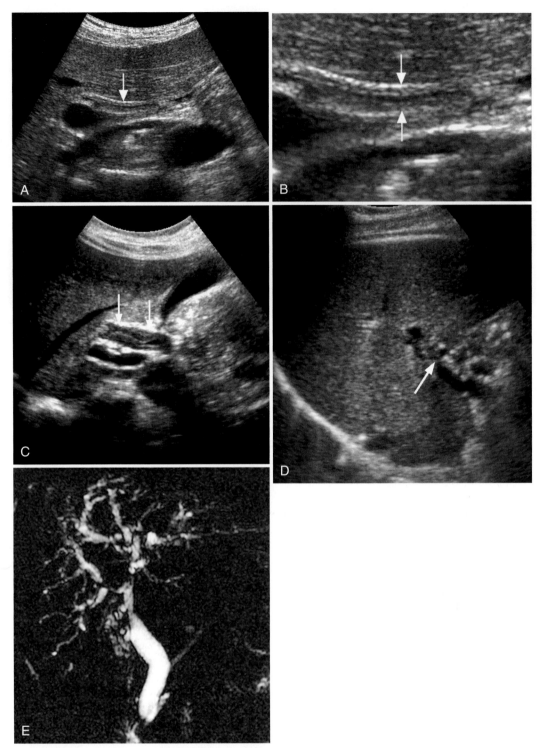

FIGURE 17-7. Bile duct: recurrent sclerosing cholangitis in three patients. *Patient 1:* **A** and **B,** Transverse sonograms at different magnifications show diffuse thickening and beading of the common hepatic duct *(arrows). Patient 2:* **C,** Transverse sonogram shows grossly thick-walled common hepatic duct *(arrows). Patient 3:* **D,** Transverse sonogram shows stricture *(arrow)* in the mid common hepatic duct. **E,** Correlative MRCP image shows multifocal strictures in the intrahepatic and extrahepatic bile ducts, resulting in diffuse beading of the biliary tree. *(**A** and **B** from Crossin J, Muradali D, Wilson SR. Ultrasound of liver transplants: normal and abnormal. Radiographics 2003;23:1093-1114.)*

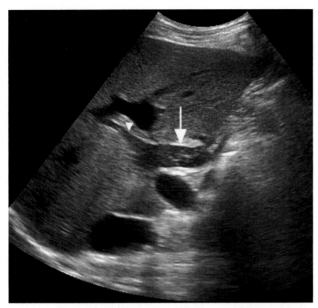

FIGURE 17-8. Bile duct: sludge. Oblique sonogram shows intraluminal sludge, secondary to ascending cholangitis, in the common bile duct *(arrow),* with extension into the right hepatic duct *(arrowhead).*

arterial supply, and a detailed clinical assessment to check for infection.

Intraductal stones are rare but may result from cyclosporine-induced changes in bile composition inciting crystal formation in the CBD, with subsequent stone development. Other causes include retained donor stones and stones secondary to biliary stasis from mechanical obstruction (e.g., stricture, dysfunctional T-tubes, mucocele formation in cystic duct remnant, kinking in redundant CBD)[23-25] (Fig. 17-9).

Dysfunction of the Sphincter of Oddi

In a minority of patients who have undergone a biliary end-to-end anastomosis, hepatic dysfunction is observed in the presence of diffuse dilation of the donor and recipient bile ducts in the absence of biliary stenosis. The cause of this is uncertain but may be related to devascularization or denervation of the ampulla of Vater, resulting in dysfunction of the sphincter of Oddi. Patients are usually treated with ERCP-guided sphincterotomy, which has been shown to normalize LFTs and decompress the biliary tree.[11,14]

Arterial Complications

At explantation, extrahepatic arterial vessels that supply the liver, such as the parabiliary arteries, are disrupted.[26] This results in the transplanted hepatic artery becoming the only arterial blood supply to intrahepatic biliary epithelium. Any compromise of the hepatic arterial perfusion can result in biliary ischemia and, potentially, biliary

necrosis. Biliary necrosis is incompatible with graft survival and is an absolute indication for retransplantation, but uncomplicated biliary ischemia (i.e., no necrosis) may be reversible if hepatic arterial flow can be reinstituted.[27] The detection of hepatic arterial dysfunction before the development of biliary necrosis is paramount in the management of liver transplant patients.

Hepatic Artery Thrombosis

Hepatic artery thrombosis is the most significant vascular complication of liver transplantation, with an incidence of 2.5% to 6.8% and mortality as high as 35%.[28] If retransplantation is not performed for these patients, mortality can increase to 73%.[29]

The pathophysiology is often difficult to decipher. Risk factors include patients requiring complex vascular reconstruction (caused by multiple arterial supply to the liver or small donor and recipient vessels), rejection, severe stenosis, increased cold ischemic time of the donor liver, and ABO blood type incompatibility.[8,30]

After transplantation, the donor bile duct is entirely dependent on the transplanted hepatic artery, particularly the right, for its arterial blood supply. Therefore, patients with hepatic artery thrombosis can present clinically with delayed biliary leak, fulminant hepatic failure, or intermittent episodes of sepsis thought to be secondary to liver abscess formation within infarcted tissue.[30] However, the precise clinical presentation, imaging findings, and patient outcome are related to the **timing of thrombosis** of the hepatic artery. Hepatic artery thrombosis occurring within 1 month of transplantation can be classified as **early** hepatic artery thrombosis. This is often associated with biliary tract necrosis, bacteremia, acute fulminant hepatic failure, and a high incidence of patient morbidity.[29] Gray-scale sonography may show the hepatic artery at the porta hepatis, however, *no flow* is detected on color or spectral Doppler in the hilum or parenchyma.

Hepatic artery thrombosis occurring after 1 month of transplantation can be classified as **late** hepatic artery thrombosis. This is usually associated with a milder clinical course, with patients remaining either asymptomatic for months to years or showing an insidious course eventually presenting with biliary tract complications, relapsing fevers or bacteremia. It is thought that the development of collateral arterial vessels, as early as 2 weeks after surgery, accounts for the survival of the transplant in these patients. Although resection of all vascular connections in the transplant can hinder development of collateral circulation, arterial collateral vessels could develop from the angiogenic potential of the omentum and mesentery. On ultrasound, a **tardus-parvus arterial waveform** (RI <0.5; AT >100 msec) is detected within the hepatic parenchyma (Fig. 17-10). Within the hilum, no arterial flow is demonstrated, or if periportal arterial collaterals are present, a tardus-parvus waveform may be

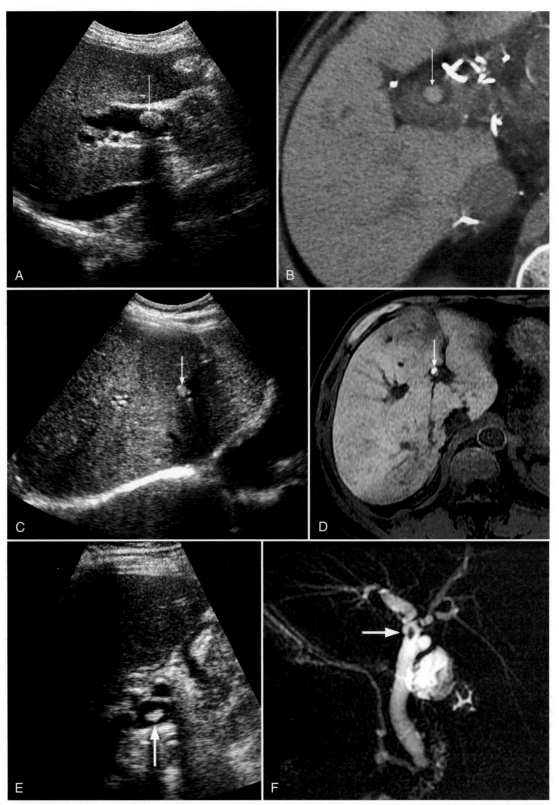

FIGURE 17-9. Bile duct: stones. A, Sonogram, and **B,** correlative non-contrast-enhanced CT scan, show the presence of a large obstructing stone *(arrow)* in the common hepatic duct. **C,** Transverse sonogram shows an echogenic focus *(arrow)* consistent with an intraductal calculus in this patient with recurrent primary sclerosing cholangitis. **D,** Corresponding axial SPGR TI-weighted pre-gadolinium-enhanced MR image shows intraductal high-frequency signal *(arrow)* consistent with a stone. **E,** Transverse sonogram at level of the common hepatic duct shows a nonshadowing echogenic focus *(arrow)* in the duct, consistent with a soft stone. **F,** Corresponding radial T2-weighted MR image shows a well-defined filling defect *(arrow),* confirming the presence of a calculus within the proximal common duct.

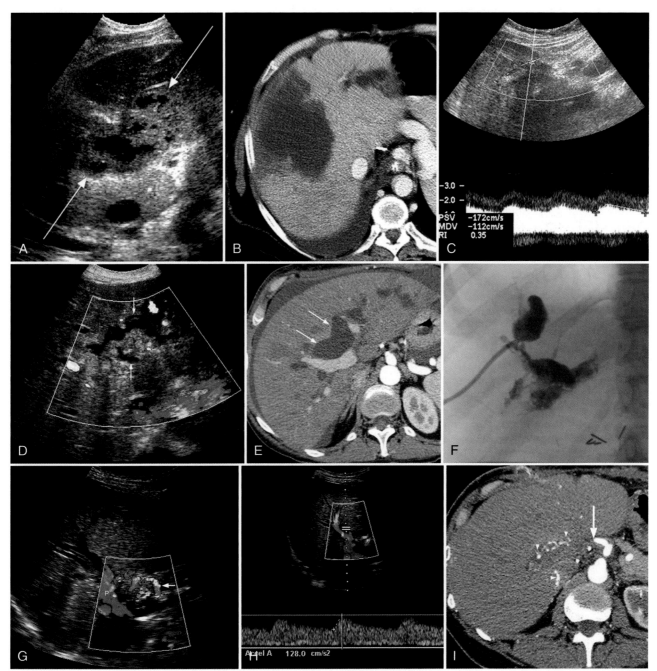

FIGURE 17-10. Hepatic artery: thrombosis in three patients. *Patient 1:* **A,** Transverse sonogram shows a right lobe infarct appearing as a solid-cystic region *(arrows),* resulting from hepatic arterial thrombosis. **B,** Corresponding CT scan shows the infarct as a low-attenuating wedge-shaped region. **C,** On spectral Doppler, no flow could be detected in the main hepatic artery. A tardus-parvus waveform detected within the liver indicates an upstream hepatic arterial problem; in this case, hepatic artery thrombosis with collateral arterial vessels supplying the hepatic tissue. *Patient 2:* **D,** Transverse sonogram shows a greatly distended bile duct *(arrows)* with echogenic material within the lumen secondary to sloughed mucosa and blood. **E,** Corresponding CT scan shows dramatically dilated intrahepatic bile ducts *(arrows).* The biliary necrosis is less well appreciated on CT. **F,** Percutaneous cholangiogram shows contrast filling shaggy, intrahepatic ducts with multiple filling defects. The filling defects correspond to the sloughed biliary mucosa. *Patient 3:* **G,** Transverse sonogram demonstrates multiple collateral vessels *(arrow)* at the porta hepatis (*P,* main portal vein). **H,** Spectral Doppler sonogram within the liver shows a tardus-parvus waveform. **I,** CT angiogram shows occlusion of the hepatic artery *(arrow)* caused by acute thrombosis. Multiple arterial collateral vessels *(arrowheads)* are identified, as seen on **G.**

detected. Therefore, demonstration of arterial flow in the hepatic parenchyma does not exclude the presence of hepatic arterial thrombosis, and meticulous inspection of the parenchymal waveform is warranted[29,30] (Fig. 17-10).

Occasionally, a false-positive diagnosis of hepatic artery thrombosis may occur with severe hepatic edema, systemic hypotension, and high-grade hepatic artery stenosis.[8] In situations with poor visibility of the porta hepatis because of abdominal girth or overlying bowel gas, lack of detectable flow within the hepatic artery should be viewed with caution and confirmed on computed tomography angiography (CTA).

Hepatic Artery Stenosis

Hepatic artery stenosis has been reported in up to 11% of transplant recipients and most often occurs at, or within a few centimeters of, the surgical anastomosis. Risk factors for development of stenosis include faulty surgical technique, clamp injury, rejection, and intimal trauma caused by perfusion catheters.[27] Clinically, patients may present with biliary ischemia or abnormal LFTs.

Doppler ultrasound may provide direct or indirect evidence of hepatic artery stenosis. **Direct** evidence involves identifying and localizing a hemodynamically significant narrowing within the vessel. The porta hepatis should be initially screened with color Doppler ultra-sound to detect a focal region of color aliasing within the hepatic artery, which would indicate the presence of high-velocity turbulent flow produced by the stenotic segment. If the stenosis is hemodynamically significant, spectral tracing will reveal peak systolic velocity (PSV) of greater than 2 to 3 m/sec, with associated turbulent flow distally. **Indirect** evidence of hepatic artery stenosis includes a tardus-parvus waveform anywhere within the hepatic artery (RI <0.5; AT >100 msec). This waveform suggests the presence of a more proximally located stenotic region.[27] Indirect evidence of stenosis is much more common in clinical practice than documentation of the stenosis itself (Figs. 17-11 and 17-12).

The presence of an intraparenchymal tardus-parvus waveform indicates alterations in the intrahepatic arterial bed from impaired arterial perfusion of the liver. Although is detected most often in patients with hepatic artery stenosis, tardus-parvus waveform may also result from collateral vessels arising from hepatic artery thrombosis or, less frequently, from severe aortoiliac atherosclerosis. Therefore, an intraparenchymal tardus-parvus waveform cannot distinguish between hepatic artery stenosis and thrombosis if the hepatic arterial trunk is not visualized and meticulously interrogated.[31]

Mild degrees of hepatic artery narrowing may also be present without Doppler abnormalities. Therefore, if clinical suspicion is high, a normal Doppler study should not preclude further investigation with other cross-sectional techniques (e.g., CTA, formal angiography),

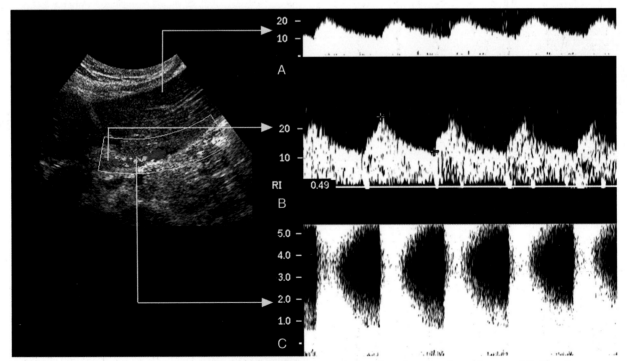

FIGURE 17-11. Hepatic artery stenosis: Doppler features. A, Intrahepatic spectral waveform, and **B,** hepatic artery waveform, at porta hepatis show a prolonged acceleration time and low resistance, a tardus-parvus waveform, suggesting an upstream problem. **C,** Spectral waveform at the anastomosis shows high-velocity flow greater than 400 cm/sec. The corresponding color Doppler sonogram shows aliasing as turquoise and yellow between the red and blue at the stenosis, with turbulence beyond.

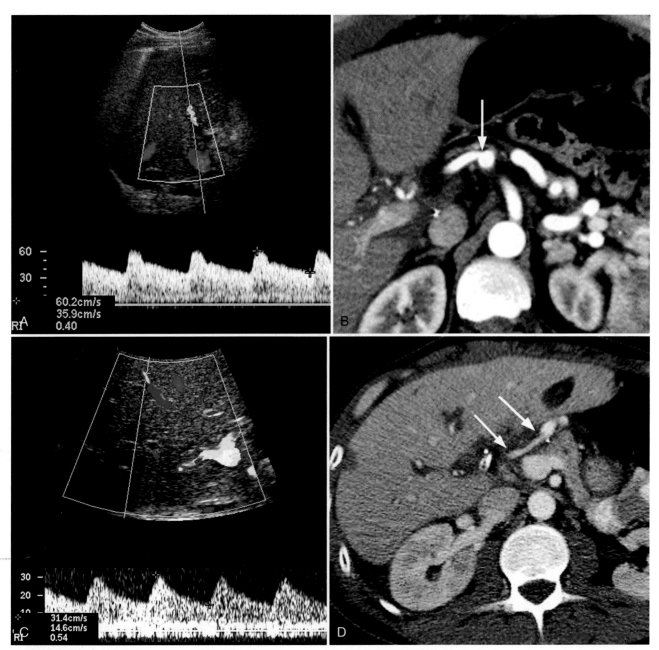

FIGURE 17-12. Hepatic artery stenosis in two patients. *Patient 1:* **A,** Intraparenchymal spectral Doppler ultrasound shows a low-resistance waveform (RI = 0.4). **B,** Corresponding contrast-enhanced CT angiogram shows subtle stenosis of the proximal hepatic artery *(arrow). Patient 2:* **C,** Intraparenchymal spectral Doppler shows a tardus-parvus, low-resistance waveform with a delayed acceleration time of 120 msec. **D,** Corresponding CT angiogram shows long stenosis of the hepatic artery *(between arrows).*

although the stenosis, if detected, may be mild in these patients.

Elevated Hepatic Arterial Resistive Index

In the early postoperative period, a normal hepatic artery may display a high-resistance arterial flow (RI > 0.8) or a complete lack of flow in diastole (RI = 1.0) on Doppler interrogation. In these patients the flow within the hepatic artery usually returns to normal in a few days.

The etiology of this waveform is uncertain, although it may be related to older donor age or prolonged cold ischemic time of the graft. A high RI of the hepatic artery on Doppler assessment has no clinical relevance and should not be misinterpreted as a sign of a hepatic artery abnormality.[32]

Hepatic Artery Pseudoaneurysms

Hepatic artery pseudoaneurysms are uncommon complications of transplantation (1%) and occur most frequently at the vascular anastomosis or as a result of prior angioplasty. **Intrahepatic** pseudoaneurysms are rare, usually peripherally located, and associated with percutaneous needle biopsies, infection, or biliary procedures. Intrahepatic aneurysms are often asymptomatic but can cause life-threatening arterial hemorrhage or, in mycotic pseudoaneurysms, produce fistulas between the aneurysm and the biliary tree or portal veins.[8] **Extrahepatic** pseudoaneurysms occur at the donor-recipient arterial anastomosis and may be caused by infection or technical failure.

Gray-scale ultrasound of hepatic artery pseudoaneurysms shows a cystic (anechoic) structure, typically following the course of the hepatic artery, with intense swirling flow on color Doppler and a disorganized spectral waveform (Fig. 17-13). Management options are dictated by the location of the pseudoaneurysm. Extrahepatic pseudoaneurysms may be treated by surgery, transcatheter embolization, or stent insertion, whereas intrahepatic pseudoaneurysms are often treated with endovascular coil embolization.

Celiac Artery Stenosis

Celiac artery stenosis may be caused by **atheromatous disease** or impingement of the celiac axis by the **median arcuate ligament** of the diaphragm. If severe, celiac stenosis can result in decreased arterial flow to the allograft. Patients are often asymptomatic before transplantation, presumably because of rich collateral networks, usually through the pancreaticoduodenal arcade. After transplantation, patients may become symptomatic, presenting with evidence of biliary ischemia and abnormalities in serum LFTs, a result of the greater flow demand imposed on the celiac artery by the newly transplanted liver.

Doppler ultrasound may be normal or may reveal a low-resistance tardus-parvus waveform in the transplanted hepatic artery and high-velocity jet across the celiac stenosis. Patients are treated with division of the median arcuate ligament or, in the case of atheromatous disease, an aortohepatic interposition bypass graft[33,34] (Fig. 17-14).

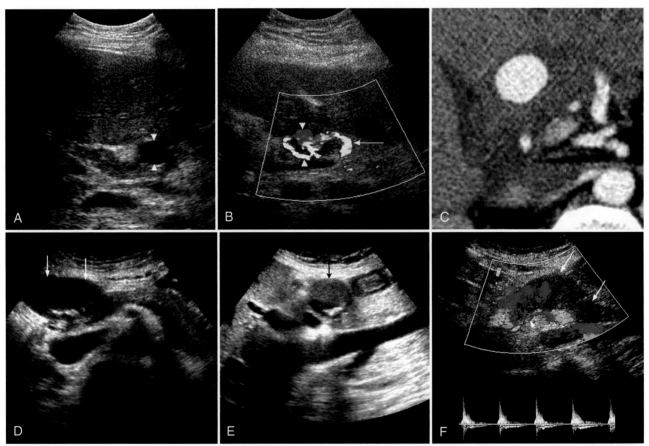

FIGURE 17-13. Hepatic artery pseudoaneurysms in two patients. *Patient 1:* **A,** Gray-scale sonogram shows a small cystic mass close to the porta hepatis *(arrowheads).* **B,** Color Doppler ultrasound confirms vascularity within the pseudoaneurysm *(arrowheads)* arising from the hepatic artery *(arrow).* **C,** Corresponding enhanced CT scan confirms the pseudoaneurysm arising at the hepatic artery anastomosis. *Patient 2:* **D,** Transverse, and **E,** sagittal, sonograms show a midline oval-shaped mass *(arrows).* **F,** On color and spectral Doppler ultrasound, disorganized flow is identified in a portion of the mass, representing a partially thrombosed pseudoaneurysm. Arrows mark the thrombosed portion of the pseudoaneurysm. *(A, B, and C from Crossin J, Muradali D, Wilson SR. Ultrasound of liver transplants: normal and abnormal. Radiographics 2003;23:1093-1114.)*

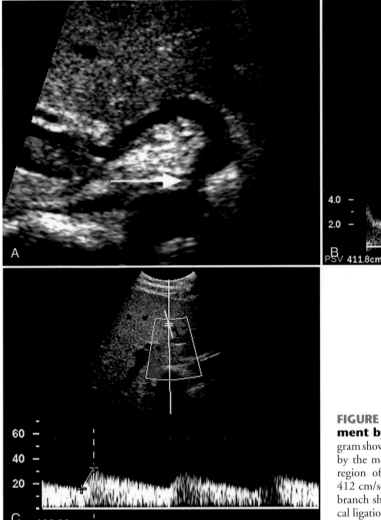

FIGURE 17-14. Celiac artery stenosis: impingement by median arcuate ligament. A, Transverse sonogram shows narrowing of the celiac artery secondary to impingement by the median arcuate ligament *(arrow)*. **B,** Spectral trace of the region of narrowing shows elevated peak systolic velocities of 412 cm/sec. **C,** Spectral trace of left lobe intrahepatic arterial branch shows low-resistance tardus-parvus waveform. After surgical ligation of the median arcuate ligament, the spectral waveforms returned to normal.

Portal Vein Complications

Portal vein **stenosis** or **thrombosis** is uncommon, with a reported incidence of 1% to 13%.[30,35,36] Risk factors include faulty surgical technique, misalignment of vessels, excessive vessel length, hypercoagulable states, and previous portal vein surgery.[30] Factors extrinsic to the portal vein may also contribute, such as increased downstream resistance caused by a suprahepatic stricture of the IVC or diminished portal venous blood flow. Clinical presentations include hepatic failure and signs of portal hypertension (gastrointestinal hemorrhage from varices or massive ascites).

Gray-scale ultrasound of **portal vein stenosis** may show narrowing of the vessel lumen, usually at the anastomosis. Doppler interrogation shows a focal region of color aliasing, reflecting turbulent, high-velocity flow, with a threefold to fourfold velocity increase at the site of stenosis relative to the prestenotic segment on spectral interrogation (Fig. 17-15). Chong et al.[37] showed that

elevated portal vein anastomotic velocities greater than 125 cm/sec, or a velocity ratio of 3:1 at the anastomosis, was greater than 95% specific for portal vein stenosis.

True portal vein stenosis must be distinguished from a **pseudostenosis** of the portal vein. This entity is seen when the recipient portal vein is larger than the donor portal vein and no associated differential gradient exists across the site of narrowing.

Portal vein thrombosis presents as echogenic solid material within the portal vein lumen (Figs. 17-16 and 17-17). In the acute state the thrombus may be anechoic, making detection difficult on gray-scale ultrasound. In this scenario the thrombus is only evident by the lack of portal venous flow on color and spectral Doppler, emphasizing the necessity for careful gray-scale and Doppler assessment of the entire portal venous system. As with portal vein thrombosis in the native liver, the thrombus may decrease in size and eventually recanalize, showing multiple venous flow channels within the thrombus. Treatment of portal vein thrombosis or ste-

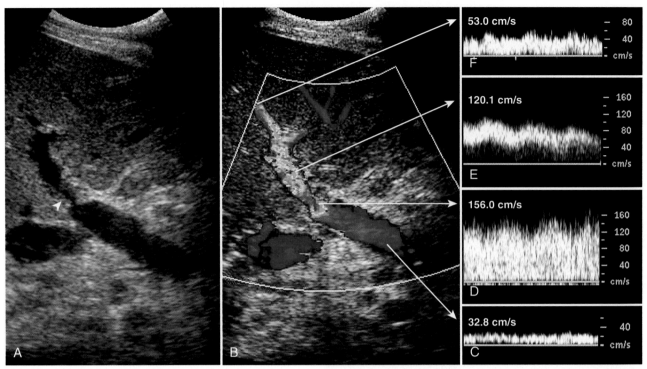

FIGURE 17-15. Portal vein stenosis: anastomotic stricture. A, Gray-scale sonogram of main portal vein shows narrowing at the anastomosis *(arrowhead)*. **B,** Color Doppler shows aliasing at the region of stenosis caused by high-velocity turbulent flow. **C,** Spectral Doppler shows velocities of 32.8 cm/sec proximal to the stenosis. **D,** Velocities at the stenosis are elevated at 156 cm/sec. **E,** Poststenotic high-velocity turbulent flow is identified, measuring 120.1 cm/sec. **F,** Beyond the turbulent flow, velocities of 53 cm/sec are obtained. This represents a threefold increased velocity gradient across the anastomosis, indicating that the stenosis is hemodynamically significant.

nosis includes thrombectomy, segmental portal vein resection, percutaneous thrombolysis, stent placement, and balloon angioplasty.

Inferior Vena Cava Complications

Stenosis of the IVC is a rare complication of liver transplantation and may occur at the suprahepatic or infrahepatic anastomosis. IVC stenosis occurs more frequently in pediatric recipients and patients undergoing retransplantation.[38] Causes of IVC stenosis include anastomotic discrepancy, IVC kinking, fibrosis, or neointimal hyperplasia. On gray-scale ultrasound, the IVC may show obvious narrowing at the site of anastomosis, associated with a focal region of aliasing on color Doppler. On spectral interrogation, a threefold to fourfold greater velocity gradient is observed across the stenosis compared with the prestenotic segment. The hepatic veins may show reversal of flow or may lose their normal phasicity, with a monophasic waveform[8] (Figs. 17-18 and 17-19).

Thrombosis of the IVC has been reported in less than 3% of recipients and is caused by technical difficulties at surgery, hypercoagulable states, or compression from adjacent fluid collections.[26,38] Gray-scale ultrasound shows echogenic thrombus within the IVC that may

continue into the hepatic veins. In cases of recurrent HCC, tumor thrombus may extend from the hepatic veins into the IVC (Fig. 17-20).

Hepatic Vein Stenosis

Hepatic vein stenosis occurs with a frequency of 1% in **orthotopic liver transplant** and 2% to 5% in **living donor transplants.** This discrepancy in frequency rate is primarily related to different surgical techniques. In orthotopic liver transplants, an anastomosis is performed between the donor and recipient IVC without touching the hepatic veins. In living donor transplants, however, the donor hepatic vein is anastomosed to either the hepatic vein stump or the IVC of the recipient. This results in the hepatic veins being rigidly fixed in position, such that any movement of the graft produces a buckling and narrowing of the hepatic veins. In addition, progressive growth of partial liver grafts after surgery may result in stretching or twisting of the hepatic veins, further contributing to narrowing of the venous outlet.[39,40]

Clinically, hepatic vein stenosis may present with liver congestion, hepatomegaly, ascites, and pleural effusions. Hepatic venous obstruction in the **early postoperative state** is a surgical emergency, and reoperation is usually necessary for correction or for retransplantation,

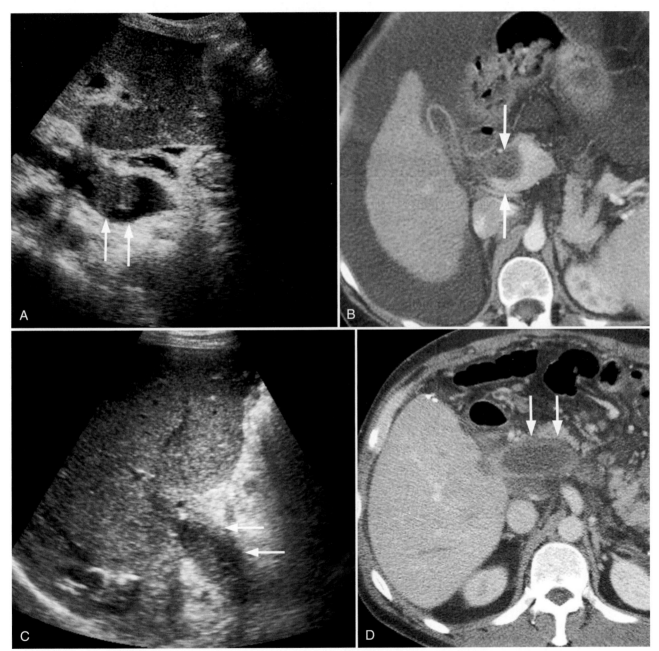

FIGURE 17-16. Portal vein: bland thrombus in two patients. *Patient 1:* **A,** Transverse sonogram, and **B,** corresponding contrast-enhanced CT scan, show nonocclusive thrombus in the main portal vein *(arrows). Patient 2:* **C,** Sagittal sonogram, and **D,** corresponding contrast-enhanced CT scan, show occlusive thrombus in the main portal vein *(arrows).*

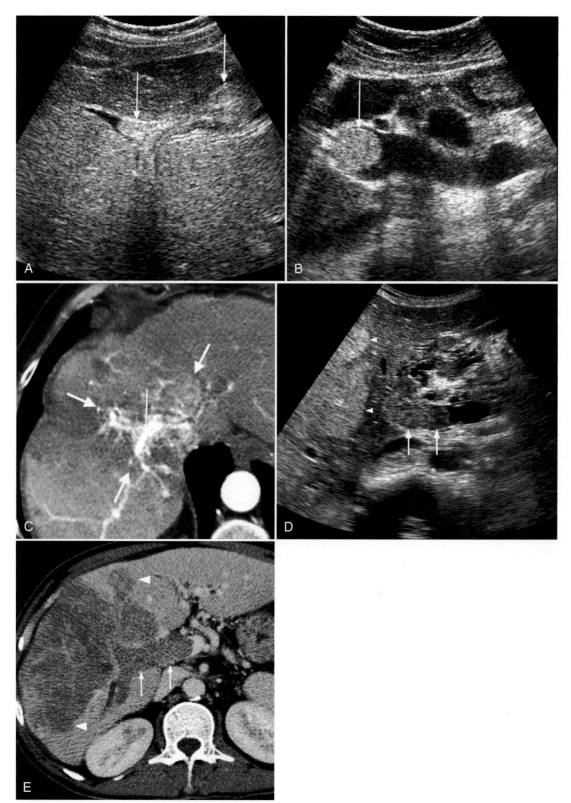

FIGURE 17-17. Portal vein: malignant thrombus in two patients. *Patient 1:* **A,** Transverse sonogram of malignant thrombus *(arrows)* in right portal vein, with **B,** extension into main portal vein *(arrow)*. **C,** Triphasic CT scan of the liver shows the recurrent hepatocellular carcinoma *(arrows)* that accounts for the portal vein thrombus. *Patient 2:* **D,** Transverse sonogram demonstrates malignant thrombus in the main portal vein *(arrows)*. The background liver is extremely abnormal, with a large echogenic mass *(arrowheads)*. **E,** Portal venous phase of a triphasic CT confirms recurrent hepatocellular carcinoma *(arrowheads)* accompanied by expansile, enhancing malignant thrombus in the main portal vein *(arrows)*. *(A, B, and C from Crossin J, Muradali D, Wilson SR. Ultrasound of liver transplants: normal and abnormal. Radiographics 2003;23:1093-1114.)*

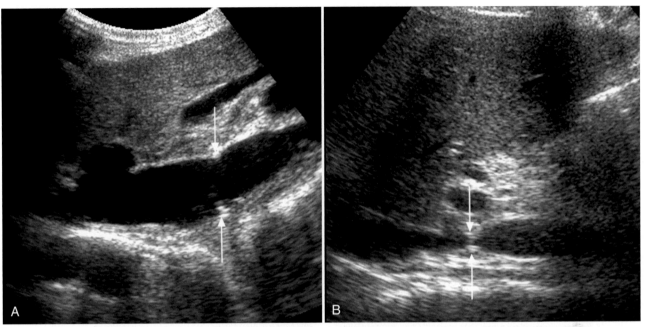

FIGURE 17-18. Inferior vena cava (IVC) infrahepatic anastomosis: normal and abnormal in two patients.
Sagittal sonograms of IVC show **A,** a normal caliber at the anastomosis *(arrows)*, and **B,** narrowing at the anastomosis *(arrows)*.

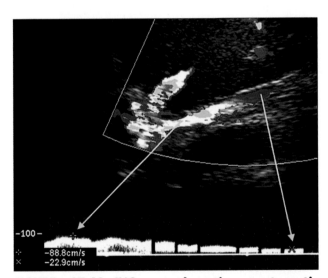

FIGURE 17-19. IVC suprahepatic anastomotic stricture. Sagittal color Doppler sonogram of a stenosed segment of the IVC shows aliasing produced by high-velocity turbulent flow in both the IVC and the hepatic vein. Spectral tracing shows a greater than threefold velocity increase at the stenotic region *(left arrow).*

if substantial hepatic necrosis has occurred. **Late-onset hepatic venous obstruction** may be associated with a more insidious deterioration in liver function. These patients may benefit from metallic stent insertion or balloon venoplasty, because surgical correction is often difficult as a result of fibrotic changes around the anastomotic sites.[39,40]

Direct signs of hepatic vein stenosis include focal narrowing on gray-scale ultrasound associated with turbulent flow on color and spectral Doppler interrogation (Fig. 17-21). A persistent, monophasic spectral waveform is suggestive of, but not diagnostic of, hepatic vein stenosis; monophasic waveforms may also be present in normal, nonobstructed hepatic veins. However, the presence of a triphasic or biphasic waveform rules out substantial hepatic vein stenosis.[40]

Extrahepatic Fluid Collections

Perihepatic fluid collections and ascites are frequently observed after transplantation. In the early postoperative period, a small amount of free fluid or a right pleural effusion may be observed, but these usually resolve in a few weeks. **Fluid collections** and **hematomas** are common in the areas of vascular anastomosis (hepatic hilum and adjacent to IVC) and biliary anastomosis, in the lesser sac, and in the perihepatic and subhepatic spaces.[7] Because the peritoneal reflections surrounding the liver are ligated at transplantation, fluid collections can occur around the **bare area** of the liver, a location not encountered in the preoperative liver[5] (Fig. 17-22).

Ultrasound is highly sensitive in detecting these fluid collections, although it lacks specificity because bile, blood, pus, and lymphatic fluid may all have a similar sonographic appearance. The presence of internal echoes in a fluid collection, although nonspecific, suggests blood or infection. Particulate ascites may also be observed in peritoneal carcinomatosis, although this would seem less likely in the transplant recipient population.[5]

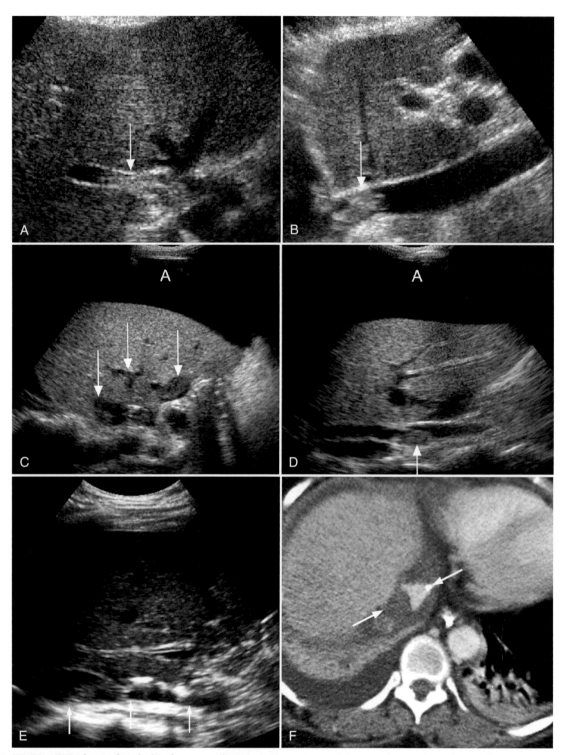

FIGURE 17-20. IVC thrombosis in three patients. A, Transverse, and **B,** sagittal, sonograms show malignant IVC and hepatic vein thrombus *(arrows)* in a patient with recurrent hepatocellular carcinoma after transplantation. **C,** Transverse sonogram of the hepatic veins, and **D,** sagittal sonogram of IVC, show bland thrombus *(arrows)* in each; *A,* ascites. **E,** Sagittal sonogram, and **F,** corresponding contrast-enhanced CT scan, show bland thrombus in the IVC *(arrows). (A and B from Crossin J, Muradali D, Wilson SR. Ultrasound of liver transplants: normal and abnormal. Radiographics 2003;23:1093-1114.)*

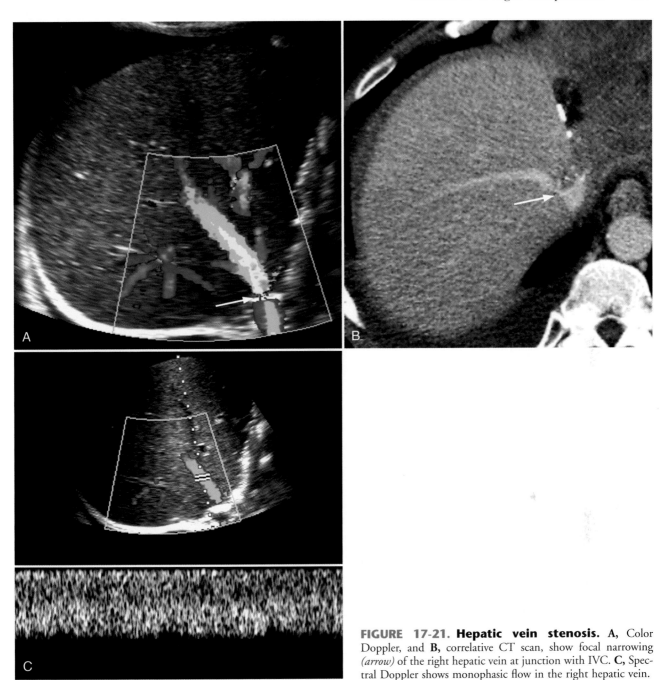

FIGURE 17-21. **Hepatic vein stenosis. A,** Color Doppler, and **B,** correlative CT scan, show focal narrowing *(arrow)* of the right hepatic vein at junction with IVC. **C,** Spectral Doppler shows monophasic flow in the right hepatic vein.

Adrenal Hemorrhage

Right-sided adrenal hemorrhage may be observed in the immediate postoperative period and results from (1) venous engorgement caused by ligation of the right adrenal vein during the removal of a portion of the IVC or (2) a coagulopathy caused by the patient's preexisting liver disease.[26] On ultrasound, adrenal hemorrhage may present as a hypoechoic nodular structure or as a fluid collection in the right suprarenal region (Fig. 17-23).

Intrahepatic Fluid Collections

Sterile postoperative fluid collections are often located along the falciform ligament and ligamentum venosum, usually appearing as fluid-filled anechoic structures surrounding the echogenic ligaments (Fig. 17-24). **Bilomas** may present as a hypoechoic, round structure or a complex cyst. **Intraparenchymal hematomas** may result from the transplant surgery, percutaneous biopsy or may be a sequela of donor trauma (e.g., motor vehicle crash).

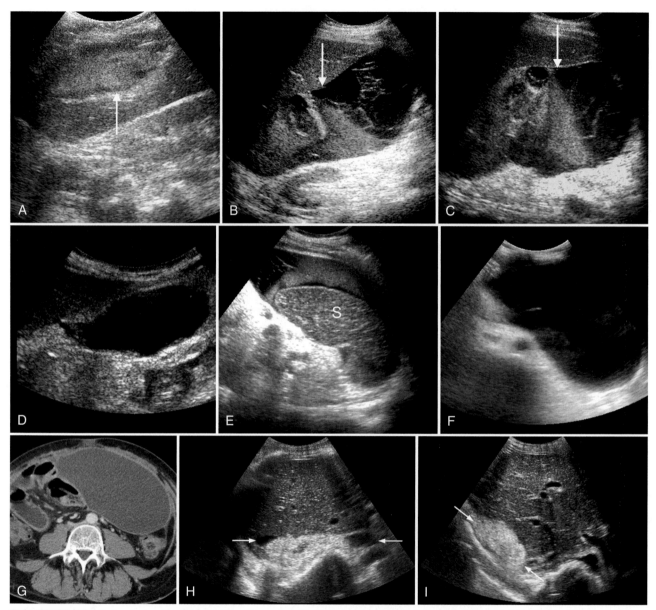

FIGURE 17-22. Extrahepatic fluid collection. A to D, Hematoma at surgical margin of a right lobe in living related transplant. **A,** Transverse sonogram shows acute hematoma that appears echogenic, heterogeneous, and solid. **B** and **C,** Hematoma liquefies after 3 weeks, with internal strands and a fluid-debris level. **D,** After 2 months, further liquefaction of the hematoma appears as a smaller, anechoic collection. Arrows mark boundary of hematomas with liver. **E,** Sagittal sonogram shows **hemoperitoneum** around spleen *(S),* with fluid-fluid level and internal strands. **F** and **G, Anastomotic leak from roux-en-Y.** Transverse sonogram and correlative CT scan show large fluid collection in the left lower quadrant. **H** and **I, Biloma secondary to anastomotic leak.** Sagittal sonogram and transverse sonogram show complex subphrenic echogenic collection *(arrows).*

Abscess versus Infarct

In the early stages, it may be difficult to differentiate a liver abscess from an infarct. Initially, both abscesses and infarcts may appear as a subtle, hypoechoic region, associated with a localized coarsening of the parenchymal echotexture. **Infarcts** may subsequently organize into avascular round or wedge-shaped lesions, which can eventually develop central hypoechoic areas reflecting liquefaction and necrosis. A focal liver infarct should be

diagnosed with accompanying Doppler evidence of hepatic arterial compromise.

As with infarcts, the ultrasound appearance of a **liver abscess** also varies with its maturation. The classic appearance of a mature transplant liver abscess is a complex, cystic structure with thick, irregular walls and particulate internal fluid, with or without associated septations.

Both infarcts and abscesses may contain bubbles of air, occurring as bright echogenic foci with or without

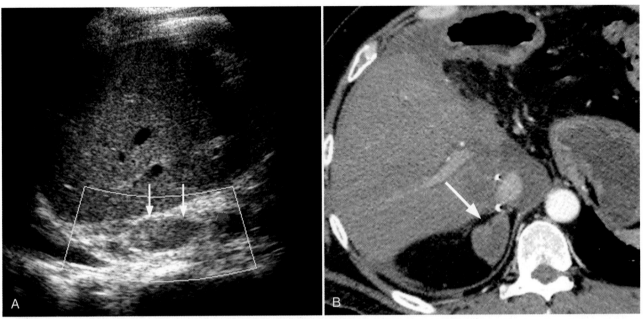

FIGURE 17-23. **Right adrenal hemorrhage.** **A**, Sagittal sonogram, and **B**, CT scan, show a small right adrenal mass *(arrows)*.

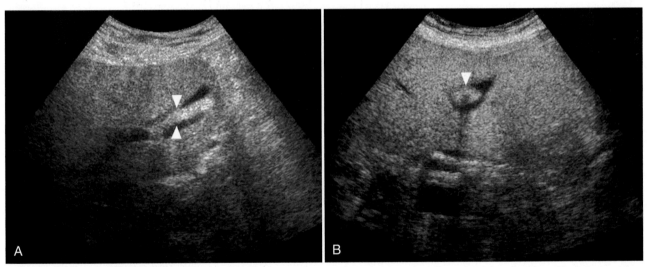

FIGURE 17-24. **Intrahepatic fluid collection.** **A**, Transverse, and **B**, sagittal, sonograms show anechoic fluid surrounding echogenic falciform ligament *(arrowheads)*.

posterior acoustic shadowing (Fig. 17-25). Occasionally, bubbles of air within the lumen of an intraparenchymal abscess can be confused with benign pneumobilia or may be mistaken for air outside the liver within the gastrointestinal tract. A high index of suspicion is critical in patients at risk for either abscess or infarct to avoid these misinterpretations.

Intrahepatic Solid Masses

The differential diagnosis of a solitary mass in the transplanted liver is similar to that in the native liver.

For example, benign lesions, such as hemangiomas and cysts, are relatively common in the transplanted liver, with the same range of appearances as described for the native liver. However, several pathologies unique to the transplanted liver may also present with a solid or complex mass on gray-scale ultrasound, including infarcts (Fig. 17-26), abscesses, hematomas, recurrent/metastatic HCC, and posttransplant lymphoproliferative disorder.

Recurrent hepatocellular carcinoma is a serious complication that can potentially develop posttransplantation in patients with a preoperative history of end-stage

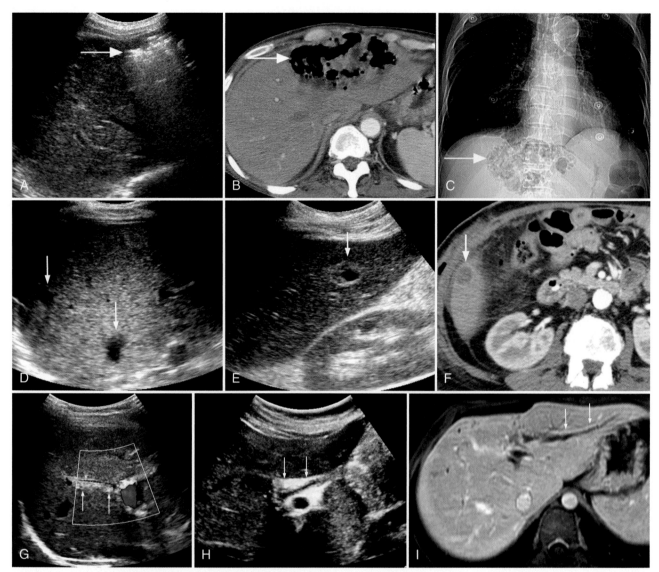

FIGURE 17-25. Liver infections in three patients: solitary abscess. A to **C, Air-containing abscess** *(arrows)* in segment IV of liver. **A,** Transverse ultrasound; **B,** CT scan; and **C,** plain film show air within the abscess, on ultrasound appearing as an echogenic interface associated with dirty shadowing. **D** to **F, Multifocal abscess. D,** Transverse, and **E,** sagittal, sonograms show multiple small parenchymal collections *(arrows)*. **F,** Corresponding CT scan shows subtle rim enhancement *(arrow)*. **G** to **I, Ascending cholangitis. G,** Transverse sonogram shows increased periductal echogenicity *(arrows)* of a right intrahepatic bile duct. **H,** Oblique sonogram shows thickening of the common hepatic duct, with increased echogenicity of the periductal fat *(arrows)*. **I,** T1-weighted contrast-enhanced MR image shows periductal enhancement *(arrows)*.

cirrhosis with known or occult hepatomas. The most common site of recurrent HCC is the lung, presumably caused by embolization with tumor cells through the hepatic veins before or during transplantation. The second most common location of recurrent hepatomas is within the allograft, followed by regional or distant lymph nodes. Early detection of **recurrent hepatomas** in the transplanted liver is essential to facilitate early resection, ablation, or chemotherapy[26,41] (Fig. 17-27). As in the general population, transplant recipients might develop any type of primary or secondary neoplasm within the liver.

RENAL TRANSPLANTATION

Transplantation is the treatment of choice for many patients with **chronic renal failure** (CRF) severe enough to warrant dialysis. The only contraindications for transplantation are unsuitability for general anesthesia or surgery, preexisting infection or malignancy, and a risk of recurrent renal disease (e.g., active vasculitis or oxalosis). Before transplantation, a suitable donor must be obtained with appropriate human lymphocyte antigen (HLA) matching with the recipient.[42]

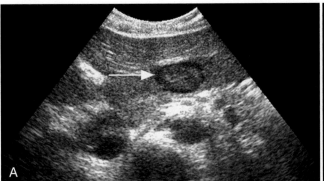
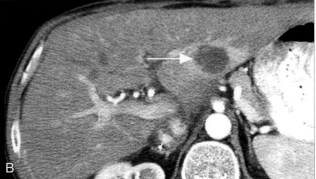

FIGURE 17-26. Atypical infarct. A, Transverse sonogram shows an atypical infarct *(arrow)* appearing as a round mass associated with a surrounding hypoechoic halo. **B,** Correlative CT scan shows that the infarct *(arrow)* is avascular, with a surrounding parenchymal blush. *(From Crossin J, Muradali D, Wilson SR. Ultrasound of liver transplants: normal and abnormal. Radiographics 2003;23:1093-1114.)*

As the number of patients with CRF continues to rise, the major limitation for expanding transplant programs is the continuing shortage of suitable donor kidneys. This organ shortage has resulted in an increasing number of renal transplantations from living related donors. These donors may include family members or close friends with a long-standing relationship with the recipient. The average life expectancy for a cadaveric allograft is 7 to 10 years, whereas that for a live donor allograft is 15 to 20 years.[42]

Regardless of whether a cadaveric or live donor allograft is used, the cost-benefit of a functioning successful transplant far outweighs that of a patient with persistent CRF, so multiple health care resources are targeted to ensure that high rates of success. Ultrasound is the most valuable noninvasive imaging modality in monitoring the renal transplant.

Surgical Technique

Detailed sonography of the renal transplant requires knowledge of the surgical procedure used in most institutions as well as the postsurgical anatomic relationships. The right or left lower quadrant is selected for the incision, based on the patient's prior surgical history and the surgeon's preference. Usually, the right lower quadrant is selected because the right iliac vein is more superficial and horizontal on this side of the pelvis, facilitating creation of a vascular anastomosis.[43,44]

The type of **arterial anastomosis** used depends on whether the allograft is cadaveric or living related and on the number and size of donor renal arteries. In patients with cadaveric transplants, the donor artery, along with a portion of the aorta (Carrel patch) is anastomosed end to side to the external iliac artery. In patients with living donor transplants, the donor renal artery is anastomosed to either the internal iliac artery (end to end) or the external iliac artery (end to side) of the recipient. Multiple donor arteries of similar size may be joined together with a side-to-side anastomosis to form a common

ostium. Alternatively, multiple arteries may be anastomosed as a Carrel patch, or anastomosed separately to the external iliac artery.[43,44]

The **donor renal vein** is almost always anastomosed end to side to the external iliac vein. In the case of multiple renal veins, the smaller veins are usually ligated, resulting in a single donor vein.[44]

The **ureter** is usually anastomosed to the superolateral wall of the urinary bladder through a neocystostomy. Several techniques are used to create a neocystostomy, but the basic procedure involves tunneling the ureter through the bladder wall to prevent reflux to the transplant. For patients undergoing repeat surgery on the collecting system and those with complex surgeries, the recipient's ureter may be used as a conduit to the bladder[43] (Fig. 17-28).

Because of the chronic shortage of donor organs, **paired cadaveric kidneys** from young (<5 years old) donors may be transplanted en bloc in an attempt to provide a functional renal mass, analogous to the renal mass of a single cadaveric kidney transplanted from an adult. At harvesting, both kidneys are removed en bloc with preservation of the ureters, main renal arteries and veins, as well as segments of the suprarenal and infrarenal abdominal aorta and IVC. The donor aorta and IVC are oversewn just cephalad to the origin of the renal arteries and veins, and the caudal ends anastomosed end to side to the recipient's external iliac artery and vein. The donor ureters are implanted into the urinary bladder through individual or common ureteroneocystostomies.[45] This surgery is more common in the pediatric population than in adults (Fig. 17-28).

Normal Renal Transplant Ultrasound

Gray-Scale Assessment

Sonography of the renal transplant is usually easily performed because of the superficial location of the kidney

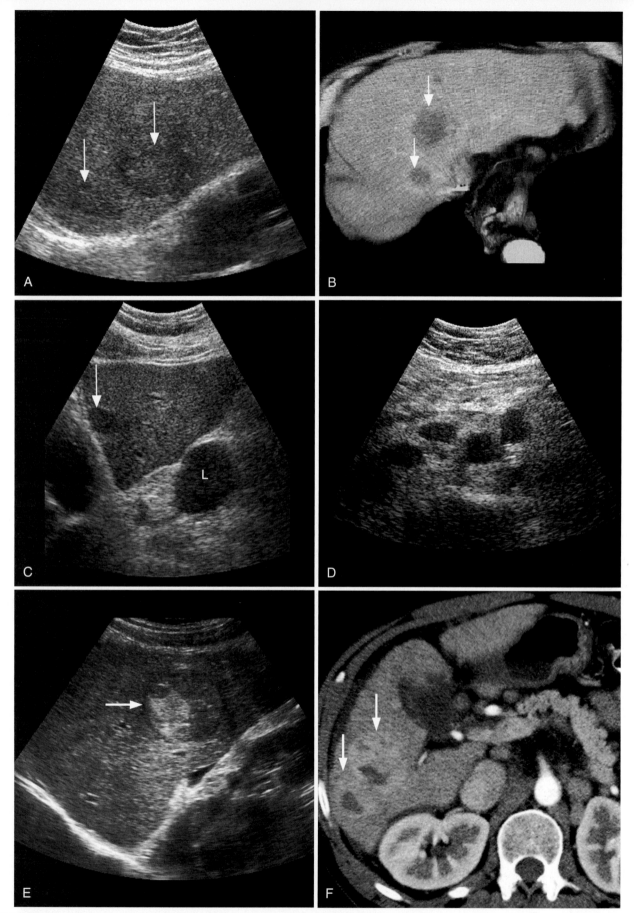

FIGURE 17-27. Recurrent hepatocellular carcinoma (HCC) in two patients. *Patient 1:* **A,** Transverse sonogram shows two malignant-appearing masses *(arrows)* secondary to recurrent HCC. **B,** Correlative arterial phase CT scan shows peripheral enhancement of the masses *(arrows).* **C,** Sagittal sonogram shows a third HCC in the medial segment of the left lobe *(arrow)* and a large metastatic lymph node *(L).* **D,** Transverse midline sonogram shows multiple enlarged metastatic lymph nodes. *Patient 2:* **E,** Sagittal sonogram shows solid mass *(arrow)* with echogenic and hypoechoic regions. **F,** Correlative arterial phase CT scan shows hypervascular masses *(arrows),* consistent with recurrent hepatocellular carcinoma. *(A to D from Crossin J, Muradali D, Wilson SR. Ultrasound of liver transplants: normal and abnormal. Radiographics 2003;23:1093-1114.)*

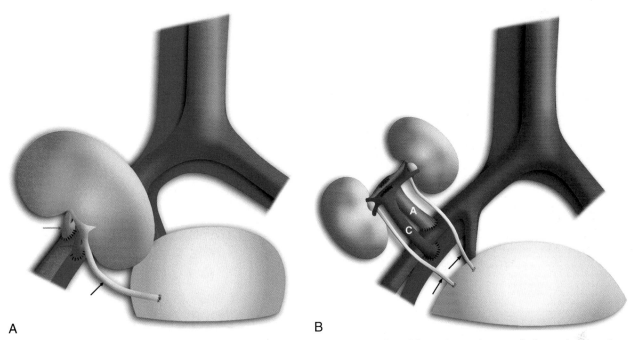

A   B

FIGURE 17-28. Renal transplant surgery: A, Single cadaveric transplant. The main renal artery *(red arrow)* and main renal vein *(purple arrow)* are anastomosed to the external iliac artery and vein, respectively. The ureter *(black arrow)* is anastomosed to the superolateral bladder wall. **B,** Double cadaveric transplant. The aorta *(A)* and IVC *(C)* are anastomosed to the external iliac artery and vein, respectively. The ureters *(black arrows)* are anastomosed to the superolateral bladder wall.

in either the right or the left lower quadrant. Because the allograft is held in place by its pedicle, a variety of orientations may be encountered. Most often, the kidney is aligned with its long axis parallel to the surgical incision, with the hilum oriented inferiorly and posteriorly. Occasionally, in obese patients, the long axis may lie in an anterior-to-posterior plane.[46]

Longitudinal and transverse (width × depth) measurements of the transplant should be obtained with the kidney imaged through the hilum in the sagittal and transverse planes, respectively. Although there are no normative data for comparison, these measurements serve as a useful baseline for future reference to assess for interval changes in volume of the allograft. The normal kidney may hypertrophy by up to 15% within the first 2 weeks after surgery, and eventually may increase in volume by 40%, with the final size attained at about 6 months.[47-49]

The transplanted kidney appears morphologically similar to the native kidney, with many of the subtle differences attributed to the improved resolution from proximity of the allograft to the skin surface (Fig. 17-29). The normal renal cortex is well defined, hypoechoic, and easily differentiated from the highly reflective, central echogenic renal sinus fat. Apart from this improved corticomedullary differentiation, the renal pyramids of the allograft are more easily visualized than in the native kidney, appearing as wedge-shaped structures that are hypoechoic to the surrounding parenchyma.[42]

The sonographer should always be aware that the transplanted kidney might show intrinsic pathology in

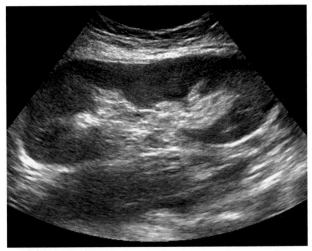

FIGURE 17-29. Normal gray-scale ultrasound of renal transplant.

the donor kidney. In our clinical practice, we have observed a host of donor pathologies in the transplanted kidney, including benign cysts, angiomyolipomas, and medullary sponge kidney (Figs. 17-30 and 17-31).

Doppler Assessment

Color Doppler gives a global assessment of the intraparenchymal perfusion and is useful in localizing the main

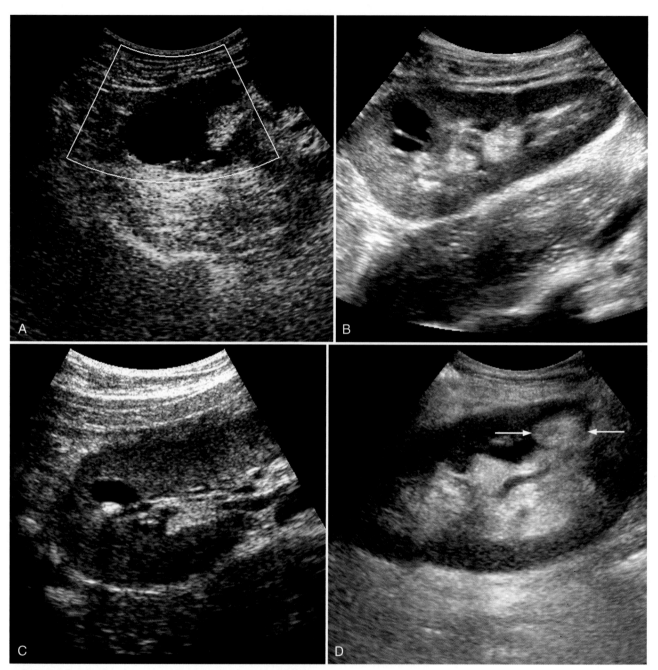

FIGURE 17-30. Benign renal cysts in four patients. Sagittal sonograms of transplant kidneys. **A,** Simple upper-pole cyst, which is avascular on color Doppler ultrasound. **B,** Upper-pole cyst with a single thin strand. **C,** Milk of calcium cyst with dependent calcification. **D,** Marsupialized renal cyst *(arrows)* presenting as an echogenic mass.

renal artery and vein. The renal parenchyma should be screened initially with color Doppler to check for focal regions of hypoperfusion and locate the interlobar arteries for spectral interrogation.[42]

Spectral traces of the interlobar arteries should be obtained from the upper-pole, middle-pole, and lower-pole regions with low filter settings, maximal gain, and the smallest scale demonstrating the peak systolic velocity. The normal waveform is low impedance with a brisk upstroke and continuous diastolic flow; RI of 0.6 to 0.8 is normal. Provided that flow in the recipient common iliac artery is normal, the velocity of the transplanted main renal artery should be less than 200 cm/sec (Fig. 17-32). An intraparenchymal RI of 0.8 to 0.9 is considered equivocal, and greater than 0.9 is classified as abnormal, suggesting increased intraparenchymal resistance. Overall, an elevated resistive index is a nonspecific marker of transplant dysfunction and is not helpful in determining the cause of the dysfunction[50] (Fig. 17-33).

The intraparenchymal and extraparenchymal renal veins show either monophasic continuous flow or pha-

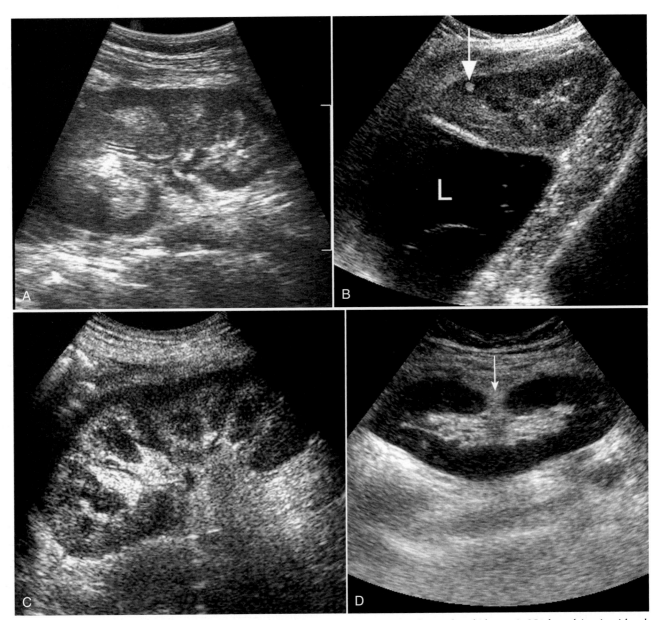

FIGURE 17-31. Donor pathology in four patients. Sagittal sonograms of transplant kidneys. **A,** Nephrocalcinosis with calcifications in the renal medulla. **B,** Tiny angiomyolipoma *(arrow); L,* lymphocele. **C,** Anderson-Carr morphology with echogenic borders around the medullary pyramids. **D,** Midpole scar *(arrow).*

sicity with the cardiac cycle. There are no accepted normal peak velocity values for these vessels. Documentation of the presence or absence of flow within the transplant and main renal vein, with an appropriate velocity gradient across the venous anastomosis, is of prime importance in the management of these patients.

Abnormal Renal Transplant

Renal transplants are routinely evaluated with sonography as either a component of a screening protocol or a workup for renal dysfunction based on a rising serum creatinine level or a decreased urine output. Postopera-

tive complications have been reported in up to 20% of renal transplant recipients.[44] When encountered in a graft with a clinical suspicion of dysfunction, the sonographer should approach the possible etiologies in terms of (1) parenchymal pathology, (2) prerenal causes, and (3) postrenal complications. Parenchymal transplant pathology includes acute tubular necrosis, acute and chronic rejection, and infection. Prerenal problems include all factors affecting blood flow to the kidney or venous drainage from the graft. Postrenal complications include intrinsic or extrinsic lesions that can obstruct either a component of the calyceal system or the transplanted ureter.

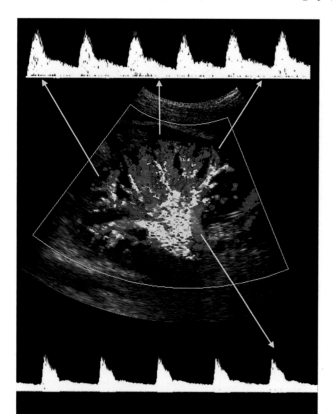

FIGURE 17-32. Normal renal transplant Doppler. Color Doppler shows flow throughout kidney *(top)*. Intrarenal spectral traces of upper, middle, and lower poles show a resistive index of less than 0.8 and continuous flow throughout diastole. The main renal artery shows continuous flow with peak velocities less than 200 cm/sec *(bottom)*.

Parenchymal Pathology

Acute Tubular Necrosis and Acute Rejection

Acute tubular necrosis (ATN) results from donor organ ischemia either prior to vascular anastomosis or secondary to perioperative hypotension. It is most common in the early postoperative period and is the major cause of delayed graft function (defined as the need for dialysis within the first week of transplantation).[43,51] In patients requiring dialysis, recovery is usually in the first 2 weeks of transplantation but may be delayed by up to 3 months. ATN occurs in most cadaveric grafts and is observed infrequently in living related renal transplants because of the relatively short cold ischemic time of the donor kidney.[42]

Transplants affected by **hyperacute rejection** are rarely imaged because graft failure occurs immediately at the vascular anastomosis during surgery.[43] **Acute rejection** occurs in up to 40% of patients in the early transplant period, peaking at 1 to 3 weeks after surgery, and is an adverse long-term prognostic indicator. Most patients with acute rejection are asymptomatic, but a small proportion may present with flulike symptoms, malaise, fever, and graft tenderness. Provided that the diagnosis can be rapidly established, acute rejection usually can be promptly reversed with high-dose steroids or antibiotic therapy.[42,52]

The imaging features of ATN and acute rejection are almost identical on gray-scale and Doppler ultrasound. Both conditions can produce increases in length and cross-sectional areas of the allograft. However, precise volumetric comparisons between interval studies can prove difficult; subtle changes in measurements have not been adopted as a strong clinical sign of potential dysfunction. Other gray-scale findings include increased cortical thickness, increased or decreased cortical echogenicity, reduction of the corticomedullary differentiation, loss of the renal sinus echoes, and prominence of the pyramids (Fig. 17-34).

Color Doppler assessment may be normal or may occasionally show diffuse decreased blood flow. The resistive index of the intraparenchymal arteries is also nonspecific in these conditions and may be normal or elevated. In severe cases, there may be a complete lack of flow in diastole or a reversal of diastolic flow[42] (Fig. 17-35). Despite the lack of specificity of gray-scale and Doppler ultrasound in these acute conditions, **serial spectral Doppler** measurements, in combination with clinical assessments and biochemical findings, provide a useful guide to the clinician in terms of monitoring the allograft function and in determining the need for percutaneous biopsy.

Chronic Rejection

Chronic rejection is defined as a reduction in allograft function starting at least 3 months after transplantation in association with fibrous intimal thickening, interstitial fibrosis, and tubular atrophy on histology. It is the most common cause of late graft loss. The most frequent predisposing risk factor for development of chronic rejection is recurrent previous episodes of acute rejection.[42,43] On ultrasound, there is progressive thinning of the renal cortex, prominence of the central renal sinus fat, and a reduction in the overall size of the transplant. **Dystrophic calcifications** may be seen scattered throughout the residual parenchyma. In the end-stage renal transplant, the entire renal cortex can become calcified, appearing as a sharp echogenic interface associated with clean distal shadowing (Fig. 17-36).

Infection

Transplant pyelonephritis can result from an ascending infection, hematologic seeding, or contiguous spread from an adjacent infected fluid collection. Ultrasound findings include a focal or diffusely granular, echogenic renal cortex associated with loss of the corticomedullary junction; increased echogenicity and thickening of the perirenal fat secondary to extension of inflammation or

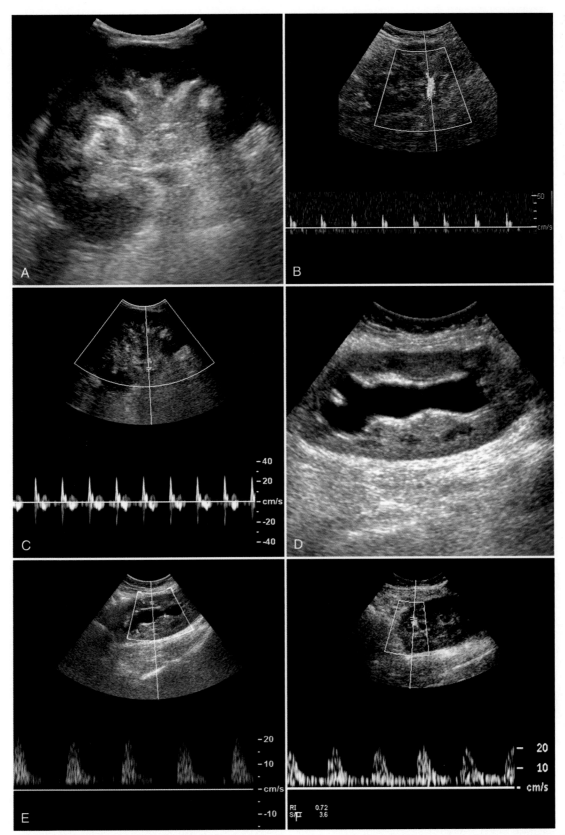

FIGURE 17-33. Elevated resistive indices in two patients. A to C, Acute rejection. A, Sagittal sonogram shows increased cortical echogenicity. **B,** Spectral Doppler ultrasound done initially shows no flow in diastole and thus a resistive index (RI) of 1.0. **C,** Follow-up spectral Doppler ultrasound 1 week later shows reversal of flow in diastole, which coincided with the clinical deterioration of the patient. **D to F, Collecting system obstruction. D,** Sagittal scan shows grade 3 pelvocaliectasis, secondary to ureteral stricture *(not shown).* **E,** Spectral Doppler shows RI of 1.0. **F,** Spectral Doppler ultrasound performed after resolution of the pelvocaliectasis shows a normal RI of 0.72.

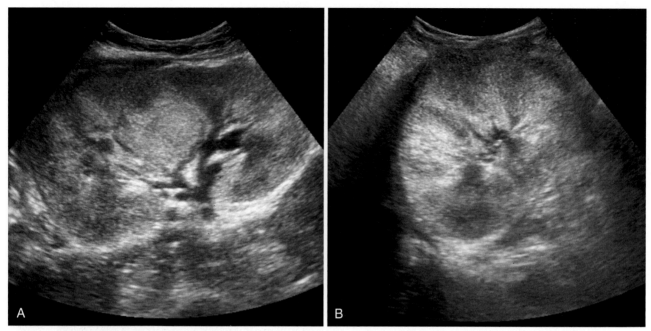

FIGURE 17-34. Acute tubular necrosis. A, Sagittal, and **B,** transverse, sonograms show increased cortical thickness and echogenicity as well as loss of the normal corticomedullary differentiation.

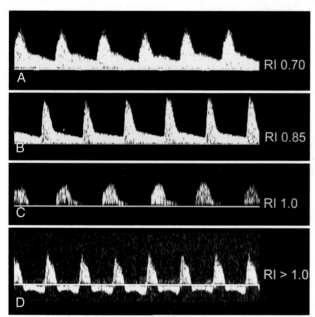

FIGURE 17-35. Intrarenal spectral waveforms in four patients. A, Normal waveform shows resistive index (RI) of 0.70. **B,** RI in a gray zone (0.85). **C,** RI elevated (1.0) with no flow in diastole. **D,** Elevated RI (>1.0) with reversal of flow in diastole. This is seen with severely increased vascular resistance in the kidney from rejection or renal vein thrombosis.

infection into the surrounding tissue; and uroepithelial thickening (Fig. 17-37).

Pyonephrosis may occur occasionally in a chronically obstructed transplanted kidney. In the early stages, the lumen of the dilated collecting system appears anechoic.

Once the lumen becomes filled with purulent material, low-level echoes develop within the calyceal system and ureter, sometimes associated with fluid-debris levels. Echogenic material within the collecting system may also result from intraluminal blood or other filling defects, or it may be artifactual as a result of scatter or side-lobe artifact (Fig. 17-37).

Abscesses can arise from infection of a previously sterile collection. On ultrasound, abscesses appear as a complex cystic structure and may be associated with fluid-fluid levels or intraluminal air (Fig. 17-38).

Air can be observed within the collecting system in **emphysematous pyelonephritis,** appearing as a bright echogenic focus with distal dirty shadowing. **Milk of calcium cysts** can produce dirty shadowing, mimicking an intrarenal abscess. Scanning the patient in a decubitus position allows for differentiation; air rises to the nondependent portion of the lumen, whereas milk of calcium does not (Fig. 17-39).

Prerenal Vascular Complications

Arterial Thrombosis

Renal artery thrombosis occurs in less than 1% of transplants, usually within the first month of surgery, and is often initially asymptomatic. The most common cause is hyperacute or acute rejection, which results in occlusion of the intraparenchymal arterioles with retrograde main renal artery thrombosis. Other predisposing factors include a young pediatric donor kidney, atherosclerotic emboli, acquired renal artery stenosis, hypotension,

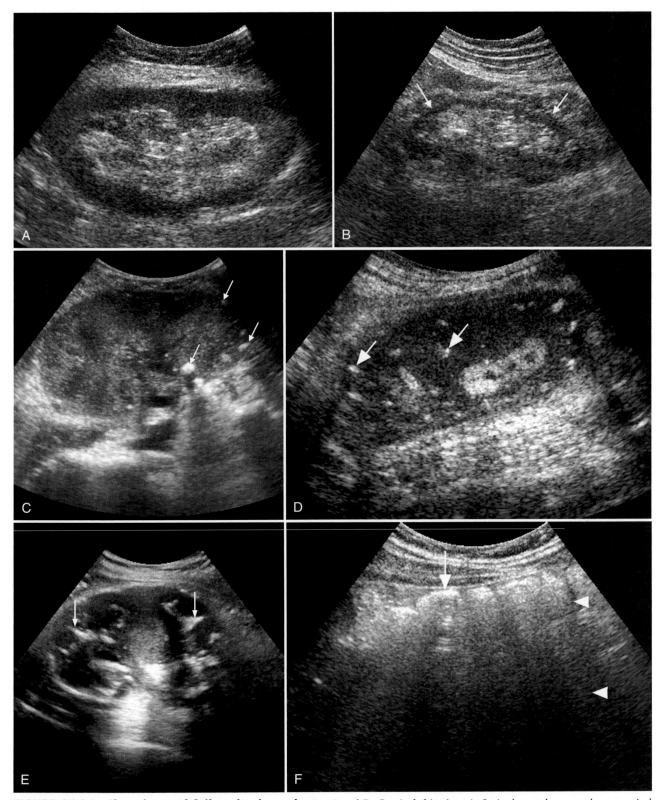

FIGURE 17-36. Chronic renal failure in six patients. A and **B, Cortical thinning. A,** Sagittal scan shows moderate cortical thinning with abundant renal sinus fat. **B,** With progression, the kidney *(arrows)* becomes smaller and the cortex thinner. **C** to **F, Dystrophic calcifications.** Sagittal sonograms show **C,** a few punctuate peripheral cortical calcifications *(arrows);* **D,** multiple peripheral and central cortical calcifications *(arrows);* and **E,** linear calcifications that extend from the peripheral to deep cortex *(arrows).* **F,** The end-stage kidney becomes calcified, appearing as an echogenic interface *(arrow)* associated with dirty shadowing *(arrowheads).* The kidney is frequently not identified on sonography at this stage.

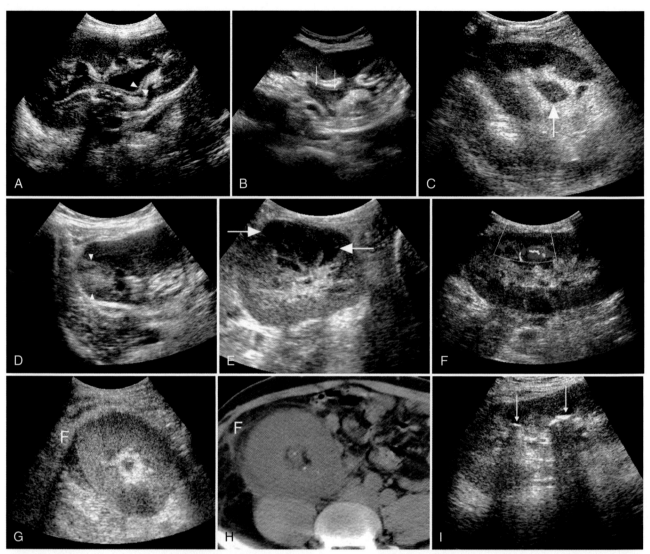

FIGURE 17-37. Renal transplant related infections. A, Uroepithelial thickening. Sagittal sonogram shows mild uroepithelial thickening *(arrowheads).* **B,** Sagittal scan shows mild uroepithelial thickening *(arrows)* surrounding a mildly dilated collecting system with internal echoes, secondary to early pyonephrosis. **C,** Transverse sonogram shows moderate to severe uroepithelial thickening *(arrow),* which can be misinterpreted as a mass in the renal pelvis. **D** to **F, Focal pyelonephritis. D,** Sagittal sonogram shows subtle, focal echogenic region in the upper-pole cortex *(arrowheads).* **E,** Intraparenchymal phlegmon appearing as a hypoechoic mass within the renal cortex *(arrows).* **F,** On color Doppler, the phlegmon seen in image **E** is vascular. **G** and **H, Diffuse pyelonephritis. G,** Transverse sonogram shows a generous kidney with echogenic granular renal cortex, surrounded by inflamed echogenic perinephric fat *(F).* **H,** Corresponding CT scan shows inflamed fat *(F)* as perinephric streaking. **I, Emphysematous pyelonephritis.** Sagittal sonogram shows air *(arrows)* within collecting system, appearing as bright, echogenic linear foci with distal dirty shadowing.

vascular kinking, cyclosporine, hypercoagulable states, intraoperative vascular trauma, and poor intimal anastomosis.[53]

Global infarction of the allograft occurs when there is occlusive thrombosis of the main renal artery, with no perfusion to the renal parenchyma. On gray-scale ultrasound, the kidney may appear diffusely hypoechoic and enlarged. On color and spectral Doppler ultrasound, complete absence of arterial and venous flow distal to the occlusion, within both the hilar and the intraparenchymal vessels, is observed. Although surgical thrombectomy with arterial repair is often attempted, nephrectomy is frequently indicated in these patients.[44]

Segmental infarction of the allograft may occur in transplants with a single main renal artery with thrombosis of a major arterial branch (Fig. 17-40), in transplants with multiple renal arteries where a single artery is thrombosed, and in patients with systemic vasculitis. On gray-scale sonography, a segmental infarct may appear as a poorly defined hypoechoic region, a hypoechoic mass, or a hypoechoic mass with a well-defined echogenic wall. On Doppler sonography, the infarcted region appears as a wedge-shaped area devoid of flow on color or spectral interrogation.[54] Interpretation of the gray-scale and Doppler findings should not be influenced by urine output of the allograft or

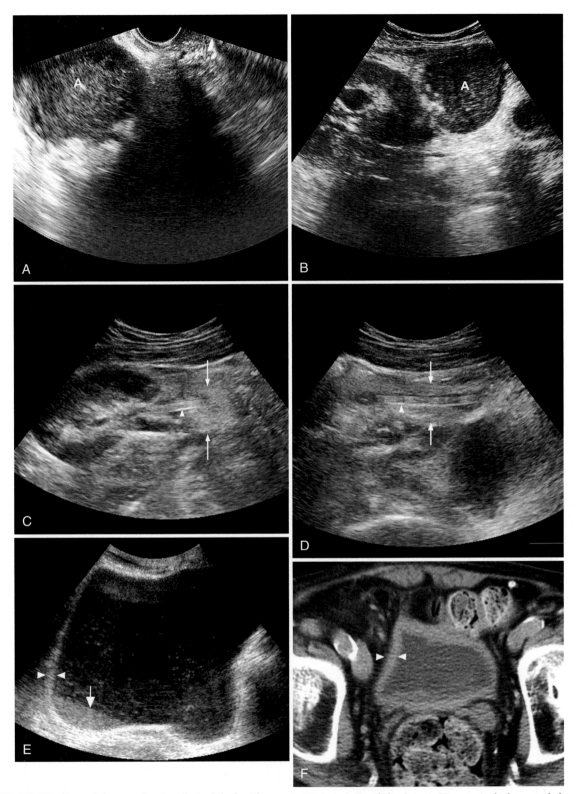

FIGURE 17-38. Renal transplant related infections. A, Perirenal *Candida* abscess. Transvaginal ultrasound shows right adnexal abscess *(A)* with diffuse internal echoes in a patient presenting with right lower quadrant pain. **B,** Corresponding transabdominal sagittal scan shows that the abscess *(A)* abuts the lower pole of the transplant. **C and D, Ureteritis.** Sagittal sonograms of proximal **(C)** and midline **(D)** ureter show inflamed echogenic periureteral fat *(arrows)* secondary to an infected ureteral stent *(arrowhead)*. **E and F, Cystitis. E,** Transverse sonogram shows internal echoes and fluid-debris level *(arrow)* in urinary bladder, secondary to cystitis. Bladder wall thickening *(arrowheads)* is identified on both ultrasound and **F,** corresponding CT scan.

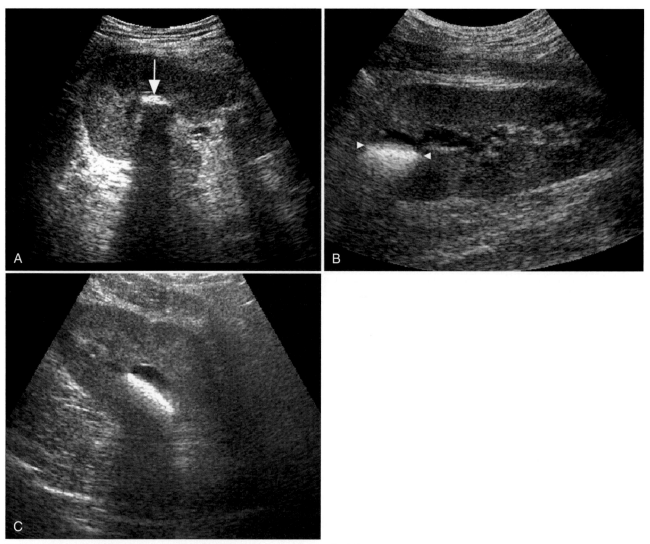

FIGURE 17-39. Mimicker of emphysematous pyelonephritis. A, Emphysematous pyelonephritis. Transverse scan shows air in collecting system *(arrow)*. **B, Milk of calcium cyst.** Supine sonogram shows layering of the calcification *(arrowheads)* in the cyst, producing dirty shadowing. **C,** Scanning this patient in a decubitus position changes the orientation of the layering of calcium to the most dependent portion of the cyst, allowing for differentiation from an air-filled collection.

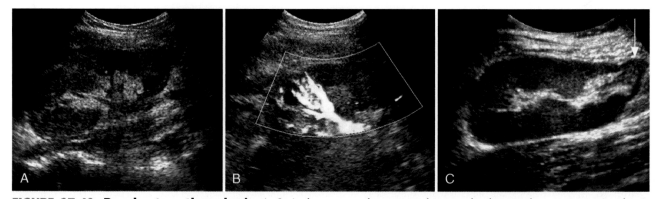

FIGURE 17-40. Renal artery thrombosis. A, Sagittal sonogram shows normal gray-scale ultrasound on postoperative day 1. **B,** However, power Doppler shows no flow in the lower pole due to thrombosis of a segmental artery. **C,** Three months later, there is secondary scarring of the entire lower pole *(arrow).*

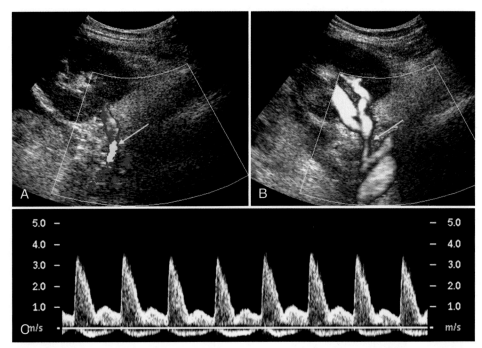

FIGURE 17-41. Renal artery stenosis: donor portion. A, Color Doppler ultrasound of donor renal artery anastomosis shows focal area of aliasing *(arrow)*. **B,** Power Doppler shows area of narrowing in this region *(arrow)*. **C,** Spectral Doppler shows elevated angle-corrected velocities at the site of the arrow, greater than 400 cm/sec.

laboratory data, because segmental infarction may occur in the presence of preserved renal function.

The absence of blood flow on Doppler interrogation in the kidney parenchyma may be observed in conditions other than arterial thrombosis, including **hyperacute rejection** and **renal vein thrombosis.** In these conditions, however, the main renal artery is patent on spectral Doppler ultrasound and may exhibit reversal of diastolic flow.[42]

Renal Artery Stenosis

Renal artery stenosis, the most common vascular complication of transplantation, occurs in up to 10% of patients within the first year and should be suspected in cases of severe hypertension refractory to medical therapy. Stenosis may occur in one of three regions of the transplanted artery: the **donor** portion (Fig. 17-41), most frequently observed in end-to-side anastomoses and thought to arise from either rejection or difficult surgical technique; the **recipient** portion (Fig. 17-42), which is more uncommon and usually the result of intraoperative clamp injury or intrinsic atherosclerotic disease; and at the **anastomosis** (Fig. 17-43), which is more frequent in end-to-end anastomoses and is directly related to surgical technique or may be secondary to rejection.[53,55,56]

Initially, color Doppler ultrasound should be used to detect the precise location of the anastomosis, as well as to document focal regions of aliasing, which would indi-

cate the presence of high-velocity turbulent flow and serve as a guide for meticulous spectral interrogation. A spectral trace should then be performed at the anastomosis and in any area where color aliasing was detected to determine the peak systolic velocity in that region. A PSV greater than 200 cm/sec, in the presence of distant turbulent flow, is suspicious for renal artery stenosis. However, high velocities in the renal artery may be secondary to changes in the external iliac artery. Therefore, the renal artery/external iliac artery PSV ratio may be calculated to determine if renal artery velocity measurements are a result of narrowing or high flow rates from the external iliac artery. In addition, within the renal parenchyma, a tardus-parvus spectral waveform may be observed when interrogating the intraparenchymal arteries in patients with renal artery stenosis.[44,54] If no flow abnormality is detected within the main renal artery after color and spectral Doppler interrogation, significant stenosis can be excluded.[57]

In summary, Doppler criteria for renal artery stenosis include color aliasing at the stenotic segment, PSVs greater than 200 cm/sec, distal turbulent flow, and a velocity gradient between the renal artery and external iliac artery greater than 2:1.

Intraparenchymal arterial stenosis may be observed in chronic rejection as a result of scarring in the tissues surrounding the involved vessels. On spectral Doppler ultrasound, a prolonged acceleration time may be observed in the segmental and interlobar arteries, with a normal main renal artery waveform.[43]

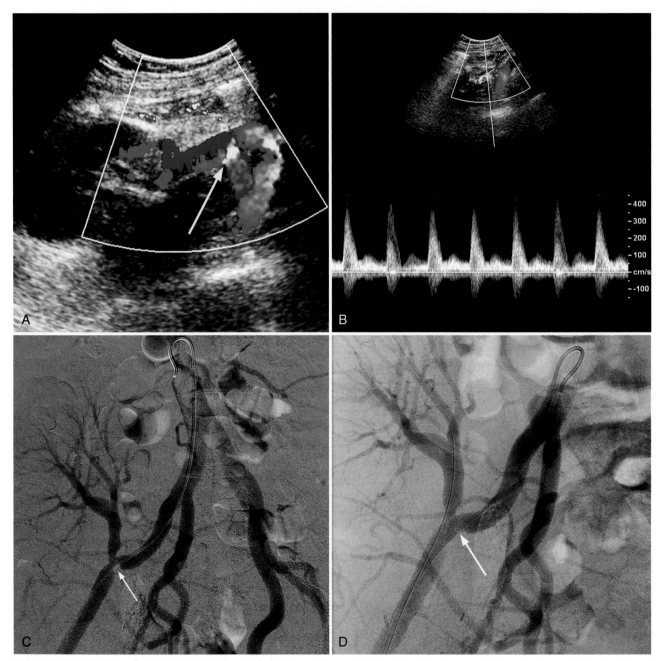

FIGURE 17-42. Renal artery stenosis: recipient portion. A, Color Doppler ultrasound shows focal area of aliasing *(arrow)* proximal to the renal artery anastomosis. **B,** Spectral Doppler of the region of aliasing seen in image **A** shows angle-corrected peak velocities of 400 cm/sec. **C,** Angiography shows a focal area of stenosis *(arrow)* arising from the external iliac artery. **D,** Angiogram performed after angioplasty shows resolution of the stenotic region *(arrow).*

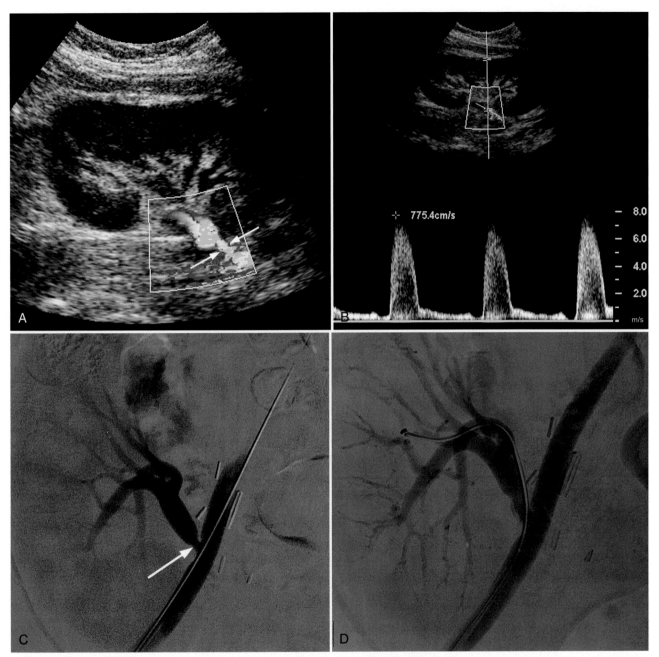

FIGURE 17-43. Renal artery stenosis: anastomosis. A, Color Doppler ultrasound shows focal area of narrowing and aliasing at the anastomosis *(arrows).* **B,** Spectral Doppler at the anastomosis shows elevated angle-corrected velocity of 775.4 cm/sec. **C,** Renal arterial angiogram confirms stenosis at the anastomosis *(arrow).* **D,** Angiogram performed after angioplasty shows resolution of the anastomotic stenosis.

Treatment options for renal artery stenosis include percutaneous transluminal angioplasty, endovascular stent placement, and surgery. Surgical management of these transplants involves resection and revision of the stenosis with insertion of a patch graft at the stenotic segment.[44]

A **false-positive Doppler diagnosis** of renal artery stenosis may occur if there is an abrupt turn in the main renal artery, if the artery is severely tortuous, or if there are errors in Doppler technique (Fig. 17-44). Inadvertent compression of the main renal artery by the sonog-rapher while performing spectral interrogation may also produce transient narrowing of the artery and elevated PSV readings.

Venous Thrombosis

Occlusive renal vein thrombosis is slightly more common than arterial thrombosis, occurring in up to 4% of transplants, and is associated with acute pain, swelling of the allograft, and an abrupt cessation of renal function between the third and eighth postoperative day. Risk

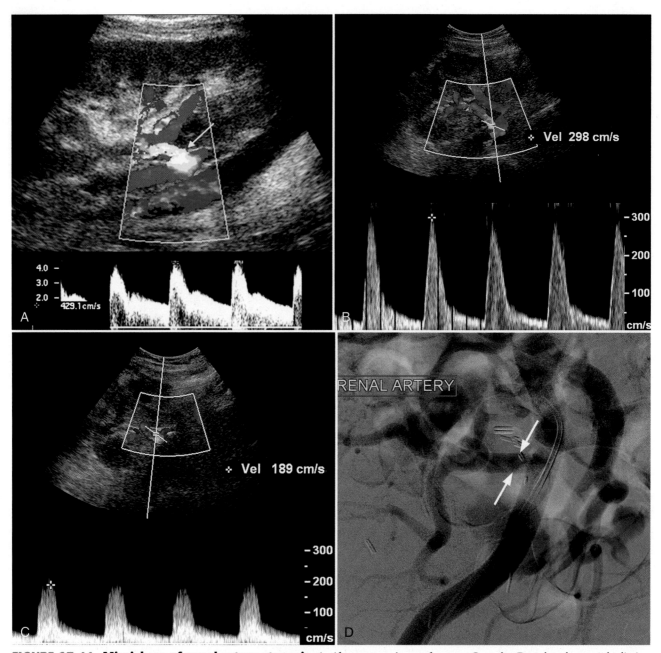

FIGURE 17-44. Mimickers of renal artery stenosis. A, Abrupt turn in renal artery. On color Doppler ultrasound, aliasing is identified in this region *(arrow),* with peak systolic velocities of 429 cm/sec on spectral Doppler. **B to D, Misaligned angle correction. B,** Initial spectral Doppler shows elevated renal artery anastomotic velocity of 298 cm/sec. This elevated velocity reading is artifactual because the spectral angle correction is not aligned with the direction of the renal artery. **C,** Follow-up spectral Doppler ultrasound shows a normal renal artery velocity of 189 cm/sec, with appropriate angle correction in the direction of the artery. **D,** Renal angiogram confirms a normal renal artery *(arrows)* with no evidence of stenosis.

factors include technical difficulties at surgery, hypovolemia, propagation of femoral or iliac thrombosis, and compression by fluid collections.[53,58]

On gray-scale ultrasound, the allograft may appear enlarged, and in rare cases, intraluminal thrombus may be detected in a dilated main renal vein or within the intraparenchymal venous system. More consistently, spectral and color Doppler ultrasound show a lack of venous flow in the renal parenchyma, absence of flow in the main renal vein, and reversal of diastolic flow in the

main renal artery, as well as sometimes in the intraparenchymal arteries[59,60] (Fig. 17-45). The sonographer should be aware that **reversal of flow in diastole in the main renal artery** or the intraparenchymal arterial branches is highly suggestive of renal vein thrombosis *only in the absence of venous flow* in the renal parenchyma and main renal vein.

Reversed diastolic arterial flow, *with preservation of venous flow,* is a nonspecific finding indicating extremely high vascular resistance in the small intrarenal vessels or

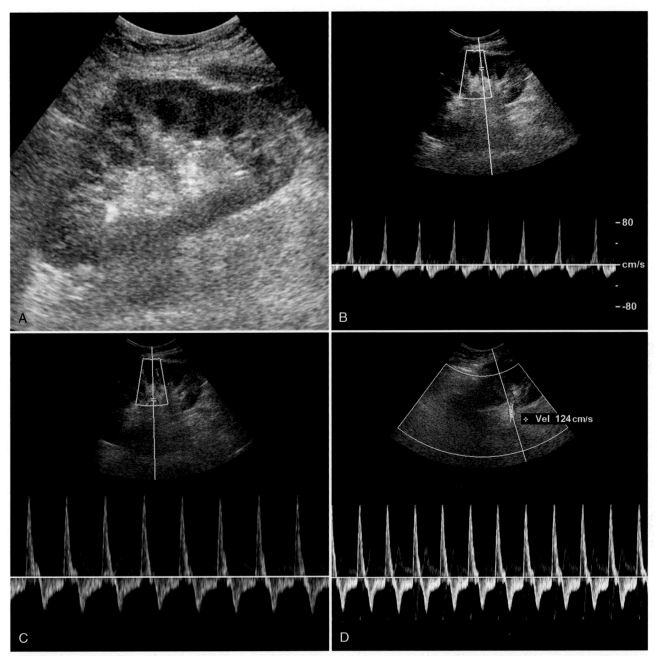

FIGURE 17-45. Renal vein thrombosis. A, Sagittal sonogram shows increased cortical echogenicity with a coarse echotexture. **B to D,** Spectral Doppler ultrasound images of cortical arteries **(B),** renal sinus arterial branches **(C),** and main renal artery **(D)** show reversal of flow in diastole. No venous flow was detected in the transplant.

main hilar vessels. The outcome for these patients is generally poor, with reported allograft loss rates of 33% to 55%. Potential causes of reversed diastolic flow in these patients include acute rejection, ATN, peritransplant hematomas (compressing renal graft or hilar vessels) and glomerulosclerosis.[61]

Renal Vein Stenosis

Renal vein stenosis most often occurs from perivascular fibrosis or external compression by adjacent fluid collections. The renal cortex appears either normal or hypoechoic, and on color Doppler, aliasing is identified at the stenotic region because of focal, high-velocity turbulent flow. On spectral Doppler sonography, a threefold to fourfold increase in velocity across the region of narrowing indicates a hemodynamically significant stenosis[57] (Fig. 17-46).

Postrenal Collecting System Obstruction

Collecting system obstruction is unusual in renal transplants, occurring in less than 5% of patients.[43,57] Because

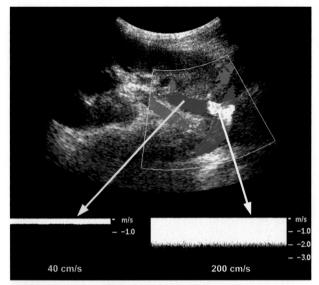

FIGURE 17-46. Renal vein stenosis. Color Doppler of renal vein anastomosis shows focal area of aliasing *(white arrow).* Spectral interrogation in region of aliasing shows velocities of 200 cm/sec. Spectral interrogation proximal to aliasing shows velocities of 40 cm/sec *(yellow arrow),* indicating a hemodynamically significant stenosis of the renal vein.

the allograft is denervated, the collecting system dilates without clinical signs of pain or discomfort. The diagnosis is often made as an incidental finding on routine screening sonography or in the workup of the transplant patient for asymptomatic deterioration of renal function parameters.

The most common cause of **ureteral obstruction** is from ischemic strictures, usually involving the terminal ureter at the ureterovesical junction. The transplanted ureter is particularly susceptible to ischemic events because of its limited vascular supply from the renal artery. The ureterovesical junction is usually the region of most pronounced involvement because it is farthest anatomically from the renal hilum, where the ureteral branch originates.[44] Other causes of ureteral obstruction include strictures from iatrogenic injury, intraluminal lesions (e.g., stones, blood clots, sloughed papillae), perigraft fibrosis, and ureteral kinking (Figs. 17-47 and 17-48). Extrinsic compression of the ureter from peritransplant collections can also result in collecting system obstruction.

Evaluation of the collecting system with fundamental gray-scale imaging may be difficult because of side-lobe

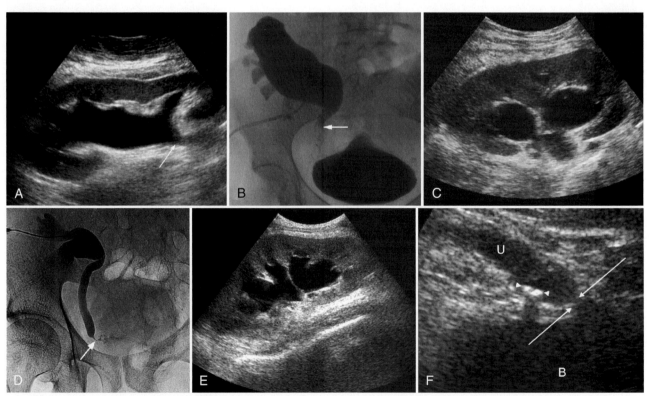

FIGURE 17-47. Ureteral strictures. A, Sagittal sonogram, and **B,** percutaneous nephrostogram, show grade 3 pelvocaliectasis secondary to a stricture at the **ureteropelvic junction** *(arrow).* **C,** Sagittal sonogram shows grade 4 pelvocaliectasis. The distal ureter was not seen on ultrasound. **D,** Percutaneous nephrostogram shows a stricture at the **ureterovesicular junction** *(arrow).* **E,** Sagittal sonogram shows grade 3 pelvocaliectasis, produced by **F,** a stricture at the **ureterovesicular junction** *(arrows); arrowheads,* tiny nonobstructing stone; *B,* bladder; *U,* ureter.

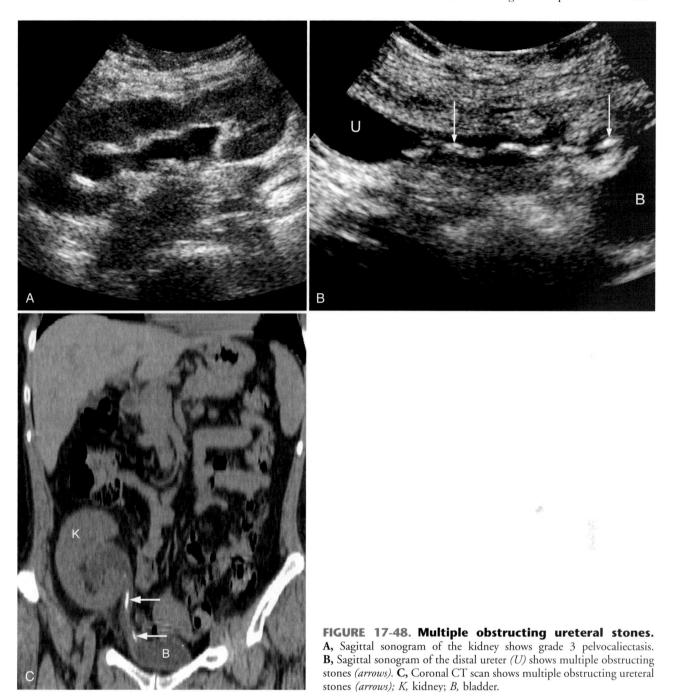

FIGURE 17-48. Multiple obstructing ureteral stones.
A, Sagittal sonogram of the kidney shows grade 3 pelvocaliectasis.
B, Sagittal sonogram of the distal ureter *(U)* shows multiple obstructing
stones *(arrows).* **C,** Coronal CT scan shows multiple obstructing ureteral
stones *(arrows); K,* kidney; *B,* bladder.

and scatter artifact, which can potentially obscure
optimal evaluation of the calyceal system and ureter.
Harmonic imaging, however, uses a narrower ultrasound
beam with smaller side lobes and is less susceptible to
scatter artifact. These parameters make harmonic imaging
ideal for evaluating anechoic structures, such as the renal
collecting system for regions of subtle dilation, and the
presence of **small intraluminal stones** (Fig. 17-49).

Mild pelvocaliectasis may be secondary to nonobstructive causes such as overhydration, decreased ureteric
tone (from denervation of transplant), and ureteric-ves-
ical reflux or can occur transiently in the immediate

postoperative period from perianastomotic edema.[43,62] In
addition, multiple parapelvic cysts can mimic a dilated
collecting system (Fig. 17-50).

Arteriovenous Malformations and Pseudoaneurysms

Intraparenchymal arteriovenous malformations (AVMs)
result from vascular trauma to both artery and vein
during percutaneous biopsies and are usually asymptomatic with little clinical significance. Because most of these
are small and resolve spontaneously, the precise inci-

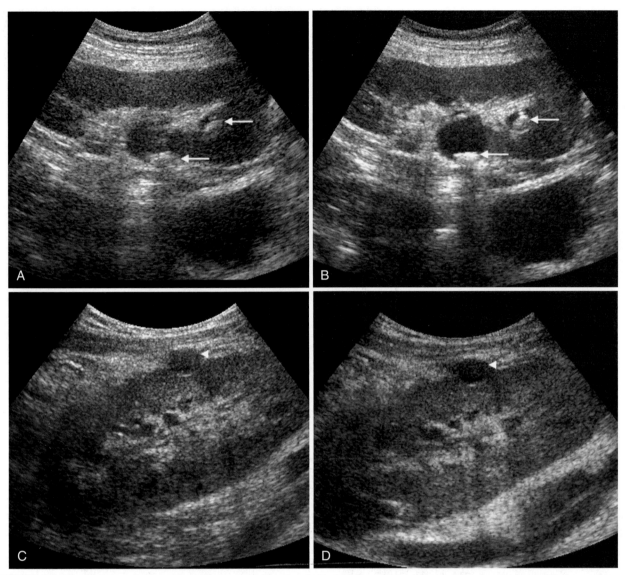

FIGURE 17-49. Harmonic imaging in two patients. A, Sagittal fundamental image shows barely detectable stones *(arrows)* and a dilated collecting system. **B,** Harmonic image shows improved resolution of stones *(arrows),* now seen associated with distal acoustic shadowing, within anechoic dilated collecting system. **C,** Fundamental image shows cortical cyst *(arrowhead)* with internal echoes and minimal through transmission. **D,** Harmonic image shows cyst *(arrowhead)* to be anechoic and simple, now associated with an appropriate amount of through-transmission.

dence of posttransplant AVMs is unknown, although rates of 1% to 18% have been reported. In rare cases, large AVMs may present with bleeding, high-output cardiac failure, or decreased renal perfusion caused by the large shunt. In these patients, treatment usually involves percutaneous embolization therapy.[42]

Gray-scale ultrasound may not reveal small AVMs. Color Doppler sonography shows a focal region of aliasing with a myriad of intense colors, often associated with a prominent feeding artery or draining vein. Turbulent flow within the AVM produces vibration of the perivascular tissues, resulting in these tissues being assigned a color signal outside the borders of the renal vasculature. Spectral Doppler ultrasound is typical of that for all AVMs, with low-resistance, high-velocity flow and dif-

ficulty differentiating between artery and vein within the malformation. If a dominant draining vein is detected, the waveform may be pulsatile or arterialized[53,62-64] (Fig. 17-51).

On color Doppler ultrasound, focal regions of cortical dystrophic calcifications or small stones can mimic an AVM by producing an intense color signal known as a **twinkling artifact.**[65] These artifacts can be differentiated from a true AVM on spectral tracing because both calcifications and stones produce characteristic linear bands on spectral interrogation. In our clinical experience, we have also observed a linear band of color posterior to these regions of calcium that extend to the limits of the color box. We have not observed this phenomenon with AVMs and have found it a useful tool in

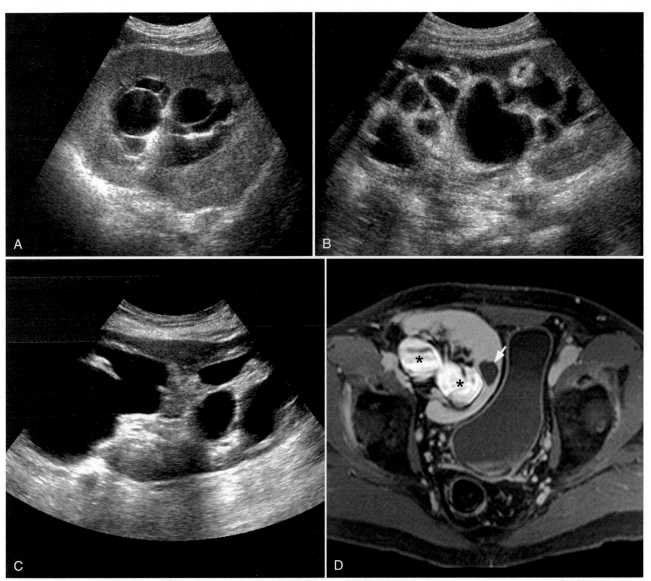

FIGURE 17-50. Parapelvic cysts versus pelvocaliectasis in two patients. *Patient 1:* **Parapelvic cysts. A,** Transverse, and **B,** sagittal, sonograms show multiple parapelvic cysts mimicking pelvocaliectasis. *Patient 2:* **Grade 3 pelvocaliectasis mimicking parapelvic cysts. C,** Sagittal sonogram shows multiple anechoic structures in the central aspect of the kidney, initially interpreted as multiple parapelvic cysts. **D,** Contrast-enhanced MRI shows contrast filling grossly dilated calyces (*). A single parapelvic cyst *(arrow)* is present.

differentiating vascular malformations from focal calcifications (Fig. 17-52).

Pseudoaneurysms result from vascular trauma to the arterial system during percutaneous biopsy or, more frequently, occur at the site of the vascular anastomosis. Pseudoaneurysms may be intrarenal or extrarenal in location (Figs. 17-53 and 17-54). On gray-scale sonography, pseudoaneurysms can mimic a simple or complex cyst. On color Doppler ultrasound, flow can easily be obtained in the lumen of patent pseudoaneurysms, often with a swirling pattern, whereas on spectral Doppler, a central to-and-fro waveform or a disorganized arterial tracing may be obtained.[43] **We suggest that any cyst identified in the renal parenchyma, or in the region of the** **hilum, be assessed with color Doppler to exclude the possibility of a pseudoaneurysm.**

Fluid Collections

Perinephric collections are demonstrated in up to 50% of transplant recipients.[66,67] The most common collections include hematoma, urinoma, lymphocele, and abscess. The ultrasound appearances of these peritransplant collections are often nonspecific, and clinical findings are warranted to determine their etiology. However, the presence of air within a perirenal collection, without a history of recent percutaneous intervention, is highly suggestive of an **abscess.** The size and location of each

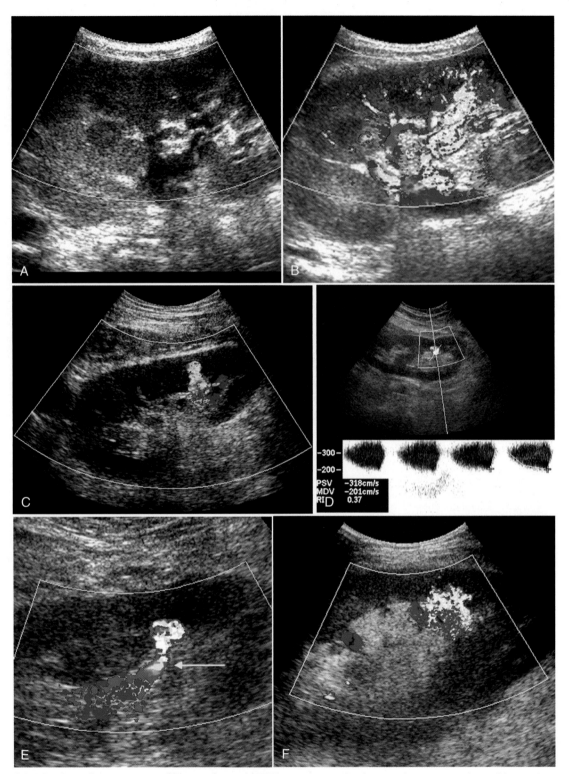

FIGURE 17-51. Arteriovenous malformations (AVM). A, Gray-scale ultrasound; AVM not detectable. **B,** Corresponding color Doppler image shows large AVM. **C,** Sagittal sonogram shows lower-pole AVM. **D,** Spectral Doppler of AVM in image **C** shows high-velocity, low-resistance waveform. **E,** Sagittal sonogram shows AVM with feeding vessel *(arrow)*. **F,** Sagittal scan shows lower-pole AVM with surrounding tissue vibration.

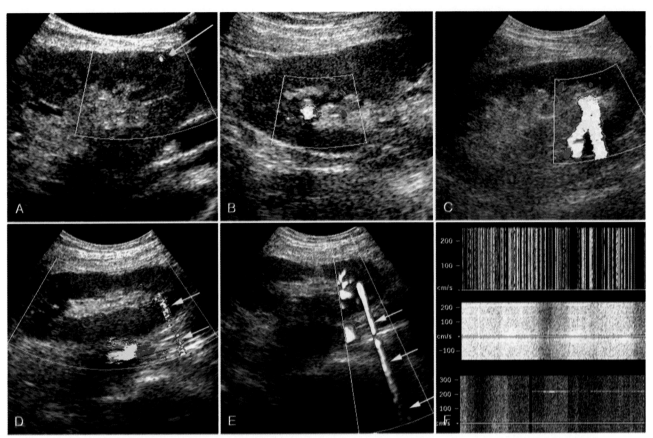

FIGURE 17-52. Arteriovenous malformation: mimicker. A to **C,** Sagittal sonograms show **twinkling artifact** produced by **A,** lower-pole dystrophic cortical calcification *(arrow);* **B,** upper-pole stone; and **C,** lower-pole stone. **D** to **F, Differentiation from AVM.** On **D,** color Doppler and **E,** power Doppler, color artifact *(arrows)* may be seen posterior to border of kidney. Size of twinkling artifact varies with size of the color box. **F,** On spectral Doppler ultrasound, the twinkling artifact shows linear bands as on these three spectral traces.

collection should be documented on baseline scans because an increase in size may indicate the need for surgical intervention.

Postoperative **hematomas** are variable in size but are often small, perirenal in location, insignificant clinically, and resolve spontaneously.[62] Their ultrasound appearance depends on the age of the collection. Acutely, hematomas appear as an echogenic heterogeneous solid mass. With time they liquefy, becoming a complex cystic structure with internal echoes, strands, or septations. Postbiopsy hematomas have a similar morphology as their postoperative counterparts (Figs. 17-55 and 17-56).

Urine leaks, or **urinomas,** have been reported in up to 6% of renal transplants and occur within the first 2 weeks after surgery.[42] They are usually secondary to either anastomotic leaks or ureteric ischemia. Rarely, urinomas can result from high-grade collecting system obstruction (Fig. 17-57). On sonography, urinomas are well defined and anechoic, may be associated with hydronephrosis, and in some cases can increase rapidly in size.[54] Large urine leaks may result in widespread extravasation and gross intraperitoneal urinary ascites.

Lymphoceles result from surgical disruption of the iliac lymphatics and have been reported in up to 20% of patients. They most often occur 4 to 8 weeks after surgery but may develop years after transplantation. Although most are discovered incidentally and are asymptomatic, lymphoceles are the most common fluid collection to result in ureteric obstruction. Lymphoceles can become infected or can obstruct venous drainage, resulting in edema of the lower limb, scrotum, or labia.[43] Symptomatic collections are drained (surgically or percutaneously) or undergo marsupialization. On sonography, lymphoceles are well-defined collections that are anechoic or that may contain fine internal strands (Figs. 17-58 and 17-59).

PANCREAS TRANSPLANTATION

Pancreatic transplantation is performed in select patients who have major complications related to type 1 diabetes. Pancreas transplant represents the only form of self-regulating endocrine replacement therapy, with more than 80% of recipients becoming free of exogenous

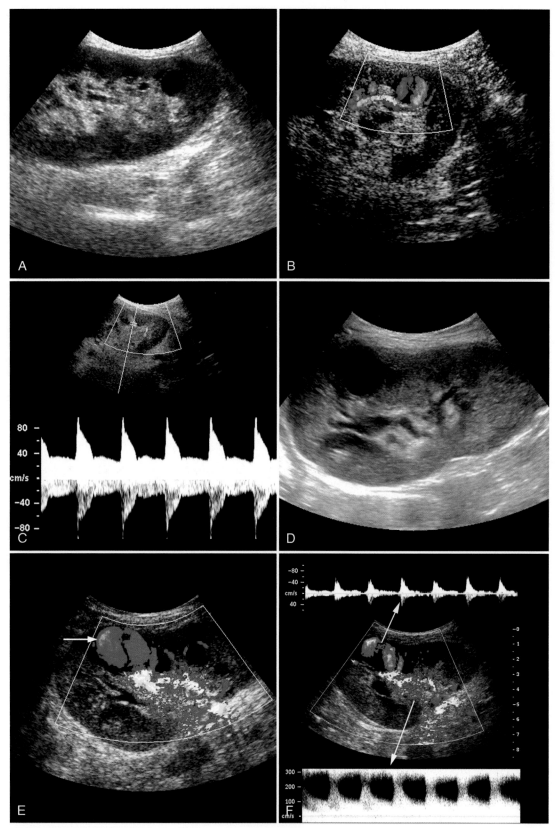

FIGURE 17-53. Intrarenal pseudoaneurysms in two patients. *Patient 1:* **A,** Sagittal sonogram shows lower-pole anechoic structure, mimicking a simple cyst. **B,** On color Doppler ultrasound, however, swirling flow is identified in this structure, indicating that it represents a pseudoaneurysm. **C,** Spectral Doppler ultrasound shows disorganized swirling flow within the pseudoaneurysm identified on image **B.** *Patient 2:* **D,** Sagittal sonogram shows upper-pole anechoic structure. **E,** On color Doppler ultrasound, swirling flow is identified in the anechoic structure identified on image **D** *(arrow).* This is adjacent to a large central AVM. **F,** Spectral Doppler ultrasound shows disorganized flow in the pseudoaneurysm *(yellow arrow)* and low-resistance high-velocity flow in the central AVM *(white arrow).*

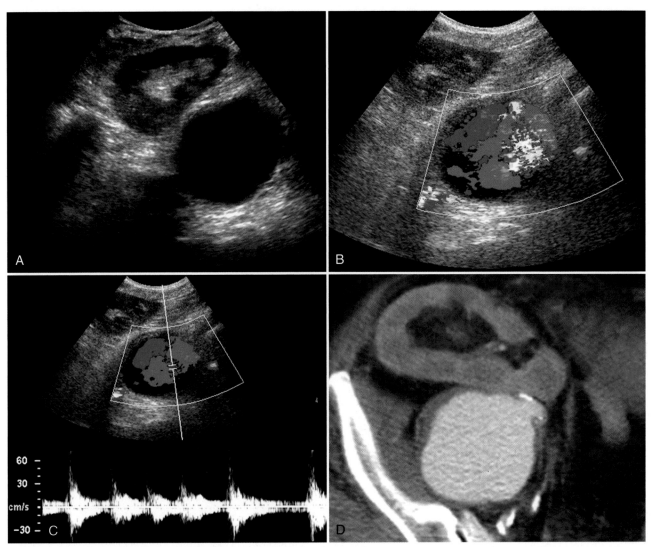

FIGURE 17-54. Extrarenal pseudoaneurysm of renal artery. A, Transverse sonogram shows anechoic structure adjacent to renal hilum. **B,** Color Doppler ultrasound shows that this structure contains swirling flow and represents a pseudoaneurysm. **C,** Spectral Doppler ultrasound shows disorganized internal flow within pseudoaneurysm. **D,** CT scan shows pseudoaneurysm arising from site of renal artery anastomosis.

insulin requirements within 1 year of surgery. Since 1988 in the United States, more than 15,000 kidney-pancreas transplants and 6000 pancreas transplants have been performed, with 1-year patient survival greater than 90%.[3,4]

Surgical Technique

Since the first pancreas transplant was performed in 1966, several surgical techniques have been described. The two most common pancreatic transplant surgeries involve transplantation of the entire gland, with an arterial anastomosis to the recipient common iliac artery. However, the techniques differ primarily in their exocrine drainage.[3,68]

The more traditional surgery, **exocrine bladder drainage**, involves anastomosing the donor duodenum to the urinary bladder and the donor portal vein to the recipient external iliac vein (systemic venous-endocrine drainage)[68] (Fig. 17-60). The chronic loss of pancreatic secretions into the bladder can result in problems with dehydration, metabolic acidosis, local bladder irritation, and allograft pancreatitis.[3]

A more recent technique, **exocrine enteric drainage,** is becoming more widely utilized and involves anastomosing the donor duodenum to a Roux-en-Y loop of jejunum. The endocrine drainage is either systemic (anastomosis of donor portal vein to right common iliac vein or distal IVC) or portal venous (anastomosis of donor portal vein to superior mesenteric vein) (Fig. 17-61). This type of surgery provides a more physiologic transplant than the more traditional techniques and is not associated with dehydration or metabolic acidosis. In addition, it provides more appropriate glycemic control, with lower fasting insulin levels, and may be

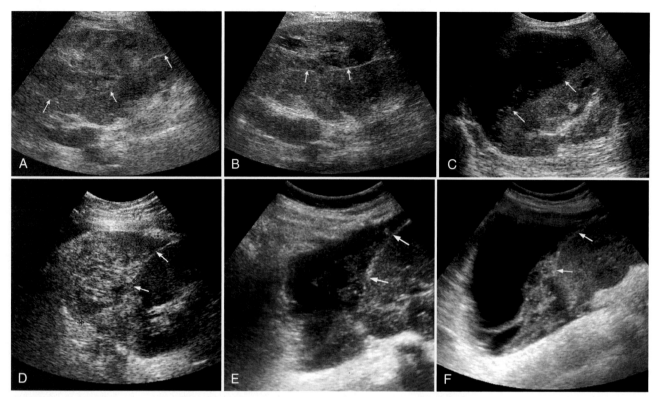

FIGURE 17-55. Renal transplant hematomas in two patients. A, Subcapsular hematoma secondary to biopsy. Sagittal sonogram shows acute hematoma appearing as solid heterogeneous structure. **B,** After 1 week, cystic regions develop within the hematoma. **C,** After 1 month, hematoma liquefies and is larger because of a hyperosmolar effect. **D to F, Postoperative perirenal hematoma. D,** Sagittal sonogram shows hematoma 1 day after surgery, appearing as a solid echogenic heterogeneous mass. **E,** Four weeks later, hematoma begins to liquefy, with interspersed solid components. **F,** Six weeks later, hematoma is almost completely liquefied; arrows mark the junction of the hematoma and renal cortex.

TABLE 17-1. SURGICAL TECHNIQUES FOR PANCREATIC TRANSPLANTATION

	Systemic Venous-Bladder Drainage	Portal Venous-Enteric Drainage
Location	Right lower quadrant	Right upper quadrant
Pancreatic orientation	Head caudad	Tail caudad
Arterial supply	Y-shaped donor arterial graft anastomosed to recipient common iliac artery	Donor splenic artery to recipient common iliac artery
Venous drainage	Donor portal vein is attached to external iliac vein	Donor portal vein anastomosed to superior mesenteric vein
Endocrine drainage	Systemic venous	Portal venous
Exocrine drainage	En bloc donor duodenal stump to recipient bladder	Duodenal segment anastomosed to Roux-en-Y loop of jejunum

associated with a lower incidence of transplant rejection than the more traditional systemic venous-bladder drainage allografts.[3,69] Table 17-1 shows the major differences between two types of pancreatic transplants (exocrine bladder drainage and exocrine enteric drainage).

Normal Pancreas Transplant Ultrasound

To perform an ultrasound assessment of a transplanted pancreas, the sonographer should be aware of the surgical technique used, the position of the allograft in the abdomen at surgery, and the sites of vascular anastomosis. This often entails a detailed review of the intraoperative surgical notes or discussion with the surgeon before scanning the patient.

Systemic venous-bladder drainage transplants are usually located in the right lower quadrant and may show a diagonal or horizontal axis. **Portal venous-enteric drainage** transplants are usually in the right upper quadrant or right paramedian region with a vertical axis. In

Text continued on p. 694.

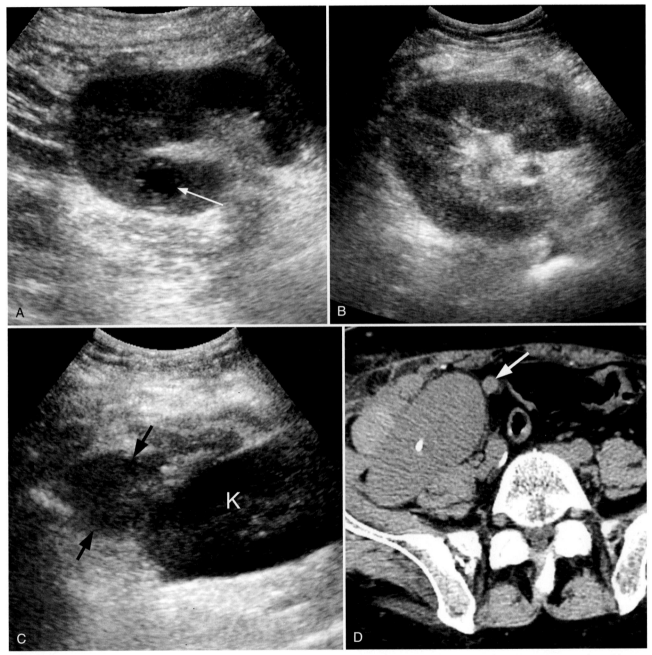

FIGURE 17-56. Atypical hematomas in two patients. *Patient 1:* **A,** Transverse sonogram shows an intraparenchymal hematoma presenting as an anechoic cyst with mildly irregular walls *(arrow).* **B,** Eight months later, the cyst resolves. *Patient 2:* **C,** Sagittal sonogram shows a hypoechoic solid-appearing mass *(arrows)* abutting the upper pole of the transplant kidney *(K).* **D,** Follow-up CT scan shows that this represents a hematoma *(arrow).*

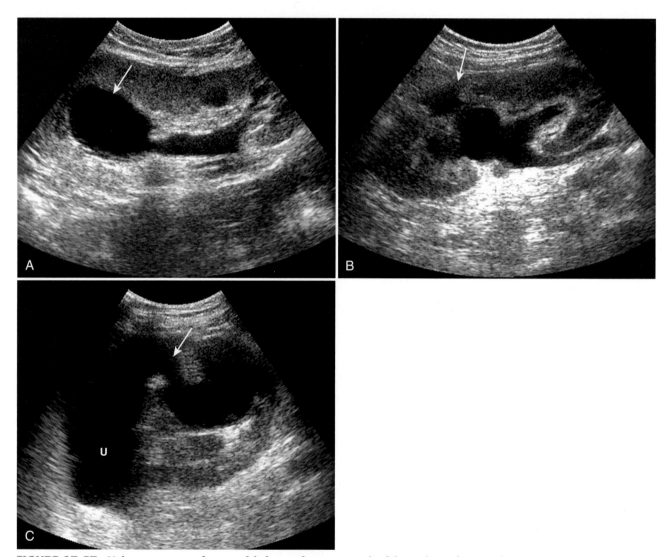

FIGURE 17-57. Urinoma secondary to high-grade uterovesical junction obstruction. A, Sagittal sonogram shows dilation of upper-pole calyx *(arrow)*. **B,** Dilation eventually ruptures through the adjacent cortex *(arrow)*. **C,** Obstruction forms a cortical defect *(arrow)* and subsequently a perinephric urinoma *(U)*.

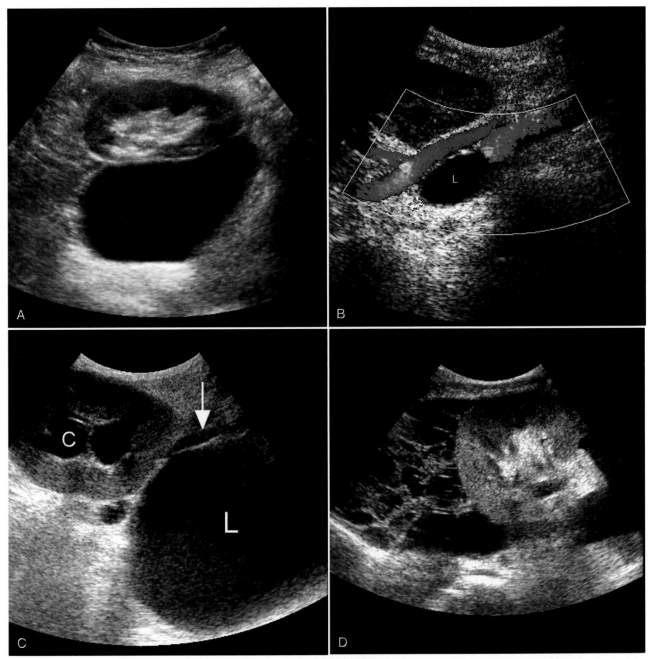

FIGURE 17-58. Sterile lymphoceles in four patients. A, Sagittal sonogram shows large, simple lymphocele abutting the transplant. **B,** Sagittal scan shows small lymphocele *(L)* adjacent to the external iliac artery and vein. **C,** Anechoic lymphocele *(L)* causes obstruction of the midureter *(arrow)* and dilation of the calyceal system *(C)*. **D,** Transverse sonogram shows septated perinephric lymphocele.

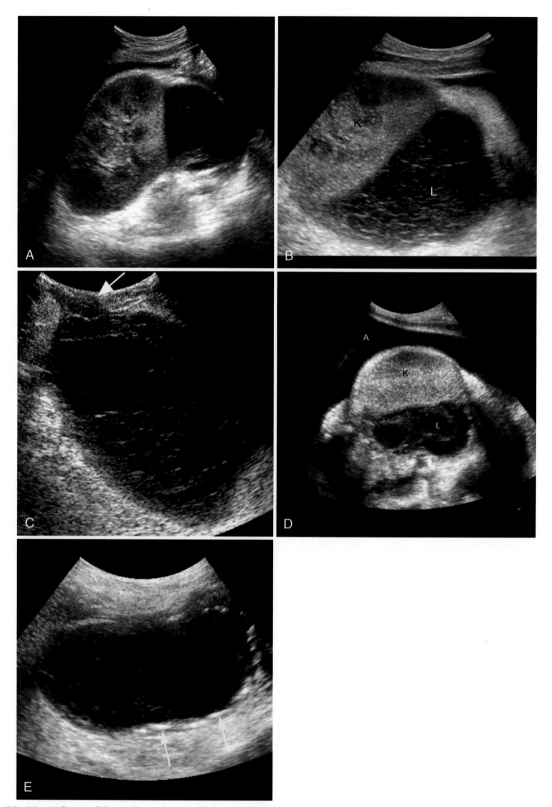

FIGURE 17-59. Infected lymphoceles in five patients. Sagittal sonograms show infected lymphoceles with **A,** a few thin internal strands; **B,** multiple internal strands; **C,** internal strands, draining to the skin through a cutaneous fistula *(arrow);* **D,** thick septations and internal echoes; and **E,** internal echoes and punctate wall calcifications *(arrows); L,* lymphocele; *K,* kidney; *A,* ascites.

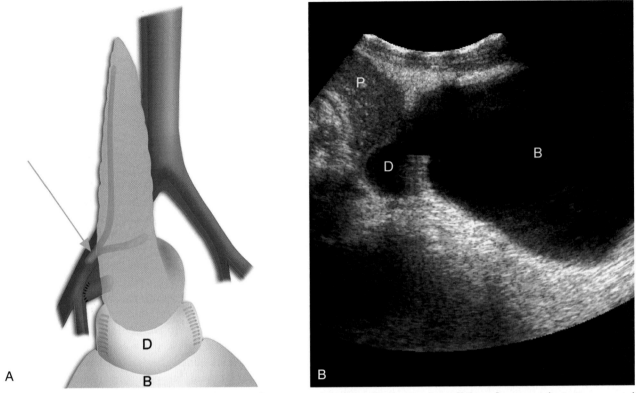

FIGURE 17-60. Pancreas transplant: systemic venous-bladder drainage (traditional surgery). A, Donor portal vein *(purple)* is anastomosed to the external iliac vein, and donor artery Y graft *(coral arrow)* to the external iliac artery. Duodenal stump *(D)* is anastomosed to the bladder *(B)*. **B,** Sagittal sonogram shows duodenal stump anastomosed to the bladder *(B); P,* pancreas.

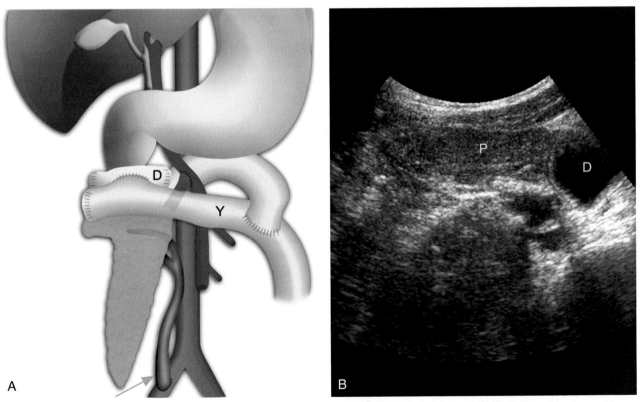

FIGURE 17-61. Pancreas transplant: portal venous-enteric drainage (new technique). A, Donor portal vein *(purple)* is anastomosed to the superior mesenteric vein *(blue),* and donor artery *(arrow)* is anastomosed to the common iliac artery. Duodenal stump *(D)* is anastomosed to a Roux-en-Y *(Y)*. **B,** Transverse sonogram shows pancreas transplant *(P)* with fluid-filled duodenal stump *(D).*

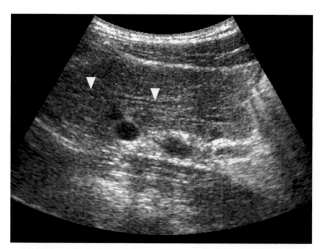

FIGURE 17-62. Normal pancreas transplant. Gray-scale ultrasound of pancreas transplant shows normal echogenicity and echotexture of allograft, with nondilated pancreatic duct (*arrowheads*).

both cases the allograft may be difficult to visualize because of overlying bowel gas; however, meticulous scanning with intermittent compression of the overlying intraluminal gas is frequently successful in visualizing the transplant. In our experience, although the normal pancreatic transplant may be obscured, both inflammation of the graft and perigraft fluid collections facilitate pancreatic visualization.

The normal allograft retains its normal gray-scale morphology with well-defined margins; a homogeneous echotexture, isoechoic or minimally echogenic to liver; and a thin, nondilated pancreatic duct (Fig. 17-62). The peripancreatic fat shows a normal echogenicity. Occasionally, a trace amount of peripancreatic fluid may be observed and usually resolves without complication. Color Doppler ultrasound is useful for locating the mesenteric vessels, particularly when the graft is poorly visualized because of overlying bowel gas. Spectral Doppler sonography of the normal graft shows continuous monophasic venous flow and low-resistance arterial waveforms.

Abnormal Pancreas Transplant

Vascular Thrombosis

Graft thrombosis, including both venous and arterial thrombosis, occurs with a reported incidence of 2% to 19% and is the second leading cause of transplant loss, after rejection. Pancreatic transplants are more vulnerable to graft thrombosis than renal transplants because the rate of blood flow in the transplanted pancreas is slower than that in a transplanted kidney.[70,71]

Although the clinical signs and symptoms of graft thrombosis are nonspecific, detection of vascular thrombosis is imperative for both salvaging the transplant and preventing life-threatening sequelae, such as sepsis and cardiovascular collapse. Venous thrombosis, which occurs with an estimated incidence of 5%, is a particular concern because of the increased risk of hemorrhagic pancreatitis, tissue necrosis, infection, thrombus propagation, and pulmonary embolism.[71]

Graft thrombosis can be categorized as early or late, depending on the time of diagnosis after surgery. **Early** graft thrombosis occurs within 1 month of transplantation and is secondary to either microvascular injury during preservation of the graft or technical error during surgery. **Late** graft thrombosis occurs 1 month after transplant surgery and is usually caused by **alloimmune arteritis,** in which gradual occlusion of the small blood vessels eventually culminates in complete proximal vessel occlusion.[70] Other technical factors predisposing to graft thrombosis include coagulopathies, long preservation time, poor donor vessels, left-sided graft placement resulting in a deeper anastomosis, and the use of a venous extension graft.[71]

On ultrasound, occlusive or nonocclusive thrombus may be visualized within the lumen of the transplanted arteries or veins (Fig. 17-63). We have also observed several cases of thrombus occurring at the suture line of blind-ending arteries or veins (Fig. 17-64). On spectral Doppler, no arterial flow is detected in transplants with occlusive arterial thrombus. In grafts with occlusive venous thrombus, a lack of venous flow is detected on spectral tracing, with high-resistance arterial flow showing either no flow in diastole (RI = 1) or reversal of diastolic flow.[71] Surgically ligated arteries containing thrombus may show a cyclic pattern of flow adjacent to the thrombus, which we presume is secondary to local eddy currents, with a normal arterial waveform more proximally.

Arteriovenous Fistula and Pseudoaneurysms

Arteriovenous fistulas and pseudoaneurysms are rare complications of pancreatic transplants and may be related to the blind ligation of mesenteric vessels along the inferior border of the pancreas during retrieval. In some patients, mycotic pseudoaneurysms may occur in the setting of graft infection.[72]

On gray-scale ultrasound, **arterial malformations** may not be detectable. On color Doppler sonography, however, a mosaic of intense colors may be identified, produced by the tangle of vessels within the malformation and adjacent tissue vibration. Spectral Doppler ultrasound reveals high-velocity, low-resistance flow within the lesion, which is typical of arteriovenous shunting (Fig. 17-65). On gray-scale ultrasound, **pseudoaneurysms** usually appear as anechoic spherical structures, although mural-based intraluminal thrombus may be detected. On spectral Doppler ultrasound, the classic to-and-fro pattern may be observed.

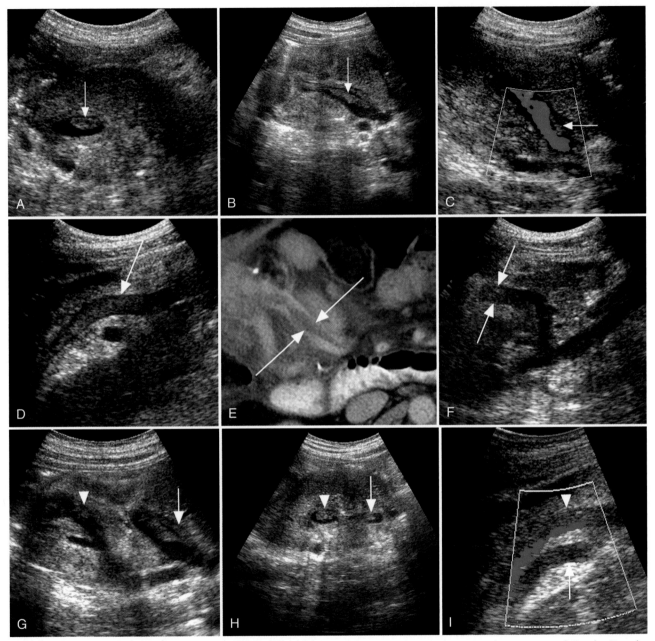

FIGURE 17-63. Graft thrombosis in different patients. A, Transverse sonogram; **B,** sagittal sonogram; and **C,** color Doppler image, show nonocclusive venous thrombus *(arrows).* **D,** Gray-scale ultrasound *(arrow),* and **E,** correlative CT scan *(arrows),* show nonocclusive venous thrombus. **F,** Sagittal sonogram shows occlusive arterial thrombus *(arrows).* **G,** Sagittal sonogram; **H,** transverse sonogram; and **I,** color Doppler image, show nonocclusive venous *(arrowhead)* and arterial *(arrow)* thrombus in the same transplant.

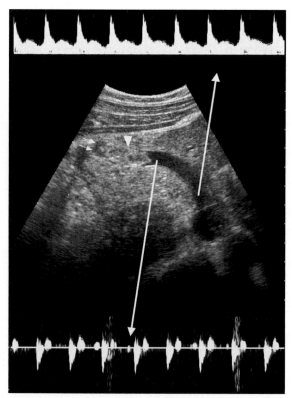

FIGURE 17-64. Thrombus adjacent to suture line.
Echogenic thrombus *(arrowhead)* at suture line *(small arrows)* of blind-ending ligated artery. Spectral trace adjacent to thrombus shows to-and-fro waveform *(bottom),* whereas spectral trace *(top)* more distally is normal.

Rejection

Rejection is the most common cause of pancreatic graft loss after transplantation. Early recognition of transplant rejection remains a challenge because clinical parameters used to evaluate pancreas graft dysfunction have low sensitivity and specificity in detection of rejection. In particular, there is no individual biochemical marker that would permit acute rejection to be distinguished from vascular thrombosis or pancreatitis.

On gray-scale ultrasound, the allograft may appear hypoechoic or may contain multiple anechoic regions, and the parenchymal echotexture may be patchy and heterogeneous[73,74] (Fig. 17-66). The utility of arterial resistive indices (RIs) as an indicator of rejection appears controversial. It has been shown that RIs of the arteries supplying the pancreatic transplant cannot differentiate allografts with mild or moderate rejection from normal transplants without rejection.[75] The reason may be that the pancreatic transplant does not contain a discrete investing capsule, and therefore swelling from transplant rejection may not necessarily result in increased parenchymal pressures or elevated vascular resistance.[76] Grossly elevated RIs greater than 0.8 have been observed in pancreatic allografts with biopsy-proven acute severe rejection. Although these elevated RIs may be sensitive, they are not specific in the detection of severe pancreatic transplant rejection.[75]

Pancreatitis

Almost all patients develop symptoms of pancreatitis immediately after surgery, presumably caused by preservation injury and ischemia.[76] Other causes of pancreatitis include partial or complete occlusion of the pancreatic duct, poor perfusion of the allograft, and in those patients with systemic venous-bladder drainage, reflux-related pancreatitis.[73]

The ultrasound appearance of pancreatitis in the allograft is **similar to that of pancreatitis in the native gland** (Fig. 17-67). Gray-scale findings include a normal-sized or bulky edematous pancreas, poorly defined margins, increased echogenicity of the peripancreatic fat secondary to surrounding inflammation, peripancreatic fluid, and thickening of the adjacent gut wall. In cases of pancreatitis resulting from ductal obstruction, a dilated pancreatic duct may be observed.[73,76] In nonacute cases of pancreatitis, pseudocysts adjacent to or distal from the transplant may be identified, usually appearing as a complex cystic structure.

Fluid Collections

Peripancreatic transplant-related fluid collections may be associated with an increased likelihood of loss of allograft function and overall increased mortality and morbidity in the recipient. Early diagnosis and characterization of these collections are imperative, because treatment in the acute stages has been associated with improved graft function and decreased recipient morbidity.[77]

In the immediate postoperative period, peritransplant fluid may be caused by leakage of pancreatic fluid from transected ductules and lymphatics, an inflammatory exudate, blood, or urine (Fig. 17-68). These collections may require either close serial imaging follow-up or drainage, depending on the clinical status of the patient.

Duodenal leaks in **systemic venous-bladder drainage** transplants occur from dehiscence of the duodenal-bladder anastomosis and result in the formation of urinomas, frequently at the medial aspect of the transplant. Urinomas may also result from infection or necrosis of the graft.[77]

Duodenal leaks in **portal venous-enteric drainage** transplants occur at the blind end of the donor duodenum or from the anastomosis with the recipient Roux-en-Y loop. On ultrasound, gross ascites, duodenal wall thickening, or free intraperitoneal air may be observed in patients with breakdown of the duodenal anastomoses. These leaks may result in overwhelming sepsis and can be life threatening. Furthermore, the presence of digestive enzymes in contact with the graft may lead to significant tissue necrosis.[76]

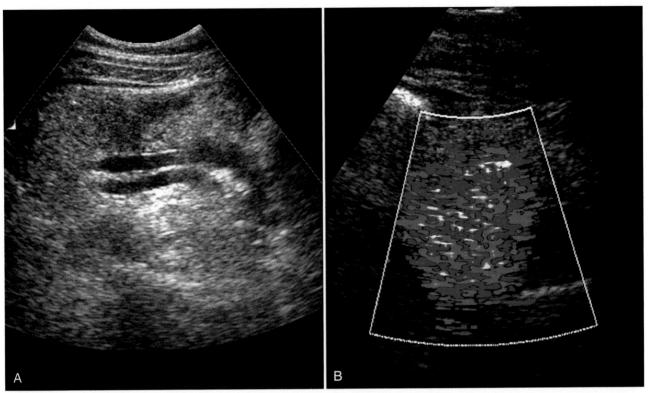

FIGURE 17-65. Pancreas transplant arteriovenous malformation (AVM). A, Transverse gray-scale ultrasound shows no abnormality. **B,** Color Doppler ultrasound, however, shows an intense mosaic of color within the pancreas, secondary to a parenchymal AVM.

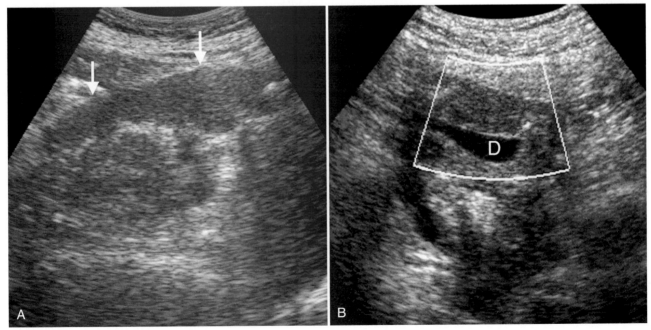

FIGURE 17-66. Pancreas transplant rejection. A, Transverse sonogram shows hypoechoic pancreas *(arrows)*. The pancreatic parenchyma is also atrophied. **B,** Oblique sonogram shows dilated pancreatic duct *(D)* secondary to surrounding parenchymal atrophy.

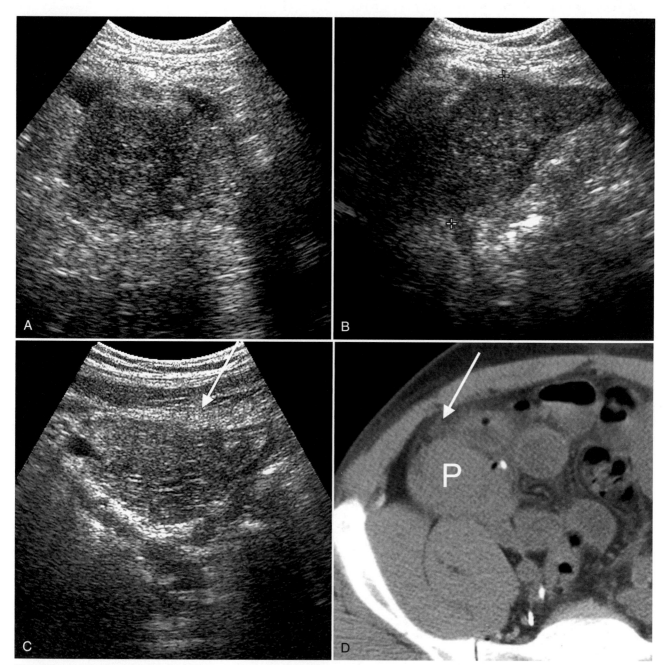

FIGURE 17-67. Pancreatitis. A, Transverse, and **B,** oblique, images show bulky, edematous allograft. **C,** Oblique ultrasound shows echogenic inflamed peripancreatic fat *(arrow).* **D,** This appears as "stranding" in the peripancreatic fat on CT *(arrow); P,* pancreas transplant.

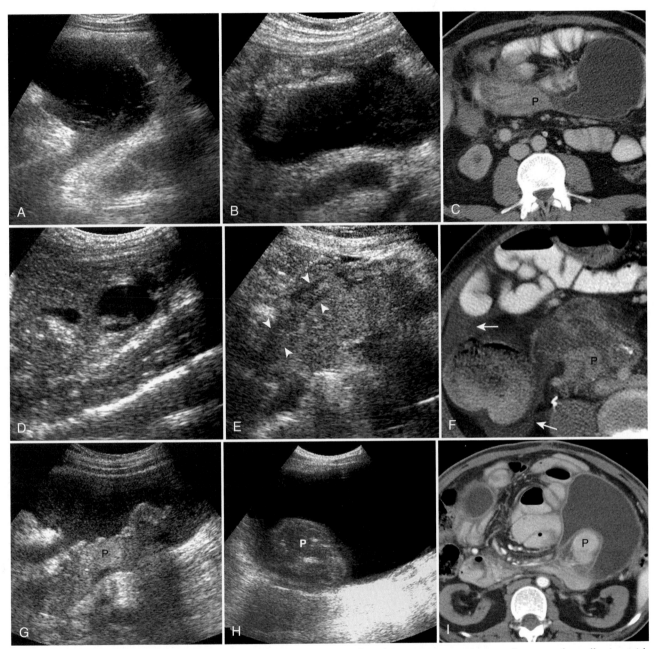

FIGURE 17-68. Fluid collections. A to **C, Hematoma. A,** Sagittal, and **B,** transverse, sonograms show complex collection with internal echoes and strands. **C,** Correlative CT scan shows hematoma in left upper quadrant that extends to pancreas *(P).* **D** to **I, Pseudocysts in three patients.** *Patient 1:* **D,** Sagittal sonogram shows complex epigastric cyst with internal septation. *Patient 2:* **E,** Sagittal sonogram shows complex collection adjacent to pancreas *(arrowheads).* **F,** Correlative CT scan shows collection extending into pancreatic head *(P)* and associated with free fluid *(arrows).* *Patient 3:* **G,** Sagittal sonogram shows large pseudocyst with internal echoes surrounding pancreatic tail *(P).* **H** and **I, Seroma.** Transverse sonogram and correlative CT scan show large, anechoic cystic structure surrounding pancreatic body *(P).* The wall enhanced on CT scan. The collection was sterile on aspiration.

Patients with pancreatic transplants are also susceptible to **infection** because of their immunosuppressive therapy, as well as their underlying diabetes mellitus. Abscesses are occasionally identified and are often associated with hematomas, urinary tract infections, and pancreatitis. Although gas within a fluid collection may indicate the presence of a gas-forming organism, bubbles of air within a collection may also result from the presence of a fistula or tissue necrosis in cases of vascular thrombosis. In the posttransplant period, the development of a new collection or change in the sonographic morphology of the collection may result from a variety of etiologies, including infection; malfunction of the pancreatic duct, stent, or external drain; hemorrhage; or associated tissue infarction.[77]

Miscellaneous Complications

Other complications of pancreatic transplants include intussusception of the Roux-en-Y loop, small bowel obstruction from adhesions or adjacent graft pancreatitis, and panniculitis.

POSTTRANSPLANT LYMPHOPROLIFERATIVE DISORDER

Lymphoproliferative disorders represent a range of conditions that can occur in any patient with an underlying primary or secondary immunodeficiency. Because patients with solid-organ transplants are chronically immunosuppressed, they are at risk for developing posttransplant lymphoproliferative disorder (PTLD). Regardless of the type of lymphoproliferative disorder affecting the patient, the pathogenesis of the condition is the same in all cases.[78]

Most patients with PTLD are actively infected with the **Epstein-Barr virus,** which induces proliferation of B lymphocytes. In the immunocompetent host, this B-cell proliferation is regulated by multiple mechanisms, many of which are mediated by T lymphocytes. However, if the host is immunosuppressed, with a deficiency in the T-cell defenses, proliferation of B cells may continue to produce a polyclonal or monoclonal lymphoproliferative disorder.[78,79]

Posttransplant lymphoproliferative disorder accounts for up to 20% of tumors in solid-organ transplantation.[80] The risk of development of PTLD, as well as the patient's prognosis, is determined by the *degree* of immunosuppressive therapy rather than the type of drug used. The aggressive immunosuppressive therapy required to prevent heart-lung transplant rejection has resulted in a reported incidence of PTLD as high as 4.6% in these patients. However, the milder immunosuppression used in patients with liver transplant or renal transplant has resulted in a lower incidence of PTLD, reported as 2.2% and 1%, respectively.[79,81]

Although PTLD may occur as early as 1 month after transplantation, the type of immunosuppression used appears to have some relationship to onset of disease. If cyclosporine is the medication used, the average length of time for development of PTLD is 15 months, whereas for azathioprine, the average is 48 months.[81,82]

Lymphoproliferative disorders tend to develop in the allograft organ, presumably related to chronic antigenic stimulation from the graft tissue, which may attract the proliferating B lymphocytes to the region of the transplant. PTLD also tends to arise in the lymphatic tissue in the periportal regions and around the anastomotic sites, occurring as masses that engulf and surround the hilar vessels in both liver and kidney transplants.[78,81]

In addition to affecting the allograft and surrounding tissues, PTLD has been described in almost all organ systems, with extranodal disease (81%) more common than lymphadenopathy (22%). The most frequent areas of involvement include the abdomen, thorax, cervical lymph nodes, and lymphatic tissue of the oropharynx. The liver is the most common site of intra-abdominal involvement, occurring in up to 69% of patients with PTLD. Enteric involvement typically involves the distal small bowel and proximal colon, with a propensity for ulceration and spontaneous perforation. In rare cases, intraosseous lesions may be present, with imaging features on computed tomography (CT) and magnetic resonance imaging (MRI) similar to metastatic disease, infection, or primary bone lymphoma. Overall, PTLD should be considered in the differential diagnosis of **any transplant patient presenting with lymphadenopathy or a new lesion within a solid viscus or the skeletal system.**[78,81,83,84]

On ultrasound, the masses produced by PTLD are usually hypoechoic or are of mixed echogenicity, with sizes ranging from 3 to 6 cm at diagnosis.[81] Calcifications may be seen in the mass secondary to tumor necrosis or treatment. Masses that develop around the anastomotic site have the potential to encase the hilar vessels and extrinsically compress the transplanted artery and vein. Renal hilar masses may also obstruct the ureter, causing postrenal obstruction and necessitating placement of a drainage catheter.[81] The involved lymph nodes have an abnormal appearance, showing a hypoechoic thickened cortex with an absent or a flattened fatty hilum (Figs. 17-69 to 17-72). Pancreatic PTLD tends to produce diffuse glandular enlargement, with an appearance that is indistinguishable from pancreatitis or rejection.[85]

The initial therapy for lymphoproliferative disorders is a reduction of immunosuppressive therapy. This is often successful for cases of polyclonal PTLD and in some cases of monoclonal disease. If this treatment option fails, chemotherapy is instituted.[78,79]

Text continued on p. 705.

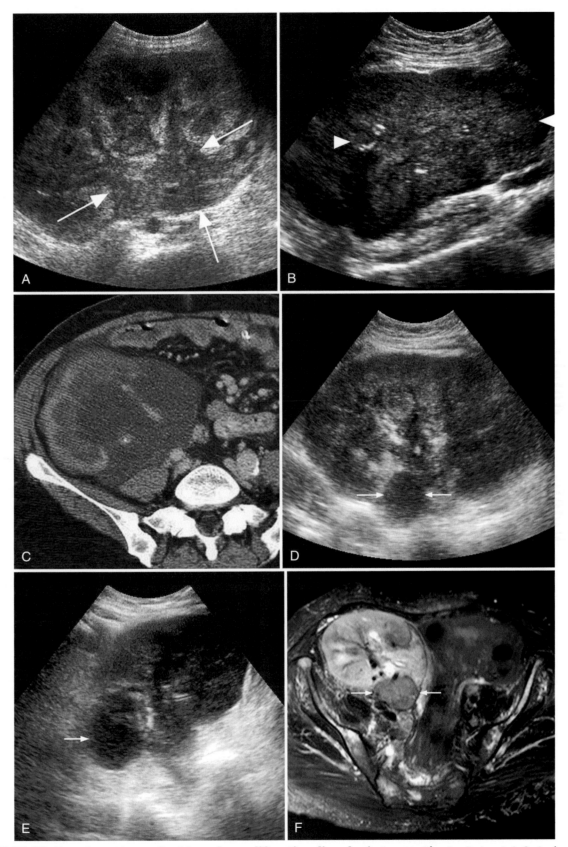

FIGURE 17-69. Renal posttransplant lymphoproliferative disorder in two patients. *Patient 1:* **A,** Sagittal sonogram shows infiltrative mass *(arrows)* in renal hilum. **B,** Six months later, the mass *(arrowheads)* has infiltrated into the renal cortex. **C,** Correlative CT scan shows hilar mass infiltrating into renal cortex. *Patient 2:* **D,** Sagittal, and **E,** transverse, sonograms show a hypoechoic to anechoic structure with low-level echoes *(arrows)* in the renal hilum that could be interpreted as a complex cyst. **F,** Contrast-enhanced MR scan shows that this structure represents a solid mass *(arrows)*.

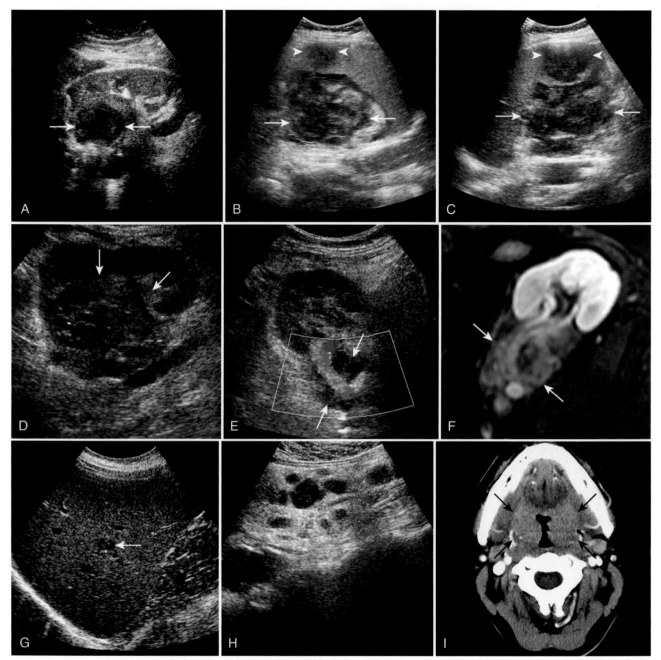

FIGURE 17-70. Renal posttransplant lymphoproliferative disorder (PTLD): extrarenal manifestations in two patients. *Patient 1:* **A,** Sagittal sonogram shows a hypoechoic renal hilar mass *(arrows).* **B,** Sagittal, and **C,** transverse, sonograms of the spleen show a mass in the hilum *(arrows)* as well as an intraparenchymal mass *(arrowheads). Patient 2:* **D,** Sagittal sonogram shows hilar mass *(arrows).* **E,** Transverse sonogram shows that mass *(arrows)* encases transplanted renal artery. **F,** Correlative MRI shows hilar mass *(arrows)* encasing renal vessels. **G,** Transverse sonogram shows malignant-appearing hepatic nodule *(arrow).* **H,** Sagittal sonogram shows malignant lymphadenopathy. **I,** CT scan shows tonsillar adenopathy in Walder's ring *(arrows)* secondary to PTLD.

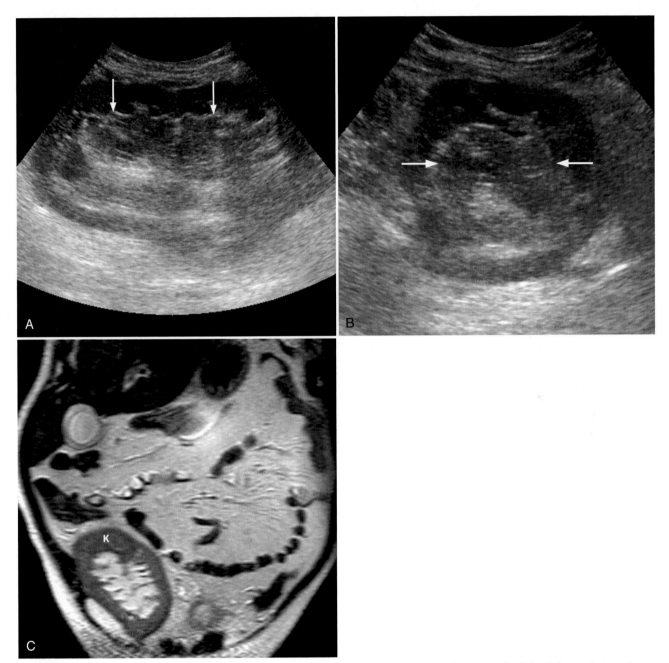

FIGURE 17-71. Renal PTLD: mimicker. A, Sagittal, and **B,** transverse, sonograms show a poorly defined, hypoechoic region in the renal sinus *(arrows)*, potentially representing an infiltrative mass. **C,** Correlative MR scan shows that the hypoechoic region represents sinus fat; *K,* kidney.

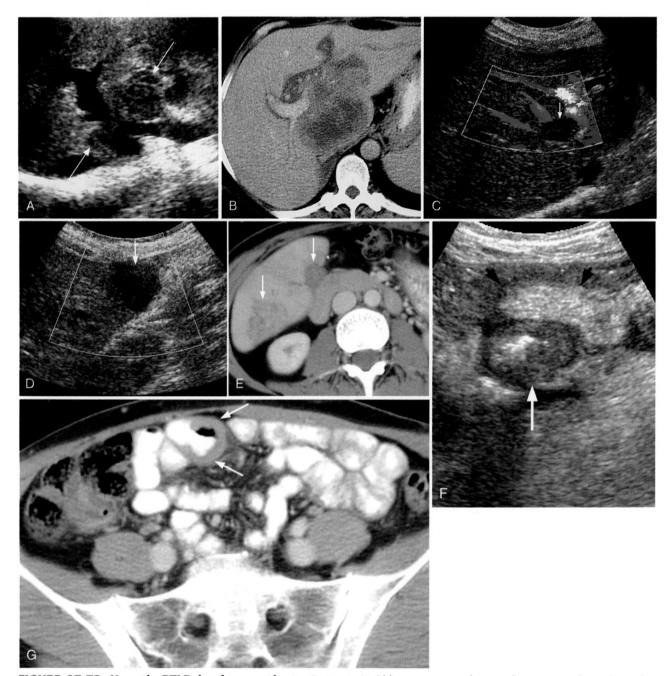

FIGURE 17-72. Hepatic PTLD in three patients. *Patient 1:* **A,** Oblique sonogram shows malignant mass *(arrows)* encasing and narrowing main portal vein. **B,** Correlative CT scan shows mass infiltrating liver. *Patient 2:* **C,** Transverse, and **D,** sagittal, color Doppler sonograms show avascular solid nodules *(arrow).* **E,** Correlative CT scan shows solid hypovascular masses *(arrows).* *Patient 3:* **F,** Transverse sonogram shows thick-walled gut *(white arrow)* adjacent to inflamed echogenic fat *(black arrows).* **G,** Correlative CT scan shows thick-walled loop of small bowel *(arrows).*

References

1. Takemoto S, Terasaki PI, Cecka JM, et al. Survival of nationally shared, HLA-matched kidney transplants from cadaveric donors. The UNOS Scientific Renal Transplant Registry. N Engl J Med 1992;327:834-839.
2. Berthoux FC, Jones EH, Mehls O, Valderrabano F. Transplantation report. 1. Renal transplantation in recipients aged 60 years or older at time of grafting. The EDTA-ERA Registry. European Dialysis and Transplant Association–European Renal Association. Nephrol Dial Transplant 1996;11(Suppl 1):37-40.
3. Cattral MS, Bigam DL, Hemming AW, et al. Portal venous and enteric exocrine drainage versus systemic venous and bladder exocrine drainage of pancreas grafts: clinical outcome of 40 consecutive transplant recipients. Ann Surg 2000;232:688-695.

Liver Transplantation
4. Data from the Organ Procurement and Transplantation Network and the US Scientific Registry of Transplant Recipients. In United Network for Organ Sharing and Scientific Registry Data. Oct 18, 2008.
5. Crossin JD, Muradali D, Wilson SR. Ultrasound of liver transplants: normal and abnormal. Radiographics 2003;23:1093-1114.
6. Mazzaferro V, Regalia E, Doci R, et al. Liver transplantation for the treatment of small hepatocellular carcinomas in patients with cirrhosis. N Engl J Med 1996;334:693-699.
7. Quiroga S, Sebastia MC, Margarit C, et al. Complications of orthotopic liver transplantation: spectrum of findings with helical CT. Radiographics 2001;21:1085-1102.
8. Nghiem HV. Imaging of hepatic transplantation. Radiol Clin North Am 1998;36:429-443.
9. Kamel IR, Kruskal JB, Raptopoulos V. Imaging for right lobe living donor liver transplantation. Semin Liver Dis 2001;21:271-282.
10. Wolfsen HC, Porayko MK, Hughes RH, et al. Role of endoscopic retrograde cholangiopancreatography after orthotopic liver transplantation. Am J Gastroenterol 1992;87:955-960.
11. Keogan MT, McDermott VG, Price SK, et al. The role of imaging in the diagnosis and management of biliary complications after liver transplantation. AJR Am J Roentgenol 1999;173:215-219.
12. Letourneau JG, Castaneda-Zuniga WR. The role of radiology in the diagnosis and treatment of biliary complications after liver transplantation. Cardiovasc Interv Radiol 1990;13:278-282.
13. Barton P, Maier A, Steininger R, et al. Biliary sludge after liver transplantation. 1. Imaging findings and efficacy of various imaging procedures. AJR Am J Roentgenol 1995;164:859-864.
14. Miller WJ, Campbell WL, Zajko AB, et al. Obstructive dilatation of extrahepatic recipient and donor bile ducts complicating orthotopic liver transplantation: imaging and laboratory findings. AJR Am J Roentgenol 1991;157:29-32.
15. Zajko AB, Campbell WL, Bron KM, et al. Cholangiography and interventional biliary radiology in adult liver transplantation. AJR Am J Roentgenol 1985;144:127-133.
16. Sheng R, Zajko AB, Campbell WL, Abu-Elmagd K. Biliary strictures in hepatic transplants: prevalence and types in patients with primary sclerosing cholangitis vs those with other liver diseases. AJR Am J Roentgenol 1993;161:297-300.
17. Ward EM, Wiesner RH, Hughes RW, Krom RA. Persistent bile leak after liver transplantation: biloma drainage and endoscopic retrograde cholangiopancreatographic sphincterotomy. Radiology 1991;179:719-720.
18. McDonald V, Matalon TA, Patel SK, et al. Biliary strictures in hepatic transplantation. J Vasc Interv Radiol 1991;2:533-538.
19. Yeh BM, Coakley FV, Westphalen AC, et al. Predicting biliary complications in right lobe liver transplant recipients according to distance between donor's bile duct and corresponding hepatic artery. Radiology 2007;242:144-151.
20. Sheng R, Sammon JK, Zajko AB, Campbell WL. Bile leak after hepatic transplantation: cholangiographic features, prevalence, and clinical outcome. Radiology 1994;192:413-416.
21. Gow PJ, Chapman RW. Liver transplantation for primary sclerosing cholangitis. Liver 2000;20:97-103.
22. Chen LY, Goldberg HI. Sclerosing cholangitis: broad spectrum of radiographic features. Gastrointest Radiol 1984;9:39-47.
23. Ciaccia D, Branch MS. Disorders of the biliary tree related to liver transplantation. In: DiMarino AJBS, editor. Gastrointestinal diseases:

an endoscopic approach. Boston: Blackwell Scientific; 1997. p. 918-927.
24. Zajko AB, Campbell WL, Bron KM, et al. Diagnostic and interventional radiology in liver transplantation. Gastroenterol Clin North Am 1988;17:105-143.
25. Starzl TE, Putnam CW, Hansbrough JF, et al. Biliary complications after liver transplantation: with special reference to the biliary cast syndrome and techniques of secondary duct repair. Surgery 1977; 81:212-221.
26. Ito K, Siegelman ES, Stolpen AH, Mitchell DG. MR imaging of complications after liver transplantation. AJR Am J Roentgenol 2000;175:1145-1149.
27. Dodd 3rd GD, Memel DS, Zajko AB, et al. Hepatic artery stenosis and thrombosis in transplant recipients: Doppler diagnosis with resistive index and systolic acceleration time. Radiology 1994;192: 657-661.
28. Horrow MM, Blumenthal BM, Reich DJ, Manzarbeitia C. Sonographic diagnosis and outcome of hepatic artery thrombosis after orthotopic liver transplantation in adults. AJR Am J Roentgenol 2007;189:346-351.
29. Gunsar F, Rolando N, Pastacaldi S, et al. Late hepatic artery thrombosis after orthotopic liver transplantation. Liver Transplant 2003; 9:605-611.
30. Wozney P, Zajko AB, Bron KM, et al. Vascular complications after liver transplantation: a 5-year experience. AJR Am J Roentgenol 1986; 147:657-663.
31. De Gaetano AM, Cotroneo AR, Maresca G, et al. Color Doppler sonography in the diagnosis and monitoring of arterial complications after liver transplantation. J Clin Ultrasound 2000;28:373-380.
32. Garcia-Criado A, Gilabert R, Salmeron JM, et al. Significance of and contributing factors for a high resistive index on Doppler sonography of the hepatic artery immediately after surgery: prognostic implications for liver transplant recipients. AJR Am J Roentgenol 2003; 181:831-838.
33. Dravid VS, Shapiro MJ, Needleman L, et al. Arterial abnormalities following orthotopic liver transplantation: arteriographic findings and correlation with Doppler sonographic findings. AJR Am J Roentgenol 1994;163:585-589.
34. Fukuzawa K, Schwartz ME, Katz E, et al. The arcuate ligament syndrome in liver transplantation. Transplantation 1993;56:223-224.
35. Langnas AN, Marujo W, Stratta RJ, et al. Hepatic allograft rescue following arterial thrombosis: role of urgent revascularization. Transplantation 1991;51:86-90.
36. Raby N, Karani J, Thomas S, et al. Stenoses of vascular anastomoses after hepatic transplantation: treatment with balloon angioplasty. AJR Am J Roentgenol 1991;157:167-171.
37. Chong WK, Beland JC, Weeks SM. Sonographic evaluation of venous obstruction in liver transplants. AJR Am J Roentgenol 2007;188:W515-W521.
38. Pfammatter T, Williams DM, Lane KL, et al. Suprahepatic caval anastomotic stenosis complicating orthotopic liver transplantation: treatment with percutaneous transluminal angioplasty, Wallstent placement, or both. AJR Am J Roentgenol 1997;168:477-480.
39. Kubo T, Shibata T, Itoh K, et al. Outcome of percutaneous transhepatic venoplasty for hepatic venous outflow obstruction after living donor liver transplantation. Radiology 2006;239:285-290.
40. Ko EY, Kim TK, Kim PN, et al. Hepatic vein stenosis after living donor liver transplantation: evaluation with Doppler ultrasound. Radiology 2003;229:806-810.
41. Ferris JV, Baron RL, Marsh Jr JW, et al. Recurrent hepatocellular carcinoma after liver transplantation: spectrum of CT findings and recurrence patterns. Radiology 1996;198:233-238.

Renal Transplantation
42. Baxter GM. Ultrasound of renal transplantation. Clin Radiol 2001; 56:802-818.
43. Brown ED, Chen MY, Wolfman NT, et al. Complications of renal transplantation: evaluation with ultrasound and radionuclide imaging. Radiographics 2000;20:607-622.
44. Kobayashi K, Censullo ML, Rossman LL, et al. Interventional radiologic management of renal transplant dysfunction: indications, limitations, and technical considerations. Radiographics 2007;27:1109-1130.
45. Memel DS, Dodd 3rd GD, Shah AN, et al. Imaging of en bloc renal transplants: normal and abnormal postoperative findings. AJR Am J Roentgenol 1993;160:75-81.

46. O'Neill WC, Baumgarten DA. Ultrasonography in renal transplantation. Am J Kidney Dis 2002;39:663-678.
47. Lachance SL, Adamson D, Barry JM. Ultrasonically determined kidney transplant hypertrophy. J Urol 1988;139:497-498.
48. Babcock DS, Slovis TL, Han BK, et al. Renal transplants in children: long-term follow-up using sonography. Radiology 1985;156:165-167.
49. Absy M, Metreweli C, Matthews C, Al Khader A. Changes in transplanted kidney volume measured by ultrasound. Br J Radiol 1987; 60:525-529.
50. Tublin ME, Bude RO, Platt JF. The resistive index in renal Doppler sonography: where do we stand? AJR Am J Roentgenol 2003;180:885-892 (review).
51. Rigg KM. Renal transplantation: current status, complications and prevention. J Antimicrob Chemother 1995;36(Suppl B):51-57.
52. Pirsch JD, Ploeg RJ, Gange S, et al. Determinants of graft survival after renal transplantation. Transplantation 1996;61:1581-1586.
53. Dodd 3rd GD, Tublin ME, Shah A, Zajko AB. Imaging of vascular complications associated with renal transplants. AJR Am J Roentgenol 1991;157:449-459.
54. Akbar SA, Jafri SZ, Amendola MA, et al. Complications of renal transplantation. Radiographics 2005;25:1335-1356.
55. Jordan ML, Cook GT, Cardella CJ. Ten years of experience with vascular complications in renal transplantation. J Urol 1982;128:689-692.
56. Hanto DW, Simmons RL. Renal transplantation: clinical considerations. Radiol Clin North Am 1987;25:239-248.
57. Tublin ME, Dodd 3rd GD. Sonography of renal transplantation. Radiol Clin North Am 1995;33:447-459.
58. Penny MJ, Nankivell BJ, Disney AP, et al. Renal graft thrombosis: a survey of 134 consecutive cases. Transplantation 1994;58:565-569.
59. Baxter GM, Morley P, Dall B. Acute renal vein thrombosis in renal allografts: new Doppler ultrasonic findings. Clin Radiol 1991;43:125-127.
60. Reuther G, Wanjura D, Bauer H. Acute renal vein thrombosis in renal allografts: detection with duplex Doppler ultrasound. Radiology 1989;170:557-558.
61. Lockhart ME, Wells CG, Morgan DE, et al. Reversed diastolic flow in the renal transplant: perioperative implications versus transplants older than 1 month. AJR Am J Roentgenol 2008;190:650-655.
62. Pozniak MA, Dodd 3rd GD, Kelcz F. Ultrasonographic evaluation of renal transplantation. Radiol Clin North Am 1992;30:1053-1066.
63. Middleton WD, Kellman GM, Melson GL, Madrazo BL. Postbiopsy renal transplant arteriovenous fistulas: color Doppler ultrasound characteristics. Radiology 1989;171:253-257.
64. Huang MW, Muradali D, Thurston WA, et al. Uterine arteriovenous malformations: gray-scale and Doppler ultrasound features with MR imaging correlation. Radiology 1998;206:115-123.
65. Rahmouni A, Bargoin R, Herment A, et al. Color Doppler twinkling artifact in hyperechoic regions. Radiology 1996;199:269-271.
66. Letourneau JG, Day DL, Ascher NL, Castaneda-Zuniga WR. Imaging of renal transplants. AJR Am J Roentgenol 1988;150:833-838.
67. Silver TM, Campbell D, Wicks JD, et al. Peritransplant fluid collections: ultrasound evaluation and clinical significance. Radiology 1981;138:145-151.

Pancreas Transplantation

68. Pozniak MA, Propeck PA, Kelcz F, Sollinger H. Imaging of pancreas transplants. Radiol Clin North Am 1995;33:581-594.
69. Freund MC, Steurer W, Gassner EM, et al. Spectrum of imaging findings after pancreas transplantation with enteric exocrine drainage. Part 1. Posttransplantation anatomy. AJR Am J Roentgenol 2004; 182:911-917.
70. Krebs TL, Daly B, Wong JJ, et al. Vascular complications of pancreatic transplantation: MR evaluation. Radiology 1995;196:793-798.
71. Foshager MC, Hedlund LJ, Troppmann C, et al. Venous thrombosis of pancreatic transplants: diagnosis by duplex sonography. AJR Am J Roentgenol 1997;169:1269-1273.
72. Hagspiel KD, Nandalur K, Burkholder B, et al. Contrast-enhanced MR angiography after pancreas transplantation: normal appearance and vascular complications. AJR Am J Roentgenol 2005;184:465-473.
73. Patel B, Markivee CR, Mahanta B, et al. Pancreatic transplantation: scintigraphy, ultrasound, and CT. Radiology 1988;167:685-687.
74. Yuh WT, Wiese JA, Abu-Yousef MM, et al. Pancreatic transplant imaging. Radiology 1988;167:679-683.
75. Aideyan OA, Foshager MC, Benedetti E, et al. Correlation of the arterial resistive index in pancreas transplants of patients with transplant rejection. AJR Am J Roentgenol 1997;168:1445-1447.
76. Heyneman LE, Keogan MT, Tuttle-Newhall JE, et al. Pancreatic transplantation using portal venous and enteric drainage: the postoperative appearance of a new surgical procedure. J Comput Assist Tomogr 1999;23:283-290.
77. Patel BK, Garvin PJ, Aridge DL, et al. Fluid collections developing after pancreatic transplantation: radiologic evaluation and intervention. Radiology 1991;181:215-220.

Posttransplant Lymphoproliferative Disorder

78. Donnelly LF, Frush DP, Marshall KW, White KS. Lymphoproliferative disorders: CT findings in immunocompromised children. AJR Am J Roentgenol 1998;171:725-731,
79. Nalesnik MA, Makowka L, Starzl TE. The diagnosis and treatment of posttransplant lymphoproliferative disorders. Curr Probl Surg 1988;25:367-372.
80. Penn I. Cancers complicating organ transplantation. N Engl J Med 1990;323:1767-1769.
81. Vrachliotis TG, Vaswani KK, Davies EA, et al. CT findings in posttransplantation lymphoproliferative disorder of renal transplants. AJR Am J Roentgenol 2000;175:183-188.
82. Dodd 3rd GD, Greenler DP, Confer SR. Thoracic and abdominal manifestations of lymphoma occurring in the immunocompromised patient. Radiol Clin North Am 1992;30:597-610.
83. Pickhardt PJ, Siegel MJ. Abdominal manifestations of posttransplantation lymphoproliferative disorder. AJR Am J Roentgenol 1998; 171:1007-1013.
84. Kaushik S, Fulcher AS, Frable WJ, May DA. Posttransplantation lymphoproliferative disorder: osseous and hepatic involvement. AJR Am J Roentgenol 2001;177:1057-1059.
85. Meador TL, Krebs TL, Cheong JJ, et al. Imaging features of posttransplantation lymphoproliferative disorder in pancreas transplant recipients. AJR Am J Roentgenol 2000;174:121-124.

Part III

Small Parts, Carotid Artery, and Peripheral Vessel Sonography

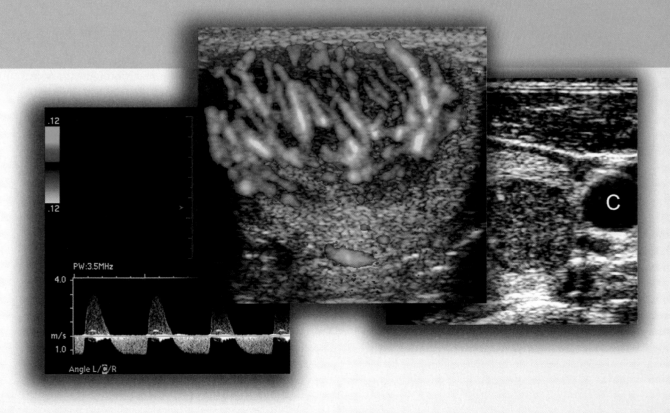

CHAPTER 18

The Thyroid Gland

*Luigi Solbiati, J. William Charboneau, Carl C. Reading,
E. Meredith James, and Ian D. Hay*

Chapter Outline

*B*ecause of the superficial location of the thyroid gland, high-resolution real-time gray-scale and color Doppler sonography can demonstrate normal thyroid anatomy and pathologic conditions with remarkable clarity. As a result, ultrasound plays an increasingly important role in the diagnostic evaluation of thyroid disease, although it is only one of several diagnostic methods currently available. To use ultrasound effectively and economically, it is important to understand its current capabilities and limitations.

INSTRUMENTATION AND TECHNIQUE

High-frequency transducers (7.5-15.0 MHz) currently provide both deep ultrasound penetration—up to 5 cm—and high-definition images, with a resolution of 0.5 to 1.0 mm. No other imaging method can achieve this degree of spatial resolution. Linear array transducers with either rectangular or trapezoidal scan format are preferred to sector transducers because of the wider near field of view and the capability to combine high-frequency gray-scale and color Doppler images. The thyroid gland is one of the most vascular organs of the body. As a result, Doppler examination may provide useful diagnostic information in some thyroid diseases.

Two newer techniques used for the sonographic study of the thyroid gland are contrast-enhanced sonography and sonoelastography. **Contrast-enhanced sonography** using second-generation contrast agents and very low mechanical index can provide useful information for the diagnosis of select cases of nodular disease and for ultrasound-guided therapeutic procedures. **Sonoelastogra-**

phy is based on the principle that when body tissues are compressed, the softer parts deform more easily than the harder parts. The amount of displacement at various depths is determined by the ultrasound signals reflected by tissues before and after they are compressed, and the corresponding strains are calculated from these displacements and displayed visually. This technique, already proven useful for the diagnosis of breast lesions, is now being applied to thyroid nodules (see later discussion).

The patient is typically examined in the supine position, with the neck extended. A small pad may be placed under the shoulders to provide better exposure of the neck, particularly in patients with a short, stocky habitus. The thyroid gland must be examined thoroughly in both transverse and longitudinal planes. Imaging of the lower poles can be enhanced by asking the patient to swallow, which momentarily raises the thyroid gland in the neck. The entire gland, including the isthmus, must be examined. The examination must also be extended laterally to include the region of the carotid artery and jugular vein in order to identify enlarged jugular chain lymph nodes, superiorly to visualize submandibular adenopathy, and inferiorly to define any pathologic supraclavicular lymph nodes.

In addition to the images recorded during the examination, some operators include in the permanent record a diagrammatic representation of the neck showing the location(s) of any abnormal findings (Fig. 18-1). This cervical "map" helps to communicate the anatomic relationships of the pathology more clearly to the referring clinician and the patient. It also serves as a useful reference for the radiologist and sonographer for follow-up examinations.

ANATOMY

The thyroid gland is located in the anteroinferior part of the neck (infrahyoid compartment) in a space outlined by muscle, trachea, esophagus, carotid arteries, and jugular veins (Fig. 18-2). The thyroid gland is made up of **two lobes** located along either side of the trachea and connected across the midline by the **isthmus,** a thin structure draping over the anterior tracheal wall at the

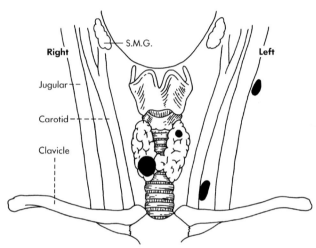

FIGURE 18-1. Cervical "map." Such diagrams help communicate relationships of pathology to clinicians and serve as a reference for follow-up examinations; *S.M.G.,* submandibular gland.

level of the junction of the middle and lower thirds of the thyroid gland. From 10% to 40% of normal patients have a small thyroid **(pyramidal)** lobe arising superiorly from the isthmus and laying in front of the thyroid cartilage.[1] It can be regularly visualized in younger patients, but it undergoes progressive atrophy in adulthood and becomes invisible. The size and shape of the thyroid lobes vary widely in normal patients. In tall individuals the lateral lobes have a longitudinally elongated shape on the sagittal scans, whereas in shorter individuals the gland is more oval. In the newborn the thyroid gland is 18 to 20 mm long, with an anteroposterior (AP) diameter of 8 to 9 mm. By 1 year of age, the mean length is 25 mm and AP diameter is 12 to 15 mm.[2] In adults the mean length is approximately 40 to 60 mm, with mean AP diameter of 13 to 18 mm. The mean thickness of the isthmus is 4 to 6 mm.[3]

Sonography is an accurate method for calculating **thyroid volume.** In about one third of cases, the sonographic measurement of volume differs from the estimated physical size on examination.[4] Thyroid volume measurements may be useful for goiter size determination to assess the need for surgery, permit calculation of the dose of iodine 131 (^{131}I) needed for treating thyrotoxicosis, and evaluate response to suppression treatments.[5] Thyroid volume can be calculated with linear parameters or more precisely with mathematical formulas. Among the linear parameters, the AP diameter is the most precise because it is relatively independent of possible dimensional asymmetry between the two lobes. When the AP diameter is more than 2 cm, the thyroid gland may be considered "enlarged."

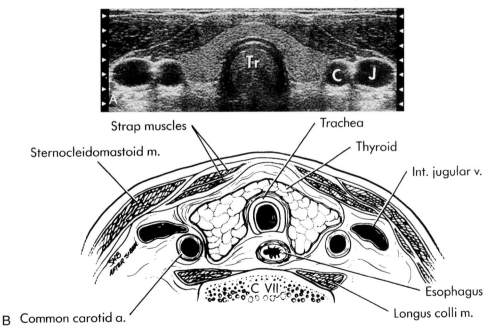

FIGURE 18-2. Normal thyroid gland. A, Transverse sonogram made with 7.5-MHz linear array transducer. **B,** Corresponding anatomic drawing; *Tr,* tracheal air shadow; *C,* common carotid artery; *J,* jugular vein. *(From James EM, Charboneau JW: High-frequency (10 MHz) thyroid ultrasonography. Semin Ultrasound, CT, MR 1985;6:294-309.)*

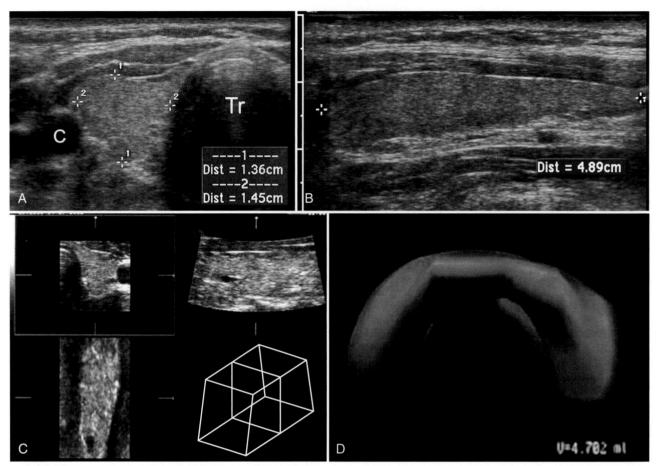

FIGURE 18-3. Volume measurement of thyroid gland. A, Transverse, and **B,** longitudinal, images show calipers at the boundaries of thyroid gland; *Tr,* trachea air shadow; *C,* carotid artery. The calculated thyroid volume is based on the ellipsoid formula with a correction factor (length × width × thickness × 0.52 for each lobe). In this case, the volume is 10 mL (or grams), which is within normal limits for this female patient. **C,** Images from real-time 3-D study of normal thyroid lobe, visualized simultaneously in axial *(top left),* longitudinal *(top right),* and coronal *(bottom left)* planes. **D,** Volumetric reconstruction of gland.

The most common mathematical method to calculate thyroid volume is based on the ellipsoid formula with a correction factor (length × width × thickness × 0.529 for each lobe)[6] (Fig. 18-3, *A* and *B*). Using this method, the mean estimated error is approximately 15%. The most precise mathematical method is the integration of the cross-sectional areas of the thyroid gland, achieved through evenly spaced sonographic scans.[7] With this method, the mean estimated error is 5% to 10%.[8] Modern three-dimensional (3-D) ultrasound technology allows one to obtain simultaneously the three orthogonal planes of thyroid lobes and then to calculate the volume either automatically or manually[9] (Fig. 18-3, *C* and *D*).

In neonates, thyroid volume ranges from 0.40 to 1.40 mL, increasing by 1.0 to 1.3 mL for each 10 kg of body weight, up to a normal volume in adults of 10 to 11 ± 3 mL.[7] Thyroid volume is generally larger in patients living in regions with iodine deficiency and in patients who have acute hepatitis or chronic renal failure. Volume is smaller in patients who have chronic hepatitis or have been treated with thyroxine or radioactive iodine.[5,7]

Normal thyroid parenchyma has a homogeneous, medium-level to high-level echogenicity that makes detection of focal cystic or hypoechoic thyroid lesions relatively easy in most cases (see Fig. 18-2). The thin, hyperechoic line around the thyroid lobes is the **capsule,** which is often identifiable on ultrasound. It may become calcified in patients who have uremia or disorders of calcium metabolism. With currently available high-sensitivity Doppler instruments, the rich vascularity of the gland can be seen homogeneously distributed throughout the entire parenchyma (Fig. 18-4). The **superior thyroid artery and vein** are found at the upper pole of each lobe. The **inferior thyroid vein** is found at the lower pole (Fig. 18-5), and the **inferior thyroid artery** is located posterior to the lower third of each lobe. The mean diameter of the arteries is 1 to 2 mm; the lower veins can be up to 8 mm in diameter. Normally, peak systolic velocities reach 20 to 40 cm/sec in the major thyroid arteries and 15 to 30 cm/sec in intraparenchymal arteries. These are the highest velocities found in blood vessels supplying superficial organs.

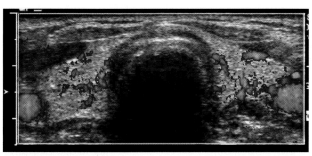

FIGURE 18-4. Normal thyroid vascularity on power Doppler ultrasound.

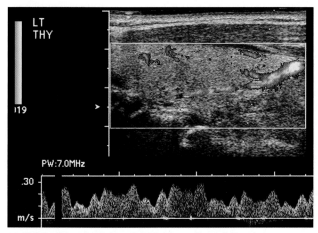

FIGURE 18-5. Normal inferior thyroid vein. Longitudinal power Doppler image shows a large inferior thyroid vein with associated normal venous spectral waveform.

The **sternohyoid** and **omohyoid muscles** (strap muscles) are seen as thin, hypoechoic bands anterior to the thyroid gland (see Fig. 18-2). The **sternocleidomastoid muscle** is seen as a larger oval band that lies lateral to the thyroid gland. An important anatomic landmark is the **longus colli muscle,** located posterior to each thyroid lobe, in close contact with the prevertebral space.

The **recurrent laryngeal nerve** and the inferior thyroid artery pass in the angle between the trachea, esophagus, and thyroid lobe. On longitudinal scans, the recurrent laryngeal nerve and inferior thyroid artery may be seen between the thyroid lobe and esophagus on the left and between the thyroid lobe and longus colli muscle on the right. The **esophagus,** primarily a midline structure, may be found laterally and is usually on the left side. It is clearly identified by the target appearance of bowel in the transverse plane and by its peristaltic movements when the patient swallows.

CONGENITAL THYROID ABNORMALITIES

Congenital conditions of the thyroid gland include **aplasia** of one lobe or the whole gland, varying degrees

of **hypoplasia,** and **ectopia** (Fig. 18-6). Sonography can be used to help establish the diagnosis of hypoplasia by demonstrating a diminutively sized gland. High-frequency ultrasound can also be used in the study of **congenital hypothyroidism** (CH), a relatively common disorder occurring in about 1 in 3000 to 4000 live births. Determining the cause of CH (dysgenesis, dyshormonogenesis, or pituitary/hypothalamic hypothyroidism) is clinically important because prognosis and therapy differ. Early initiation of therapy can prevent mental retardation and delayed bone development.[10,11]

Measurement of thyroid lobes can be used to differentiate aplasia (absent gland) from goitrous hypothyroidism (gland enlargement). Radionuclide scans are more often used to detect ectopic thyroid tissue (e.g., in a lingual or suprahyoid position).

NODULAR THYROID DISEASE

Many thyroid diseases can present clinically with one or more thyroid nodules. Such nodules represent common and controversial clinical problems. Epidemiologic studies estimate that 4% to 7% of adults in the United States have palpable thyroid nodules, with women affected more frequently than men.[12,13] Exposure to ionizing radiation increases the incidence of benign and malignant nodules, with 20% to 30% of a radiation-exposed population having palpable thyroid disease.[14,15]

Although nodular thyroid disease is relatively common, **thyroid cancer** is rare and accounts for less than 1% of all malignant neoplasms.[16] The overwhelming majority of thyroid nodules are benign. The clinical challenge is to distinguish the few clinically significant malignant nodules from the many benign nodules and thus identify patients who need surgical excision. This task is complicated because nodular disease of the thyroid gland often is clinically occult (<10-15 mm), although it can be readily detected by high-resolution sonography. The important question of how to manage these small nodules discovered incidentally by sonography is addressed later in this chapter.

NODULAR THYROID DISEASE: SONOGRAPHIC EVALUATION

Determine location of palpable neck mass (e.g., thyroid or extrathyroid).

Characterize benign versus malignant nodule features.

Detect occult nodule in patient with history of head and neck irradiation or MEN II syndrome.

Determine extent of known thyroid malignancy.

Detect residual, recurrent, or metastatic carcinoma.

Guide fine-needle aspiration of thyroid nodule or cervical lymph nodes.

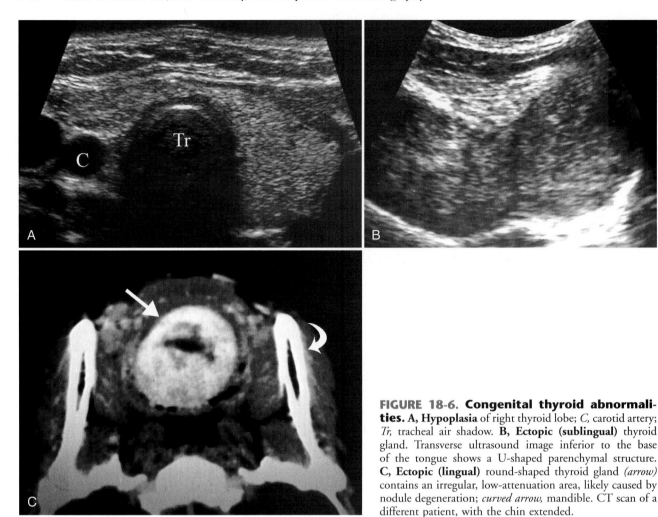

FIGURE 18-6. Congenital thyroid abnormalities. A, Hypoplasia of right thyroid lobe; *C,* carotid artery; *Tr,* tracheal air shadow. **B, Ectopic (sublingual)** thyroid gland. Transverse ultrasound image inferior to the base of the tongue shows a U-shaped parenchymal structure. **C, Ectopic (lingual)** round-shaped thyroid gland *(arrow)* contains an irregular, low-attenuation area, likely caused by nodule degeneration; *curved arrow,* mandible. CT scan of a different patient, with the chin extended.

Pathologic Features and Sonographic Correlates

Hyperplasia and Goiter

Approximately 80% of nodular thyroid disease is caused by **hyperplasia** of the gland and occurs in up to 5% of any population.[17] Its etiology includes **iodine deficiency** (endemic), **disorders of hormonogenesis** (hereditary familial forms), and **poor utilization of iodine** as a result of medication. When hyperplasia leads to an overall increase in size or volume of the gland, the term **goiter** is used. The peak age of patients with goiter is 35 to 50 years, and women are affected three times more often than men.

Histologically, the initial stage is cellular hyperplasia of the thyroid acini, followed by micronodule and macronodule formation, often indistinguishable from normal thyroid parenchyma, even at histology. Hyperplastic nodules often undergo liquefactive degeneration with the accumulation of blood, serous fluid, and colloid substance (Fig. 18-7; **Video 18-1**). Pathologi-

cally, they are often referred to as **hyperplastic, adenomatous,** or **colloid** nodules. Many (if not all) cystic thyroid lesions are hyperplastic nodules that have undergone extensive liquefactive degeneration. Pathologically, true epithelial-lined cysts of the thyroid gland are rare. In the course of this cystic degenerative process, **calcification,** which is often coarse and perinodular, may occur.[5,18] Hyperplastic nodule function may have decreased, may have remained normal, or may have increased (toxic nodules).

Sonographically, most hyperplastic or adenomatous nodules are **isoechoic** compared to normal thyroid tissue (Fig. 18-8, *A*), but may become **hyperechoic** because of the numerous interfaces between cells and colloid substance[5,19] (Fig. 18-8, *B* and *C*). Less frequently, a hypoechoic spongelike or **honeycomb** pattern is seen (Fig. 18-9; **Video 18-2**). When the nodule is isoechoic or hyperechoic, a thin peripheral **hypoechoic halo** is typically seen, most likely caused by perinodular blood vessels and mild edema or compression of the adjacent normal parenchyma. Perinodular blood vessels are typically detected by color Doppler sonography, and with

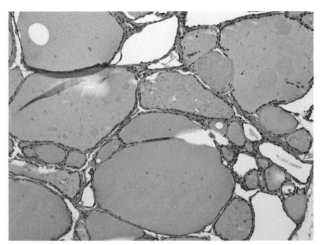

FIGURE 18-7. Histology of hyperplastic (adenomatous) change of thyroid gland. Histologic specimen shows many large dilated follicles that are filled with colloid material.

current high-sensitivity Doppler technology, intranodular vascularity can also be seen.[5,20,21] **Hyperfunctioning** (autonomous) nodules often exhibit an abundant perinodular and intranodular vascularity; however, because of the hypervascular pattern shown in most solid thyroid nodules on high-sensitivity Doppler systems, this feature does not allow detection of hyperfunctioning nodules within multinodular goiters with sonography.[20,21]

The degenerative changes of goitrous nodules correspond to their sonographic appearances (Fig. 18-10). Purely anechoic areas are caused by **serous or colloid fluid.** Echogenic fluid or moving fluid-fluid levels correspond to **hemorrhage.**[22] Bright echogenic foci with **comet-tail artifacts** are likely caused by **microcrystals** or aggregates of colloid substance, which may also move slowly, like snowflakes, within the fluid collection.[23] **Thin, intracystic septations** probably correspond to attenuated strands of thyroid tissue and appear

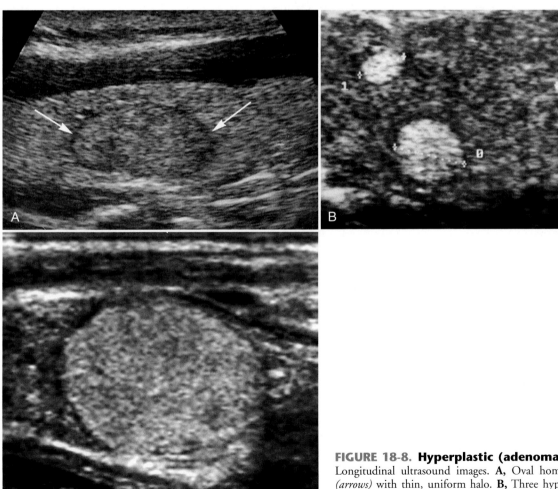

FIGURE 18-8. Hyperplastic (adenomatous) nodule. Longitudinal ultrasound images. **A,** Oval homogeneous nodule *(arrows)* with thin, uniform halo. **B,** Three hyperechoic nodules, typical of hyperplasia. **C,** Solitary hyperechoic nodule, which was benign on fine-needle aspiration biopsy.

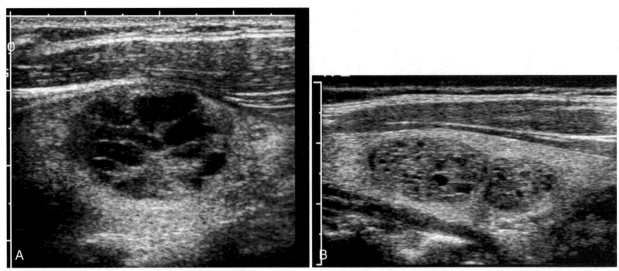

FIGURE 18-9. Benign nodule feature. Longitudinal images. Extensive honeycomb-like or cystic changes, with nodules showing **A,** larger cystic spaces, and **B,** smaller cystic spaces. These features indicate a very high probability of a benign process.

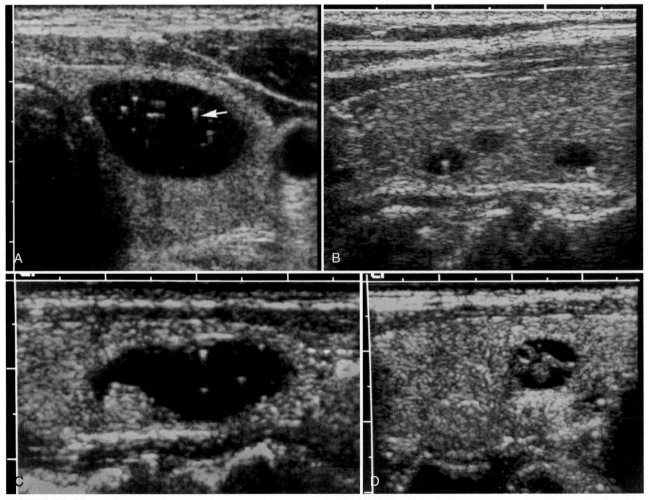

FIGURE 18-10. Colloid cysts. Transverse (**A**) and longitudinal (**B, C,** and **D**), images of four patients show the typical appearance of colloid cysts. Some of the nodules have tiny echogenic foci that are thought to be microcrystals. A few of these foci are associated with comet-tail artifacts (*arrow* in **A**) posteriorly. Nodules that are mostly cystic, such as these, are considered benign. Colloid cysts often contain internal echoes.

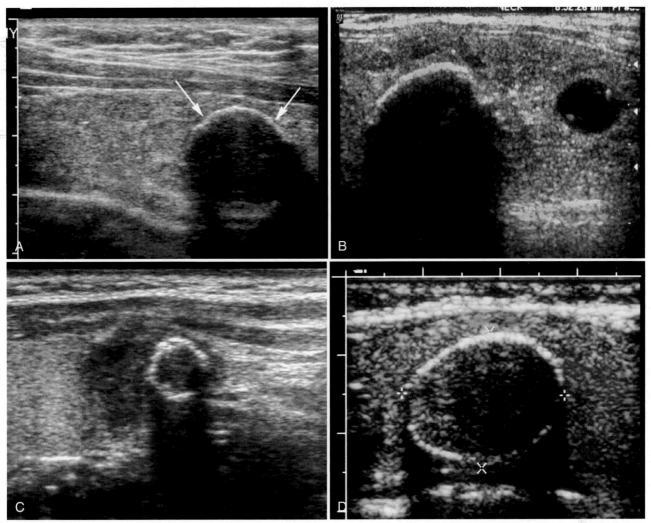

FIGURE 18-11. "Eggshell" calcification. Peripheral (eggshell) calcification was previously thought to indicate a benign nodule, but malignant nodules may have the appearance shown on these longitudinal images. **A,** Coarse peripheral calcification *(arrows)* casts a large acoustic shadow. **B,** Eggshell calcification and a typical appearance of colloid cyst on the right side in another patient. **C,** Hypoechoic solid mass caused by papillary carcinoma surrounds area of eggshell calcification. **D,** Peripheral shell (eggshell) calcification.

completely avascular on color Doppler ultrasound. These degenerative processes may also lead to the formation of calcifications, which may be either **thin, peripheral shells** ("eggshell") or **coarse, highly reflective foci** with associated acoustic shadows, scattered throughout the gland[8] (Fig. 18-11).

Intracystic solid projections, or papillae, usually containing color Doppler signals, may appear similar to the rare cystic papillary thyroid carcinoma.[21,22] In some cases, sonography and color Doppler imaging cannot differentiate the septations of colloid hyperplastic nodules from the vegetations seen in papillary carcinomas; before moving to aspiration cytology studies, contrast-enhanced sonography with second-generation microbubbles and nondisruptive imaging can be used. **Benign septa** do not show enhancement (and "disappear" in harmonic mode) (Fig. 18-12, *A* and *B*), whereas **malignant vegetations** show intense enhancement in arterial phase with relatively fast washout (Fig. 18-12, *C* and *D*).

Adenoma

Adenomas represent only 5% to 10% of all nodular disease of the thyroid and are seven times more common in women than men.[5] Most result in no thyroid dysfunction; a minority (<10%) hyperfunction, develop autonomy and may cause thyrotoxicosis. Most adenomas are solitary, but may also develop as part of a multinodular process.

The **benign follicular adenoma** is a true thyroid neoplasm, characterized by compression of adjacent tissues and fibrous encapsulation. Various subtypes of follicular adenoma include the **fetal adenoma, Hürthle cell adenoma,** and **embryonal adenoma,** each distinguished according to the type of cell proliferation. The cytologic features of follicular adenomas are generally indistinguishable from those of follicular carcinoma. Vascular and capsular invasion are the hallmarks of **follicular carcinoma,** identified by histologic rather than cytologic analysis. Needle biopsy is therefore not a reli-

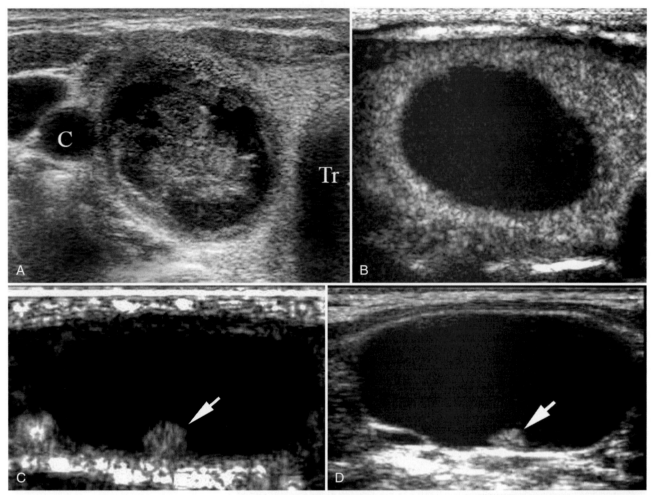

FIGURE 18-12. Contrast-enhanced sonography to differentiate benign from malignant fluid-filled thyroid nodules with internal septations or solid projections. A, Conventional B-mode sonogram of right thyroid lobe demonstrates large, mixed solid and cystic nodule; *Tr,* tracheal air shadow; *C,* common carotid artery. **B,** Contrast-enhanced sonogram. After administration of contrast material, the internal contents are no longer visible because they lack enhancement, indicating that the contents were likely colloid and blood products. **C,** Conventional B-mode sonogram in longitudinal plane demonstrates a nodule *(arrow)* arising from the posterior wall. **D,** Contrast-enhanced longitudinal sonogram shows that the nodule remains visible, indicating enhancement after contrast enhancement. The lesion was a cystic papillary carcinoma.

able method to distinguish between follicular carcinoma and cellular adenoma. Therefore, such tumors are usually surgically removed.

Sonographically, adenomas are usually solid masses that may be hyperechoic, isoechoic, or hypoechoic (Fig. 18-13; **Video 18-3**). They often have a thick, smooth peripheral hypoechoic halo resulting from the fibrous capsule and blood vessels, which can be readily seen by color Doppler imaging. Often, vessels pass from the periphery to the central regions of the nodule, sometimes creating a "spoke and wheel" appearance. This vascular pattern is usually seen in both hyperfunctioning and poorly functioning adenomas and thus does not allow the detection of hyperfunctioning lesions.

Carcinoma

Most **primary thyroid cancers** are of epithelial origin and are derived from follicular or parafollicular cells.[16]

Malignant thyroid tumors of mesenchymal origin are exceedingly rare, as are metastases to the thyroid. Most thyroid cancers are well differentiated, and papillary carcinoma (including so-called mixed papillary and follicular carcinoma) accounts for 75% to 90% of all cases.[16,24] In contrast, medullary, follicular, and anaplastic carcinomas (combined) represent only 10% to 25% of all thyroid carcinomas currently diagnosed in North America.

Papillary Carcinoma of Thyroid. Although it can occur in patients of any age, prevalence of papillary thyroid carcinoma peaks in both the third and the seventh decade of life.[16] Women are affected more often than men. On microscopic examination, the tumor is multicentric within the thyroid gland in at least 20% of cases.[25] Round, laminated calcifications (**psammoma bodies**) in the cytoplasm of papillary cancer cells are seen in approximately 35% of patients. The major route of spread of papillary carcinoma is through the lymphatics

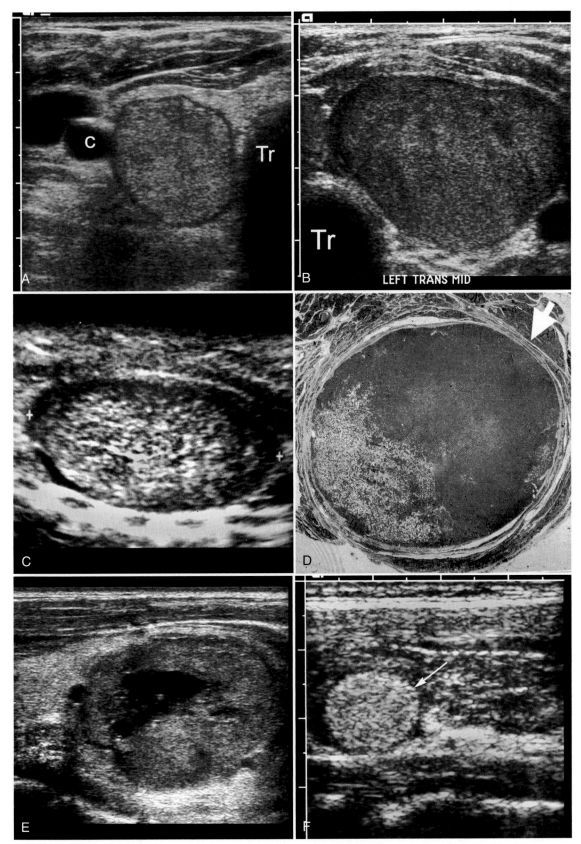

FIGURE 18-13. Benign follicular adenoma: spectrum of appearances. Transverse images of **A,** right lobe, and **B,** left lobe, of thyroid gland in two patients show homogeneous, hypoechoic, round to oval masses with a surrounding thin halo, the capsule of the adenoma; *Tr,* tracheal air shadow; *C,* carotid artery. **C,** Longitudinal image shows oval hyperechoic lesion with thick peripheral halo. **D,** Histology of lesion in **C.** Note the uniform capsule *(arrow)* of the mass. **E,** Longitudinal image shows oval mass with internal cystic component. **F,** Longitudinal image shows round, hyperechoic homogeneous mass *(arrow)* in patient with Hashimoto's thyroiditis.

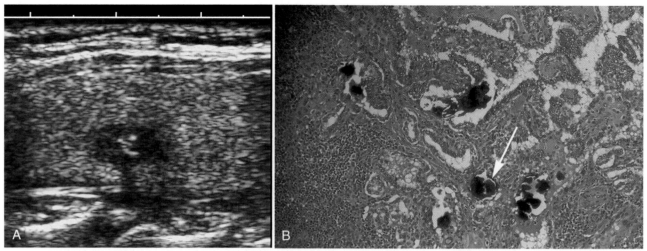

FIGURE 18-14. Papillary carcinoma: small cancer with microscopic correlation. A, Longitudinal image shows 7-mm, hypoechoic solid nodule containing microcalcifications. **B,** Microscopic pathologic image shows microcalcifications, or "psammoma bodies" *(arrow).*

to nearby cervical lymph nodes. In fact, a patient with papillary thyroid cancer may present with enlarged cervical nodes and a palpably normal thyroid gland.[26,27] Interestingly, the presence of nodal metastasis in the neck generally does not appear to worsen the prognosis for this malignancy. Distant metastases are very rare (2%-3%) and occur mostly in the mediastinum and lung. After 20 years, the cumulative mortality from papillary thyroid cancer is typically only 4% to 8%.[26]

Papillary carcinoma has peculiar histologic (fibrous capsule, microcalcifications) and cytologic ("ground glass" nuclei, cytoplasmic inclusions in nucleus, indentations of nuclear membrane) features, which often allow a relatively easy pathologic diagnosis.[28] In particular, microcalcifications, which result from the deposition of calcium salts in the psammoma bodies, are frequently present in both the primary tumor and the cervical lymph node metastases[27,29] (Fig. 18-14).

Similar to the pathologic features, sonographic characteristics of papillary carcinoma usually are relatively distinctive, as follows (Figs. 18-15 and 18-16):

- Hypoechogenicity (90% of cases), resulting from closely packed cell content, with minimal colloid substance.
- Microcalcifications, appearing as tiny, punctate hyperechoic foci, either with or without acoustic shadows **(Videos 18-4 and 18-5).** In rare, but usually aggressive cases of papillary carcinomas of childhood, microcalcifications may be the only sonographic sign of the neoplasm, even without evidence of a nodular lesion[18,21,30,31] (Fig. 18-15, *B*).
- Hypervascularity (90% of cases), with disorganized vascularity, mostly in well-encapsulated forms[31] (Fig. 18-16).
- Cervical lymph node metastases, which may contain tiny, punctate echogenic foci caused by microcalcifications (Fig. 18-17). These are mainly

located in the caudal half of the deep jugular chain. Occasionally, metastatic nodes may be cystic as a result of extensive degeneration (Fig. 18-17, *H*).

Cystic nodal metastases show a thickened outer wall, internal nodularity, and septations in most cases, although they may appear purely cystic in younger patients.[27] Cystic lymph node metastases in the neck occur almost exclusively in association with papillary thyroid carcinoma, but occasionally with nasopharyngeal carcinomas.[32] On power Doppler sonography, noncystic nodes often show diffuse hypervascularity with tortuous vessels, arteriovenous (AV) shunts, and high vascular resistance (RI > 0.8). In some cases, however, these nodes may show only prominent hilar vascularity, similar to that of reactive nodes and low resistive indices (RIs).[31]

Papillary carcinoma rarely displays extensive cystic change (Fig. 18-18). In our review of the amount of cystic change found in 360 thyroid carcinomas, a large amount of cystic change occurred in less than 3% of cases.[33] The overwhelming majority of papillary carcinomas appear as a predominantly solid mass. **Invasion of adjacent muscles** is infrequently visualized by ultrasound but indicates that the mass is malignant (Fig. 18-19). A **follicular variant** accounts for 10% of cases of papillary carcinoma and appears similar to a follicular neoplasm on gross pathologic inspection and ultrasound (Fig. 18-20). High-power microscopic studies show that the nuclear features are those of papillary carcinoma, and it is classified as a "follicular variant of papillary carcinoma." The clinical course and treatment are the same as for typical papillary thyroid carcinoma.

Papillary microcarcinoma is a rare, nonencapsulated sclerosing tumor measuring 1 cm or less in diameter (Fig. 18-21). Most patient (80%) present with enlarged cervical nodes and a palpably normal thyroid gland.[26,28] Papillary microcarcinoma can be imaged by high-frequency

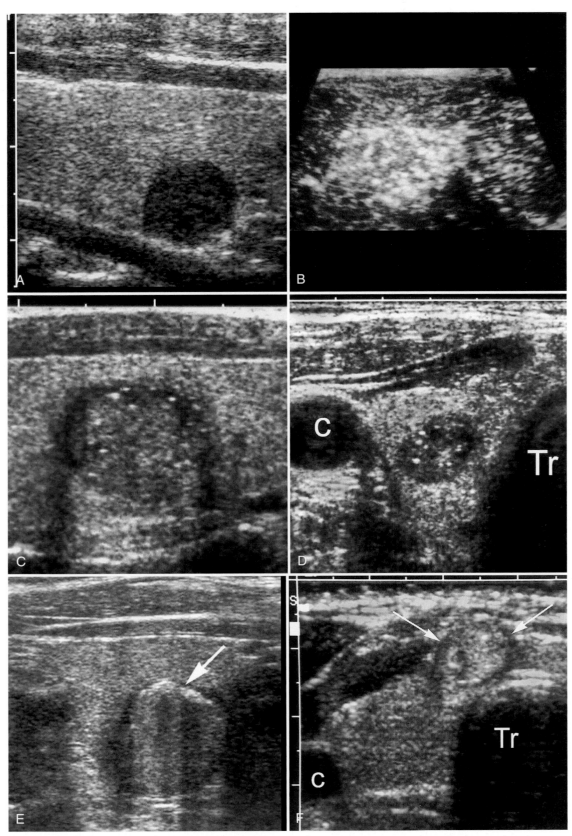

FIGURE 18-15. Papillary thyroid carcinoma: spectrum of appearances. A, Longitudinal image demonstrates extremely hypoechoic solid nodule without evidence of calcification. **B,** Longitudinal image of the thyroid of a 6-year-old patient shows extensive diffuse microcalcifications without discrete mass. This is a very rare appearance and is more often encountered in children than adults. **C,** Longitudinal, and **D,** transverse, images show hypoechoic nodules that contain echogenic foci caused by microcalcification; *Tr,* tracheal air shadow; *C,* carotid artery. **E,** Longitudinal image shows hypoechoic solid nodule with thick, irregular halo and linear calcifications at anterior margin *(arrow).* **F,** Transverse image shows heterogeneous but isoechoic mass in the isthmus *(arrows)* that contains microcalcifications and has a thick, irregular halo; *Tr,* tracheal air shadow; *C,* carotid artery.

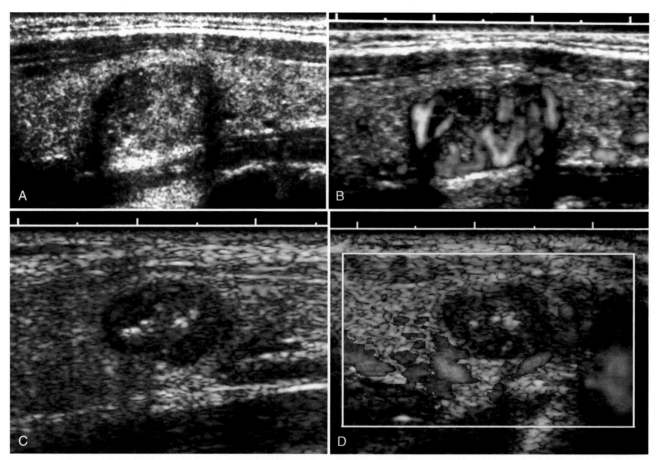

FIGURE 18-16. Papillary carcinoma: power Doppler appearances. Blood flow within cancer is often, but not always, increased. **A,** Longitudinal image shows 1.5-cm nodule with a thick, irregular halo. **B,** Power Doppler image shows that nodule is hyper-vascular and has flow in the center and at the periphery. **C,** Longitudinal image shows hypoechoic nodule with microcalcifications. **D,** Power Doppler image shows no blood flow within the cancer.

ultrasound in approximately 70% of cases, either as a small, hyperechoic patch (fibrotic-like) under the capsule with thickening and retraction of the capsule, or as a minute hypoechoic nodule with blurred irregular outline with no visible microcalcifications, but often with intense vascular signals within and around the lesion.

Follicular Carcinoma. Follicular carcinoma is the second subtype of well-differentiated thyroid cancer. It accounts for 5% to 15% of all cases of thyroid cancer, affecting women more often than men.[16] The two vari-ants of follicular carcinoma differ greatly in histology and clinical course.[16,24,28] The **minimally invasive** fol-licular carcinomas are encapsulated, and only the histo-logic demonstration of focal invasion of capsular blood vessels of the fibrous capsule itself permits differentiation from follicular adenoma. The **widely invasive** follicular carcinomas are not well encapsulated, and invasion of the vessels and the adjacent thyroid is more easily dem-onstrated. Both variants of follicular carcinoma tend to spread through the bloodstream rather than the lym-phatics, and distant metastases to bone, lung, brain, and liver are more likely than metastases to cervical lymph nodes. The widely invasive follicular carcinoma variant metastasizes in about 20% to 40% of cases, and the minimally invasive metastasizes in only 5% to 10%. Mortality from follicular carcinoma is 20% to 30% at 20 years postoperatively.[16,26]

No unique sonographic features allow differentiation of follicular carcinoma from adenoma, which is not sur-prising, given the cytologic and histologic similarities of these two tumors (Figs. 18-22 and 18-23). Similarly, fine-needle aspiration is not reliable in differentiating benign from malignant follicular neoplasms because the pathologic diagnosis is not based on cellular appearance but rather on capsular and vascular invasion. Therefore, most follicular nodules must be surgically removed for accurate pathologic diagnosis. Features that suggest fol-licular carcinoma are rarely seen but include irregular tumor margins, a thick irregular halo, and a tortuous or chaotic arrangement of internal blood vessels on color Doppler imaging.[20,34]

Medullary Carcinoma. Medullary carcinoma accounts for about 5% of all malignant thyroid diseases. It is derived from the parafollicular cells, or C cells, and

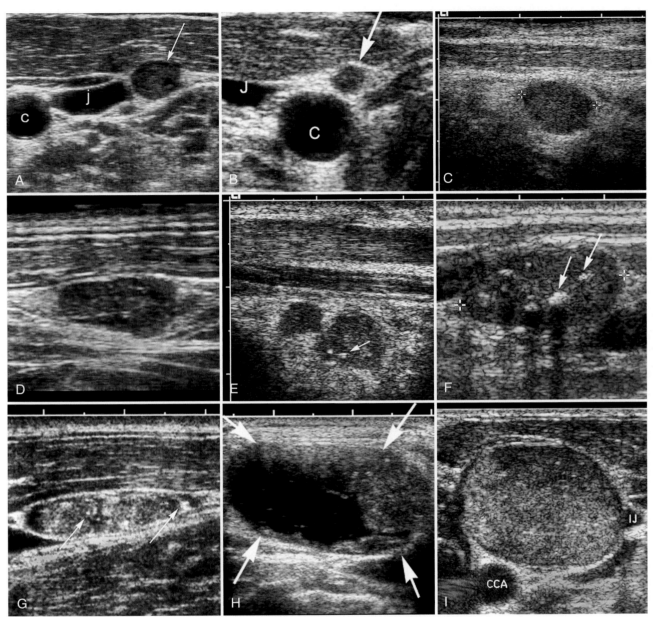

FIGURE 18-17. Metastases involving cervical lymph nodes: spectrum of appearances. A and **B,** Transverse images near the carotid artery *(C)* and jugular vein *(J)* show small, round, hypoechoic lymph nodes *(arrows)*. Despite their small size (~4 mm), the round shape and the hypoechoic appearance are highly indicative of metastasis. **C** and **D,** Longitudinal images show oval hypoechoic nodes. **E,** Longitudinal image of thyroid bed after thyroidectomy shows two abnormal lymph nodes, one of which contains microcalcifications *(arrow)*. **F** and **G,** Longitudinal images show heterogeneous lymph nodes containing calcification *(arrows)*. **H,** Longitudinal image shows a large lymph node *(arrows)* containing cystic change. Cystic change in a cervical lymph node is almost always caused by metastatic papillary carcinoma. **I,** Transverse image shows a large, round lymph node between the internal jugular vein *(IJ)* and the common carotid artery *(CCA)*.

FOLLICULAR THYROID CARCINOMA: SONOGRAPHIC FEATURES

Irregular tumor margins
Thick, irregular halo
Tortuous or chaotic arrangement of internal blood
  vessels

typically secretes the hormone **calcitonin,** which can be a useful serum marker. This cancer is frequently familial (20%) and is an essential component of the **multiple endocrine neoplasia (MEN) type II syndromes.**[35] The disease is multicentric and/or bilateral in about 90% of the familial cases[16] (Fig. 18-24). There is a high incidence of metastatic involvement of lymph nodes. The prognosis for patients with medullary cancer is somewhat worse than for follicular cancer.

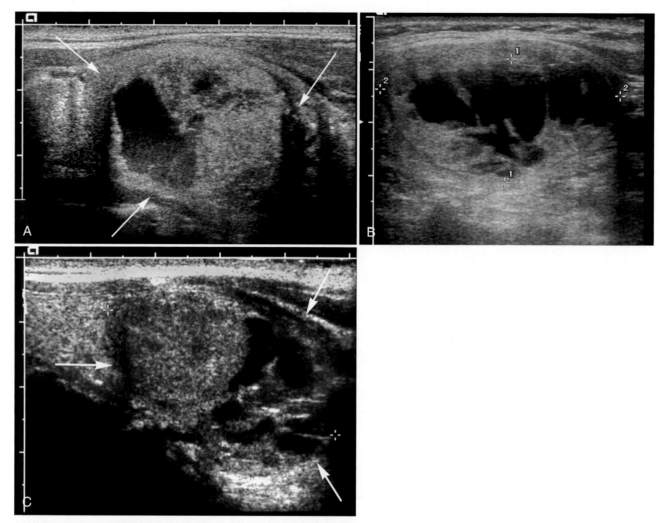

FIGURE 18-18. Papillary thyroid carcinoma: atypical. Three examples of moderate to marked cystic degeneration of papillary carcinoma. In the authors' experience, less than 5% of papillary carcinoma has this appearance of a large amount of cystic change. More than 90% of papillary thyroid carcinomas are uniformly solid masses. **A, B,** and **C,** Longitudinal images show three large nodules *(arrows, cursors)* that display extensive cystic change.

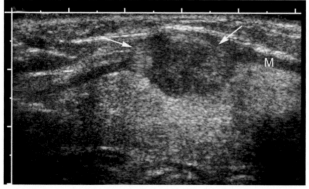

FIGURE 18-19. Papillary carcinoma invades muscle. Longitudinal image shows hypoechoic mass arising from anterior surface of the thyroid. This mass invades *(arrows)* adjacent strap muscle *(M).* Muscular invasion is very rare.

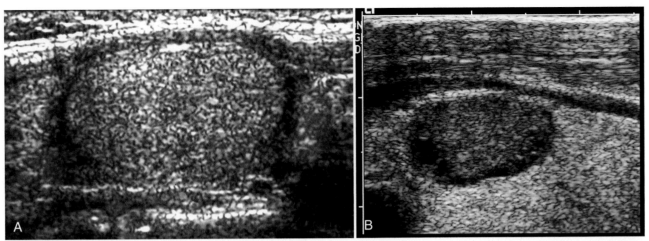

FIGURE 18-20. Atypical papillary thyroid carcinoma. Longitudinal images show two examples of the follicular variant of papillary thyroid carcinoma. **A,** oval isoechoic and **B,** hypoechoic mass that looks similar to the typical ultrasound appearance of a follicular neoplasm. This follicular variant is uncommon, accounting for 10% of cases of papillary carcinoma. The clinical course and treatment are the same as that of typical papillary thyroid carcinoma.

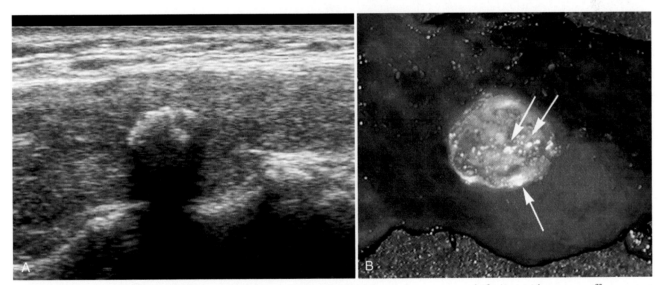

FIGURE 18-21. Atypical papillary carcinoma. A, Longitudinal image shows coarse calcification without mass effect, seen at the periphery and internally. **B,** Gross pathologic specimen of **A** shows round nodule that contains multiple areas of grossly visible calcifications *(arrows)*. This is a rare sclerosing form of papillary carcinoma that contains a large amount of fibrosis and calcification.

The sonographic appearance of medullary carcinoma is usually similar to that of papillary carcinoma and is seen most often as a hypoechoic solid mass. Calcifications are often seen (histologically caused by calcified nests of amyloid substance) and tend to be more coarse than the calcifications of typical papillary carcinoma[36] (Fig. 18-25). Calcifications can be seen not only in the primary tumor but also in lymph node metastases and even in hepatic metastases.

Anaplastic Thyroid Carcinoma. Anaplastic thyroid carcinoma is typically a disease of elderly persons; it represents one of the most lethal of solid tumors. Although it accounts for less than 2% of all thyroid cancers, it carries the worst prognosis, with a 5-year mortality rate of more than 95%.[37] The tumor typically presents as a rapidly enlarging mass extending beyond the gland and invading adjacent structures. It is often inoperable at presentation. Anaplastic carcinomas may often be associated with papillary or follicular carcinomas, presumably representing a dedifferentiation of the neoplasm. They tend not to spread via the lymphatics but instead are prone to aggressive local invasion of muscles and vessels.[28]

Sonographically, anaplastic thyroid carcinomas are usually hypoechoic and often encase or invade blood

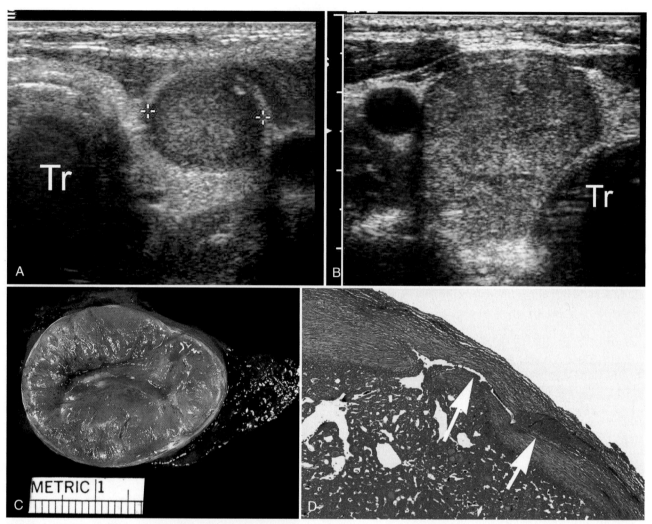

FIGURE 18-22. Follicular neoplasms: benign and malignant in same patient. A, Left lobe, and **B,** right lobe, of the thyroid show round, homogeneous hypoechoic masses that appear identical except for size differences on transverse images; *Tr,* tracheal air shadow. The smaller mass was malignant and the larger mass benign. **C,** Gross pathologic specimen of follicular neoplasm shows a homogeneous tumor with a thin capsule. This capsule is present in both benign and malignant follicular neoplasms and is often seen on ultrasound. **D,** Microscopic appearance of the capsule shows invasion of the follicular cells into the capsule *(arrows).* This is one of the microscopic features that allows a pathologic diagnosis of malignancy but is not visible by ultrasound.

ANAPLASTIC THYROID CARCINOMA: SONOGRAPHIC FEATURES

Large, hypoechoic mass
Encase or invade blood vessels
Invade neck muscles

vessels and neck muscles (Fig. 18-26). Often these tumors cannot be adequately examined by ultrasound because of their large size. Instead, computed tomography (CT) or magnetic resonance imaging (MRI) of the neck usually demonstrates the extent of disease more accurately.

Lymphoma

Lymphoma accounts for approximately 4% of all thyroid malignancies. It is mostly of the non-Hodgkin's type and usually affects older women. The typical clinical sign is a rapidly growing mass that may cause symptoms of obstruction such as dyspnea and dysphagia.[38] In 70% to 80% of patients, lymphoma arises from a preexisting chronic lymphocytic thyroiditis (Hashimoto's thyroiditis) with subclinical or overt hypothyroidism. The prognosis is highly variable and depends on the stage of the disease. Five-year survival ranges from almost 90% in early-stage cases to less than 5% in advanced, disseminated disease.

Sonographically, lymphoma of the thyroid appears as an extremely hypoechoic and lobulated mass. Large areas of cystic necrosis may occur, as well as encasement of

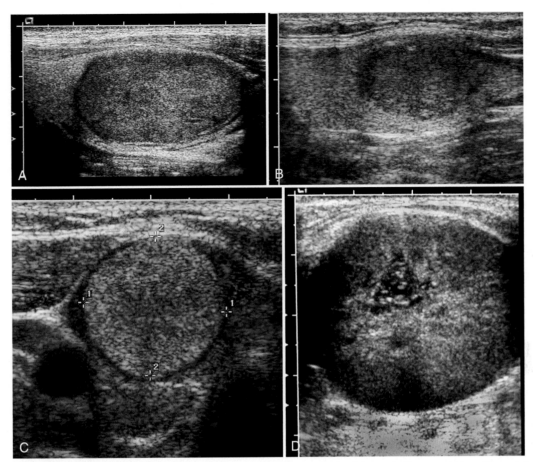

FIGURE 18-23. Malignant follicular neoplasms. A and **B,** Longitudinal images of two patients with oval homogeneous hypoechoic masses. **C** and **D,** Transverse images of two other patients with round homogeneous masses. These four carcinomas appear identical to the benign follicular neoplasms (see Fig. 18-13), and surgical removal is required to exclude or establish malignancy of most follicular tumors.

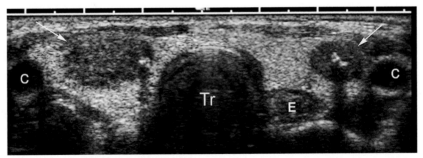

FIGURE 18-24. Multicentric medullary thyroid carcinoma. Transverse dual image in patient with multiple endocrine neoplasia type II (MEN II) shows bilateral hypoechoic masses *(arrows)* that contain areas of coarse calcification; *C,* carotid arteries; *Tr,* trachea; *E,* esophagus.

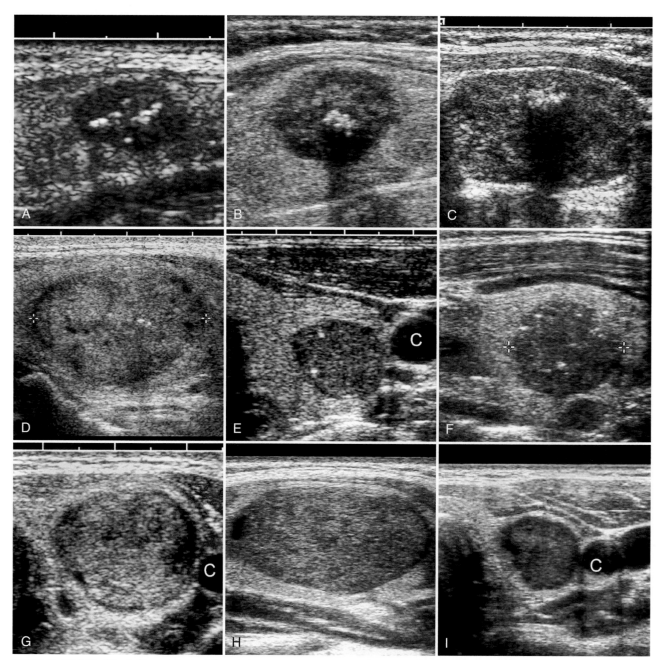

FIGURE 18-25. Medullary thyroid carcinoma: spectrum of appearances. A to **C,** Hypoechoic solid nodules with coarse internal calcifications. **D, E,** and **F,** Hypoechoic solid nodules with fine internal calcifications. **G, H,** and **I,** Hypoechoic solid nodules without calcification and with a similar appearance as follicular neoplasms; *C,* carotid artery.

adjacent neck vessels[39] (Fig. 18-27). On color Doppler imaging, both nodular and diffuse thyroid lymphomas may appear mostly hypovascular or may show blood vessels with chaotic distribution and AV shunts. The adjacent thyroid parenchyma may be heterogeneous as a result of associated chronic thyroiditis.[40]

Thyroid Metastases

Metastases to the thyroid are infrequent, occurring late in the course of neoplastic diseases as the result of hematogenous spread or less frequently a lymphatic route.

Metastases usually are from **melanoma** (39%), **breast** (21%), and **renal cell** (10%) carcinoma. Metastases may appear as solitary, well-circumscribed nodules or as diffuse involvement of the gland. On sonography, thyroid tumors are solid, homogeneously hypoechoic masses, without calcifications[41] (Fig. 18-28).

Fine-Needle Aspiration Biopsy

Once a thyroid nodule has been detected, the fundamental challenge is to determine if it is benign or malignant. Short of surgical excision, several methods for nodule

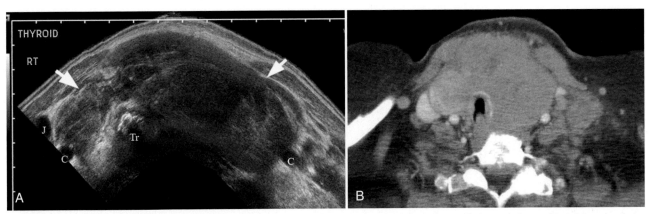

FIGURE 18-26. Anaplastic thyroid carcinoma. A, Transverse image shows large hypoechoic mass *(arrows)* involving the entire gland, greater on the left, which causes deviation of the trachea to the right; *Tr,* tracheal air shadow; *C,* common carotid artery; *J,* jugular vein. **B,** Contrast-enhanced CT scan of the patient shows the large mass and its relationship to adjacent structures.

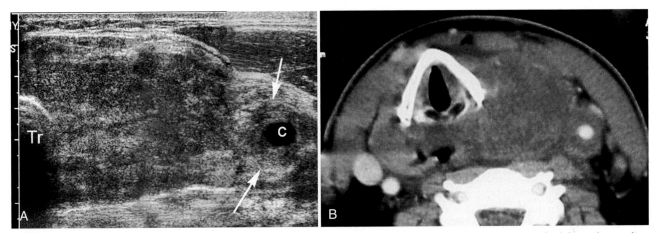

FIGURE 18-27. Lymphoma. A, Transverse image of left lobe of the thyroid shows diffuse mass enlarging the lobe and extending into the soft tissues *(arrows)* surrounding the common carotid artery *(c); Tr,* tracheal air shadow. **B,** Contrast-enhanced CT scan shows a hypovascular mass in the left thyroid lobe and soft tissue encasement of the carotid artery.

characterization are in common use, including radionuclide imaging, sonography, and fine-needle aspiration (FNA) biopsy. Each of these techniques has advantages and limitations, and the choice in any specific clinical setting depends largely on available instrumentation and expertise.

It is generally recognized that FNA biopsy is the most effective method for diagnosing malignancy in a thyroid nodule.[42-44] In many clinical practices, FNA under direct palpation is the first diagnostic examination performed on any clinically palpable nodule. Neither isotopic nor sonographic imaging is used routinely, instead reserved for special situations or difficult cases. FNA has had a substantial impact on the management of thyroid nodules because it provides more direct information than any other available diagnostic technique. It is safe, inexpensive, and results in better selection of patients for surgery. The successful use of FNA in clinical practice, however, depends heavily on the presence of an experienced aspirationist and an expert cytopathologist.

Fine-needle thyroid aspirates are often classified cytopathologically into the following four categories:
1. Negative (no malignant cells)
2. Positive for malignancy
3. Suggestive of malignancy
4. Nondiagnostic

If a nodule is classified in either of the first two categories, the results are highly sensitive and specific.[44] The major limitation of the technique is the lack of specificity in the third group, whose results are suggestive of malignancy, primarily because of the inability to distinguish follicular or Hürthle cell adenomas from their malignant counterparts. In these cases, surgical excision is required for diagnosis. In addition, up to 20% of aspirates may be nondiagnostic, approximately half of which result from inadequate cell sampling of cystic lesions. In these cases, repeat FNA under sonographic guidance can be performed for **selective sampling** of the solid elements of the mass. In the world literature, FNA of thyroid nodules has a sensitivity range of 65% to 98% and specificity of

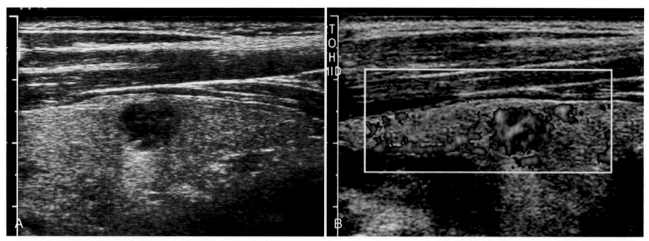

FIGURE 18-28. Thyroid metastasis from renal cell carcinoma. A, Longitudinal (gray scale), and **B,** power Doppler, images show a 1-cm solid vascular mass.

TABLE 18-1. DIAGNOSTIC YIELD OF THYROID FINE-NEEDLE ASPIRATION (FNA)

SERIES	NO. OF CASES	FN RATE	FP RATE	SENSITIVITY	SPECIFICITY
Hawkins et al.[46]	1399	2.4%	4.6%	86%	95%
Khafagi et al.[47]	618	4.1%	7.7%	87%	72%
Hall et al.[48]	795	1.3%	3.0%	84%	90%
Altavilla et al.[49]	2433	6.0%	0.0%	71%	100%
Gharib and Goellner[45]	10,971	2.0%	0.7%	98%	99%
Ravetto et al.[50]	2014	11.2%	0.7%	89%	99%

Modified from Gharib H, Goellner JR. Fine-needle aspiration biopsy of the thyroid: an appraisal. Ann Intern Med 1993; 118:282-289.
   FN, False-negative; *FP,* False-positive.

72% to 100%, with a false-negative rate of 1% to 11% and a false-positive rate of 1% to 8%[45-51] (Table 18-1). In a recent study based on more than 5000 cytologic examinations, the most frequent cause of false-negative findings was the failure to recognize the follicular variant of papillary carcinoma.[51] In our practices, the overall accuracy of FNA exceeds 95%, and therefore it is currently the most accurate and cost-effective method for initial evaluation of patients with nodular thyroid disease. Since the introduction of FNA into routine clinical practice, the percentage of patients undergoing thyroidectomy has significantly decreased (to ~25%), and the cost of thyroid nodule care has been reduced by 25%.[45]

The evaluation of thyroid nodules primarily by FNA is common in North America and northern Europe. In other European countries and Japan, where goiter is prevalent, the initial evaluation often relies on radionuclide and sonographic imaging because of the need to select nodules that must undergo FNA.

Sonographic Applications

Although FNA is the most reliable diagnostic method for evaluating clinically palpable thyroid nodules, high-resolution sonography has four primary clinical applications, as follows[52-54]:

• Detection of thyroid and other cervical masses before and after thyroidectomy.
• Differentiation of benign from malignant masses on the basis of their sonographic appearance.
• Guidance for FNA biopsy.
• Guidance for the percutaneous treatment of nonfunctional and hyperfunctioning benign thyroid nodules and of lymph node metastases from papillary carcinoma.

Detection of Thyroid Masses

A practical use of sonography is to establish the precise anatomic location of a palpable cervical mass. The determination of whether such a mass is within or adjacent to the thyroid cannot always be made on the basis of the physical examination alone. Sonography can readily differentiate thyroid nodules from other cervical masses, such as cystic hygromas, thyroglossal duct cysts, and enlarged lymph nodes. Alternatively, sonography may help to confirm the presence of a thyroid nodule when the findings on physical examination are equivocal.

Sonography may be used to detect occult thyroid nodules in patients who have a **history of head and neck irradiation** during childhood as well as for those with a **family history of MEN II syndrome;** both groups have a known increased risk for development of thyroid malignancy. If a nodule is discovered, a biopsy can be performed under sonographic guidance. It is unknown, however, whether the detection of a thyroid cancer before it becomes clinically palpable will change the ultimate clinical outcome for a given patient.

In the past, when thyroid nodules were evaluated primarily with isotope scintigraphy, it was generally accepted that a "solitary cold" nodule carried a probability of malignancy of 15% to 25%, whereas a "cold" nodule in a multinodular gland was malignant in less than 1% of cases.[55] However, benign goiter is multinodular in 70% to 80% of cases, and 70% of nodules considered "solitary" on scintigraphy or physical examination are actually *multiple* when assessed with high-frequency ultrasound[22,56] (Fig. 18-29).

It has been suggested, therefore, that sonography may be used to detect additional occult nodules in patients with clinically solitary lesions, thereby implying that the dominant palpable mass is benign. Such a conclusion is unwarranted, however, because pathologically, benign nodules often coexist with malignant nodules. In a series of 1500 consecutive patients undergoing surgery for papillary carcinoma, 33% had coexistent benign nodules at surgery.[57] In addition, papillary thyroid cancer is recognized to be multicentric in at least 20% of cases and occult (<1.5 cm in diameter) in up to 48% of cases.[24,55] In a previous study, almost two thirds (64%) of patients with thyroid cancer had at least one nodule in addition to the dominant nodule detected sonographically.[58] Pathologically, these extra nodules can be benign or malignant. Therefore, in patients with a clinically solitary nodule, the sonographic detection of a few additional nodules is not a reliable sign for excluding malignancy.

An ultrasound-guided FNA biopsy is performed for patients with **multinodular goiter** when there is a dominant nodule. A **dominant nodule** is the largest nodule or has ultrasound features different from the other nodules or features suggestive of carcinoma.

In patients with known thyroid cancer, sonography can be useful to **determine the extent of disease,** both preoperatively and postoperatively. In most patients a sonographic examination is not performed routinely before thyroidectomy, but it can be useful in those with large cervical masses for evaluation of nearby structures, such as the carotid artery and internal jugular vein for evidence of direct invasion or encasement by the tumor. Alternatively, in patients who present with cervical lymphadenopathy caused by papillary thyroid cancer but

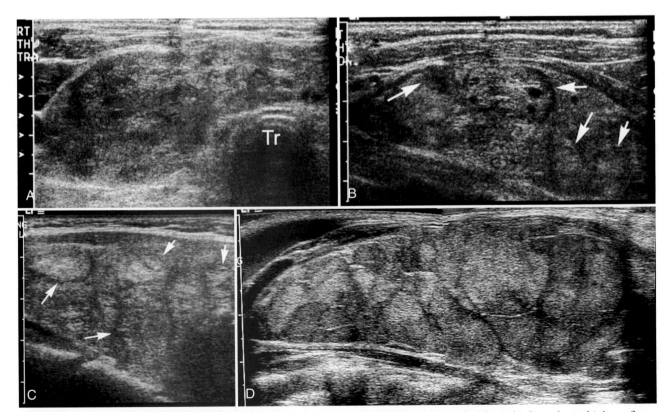

FIGURE 18-29. Multinodular goiter. A, Transverse image shows enlargement of the right lobe and isthmus by multiple confluent hypoechoic and hyperechoic nodules; *Tr,* tracheal air shadow. **B** and **C,** Longitudinal images show multiple confluent nodules *(arrows).* **D,** Longitudinal dual image shows enlargement of a lobe by multiple nodules.

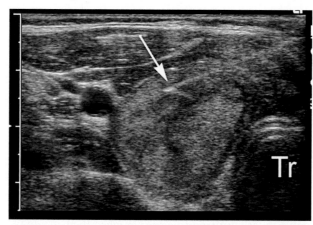

FIGURE 18-30. Fine-needle aspiration of thyroid nodule caused by follicular neoplasm. Transverse image shows a large nodule replacing the right thyroid lobe; *Tr*, tracheal air shadow. The tip of the 25-gauge needle is highly visible *(arrow)*, and the shaft of the needle is faintly visible.

TABLE 18-2. RELIABILITY OF SONOGRAPHIC FEATURES IN DIFFERENTIATION OF BENIGN FROM MALIGNANT THYROID NODULES

	Pathologic Diagnosis	
FEATURE	**BENIGN**	**MALIGNANT**
Shape		
Wider than tall	+++	++
Taller than wide	+	++++
Internal Contents		
Purely cystic content	++++	+
Cystic with thin septa	++++	+
Mixed solid and cystic	+++	++
Comet-tail artifact	+++	+
Echogenicity		
Hyperechoic	++++	+
Isoechoic	+++	++
Hypoechoic	+++	+++
Markedly hypoechoic	+	++++
Halo		
Thin halo	++++	++
Thick, incomplete halo	+	+++
Absent	+	+++
Margin		
Well defined	+++	++
Poorly defined	++	+++
Spiculated	+	++++
Calcification		
Eggshell calcification	+++	++
Coarse calcification	+++	+
Microcalcification	++	++++
Doppler		
Peripheral flow pattern	+++	++
Internal flow pattern	++	+++
Sonoelastography		
Patterns 1 and 2	++++	+
Patterns 3 and 4	+	+++

Data from authors' experience and literature reports.
+, Rare (<1%); ++, low probability (<15%); +++, intermediate probability (16%-84%); ++++, high probability (>85%).

in whom the thyroid gland is palpably normal, sonography may be used preoperatively to detect an occult, nonpalpable primary focus within the gland.

After partial or near-total thyroidectomy for carcinoma, sonography is the preferred method for follow-up, by detecting **residual, recurrent, or metastatic disease** in the neck.[59] In patients who have had subtotal thyroidectomy, the sonographic appearance of the remaining thyroid tissue may serve as an important factor in deciding whether complete thyroidectomy is recommended. If a mass is identified, its nature can be determined by ultrasound-guided FNA (Fig. 18-30). If no masses are seen, the clinician may choose to follow the patient with periodic sonographic studies. For patients who have had total or near-total thyroidectomy, sonography has proved to be more sensitive than physical examination in detecting recurrent disease within the thyroid bed or metastatic disease in cervical lymph nodes.[60] Patients with a history of thyroid cancer often undergo periodic sonographic examinations of the neck to detect nonpalpable recurrent or metastatic disease. When a mass is identified, FNA under sonographic guidance can establish a diagnosis of malignancy and help in surgical planning.

Differentiation of Benign and Malignant Nodules

According to several reports, for the differentiation of benign versus malignant thyroid nodules, sonography has sensitivity rates of 63% to 94%, specificity of 61% to 95%, and overall accuracy of 78% to 94%.[4,5,61-67] Currently, no single sonographic criterion distinguishes benign thyroid nodules from malignant nodules with complete reliability.[5,61-63,67] Nevertheless, certain sonographic features are seen more often with one type of histology or another type, thus establishing general diagnostic trends[34] (Table 18-2).

The fundamental anatomic features of a thyroid nodule on high-resolution sonography are as follows:
• Internal consistency (solid, mixed solid and cystic, or purely cystic)
• Echogenicity relative to adjacent thyroid parenchyma
• Margin
• Shape
• Presence and pattern of calcification
• Peripheral sonolucent halo
• Presence and distribution of blood flow signals

Internal Contents. In our experience, approximately 70% of thyroid nodules are solid, whereas the remaining 30% exhibit various amounts of cystic change. A nodule that has a significant cystic component is usually a **benign adenomatous (colloid) nodule** that has undergone degeneration or hemorrhage. When detected by older, lower-resolution ultrasound machines, these lesions were called "cysts" because the presence of internal debris and a thick wall could not be appreciated. Pathologically, a true epithelium-lined, simple thyroid cyst is extremely rare. Virtually all cystic thyroid lesions seen with high-resolution ultrasound demonstrate some wall irregularity and internal solid elements or debris caused by nodule degeneration (see Figs. 18-9 and 18-10). When high-frequency gray-scale sonography and color Doppler imaging cannot differentiate debris and septa from neoplastic intracystic vegetations, contrast-enhanced sonography can sometimes resolve the problem by demonstrating the arterial enhancement in tumoral projections and the complete lack of enhancement of benign septa and debris (see Fig. 18-12, *A* and *B*). **Comet-tail artifacts** are frequently encountered in cystic thyroid nodules and are likely related to the presence of microcrystals (see Fig. 18-10). In a published series of 100 patients presenting with this feature, FNA biopsy was benign in all cases.[23] These comet-tail artifacts can be located in the cyst walls and internal septations or in the cyst fluid. When a more densely echogenic fluid is gravitationally layered in the posterior portion of a cystic cavity, the likelihood of hemorrhagic debris is very high. Frequently, patients with hemorrhagic debris present clinically with a rapidly growing, often tender neck mass. The **spongiform appearance** of thyroid nodules, related to the presence of tiny colloid changes, is an extremely uncommon finding in malignant nodules, particularly when it is associated with other findings such as well-defined margins and isoechogenicity. This pattern is highly predictive of a benign nodule (see Fig. 18-9).

Papillary carcinomas may rarely exhibit varying amounts of cystic change and appear almost indistinguishable from benign cystic nodules.[68-70] In cystic papillary carcinomas, however, the frequent sonographic detection of a solid elements or projections (≥1 cm with blood flow signals and/or microcalcifications) into the lumen can lead to suspicion of malignancy (see Fig. 18-18). Cervical metastatic lymph nodes from either a solid or a cystic primary papillary cancer may also demonstrate a cystic pattern; this is likely pathognomonic of malignant adenopathy.

Shape. A taller-than-wide shape, in which the AP diameter is equal or less than its transverse diameter on a transverse or longitudinal plane, is specific for differentiating malignant nodules from benign nodules, likely because malignant neoplasms (taller than wide) grow across normal tissue planes, whereas benign nodules grow parallel to normal tissue planes.[61,67,68]

Echogenicity. Thyroid cancers are usually hypoechoic relative to the adjacent normal thyroid parenchyma (see Fig. 18-15). Unfortunately, many benign thyroid nodules are also hypoechoic. In fact, most **hypoechoic nodules** are benign because benign nodules are so much more common than malignant nodules. As recently observed, however, marked hypoechogenicity is highly specific for diagnosing malignant nodules, whereas the

hypoechogenicity often found in benign lesions is usually less marked.[67] A predominantly **hyperechoic nodule,** although relatively uncommon, is more likely to be benign.[22] The **isoechoic nodule,** visible because of a peripheral sonolucent rim that separates it from the adjacent normal parenchyma, has an intermediate to low risk of malignancy. Isoechogenicity has low sensitivity but high specificity and positive predictive value for the diagnosis of benign nodules.[67]

Halo. A peripheral sonolucent halo that completely or incompletely surrounds a thyroid nodule may be present in 60% to 80% of benign nodules and 15% of thyroid cancers.[22,71] Histologically, it is thought to represent the capsule of the nodule, but hyperplastic nodules that have no capsule often have this sonographic feature. The hypothesis that it represents compressed normal thyroid parenchyma seems acceptable, especially for rapidly growing thyroid cancers, which often have thick, irregular, and incomplete halos (see Fig. 18-15, *C*) that are hypovascular or avascular on color Doppler scans. Color and power Doppler imaging demonstrates that the thin, complete peripheral halo, which is strongly suggestive of benign nodules, represents blood vessels coursing around the periphery of the lesion, the "basket pattern."

Margin. Benign thyroid nodules tend to have sharp, well-defined margins, whereas malignant lesions tend to have irregular, spiculated, or poorly defined margins. For any given nodule, however, the appearance of the outer margin cannot reliably predict the histologic features because many exceptions to these general trends have been identified, even if the association of spiculated margins with malignant nodules has recently been demonstrated as highly specific.[67]

Calcification. Calcification can be detected in about 10% to 15% of all thyroid nodules, but the location and pattern of the calcification have a more predictive value in distinguishing benign from malignant lesions.[22] **Peripheral shell (eggshell) calcification**, although rarely present, has traditionally been considered a characteristic of a benign nodule (see Fig. 18-11). As recently reported, however, **thickened and interrupted peripheral calcifications**, particularly if associated with hypoechoic halo, have very high sensitivity for the diagnosis of malignant nature.[72,73] Scattered echogenic foci of calcification with or without associated acoustic shadows are more common. When these calcifications are **large and coarse** (usually related to fibrosis and degeneration), the nodule is more likely to be a benign nodule, with long disease duration. When the calcifications are **fine and punctate**, however, malignancy is more likely. Pathologically, these fine calcifications may be caused by psammoma bodies, typically seen in papillary cancers (see Figs. 18-14 and 18-15).

Medullary thyroid carcinomas often exhibit bright echogenic foci either within the primary tumor or within metastatically involved cervical lymph nodes.[35] The larger echogenic foci are usually associated with acoustic shadowing (see Fig. 18-25). Pathologically, these densities are caused by reactive fibrosis and calcification around amyloid deposits, which are characteristic of medullary carcinoma. In the appropriate clinical setting (e.g., MEN II syndrome, increased serum calcitonin level), the finding of echogenic foci within a hypoechoic thyroid nodule or a cervical node can be highly suggestive of medullary carcinoma.

Kakkos et al.[74] found a strong association between sonographically detected thyroid calcifications and thyroid malignancy, particularly in young patients or those with a solitary thyroid nodule. Patients younger than 40 with calcified nodules constitute a high-risk group, four times more likely to harbor thyroid malignancies than patients of the same age but without intranodular calcifications. Similarly, the presence of calcifications within a solitary nodule increases the incidence of malignancy. Therefore, these patients must be further evaluated or followed.

According to multiple studies of the various sonographic features seen in thyroid nodules, **microcalcifications** show the highest accuracy (76%), specificity (93%), and positive predictive value (70%) for malignancy as a single sign. However, sensitivity is low (36%) and insufficient to be reliable for detection of malignancy.[30,32,67,74]

Doppler Flow Pattern. It is well known from histologic studies that most hyperplastic nodules are hypovascular lesions and are less vascular than normal thyroid parenchyma. On the contrary, most **well-differentiated thyroid carcinomas** are generally hypervascular, with irregular tortuous vessels and AV shunting (see Fig. 18-16). **Poorly differentiated and anaplastic carcinomas** are often hypovascular because of the extensive necrosis associated with their rapid growth (see Fig. 18-26).

Quantitative analysis of flow velocities is not accurate in differentiating benign from malignant nodules, so the only Doppler feature that may be useful is the distribution of vessels. With current technology, no thyroid nodule appears totally avascular or extremely hypovascular on color and power Doppler imaging. The two main categories of vessel distribution are nodules with peripheral vascularity and nodules with internal vascularity (with or without a peripheral component).[20,21,75] Past studies demonstrated that 80% to 95% of hyperplastic, goitrous, and adenomatous nodules display **peripheral vascularity,** whereas 70% to 90% of thyroid malignancies display **internal vascularity,** with or without a peripheral component.[5,18,75-77] In addition, the resistive index (RI) of intranodular vessels was significantly higher in malignant nodules. Consequently, the vascular pattern and RI provide high sensitivity (92.3%) and specificity (88%) for the differentiation between benign and malignant tumors.[77] According to other reports, however, color Doppler imaging was not a reliable aid in the sonographic diagnosis of thyroid nodules.[78-80] With the current generation of Doppler instruments, which have extremely high sensitivity to blood flow, the overlapping of the two populations of nodules significantly increased, significantly reducing the diagnostic reliability of Doppler findings.[81]

Findings on gray-scale and color Doppler ultrasound become highly predictive for malignancy only when multiple signs are simultaneously present in a nodule.[61,63,67] In a series the combination of **absent halo sign plus microcalcifications plus intranodular flow pattern** achieved a 97.2% specificity for the diagnosis of thyroid malignancy.[61] In a recent report the presence of at least one malignant sonographic finding (taller-than-wide shape, spiculated margin, marked hypoechogenicity, microcalcification and macrocalcification) had sensitivity of 83.3%, specificity of 74.0%, and diagnostic accuracy of 78.0%.[67] The presence of other findings (e.g., rim calcification) showed no statistical significance in the differentiation of a malignant nodule from a benign nodule.

Sonoelastography

Recently, a new sonographic technique called **sonoelastography** (or **elastosonography**) has been applied to the study of thyroid nodules, following the results achieved for breast nodules. Sonoelastography provides information on tissue elasticity, based on the premise that pathologic processes such as cancer alter the physical characteristics of the involved tissue. Sonoelastographic measurements are performed during the ultrasound examination, using the same ultrasound machine and the same transducer. The operator exerts light pressure with the probe and selects the portion of the image that includes the nodule to be evaluated. The purpose is to acquire two sonographic images (before and after tissue compression) and track tissue displacement by assessing the propagation of the beam, providing accurate measurement of tissue distortion.[82,83]

The ultrasound elastogram is displayed over the typical B-mode gray-scale ultrasound scan in a color scale and classified by using the elasticity score.[84] To minimize interobserver and intraobserver variability, the freehand compression applied on the neck region is standardized by real-time measurement displayed on a numeric scale to maintain an intermediate level optimal for **elastographic evaluation.** Four elastographic patterns have been classified as follows[82,83,85]:

Pattern 1: Elasticity in the whole nodule (Fig. 18-31).
Pattern 2: Elasticity in a large part of the nodule, with inconstant appearance of anelastic areas (Fig. 18-32).
Pattern 3: Constant presence of large anelastic areas at the periphery (Fig. 18-33).
Pattern 4: Uniformly anelastic (Fig. 18-34).

In recent literature reports, 78% to 100% of benign nodules had a score of 1 to 2, whereas 88% to 96% of malignant nodules had a score of 3 to 4. Sensitivity was

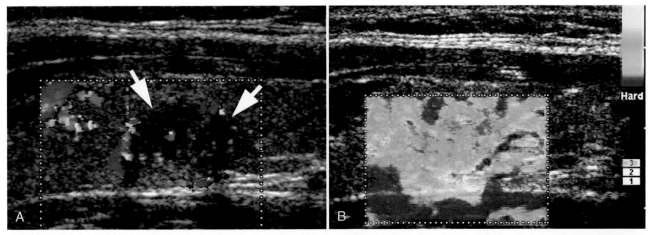

FIGURE 18-31. Use of ultrasound elastography on thyroid nodule: benign nodular hyperplasia (pattern 1). A, Conventional longitudinal B-mode sonogram with color Doppler shows a hypoechoic solid nodule *(arrows)* with peripheral halo, internal comet-tail artifacts, and perilesional blood flow pattern. **B,** Longitudinal ultrasound elastography at same location demonstrates a "soft" color pattern 1.

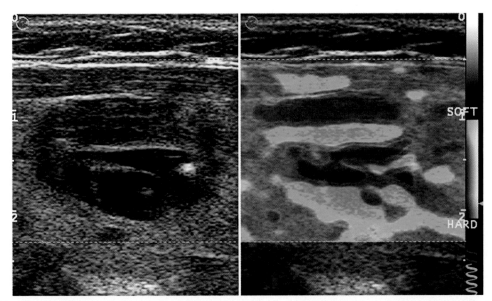

FIGURE 18-32. Use of ultrasound elastography on thyroid nodule: benign nodular hyperplasia with cystic changes (pattern 2). Left half of image shows a cystic, poorly defined nodule on conventional B-mode gray-scale sonogram. Right half of sonoelastogram of the nodule shows a predominantly elastic *(green)* pattern with a few internal anelastic bandlike areas.

82% to 97%, specificity 78% to 100%, positive predictive value 64% to 81%, and negative predictive value 91% to 98%.[83-88]

Specificity and sensitivity are relatively independent of the nodule's size. However, the best accuracy is achieved in small nodules and when FNA biopsy is nondiagnostic or suggests a follicular lesion, provided the nodule is solid and devoid of coarse calcifications.

Guidance for Needle Biopsy

Sonographically guided percutaneous needle biopsy of cervical masses has become an important technique in many clinical situations. Its main advantage is that it

affords continuous real-time visualization of the needle, a crucial requirement for the biopsy of small lesions. Most physicians use a 25-gauge needle employing either capillary action or minimal suction with a syringe **(Video 18-6).** There are reports of the usefulness of large-gauge, automated cutting needles for improved pathologic diagnosis.[89,90]

Sonographic guidance is generally suggested for all thyroid aspiration biopsies, but it is strongly recommended in three settings. The first situation is the questionable or inconclusive physical examination when a nodule is suggested but cannot be palpated with certainty. In these patients, sonography is used to confirm the presence of a nodule and to provide guidance for

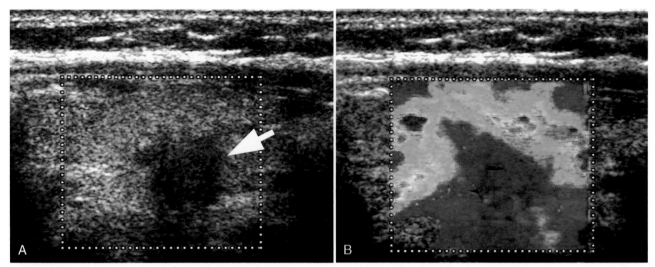

FIGURE 18-33. Use of ultrasound elastography on thyroid nodule: papillary thyroid carcinoma (pattern 3). A, Conventional longitudinal B-mode sonogram demonstrates a hypoechoic papillary carcinoma with irregular, poorly defined margins *(arrow).* **B,** Ultrasound elastography shows a predominantly anelastic *(blue)* pattern with a few small, elastic *(green)* areas in the posterior portion.

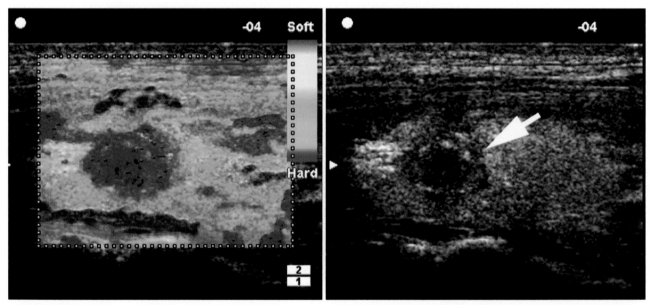

FIGURE 18-34. Use of ultrasound elastography on thyroid nodule: papillary thyroid carcinoma (pattern 4). Right half of image shows a hypoechoic solid nodule *(arrow)* with microcalcifications, typical of papillary carcinoma. Left half of image shows that on ultrasound elastography, the nodule is almost entirely anelastic *(blue)* pattern 4. The small, elastic areas seen in the posterior portion of the lesion are artifacts caused by pulsations of the underlying carotid artery.

accurate biopsy. The second setting involves patients at high risk for thyroid cancer with a normal gland on physical examination but a sonographically demonstrated nodule. This group includes patients with a previous history of head and neck irradiation, a positive family history of MEN II syndrome, or a previous subtotal thyroid resection for malignancy. The third situation for ultrasound FNA guidance involves patients who had a nondiagnostic or inconclusive biopsy performed under direct palpation. Usually about 20% of specimens obtained by palpation guidance are cytologically incon-clusive, most often because of the aspiration of nondiagnostic fluid from cystic lesions. Sonography may be used in these cases to guide the needle selectively into a solid portion of the mass. The diagnostic accuracy of FNA is very high, with sensitivity of approximately 85% and specificity of 99% in centers with extensive experience using these procedures.[43-50,91]

In patients who have undergone a previous thyroid resection for carcinoma, sonographically guided FNA has become an important method in the early diagnosis of recurrent or metastatic disease in the neck. In patients

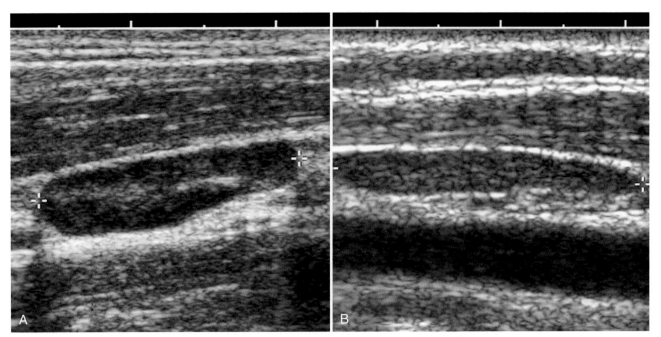

FIGURE 18-35. Normal cervical lymph nodes: elongated shape is typical. Longitudinal images. **A,** Slender node is homogeneous except for central echogenic hilum. **B,** Normal homogeneous slender node near the jugular vein without a visible hilum.

who have undergone hemithyroidectomy for a benign nodule, with the detection of one or more foci of occult malignant tumor in the surgical specimen, ultrasound evaluation of the contralateral lobe is warranted to exclude the existence of a residual nodule.

Cervical lymph nodes, both normal and abnormal, can be readily visualized by high-resolution sonography. They tend to lie along the internal jugular chain, extending from the level of the clavicles to the angle of the mandible, or to be in the region of the thyroid bed. **Benign cervical lymph nodes** usually have a slender, oval shape and often exhibit a central echogenic band that represents the fatty hilum (Fig. 18-35). **Malignant lymph nodes,** on the other hand, are more often located in the lower third of the neck and are usually rounder and have no echogenic hilum, presumably because of obliteration by tumor infiltration (see Fig. 18-17). Although often hypoechoic, malignant nodes may be diffusely echogenic, may be heterogeneous, and may contain calcifications and cystic changes. Calcifications can be seen in nodal metastases from papillary and medullary thyroid malignancies, and cystic changes are very characteristic in metastatic papillary carcinoma.[92] In addition, Lyshchik et al.[93] recently reported that at sonoelastography, cervical lymph nodes with a strain index greater than 1.5 are usually malignant (85% sensitivity and 98% specificity).

When the differentiation between benign and malignant lymph nodes is not feasible with sonography, FNA under sonographic guidance is often used. In our experience, biopsy can be done with a high degree of accuracy in cervical nodes that are as small as 0.5 cm in diameter[60] (Fig. 18-36). In addition to cytologic analysis, the "washout" of the aspirate can be sent for thyroglobulin assay, which is highly accurate for the diagnosis of metastatic papillary and follicular cancer.[94]

Guidance for Percutaneous Treatment

Ethanol Injection of Benign Cystic Thyroid Lesions. Lesions containing fluid (usually colloid cysts) account for 31% of thyroid nodules found on sonography, but less than 1% of these are pure epithelial-lined cysts.[5] Management of cystic thyroid nodules relies first on FNA biopsy to rule out malignancy. Simple aspiration may result in permanent shrinkage of the lesion, but the recurrence rate after aspiration is high, 10% to 80%, depending on the number of aspirations and the cyst volume; the greater the volume, the greater the recurrence risk.[95,96]

Prevention of cyst recurrence requires intranodular injection of a sclerosing agent. Ethanol has been used successfully for the past 20 years, with accurate placement using real-time sonographic guidance. Ethanol is distributed within tissues by diffusion and induces cellular dehydration and protein denaturation, followed by coagulation necrosis and reactive fibrosis. The cyst fluid is completely aspirated with a fine needle, and then sterile 95% ethanol is injected under ultrasound guidance, in an amount varying from 30% to 60% (according to different experiences) of the aspirated fluid[97,98] (Fig. 18-37). Subsequently, ethanol can be either reaspirated in 1 to 2 days or permanently left in place. In large cystic cavities, this procedure can be repeated once or twice after several weeks. The volume reduction of the cyst is more significant if a larger

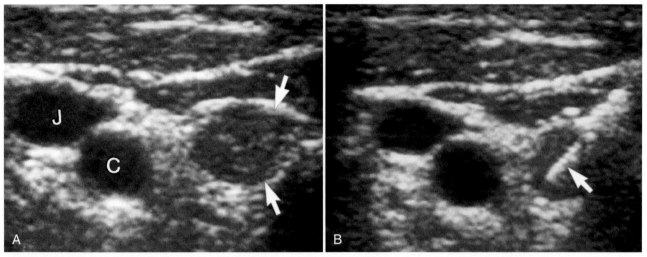

FIGURE 18-36. Biopsy of recurrent papillary carcinoma in thyroid bed after thyroidectomy. A, Transverse scan of right side of the neck shows a 1-cm solid mass *(arrows)* medial to carotid artery *(C)* and jugular vein *(J).* **B,** Sonographically guided fine-needle aspiration with needle seen within mass *(arrow).*

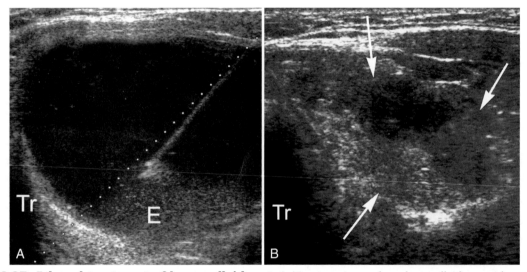

FIGURE 18-37. Ethanol treatment of large colloid cyst. A, Transverse image shows large colloid cyst with needle. Injected ethanol appears as low-level echoes *(E); Tr,* tracheal air shadow. **B,** Follow-up image 1 month later shows that the large cystic component has mostly resolved, leaving a slightly enlarged residual gland *(arrows).*

amount of ethanol is injected; thus a relationship exists between the volume of ethanol instilled and the ablative effect.

Ethanol injection is usually well tolerated by the patient. Transient mild to moderate local pain is the most common complication, a result of ethanol leaking into subcutaneous tissue. Rare complications of **ethanol sclerotherapy** are transient hyperthyroidism, hoarseness, hematoma, and dyspnea.

Reported success rates (total disappearance or volume reduction greater than 70% of initial volume) of this

treatment range from 72% to 95% at long-term follow-up,[97-100] achieved without a change in thyroid function. Ethanol injection is considered the percutaneous treatment of choice for cystic lesions of the thyroid gland at some institutions.

Ethanol Injection of Autonomously Functioning Thyroid Nodules. Thyroid nodules with independent secretory and proliferative activity are defined as **autonomous** thyroid nodules. On radionuclide scans, these nodules appear "hot," in contrast to the low or absent extranodular uptake, likely related to the avidity of iodine trapping and the degree of thyroid hyperfunction. Patients may be toxic or nontoxic, depending on the amount of thyroid hormones secreted. The level of hyperthyroidism is usually proportional to the nodule volume. Therefore, autonomous thyroid nodules can cause a range of functional abnormalities, from euthyroidism (compensated) to subclinical hyperthyroidism (pretoxic) and clinical hyperthyroidism (toxic).

The currently available treatments of autonomous nodules include surgery and radioactive iodine therapy. Surgery is effective but has the disadvantage of intrinsic anesthesiologic and surgical risks. Radioactive iodine therapy may require repeated sessions before achieving euthyroidism.

Percutaneous ethanol injection under ultrasound guidance, first proposed by Livraghi et al.[101] in 1990, is an alternative therapy. The diffusion of ethanol causes direct damage. Cell dehydration is followed by immediate coagulation necrosis and subsequent fibrotic changes. Sterile 95% ethanol is injected through a 21- or 22-gauge spinal needle with closed conical tip and three terminal side holes. This allows the injection of a large amount of ethanol, reduces the total number of sessions, increases the treated volume, and minimizes the risk of laryngeal nerve damage because of the lateral diffusion of ethanol. Several treatment sessions are needed (usually four to eight), generally performed at 2-day to 2-week intervals. The total amount of ethanol delivered is usually 1.5 times the nodular volume.

Color Doppler imaging and, if available, contrast-enhanced sonography are extremely valuable to assess the results of ethanol injection. The reduction (up to complete disappearance) of vascularity and contrast enhancement is directly related to the ethanol-induced necrosis. In addition, residual vascularity after treatment can be targeted to achieve complete ablation.[102] **Complete cure** is defined as normalization of serum free thyroid hormones and serum thyrotropin and scintigraphic reactivation of extranodular tissue. **Partial cure** occurs when serum free thyroid hormones and thyrotropin levels are normalized, but the nodule is still visible at scintigraphy.[101,103]

Percutaneous ethanol injection is generally well tolerated. The common side effect is a brief burning sensation or moderate pain at the injection site, radiating to the mandibular or retroauricular regions. The slow withdrawal of the needle and use of the multihole needle reduce this side effect. In some patients with larger nodules, when the amount of necrosis is high, fever lasting 2 to 3 days develops after the initial treatments. The only important complication is transient damage of the recurrent laryngeal nerve, reported 1% to 4% of cases.[81,84] Nerve damage is induced chemically or by compression. Full nerve recovery is likely because, in contrast to surgery, there is no anatomic nerve interruption.

Efficacy of response is inversely proportional to the nodule volume; the smaller the nodule, the more complete the response. Complete cure is reported to be achieved in 68% to 100% of pretoxic nodules and 50% to 89% of toxic nodules.[101-106] Ultrasound-guided percutaneous ethanol injection is the treatment of choice in older patients with contraindications to surgery, in pregnant patients, and in patients with large autonomous nodules (>40 mL), in addition to medical treatment to obtain euthyroidism more rapidly.

Recently, the use of **radiofrequency ablation** (RFA) with either internally cooled or multipronged electrodes has been reported in the treatment of autonomously functioning thyroid nodules, mostly for large nodules causing compressive symptoms. A significant decrease in size (≥50%) of the treated lesions was reported in all cases, and complete normalization of thyroid function was achieved in 24% to 44% of patients.[107,108]

Percutaneous Treatment of Solitary Solid Benign "Cold" Thyroid Nodules. In patients with solitary solid, biopsy-proven, benign "cold" thyroid nodules, ethanol injection, interstitial laser photocoagulation, and RFA have been proposed as ultrasound-guided percutaneous treatments, to achieve marked shrinkage of the nodule to a small, fibrous-calcified mass. With percutaneous ethanol injection, a mean nodule volume reduction of 84% (range, 73%-98%) has been reported after 3 to 10 treatments.[109] With low-power interstitial laser photocoagulation, mean thyroid nodule volumes decreased by 40% to 50% after 6 months, with improvement of local clinical symptoms in approximately 80% of patients and no side effects.[110-112]

Radiofrequency ablation with internally cooled electrodes and low power (20-70 W) has also been employed for the treatment of benign cold thyroid nodules, with only one ablation session for a single nodule. A significant volume reduction of the treated nodules without adverse effects has been reported at follow-up, but studies with longer follow-up are needed to assess efficacy and safety.[113] RFA and ethanol injection have been proposed for the treatment of recurrent disease and metastatic lymph nodes in patients who have previously undergone surgery.[114]

Percutaneous Ethanol Injection of Cervical Nodal Metastases from Papillary Carcinoma. Percutaneous ethanol injection (PEI) is an effective and safe method of treatment for limited lymph node metastasis from thyroid cancer. In a 2002 report from the Mayo Clinic, 14 patients who had undergone thyroidectomy for papillary thyroid carcinoma (PTC) presented with 29 metastatic lymph nodes on follow-up sonographic imaging.[115] Each node was treated with direct injection of ethanol using ultrasound guidance. Follow-up examination at 2 years showed a 95% decrease in the size of treated nodes. There were no major complications (e.g., recurrent laryngeal nerve palsy, bleeding) in the Mayo Clinic series or in 187 patients with papillary cancer nodes treated

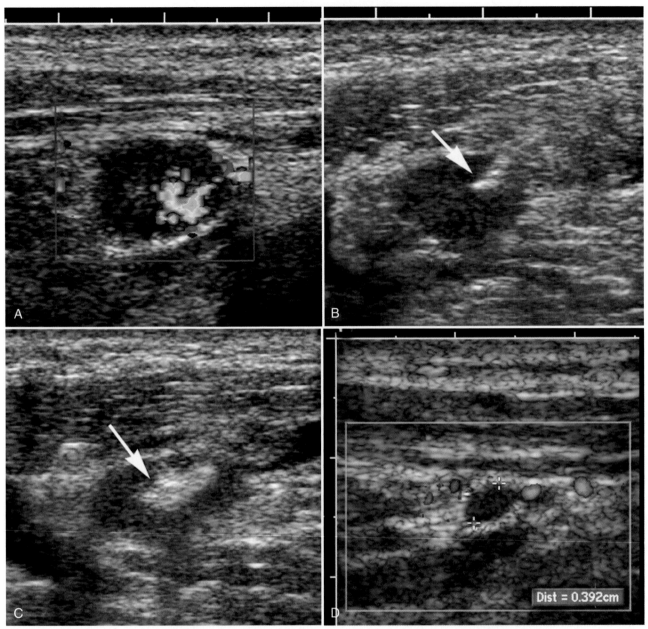

FIGURE 18-38. Ethanol treatment of thyroid metastasis in a cervical lymph node. A, Longitudinal color Doppler image shows a round, 1.6-cm, pathologic-appearing node with moderate vascularity. **B,** The tip of a 25-gauge needle *(arrow)* is in the lymph node. **C,** The ethanol effect is visible as a focal hyperechoic area *(arrow)* at injection and is caused by microbubbles that form from the interaction of ethanol with the tissues. This hyperechoic appearance will last from several seconds to several minutes and will be followed by a normal or near-normal appearance. During the injection, the hyperechogenicity is a useful marker to identify the areas treated. **D,** Follow-up power Doppler image 6 months after ethanol injection shows that the lymph node has dramatically decreased in size (0.4 cm) and is no longer vascular. No further therapy is needed except to follow every 6 to 12 months to confirm lack of change.

with PEI at the Ito Hospital in Japan.[116] Kim et al.[117] reported similar excellent results in 27 PTC patients with 47 neck recurrences; all treated lesions significantly decreased in volume (mean, 93.6%). They concluded that PEI offered an alternative for controlling neck recurrence of PTC in select patients who were poor surgical candidates.

The PEI technique is similar to the method used for percutaneous ethanol therapy of parathyroid adenomas. A 25-gauge needle is attached to a tuberculin syringe containing up to 1 mL of 95% ethanol. The needle is placed with ultrasound guidance using a freehand technique that allows fine positioning of the needle within the node (Fig. 18-38). Each node is injected in several sites. The portion of the node that is injected becomes hyperechoic due to the formation of microbubbles of gas. After usually less than 1 minute, the hyperechoic zone decreases. The needle is repositioned in the node, and several injections are made until the node appears adequately treated. Patients may experience mild to moderate pain at injection, but this resolves within minutes. For small nodes about 5 mm in diameter, a single injection may be sufficient. For larger nodes, a reinjection the following day is needed for complete therapy. Follow-up ultrasound at 3 to 6 months will show a reduction in size of the node in most cases. If blood flow was visualized in the node before therapy, it will often be significantly decreased or absent on follow-up. If on follow-up the size of the node has not decreased, or if there is residual blood flow on power Doppler examination, a repeat injection is performed.

Although since 1993 we have successfully treated recurrent neck nodal metastases from both Hürthle cell cancer and medullary thyroid cancer, we believe PEI is optimally employed in select patients with PTC, particularly those who had multiple prior neck surgeries and who proved to be refractory to repeated applications of therapeutic radioactive iodine. The majority of our PEI-treated patients at Mayo have proved to be pTNM stage I PTC, whose cause-specific survival approaches 100% but whose quality of life is diminished by multiple neck nodal recurrences. Of 35 such patients treated from 1993 to 2004, 52% of their 56 PEI-treated nodes completely disappeared, while the remaining 48% were identifiable, were significantly reduced in size, and had no Doppler flow. These stage I patients were followed on average for 5.6 years (range, 3-14 years); there was no documented regrowth of any PEI-treated nodes, and no treated node required further surgical intervention. At latest follow-up, the median serum thyroglobulin (tumor marker) level was almost undetectable at 0.3 ng/mL, and none of the 35 patients had hoarseness after successful PEI treatment.[118]

The Incidentally Detected Nodule

Although using high-frequency sonography to detect small, nonpalpable thyroid nodules may be beneficial in certain clinical settings, it may actually introduce problems in other situations. What should one do with the many thyroid nodules detected incidentally during carotid, parathyroid, and other sonographic examinations of the neck? The goal should be to avoid extensive and costly evaluations in the majority of patients with benign disease, without missing the minority of patients who have clinically significant thyroid cancer (Table 18-3). Understanding the challenge of selecting nodules for workup requires background information in the following four areas:

EVALUATION OF NODULES INCIDENTALLY DETECTED BY SONOGRAPHY

Nodules less than 1.5 cm
• Followed by palpation at next physical examination.
Nodules greater than 1.5 cm
• Evaluation, usually by FNA.
Nodules that have malignant features
• Evaluation by FNA.

FNA, Fine-needle aspiration.

TABLE 18-3. PREVALENCE OF THYROID NODULES

METHOD OF DETECTION	PATIENTS (%)
Autopsy	49
Sonography	41
Palpation	7
Occult cancer (autopsy)	2
Cancer incidence (annual)	0.005

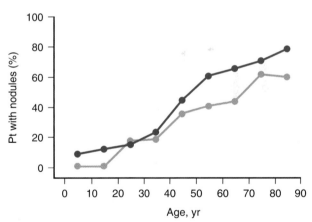

FIGURE 18-39. Prevalence of thyroid nodules on autopsy and sonography. Autopsy *(blue circles)* revealed thyroid nodules on average in 49% of patients in 1955, and sonography *(orange circles)* detected thyroid nodules in 41% in 1985, with both shown here as a function of patient age. *(From Horlocker TT, Hay JE, James EM, et al. Prevalence of incidental nodular thyroid disease detected during high-resolution parathyroid ultrasonography. In Medeiros-Neto G, Gaitlin E, editors. Frontiers in thyroidology. Vol 2. New York, 1986, Plenum, pp 1309-1312.)*

1. **The epidemic of thyroid nodules has resulted mostly from ultrasound imaging.**

On physical palpation, an estimated 7% of the North American population has at least one thyroid nodule. In contrast, there is an "epidemic" of thyroid nodules detected by ultrasound, with studies showing up to 67% of patients having a nodule.[119] Our study of 1000 consecutive patients imaged with 10-MHz ultrasound transducers showed a prevalence of 41%.[120] This study also showed an increasing prevalence with advancing age, which parallels autopsy rates of prevalence compared with patient age (Fig 18-39).

From these studies it is reasonable to estimate that more than 100 million Americans have thyroid nodules on ultrasound. The problem of the high rate of incidentally detected thyroid nodules, the so called "incidentaloma," has led some to ask if it is "time to turn off the ultrasound machines."[121] The morbidity and cost to patients and society from workup of these nodules may far outweigh the benefit of detecting an occult thyroid cancer, because the vast majority of thyroid cancers behave in a benign manner. Specifically, patients with PTC have a 99% 10-year survival and approximately a 95% overall 30-year survival.[57,122]

2. The incidence of thyroid cancer is increasing.

Over 50 years ago, pathologists reported that clinically insignificant thyroid cancer was a common finding at autopsy. In the 1980s, Harach et al.[123] studied thinly sectioned thyroid glands at autopsy and found that 36% had occult thyroid cancer. They stated that had they sectioned the glands even more finely, almost every person would harbor a thyroid cancer. They concluded that occult PTC was a "normal" finding at autopsy.

Over the last three decades, the reported incidence of thyroid cancer in North America has more than doubled.[124] This raises the question whether the increase is caused by a real increased incidence of thyroid cancer or if it is simply a result of an increased rate of detection by diagnostic imaging methods such as ultrasound. Analyzing the data, Davies and Welch[124] found that the increased incidence resulted from increased detection of subclinical disease rather than from an increase in the true occurrence of thyroid cancer. Their work showed that PTC accounts for virtually the entire increase in incidence (Fig. 18-40). They also showed that the increased rate of detection is caused by small, subclinical thyroid cancer (Fig. 18-41). Furthermore, although the prevalence of thyroid cancer more than doubled over 30 years, the mortality rate remained unchanged (Fig. 18-42). According to Ross,[125] "Considering the anxiety, costs and complications suffered by many of these patients, one can reasonably question the benefits of increased cancer detection."

3. What are the costs of frequent use of FNA biopsy for management of incidentally detected thyroid nodules?

If FNA biopsy were used as the automatic next step after nodule detection, the costs to patients and society would be great. Whereas FNA biopsy is considered the "gold standard" for nodule diagnosis, it is an imperfect technique for many reasons. First, the results are nondiagnostic in 10% to 20% of cases.[91,126] Second, there is a

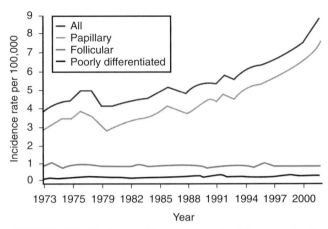

FIGURE 18-40. Thyroid cancer: incidence. Graph shows the increasing incidence of thyroid cancer in North America during the past three decades. Note that the type of thyroid malignancy is almost entirely caused by papillary carcinoma. The increasing incidence results from the increased rate of detection by diagnostic imaging methods such as ultrasound, rather than from an increase in the true occurrence of thyroid cancer.

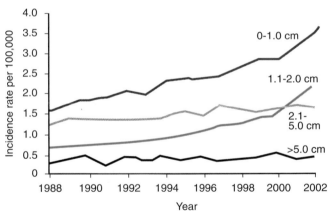

FIGURE 18-41. Thyroid cancer: incidence by size of tumor. Note that the increased incidence of thyroid carcinoma is primarily the result of the detection of smaller tumors.

false-negative rate of 3% to 5%.[127] Third, interpretive skills vary widely regarding cytopathology of the thyroid nodule. Unfortunately, in less experienced centers, the report of "follicular cells are present, cannot exclude follicular neoplasm" occurs more frequently than in centers with greater interpretive experience. This report typically leads to the need for surgical excision. Given these considerations, an estimated 18% of all patients who have FNA biopsy ultimately undergo surgery for nodule excision based on positive, suspicious, or nondiagnostic

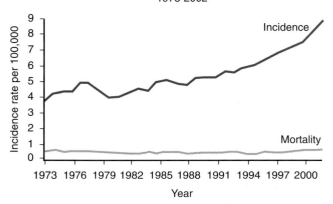

THYROID CANCER INCIDENCE AND MORTALITY
1973-2002

FIGURE 18-42. Thyroid cancer: incidence versus mortality. Although the rate of occurrence of thyroid cancer has more than doubled in the last 30 years, the mortality rate is unchanged over that period.

DIFFUSE THYROID DISEASES

Acute suppurative thyroiditis
Subacute granulomatous thyroiditis
Hashimoto's thyroiditis (chronic lymphocytic thyroiditis)
Adenomatous or colloid goiter
Painless (silent) thyroiditis

results, and most of these nodules are benign.[91,128,129] Of these surgical patients, only 15% to 32% have cancer.[91,128] Therefore, the majority of patients who have surgery for thyroid nodule excision will have had an operation for clinically insignificant, benign nodular disease.

The potential cost of the FNA biopsy workup of these nodules must be considered. For discussion purposes, assume that 1 million of the estimated 300 million people in the United States undergo a high-frequency ultrasound thyroid examination, and that one or more thyroid nodules are detected in approximately 40%. Therefore, 400,000 people will have one or more thyroid nodules detected by ultrasound imaging. Assuming a cost of approximately $1500 for an ultrasound-guided FNA and cytologic analysis, $600 million could theoretically be spent to exclude or detect thyroid cancer in this group. If 18% of these FNA biopsies result in suspicious or nondiagnostic results, 72,000 procedures could occur at a cost of almost $20,000 each, for an additional cost of $1.44 billion. Finally, approximately 5%, or almost 3600 patients, could experience significant postsurgical morbidity, including hoarseness, hypoparathyroidism, and long-lasting pain.[130] Clearly, this type of aggressive management of thyroid nodules would entail massive health care expenditures and could have an extremely negative clinical impact.[131]

4. **Which incidentally discovered nodules should be pursued?**

Because of the many nodules detected on ultrasound, the therapeutic approach should allow most patients with clinically significant cancers to go on to further investigations. More importantly, it should allow most patients with benign lesions to avoid further costly, potentially harmful workup. With this goal in mind, many practices, including ours, have found that it is both impractical and imprudent to pursue the diagnosis for most of the small nodules detected incidentally on ultrasound. If technically possible, we usually obtain FNA biopsy of lesions that exhibit sonographic features strongly associated with malignancy, such as marked hypoechogenicity, taller-than-wide shape, and thick irregular margins, as well as lesions containing microcalcifications.

DIFFUSE THYROID DISEASE

Several thyroid diseases are characterized by diffuse rather than focal involvement. This usually results in generalized enlargement of the gland **(goiter)** and no palpable nodules. Specific conditions that produce such diffuse enlargement include chronic autoimmune lymphocytic thyroiditis (Hashimoto's thyroiditis), colloid or adenomatous goiter, and Graves' disease. These conditions are usually diagnosed on the basis of clinical and laboratory findings and occasionally FNA biopsy. Sonography is seldom indicated. However, high-resolution sonography can be helpful when the underlying diffuse disease causes **asymmetrical** thyroid enlargement, which suggests a mass in the larger lobe. The sonographic finding of generalized parenchymal abnormality may alert the clinician to consider diffuse thyroid disease as the underlying cause. FNA, with sonographic guidance if necessary, can be performed if a nodule is detected. Recognition of diffuse thyroid enlargement on sonography can often be facilitated by noting the thickness of the isthmus, normally a thin bridge of tissue measuring only a few millimeters in AP dimension. With diffuse thyroid enlargement, the isthmus may be up to 1 cm or more in thickness.

Each type of thyroiditis, including acute suppurative thyroiditis, subacute granulomatous thyroiditis (de Quervain's disease), and chronic lymphocytic thyroiditis (Hashimoto's disease) has distinctive clinical and laboratory features.[132] **Acute suppurative thyroiditis** is a rare inflammatory disease usually caused by bacterial infection and affecting children. Sonography can be useful in select patients to detect the development of a frank thyroid abscess. The infection usually begins in the perithyroidal soft tissues. On ultrasound images, an abscess is seen as a poorly defined, hypoechoic heterogeneous

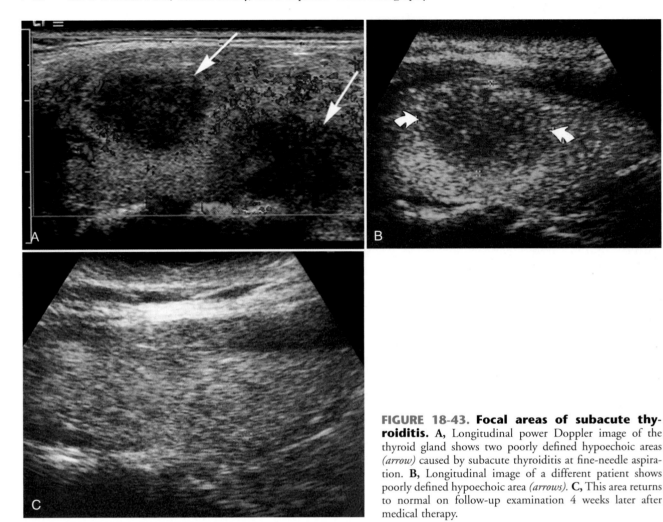

FIGURE 18-43. Focal areas of subacute thyroiditis. A, Longitudinal power Doppler image of the thyroid gland shows two poorly defined hypoechoic areas *(arrow)* caused by subacute thyroiditis at fine-needle aspiration. **B,** Longitudinal image of a different patient shows poorly defined hypoechoic area *(arrows).* **C,** This area returns to normal on follow-up examination 4 weeks later after medical therapy.

mass with internal debris, with or without septa and gas. Adjacent inflammatory nodes are often present.

Subacute granulomatous thyroiditis or de Quervain's disease, is a spontaneously remitting inflammatory disease probably caused by viral infection. The clinical findings include fever, enlargement of the gland, and pain on palpation. Sonographically, the gland may appear enlarged and hypoechoic, with normal or decreased vascularity caused by diffuse edema of the gland, or the process may appear as focal hypoechoic regions[133,134] (Fig. 18-43). Although usually not necessary, sonography can be used to assess evolution of de Quervain's disease after medical therapy.

The most common type of thyroiditis is **chronic autoimmune lymphocytic thyroiditis, or Hashimoto's thyroiditis.** It typically occurs as a painless, diffuse enlargement of the thyroid gland in a young or middle-aged woman, often associated with hypothyroidism. It is the most common cause of hypothyroidism in North America. Patients with this autoimmune disease develop antibodies to their own thyroglobulin as well as to the major enzyme of thyroid hormonogenesis, thyroid peroxidase (TPO). The typical sonographic appearance of Hashimoto's thyroiditis is diffuse, coarsened, parenchymal echotexture, generally more hypoechoic than a normal thyroid[130] (Fig. 18-44). In most cases the gland is enlarged. Multiple, discrete **hypoechoic micronodules** from 1 to 6 mm in diameter are strongly suggestive of chronic thyroiditis; this appearance has been called **micronodulation** (Fig. 18-44; **Video 18-7**). Micronodulation is a highly sensitive sign of chronic thyroiditis, with a positive predictive value of 94.7%.[135] Histologically, micronodules represent lobules of thyroid parenchyma that have been infiltrated by lymphocytes and plasma cells. These lobules are surrounded by multiple linear echogenic fibrous septations (Fig. 18-45). These fibrotic septations may give the parenchyma a "pseudolobulated" appearance. Both benign and malignant thyroid nodules may coexist with chronic lymphocytic thyroiditis, and FNA is often necessary to establish the final diagnosis[136] (Figs. 18-46 to 18-48). As with other autoimmune disorders, there is an increased risk of malignancy, with a B-cell malignant lymphoma most often arising within the gland.

The vascularity on color Doppler imaging is normal or decreased in most patients with the diagnosis of

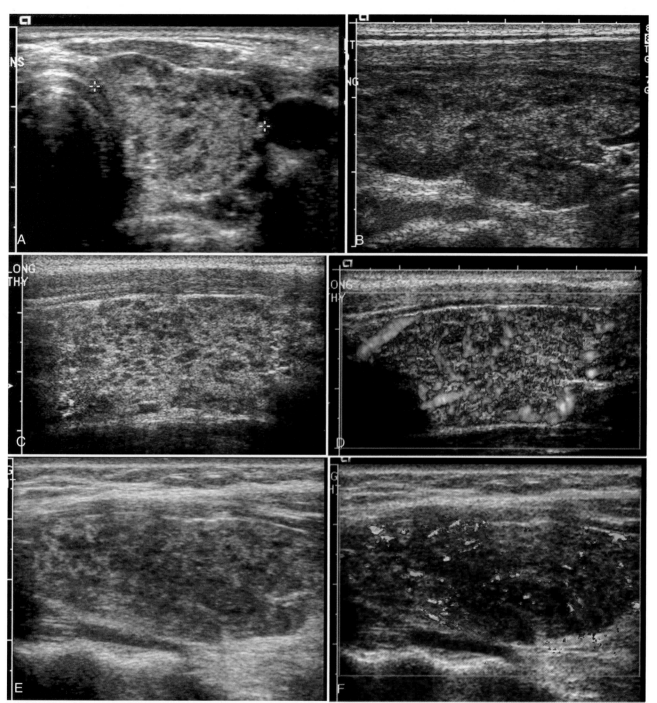

FIGURE 18-44. Hashimoto's thyroiditis: micronodularity. A, Transverse, and **B,** longitudinal, images of the left lobe demonstrate multiple small hypoechoic nodules that are lymphocyte infiltration of the parenchyma. **C** and **D,** Longitudinal images of another patient show multiple tiny hypoechoic nodules and increased flow on power Doppler. This increased flow may indicate an acute phase of the thyroiditis. **E** and **F,** Longitudinal images of a different patient show multiple tiny hypoechoic nodules and decreased flow on color Doppler scan. The blood flow is normal or diminished in most cases of Hashimoto's thyroiditis.

Hashimoto's thyroiditis (see Fig. 18-44). Occasionally, hypervascularity similar to the "thyroid inferno" of Graves' disease occurs. One study suggested that hypervascularity occurs when hypothyroidism develops, perhaps related to stimulation from the associated high serum levels of thyrotropin (TSH).[137] Often, cervical lymphadenopathy is present, most evident near the lower pole of the thyroid gland (Fig. 18-49). The end stage of chronic thyroiditis is atrophy, when the thyroid gland is small, with poorly defined margins and heterogeneous texture caused by progressive fibrosis. Blood flow signals are absent. Occasionally, discrete nodules occur, and FNA biopsy is needed to establish the diagnosis.[136]

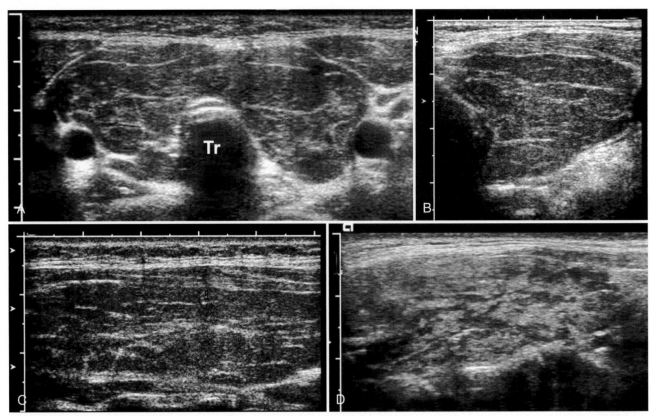

FIGURE 18-45. Hashimoto's thyroiditis: coarse septations. A, Transverse dual image of the thyroid shows marked diffuse enlargement of both lobes and the isthmus. Multiple linear bright echoes throughout the hypoechoic parenchyma are caused by lymphocytic infiltration of the gland with coarse septations from fibrous bands. *Tr,* Tracheal air shadow. **B,** Transverse, and **C,** longitudinal, images of another patient demonstrate linear echogenic septations throughout the gland. **D,** Longitudinal image of another patient shows thicker echogenic linear areas that separate hypoechoic regions.

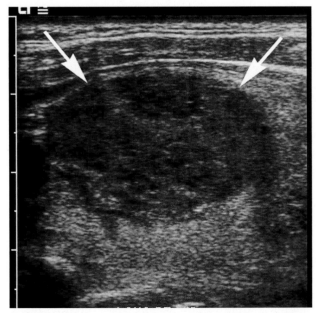

FIGURE 18-46. Hashimoto's thyroiditis: nodule. Longitudinal image shows a discrete hypoechoic nodule *(arrows)* that proved to be Hashimoto's thyroiditis at fine-needle aspiration biopsy.

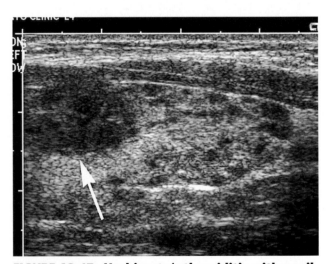

FIGURE 18-47. Hashimoto's thyroiditis with papillary thyroid cancer. Longitudinal image shows classic Hashimoto's thyroiditis (micronodularity) and a hypoechoic dominant nodule *(arrow)* in the upper pole caused by papillary thyroid carcinoma. A dominant nodule in Hashimoto's thyroiditis should be considered "indeterminate" and fine-needle aspiration performed.

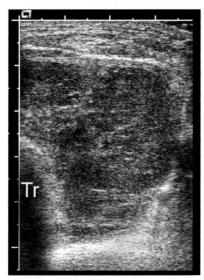

FIGURE 18-48. Lymphoma in Hashimoto's thyroiditis. Transverse image of the left lobe shows diffuse hypoechoic enlargement caused by lymphoma in a gland with Hashimoto's thyroiditis; *Tr,* tracheal air shadow.

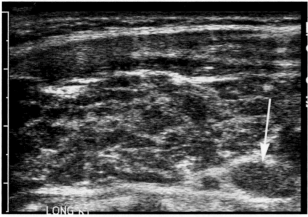

FIGURE 18-49. Hashimoto's thyroiditis with hyperplastic enlarged lymph nodes. Longitudinal image shows micronodularity of Hashimoto's thyroiditis and an enlarged lymph node *(arrow)* inferior to the lower pole.

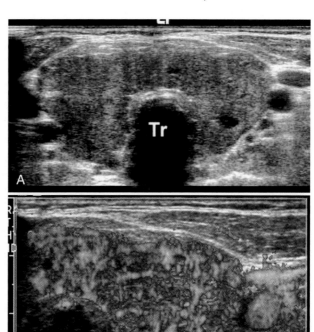

FIGURE 18-50. Hyperthyroidism: Graves' disease. **A,** Transverse dual image of the thyroid gland shows marked diffuse enlargement of both thyroid lobes and the isthmus. The gland is diffusely hypoechoic. **B,** Transverse color Doppler image of the left lobe shows increased vascularity, indicating an acute stage of the Graves' disease process; *Tr,* trachea.

Painless (silent) thyroiditis has the typical histologic and sonographic pattern of chronic autoimmune thyroiditis (hypoechogenicity, micronodulation, and fibrosis), but clinical findings resemble classic subacute thyroiditis, with the exception of node tenderness. Moderate hyperthyroidism with thyroid enlargement usually occurs in the early phase, in some cases followed by hypothyroidism of variable degree. In postpartum thyroiditis the progression to hypothyroidism is more common. In most cases the disease spontaneously remits within 3 to 6 months, and the gland may return to a normal appearance.

Although the appearance of diffuse parenchymal inhomogeneity and micronodularity is typical of Hashimoto's thyroiditis, other diffuse thyroid diseases, most frequently **multinodular** or **adenomatous goiter,** may have a similar sonographic appearance. Most patients with adenomatous goiter have multiple discrete nodules separated by otherwise normal-appearing thyroid parenchyma (see Fig. 18-29); others have enlargement with rounding of the poles of the gland, diffuse parenchymal inhomogeneity, and no recognizable normal tissue. Adenomatous goiter affects women three times more often than men.

Graves' disease is a common diffuse abnormality of the thyroid gland and is usually biochemically characterized by hyperfunction (thyrotoxicosis). The echotexture may be more inhomogeneous than in diffuse goiter, mainly because of numerous large, intraparenchymal vessels. Further, especially in young patients, the parenchyma may be diffusely hypoechoic because of the extensive lymphocytic infiltration or the predominantly cellular content of the parenchyma, which becomes almost devoid of colloid substance. Color Doppler sonography often demonstrates a hypervascular pattern referred to as the **thyroid inferno** (Fig. 18-50). Spectral Doppler will often demonstrate peak systolic velocities exceeding 70 cm/sec, which is the highest velocity found

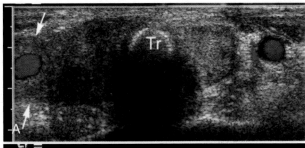

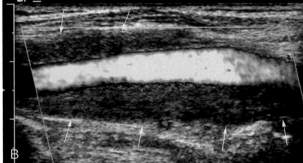

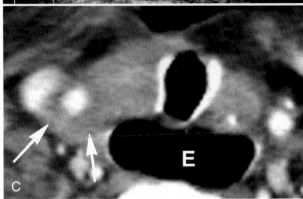

FIGURE 18-51. Reidel's struma (invasive fibrous thyroiditis). A, Transverse dual-color Doppler ultrasound image of the thyroid shows a diffuse hypoechoic process in the right lobe extending around the common carotid artery *(arrows); Tr,* trachea. **B,** Longitudinal power Doppler image of the right common carotid artery shows a hypoechoic soft tissue mass *(arrows)* encasing the vessel. **C,** Contrast-enhanced CT scan shows mild enlargement of the right thyroid lobe and soft tissue thickening *(arrows)* around the right common carotid artery. Incidentally noted is dilation of the air-filled esophagus *(E).*

in thyroid disease. There is no correlation between the degree of thyroid hyperfunction assessed by laboratory studies and the extent of hypervascularity or blood flow velocities. Previous studies have shown that Doppler analysis can be used to monitor therapeutic response in patients with Graves' disease.[138] A significant decrease in flow velocities in the superior and inferior thyroid arteries after medical treatment has been reported.

The rarest type of inflammatory thyroid disease is **invasive fibrous thyroiditis,** also called **Riedel's struma.**[132] This disease primarily affects women and often progresses to complete destruction of the gland. Some cases may be associated with mediastinal or retroperitoneal fibrosis or sclerosing cholangitis. In the few

cases of invasive fibrous thyroiditis examined sonographically, the gland was diffusely enlarged and had an inhomogeneous parenchymal echotexture. The primary reason for sonography is to check for extrathyroid extension of the inflammatory process, with encasement of the adjacent vessels (Fig. 18-51). Such information can be particularly useful in surgical planning. Open biopsy is generally required to distinguish this condition from anaplastic thyroid carcinoma. The sonographic findings in these two diseases may be identical.

References

Anatomy

1. Rogers WM. Anomalous development of the thyroid. In: Werner SC, Ingbar SH, editors. The thyroid. New York: Harper & Row; 1978. p. 416-420.
2. Toma P, Guastalla PP, Carini C, et al. Collo [The neck]. In: Fariello G, Perale R, Perri G, et al, editors. Ecografia Pediatrica. Milan: Ambrosiana; 1992. p. 139-162.
3. Solbiati L. La tiroide e le paratiroidi [The thyroid and the parathyroid]. In: Rizzatto G, Solbiati L, editors. Anatomia Ecografica: quadri normali, varianti e limiti con il patologico. Milan: Masson; 1992. p. 35-45.
4. Jarlov AE, Hegedus L, Gjorup T, Hansen JE. Accuracy of the clinical assessment of thyroid size. Dan Med Bull 1991;38:87-89.
5. Kerr L. High-resolution thyroid ultrasound: the value of color Doppler. Ultrasound Q 1994;12:21-43.
6. Shabana W, Peeters E, De Maeseneer M. Measuring thyroid gland volume: should we change the correction factor? AJR Am J Roentgenol 2006;186:234-236.
7. Hegedus L, Perrild H, Poulsen LR, et al. The determination of thyroid volume by ultrasound and its relationship to body weight, age, and sex in normal subjects. J Clin Endocrinol Metab 1983; 56:260-263.
8. Solbiati L, Osti V, Cova L, et al. The neck. In: Meire H, Cosgrove D, editors. Abdominal and general ultrasound. Edinburgh: Churchill Livingstone; 2001. p. 699-737.
9. Brandl H, Gritzky A, Haizinger M. 3D ultrasound: a dedicated system. Eur Radiol 1999;9(Suppl 3):331-333.

Congenital Thyroid Abnormalities

10. Ueda D, Mitamura R, Suzuki N, et al. Sonographic imaging of the thyroid gland in congenital hypothyroidism. Pediatr Radiol 1992; 22:102-105.
11. Chang YW, Hong HS, Choi DL. Sonography of the pediatric thyroid: a pictorial essay. J Clin Ultrasound 2009;37:149-157.

Nodular Thyroid Disease

12. Rojeski MT, Gharib H. Nodular thyroid disease: evaluation and management. N Engl J Med 1985;313:428-436.
13. Van Herle AJ, Rich P, Ljung BM, et al. The thyroid nodule. Ann Intern Med 1992;96:221-232.
14. Favus MJ, Schneider AB, Stachura ME, et al. Thyroid cancer occurring as a late consequence of head-and-neck irradiation: evaluation of 1056 patients. N Engl J Med 1976;294:1019-1025.
15. DeGroot LJ, Reilly M, Pinnameneni K, Refetoff S. Retrospective and prospective study of radiation-induced thyroid disease. Am J Med 1983;74:852-862.
16. Grebe SK, Hay ID. Follicular cell–derived thyroid carcinomas. Cancer Treat Res 1997;89:91-140.
17. Hennemann G. Non-toxic goitre. Clin Endocrinol Metab 1979;8:167-179.
18. Solbiati L, Cioffi V, Ballarati E. Ultrasonography of the neck. Radiol Clin North Am 1992;30:941-954.
19. Muller HW, Schroder S, Schneider C, Seifert G. Sonographic tissue characterisation in thyroid gland diagnosis: a correlation between sonography and histology. Klin Wochenschr 1985;63:706-710.
20. Lagalla R, Caruso G, Midiri M, et al. Echo Doppler-couleur et pathologie thyroidienne. JEMU 1992;13:44-47.

21. Solbiati L, Ballarati E, Cioffi V. Contribution of color-flow mapping to the differential diagnosis of the thyroid nodules. Radiological Society of North America; 1991 [abstract].

22. Solbiati L, Volterrani L, Rizzatto G, et al. The thyroid gland with low uptake lesions: evaluation by ultrasound. Radiology 1985;155:187-191.

23. Ahuja A, Chick W, King W, Metreweli C. Clinical significance of the comet-tail artifact in thyroid ultrasound. J Clin Ultrasound 1996;24:129-133.

24. Schlumberger MJ, Filetti S, Hay ID. Nontoxic goiter and thyroid neoplasia. In: Larsen PR, Kronenberg HM, Melmed S, et al, editors. Williams textbook of endocrinology. 10th ed. Philadelphia: Saunders; 2003. p. 457-490.

25. Black BM, Kirk Jr TA, Woolner LB. Multicentricity of papillary adenocarcinoma of the thyroid: influence on treatment. J Clin Endocrinol Metab 1960;20:130-135.

26. Hay ID, McConahey WM, Goellner JR. Managing patients with papillary thyroid carcinoma: insights gained from the Mayo Clinic's experience of treating 2,512 consecutive patients during 1940 through 2000. Trans Am Clin Climatol Assoc 2002;113:241-260.

27. Wunderbaldinger P, Harisinghani MG, Hahn PF, et al. Cystic lymph node metastases in papillary thyroid carcinoma. AJR Am J Roentgenol 2002;178:693-697.

28. Pilotti S, Pierotti MA. Classificazione istologica e caratterizzazione molecolare dei tumori dell'epitelio follicolare della tiroide. Argomenti Oncol 1992;13:365-380.

29. Holtz S, Powers WE. Calcification in papillary carcinoma of the thyroid. Am J Roentgenol Radium Ther Nucl Med 1958;80:997-1000.

30. Brkljacic B, Cuk V, Tomic-Brzac H, et al. Ultrasonic evaluation of benign and malignant nodules in echographically multinodular thyroids. J Clin Ultrasound 1994;22:71-76.

31. Ahuja AT, Ying M, Yuen HY, Metreweli C. Power Doppler sonography of metastatic nodes from papillary carcinoma of the thyroid. Clin Radiol 2001;56:284-288.

32. Solbiati L, Ierace T, Lagalla R, et al. Reliability of high-frequency US and color Doppler US of thyroid nodules: Italian multicenter study of 1,042 pathologically confirmed cases—which role for scintigraphy and biopsy? Radiological Society of North America, 1995 [abstract].

33. Henrichsen T, Reading CC, Charboneau JW, et al. Cystic change in thyroid carcinoma: incidence and estimated volume in 360 carcinomas. J Clin Ultrasound (at press).

34. Solbiati L, Livraghi T, Ballarati E, et al. Thyroid gland. In: Solbiati L, Rizzatto G, editors. Ultrasound of superficial structures. Edinburgh: Churchill Livingstone; 1995. p. 49-85.

35. Chong GC, Beahrs OH, Sizemore GW, Woolner LH. Medullary carcinoma of the thyroid gland. Cancer 1975;35:695-704.

36. Gorman B, Charboneau JW, James EM, et al. Medullary thyroid carcinoma: role of high-resolution ultrasound. Radiology 1987;162:147-150.

37. Nel CJ, van Heerden JA, Goellner JR, et al. Anaplastic carcinoma of the thyroid: a clinicopathologic study of 82 cases. Mayo Clin Proc 1985;60:51-58.

38. Hamburger JI, Miller JM, Kini SR. Lymphoma of the thyroid. Ann Intern Med 1983;99:685-693.

39. Kasagi K, Hatabu H, Tokuda Y, et al. Lymphoproliferative disorders of the thyroid gland: radiological appearances. Br J Radiol 1991;64:569-575.

40. Takashima S, Morimoto S, Ikezoe J, et al. Primary thyroid lymphoma: comparison of CT and US assessment. Radiology 1989;171:439-443.

41. Ahuja A, Evans R. The thyroid and parathyroid. In: Practical head and neck ultrasound. London: GMM; 2000.

42. Feld S, Barcia M, Baskic HJ, et al. AACE clinical practice guidelines for the diagnosis and management of thyroid nodules. Endocr Pract 1996;2:78-84.

43. Miller JM. Evaluation of thyroid nodules: accent on needle biopsy. Med Clin North Am 1985;69:1063-1077.

44. Hamberger B, Gharib H, Melton 3rd LJ, et al. Fine-needle aspiration biopsy of thyroid nodules: impact on thyroid practice and cost of care. Am J Med 1982;73:381-384.

45. Gharib H, Goellner JR. Fine-needle aspiration biopsy of the thyroid: an appraisal. Ann Intern Med 1993;118:282-289.

46. Hawkins F, Bellido D, Bernal C, et al. Fine-needle aspiration biopsy in the diagnosis of thyroid cancer and thyroid disease. Cancer 1987;59:1206-1209.

47. Khafagi F, Wright G, Castles H, et al. Screening for thyroid malignancy: the role of fine-needle biopsy. Med J Aust 1988;149:302-303, 6-7.

48. Hall TL, Layfield LJ, Philippe A, Rosenthal DL. Sources of diagnostic error in fine-needle aspiration of the thyroid. Cancer 1989;63:718-725.

49. Altavilla G, Pascale M, Nenci I. Fine-needle aspiration cytology of thyroid gland diseases. Acta Cytol 1990;34:251-256.

50. Ravetto C, Spreafico G, Colombo L. [Cytological examination using needle aspiration in the early diagnosis of thyroid neoplasms: comparison of clinical and scintigraphic data]. Recenti Prog Med 1977;63:258-274.

51. Sangalli G, Serio G, Zampatti C, et al. Fine-needle aspiration cytology of the thyroid: a comparison of 5469 cytological and final histological diagnoses. Cytopathology 2006;17:245-250.

52. James EM, Charboneau JW. High-frequency (10 MHz) thyroid ultrasonography. Semin Ultrasound CT MR 1985;6:294-309.

53. Scheible W, Leopold GR, Woo VL, Gosink BB. High-resolution real-time ultrasonography of thyroid nodules. Radiology 1979;133:413-417.

54. Simeone JF, Daniels GH, Mueller PR, et al. High-resolution real-time sonography of the thyroid. Radiology 1982;145:431-435.

55. Brown CL. Pathology of the cold nodule. Clin Endocrinol Metab 1981;10:235-245.

56. Brander A, Viikinkoski P, Nickels J, Kivisaari L. Thyroid gland: ultrasound screening in middle-aged women with no previous thyroid disease. Radiology 1989;173:507-510.

57. Hay ID. Papillary thyroid carcinoma. Endocrinol Metab Clin North Am 1990;19:545-576.

58. Hay ID, Reading CC, Weiland LH, et al. Clinicopathologic and high-resolution ultrasonographic evaluation of clinically suspicious or malignant thyroid disease. In: Medeiros-Neto G, Gaitan E, editors. Frontiers in thyroidology. New York: Plenum; 1986.

59. Simeone JF, Daniels GH, Hall DA, et al. Sonography in the follow-up of 100 patients with thyroid carcinoma. AJR Am J Roentgenol 1987;148:45-49.

60. Sutton RT, Reading CC, Charboneau JW, et al. Ultrasound-guided biopsy of neck masses in postoperative management of patients with thyroid cancer. Radiology 1988;168:769-772.

61. Kim EK, Park CS, Chung WY, et al. New sonographic criteria for recommending fine-needle aspiration biopsy of nonpalpable solid nodules of the thyroid. AJR Am J Roentgenol 2002;178:687-691.

62. Koike E, Noguchi S, Yamashita H, et al. Ultrasonographic characteristics of thyroid nodules: prediction of malignancy. Arch Surg 2001;136:334-337.

63. Rago T, Vitti P, Chiovato L, et al. Role of conventional ultrasonography and color flow Doppler sonography in predicting malignancy in "cold" thyroid nodules. Eur J Endocrinol 1998;138:41-46.

64. Watters DA, Ahuja AT, Evans RM, et al. Role of ultrasound in the management of thyroid nodules. Am J Surg 1992;164:654-657.

65. Okamoto T, Yamashita T, Harasawa A, et al. Test performances of three diagnostic procedures in evaluating thyroid nodules: physical examination, ultrasonography and fine-needle aspiration cytology. Endocr J 1994;41:243-247.

66. Leenhardt L, Tramalloni J, Aurengo H, et al. [Echography of thyroid nodules: the echography specialist facing the clinician's requirements]. Presse Med 1994;23:1389-1392.

67. Moon WJ, Jung SL, Lee JH, et al. Benign and malignant thyroid nodules: ultrasound differentiation—multicenter retrospective study. Radiology 2008;247:762-770.

68. Alexander EK, Marqusee E, Orcutt J, et al. Thyroid nodule shape and prediction of malignancy. Thyroid 2004;14:953-958.

69. Hammer M, Wortsman J, Folse R. Cancer in cystic lesions of the thyroid. Arch Surg 1982;117:1020-1023.

70. Livolsi A. Pathology of thyroid disease. In: Falj SA, editor. Thyroid disease: endocrinology, surgery, nuclear medicine and radiotherapy. Philadelphia: Lippincott-Raven; 1997. p. 65-104.

71. Propper RA, Skolnick ML, Weinstein BJ, Dekker A. The non-specificity of the thyroid halo sign. J Clin Ultrasound 1980;8:129-132.

72. Kim BM, Kim MJ, Kim EK, et al. Sonographic differentiation of thyroid nodules with eggshell calcifications. J Ultrasound Med 2008;27:1425-1430.

73. Park M, Shin JH, Han BK, et al. Sonography of thyroid nodules with peripheral calcifications. J Clin Ultrasound 2009;37:324-328.

74. Kakkos SK, Scopa CD, Chalmoukis AK, et al. Relative risk of cancer in sonographically detected thyroid nodules with calcifications. J Clin Ultrasound 2000;28:347-352.

75. Fobbe F, Finke R, Reichenstein E, et al. Appearance of thyroid diseases using colour-coded duplex sonography. Eur J Radiol 1989;9:29-31.

76. Argalia G, D'Ambrosio F, Lucarelli F, et al. [Echo Doppler in the characterization of thyroid nodular disease]. Radiol Med 1995;89:651-657.

77. Chammas MC, Gerhard R, de Oliveira IR, et al. Thyroid nodules: evaluation with power Doppler and duplex Doppler ultrasound. Otolaryngol Head Neck Surg 2005;132:874-882.

78. Spiezia S, Colao A, Assanti AP, et al. [Usefulness of color echo Doppler with power Doppler in the diagnosis of hypoechoic thyroid nodules: work in progress]. Radiol Med 1996;91:616-621.

79. Clark KJ, Cronan JJ, Scola FH. Color Doppler sonography: anatomic and physiologic assessment of the thyroid. J Clin Ultrasound 1995;23:215-223.

80. Shimamoto K, Endo T, Ishigaki T, et al. Thyroid nodules: evaluation with color Doppler ultrasonography. J Ultrasound Med 1993;12:673-678.

81. Frates MC, Benson CB, Doubilet PM, et al. Can color Doppler sonography aid in the prediction of malignancy of thyroid nodules? J Ultrasound Med 2003;22:127-131; quiz 132-134.

82. Rago T, Vitti P. Role of thyroid ultrasound in the diagnostic evaluation of thyroid nodules. Best Pract Res Clin Endocrinol Metab 2008;22:913-928.

83. Rubaltelli L, Corradin S, Dorigo A, et al. Differential diagnosis of benign and malignant thyroid nodules at elastosonography. Ultraschall Med 2009;30:175-179.

84. Ueno E, Ito A. Diagnosis of breast cancer by elasticity imaging. Eizo Joho Medical 2004;36:2-6.

85. Ferrari FS, Megliola A, Scorzelli A, et al. Ultrasound examination using contrast agent and elastosonography in the evaluation of single thyroid nodules: preliminary results. J Ultrasound 2008;11:47-54.

86. Hong Y, Liu X, Li Z, et al. Real-time ultrasound elastography in the differential diagnosis of benign and malignant thyroid nodules. J Ultrasound Med 2009;28:861-867.

87. Lyshchik A, Higashi T, Asato R, et al. Thyroid gland tumor diagnosis at ultrasound elastography. Radiology 2005;237:202-211.

88. Rago T, Santini F, Scutari M, et al. Elastography: new developments in ultrasound for predicting malignancy in thyroid nodules. J Clin Endocrinol Metab 2007;92:2917-2922.

89. Quinn SF, Nelson HA, Demlow TA. Thyroid biopsies: fine-needle aspiration biopsy versus spring-activated core biopsy needle in 102 patients. J Vasc Interv Radiol 1994;5:619-623.

90. Taki S, Kakuda K, Kakuma K, et al. Thyroid nodules: evaluation with ultrasound-guided core biopsy with an automated biopsy gun. Radiology 1997;202:874-877.

91. Goellner JR, Gharib H, Grant CS, Johnson DA. Fine-needle aspiration cytology of the thyroid, 1980 to 1986. Acta Cytol 1987;31:587-590.

92. Kuna SK, Bracic I, Tesic V, et al. Ultrasonographic differentiation of benign from malignant neck lymphadenopathy in thyroid cancer. J Ultrasound Med 2006;25:1531-1537; quiz 1538-1540.

93. Lyshchik A, Higashi T, Asato R, et al. Cervical lymph node metastases: diagnosis at sonoelastography—initial experience. Radiology 2007;243:258-267.

94. Snozek CL, Chambers EP, Reading CC, et al. Serum thyroglobulin, high-resolution ultrasound, and lymph node thyroglobulin in diagnosis of differentiated thyroid carcinoma nodal metastases. J Clin Endocrinol Metab 2007;92:4278-4281.

95. Miller JM, Hamburger JI, Taylor CI. Is needle aspiration of the cystic thyroid nodule effective and safe treatment? In: Hamburger JI, Miller JM, editors. Controversies in clinical thyroidology. New York: Springer-Verlag; 1981.

96. Verde G, Papini E, Pacella CM, et al. Ultrasound-guided percutaneous ethanol injection in the treatment of cystic thyroid nodules. Clin Endocrinol (Oxford) 1994;41:719-724.

97. Yasuda K, Ozaki O, Sugino K, et al. Treatment of cystic lesions of the thyroid by ethanol instillation. World J Surg 1992;16:958-961.

98. Antonelli A, Campatelli A, Di Vito A, et al. Comparison between ethanol sclerotherapy and emptying with injection of saline in treatment of thyroid cysts. Clin Invest 1994;72:971-974.

99. Lee SJ, Ahn IM. Effectiveness of percutaneous ethanol injection therapy in benign nodular and cystic thyroid diseases: long-term follow-up experience. Endocr J 2005;52:455-462.

100. Raggiunti B, Fiore G, Mongia A, et al. A 7-year follow-up of patients with thyroid cysts and pseudocysts treated with percutaneous ethanol injection: volume change and cost analysis. J Ultrasound 2009;12:107-111.

101. Livraghi T, Paracchi A, Ferrari C, et al. Treatment of autonomous thyroid nodules with percutaneous ethanol injection: preliminary results: work in progress. Radiology 1990;175:827-829.

102. Cerbone G, Spiezia S, Colao A, et al. Percutaneous ethanol injection under power Doppler ultrasound assistance in the treatment of autonomously functioning thyroid nodules. J Endocrinol Invest 1999;22:752-759.

103. Goletti O, Monzani F, Caraccio N, et al. Percutaneous ethanol injection treatment of autonomously functioning single thyroid nodules: optimization of treatment and short-term outcome. World J Surg 1992;16:784-789; discussion 789-790.

104. Livraghi T, Paracchi A, Ferrari C, et al. Treatment of autonomous thyroid nodules with percutaneous ethanol injection: 4-year experience. Radiology 1994;190:529-533.

105. Ozdemir H, Ilgit ET, Yucel C, et al. Treatment of autonomous thyroid nodules: safety and efficacy of sonographically guided percutaneous injection of ethanol. AJR Am J Roentgenol 1994;163:929-932.

106. Pacella CM, Papini E, Bizzarri G, et al. Assessment of the effect of percutaneous ethanol injection in autonomously functioning thyroid nodules by colour-coded duplex sonography. Eur J Radiol 1995;5:395-400.

107. Baek JH, Moon WJ, Kim YS, et al. Radiofrequency ablation for the treatment of autonomously functioning thyroid nodules. World J Surg 2009;33:1971-1977.

108. Deandrea M, Limone P, Basso E, et al. Ultrasound-guided percutaneous radiofrequency thermal ablation for the treatment of solid benign hyperfunctioning or compressive thyroid nodules. Ultrasound Med Biol 2008;34:784-791.

109. Goletti O, Monzani F, Lenziardi M, et al. Cold thyroid nodules: a new application of percutaneous ethanol injection treatment. J Clin Ultrasound 1994;22:175-178.

110. Dossing H, Bennedbaek FN, Karstrup S, Hegedus L. Benign solitary solid cold thyroid nodules: ultrasound-guided interstitial laser photocoagulation—initial experience. Radiology 2002;225:53-57.

111. Pacella CM, Bizzarri G, Spiezia S, et al. Thyroid tissue: ultrasound-guided percutaneous laser thermal ablation. Radiology 2004;232:272-280.

112. Papini E, Guglielmi R, Bizzarri G, et al. Treatment of benign cold thyroid nodules: a randomized clinical trial of percutaneous laser ablation versus levothyroxine therapy or follow-up. Thyroid 2007;17:229-235.

113. Jeong WK, Baek JH, Rhim H, et al. Radiofrequency ablation of benign thyroid nodules: safety and imaging follow-up in 236 patients. Eur Radiol 2008;18:1244-1250.

114. Dupuy DE, Monchik JM, Decrea C, Pisharodi L. Radiofrequency ablation of regional recurrence from well-differentiated thyroid malignancy. Surgery 2001;130:971-977.

115. Lewis BD, Hay ID, Charboneau JW, et al. Percutaneous ethanol injection for treatment of cervical lymph node metastases in patients with papillary thyroid carcinoma. AJR Am J Roentgenol 2002;178:699-704.

116. Fukunari N. PEI therapy for thyroid lesions. Biomed Pharmacother 2002;56:79-82.

117. Kim BM, Kim MJ, Kim EK, et al. Controlling recurrent papillary thyroid carcinoma in the neck by ultrasonography-guided percutaneous ethanol injection. Eur Radiol 2008;18:835-842.

118. Hay ID, Reading CC, Charboneau JW. Long-term efficacy of ultrasound-guided percutaneous ethanol ablation of recurrent neck nodal metastases in patients with pTNM stage 1 papillary thyroid carcinoma. Thyroid 2005;15:S2-S3.

119. Mazzaferri EL. Managing small thyroid cancers. JAMA 2006;295:2179-2182.

120. Horlocker T, Hay I, James E. Prevalence of incidental nodular thyroid disease detected during high-resolution parathyroid ultrasonography. In: Medeiros-Neto G, Gaitan E, editors. Frontiers in thyroidology. New York: Plenum; 1986. p. 1209-1312.

121. Cronan JJ. Thyroid nodules: is it time to turn off the ultrasound machines? Radiology 2008;247:602-604.

122. Hay ID, Bergstralh EJ, Goellner JR, et al. Predicting outcome in papillary thyroid carcinoma: development of a reliable prognostic scoring system in a cohort of 1779 patients surgically treated at one institution during 1940 through 1989. Surgery 1993;114:1050-1057; discussion 1057-1058.

123. Harach HR, Franssila KO, Wasenius VM. Occult papillary carcinoma of the thyroid: a "normal" finding in Finland—a systematic autopsy study. Cancer 1985;56:531-538.

124. Davies L, Welch HG. Increasing incidence of thyroid cancer in the United States, 1973–2002. JAMA 2006;295:2164-2167.

125. Ross DS. Predicting thyroid malignancy [editorial]. J Clin Endocrinol Metab 2006;91:4253-4255.

126. Burch HB. Evaluation and management of the solid thyroid nodule. Endocrinol Metab Clin North Am 1995;24:663-710.

127. Goellner J. Fine-needle aspiration of the thyroid gland. In: Erosan YS, Bonfiglio TA, editors. Fine-needle aspiration of subcutaneous organs and masses. Philadelphia: Lippincott-Raven; 1996. p. 81-98.

128. Haas S, Trujillo A, Kunstle J. Fine-needle aspiration of thyroid nodules in a rural setting. Am J Med 1993;94:357-361.

129. Spiliotis J, Scopa CD, Gatopoulou C, et al. Diagnosis of thyroid cancer in southwestern Greece. Bull Cancer 1991;78:953-959.

130. Songun I, Kievit J, Wobbes T, et al. Extent of thyroidectomy in nodular thyroid disease. Eur J Surg 1999;165:839-842.

131. Reading CC, Charboneau JW, Hay ID, Sebo TJ. Sonography of thyroid nodules: a "classic pattern" diagnostic approach. Ultrasound Q 2005;21:157-165.

Diffuse Thyroid Disease

132. Hay ID. Thyroiditis: a clinical update. Mayo Clin Proc 1985;60: 836-843.

133. Adams H, Jones MC. Ultrasound appearances of de Quervain's thyroiditis. Clin Radiol 1990;42:217-218.

134. Birchall IW, Chow CC, Metreweli C. Ultrasound appearances of de Quervain's thyroiditis. Clin Radiol 1990;41:57-59.

135. Yeh HC, Futterweit W, Gilbert P. Micronodulation: ultrasonographic sign of Hashimoto thyroiditis. J Ultrasound Med 1996; 15:813-819.

136. Takashima S, Matsuzuka F, Nagareda T, et al. Thyroid nodules associated with Hashimoto thyroiditis: assessment with ultrasound. Radiology 1992;185:125-130.

137. Lagalla R, Caruso G, Benza I, et al. [Echo color Doppler in the study of hypothyroidism in the adult]. Radiol Med 1993;86:281-283.

138. Castagnone D, Rivolta R, Rescalli S, et al. Color Doppler sonography in Graves' disease: value in assessing activity of disease and predicting outcome. AJR Am J Roentgenol 1996;166:203-207.

CHAPTER 19

The Parathyroid Glands

Bonnie J. Huppert and Carl C. Reading

Chapter Outline

High-frequency sonography is a well-established, noninvasive imaging method used in the evaluation and treatment of patients with parathyroid disease. Sonography is often used for the preoperative localization of enlarged parathyroid glands or adenomas in patients with hyperparathyroidism. Ultrasound is also used to guide the percutaneous biopsy of suspected parathyroid adenomas or enlarged glands, particularly in patients with persistent or recurrent hyperparathyroidism, as well as in some patients with suspected ectopic glands. In select patients, sonography can be used to guide the percutaneous ethanol ablation of parathyroid adenomas as an alternative to surgical treatment.

EMBRYOLOGY AND ANATOMY

The paired superior and inferior parathyroid glands have different embryologic origins, and knowledge of their development aids in understanding their ultimate anatomic locations.[1-3] The **superior parathyroid glands** arise from the paired fourth branchial pouches (clefts), along with the lateral lobes of the thyroid gland. Minimal migration occurs during fetal development, and the superior parathyroids usually remain associated with the posterior aspect of the middle to upper portion of the thyroid gland. The majority of superior parathyroid glands (>80%) are found at autopsy within a 2-cm area

located just superior to the crossing of the recurrent laryngeal nerve and the inferior thyroid artery.[4]

The **inferior parathyroid glands** arise from the paired third branchial pouches, along with the thymus.[2] During fetal development, these "parathymus glands" migrate caudally along with the thymus in a more anterior plane than their superior counterparts, bypassing the superior glands to become the inferior parathyroid glands.[3] Because of their greater caudal migration, the inferior parathyroid glands are more variable in location than the superior glands and can be found anywhere from the angle of the mandible to the pericardium. The majority of inferior parathyroid glands (>60%) come to rest at or just inferior to the posterior aspect of the lower pole of the thyroid[4] (Fig. 19-1).

A significant percentage of parathyroid glands lie in relatively or frankly **ectopic** locations in the neck or mediastinum. Symmetry to fixed landmarks occurs in 70% to 80%, so side-to-side comparisons can often be made.[3,4] The ectopic superior parathyroid gland usually lies posterior to the esophagus or in the tracheoesophageal groove, in the retropharyngeal space, or has continued its descent from the posterior neck into the posterosuperior mediastinum.[5,6] Superior glands are less often found higher in the neck, near the superior extent of the thyroid, or rarely, surrounded by thyroid tissue within the thyroid capsule.[4] The inferior parathyroid gland is more frequently ectopic than its superior

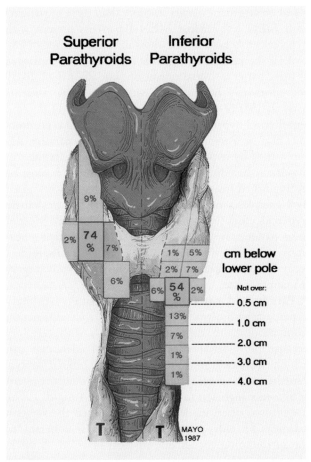

FIGURE 19-1. Location of parathyroid glands. Frequency of the location of normal superior and inferior parathyroid glands. Anatomic drawing from 527 autopsies. *T,* Thymus. *(Modified from Gilmour JR. The gross anatomy of the parathyroid glands. J Pathol 1938;46:133-148.)*

counterpart.[4,6] About 25% of the inferior glands fail to completely dissociate from the thymus and continue to migrate in an anterocaudal direction and are found in the low neck along the thyrothymic ligament or embedded within or adjacent to the thymus in the low neck and anterosuperior mediastinum. Less common ectopic positions of the inferior parathyroid glands include an undescended position high in the neck anterior to the carotid bifurcation associated with a remnant of thymus, and lower in the neck along or within the carotid sheath.[7] In other rare cases, ectopic glands have also been reported in the mediastinum posterior to the esophagus or carina, in the aortopulmonic window, within the pericardium, or even far laterally within the posterior triangle of the neck.

Most adults have four parathyroid glands, two superior and two inferior, each measuring about 5 × 3 × 1 mm and weighing on average 35 to 40 mg (range, 10-78 mg).[3,8] **Supernumerary glands** (>4) may be present and result from the separation of parathyroid anlage when the glands pull away from the pouch structures during the embryologic branchial complex phase.[9,10] These supernu-

merary glands are often associated with the thymus in the anterior mediastinum, suggesting a relationship in their development with the inferior parathyroid glands.[11] Supernumerary glands have been reported in 13% of the population at autopsy studies;[3,4] however, many of these are small, rudimentary or split glands. "Proper" supernumerary glands (>5 mg and located well away from the other four glands) are found in 5% of cases. The presence of fewer than four parathyroid glands is rare clinically, but has been reported in 3% at autopsy.

Normal parathyroid glands vary from a yellow to a red-brown color, depending on the degree of vascularity and the relative content of yellow parenchymal fat and chief cells.[8] The chief cells are the primary source for the production of **parathyroid hormone (PTH, parathormone)**. The percentage of glandular fat typically increases with age or with disuse atrophy. Hyperfunctioning glands resulting from adenomas or hyperplasia contain relatively little fat and are vascular, thus more reddish. The glands are generally oval or bean shaped but may be spherical, lobular, elongated, or flattened. Although normal parathyroid glands are occasionally seen with high-frequency ultrasound,[12,13] typically they are not visualized, likely because of their small size, deep location, and poor conspicuity related to increased glandular fat. **Eutopic** parathyroid glands typically derive their major blood supply from branches of the inferior thyroid artery, with a lesser and variable contribution to the superior glands from the superior thyroid artery.[3,7]

PRIMARY HYPERPARATHYROIDISM

Prevalence

Primary hyperparathyroidism is now recognized as a common endocrine disease, with prevalence in the United States of 1 to 2 per 1000 population.[14] Women are affected two to three times more frequently than men, particularly after menopause. More than half of patients with primary hyperparathyroidism are over 50 years old, and cases are rare in those under age 20.

Diagnosis

Primary hyperparathyroidism is usually suspected because an increased serum calcium level is detected on routine biochemical screening. Elevated ionized serum calcium level, hypophosphatasia, and hypercalciuria may be further biochemical clues to the disease. A serum PTH level that is "inappropriately high" for the corresponding serum calcium level confirms the diagnosis. Even when the PTH level is within the upper limits of the normal range in a hypercalcemic patient, the diagnosis of primary hyperparathyroidism should still be suspected, since hypercalcemia from other nonparathyroid causes (including malignancy) should suppress the glandular function and decrease the serum PTH level. Because of earlier detection by increasingly routine laboratory tests, the later "classic" signs of hyperparathyroidism, such as "painful bones, renal stones, abdominal groans, and psychic moans," are often not present. Many patients are now diagnosed before severe manifestations of hyperparathyroidism, such as **nephrolithiasis, osteopenia, subperiosteal resorption,** and **osteitis fibrosis cystica**. In general, patients rarely have obvious symptoms unless their serum calcium level exceeds 12 mg/dL. However, subtle nonspecific symptoms, such as muscle weakness, malaise, constipation, dyspepsia, polydipsia, and polyuria, may be elicited from these otherwise asymptomatic patients by more specific questioning.

Pathology

Primary hyperparathyroidism is caused by a **single adenoma** in 80% to 90% of cases, by **multiple gland enlargement** in 10% to 20%, and by **carcinoma** in less than 1%.[6,15,16] A solitary adenoma may involve any one of the four glands. Multigland enlargement most often results from primary parathyroid hyperplasia and less often from multiple adenomas. Hyperplasia usually involves all four glands asymmetrically, whereas multiple adenomas may involve two or possibly three glands. An adenoma and hyperplasia cannot always be reliably distinguished histologically, and the sample may be referred to as "hypercellular parathyroid" tissue. Because of this inconsistent pattern of gland involvement, and because distinguishing hyperplasia from multiple adenomas is difficult pathologically, these two entities are often histologically considered together as "multiple gland disease."[17]

Most cases of primary hyperparathyroidism are sporadic. However, **prior external neck irradiation** has been associated with the development of hyperparathyroidism in a small percentage of cases. Patients receiving **long-term lithium therapy** may also present with primary hyperparathyroidism. Up to 10% of cases may occur on a hereditary basis, most often caused by **multiple endocrine neoplasia syndrome,** type I (MEN I). This condition is an uncommon disorder that most typically follows an autosomal dominant pattern of inheritance and has a high penetrance, resulting in adenomatous parathyroid hyperplasia, as well as pancreatic islet cell tumors and pituitary adenomas. Multiple–parathyroid

gland enlargement occurs in more than 90% of patients with MEN I.[18,19] Most MEN I patients present with hypercalcemia before their third or fourth decade of life. Not all the parathyroid glands may be grossly enlarged at these patients' initial operation, but all of them likely will ultimately be involved with hyperplasia. Patients with the **MEN IIA syndrome** less frequently develop parathyroid hyperplasia. Other, rarer familial syndromes may also be associated with primary hyperparathyroidism caused by hyperplasia, adenomas, or carcinoma. An important hereditary hyperparathyroidism that must be distinguished from primary hyperparathyroidism caused by hyperplasia or adenoma is **familial hypocalciuric hypercalcemia** (benign familial hypercalcemia). Most of these patients are asymptomatic, without the complications of primary hyperparathyroidism. Parathyroidectomy does not cure the hypercalcemia, and thus surgery is inappropriate.

Parathyroid carcinoma is a rare cause of primary hyperparathyroidism.[20-23] The histologic distinction from adenoma is difficult to establish with certainty because both carcinomas and atypical adenomas can exhibit increased mitotic activity and cellular atypia. Patients with parathyroid carcinoma usually present with a very high serum calcium level (>14 mg/dL). The diagnosis is often made at operation when the surgeon discovers an enlarged, firm gland that is adherent to the surrounding tissues due to local invasion. A thick, fibrotic capsule is often present. Treatment consists of en bloc resection without entering the capsule, to prevent tumor seeding. In many cases, cure may not be possible because of the invasive and metastatic nature of the disease. Generally, death occurs not from tumor spread, but from complications associated with unrelenting hyperparathyroidism.

Treatment

No effective definitive medical therapies are available for the treatment of primary hyperparathyroidism. Short-term hypocalcemic agents include calcitonin and the bisphosphonates. **Calcimimetics** (calcium-sensing receptor agonists) such as cinacalcet and synthetic vitamin D analogs such as paricalcitol are used mainly in the treatment of secondary hyperparathyroidism.

Surgery is the only definitive treatment for primary hyperparathyroidism. Studies demonstrate that surgical cure rates by an experienced surgeon are greater than 95%, and the morbidity and mortality rates are extremely low.[24,25] Therefore, in symptomatic patients with primary hyperparathyroidism, the treatment of choice is surgical excision of the involved parathyroid gland or glands.

However, now that many cases of primary hyperparathyroidism are discovered in the early stages of the disease, some controversy exists as to whether asymptomatic patients with minimal hypercalcemia should be treated surgically, or followed medically with frequent

CAUSES OF PRIMARY HYPERPARATHYROIDISM	
Single adenoma	80%-90%
Multiple gland disease	10%-20%
Carcinoma	<1%

measurements of bone density, serum calcium levels, and urinary calcium excretion and monitoring for nephrolithiasis. A prospective 10-year clinical follow-up study reported that of 52 asymptomatic patients with primary hyperparathyroidism with calcium levels less than 11 mg/dL, 73% did well, with no evidence of disease progression. However, 27% had evidence of progression based on development of one or more indications for surgery.[26] Recommendations for the management of asymptomatic primary hyperparathyroidism have been outlined in various articles, many of which are based on the National Institutes of Health (NIH) Consensus Conference statement and its subsequent updates. However, this area continues to evolve, and approaches to treatment may differ among clinical practices.[24,25,27-30]

SONOGRAPHIC APPEARANCE

Shape

Parathyroid adenomas are typically oval or bean shaped (Fig. 19-2). As parathyroid glands enlarge, they dissect between longitudinally oriented tissue planes in the neck and acquire a characteristic oblong shape. If this process is exaggerated, they can become tubular or flattened. There is often asymmetry in the enlargement, and the cephalic and/or caudal end can be more bulbous, producing a triangular, tapering, teardrop or bilobed shape.[19,31-33]

Echogenicity and Internal Architecture

The echogenicity of most parathyroid adenomas is substantially less than that of normal thyroid tissue (Fig. 19-3). The characteristic **hypoechoic** appearance of parathyroid adenomas is caused by the uniform hypercellularity of the gland with little fat content, which leaves few interfaces for reflecting sound. Occasionally, adenomas have a heterogeneous appearance, with areas of increased and decreased echogenicity. The rare, func-

tioning parathyroid lipoadenomas are more echogenic than the adjacent thyroid gland because of their high fat content[34] (Fig. 19-3, G). A great majority of parathyroid adenomas are **homogeneously solid.** About 2% have internal cystic components resulting from **cystic degeneration** (most often) or true simple cysts (less often).[35,36] Adenomas may rarely contain internal calcification (Fig. 19-3, H and I).

Vascularity

Color flow, spectral, and power Doppler sonography of an enlarged parathyroid gland may demonstrate a hypervascular pattern with prominent diastolic flow (Fig. 19-4). An **enlarged extrathyroidal artery**, often originating from branches of the inferior thyroidal artery, may be visualized supplying the adenoma with its insertion along the long-axis pole.[37-42] A finding described in parathyroid adenomas is a **vascular arc,** which envelops 90 to 270 degrees of the mass. This vascular flow pattern may increase the sensitivity of initial detection of parathyroid adenomas and aid in confirming the diagnosis by allowing for differentiation from lymph nodes, which have a central hilar flow pattern. Asymmetric increased vascular flow may also be present in the thyroid gland adjacent to a parathyroid adenoma.

Size

Most parathyroid adenomas are 0.8 to 1.5 cm long and weigh 500 to 1000 mg. The smallest adenomas can be minimally enlarged glands that appear virtually normal during surgery but are found to be hypercellular on pathologic examination (Fig. 19-5; **Video 19-1**). Large adenomas can be 5 cm or more in length and weigh more than 10 g. Preoperative serum calcium levels are usually higher in patients with larger adenomas.[31]

Multiple Gland Disease

Multiple gland disease may be caused by diffuse hyperplasia or multiple adenomas. Individually, these enlarged

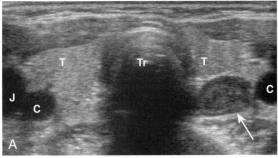
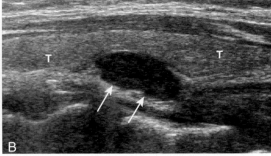

FIGURE 19-2. Typical parathyroid adenoma. A, Transverse, and, **B,** longitudinal, sonograms of a typical adenoma *(arrows)* located adjacent to the posterior aspect of the thyroid *(T); Tr,* trachea; *C,* common carotid artery; *J,* internal jugular vein.

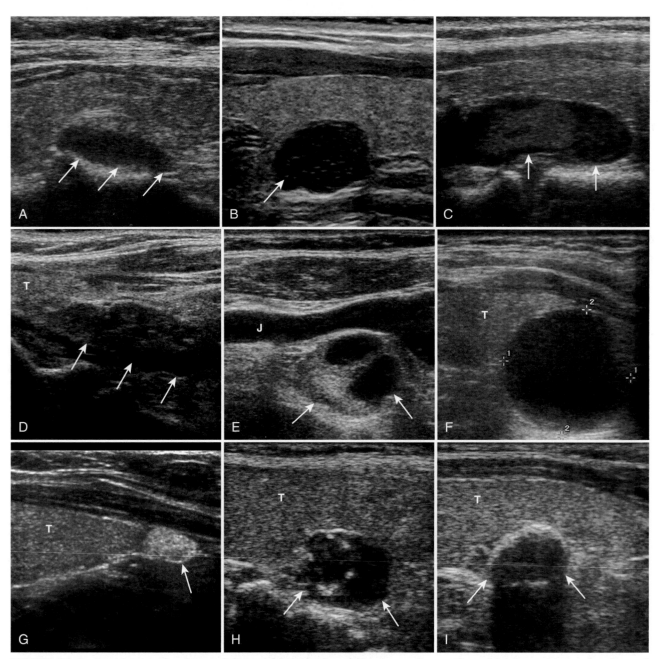

FIGURE 19-3. Spectrum of echogenicity and internal architecture of parathyroid adenomas and enlarged hyperplastic glands. Longitudinal sonograms. A, Typical homogeneous hypoechoic appearance of a parathyroid adenoma *(arrows)* with respect to the overlying thyroid tissue. **B,** Highly hypoechoic solid adenoma *(arrow).* **C,** Mixed-geographic echogenicity. The adenoma *(arrows)* is hyperechoic in its cranial portion and hypoechoic in its caudal portion. **D,** An adenoma *(arrows)* with diffusely heterogeneous echotexture adenoma *(arrows); T,* thyroid. **E,** Partial cystic change. An ectopic adenoma *(arrows)* posterior to the jugular vein *(J)* has both solid and cystic components. **F,** Completely cystic 2-cm adenoma *(cursors)* near the lower pole of the thyroid *(T).* **G,** A lipoadenoma *(arrow)* is more echogenic than the adjacent lower pole thyroid tissue *(T).* **H,** Enlarged parathyroid gland *(arrows)* with small, nonshadowing calcifications in the setting of secondary hyperparathyroidism related to chronic renal failure; *T,* thyroid. **I,** Enlarged parathyroid gland *(arrows)* with densely shadowing peripheral calcifications in the setting of secondary hyperparathyroidism; *T,* thyroid.

 glands may have the same sonographic and gross appearance as other parathyroid adenomas (Fig. 19-6; **Video 19-2**). However, the glands may be inconsistently and asymmetrically enlarged, and the diagnosis of multigland disease can be difficult to make sonographically. For example, if one gland is much larger than the others, the appearance may be misinterpreted as solitary adenomatous disease. Alternatively, if multiple glands are only minimally enlarged, the diagnosis may be missed altogether.

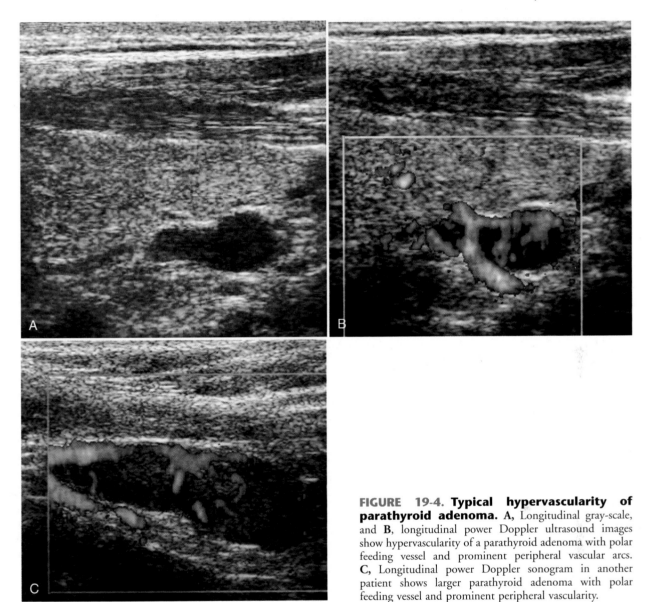

FIGURE 19-4. Typical hypervascularity of parathyroid adenoma. A, Longitudinal gray-scale, and **B,** longitudinal power Doppler ultrasound images show hypervascularity of a parathyroid adenoma with polar feeding vessel and prominent peripheral vascular arcs. **C,** Longitudinal power Doppler sonogram in another patient shows larger parathyroid adenoma with polar feeding vessel and prominent peripheral vascularity.

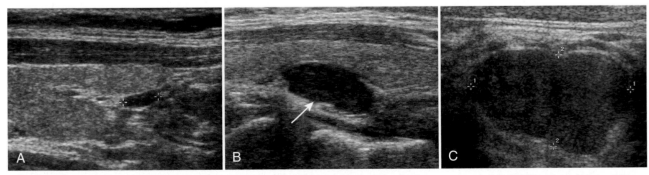

FIGURE 19-5. Spectrum of size of parathyroid adenomas. Longitudinal sonograms. **A,** Minimally enlarged, 0.5 × 0.2–cm parathyroid adenoma *(cursors)*. **B,** Typical midsized, 1.5 × 0.6–cm, 400-mg adenoma *(arrow)*. **C,** Large, 3.5 × 2–cm, >4000-mg adenoma *(cursors)*.

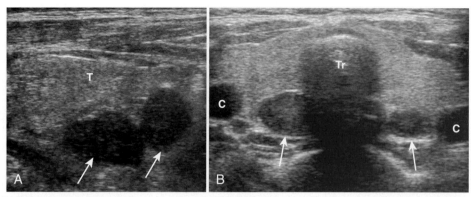

FIGURE 19-6. Multiple gland disease. A, Longitudinal sonogram of the right neck shows superior and inferior parathyroid gland enlargement *(arrows)* in the setting of secondary hyperparathyroidism, which can be difficult to distinguish from multiple adenomas; *T,* thyroid. **B,** Transverse sonogram in another patient shows enlargement of bilateral superior parathyroid glands *(arrows)* in the setting of secondary hyperparathyroidism; *Tr,* trachea; *C,* common carotid artery.

Carcinoma

Carcinomas are usually larger than adenomas.[43-45] Carcinomas often measure more than 2 cm, versus about 1 cm for adenomas (Fig. 19-7). On ultrasound, carcinomas also frequently have a lobular contour, heterogeneous internal architecture, and internal cystic components. However, large adenomas may also have these features. In many cases, prospective carcinomas are indistinguishable sonographically from large, benign adenomas.[43] Some authors report that a depth/width ratio of 1 or greater is a sonographic feature more associated with carcinoma rather than adenoma, with sensitivity and specificity of 94% and 95%, respectively.[45] Gross evidence of invasion of adjacent structures, such as vessels or muscles, is a reliable preoperative sonographic criterion for the diagnosis of malignancy, but this is an uncommon finding.

ADENOMA LOCALIZATION

Sonographic Examination and Typical Locations

The sonographic examination of the neck for parathyroid adenoma localization is performed with the patient supine. The **patient's neck is hyperextended by a pad** centered under the scapulae, and the examiner usually sits at the patient's head. **High-frequency transducers** (8-17 MHz) are used to provide optimal spatial resolution and visualization in most patients; the highest frequency possible should be used that still allows for tissue penetration to visualize the deeper structures, such as the longus colli muscles. In obese patients with thick necks or with large multinodular thyroid glands, use of a 5-MHz to 8-MHz transducer may be necessary to obtain adequate depth of penetration.

The pattern of the sonographic survey of the neck for adenoma localization can be considered in terms of the

pattern of dissection and visualization that the surgeon uses in a thorough neck exploration. The typical **superior parathyroid adenoma** is usually adjacent to the posterior aspect of the midportion of the thyroid (Fig. 19-8; **Video 19-3**). The location of the typical **inferior parathyroid adenoma** is more variable but usually lies close to the lower pole of the thyroid (Fig. 19-9; **Video 19-4**). Most of these inferior adenomas are adjacent to the posterior aspect of the lower pole of the thyroid, and the rest are in the soft tissues 1 to 2 cm inferior to the thyroid. Therefore the examination is initiated on one side of the neck, centered in the region of the thyroid gland, with the electronic focus placed deep to the thyroid. High-resolution gray-scale images are obtained in the transverse (axial) and longitudinal (sagittal) planes. Any potential parathyroid adenomas detected in the transverse scan plane must be confirmed by longitudinal imaging to prevent mistaking other structures for an adenoma.

Some authors recommend the use of **compression** of the superficial soft tissues to aid in adenoma detection.[12,41] This has been described as "graded" compression with the transducer to effect minimal deformity of the overlying subcutaneous tissues and strap muscles and increase the conspicuity of deeper, smaller adenomas (<1 cm). Color flow or power Doppler sonography is also used to assess the vascularity of any potential adenoma, aid in detection, and differentiation from other structures.[38-42] Hypervascularity may be evident with a polar insertion of a prominent extrathyroidal feeding artery, also with peripheral arcs of blood flow. After one side of the neck has been examined, a similar survey is conducted of the opposite side. However, 1% to 3% of parathyroid adenomas are frankly ectopic and not found in typical locations adjacent to the thyroid. Therefore the sonographic examination must be extended laterally along the carotid sheaths, superiorly from the level of the mandible, and inferiorly to the level of the sternal notch and clavicles. The four most common ectopic locations are considered separately next.

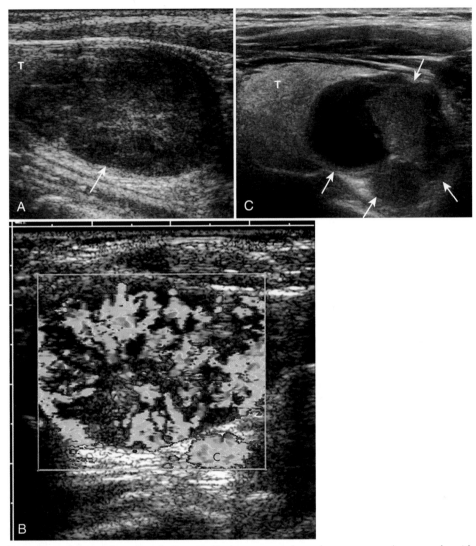

FIGURE 19-7. Parathyroid carcinoma. A, Longitudinal sonogram shows heterogeneous 4-cm parathyroid carcinoma *(arrow)* located near tip of lower pole of the left thyroid lobe *(T)*. **B,** Transverse sonogram with color Doppler flow imaging shows prominent internal vascularity of the carcinoma; **C,** common carotid artery. **C,** Longitudinal sonogram in another patient shows lobulated, solid and cystic, 4-cm parathyroid carcinoma *(arrows)* adjacent to the lower pole of the thyroid *(T)*.

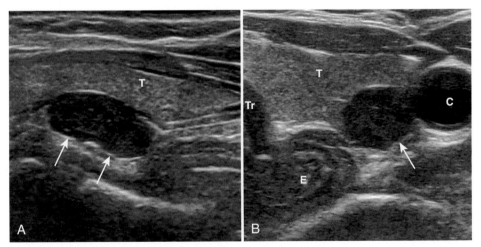

FIGURE 19-8. Superior parathyroid adenoma. A, Longitudinal, and **B,** transverse, sonograms show an adenoma *(arrows)* adjacent to the posterior aspect of the midportion of the left lobe of the thyroid *(T); C,* common carotid artery; *E,* esophagus; *J,* internal jugular vein; *Tr,* trachea.

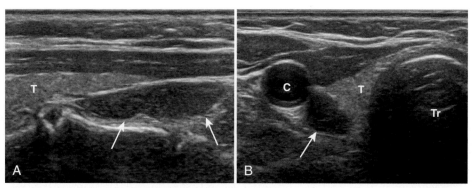

FIGURE 19-9. Inferior parathyroid adenoma. A, Longitudinal, and **B,** transverse, sonograms show an adenoma *(arrows)* adjacent to lower pole of right lobe of the thyroid *(T); C,* common carotid artery; *Tr,* trachea.

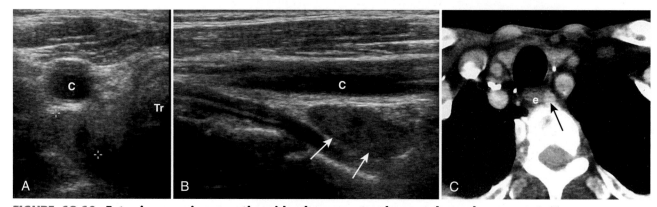

FIGURE 19-10. Ectopic superior parathyroid adenoma: tracheoesophageal groove. A, Transverse sonogram reveals an adenoma *(cursors)* arising from the right tracheoesophageal groove located posteriorly in the neck. The patient's head is turned to the left, which deviates the adenoma laterally and aids in visualization. *C,* Common carotid artery; *Tr,* trachea. **B,** Corresponding longitudinal sonogram shows the ectopic superior parathyroid adenoma *(arrows)* posterior in the low neck adjacent to the cervical spine; *C,* common carotid artery. **C,** CT scan of the low neck/upper mediastinum in another patient shows an ectopic adenoma *(arrow)* in the left tracheoesophageal groove adjacent to the esophagus *(e).*

Ectopic Locations

Retrotracheal/Retroesophageal Adenoma

 Superior adenomas tend to enlarge between tissue planes that extend toward the posterior mediastinum; the most common location of an ectopic superior adenoma is deep in the neck, posterior or posterolateral to the trachea or esophagus (Fig. 19-10; **Video 19-5**). Acoustic shadowing from air in the trachea can make evaluation of this area difficult. The transducer should be angled medially to visualize the tissues posterior to the trachea. Often the adenoma protrudes slightly from behind the trachea, and only a portion of the mass will be visible. **Turning the patient's head to the opposite side** will accentuate the protrusion and provide better accessibility to the retrotracheal area. This process is then repeated on the other side of the neck to visualize the contralateral aspect of the retrotracheal area. This process is analogous to the maneuver that a surgeon uses to run a fingertip behind the trachea in an attempt to palpate a retrotracheal

adenoma. Maximal turning of the head also often causes the esophagus to move to the opposite side of the trachea as it becomes compressed between the trachea and the cervical spine. If the examiner sees the esophagus move completely from one side of the trachea to the opposite side during maximal head turning, the esophagus has effectively "swept" the retrotracheal space and will have pushed any parathyroid adenoma in this location out from behind the trachea.

Mediastinal Adenoma

The most common location for ectopic inferior parathyroid adenomas is low within the neck or in the antero-superior mediastinum[4,6,46,47] (Fig. 19-11). Parathyroid adenomas are sufficiently hypoechoic that they may be visualized as discrete structures separate from the thymus and surrounding tissues. To visualize this area optimally, the **patient's neck is maximally hyperextended.** With this technique and the transducer angled posterior and caudal to the clavicular heads, sonographic visualization is often possible to the level of the brachiocephalic veins.

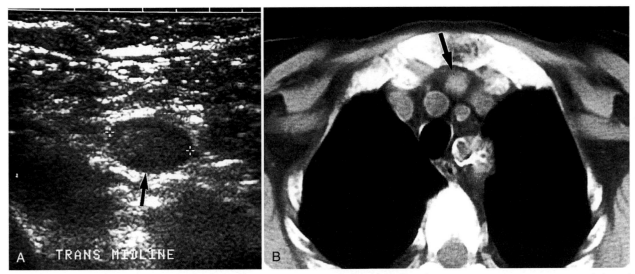

FIGURE 19-11. Ectopic parathyroid adenoma: anterosuperior mediastinum. A, Transverse sonogram angled caudal to the clavicles shows an oval, 1-cm ectopic inferior parathyroid adenoma *(arrow)* in the soft tissues of the anterosuperior mediastinum. **B,** CT scan of the upper mediastinum shows the ectopic adenoma *(arrow)* in the anterosuperior mediastinum, deep to the manubrium and adjacent to the great vessels.

If the adenoma lies caudal to this level or far anterior, just deep to the sternum, it cannot be visualized sonographically.

Ectopic superior adenomas located in the mediastinum tend to stay in a more posterior plane than their ectopic inferior counterparts and are often not visible with traditional sonography. They usually lie deep in the low neck or posterior superior mediastinum, requiring use of a 5-MHz transducer for maximal penetration. Ectopic superior adenomas may be intimately associated with the posterior aspect of the trachea, and the head-turning maneuver described for retrotracheal adenomas in the neck can be applied here as well. With the patient's neck hyperextended and the transducer angled caudally, the posterior mediastinum may sometimes be visualized to the level of the apex of the aortic arch; adenomas lying caudal to this level cannot be visualized.

Intrathyroid Adenoma

Intrathyroid parathyroid adenomas are uncommon and have been described as either superior or inferior gland adenomas.[4,6,8] Most intrathyroid adenomas are in the posterior half of the middle to lower thyroid, are completely surrounded by thyroid tissue, and are oriented with their greatest dimension in the cephalocaudal direction (Fig. 19-12; **Video 19-6**). Intrathyroid adenomas may be overlooked at surgery because they are soft and are similar to the surrounding thyroid tissue on palpation. A thyroidotomy or subtotal lobectomy may be needed to find an intrathyroid adenoma. Sonographically, however, parathyroid adenomas usually are well visualized because they are highly **hypoechoic, in contrast to the echogenic thyroid parenchyma.** The internal architecture and appearance of these adenomas are

the same as for adenomas elsewhere in the neck. Sonographically, intrathyroid parathyroid adenomas can be similar to thyroid nodules in appearance, and percutaneous biopsy is often necessary to distinguish between these entities.

Some parathyroid adenomas may lie under the pseudocapsule or sheath that covers the thyroid gland or within a sulcus of the thyroid, but these are not usually considered to be true intrathyroid adenomas. These adenomas may be difficult for the surgeon to visualize at surgery unless this sheath is opened.[4,8] Sonographically, these may appear the same as other parathyroid adenomas that lie immediately adjacent to the thyroid, although the typical thin, echogenic capsular interface often seen between the thyroid and a parathyroid adenoma may be absent.

Carotid Sheath/Undescended Adenoma

Rare ectopic adenomas can lie in a high position superior and lateral in the neck, near the carotid bifurcation at the level of the hyoid bone and adjacent to the submandibular gland, or elsewhere within or along the carotid sheath[4,7,19,48-50] (Fig. 19-13; **Video 19-7**). These adenomas likely arise from inferior glands that are embryologically undescended, or partially descended, having come to reside within or adjacent to the carotid sheath that surrounds the carotid artery, jugular vein, and vagus nerve. They may be associated with a small amount of ectopic thymic tissue. These adenomas are frequently overlooked during surgery unless the surgeon specifically opens the carotid sheath and dissects within it.[6,7] Sonographically, these masses can appear similar to mildly enlarged lymph nodes in the jugular chain; correlative

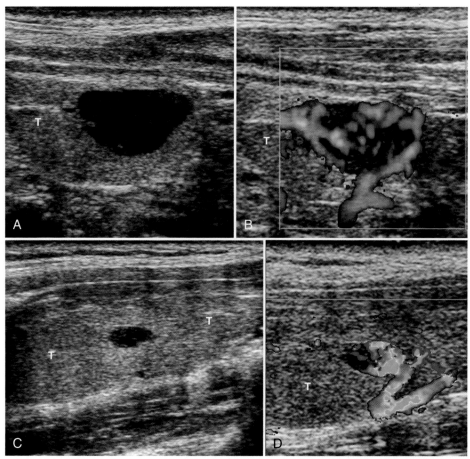

FIGURE 19-12. Ectopic parathyroid adenoma: intrathyroidal. A, Longitudinal sonogram shows hypoechoic intrathyroid parathyroid adenoma completely surrounded by thyroid tissue. *T,* Thyroid. **B,** Corresponding power Doppler image demonstrates prominent peripheral vascularity; *T,* thyroid. **C,** Longitudinal sonogram in another patient shows a subcentimeter hypoechoic intrathyroid parathyroid adenoma. *T,* Thyroid. **D,** Corresponding color Doppler flow imaging demonstrates typical hypervascularity with polar insertion of feeding vessel; *T,* thyroid.

imaging and percutaneous biopsy are often necessary for confirmation before surgery. Ectopic undescended superior gland adenomas may be present high in the neck in a parapharyngeal location, but frequently are not seen with traditional sonography.

PERSISTENT OR RECURRENT HYPERPARATHYROIDISM

Persistent hyperparathyroidism is the persistence of hypercalcemia after previous failed parathyroid surgery. This is frequently caused by an undiscovered ectopic parathyroid adenoma or unrecognized multiple gland disease, with failure to resect all the hyperfunctioning tissue during surgery.[51-53] **Recurrent hyperparathyroidism** is defined as hypercalcemia occurring after a 6-month interval of normocalcemia, resulting from the new development of hyperfunctioning parathyroid tissue from previously normal glands.[54] Recurrent hyperparathyroidism is often seen in patients with unrecognized MEN syndromes.

Because of scarring and fibrosis from previous surgery, the curative rate for repeat surgery is lower than for initial surgery; the risk of recurrent laryngeal nerve damage and postoperative hypocalcemia from hypoparathyroidism may also be greater.[55,56] Imaging before reoperation is particularly beneficial, and most care strategies recommend liberal use of imaging studies in this situation.[53,56-60] Ultrasound is an effective first-line imaging modality in the preoperative and reoperative assessment of parathyroid disease, providing anatomic localization with a relatively inexpensive, noninvasive method that avoids the use of ionizing radiation.[41,42,59,60] During sonographic evaluation of reoperative patients, specific attention is paid to the most likely ectopic parathyroid locations—those associated with a gland that was not discovered at the initial neck dissection.

A small subgroup of patients who develop recurrent hyperparathyroidism underwent previous **autotransplantation** of parathyroid tissue in conjunction with previous total parathyroidectomy, typically for complications of chronic renal failure. Hyperparathyroidism in the setting of parathyroid autotransplantation is

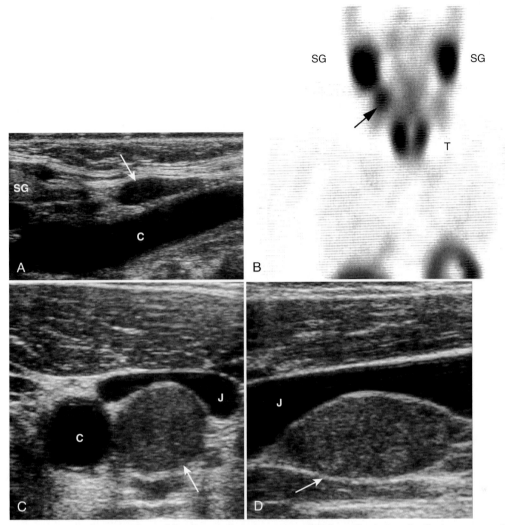

FIGURE 19-13. Ectopic parathyroid adenoma: near carotid sheath. A, Longitudinal sonogram of right side of the neck shows an ectopic undescended parathyroid adenoma *(arrow)* external to the carotid sheath, anterior to the common carotid artery *(C)*. Ultrasound-guided biopsy confirmed parathyroid tissue before surgical exploration. *SG,* Submandibular gland. **B,** Scintigraphy using technetium-99m sestamibi and coronal SPECT imaging shows a focal area of increased activity in right superior lateral neck *(arrow),* which corresponds to the ectopic adenoma; *SG,* salivary glands; *T,* thyroid. **C,** Transverse, and **D,** longitudinal, sonograms in another patient show an ectopic left inferior adenoma *(arrow)* located within the carotid sheath, posterior to the internal jugular vein *(J)*. Ultrasound-guided biopsy confirmed parathyroid tissue before surgical exploration. At surgery, the adenoma was adherent to the vagus nerve. *C,* Common carotid artery.

referred to as **graft-dependent hyperparathyroidism.** In parathyroid autotransplantation, a gland is sliced into fragments that are inserted into surgically prepared intramuscular pockets in the forearm or sternocleido-mastoid muscle. Normal-functioning autotransplanted parathyroid grafts are typically too small and similar in echotexture to the surrounding muscle to be adequately visualized sonographically. However, graft-dependent recurrent hyperparathyroidism can be imaged sono-graphically, appearing as oval, sharply marginated, hypoechoic hypervascular nodules measuring 5 to 11 mm and similar in appearance to hyperfunctioning parathyroid glands or adenomas arising in the neck[61] (Fig. 19-14). The hyperfunctioning autotransplanted fragments usually can be found by the surgeon while the

patient is under local anesthesia, and a portion of the grafted tissue can be excised to cure the hypercalcemia. Occasionally, for patients who are not candidates for repeat surgery, ultrasound-guided percutaneous ethanol injection may be used for ablation of recurrent hyper-parathyroid disease in the neck or at a graft site (see Ethanol Ablation).

SECONDARY HYPERPARATHYROIDISM

Secondary hyperparathyroidism is characterized by pro-nounced parathyroid gland hyperfunction resulting from end-organ resistance to PTH and is most often found in

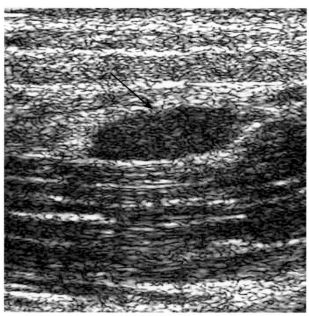

FIGURE 19-14. Graft-dependent hyperparathyroidism. Longitudinal sonogram of left forearm shows an oval, 2-cm hypoechoic nodule *(arrow)* resulting from hyperplasia of autotransplanted parathyroid tissue.

PARATHYROID ADENOMA: CAUSES OF EXAMINATION ERRORS

FALSE-POSITIVE RESULTS
Cervical lymph node
Prominent blood vessel
Esophagus
Longus colli muscle
Thyroid nodule

FALSE-NEGATIVE RESULTS
Minimally enlarged adenoma/gland
Multinodular thyroid goiter
Ectopic parathyroid adenoma

for ablation of hyperplastic parathyroid glands in patients with refractory secondary hyperparathyroidism who are not surgical candidates.

PITFALLS IN INTERPRETATION

False-Positive Examination

Normal and pathologic cervical structures, such as lymph nodes, small veins adjacent to the thyroid gland, the esophagus, the longus colli muscles, and thyroid nodules, can simulate parathyroid adenomas, producing false-positive results during neck sonography.

One source for a false-positive ultrasound study is confusion of **cervical lymph nodes** for a parathyroid adenoma.[31] Cervical lymph nodes are usually visualized sonographically in the lateral neck adjacent to the jugular vein and away from the thyroid. However, lymph nodes found adjacent to the carotid artery may occasionally simulate an ectopic adenoma. Lymph nodes may also be visualized within the central compartment near the inferior pole of the thyroid, simulating an inferior gland adenoma. Enlarged cervical lymph nodes may have an oval, hypoechoic appearance similar to parathyroid adenomas, but they often also have a central echogenic band or hilum composed of fat, vessels, and fibrous tissue, which differentiates them from parathyroid adenomas.[67] Nonetheless, ultrasound-guided biopsy may be necessary to distinguish a potential parathyroid adenoma from an atypical lymph node, particularly in the reoperative setting.

Many **small veins** lie immediately adjacent to the posterior and lateral aspects of both lobes of the thyroid, and a tortuous or segmentally dilated vein can simulate a small parathyroid adenoma. Scanning maneuvers to help establish the structure as a vein, not an adenoma, include (1) real-time imaging in multiple planes to show the tubular nature of the vein; (2) a Valsalva maneuver by the patient, which may cause transient engorgement

patients with chronic renal failure. In these patients, chronic relative hypocalcemia is the result of multiple complex factors, including decreased synthesis of the active form of vitamin D, poor calcium and vitamin D absorption, persistent hyperphosphatemia, and skeletal resistance to the actions of PTH. These factors contribute to parathyroid hyperplasia. If untreated, secondary hyperparathyroidism can result in bone demineralization, soft tissue calcification, and acceleration of vascular calcification. Surgical treatment for secondary hyperparathyroidism is less common because of the success of renal transplantation, dialysis, and medical therapy, including the newer calcimimetics. However, in symptomatic patients who are refractory to these therapies, subtotal parathyroidectomy or total parathyroidectomy with autotransplantation are surgical options.[25,62-64]

Patients with secondary hyperparathyroidism have **multiple enlarged glands.** Individually, these glands may have the same sonographic appearance as other parathyroid adenomas (see Fig. 19-6 and **Video 19-2**). However, the glands may be asymmetrically enlarged and more lobular. Although imaging is not usually necessary, sonography can be used to evaluate the severity of parathyroid hyperplasia by assessing gland enlargement.[65,66] Patients with sonographically enlarged glands tend to have significantly worse symptoms, laboratory values, and radiographic signs of secondary hyperparathyroidism than patients without gland enlargement. Sonography can also be used to aid in localization of the enlarged parathyroid glands before surgical resection for secondary hyperparathyroidism. Ultrasound-guided percutaneous ethanol injection is also a treatment option

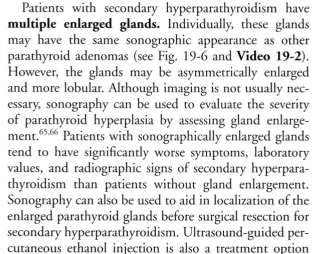

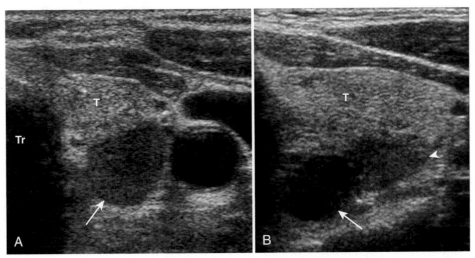

FIGURE 19-15. Thyroid nodules may simulate parathyroid adenoma. A, Transverse sonogram shows hypoechoic thyroid nodule *(arrow)* arising within the posterior aspect, left lobe of the thyroid *(T),* which could simulate a parathyroid adenoma; *Tr,* trachea. **B,** Transverse sonogram in another patient shows highly hypoechoic parathyroid adenoma *(arrow)* posterior to left lobe of the thyroid. An adjacent, slightly hypoechoic thyroid *(T)* nodule *(arrowhead)* is also present and might simulate a parathyroid adenoma.

of the vein; and (3) spectral or color Doppler sonography to show flow within the vein.

The **esophagus** may partially protrude from behind the posterolateral aspect of the trachea and simulate a mass or parathyroid adenoma (see Fig. 19-8, *B*). Turning the patient's head to the opposite side will accentuate the protrusion. Careful inspection of this structure in the transverse plane shows that it has the typical concentric ring appearance of bowel, with a peripheral hypoechoic muscular layer and the central echogenic appearance of the mucosa and intraluminal contents. Using a longitudinal scan plane helps to demonstrate the tubular nature of this structure. Real-time imaging while the patient swallows will cause a stream of brightly echogenic mucus and microbubbles to flow through the lumen, which confirms that the structure is the esophagus.

The **longus colli muscle** lies adjacent to the anterolateral aspect of the cervical spine. If viewed in the transverse plane, it appears as a hypoechoic triangular mass that can simulate a large parathyroid adenoma located posterior to the thyroid gland. However, scanning in the longitudinal plane will show that this structure is long and flat and contains longitudinal echogenic striations typical of skeletal muscle. Real-time imaging while the patient swallows can be useful because swallowing will cause movement of the thyroid gland and adjacent thyroid structures, such as a parathyroid adenoma, but the longus colli muscle, which is attached to the spine, will remain stationary. Finally, comparison with the opposite side of the neck will demonstrate similar symmetric findings because the longus colli muscles are paired structures located on both sides of the cervical spine.

Thyroid nodules are also potential causes of false-positive ultrasound and scintigraphic imaging.[31,68] If a thyroid nodule protrudes from the posterior aspect of

the thyroid, it can simulate a mass in the location of a parathyroid adenoma (Fig. 19-15). A useful sign in this situation is the thin, echogenic line of the capsular interface that separates the parathyroid adenoma (which usually arises outside the thyroid) from the thyroid gland itself. Thyroid nodules, which arise within the thyroid gland, typically do not show this tissue plane of separation.[69] Morphologically, thyroid nodules, unlike parathyroid adenomas, are often partially cystic, and some are calcified. Also, thyroid nodules often are of a heterogeneous, mixed echogenicity, whereas parathyroid adenomas are typically of a homogeneous, hypoechoic echogenicity. When a parathyroid adenoma cannot be distinguished from a thyroid nodule by imaging criteria, ultrasound-guided percutaneous biopsy may be necessary.

False-Negative Examination

Minimally enlarged adenomas, adenomas displaced posteriorly and obscured by a greatly enlarged nodular thyroid, and ectopic adenomas may cause false-negative imaging results.

Minimally enlarged adenomas or **hyperplastic glands** are a common cause of error because they can be difficult to distinguish from the thyroid and adjacent soft tissues[31,70] (see Fig. 19-5, *A,* and Video 19-1). The abnormal but minimally enlarged gland can be encountered with single adenomas or with multigland disease caused by hyperplasia. **Multinodular thyroid goiters** interfere with parathyroid adenoma detection in two ways.[31,68,70] First, the thyroid gland enlargement displaces structures located adjacent to the posterior thyroid, away from the transducer **(Video 19-8).** This can necessitate the use of 5-MHz transducers rather than higher-frequency transducers to obtain the necessary penetration, which decreases spatial resolution. Second, thyroid goiters may have a multinodular contour and irregular echotexture, which can cast refractive shadows, decrease the conspicuity and thereby hinder the detection of adjacent parathyroid gland enlargement **(Video 19-9).** Some **ectopic adenomas,** such as retrotracheal adenomas or adenomas located deep in the mediastinum, will not be visible because of acoustic shadowing from overlying air and bone.

ACCURACY IN IMAGING

Ultrasound

Sonographic imaging provides a noninvasive and economical method to localize parathyroid adenomas in the preoperative setting of primary hyperparathyroidism, without the need for patient radiation exposure.[41,42,59,60,71-80] However, the success of parathyroid ultrasound depends on the use of high-frequency, higher-resolution technology and improves with operator experience and diligence. The sensitivity of sonographic parathyroid adenoma localization in primary hyperparathyroidism varies from 74% to 89%.[40,41,59,74-77] Sensitivity also improves with the use of higher-resolution sonography and experience. The accuracy for ultrasound in detecting adenomatous disease is 74% to 94%, with a positive predictive value of 93% to 98%.[40,41,71,75,76] However, the sensitivity of ultrasound to detect ectopic mediastinal adenomas is predictably much lower, and the accuracy, sensitivity, and specificity decrease in the setting of multigland disease.[40-42,71,73,77] Therefore the success of sonographic parathyroid adenoma localization also depends on the specific characteristics of the patient population imaged, including the prevalence of multi-gland and ectopic mediastinal parathyroid disease.

As described later, ultrasound-guided **fine-needle aspiration (FNA) biopsy** is a valuable adjunct to the ultrasound examination and can be used to improve its accuracy, specificity, and sensitivity. For any suspected adenoma mass, aspirates should be sent for PTH assay, in addition to cytologic analysis.[19,56,81-86] Another advantage of ultrasound is its ability to assess for concomitant thyroid disease during the evaluation for parathyroid disease, which may further impact surgical planning.

In persistent or recurrent hyperparathyroidism, sensitivity of sonography in adenoma localization varies widely. However, sonography has demonstrated some of the highest sensitivities and accuracies of all modalities for adenoma detection in the reoperative setting, especially when combined with ultrasound-guided FNA biopsy of a suspected parathyroid adenoma.* Ultrasound augmented by FNA biopsy and PTH assay can lead to a specificity approaching 100% and a sensitivity

and accuracy of 90% and 82%, respectively.[56] It is important to understand that in most large clinical series of patients undergoing reoperation for hyperparathyroidism, the great majority of parathyroid adenomas are still found in the neck or are accessible through a neck incision.[55-57,60] Therefore a thorough ultrasound examination of the neck is important in these reoperative patients. If the adenoma is not visible sonographically, an ectopic mediastinal location must be considered. There should be a low threshold to utilize multiple imaging modalities, especially when initial imaging findings are ambiguous or the surgical risk is high.[53,56,57,60] This approach significantly improves the success rate and decreases the procedural time and cost in the reoperated patient.[53,55,56]

Other Modalities

Another imaging modality widely used for parathyroid adenoma localization is **scintigraphy** with technetium-99m (^{99m}Tc) sestamibi.[42,70,74,77,90-95] ^{99m}Tc sestamibi scintigraphy, particularly when combined with single-photon emission computed tomography (SPECT), has a sensitivity similar to or better than ultrasound.[42,58,70,74,90-96] Scintigraphy can demonstrate adenomas in areas that are missed by ultrasound, including the mediastinum and retrotracheal space. However, scintigraphy is more expensive than ultrasound and requires the use of ionizing radiation. As with ultrasound, parathyroid scintigraphy also appears to be less sensitive and accurate in multiglandular parathyroid disease, for smaller adenomas, and in the presence of multinodular thyroid disease.

Magnetic resonance imaging (MRI) is also a useful noninvasive modality in the evaluation of parathyroid disease.[42,97-101] Although more expensive than ultrasound, MRI has demonstrated particular utility in localizing mediastinal adenomas and in the evaluation of the reoperative patient.

Less common imaging modalities include **computed tomography (CT),** angiography, and venous sampling.[42,75,102] Selective **venous sampling** is more invasive, expensive, and technically demanding than other imaging modalities. However, it can be a useful technique to lateralize parathyroid disease, particularly in a high-risk reoperative setting or when previous noninvasive imaging is inconclusive.[102]

The combination of multiple preoperative imaging studies demonstrates improved sensitivity compared with single-modality evaluation. Combined imaging with ultrasound and ^{99m}Tc sestamibi scintigraphy increases the sensitivity for the preoperative diagnosis of parathyroid disease[42,74,79,90,96] (Fig. 19-16). MRI combined with ^{99m}Tc sestamibi scintigraphy increased imaging sensitivity in evaluation of recurrent or persistent hyperparathyroidism.[101]

When multiple studies are used, ultrasound is a good choice for initial preoperative imaging because of its

---

*References 53, 55, 56, 58, 60, 87-89.

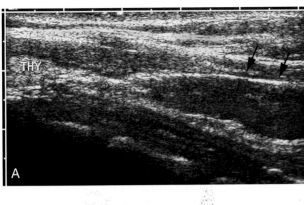

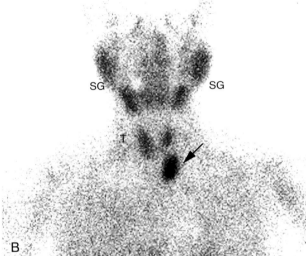

FIGURE 19-16. Correlation of ultrasound and scintigraphic imaging of parathyroid adenoma. A, Longitudinal sonogram shows a 3-cm hypoechoic adenoma *(arrows)* located inferior to tip of lower pole of the left thyroid lobe *(THY)* within the thyrothymic ligament. **B,** Planar imaging with technetium-99m sestamibi shows increased focal activity in the inferior left neck corresponding to the adenoma *(arrow)*, well below the level of the thyroid *(T)* and salivary glands *(SG)*.

noninvasiveness, relative low cost, anatomic detail, and competitive sensitivity and accuracy when used by an experienced examiner (Figs. 19-17 and 19-18).

Significance in Primary Hyperparathyroidism

Definitive cure of primary hyperparathyroidism requires surgical parathyroidectomy, which can be accomplished with a very high degree of success and minimal morbidity when performed by an experienced surgeon.[24,25,103] Historically, the standard surgical procedure involved open bilateral neck dissection with inspection of each parathyroid gland, and routine preoperative imaging was not considered necessary.

Minimally invasive surgical techniques, such as the more recently termed **minimal-access parathyroidectomy (MAP)**, are increasingly recommended and used for first-time surgery in primary hyperparathyroidism.[24,103-107] In MAP the abnormal gland or adenoma is selectively removed through a small (2 cm) incision in the neck, thereby potentially improving cosmesis, reducing complication risks, and decreasing operative time, hospital stay, and overall cost, often without sacrificing significant operative efficacy when performed by an experienced surgeon (Fig. 19-19). Moreover, postsurgical fibrosis is limited to a smaller area, thus facilitating any necessary repeat surgery in the future. The successful institution of these minimally invasive techniques is predicated on the availability of (1) **accurate preoperative imaging techniques** to direct a focused surgical approach and (2) reliable, rapid (10-15 minutes) **intraoperative parathyroid hormone (IOPTH) monitoring**, which facilitates the surgical determination of the need for further exploration.

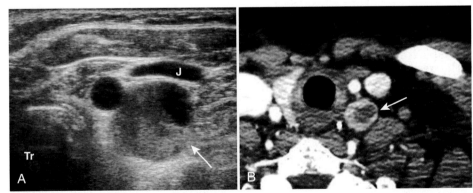

FIGURE 19-17. Correlation of ultrasound and CT imaging of parathyroid adenoma. A, Transverse sonogram shows a partially cystic ectopic supernumerary parathyroid adenoma *(arrow)* posterior to the left internal jugular vein *(J)* but external to the carotid sheath. Left superior and inferior parathyroid glands and the left thyroid lobe had previously been resected. Biopsy confirmed parathyroid tissue before repeat surgical exploration. *Tr,* Trachea. **B,** Enhanced axial CT image of the neck shows the same partially cystic parathyroid adenoma *(arrow)*.

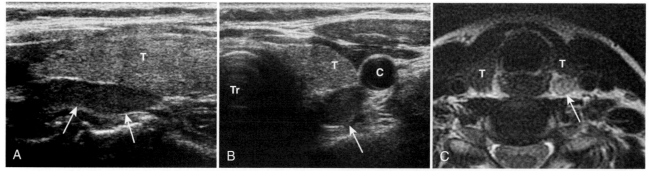

FIGURE 19-18. Correlation of ultrasound and MR imaging of parathyroid adenoma. A, Longitudinal, and, **B,** transverse, sonograms show superior parathyroid adenoma *(arrows)* posterior to upper-middle portion of left lobe of the thyroid *(T); C,* common carotid artery; *Tr,* trachea. **C,** T2-weighted fast spin-echo axial MR image of the neck shows the same left superior parathyroid adenoma *(arrow),* which appears hyperintense compared with the thyroid gland *(T).*

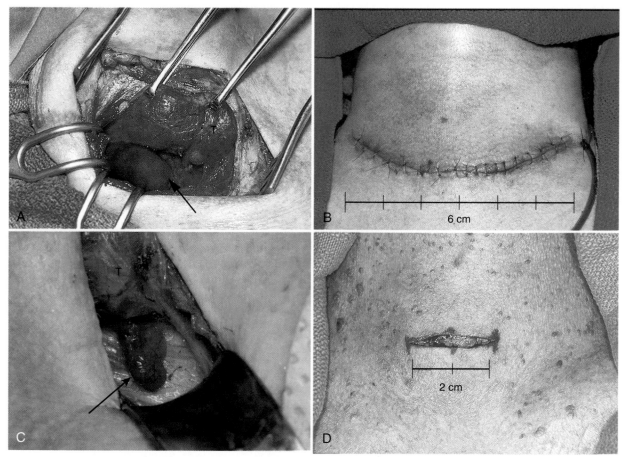

FIGURE 19-19. Comparison of surgical procedures for removal of parathyroid adenoma. A, Intraoperative photograph during bilateral neck dissection for parathyroidectomy. The thyroid gland *(T)* is retracted back and a parathyroid adenoma *(arrow)* exposed. **B,** Corresponding 6-cm "collar" incision with a surgical drain. **C,** Intraoperative photograph during minimally invasive surgery uses a much smaller incision. Parathyroid adenoma *(arrow)* is exposed adjacent to the thyroid *(T).* **D,** Minimally invasive surgical incision, approximately 2 cm. *(Photographs courtesy Geoffrey B. Thompson, MD, Mayo Clinic, Rochester, Minn.)*

Many investigators promote the use of **both anatomic and functional imaging,** such as ultrasound and ^{99m}Tc sestamibi scintigraphy, to increase the preoperative certainty of unilateral disease and aid in excluding patients with multigland disease who are not candidates for MAP.* With IOPTH monitoring the surgeon can quickly assess the success of a focused unilateral approach.

If intraoperative PTH levels fail to normalize or decrease by at least 50%, multigland disease should be suspected, and the procedure may be converted to a bilateral dissection. Proponents of preoperative imaging in primary hyperthyroidism also note that some adenomas are found lower in the neck or mediastinum, and that the initial operative approach may be changed or optimized if imaging shows parathyroid disease near the thymus.[24,56,76,80]

*References 19, 58, 71, 73-75, 90, 96.

In persistent or recurrent hyperparathyroidism, localization studies are liberally used because of the lower surgical success rate and the higher morbidity of reoperation. Preoperative localization studies in recurrent hyperparathyroidism contribute to both the success and the speed of the repeat surgery. In patients who had reexploration for persistent or recurrent hyperparathyroidism, the surgical cure rate was 88% to 89%, and it was thought that prospective localization studies contributed to this high rate of success and decreased surgical time.[53,55,56] Because most persistent and recurrent parathyroid adenomas are accessible in the neck or the upper mediastinum through a cervical incision, sonography and ^{99m}Tc sestamibi scintigraphy may be the localizing procedures of choice and, in select patients, can aid in directing a focused, minimal-access surgical approach.*

INTRAOPERATIVE SONOGRAPHY

Intraoperative sonography is occasionally a useful adjunct in the surgical detection of parathyroid adenomas, particularly in the reoperative setting.[19,108,109] Intraoperative scanning can be performed with a small, conventional, high-frequency (8-15 MHz) transducer draped with a sterile plastic sheath, or with a dedicated sterilized intraoperative transducer. Intraoperative ultrasound appears to be most useful for localizing abnormal inferior and intrathyroid parathyroid glands.[109] Correlated with preoperative imaging, intraoperative sonography can also help guide a focused surgical resection to limit tissue damage associated with exploration in the reoperated patient; it also allows directed resection of ectopic adenomas in the mediastinum, thyroid, and carotid sheath. If an abnormal parathyroid gland is detected, surgical time may be shortened.

PERCUTANEOUS BIOPSY

Sonographically guided percutaneous FNA biopsy can be used for preoperative confirmation of suspected abnormal parathyroid glands, particularly in the candidate for reoperation.[55,56,81-89] This technique can decrease the false-positive rate and increase the specificity of sonography by permitting the reliable differentiation of parathyroid adenomas from other pathologic structures, such as thyroid nodules and cervical lymph nodes. In addition to its value to the surgeon, a positive biopsy may reassure the reluctant reoperative patient. FNA biopsy is also generally obtained for diagnostic confirmation before percutaneously injected ethanol ablation of a suspected abnormal gland.

If the suspected parathyroid adenoma is in a location remote from the thyroid gland, the main differential diagnostic consideration is a lymph node. Percutaneous

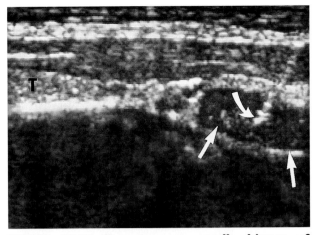

FIGURE 19-20. Percutaneous needle biopsy of parathyroid adenoma. Longitudinal sonogram shows an oval, 1.5-cm hypoechoic parathyroid adenoma *(straight arrows)* in the low neck in a patient with recurrent hyperparathyroidism. Needle biopsy *(curved arrow)* obtained parathyroid cells and an aspirate was positive for PTH, confirming that this mass was a parathyroid adenoma. *T,* Thyroid.

biopsy is performed by using a standard noncutting 25-gauge needle to obtain aspirates that contain either parathyroid cells or lymphocytes (Fig. 19-20; **Video 19-10**). **The aspirate must also be analyzed for PTH** because elevated levels indicate the presence of parathyroid tissue, even if the cytologic results are inconclusive.[19,83-86] After the aspirated material is expelled onto a slide for cytologic review, the residual sample in the needle hub is rinsed with a tiny amount of sterile saline, emptied into a tube, and placed on ice. This is repeated for each aspirate, diluting the sample for PTH assay into a total volume of 1 to 2 mL. Alternatively, three to four aspirates may be expelled and rinsed directly into a tube containing 1 to 2 mL of sterile saline, then placed on ice. If the suspected parathyroid adenoma lies adjacent to the thyroid, FNA biopsy may be necessary to differentiate parathyroid and thyroid tissue. These aspirates should also be analyzed for PTH because parathyroid and thyroid tissue can be very difficult to differentiate by cytology.[19,83-86] In addition, thyroid tissue sometimes must be traversed to access a parathyroid adenoma, causing possible sample contamination with thyroid cells.[19] A histologic specimen obtained with a small-caliber (20-22 gauge) cutting needle may provide more cellular material for analysis but usually is unnecessary if PTH assay is performed. In addition, the possibility of postbiopsy periglandular fibrosis complicating subsequent surgery may be greater with cutting-needle biopsy. FNA biopsy of suspected parathyroid adenomas is well tolerated, with few reported complications. Although a theoretic consideration, **parathymosis** (implantation of hyperfunctioning parathyroid tissue in neck or mediastinum, resulting in hypercalcemia) does not appear to be a complication of FNA biopsy.[110]

*References 42, 55, 56, 58, 60, 87.

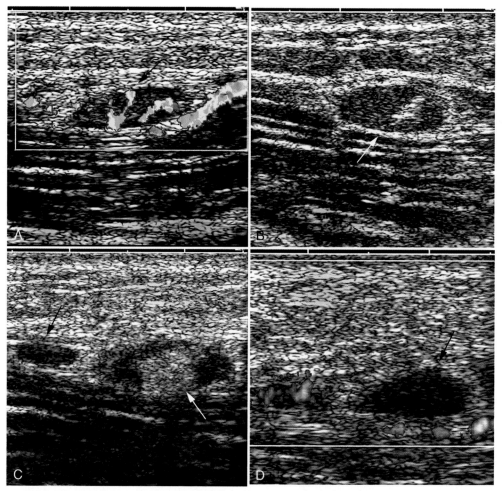

FIGURE 19-21. Ethanol ablation of hyperplastic autotransplanted parathyroid tissue. A, Color Doppler flow sonogram of the superficial forearm tissues shows a dominant vascular nodule that represents hyperfunctioning parathyroid tissue *(arrow)* in a patient with recurrent graft-dependent hyperparathyroidism. **B,** Under sonographic guidance, a needle tip *(arrow)* is placed within the nodule. **C,** Ethanol is injected into portions of the nodule, which causes the tissues adjacent to the needle tip to become transiently, brightly echogenic *(white arrow)*. A smaller, adjacent nodule of parathyroid tissue *(black arrow)* is not injected, to maintain baseline graft function. **D,** After ethanol ablation, power Doppler sonogram shows decreased vascularity in the injected nodule *(arrow)*.

ETHANOL ABLATION

Sonography can be used to guide percutaneous injection of ethanol into abnormally enlarged parathyroid glands for chemical ablation.[111-124] Ethanol ablation is most often used in postoperative patients with recurrent or persistent hyperparathyroidism who have sonographically visible, biopsy-proven hyperfunctioning parathyroid tissue, but who are poor surgical candidates.[114,117,119] Some dialysis patients with secondary hyperparathyroidism and patients with a history of multigland disease with recalcitrant recurrent hyperparathyroidism after previous subtotal surgery have also received this treatment.[114,119-124] Ethanol ablation has been shown to be very useful in patients with MEN I who have had previous subtotal parathyroidectomy and recurrent disease in their remaining residual half-gland in the neck.[114] A portion of the remaining gland can be ablated with ethanol to control

hypercalcemia and avoid repeat surgery, which has a very high complication rate of postoperative hypoparathyroidism in these patients. Autografts in patients with recurrent graft-dependent hyperparathyroidism can be similarly treated[125] (Fig. 19-21). Adenomatous hyperplasia with autonomously functioning glands **(tertiary hyperparathyroidism)** has also been treated with ultrasound-guided ethanol injection to reduce gland mass, but with unpredictable results.[126,127]

Ethanol ablation is generally performed under local anesthesia, typically after confirmation of parathyroid tissue with FNA biopsy. Under real-time ultrasound guidance, a standard 25-gauge needle attached to a 1-mL tuberculin syringe is inserted into the mass. With the tip in constant visualization, sterile 95% ethanol is injected into multiple regions of the mass, with a volume about half that of the mass, typically 0.1 to 1.0 mL. The tissue becomes highly echogenic at the moment of injection;

the echogenicity slowly disappears over 1 minute. There is also a marked decrease in vascularity of the parathyroid adenoma after alcohol injection, presumably secondary to thrombosis and occlusion of parathyroid vessels (Fig. 19-21, *D*). The injections are repeated every day or every other day until the serum calcium level reaches the normal range. In most patients, three or fewer injections are necessary. All patients undergoing parathyroid ethanol ablation require long-term close follow-up of serum calcium levels to detect subsequent hypoparathyroidism or, more often, recurrent hyperparathyroidism.

The reported adverse effects from ethanol ablation of parathyroid adenomas have been limited to temporary jaw pain during the procedure and dysphonia from vocal cord paralysis. Dysphonia is caused by recurrent laryngeal nerve palsy, which is typically a transient effect. Patients who have had prior subtotal parathyroid surgery are also theoretically at increased risk for postablation hypoparathyroidism, and conservative ablation of only a portion of the remaining gland is prudent.

The long-term efficacy of ethanol ablation as a treatment of hyperparathyroidism in patients with primary disease does not approach that of surgery.[112-115,117,119] In addition, postablation periglandular fibrosis may make future surgical procedures more difficult. Therefore, ethanol ablation as a treatment of primary hyperparathyroidism is reserved for patients who cannot or will not undergo surgery. Studies on the outcomes of ethanol ablation in primary hyperparathyroidism report that most patients had either partial or complete biochemical improvement, although many of these patients will have recurrent disease.[114,115,119] Thus, close clinical and biochemical follow-up is necessary, and repeat treatments may be required. Reasons for failure include (1) incomplete ablation of hyperfunctioning tissue within the treated adenoma and (2) residual hyperfunctioning of other untreated glands in the patient with unrecognized multigland disease.

In theory, methods of thermal tissue ablation such as radiotherapy, cryotherapy, and laser therapy, which have been used to treat tumors elsewhere in the body, could also be applied to treat parathyroid disease in the neck. These methods are limited at present by the lack of ablation devices that can precisely treat very small amounts of tissue. In patients not considered surgical candidates, there have been initial reports of successful treatment of parathyroid adenomas using ultrasound-guided percutaneous laser ablation.[128,129] However, further studies are needed to determine the usefulness of these methods of ablation in the neck in the treatment of parathyroid disease.

References

Embryology and Anatomy
1. Gilmour JR. The gross anatomy of the parathyroid glands. J Pathol 1938;46:133-148.
2. Weller Jr GL. Development of the thyroid, parathyroid and thymus glands in man. Carnegie Institution of Washington. Contributions to Embryology 1933;24:93-139.
3. Mansberger Jr AR, Wei JP. Surgical embryology and anatomy of the thyroid and parathyroid glands. Surg Clin North Am 1993;73:727-746.
4. Akerstrom G, Malmaeus J, Bergstrom R. Surgical anatomy of human parathyroid glands. Surgery 1984;95:14-21.
5. Edis AJ. Surgical anatomy and technique of neck exploration for primary hyperparathyroidism. Surg Clin North Am 1977;57:495-504.
6. Thompson NW, Eckhauser FE, Harness JK. The anatomy of primary hyperparathyroidism. Surgery 1982;92:814-821.
7. Edis AJ, Purnell DC, van Heerden JA. The undescended "parathymus": an occasional cause of failed neck exploration for hyperparathyroidism. Ann Surg 1979;190:64-68.
8. Wang C. The anatomic basis of parathyroid surgery. Ann Surg 1976;183:271-275.
9. Norris EH. The parathyroid glands and the lateral thyroid in man: their morphogenesis, histogenesis, topographic anatomy and prenatal growth. Carnegie Institution of Washington: Contributions to Embryology 1937;26:247-294.
10. Castleman B, Roth SI. Tumors of the parathyroid glands. In: Atlas of tumor pathology. Fasc 14, 2nd series. Washington, DC: Armed Forces Institute of Pathology; 1978.
11. Russell CF, Grant CS, van Heerden JA. Hyperfunctioning supernumerary parathyroid glands. an occasional cause of hyperparathyroidism. Mayo Clin Proc 1982;57:121-124.
12. Kamaya K, Quon A, Jeffrey RB. Sonography of the abnormal parathyroid gland. Ultrasound Q 2006;22:253-262.
13. Huppert BJ, Reading CC. Parathyroid sonography: imaging and intervention. J Clin Ultrasound 2007;35:144-155.

Primary Hyperparathyroidism
14. Heath 3rd H, Hodgson SF, Kennedy MA. Primary hyperparathyroidism: incidence, morbidity, and potential economic impact in a community. N Engl J Med 1980;302:189-193.
15. Van Heerden JA, Beahrs OH, Woolner LB. The pathology and surgical management of primary hyperparathyroidism. Surg Clin North Am 1977;57:557-563.
16. Wang CA. Surgery of the parathyroid glands. Adv Surg 1966;5:109-127.
17. Black 3rd WC, Utley JR. The differential diagnosis of parathyroid adenoma and chief cell hyperplasia. Am J Clin Pathol 1968;49:761-775.
18. Van Heerden JA, Kent 3rd RB, et al. Primary hyperparathyroidism in patients with multiple endocrine neoplasia syndromes: surgical experience. Arch Surg 1983;118:533-536.
19. Shawker TH. Ultrasound evaluation of primary hyperparathyroidism. Ultrasound Q 2000;16:73-87.
20. Vetto JT, Brennan MF, Woodruf J, Burt M. Parathyroid carcinoma: diagnosis and clinical history. Surgery 1993;114:882-892.
21. Delellis RA. Tumors of the parathyroid gland. In Atlas of tumor pathology. Fasc 6, 3rd series. Washington, DC: Armed Forces Institute of Pathology; 1993.
22. Shane E, Bilezikian JP. Parathyroid carcinoma: a review of 62 patients. Endocr Rev 1982;3:218-226.
23. Wynne AG, van Heerden J, Carney JA, Fitzpatrick LA. Parathyroid carcinoma: clinical and pathologic features in 43 patients. Medicine (Baltimore) 1992;71:197-205.
24. Grant CS, Thompson G, Farley D, van Heerden J. Primary hyperparathyroidism surgical management since the introduction of minimally invasive parathyroidectomy: Mayo Clinic experience. Arch Surg 2005;140:472-478; discussion 478-479.
25. Kearns AE, Thompson GB. Medical and surgical management of hyperparathyroidism. Mayo Clin Proc 2002;77:87-91.
26. Silverberg SJ, Shane E, Jacobs TP, et al. A 10-year prospective study of primary hyperparathyroidism with or without parathyroid surgery. N Engl J Med 1999;341:1249-1255.
27. US National Institutes of Health Consensus Development Conference Statement. Diagnosis and management of asymptomatic primary hyperparathyroidism. Ann Intern Med 1991;114:593-597.
28. Silverberg SJ, Bilezikian JP, Bone HG, et al. Therapeutic controversies in primary hyperparathyroidism. J Clin Endocrinol Metab 1999;84:2275-2285.

29. Irvin 3rd GL, Carneiro DM. Management changes in primary hyperparathyroidism. JAMA 2000;284:934-936.
30. Bilezikian JP, Potts Jr JT, Fuleihan Gel H, et al. Summary statement from a workshop on asymptomatic primary hyperparathyroidism: a perspective for the 21st century. J Clin Endocrinol Metab 2002; 87:5353-5361.

Sonographic Appearance

31. Reading CC, Charboneau JW, James EM, et al. High-resolution parathyroid sonography. AJR Am J Roentgenol 1982;139:539-546.
32. Randel SB, Gooding GA, Clark OH, et al. Parathyroid variants: ultrasound evaluation. Radiology 1987;165:191-194.
33. Graif M, Itzchak Y, Strauss S, et al. Parathyroid sonography: diagnostic accuracy related to shape, location, and texture of the gland. Br J Radiol 1987;60:439-443.
34. Obara T, Fujimoto Y, Ito Y, et al. Functioning parathyroid lipoadenoma: report of four cases—clinicopathological and ultrasonographic features. Endocrinol Jpn 1989;36:135-145.
35. Krudy AG, Doppman JL, Shawker TH, et al. Hyperfunctioning cystic parathyroid glands: CT and sonographic findings. AJR Am J Roentgenol 1984;142:175-178.
36. Gooding GA, Duh QY. Primary hyperparathyroidism: functioning hemorrhagic parathyroid cyst. J Clin Ultrasound 1997;25:82-84.
37. Doppman JL, Brennan MF, Kahn CR, Marx SJ. Circumscribing or periadenomal vessel: a helpful angiographic finding in certain islet cell and parathyroid adenomas. AJR Am J Roentgenol 1981;136: 163-165.
38. Gooding GA, Clark OH. Use of color Doppler imaging in the distinction between thyroid and parathyroid lesions. Am J Surg 1992;164:51-56.
39. Wolf RJ, Cronan JJ, Monchik JM. Color Doppler sonography: an adjunctive technique in assessment of parathyroid adenomas. J Ultrasound Med 1994;13:303-308.
40. Lane MJ, Desser TS, Weigel RJ, Jeffrey Jr RB. Use of color and power Doppler sonography to identify feeding arteries associated with parathyroid adenomas. AJR Am J Roentgenol 1998;171:819-823.
41. Reeder SB, Desser TS, Weigel RJ, Jeffrey RB. Sonography in primary hyperparathyroidism: review with emphasis on scanning technique. J Ultrasound Med 2002;21:539-552; quiz 553-554.
42. Johnson NA, Tublin ME, Ogilvie JB. Parathyroid imaging: technique and role in the preoperative evaluation of primary hyperparathyroidism. AJR Am J Roentgenol 2007;188:1706-1715.
43. Edmonson GR, Charboneau JW, James EM, et al. Parathyroid carcinoma: high-frequency sonographic features. Radiology 1986; 161:65-67.
44. Daly BD, Coffey SL, Behan M. Ultrasonographic appearances of parathyroid carcinoma. Br J Radiol 1989;62:1017-1019.
45. Hara H, Igarashi A, Yano Y, et al. Ultrasonographic features of parathyroid carcinoma. Endocr J 2001;48:213-217.

Adenoma Localization

46. Clark OH. Mediastinal parathyroid tumors. Arch Surg 1988; 123:1096-1100.
47. Thompson NW, Vinik AI, editors. Endocrine surgery update. New York: Grune & Stratton; 1983.
48. Fraker DL, Doppman JL, Shawker TH, et al. Undescended parathyroid adenoma: an important etiology for failed operations for primary hyperparathyroidism. World J Surg 1990;14:342-348.
49. Doppman JL, Shawker TH, Krudy AG, et al. Parathymic parathyroid: CT, ultrasound, and angiographic findings. Radiology 1985; 157:419-423.
50. Doppman JL, Shawker TH, Fraker DL, et al. Parathyroid adenoma within the vagus nerve. AJR Am J Roentgenol 1994;163:943-945.

Persistent or Recurrent Hyperparathyroidism

51. Irvin 3rd GL, Prudhomme DL, Deriso GT, et al. A new approach to parathyroidectomy. Ann Surg 1994;219:574-579; discussion 579-581.
52. Levin KE, Clark OH. The reasons for failure in parathyroid operations. Arch Surg 1989;124:911-914; discussion 914-915.
53. Grant CS, van Heerden JA, Charboneau JW, et al. Clinical management of persistent and/or recurrent primary hyperparathyroidism. World J Surg 1986;10:555-565.

54. Clark OH, Way LW, Hunt TK. Recurrent hyperparathyroidism. Ann Surg 1976;184:391-402.
55. Richards ML, Thompson GB, Farley DR, Grant CS. Reoperative parathyroidectomy in 228 patients during the era of minimal-access surgery and intraoperative parathyroid hormone monitoring. Am J Surg 2008;196:937-942; discussion 942-943.
56. Thompson GB, Grant CS, Perrier ND, et al. Reoperative parathyroid surgery in the era of sestamibi scanning and intraoperative parathyroid hormone monitoring. Arch Surg 1999;134:699-704; discussion 704-705.
57. Rodriquez JM, Tezelman S, Siperstein AE, et al. Localization procedures in patients with persistent or recurrent hyperparathyroidism. Arch Surg 1994;129:870-875.
58. Feingold DL, Alexander HR, Chen CC, et al. Ultrasound and sestamibi scan as the only preoperative imaging tests in reoperation for parathyroid adenomas. Surgery 2000;128:1103-1109; discussion 1109-1110.
59. Koslin DB, Adams J, Andersen P, et al. Preoperative evaluation of patients with primary hyperparathyroidism: role of high-resolution ultrasound. Laryngoscope 1997;107:1249-1253.
60. Ghaheri BA, Koslin DB, Wood AH, Cohen JI. Preoperative ultrasound is worthwhile for reoperative parathyroid surgery. Laryngoscope 2004;114:2168-2171.
61. Winkelbauer F, Ammann ME, Langle F, Niederle B. Diagnosis of hyperparathyroidism with ultrasound after autotransplantation: results of a prospective study. Radiology 1993;186:255-257.

Secondary Hyperparathyroidism

62. Richards ML, Wormuth J, Bingener J, Sirinek K. Parathyroidectomy in secondary hyperparathyroidism: is there an optimal operative management? Surgery 2006;139:174-180.
63. Milas M, Weber CJ. Near-total parathyroidectomy is beneficial for patients with secondary and tertiary hyperparathyroidism. Surgery 2004;136:1252-1260.
64. Leapman SB, Filo RS, Thomalla JV, King D. Secondary hyperparathyroidism: the role of surgery. Am Surg 1989;55:359-365.
65. Takebayashi S, Matsui K, Onohara Y, Hidai H. Sonography for early diagnosis of enlarged parathyroid glands in patients with secondary hyperparathyroidism. AJR Am J Roentgenol 1987;148: 911-914.
66. Gladziwa U, Ittel TH, Dakshinamurty KV, et al. Secondary hyperparathyroidism and sonographic evaluation of parathyroid gland hyperplasia in dialysis patients. Clin Nephrol 1992;38:162-166.

Pitfalls in Interpretation

67. Sutton RT, Reading CC, Charboneau JW, et al. Ultrasound-guided biopsy of neck masses in postoperative management of patients with thyroid cancer. Radiology 1988;168:769-772.
68. Karstrup S, Hegedus L. Concomitant thyroid disease in hyperparathyroidism: reasons for unsatisfactory ultrasonographical localization of parathyroid glands. Eur J Radiol 1986;6:149-152.
69. Scheible W, Deutsch AL, Leopold GR. Parathyroid adenoma: accuracy of preoperative localization by high-resolution real-time sonography. J Clin Ultrasound 1981;9:325-330.
70. Mazzeo S, Caramella D, Lencioni R, et al. Comparison among sonography, double-tracer subtraction scintigraphy, and double-phase scintigraphy in the detection of parathyroid lesions. AJR Am J Roentgenol 1996;166:1465-1470.

Accuracy in Imaging

71. Soon PS, Delbridge LW, Sywak MS, et al. Surgeon-performed ultrasound facilitates minimally invasive parathyroidectomy by the focused lateral mini-incision approach. World J Surg 2008;32: 766-771.
72. Meilstrup JW. Ultrasound examination of the parathyroid glands. Otolaryngol Clin North Am 2004;37:763-778, ix.
73. Yeh MW, Barraclough BM, Sidhu SB, et al. Two hundred consecutive parathyroid ultrasound studies by a single clinician: the impact of experience. Endocr Pract 2006;12:257-263.
74. Lumachi F, Ermani M, Basso S, et al. Localization of parathyroid tumours in the minimally invasive era: which technique should be chosen? Population-based analysis of 253 patients undergoing parathyroidectomy and factors affecting parathyroid gland detection. Endocr Relat Cancer 2001;8:63-69.

75. Van Dalen A, Smit CP, van Vroonhoven TJ, et al. Minimally invasive surgery for solitary parathyroid adenomas in patients with primary hyperparathyroidism: role of ultrasound with supplemental CT. Radiology 2001;220:631-639.

76. Haber RS, Kim CK, Inabnet WB. Ultrasonography for preoperative localization of enlarged parathyroid glands in primary hyperparathyroidism: comparison with ⁹⁹ᵐtechnetium sestamibi scintigraphy. Clin Endocrinol (Oxf) 2002;57:241-249.

77. Ruda JM, Hollenbeak CS, Stack Jr BC. A systematic review of the diagnosis and treatment of primary hyperparathyroidism from 1995 to 2003. Otolaryngol Head Neck Surg 2005;132:359-372.

78. Milas M, Stephen A, Berber E, et al. Ultrasonography for the endocrine surgeon: a valuable clinical tool that enhances diagnostic and therapeutic outcomes. Surgery 2005;138:1193-1200; discussion 1200-1201.

79. Solorzano CC, Carneiro-Pla DM, Irvin 3rd GL. Surgeon-performed ultrasonography as the initial and only localizing study in sporadic primary hyperparathyroidism. J Am Coll Surg 2006;202:18-24.

80. Van Husen R, Kim LT. Accuracy of surgeon-performed ultrasound in parathyroid localization. World J Surg 2004;28:1122-1126.

81. Solbiati L, Montali G, Croce F, et al. Parathyroid tumors detected by fine-needle aspiration biopsy under ultrasonic guidance. Radiology 1983;148:793-797.

82. Charboneau JW, Grant CS, James EM, et al. High-resolution ultrasound-guided percutaneous needle biopsy and intraoperative ultrasonography of a cervical parathyroid adenoma in a patient with persistent hyperparathyroidism. Mayo Clin Proc 1983;58:497-500.

83. Glenthoj A, Karstrup S. Parathyroid identification by ultrasonically guided aspiration cytology: is correct cytological identification possible? APMIS 1989;97:497-502.

84. Karstrup S, Glenthoj A, Hainau B, et al. Ultrasound-guided, histological, fine-needle biopsy from suspect parathyroid tumours: success-rate and reliability of histological diagnosis. Br J Radiol 1989;62:981-985.

85. Bergenfelz A, Forsberg L, Hederstrom E, Ahren B. Preoperative localization of enlarged parathyroid glands with ultrasonically guided fine-needle aspiration for parathyroid hormone assay. Acta Radiol 1991;32:403-405.

86. Sacks BA, Pallotta JA, Cole A, Hurwitz J. Diagnosis of parathyroid adenomas: efficacy of measuring parathormone levels in needle aspirates of cervical masses. AJR Am J Roentgenol 1994;163:1223-1226.

87. Reading CC, Charboneau JW, James EM, et al. Postoperative parathyroid high-frequency sonography: evaluation of persistent or recurrent hyperparathyroidism. AJR Am J Roentgenol 1985;144:399-402.

88. Gooding GA, Clark OH, Stark DD, et al. Parathyroid aspiration biopsy under ultrasound guidance in the postoperative hyperparathyroid patient. Radiology 1985;155:193-196.

89. MacFarlane MP, Fraker DL, Shawker TH, et al. Use of preoperative fine-needle aspiration in patients undergoing reoperation for primary hyperparathyroidism. Surgery 1994;116:959-964; discussion 964-965.

90. De Feo ML, Colagrande S, Biagini C, et al. Parathyroid glands: combination of ⁹⁹ᵐTc MIBI scintigraphy and ultrasound for demonstration of parathyroid glands and nodules. Radiology 2000;214:393-402.

91. Mullan BP. Nuclear medicine imaging of the parathyroid. Otolaryngol Clin North Am 2004;37:909-939, xi-xii.

92. Moka D, Voth E, Dietlein M, et al. Technetium 99m-MIBI-SPECT: a highly sensitive diagnostic tool for localization of parathyroid adenomas. Surgery 2000;128:29-35.

93. Civelek AC, Ozalp E, Donovan P, Udelsman R. Prospective evaluation of delayed technetium-99m sestamibi SPECT scintigraphy for preoperative localization of primary hyperparathyroidism. Surgery 2002;131:149-157.

94. Lorberboym M, Minski I, Macadziob S, et al. Incremental diagnostic value of preoperative ⁹⁹ᵐTc-MIBI SPECT in patients with a parathyroid adenoma. J Nucl Med 2003;44:904-908.

95. Jones JM, Russell CF, Ferguson WR, Laird JD. Pre-operative sestamibi-technetium subtraction scintigraphy in primary hyperparathyroidism: experience with 156 consecutive patients. Clin Radiol 2001;56:556-559.

96. Lumachi F, Zucchetta P, Marzola MC, et al. Advantages of combined technetium-99m-sestamibi scintigraphy and high-resolution ultrasonography in parathyroid localization: comparative study in 91 patients with primary hyperparathyroidism. Eur J Endocrinol 2000;143:755-760.

97. Kang YS, Rosen K, Clark OH, Higgins CB. Localization of abnormal parathyroid glands of the mediastinum with MR imaging. Radiology 1993;189:137-141.

98. McDermott VG, Fernandez RJ, Meakem 3rd TJ, et al. Preoperative MR imaging in hyperparathyroidism: results and factors affecting parathyroid detection. AJR Am J Roentgenol 1996;166:705-710.

99. Gotway MB, Higgins CB. MR imaging of the thyroid and parathyroid glands. Magn Reson Imaging Clin North Am 2000;8:163-182, ix.

100. Gotway MB, Leung JW, Gooding GA, et al. Hyperfunctioning parathyroid tissue: spectrum of appearances on noninvasive imaging. AJR Am J Roentgenol 2002;179:495-502.

101. Gotway MB, Reddy GP, Webb WR, et al. Comparison between MR imaging and ⁹⁹ᵐTc MIBI scintigraphy in the evaluation of recurrent of persistent hyperparathyroidism. Radiology 2001;218:783-790.

102. Reidel MA, Schilling T, Graf S, et al. Localization of hyperfunctioning parathyroid glands by selective venous sampling in reoperation for primary or secondary hyperparathyroidism. Surgery 2006;140:907-913; discussion 913.

103. Van Heerden JA, Grant CS. Surgical treatment of primary hyperparathyroidism: an institutional perspective. World J Surg 1991;15:688-692.

104. Russell CF, Laird JD, Ferguson WR. Scan-directed unilateral cervical exploration for parathyroid adenoma: a legitimate approach? World J Surg 1990;14:406-409.

105. Lorenz K, Nguyen-Thanh P, Dralle H. Unilateral open and minimally-invasive procedures for primary hyperparathyroidism: a review of selective approaches. Langenbeck Arch Surg 2000;385:106-117.

106. Udelsman R. Six hundred fifty-six consecutive explorations for primary hyperparathyroidism. Ann Surg 2002;235:665-670; discussion 670-672.

107. Palazzo FF, Delbridge LW. Minimal-access/minimally invasive parathyroidectomy for primary hyperparathyroidism. Surg Clin North Am 2004;84:717-734.

Intraoperative Sonography

108. Norton JA, Shawker TH, Jones BL, et al. Intraoperative ultrasound and reoperative parathyroid surgery: an initial evaluation. World J Surg 1986;10:631-639.

109. Kern KA, Shawker TH, Doppman JL, et al. The use of high-resolution ultrasound to locate parathyroid tumors during reoperations for primary hyperparathyroidism. World J Surg 1987;11:579-585.

Percutaneous Biopsy

110. Kendrick ML, Charboneau JW, Curlee KJ, et al. Risk of parathyromatosis after fine-needle aspiration. Am Surg 2001;67:290-293; discussion 293-294.

Ethanol Ablation

111. Charboneau JW, Hay ID, van Heerden JA. Persistent primary hyperparathyroidism: successful ultrasound-guided percutaneous ethanol ablation of an occult adenoma. Mayo Clin Proc 1988;63:913-917.

112. Karstrup S, Holm HH, Glenthoj A, Hegedus L. Nonsurgical treatment of primary hyperparathyroidism with sonographically guided percutaneous injection of ethanol: results in a selected series of patients. AJR Am J Roentgenol 1990;154:1087-1890.

113. Karstrup S, Hegedus L, Holm HH. Ultrasonically guided chemical parathyroidectomy in patients with primary hyperparathyroidism: a follow-up study. Clin Endocrinol (Oxf) 1993;38:523-530.

114. Harman CR, Grant CS, Hay ID, et al. Indications, technique, and efficacy of alcohol injection of enlarged parathyroid glands in patients with primary hyperparathyroidism. Surgery 1998;124:1011-1019; discussion 1019-1020.

115. Cercueil JP, Jacob D, Verges B, et al. Percutaneous ethanol injection into parathyroid adenomas: mid- and long-term results. Eur Radiol 1998;8:1565-1569.

116. Reading CC. Ultrasound-guided percutaneous ethanol ablation of solid and cystic masses of the liver, kidney, thyroid, and parathyroid. Ultrasound Q 1994;12:67-68.

117. Bennedbaek FN, Karstrup S, Hegedus L. Percutaneous ethanol injection therapy in the treatment of thyroid and parathyroid diseases. Eur J Endocrinol 1997;136:240-250.

118. Lewis BD, Charboneau JW, Reading CC. Ultrasound-guided biopsy and ablation in the neck. Ultrasound Q 2002;18:3-12.

119. Veldman MW, Reading CC, Farrell MA, et al. Percutaneous parathyroid ethanol ablation in patients with multiple endocrine neoplasia type 1. AJR Am J Roentgenol 2008;191:1740-1744.

120. Solbiati L, Giangrande A, De Pra L, et al. Percutaneous ethanol injection of parathyroid tumors under ultrasound guidance: treatment for secondary hyperparathyroidism. Radiology 1985;155:607-610.

121. Kakuta T, Fukagawa M, Fujisaki T, et al. Prognosis of parathyroid function after successful percutaneous ethanol injection therapy guided by color Doppler flow mapping in chronic dialysis patients. Am J Kidney Dis 1999;33:1091-1099.

122. Takeda S, Michigishi T, Takazakura E. Successful ultrasonically guided percutaneous ethanol injection for secondary hyperparathyroidism. Nephron 1992;62:100-103.

123. Kitaoka M, Fukagawa M, Ogata E, Kurokawa K. Reduction of functioning parathyroid cell mass by ethanol injection in chronic dialysis patients. Kidney Int 1994;46:1110-1117.

124. Giangrande A, Castiglioni A, Solbiati L, Allaria P. Ultrasound-guided percutaneous fine-needle ethanol injection into parathyroid glands in secondary hyperparathyroidism. Nephrol Dial Transplant 1992;7:412-421.

125. Takeda S, Michigishi T, Takazakura E. Ultrasonically guided percutaneous ethanol injection to parathyroid autografts for recurrent hyperparathyroidism. Nephron 1993;65:651-652.

126. Cintin C, Karstrup S, Ladefoged SD, Joffe P. Tertiary hyperparathyroidism treated by ultrasonically guided percutaneous fine-needle ethanol injection. Nephron 1994;68:217-220.

127. Fletcher S, Kanagasundaram NS, Rayner HC, et al. Assessment of ultrasound-guided percutaneous ethanol injection and parathyroidectomy in patients with tertiary hyperparathyroidism. Nephrol Dial Transplant 1998;13:3111-3117.

128. Bennedbaek FN, Karstrup S, Hegedus L. Ultrasound guided laser ablation of a parathyroid adenoma. Br J Radiol 2001;74:905-907.

129. Adda G, Scillitani A, Epaminonda P, et al. Ultrasound-guided laser thermal ablation for parathyroid adenomas: analysis of three cases with a three-year follow-up. Horm Res 2006;65:231-234.

CHAPTER 20

The Breast

A. Thomas Stavros

Chapter Outline

APPLICATIONS OF BREAST ULTRASOUND

There are three roles for sonography in breast imaging: (1) primary screening; (2) secondary screening (following mammography); and (3) diagnosis. Sonography currently does not have a proven role in primary breast cancer screening, but the use of sonography in **secondary screening** (after mammography, as an ancillary study), especially in women with dense breast tissue on mammography, has expanded since the last edition and continues to be investigated.

Kolb et al.,[1,2] Buchberger et al.,[3] and Kaplan[4] have all shown very promising results for sonography as a secondary breast cancer screening examination when used after primary screening mammography in patients who have dense breasts on mammography. In all four studies, sonography detected approximately three carcinomas that were missed by primary screening mammography per 1000 patients. The lesions were missed on mammography because they did not contain calcifications and were obscured by surrounding or superimposed dense tissues on the mammogram. Three per 1000 patients is the mammographic detection rate expected

for interval cancers in previously screened mammography patients and suggests that sonography might be very useful as a secondary screening tool in patients who have dense breasts on mammography. Additionally, the maximum diameter of, and the prognosis for, lesions detected only by ultrasound are similar to lesions found by mammographic screening, and the cost per cancer detected is similar to that of mammography.

The American College of Radiology Imaging Network whole-breast ultrasound screening trial (ACRIN 6666) was designed to assess the role of bilateral whole-breast screening ultrasound in a group of patients at increased risk for breast cancer and with dense breast tissue on mammography. Each patient had three scans over 3 years in addition to mammography. The results of the first prevalence scan show that ultrasound detected 4.2 cancers per 1000, more than were detected by mammography, but at a high cost in benign biopsies compared to mammography. Hand-held whole-breast ultrasound screening led to biopsies in 5% of patients, but only 8.8% of the biopsies were positive. I expect that results from the second and third studies in the ACRIN 6666 trial will be better than for the prevalence study. Screening is not the same as diagnosis, and it takes time, even for an expert at diagnostic ultrasound, to learn to screen using ultrasound. The rules of interpretation are different for screening and diagnosis. The pretest probability is much lower in a screening population than in a diagnostic population, so the posttest probability of cancer is also lower. Findings that might be viewed with suspicion in a patient with a palpable lump or suspicious mammographic abnormality must be ignored in a screening setting. It takes time to learn this. In my experience as an investigator in the ACRIN 6666 trial, the callback rate from screening ultrasound decreased with the second and third screenings, whereas the detection rate actually improved. We believe that with increasing experience, screening ultrasound data will improve.

Despite the results of many hand-held screening ultrasound studies, however, we do not believe that the United States has adequate physician/sonographer resources for hand-held ultrasound screening because of a chronic shortage of breast radiologists, mammographers, and breast sonographers. Thus, widespread screening will require improvement not only in callback and negative biopsy rates, but also in automation. This realization has led to renewed interest in automated approaches to breast ultrasound screening. Several dedicated automated breast ultrasound machines are being developed, but no data from automated scanners have yet been published. Most automated approaches utilize three-dimensional (3-D) ultrasound, but most experience is with hand-held two-dimensional (2-D) ultrasound, so much work remains on 3-D ultrasound. One automated device employs automated 2-D scans that are stored in video rather than a 3-D matrix. The unpublished data report a 7.2:1000 detection rate, double the mammography detection rate of 3.6:1000 in a prevalence screening. Thus, the increased detection rate over mammography is comparable to that of the hand-held screening studies previously mentioned. The automated scanner was better than hand-held ultrasound in the percentage of cancers detected less than 10 mm in maximum diameter, which was three times higher in the ultrasound-detected group than the mammography-detected group. Previous hand-held studies have found similar sizes in sonographically and mammographically detected cancers, but not better. Thus, the results of one study are encouraging for an automated approach to whole-breast ultrasound screening.

To date, breast ultrasound is not approved for screening, so there are no billing codes or reimbursement available. Most whole-breast examinations are extensions of targeted diagnostic scans. More data, particularly from automated scanners, and more years of experience will be necessary before codes and reimbursement for screening breast ultrasound are approved.

The approved and most widespread role for breast ultrasound is **diagnosis.** This is usually performed in a targeted fashion following mammography and clinical examination, to provide a more specific diagnosis than can be obtained from mammography or examination

alone. Palpable masses and mammographic abnormalities constitute the most common indications for targeted diagnostic breast ultrasound. Specific goals of targeted diagnostic sonography are to prevent biopsies and short-interval follow-up mammography of benign lesions, to guide interventions of all types, to give feedback that improves clinical and mammographic skills, and to find malignancies missed on mammography.

SONOGRAPHIC EQUIPMENT

Breast ultrasound requires high-frequency transducers that are optimized for near-field imaging. Transducers used for breast sonography are usually electronically focused linear arrays. All the organizations involved in accreditation of breast sonography—American Cancer Society (ACS), American College of Radiology (ACR), and American Institute of Ultrasound in Medicine (AIUM)—require a minimum transducer frequency of 7 megahertz (MHz). These linear arrays can be electronically focused along the long axis of the transducer, but not along the short axis (unless they are of 1.5-dimensional or matrix array transducers). Focusing in the short axis requires that a fixed acoustic lens be placed when the transducer is constructed. The focal length of the short-axis lens varies with transducer frequency and the application for which the transducer will typically be used, being deeper for lower frequencies and shallower for higher frequencies. Transducers of 5 MHz typically are used for peripheral vascular ultrasound, not near-field imaging, and are focused too deeply (3.5-4.0 cm, usually in chest wall) for breast ultrasound. When the focal length of the transducer is in the chest wall, small lesions in the middle and near portions of the breast may be subject to volume averaging. **Volume averaging** can alter the echogenicity so much that cystic lesions falsely appear solid and hypoechoic solid lesions become isoechoic and inconspicuous. The 7.5 to 12–MHz transducers that are usually employed in breast ultrasound are focused at 1.5 to 2.0 cm of depth, an ideal focal length for breast ultrasound, minimizing volume averaging (Fig. 20-1). However, even transducers that are focused in the midbreast in the short axis can result in volume averaging for small, superficially located lesions, unless a thin, acoustic standoff pad or a standoff of gel is used (Fig. 20-2).

A good general rule for breast ultrasound is that the lesions that appear to be just under the skin on the mammogram, or that are palpable and "pea sized" or smaller, are those that are most prone to volume averaging and that should routinely be imaged through an **acoustic standoff.** In some patients, simply scanning with lighter compression can alter the position of the short-axis focal zone enough to obviate the need for a standoff. A 1.5-dimensional array transducer can be focused electronically in the short axis as well as in the long axis and

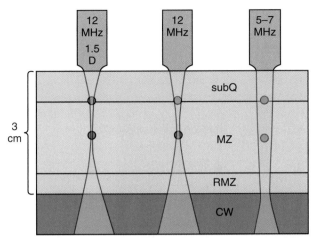

FIGURE 20-1. Short-axis views of three transducers used for breast ultrasound. *Left,* 12-MHz 1.5-D (1.5-dimensional, or matrix, array) transducer; *middle,* 12-MHz 1-D (one-dimensional array) transducer; *right,* 5-MHz to 7-MHz 1-D array transducer. Transducers that are **1-D array** have an acoustic lens in the short axis of the probe that has a fixed focal length, determined by the most frequent use of the transducer. **Linear array** transducers that have frequencies in the 5 to 7–MHz range *(right)* are designed for vascular imaging, not breast imaging. The fixed, short-axis focal depth is about 3 to 4 cm, the depth of carotid and femoral vessels in most patients. These transducers are focused too deep for breast ultrasound. Small lesions at 1.5 cm, in the center of the mammary zone in most patients, will frequently be subject to volume averaging with surrounding tissues. This can result in mischaracterization and false negatives. Small cysts can falsely appear solid, and small, subtle, hypoechoic solid nodules can falsely appear isoechoic and indistinguishable from surrounding tissues. Lesions closer to the skin are even more subject to volume averaging, mischaracterization, and false negatives. The typical 12-MHz 1-D array transducer *(middle)* has a short-axis focal length of 1.5 to 2.0 cm, ideal for breast ultrasound. A small lesion at 1.5 cm of depth will be wider than the ultrasound beam, will not be subject to volume averaging, and can accurately be detected and characterized. However, even with 12-MHz 1-D array transducers, lesions in the near field, less than 10 mm from the skin, can be subject to volume averaging because the beam has not yet become fully focused. An acoustic standoff of gel or a standoff pad may be necessary in such cases. In general, these are skin lesions or lesions that are palpable and pea-sized or smaller or lesions that appear to be just under the skin on mammography. The 12-MHz matrix array transducers *(left)* have adjustable short-axis focal zones. The beam is focused more tightly, the beam is narrower, and the beam becomes tightly focused at a shallower depth. Even near-field lesions can be scanned without volume averaging and without using an acoustic standoff, and both characterization and detection are better than with 1-D array transducers. *MZ,* Mammary zone; *RMZ,* retromammary zone; *CW,* chest wall; *subQ,* subcutaneous.

can reduce, but not eliminate, difficulties with near-field volume averaging (see Fig. 20-1, *left* transducer). Choosing the correct transducer is important, but equally important is controlling the depth of the **focal zone** position. Current ultrasound machines focus the transducer continuously at all depths on receiving the beam. However, the user must still choose the depth at which the machine focuses the transmitted ultrasound beam

(transmit focal zone). This is shown by "carrots" of various shapes. These should be placed at or just deep to the depth of any lesion being characterized. In survey mode, when looking for a lesion at an unknown depth, multiple focal zones are usually best. Mispositioned focal zones can lead to severe volume averaging and mischaracterization of even midsized lesions, particularly if the focal zones are positioned much too deeply (Fig. 20-3).

Split-screen imaging capability is invaluable in breast imaging. Split-screen images are most frequently used to compare mirror-image locations in the right and left breasts to document that **asymmetrical fibroglandular tissue** causes either a mammographic asymmetry or a palpable lump (Fig. 20-4). Split-screen imaging can also be used to document dynamic events, such as compressibility and mobility, on a single freeze-frame image and in simultaneous mode, to show both the gray-scale image on one side and the color or power Doppler image on the other.

Multiple lesions and lesions larger than the width of the transducer require special techniques for demonstration. Of several methods for demonstrating larger fields of view, one can use combined split-screen images, virtual convex imaging, or extended–field of view imaging (Fig. 20-5). A picture archiving and communication system (PACS) can be useful not only for filmless interpretation and archiving images, but also for digitally storing video loops, the most efficient and esthetically pleasing method of documenting dynamic events.

BREAST ANATOMY AND PHYSIOLOGY

The breast is a modified sweat gland that is composed of 15 to 20 lobes that are not well delineated from each other, that overlap, and that vary greatly in size and distribution. Each lobe consists of parenchymal elements (lobar duct, smaller branch ducts, and lobules) and supporting stromal tissues (compact interlobular stromal fibrous tissue, loose periductal and intralobular stromal fibrous tissue, and fat). The functional unit of the breast is the **terminal ductolobular unit** (TDLU), which consists of a lobule and its extralobular terminal duct. Each lobule consists of the intralobular segment of the terminal duct, ductules, and loose intralobular stromal fibrous tissue. TDLUs are important because they are the site of origin of most breast pathology and of **aberrations of normal development and involution** (ANDIs).

Most breast carcinomas are thought to arise in the terminal duct near the junction of the intralobular and extralobular segments. Lobar ducts give rise to much less pathology than do TDLUs—mainly large **duct papillomas** and the **duct ectasia–periductal mastitis complex.** However, most **invasive ductal carcinomas** have ductal carcinoma in situ components that can use the ductal system as conduits for growth into other parts

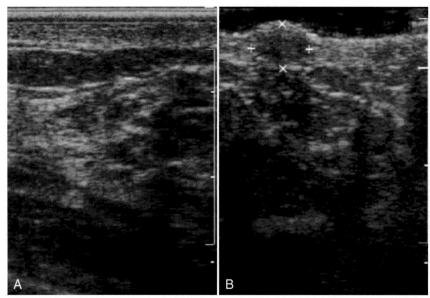

FIGURE 20-2. Value of standoff pad. Even with adequate high frequency 1-D array transducers that have appropriate short-axis acoustic lens focal lengths of 1.5 cm an acoustic standoff may be necessary when the lesion is very superficial in location. **A,** Sebaceous cyst presented as BB-sized palpable lump. It is not visible without an acoustic standoff. **B,** With a thick layer of acoustic gel as a standoff, the lesion can be clearly seen to originate from the skin.

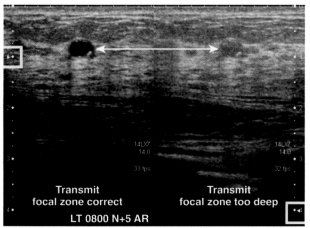

FIGURE 20-3. Importance of proper positioning of long-axis transmission focal zones. This split-screen image shows a small, benign cyst with milk of calcium. The left image was obtained with the transmit focal zone appropriately placed at the level of the cyst. There is no volume averaging, and the cyst is accurately characterized. The image on the right was obtained with the focal zone intentionally positioned far too deeply. Because the ultrasound beam is not appropriately focused in its long axis, on beam transmission at the depth of the cyst, the cyst is subject to volume averaging with surrounding tissues, which falsely makes it appear to be solid and isoechoic.

of the breast. Each segmental duct has several rows of TDLUs arising from it. Anterior TDLUs tend to have long extralobular terminal ducts, whereas posterior TDLUs tend to have shorter extralobular terminal ducts. Some TDLUs lie at the distal end of the ductal system

and are horizontally oriented. Anterior TDLUs are more numerous than posterior and terminal TDLUs, and over time, the posterior TDLUs tend to regress, leaving a progressively larger percentage of anterior TDLUs. Because anterior TDLUs greatly outnumber posterior TDLUs, most breast pathology that arises from TDLUs occurs in the superficial half of the mammary zone, just deep to the anterior mammary fascia.

The breast can be divided into three zones, from superficial to deep (Fig. 20-6). The most superficial zone is the **premammary zone,** or **subcutaneous zone,** which lies between the skin and the anterior mammary fascia. The premammary zone is really part of the integument, and processes that arise primarily within the premammary zone are usually not true breast lesions. Rather, these are lesions of the skin and/or subcutaneous tissues that are identical to those arising from skin and subcutaneous tissues covering any other part of the body (e.g., lipomas, sebaceous cysts). The **mammary zone** is the middle zone and lies between the anterior mammary fascia and the posterior mammary fascia. It contains the lobar ducts, their branches, most of the TDLUs, and most of the fibrous stromal elements of the breast. The deepest of the zones is the **retromammary zone.** It mainly contains fat, blood vessels, and lymphatics and is usually much less apparent on sonograms than on mammograms because sonographic compression flattens the retromammary zone against the chest wall. This differs greatly from mammography, where mammographic compression pulls the retromammary fat away from the

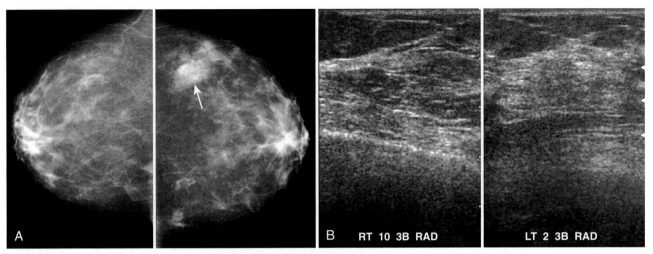

FIGURE 20-4. Value of split-screen mirror ultrasound image. A, Mammography of both breasts showed a focal asymmetrical density in the left breast, upper outer quadrant on the craniocaudal (CC) view *(arrow)*. **B,** Split-screen mirror-image ultrasound images show focal fibrous tissue in the upper outer quadrant of the left breast that is markedly asymmetrical with the thickness of tissue in the mirror-image upper outer quadrant location of the right breast. This collection of asymmetrical fibrous tissue is the cause of the mammographic asymmetry.

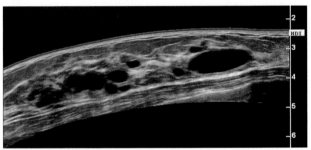

FIGURE 20-5. Extended–field of view (FOV) images. Extended-FOV images can be helpful in demonstrating very large lesions, multifocal and multicentric malignant lesions, lymph node levels, implant integrity, or as in this case, extensive fibrocystic change with numerous cysts of variable size within the breast.

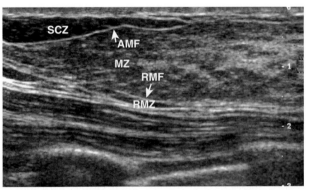

FIGURE 20-6. Three zones of the breast. The premammary or subcutaneous zone *(scz)*, mammary zone *(mz)*, and retromammary zone *(rmz)*. The mammary zone is where most of the ducts and lobules of the breast that give rise to breast pathology lie. The mammary zone is enveloped in thick, tough fascia. Anteriorly it is delineated from the subcutaneous fat by the premammary or anterior mammary fascia *(amf)* and posteriorly from the retromammary fat by the posterior or retromammary fascia *(rmf)*. The anterior mammary fascia is continuous with Cooper's ligaments, with each ligament being formed by two apposed layers of anterior mammary fascia. The retromammary zone is compressed during real-time sonography in the recumbent position and is relatively small and inapparent in comparison to its appearance on mammography.

chest wall and expands it in the anteroposterior (AP) direction. Because most breast pathology arises from TDLUs and, to a lesser extent, from the mammary ducts, and because most of the ducts and lobules lie within the mammary zone, most true breast pathology arises from the mammary zone. Although lesions that arise within the premammary or retromammary zone are usually skin lesions, true breast lesions that arise within the mammary zone can secondarily involve the premammary and retromammary tissues.

The **mammary fascia** that envelops the mammary zone is tough and is relatively more resistant to invasive malignancy than are loose, stromal fibrous tissues. The anterior mammary fascia is continuous with **Cooper's ligaments**. At the point where it is continuous with a ligament, the anterior mammary fascia continues superficially obliquely through the subcutaneous fat, attaches

to superficial fascia, and then courses back down through the subcutaneous fat, where it continues on as anterior mammary fascia. Each Cooper's ligament is composed of two closely applied layers of anterior mammary fascia with a potential space inferiorly, where the two layers separate and course away from each other as anterior mammary fasciae (Fig. 20-7). This affects the sonographic appearance of invasive malignancies, as discussed later.

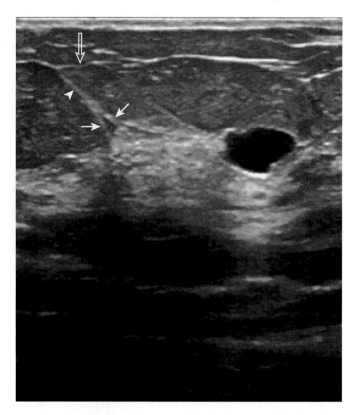

FIGURE 20-7. Mammary fasciae and Cooper's ligaments. Two layers of anterior mammary fascia *(arrows)* form the bases of a Cooper's ligament *(white arrowhead)*, which inserts into superficial fascia *(open arrow)*. Invasive malignancies often develop angles as they invade the base of Cooper's ligaments.

The normal anatomic structures of the breast span a spectrum of echogenicities, from midlevel gray to intensely hyperechoic. **Hyperechoic** normal structures include compact interlobular stromal fibrous tissue, anterior and posterior mammary fasciae, Cooper's ligaments, and skin. Duct walls, when visible, also appear hyperechoic. Normal structures that have midlevel echogenicity **(isoechoic)** include fat, epithelial tissues in ducts and lobules, and loose, intralobular and periductal, stromal fibrous tissue. **Water density tissue** on mammography corresponds to a variety of different normal tissues that can be shown sonographically. Dense interlobular stromal fibrous tissue, loose periductal or intralobular stromal fibrous tissue, and epithelial elements in ducts and lobules all appear to be of equal density mammographically. **Mammographically dense tissue** can correspond to purely hyperechoic, purely isoechoic, or mixed hyperechoic and isoechoic tissues on sonography (Fig. 20-8). Most contain mixtures of fibrous and glandular elements interspersed with variable amounts of fat (Fig. 20-9). Over time, atrophy tends to occur more rapidly in the areas of the mammary zone that lie between Cooper's ligaments, leaving progressively more of the residual fibroglandular elements within these ligaments (Fig. 20-10).

Normal mammary ducts that are not ectatic can appear in two ways sonographically. A mammary duct can appear purely isoechoic when the centrally located hyperechoic duct wall cannot be visualized because

of poor angle of incidence or suboptimal transducer resolution—when only the loose periductal stromal fibrous tissue is visible. A mammary duct can also be shown as a central, bright echo surrounded by isoechoic loose stromal fibrous tissue when the apposed walls of the central duct can be optimally demonstrated (Fig. 20-11, *A*). It is common for a single duct to have both sonographic appearances, depending on the angle of incidence with the duct walls. Variable degrees of **ductal ectasia** become increasingly common with age, particularly within the lactiferous sinus portion of the lobar duct in the subareolar region. In **ectatic ducts,** anechoic or hypoechoic fluid separates the two duct walls and compresses the loose periductal stromal tissues to variable degrees (Fig. 20-11, *B* and *C*). Duct ectasia occurs in up to 50% of women over age 50 and usually is asymptomatic. In certain patients, however, ductal ectasia may be associated with nipple discharge or may lead to periductal mastitis and its acute and chronic complications.

The ducts within the nipple and immediate subareolar regions are poorly seen when scanned from straight anteriorly because they course almost parallel to the beam in those locations. However, special maneuvers designed to improve the angle of incidence enable adequate demonstration of the entire mammary duct throughout the subareolar region, even within the nipple when necessary. These maneuvers include the **peripheral compression technique, two-handed compression**

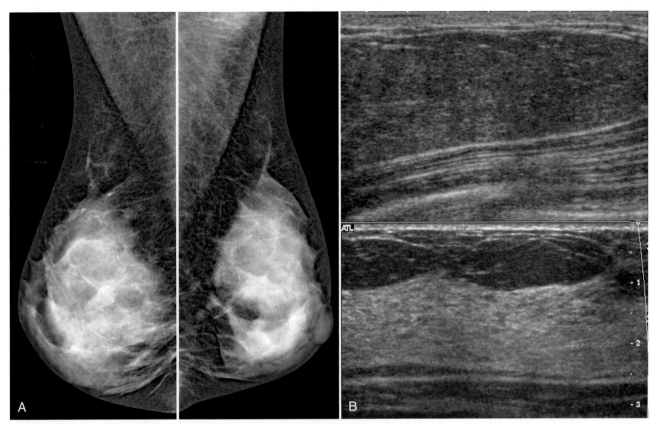

FIGURE 20-8. Dense breast tissue: radiographic-sonographic correlation. Radiographically dense (water density) tissue on mammograms (**A**) can correspond to two different types of tissue on sonography: **B,** almost-isoechoic glandular tissue, and **C,** intensely hyperechoic interlobular stromal fibrous tissue.

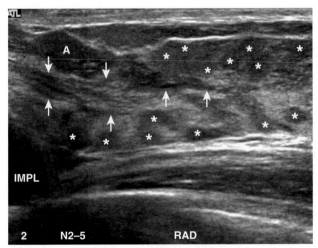

FIGURE 20-9. Water density breast tissue. Most water density tissue on mammography is not pure fibrous or glandular tissue, but a mixture of hyperechoic interlobular stromal fibrous tissue and isoechoic glandular or loose periductal and intralobular stromal tissue. Note that the lobar duct is mildly ectatic (*arrows*). The round or taller-than-wide isoechoic elements (*asterisk*) within the peripheral segments of the mammary zone represent epithelial and loose stromal tissues within terminal ductolobular units (TDLUs). Note that TDLUs are more numerous and prominent anteriorly than they are posteriorly.

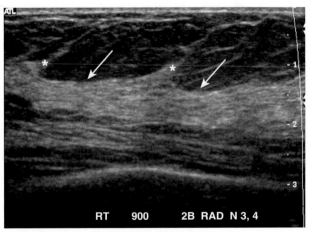

FIGURE 20-10. Breast atrophy. With advancing age, and particularly after full-term pregnancy and breastfeeding, the fibroglandular elements of the breast regress more rapidly in the areas of the mammary zone (*arrows*) that lie between Cooper's ligaments than in the area within the ligaments. This eventually can leave much or all of the residual breast tissue entrapped within Cooper's ligaments (*asterisk*).

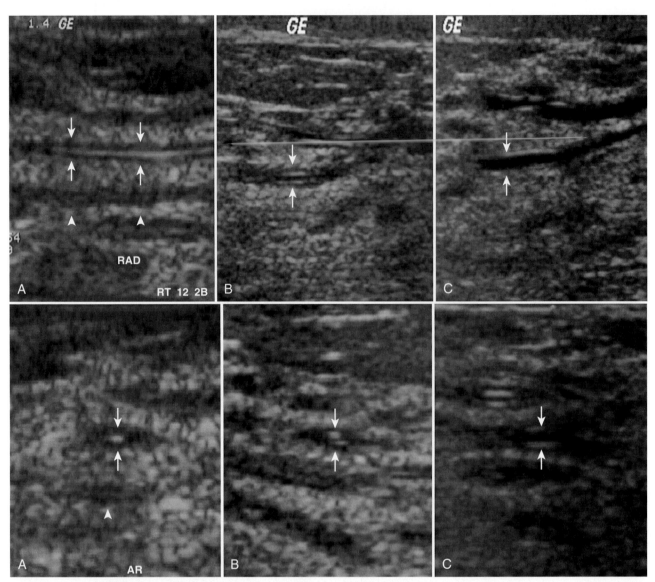

FIGURE 20-11. Mammary duct: spectrum of normal appearances. A, With high spatial resolution, 90-degree angle of incidence, and perfect centering, the duct appears to be composed of a central echogenic line *(arrows)* that represents the apposed walls of the collapsed mammary duct. The surrounding isoechoic tissue represents loose periductal stromal tissue. Unfortunately, only a minority of the ducts seen have this trilaminar appearance in the long axis and targetoid appearance in the short axis. Ducts that are slightly out of focus, coursing at an angle, or not perfectly centered within the beam have a different appearance. The deeper duct *(arrowheads)* is too deep for the short-axis focal length of the transducer. The central echo that represents the apposed walls of the collapsed duct is not seen. Only the isoechoic loose periductal stromal tissue can be identified. **B,** This mildly ectatic duct *(arrows)* is shown in long axis *(upper image)* and short axis *(lower image)*. The duct is now represented by two hyperechoic lines that represent the anterior and posterior walls of the duct separated by secretions within the duct lumen. **C,** This severely ectatic duct *(arrows)* is shown in long axis *(upper image)* and short axis *(lower image)*. As the degree of ductal ectasia increases, the walls of the duct become more separated, and the loose periductal stromal tissue becomes more compressed and less apparent. In severe ductal ectasia the periductal loose stromal tissue may no longer be visible.

technique, and **rolled nipple technique.** These maneuvers are most useful when evaluating patients with nipple discharge (Fig. 20-12) and in assessing malignant nodules for extensive intraductal involvement growing within the duct toward the nipple. The two-handed compression technique is also useful in assessing gynecomastia.

Individual TDLUs may be sonographically visible—under ideal conditions—as small isoechoic structures. Normal TDLUs are about 2 mm in diameter but may

be as large as 5 mm in patients with **fibrocystic change, adenosis,** or other ANDIs (Fig. 20-13). In patients who are pregnant or lactating and in patients with adenosis, not only are TDLUs enlarged, but they are also increased in number. In certain cases, TDLUs become large and numerous enough to form continuous sheets of isoechoic tissue. The variable prominence of TDLUs creates a continuous spectrum in the appearance of breast tissue from TDLUs that are not visible to breasts that appear

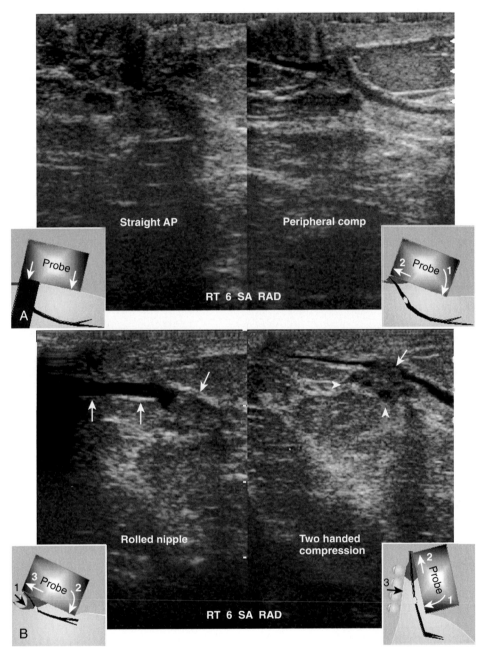

FIGURE 20-12. Maneuvers for demonstrating subareolar and intranipple mammary ducts. A, *Left image,* The subareolar ducts are difficult to assess from a straight anterior approach because shadowing arises from the nipple and areola and the tissue planes of the nipple are parallel to the ultrasound beam. *Right image,* **Peripheral compression technique**. With vigorous compression on the peripheral end of the transducer and sliding it over the nipple to push the nipple to the side, shadowing can be minimized, and the angle of incidence of the beam with the subareolar ducts can be improved. Lesions that lie in the immediate subareolar region *(arrow)* can often be demonstrated. **B,** *Left image,* **Rolled nipple technique** is the best way to demonstrate the ducts within the nipple and if a lesion extends into the nipple from the subareolar ducts. **B,** *Right image,* **Two-handed compression technique** further improves the angle of incidence with the subareolar ducts and helps assess the compressibility of the ducts. This can help to distinguish echogenic, inspissated secretions from intraductal papillary lesions and determine whether the lesion *(arrows)* has penetrated through the duct wall *(arrowheads)*. The rolled nipple technique shows that this malignant intraductal papillary lesion does not extend into the intranipple segment of the duct, but the two-handed compression maneuver shows that it has invaded through the posterior duct wall and is forming angles within the periductal tissues.

to be totally isoechoic (Fig. 20-14). This most often occurs anteriorly, where lobules are most numerous, but in certain cases can fill and distend the entire mammary zone. One of the most valuable features of high-frequency coded **harmonic imaging** is that it tends to make pathologic solid nodules appear relatively more hypoechoic and conspicuous in a background of isoechoic tissues, reducing the chance that such a nodule will not be detected and distinguished from normal lobules.

Lymphatic drainage from most of the breast is from deep to superficial, toward the subdermal lymphatic network, then to the periareolar plexus (Sappey's plexus),

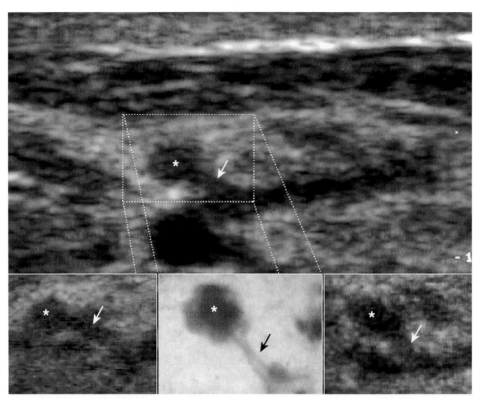

FIGURE 20-13. Terminal ductolobular units (TDLUs). The TDLU includes the extralobular terminal duct and the lobule, which contains the intralobular terminal duct, ductules, and intralobular isoechoic loose stromal tissue. TDLUs present as an isoechoic structure similar to a tennis racket; the head of the racket *(asterisk)* represents the lobule, and the handle and neck of the racket *(arrows)* represent the extralobular terminal duct. Bottom center image is 3-D histology. *(Courtesy Hanne M. Jensen, MD.)*

and finally on to the axilla. Some of the deep portions of the breast, particularly medially, preferentially drain along the chest wall to the internal mammary lymph nodes. Most drainage of the breast is to the axillary lymph nodes. Most lymphatic metastases from the breast are to the axilla, with a minority occurring in the internal mammary lymph nodes. The three levels of axillary lymph nodes are determined by their location relative to the pectoralis minor muscle. Lymph nodes that lie peripheral to the inferolateral edge of the pectoralis minor are **level 1** lymph nodes; nodes that lie posterior to the pectoralis minor muscle are **level 2** lymph nodes; and nodes that lie proximal to the superomedial border of the pectoralis minor muscle are **level 3** lymph nodes or **infraclavicular nodes.** Lymphatic drainage to the axilla usually passes through level 1, then level 2, and finally to level 3 lymph nodes (Fig. 20-15). From level 3 nodes, metastases may progress to internal jugular or supraclavicular lymph nodes. **Rotter nodes** lie between the pectoralis major and pectoralis minor muscles. It is important to recognize level 2 and 3 lymph nodes and Rotter lymph node metastases, because unrecognized and untreated metastases to these lymph nodes are a frequent source of so-called chest wall recurrences.

Internal mammary nodes lie in a chain parallel to the internal mammary artery and veins along the deep side of the chest wall, just lateral to the edges of the sternum. Metastases most often involve internal mammary lymph nodes in the second and third interspaces. Using color Doppler sonography to identify the internal mammary vessels can be helpful in finding abnormal internal mammary lymph nodes. Normal internal mammary lymph nodes can be identified under ideal circumstances, but not in all patients.

A significant percentage of patients have lymph nodes that lie within the breast, **intramammary lymph nodes.** These can lie anywhere within the breast but are most common in the axillary segment just below the axilla. They usually lie within a centimeter of the posterior mammary artery, a branch of the axillary artery that extends from the axilla toward the nipple. Intramammary lymph nodes can also be found occasionally in the medial edge of the breast superficial to the internal mammary lymph nodes. These medial lymph nodes are seen much less frequently on mammography than on sonography because mammographic compression can seldom pull them far enough away from the chest wall to be mammographically visible. Medial intramammary lymph nodes can be difficult to demonstrate sonographically without the use of an acoustic standoff because of their superficial location just beneath the skin.

Breast cancer metastases can involve the **supraclavicular lymph nodes,** but these nodes are positive only

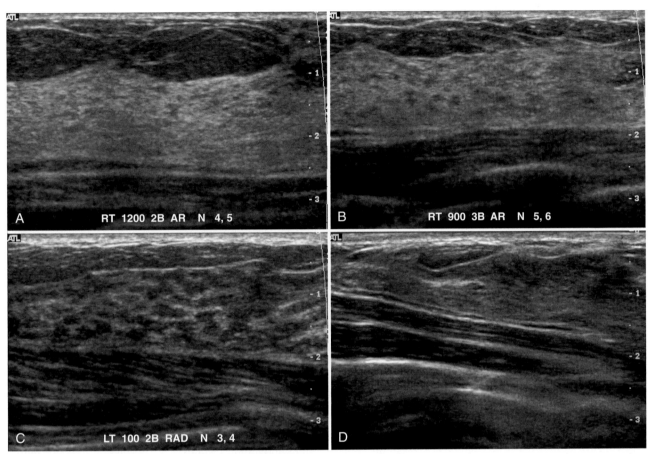

FIGURE 20-14. Variable prominence of TDLUs. A, Only a few scattered TDLUs may be visible. **B,** As TDLUs become larger and more numerous in adenosis and adenosis of pregnancy, they may almost touch each other. Because anterior TDLUs are more numerous than posterior TDLUs, these changes tend to affect the superficial aspect of the mammary zone earlier and to a greater extent than they affect its deep aspect. **C,** When lobular enlargement is pronounced, the entire superficial aspect of the mammary zone may appear isoechoic with the deep half still being hyperechoic. **D,** When lobular prominence is most pronounced, both superficial and deep aspects of the mammary zone may appear almost homogeneously isoechoic. Prominent TDLUs create an "in-between" sensitivity state for sonography that lies between that of purely hyperechoic and purely isoechoic breasts.

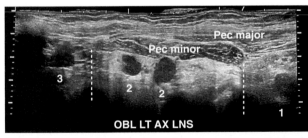

FIGURE 20-15. Pectoralis minor muscle and levels of axillary lymph nodes. Extended-FOV sonogram shows metastases to all three axillary lymph node levels on the left. The level of axillary lymph nodes is determined by the pectoralis minor muscle. Lymph nodes that lie inferior and lateral to the inferolateral edge of the pectoralis minor muscle are level 1 nodes; those that lie deep to the pectoralis minor muscle are level 2 lymph nodes; and those that lie superior and medial to the superomedial edge of the pectoralis minor muscles are level 3 (infraclavicular) lymph nodes.

when lymph node metastases are extensive. Metastases must involve levels 1, 2, and 3 axillary lymph nodes or internal mammary and internal jugular lymph nodes before reaching the supraclavicular nodes.

The first lymph node to which lymphatic drainage flows and the first node involved by metastases has been termed the **sentinel lymph node.** The location of the sentinel node varies, depending on the location of the primary tumor within the breast. The sentinel lymph node is usually a level 1 axillary lymph node, but in certain cases, it may be an intramammary node or even a level 2 node. Occasionally, the sentinel node may be an internal mammary node.

SONOGRAPHIC TECHNIQUE

Annotation

The location of a scan plane in the breast or the location of a lesion in the breast should be annotated or demonstrated compliant with ACR ultrasound BIRADS lexicon. The side (left and right), clock face position, distance from the nipple in centimeters, and transducer orientation must be recorded. Painting centimeter markers on the transducer can facilitate recording the distance from the nipple in centimeters, but the distance is usually estimated from the known lengths of linear high-frequency transducers, either 38 mm or 50 mm. The transducer orientation can be longitudinal, transverse, radial, or **antiradial,** which is orthogonal to the radial plane. The advantage of radial imaging is that the central ducts are radially oriented with respect to the nipple. Scanning in a plane that lies radial to the duct enables visualization of **ductal carcinoma in situ** (DCIS) components of lesions growing within the ductal system of the breast.

Identifying intraductal components of tumor can reduce the chances of mischaracterizing a malignant solid nodule as benign or "probably benign" and also facilitates demonstrating the true extent of DCIS components of mixed invasive and intraductal malignant lesions. The farther from the nipple a lesion lies, the less likely the duct will course in a plane that is truly radial with respect to the nipple because of tortuosity of the duct, or because the duct of interest is a branch duct that is not oriented perfectly radial. The sonographer should think of internal radial *planes* versus the external true radial plane with respect to the nipple. The internal radial plane is parallel to the long axis of the ducts in the region of interest. In particular, when assessing solid nodules, we want to know if the lesion is growing into the ducts that surround it. This can be best accomplished when the scan plane is parallel to the long axis of the ducts in the region of the solid nodule.

In addition to the ACR BIRADS lexicon mandates, we elect to record the depth of a lesion in addition to the parameters previously discussed. We use three zones: **A** for the superficial third, **B** for the middle third, and **C** for the deep third of the breast. Thus, a lesion at the 12 o'clock position of the right breast that lies 2 cm from the nipple and middle third in depth, when scanned radially would be annotated as "R 12 N2 RAD." This method of annotation is cryptic and reproducible. An icon of the right or left breast with a linear marker that demonstrates the position and orientation of the transducer is an acceptable alternative for annotation of scan location, and most ultrasound equipment manufacturers provide breast icons for this.

Documentation of Lesions

All lesions should be scanned in their entirety in two orthogonal planes to assess the surface and internal characteristics as well as shape. Hard-copy or soft-copy images should be obtained in a minimum of two orthogonal planes. These orthogonal planes could be longitudinal and transverse, but we prefer radial and antiradial

planes. Each image plane should be recorded with and without calipers. It is important to document the maximum diameter of the lesion, an important prognostic indicator. If the maximum diameter does not lie in one of the standard longitudinal, transverse, radial, or antiradial planes, an additional oblique view parallel to the long axis of the lesion should be obtained with and without calipers. Films without calipers are especially important in small lesions, where the calipers may interfere with assessment of surface characteristics.

BIRADS Risk Categories

The official **Breast Imaging Reporting and Data System (BIRADS)** ultrasound lexicon has been developed by the ACR to standardize reporting and data. We believe in using BIRADS risk categories for the final assessment of every sonogram. Because most sonograms are targeted to clinical or mammographic abnormalities that require the preceding mammogram to be characterized as "BIRADS 0" (incomplete assessment), any final assessment in a patient who has undergone diagnostic sonography will be based on combined ultrasound and mammography findings. BIRADS categories are also important to assess and improve sonographic performance. If each sonographic category carries the same risk as the corresponding mammographic BIRADS category, the rules for managing sonographic lesions may be identical to the mammographic rules for the same category. Separate rules do not need to be developed for sonography. We do not use the BIRADS 0 category after sonography except in the rare cases in which sonography is performed before mammography. BIRADS categories are **0,** incomplete assessment, needs additional evaluation; **1,** normal; **2,** benign; **3,** probably benign; **4,** suspicious; **5,** malignant; and **6,** biopsy-proven malignancy. The expected risks of malignancy for categories 1 to 5 are: BIRADS 1 and 2, 0%; BIRADS 3, 2% or less; BIRADS 4, greater than 2% and less than 95%; and BIRADS 5, 95% or greater. Because the BIRADS 4 category has such a wide range of risk (>2% to <95%), optional subcategories have been developed: 4a, 4b, and 4c.

The sonographic **BIRADS 1** category corresponds to sonographically normal tissues that cause mammographic or clinical abnormalities. The sonographic **BIRADS 2** category corresponds to benign entities and includes intramammary lymph nodes, ectatic ducts, all simple and many complicated cysts, and definitively benign solid nodules, such as lipomas and hamartomas. The **BIRADS 3** category corresponds to "probably benign" lesions that have a 2% or less risk of malignancy and includes some complicated and complex cysts, small intraductal papillomas, and a subset of fibroadenomas. We divide the large ACR **BIRADS 4** category that is termed "suspicious" into three subcategories. Rules for subdividing BIRADS 4 into the optional 4a, 4b, and 4c subcategories have not been developed. The **BIRADS 4a** category is "mildly suspicious" and carries a greater than 2% to 10% risk of malignancy. **BIRADS 4b** is "moderately suspicious" and carries a risk of greater than 10% to 50%. The **BIRADS 4c** risk of malignancy is greater than 50% to less than 95%. The **BIRADS 5** category is termed "malignant" and indicates a 95% or greater risk of malignancy.

The management rules for each category have already been developed for mammography and are quite simple. BIRADS 1 and 2 characterizations enable the patient to return to routine screening follow-up. BIRADS 3 characterization presents the patient with three choices: surgical biopsy, image-guided needle biopsy, or short-interval sonographic follow-up. Although the subdivision of the BIRADS 4 category is subjective and not defined by rules, the rules for *management* of the BIRADS 4 categories are well established. Lesions with BIRADS 4a, 4b, 4c, and 5 classifications all require biopsy. After a BIRADS category 1 sonogram, patients usually return to routine screening. After a BIRADS 2 category sonogram, management depends on the indication for the study. Patients with palpable abnormalities and a BIRADS 2 breast ultrasound undergo a clinical follow-up with palpation in 6 weeks and routine screening, unless there are clinical indications for further evaluation. Patients with a mammographic abnormality and a BIRADS 2 breast ultrasound exam usually return to routine mammographic screening. Patients with a BIRADS 3 breast ultrasound are offered the option of short-interval follow-up in 6 months or biopsy.

Diagnostic examinations in addition to mammography and ultrasound will be most helpful in patients with BIRADS 4a and perhaps a few BIRADS 4b lesions. Patients with BIRADS 2 and 3 lesions generally do not require additional imaging. Patients with BIRADS 4b, 4c, and 5 lesions will almost always proceed straight to biopsy, regardless of other imaging results.

Special Breast Techniques

Breast sonographic evaluation depends heavily on special **dynamic** and **positional** maneuvers performed during the examination. Dynamic maneuvers include **varying compression** to assess compressibility and mobility. Lesions that are more than 30% compressible are fatty with a high degree of certainty—either a normal fat lobule or a benign lipoma. Superficial venous thrombosis (Mondor's disease) requires incompressibility and lack of flow on Doppler ultrasound for diagnosis. **Ballottement** (alternating compression and compression release) can be helpful to demonstrate mobility of echoes with ectatic ducts or complex cysts. Varying compression can also eradicate artifactual shadowing from critical angle shadowing off steeply oblique tissue planes. **Heeling and toeing of the transducer** can minimize critical angle shadowing arising from Cooper's ligaments and better demonstrate the thin, echogenic capsule on the ends of

solid nodules, an important sign of a noninvasive lesion margin. Heeling and toeing can also improve the angle of incidence with duct walls, allowing better demonstration of ductal anatomy and pathology, especially in the subareolar portions of the ducts. **Doppler ultrasound assessment** of the breast depends greatly on using as little compression pressure as possible. Blood flow in a breast lesion can easily be decreased or even completely ablated if compression is too vigorous.

Positional changes are important in assessment of complex cysts. **Fluid-debris levels, milk of calcium, and fat-fluid levels** can all be shown to change sonographically between supine and upright or lateral decubitus positions. Some palpable abnormalities are clinically evident only in the upright position and therefore require that the scan be performed in the upright position. Even routine whole-breast scanning may require changing the position of the patient during the examination. Contralateral posterior oblique positions are better for evaluating the lateral half of the breast, whereas supine positioning is better for the medial half of the breast.

MAIN INDICATIONS

Most diagnostic breast ultrasound is performed in a targeted fashion to evaluate a particular palpable or mammographic abnormality.

Palpable Lumps

Sonography is very useful in evaluating palpable lumps, especially when there is dense tissue in the area of the palpable lump on mammography. Lesions that do not contain calcifications may be obscured by surrounding dense tissues on mammography. Sonography has much less to contribute to cases with only fatty density in the area of the palpable lump on mammography. It is unlikely that the mammogram missed anything significant, and the palpable lump is almost certain to be either a fat lobule or a benign lipoma in such cases. The rare exception to this general rule occurs in cases of pea-sized or smaller palpable lumps when the skin line is overpenetrated on the film-screen mammogram and thus cannot be appreciated, even with the use of a hot light. These patients may have a tiny, superficial lesion just under the skin that is not adequately shown on the mammogram. This situation is much less common on digital mammograms with current tissue equalization techniques. When the mammographic area of the palpable lump is of mixed fatty and water density, sonographic evaluation should be aggressively performed. Risk of missing a lesion mammographically is greatly reduced if the breast is fatty, but even minimal right-left asymmetries merit sonographic evaluation in such patients.

The specific goal of targeted sonographic evaluation of palpable lumps is either (1) to find normal or defini-

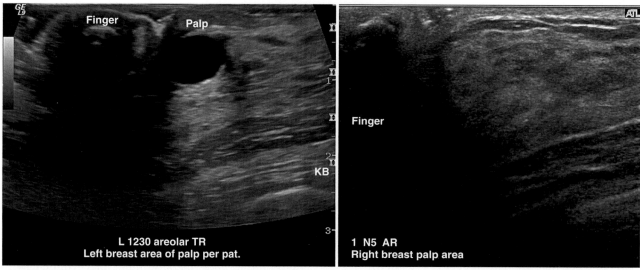

FIGURE 20-16. Marking palpable lesions during targeted diagnostic sonography is critical. *Left,* Small, simple cyst is palpated with the nonscanning index finger during imaging. *Right,* Fibroductal ridge is palpated during scanning.

tively benign causes of the lump that do not require biopsy or short-interval follow-up or (2) to find a malignant lesion that has been obscured by surrounding dense tissues on the mammogram. If sonography is to be truly effective at preventing biopsy of palpable normal breast tissues or definitively benign lesions (BIRADS 1 and 2 findings), it is essential that the abnormality be simultaneously palpated while being scanned. The image should be annotated with the word "palpable," or an image that documents the palpating finger on the lesion should be obtained (Fig. 20-16). Simply showing that normal tissue or a benign cyst exists in the same quadrant is insufficient proof that it is the cause of the palpable lump. For large lesions in compressible breasts, the operator can usually slide the nonscanning index finger under the transducer while scanning. For smaller lesions and firmer breasts, the index finger may lift the ends of the transducer so far off the skin that the lesion cannot be scanned with the finger between the transducer and skin. In such cases, trapping the lesion between the index and middle fingers and scanning the lesion while it is trapped may be useful (Fig. 20-17). For very small and superficial lesions, an opened paper clip or empty metal ballpoint pen cartridge can be used to palpate the lesion during scanning without lifting the ends of the transducer off the skin.

By aggressively scanning palpable abnormalities in patients who have dense tissue in the area of the palpable lumps, sonography should regularly detect malignant nodules that are missed by mammography. This is not an indictment of mammography, but rather indicates that understanding the limitations of mammography, with proper use of sonography in these highly select cases, can improve imaging performance in patients who have dense breasts on mammography.

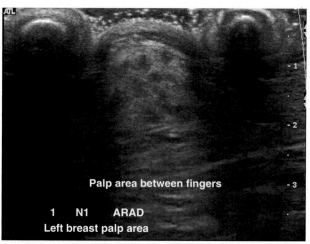

FIGURE 20-17. Finger trapping to document breast lesion. Trapping the palpable abnormality between the index and middle fingers can be helpful in documenting the cause of the "lump." In some cases, it may not be possible to palpate along the long axis of the transducer because the lesion is too small or because the breast is so small and firm that the ends of the transducers no longer touch the breast when the palpating finger has been placed between the transducer and the skin.

Sonography can prevent biopsy by showing normal or definitively benign findings. Several studies have now shown an extremely high ($\geq$99%) negative predictive value for the combination of negative mammography and normal or benign ultrasound findings. Past common wisdom that all palpable lumps need to be biopsied is no longer true. However, palpable abnormalities span a spectrum from vague thickening to "rock-hard" immovable lumps, the latter obviously engendering greater clinical concern. However, the rock-hard immovable lump would virtually *always* be associated with suspicious sonographic findings. In general, our BIRADS classification and recommendation for management are based on imaging findings, not palpability. However, in many patients with BIRADS 3 findings, who are offered a choice between short-interval follow-up and biopsy, palpability does play a role in their decision to have biopsy rather than follow-up sonography. Thus, patients whose indication for targeted sonography was a palpable lump "self-select" biopsy.

The concept of a "negative" ultrasound report in patients with palpable breast lesions is flawed. Negative sonograms imply that the breast sonographer is detached from the interpretation of the images and may not fully understand the problem for which the patient presented. Rather, all sonograms in patients with palpable lumps should be viewed as being "positive for an explanation." The positive finding can be palpable normal breast tissue or a palpable, clearly benign lesion, such as a simple cyst, but the finding *positively* and definitively explains the cause of the palpable abnormality. It is much more reassuring to the patient to be shown on the monitor that the lump palpated during the scan corresponds to a positive but normal finding, such as a ridge of normal fibroglandular tissue, than to be told her ultrasound is "negative." The positive, but normal, ultrasound engenders confidence that the breast sonographer truly understands the patient's problem, whereas a negative ultrasound engenders fear that the operator does not understand why the patient presented and might have missed something more sinister.

Mammographic Densities

Sonography is the best diagnostic tool for assessing mammographic abnormalities that do not contain suspicious calcifications. These mammographic abnormalities range from discrete masses to focal asymmetrical densities. As with palpable abnormalities, sonography will demonstrate either asymmetrical normal tissues or definitively benign abnormalities, such as simple cysts, in most mammographic abnormalities. In a smaller percentage of patients, sonography will show findings that are more suspicious or malignant appearing than suggested by mammography.

When sonography suggests that a benign abnormality, such as a simple cyst or asymmetrical normal breast tissue, causes the mammographic abnormality, it is important to be sure that the sonographic finding really explains the mammographic abnormality, and that there are not two completely different findings—a mammographic finding and a separate and incidental sonographic finding. To ensure that there is only a *single* finding and that the sonographic finding and mammographic finding are the same, the clinician must rigorously assure that the size, shape, location, and surrounding tissue density of the mammographic and sonographic findings are the same. **Mammographic-sonographic** **correlation** of size, shape, location, and surrounding tissue density is best made between the craniocaudal (CC) mammographic view and the transverse sonographic view because there is little rotation and no obliquity of the x-ray beam on the mammographic CC view. Thus, the sonographic transverse view is obtained in the exact plane of mammographic compression. The mediolateral oblique (MLO) view is obtained between 30 degrees and 60 degrees of obliquity off the true mediolateral plane and also usually involves some rotation of the breast. It is difficult to obtain an oblique sonographic plane that exactly reproduces the unknown degree of obliquity used to obtain the mammographic MLO view. The sonographic plane also cannot reproduce the rotation of the breast that may occur when obtaining an MLO mammographic view. If a mammographic lesion can only be seen on the MLO view, it is usually best to obtain a true mediolateral (ML) view, taking care not to rotate the breast during compression, and then obtain a true longitudinal ultrasound view to correlate with the mammographic ML view.

Size Correlation

Mammographic-sonographic correlation of size should take into account everything that is water density. Therefore, an oval-shaped, 3-cm, circumscribed mass might be shown to be (1) a cyst or (2) solid nodule with a thin echogenic capsule, (3) a cyst that contains a mural nodule, (4) a 3-cm collection of fibroglandular tissue, or (5) a smaller cyst or (6) solid nodule surrounded by fibroglandular tissue, where the cyst or solid nodule, together with the surrounding fibrous tissue, measures 3 cm (Fig. 20-18). All six sonographic structures would constitute a perfect mammographic-sonographic size match if all structures that appear as water density mammographically were appropriately taken into account. Measurements should be made outside-to-outside to include the capsule that surrounds the cyst or solid nodules, because the capsule is water density and will be included in the measurement of the lesion on the mammogram. Sonographic-mammographic correlation works best when the lesion is measured identically by both modalities. Mammography cannot distinguish the water density capsule from the water density lesion that it surrounds, meaning that the capsule will be included in the mammographic measurement. Therefore, the capsule must be included in the sonographic measurement of the lesion as well.

Maximum diameter is better suited for sonographic-mammographic correlation than mean diameter, because many mammographic lesions are partially compressible. To obtain the three measurements necessary for calculation of mean diameter on mammograms, two views are necessary. These views are not truly orthogonal. Only the dimensions of the lesion that are perpendicular to the axis of compression can be shown, and neither view

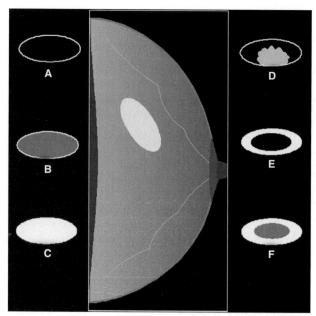

FIGURE 20-18. Importance of mammographic-sonographic correlation. Everything that is water density could contribute to the size of the mammographic lesion. Thus, a 3-cm, ovoid, circumscribed mammographic mass could represent *A*, a cyst, or *B*, a solid nodule, surrounded by a thin echogenic capsule; *C*, 3-cm collection of interlobular stromal fibrous tissue; *D*, 3-cm cyst containing a mural nodule; or *E*, smaller cyst, or *F*, solid nodule, surrounded by fibrous or glandular tissue.

shows the compressed dimension of the lesion. The two mammographic views will yield three measurements, all obtained perpendicular to the axis of compression. Sonography also requires two views to obtain the three measurements necessary for calculation of mean diameter, but these views are truly orthogonal. Whereas two of the three dimensions obtained from sonography also lie perpendicular to the axis of compression, sonography can show the compressed diameter, which is the third measurement. As a result, sonography shows **two** large diameters and **one** small diameter. Thus, lesions that appear to be spherical in shape on mammography are often oval shaped on ultrasound (Fig. 20-19). This causes the mean diameter of compressible lesions obtained from sonography to be smaller than the mean diameter of the same lesion obtained from mammography. Despite the different mean diameters obtained by mammography and sonography, the *maximum* diameters will be the same. Maximum diameter, not mean diameter, should be used for sonographic correlation of lesion size. Mean sonographic diameters can be used for short-interval follow-up of a lesion.

Shape Correlation

Sonographic-mammographic correlation of shape must consider two phenomena: **partial compressibility** and **rotary forces** applied during compression. The same phenomenon that causes the mean diameter of partially compressible lesions to appear larger on mammography than on sonography also causes a consistent shape difference between mammography and sonography. Partially compressible lesions that appear spherical on mammography are oval shaped on sonography because sonography is capable of showing the compressed diameter of the lesion, whereas mammography cannot (Fig. 20-19). When the mammographic lesion is spherical and incompressible, the shape will be spherical on sonography. Mammographic compression and sonographic compression apply different rotatory forces on lesions that are not spherical. Mammographic compression not only pulls lesions away from the chest wall, but also tends to rotate the lesion so that its long axis lies perpendicular to the chest wall. Sonographic compression will push lesions closer to the chest wall and tends to rotate the lesion's long axis parallel to the chest wall. There is typically a 90-degree difference in the orientation of the long axis of lesions between the mammogram and the sonogram (Fig. 20-20). If this rotation is not taken into account, the breast sonographer may falsely conclude that the shape of the lesion is different on the mammographic and sonographic images.

Location or Position Correlation

Because mammographic compression pulls a lesion away from the chest wall and sonographic compression pushes the lesion closer to the chest wall, lesions usually appear much closer to the chest wall on sonography than on mammography. Lesions that appear to lie several centimeters from the chest wall on mammography may appear to lie very close to the chest wall, even indenting the chest wall musculature, on sonography. Lesions that would be considered in the B zone in depth on mammograms often lie within the C zone sonographically. If this routine apparent difference in depth of lesions on mammography and sonography is not understood, the clinician might falsely conclude that the sonographic lesion lies too deep to correspond to the mammographic lesion.

Surrounding Tissue Density Correlation

The final step in correlating the sonographic and mammographic findings is assessment of the density of surrounding tissues. A lesion that protrudes into the subcutaneous fat from the mammary zone, and that is surrounded by fat superficially and water density tissue along its deep margins on the mammogram, should lie at the junction of the subcutaneous fat and mammary zone on the sonogram. It should be surrounded by subcutaneous fat along its superficial margin and by either hyperechoic fibrous tissue or isoechoic

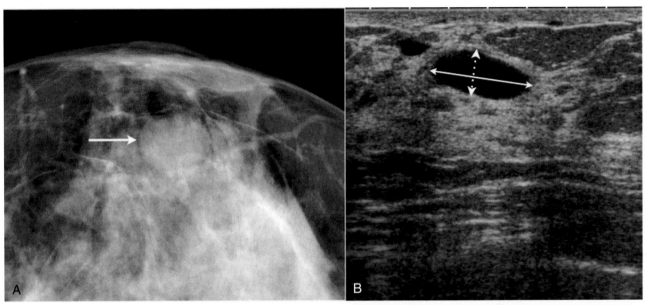

FIGURE 20-19. Lesions that appear spherical on mammography often appear elliptical on sonography.
A, Circumscribed isodense mammographic nodules appeared circular in both views (spherical) because the mammogram only demonstrates the axes of the cyst that lies perpendicular to the axis of compression and not the compressed axis. Sonography, however, does show the compressed axis. The mean diameter calculated from mammograms includes three large diameters that all lie in axes perpendicular to the axis of compression. **B,** The mean diameter calculated from the sonographic views includes two large diameters that lie perpendicular to the axis of compression *(solid arrow)* and one smaller diameter that lies parallel to the axis of compression *(dotted arrow)*. For compressible lesions, the mean diameter obtained from sonograms is often smaller than the mean diameter obtained from mammography, but the maximum diameters from mammography and sonography will be similar.

glandular tissue along its deep border on the sonogram (Fig. 20-21).

Sonographic-Mammographic Confirmation

Correlating size, shape, location, and surrounding tissue density will allow the mammographic and sonographic findings to be definitively correlated in most cases, but in some cases may fail. If it cannot be determined with absolute certainty that the mammographic and sonographic lesions are indeed the same, minimally invasive sonographic procedures can be performed to confirm the correlation. If sonography shows the suspect mammographic lesion to be cystic, ultrasound-guided cyst aspiration can be performed and the mammogram repeated to see if the mammographic lesion has disappeared. If sonography shows the suspect lesion to be solid, ultrasound-guided needle localization with a removable wire can be performed and the mammogram repeated with the wire in place, to document that the sonographic lesion and mammographic lesion are indeed the same lesion.

SONOGRAPHIC FINDINGS

The sonographic findings that correlate with palpable or mammographic abnormalities can fall into several differ-

ent categories: (1) ANDIs, (2) cysts, (3) solid nodules, and (4) indeterminate (cystic vs. solid) lesions.

Normal Tissues and Variations

Normal breast tissues and variations of normal tissues, including duct ectasia, fibrocystic change, and benign proliferative disorders, can cause both mammographic and sonographic abnormalities. These changes have been termed ANDIs, aberrations of normal development and involution. ANDIs can present sonographically not only as normal tissues but as cysts and solid nodules as well, accounting for some false-positive results at biopsy. As noted earlier, because normal tissue and ANDIs can cause both palpable and mammographic abnormalities, it is best to discard the concept of a "negative ultrasound" when evaluating clinical or mammographic abnormalities. It is better to think of all sonograms as positive—positive for a definitive explanation of the clinical or mammographic abnormality. That positive finding, however, may be a ridge of palpable fibroglandular tissue or a collection of asymmetrical fibroglandular tissues that cause an asymmetrical mammographic density. Most sonographically normal tissues can be characterized as BIRADS 1. ANDIs cause a spectrum of abnormalities that can be characterized as BIRADS 2, 3, or 4.

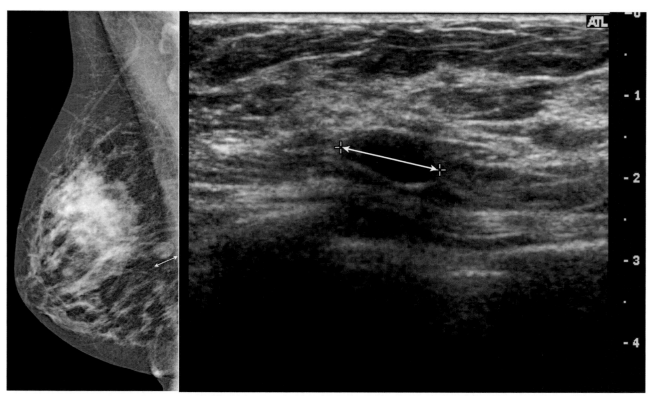

FIGURE 20-20. Mammographic-sonographic compression and lesion orientation. Mammographic compression *(left)* tends to rotate the long axis of the lesion *perpendicular* to the chest wall, whereas Sonographic compression *(right)* tends to rotate the long axis *parallel* to the chest wall. The long axes of lesions on mammography and sonography often differ by almost 90 degrees. The double-headed arrows show the long axis of the lesions.

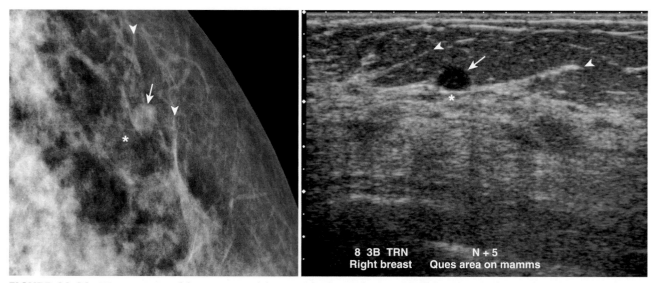

FIGURE 20-21. Mammographic-sonographic correlation of surrounding tissue density. Mammogram shows a nodule projecting between two Cooper's ligaments *(arrowheads)* and bulging anteriorly into the subcutaneous fat *(arrow)* from the mammary zone *(asterisk)* Sonogram shows that the mammographic nodule is a small cyst that protrudes out of fibrous tissue in the mammary zone (asterisk) and into the subcutaneous fat *(arrow).* It lies between two Cooper's ligaments *(arrowheads).*

Simple Cysts

The initial role of diagnostic breast sonography, to distinguish between cysts and solid nodules, remains a key role for sonography, but certainly not its only role. Demonstrating that a simple cyst causes a palpable lump or mammographic nodule is by far the most valuable finding demonstrable on sonography, because simple cysts are as definitively benign as anything that can be identified by any diagnostic imaging modality. Furthermore, the negative predictive value of a simple cyst is 100%, higher than the 99+% negative predictive value of sonographic demonstration of normal breast tissues causing mammographic or palpable abnormalities. If strict criteria for a simple cyst are met, the lesion is BIRADS 2, and no biopsy, aspiration, or follow-up is necessary. In general, we only aspirate simple cysts in cases where they are so tense that they cause severe pain. The negative predictive value of demonstrating that a simple cyst causes a palpable or mammographic abnormality is higher than demonstrating normal tissue or ANDIs as the cause. Complicated and complex cysts create a spectrum of lesions that can be characterized as BIRADS 2, 3, or 4.

Solid Nodules

Because the initial role of sonography in breast diagnosis was to distinguish between cysts and solid nodules, demonstration of a solid nodule initially was an automatic indication for biopsy. Several early sonographic studies on characterization of solid nodules reported too much overlap between the features of benign and malignant solid nodules to allow distinction between all solid malignant and all solid benign nodules. These studies were performed with older, lower-frequency, lower-resolution equipment and generally assessed only single sonographic findings. Since then, the approach to characterizing solid nodules has evolved.

The key to developing a successful algorithm for characterizing solid nodules is having realistic goals. The goal of distinguishing all benign from all malignant solid nodules was overly ambitious and not achievable. A more realistic goal is to identify a subpopulation of all solid nodules that is so likely to be benign that the patient can be offered the option of follow-up in addition to the option of biopsy. The precedent for this has been established in the mammographic literature. BIRADS 3 lesions, as they are currently defined in the mammographic literature, must have a 2% or lower risk of being malignant. To be prudent and conservative, any algorithm developed to identify the BIRADS 3 solid-nodule subgroup on sonography must adhere to strict criteria that are identical to those accepted as the standard of care in the mammographic literature.

Figure 20-22 illustrates the **heterogeneity** of breast cancer, which can be thought of as spanning a spectrum from spiculated to circumscribed lesions. Not only is breast cancer heterogeneous from one nodule to another, but it also can be heterogeneous within an individual nodule, so there is a peak of mixed circumscribed-spiculated lesions in the center of the spectrum. Any sonographic algorithm designed to identify a BIRADS 3 subgroup must consider heterogeneity.

Spiculated and circumscribed cancers differ greatly. The histologic and gross morphologic features of the

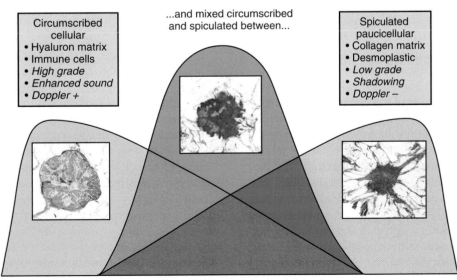

BREAST CANCER IS HETEROGENEOUS

Circumscribed
cellular
• Hyaluron matrix
• Immune cells
• *High grade*
• *Enhanced sound*
• *Doppler +*

...and mixed circumscribed
and spiculated between...

Spiculated
paucicellular
• Collagen matrix
• Desmoplastic
• *Low grade*
• *Shadowing*
• *Doppler –*

FIGURE 20-22. Malignant masses: spectrum of appearances. The appearance of breast cancer spans a spectrum from classic spiculated lesions to circumscribed carcinomas. There are also mixed spiculated and circumscribed lesions in the middle of the spectrum. Sonographic findings for circumscribed and spiculated lesions can be opposite from each other. Only by using multiple findings capable of identifying lesions at both ends of the spectrum can carcinomas be identified with the desired 98% or greater sensitivity.

spiculated and circumscribed ends of the malignant spectrum differ in cellularity, constituents of the extracellular matrix (ECM), host reaction to the tumor, and water content. Additionally, spiculated or stellate malignant lesions tend to be low to intermediate in histologic grade, whereas circumscribed lesions tend to be either special-type tumors (e.g., colloid or medullary carcinoma) or high-grade invasive ductal carcinoma. The classic **spiculated breast carcinoma** is composed of tumor cells, ECM, and desmoplastic host response to the lesion. Compared to circumscribed carcinomas, the usually low-grade spiculated carcinomas are paucicellular—a small percentage of the total volume of the lesion is composed of tumor cells. **Circumscribed carcinomas,** usually high-grade invasive ductal carcinomas, on the other hand, are highly cellular. Spiculated carcinomas have a primarily collagenous ECM, whereas circumscribed lesions have more hyaluronic acid in the matrix. Spiculated carcinomas have abundant desmoplastic host response, whereas circumscribed carcinomas manifest a primarily lymphoplasmacytic immune response. The paucicellular nature, collagenous matrix, and desmoplastic host response of spiculated malignant lesions makes them relatively *water poor,* so they often cause acoustic shadowing. The high cellularity, hydrophilic hyaluronic acid matrix, and lymphoplasmacytic response in circumscribed lesions makes them *water rich.* Not only do circumscribed lesions not cause acoustic shadowing, they usually manifest increased sound transmission.

Thus, **acoustic shadowing** helps clinicians detect lesions at the spiculated end of the spectrum and some of the mixed lesions in the middle of the spectrum, but it is much less effective at the circumscribed end of the spectrum. Because of the high tumor cellularity of circumscribed carcinomas, they elaborate abundant angiogenesis factors, and because the lymphoplasmacytic immune-inflammatory response, they also cause vasodilation in surrounding vessels. The combined tumor neovascularity and inflammatory hyperemia caused by circumscribed malignant lesions makes them hypervascular and positive on Doppler ultrasound studies. On the other hand, all living tissues have blood flow. Because spiculated lesions have relatively few tumor cells that elaborate angiogenesis factors, and because the collagen matrix and desmoplasia require little blood flow, spiculated lesions often do not have perceptibly increased flow compared to benign lesions or normal tissue. Thus, Doppler sonography is usually quite effective for detecting circumscribed cancers, but is less effective for stellate lesions. This means that, because of the heterogeneity of breast cancer, multiple different findings will be necessary to detect cancer with adequate sensitivity, some better for the circumscribed end and some better for the spiculated end of the spectrum. A set of rules is also necessary to deal with the mixed circumscribed and spiculated lesions that lie in the middle of the spectrum.

TABLE 20-1. COMPARISON OF SUSPICIOUS SONOGRAPHIC AND MAMMOGRAPHIC FINDINGS

Suspicious Mammographic Findings	Suspicious Sonographic Findings
Spiculation	Spiculation (thick, echogenic halo)
Irregular or poorly defined margins	Angular margins
Microlobulation	Microlobulation
Calcifications	Calcifications
Linear calcification pattern	Duct extension
Branching calcification pattern	Branch pattern
Mass or nodule	Taller-than-wide shape*
Asymmetrical density	Acoustic shadowing*
Developing density	Hypoechogenicity*

*Findings unique to ultrasound.

The algorithm that we use to evaluate lesions must account for internal heterogeneity by (1) assessing the surface, shape, and volume of the lesion for suspicious findings completely in two orthogonal planes (preferably radial and antiradial) and (2) ignoring benign or nonsuspicious findings in lesions that have a mixture of suspicious and nonsuspicious findings. The entire lesion must always be characterized by its most suspicious features. Table 20-1 shows the suspicious sonographic findings in solid breast nodules and compares them to suspicious mammographic findings. Note that six of the nine suspicious sonographic findings are suspicious mammographic findings that have been applied directly to sonography. Of the nine findings, only three—**taller-than-wide shape, acoustic shadowing,** and **hypoechogenicity**—are unique to sonography.

Suspicious Findings

The suspicious sonographic findings can be classified into three subgroups by morphologic features or by histopathologic features. Table 20-2 shows the suspicious findings listed by their morphologic features: **surface characteristics** (spiculation, angular margins, and microlobulations); **shapes** (taller than wide, duct extension, and branch pattern); and **internal characteristics** (acoustic shadowing, hypoechoic echotexture, and calcifications). Histologic classification can be even more useful than morphologic classification (Table 20-2). Histopathologic categories include **"hard" findings** that indicate the presence of invasion of surrounding tissues (angular margins, spiculation, thick echogenic halo, and acoustic shadowing); **"soft" findings** that indicate the presence of DCIS components of tumor (microlobulations, calcifications, duct extension and branch pattern); and **mixed findings** that can be seen in

TABLE 20-2. COMPARISON OF MORPHOLOGIC AND HISTOPATHOLOGIC FEATURES OF SUSPICIOUS SONOGRAPHIC FINDINGS

MORPHOLOGIC FEATURES	HISTOPATHOLOGIC FEATURES
Surface Characteristics	*"Hard" Findings*
Spiculation	Spiculation (halo)
Angular margins	Angular margins
Microlobulation	Acoustic shadowing
Shapes	*Mixed Findings*
Taller than wide	Hypoechogenicity
Duct extension	Taller than wide
Branch pattern	*"Soft" Findings*
Internal Characteristics	Microlobulation
Calcifications	Duct extension
Acoustic shadowing	Branch pattern
Hypoechogenicity	Microcalcifications

association with either invasive or DCIS components of tumor (hypoechoic echotexture and taller-than-wide orientation).

Including soft findings is important because the most common breast carcinoma, invasive duct carcinoma—invasive not otherwise specific (NOS) or no specific type (NST) carcinoma—usually contains DCIS components. "Soft" suspicious findings help in two ways. First, soft findings can help clinicians detect pure DCIS, which rarely develops "hard" suspicious findings. Second, including soft findings can help to detect and characterize the circumscribed invasive duct carcinomas that contain both invasive and DCIS components. In such cases, the new periphery of the lesion is where the DCIS components are located. Thus, the surface characteristics and shapes of the lesion are created by the DCIS elements of the lesion, not by the centrally located invasive components. Finally, the use of soft findings can aid in accurately staging malignant breast lesions on sonography; the DCIS components of the lesion that extend into the surrounding tissues for variable distances can be identified only by soft findings. Soft findings do increase the sensitivity of the sonographic algorithm for detecting malignant disease, but also increase the false-positive rate, especially for lesions that contain only soft findings. Lesions that demonstrate only soft findings are most likely to be benign—papillomas, fibroadenomas, and fibrocystic change (FCC). However, the risk of malignancy for solid nodules that demonstrate only soft suspicious findings is greater than 2%, requiring that such lesions be characterized as mildly suspicious (BIRADS 4a) and biopsied. Each of the individual suspicious sonographic findings has a solid histopathologic basis.

Spiculation or Thick Echogenic Halo

Spiculation (spicule) is a hard sonographic finding that corresponds to invasion of surrounding tissues and a desmoplastic host response to the lesion. Spiculation is a mammographic finding that can be directly applied to sonography (Fig. 20-23, *A*). When the spiculations are coarse, they manifest as alternating hypoechoic and hyperechoic lines that radiate perpendicular to the surface of the nodule; the **hypoechoic** components represent either fingers of invasive tumor or DCIS components of tumor extending into the surrounding tissues, and the **hyperechoic** elements represent the interfaces between the spicules and surrounding breast tissues (Fig. 20-23, *B*). In most cases, however, spicules are fine and present with only a single echogenicity. They appear to be either hyperechoic or hypoechoic depending on echogenicity of the tissue within which the lesion lies.

The spicules in malignant nodules that are surrounded by hyperechoic fibrous tissues appear hypoechoic (Fig. 20-23, *C*), whereas spicules in malignant nodules that are surrounded by fat appear hyperechoic (Fig. 20-23, *D*). The role of sonography in fat-surrounded lesions is usually to guide interventional procedures or to determine extent of disease, whereas its role in fibrous-surrounded lesions may be diagnostic because such lesions can be completely obscured by surrounding dense tissues on the mammogram. The thick, echogenic halo that surrounds some malignant solid nodules represents spiculations that are too small to demonstrate sonographically. For this reason, either frank spiculations or the presence of a thick, echogenic halo should be considered to be spiculations. The classic thick echogenic halo appears thicker along the edges of the nodule than on its anterior and posterior surfaces (Fig. 20-24); the spicules are more numerous in the coronal plane and are perpendicular to the beam along the edges of the nodule, forming strong spicular reflectors. The less common spicules that do occur on the anterior and posterior surfaces of the nodule lie nearly parallel to the sonographic beam and therefore are very weak spicular reflectors. Considering the thick echogenic halo to be a variant of frank spiculations approximately doubles the sensitivity of spiculation for malignant nodules, from 36% to 70%.

Sonographic imaging in three dimensions is very helpful at demonstrating spiculations. Most spiculations are oriented in the coronal plane, so the reconstructed coronal plane is especially helpful. Thick, echogenic halos in standard planes can often be resolved as frank spiculations in the coronal plane. This is true for hand-held and automated breast scanners (Figs. 20-25 and 20-26).

Angular Margins

Angular margins are the jagged or irregular margins discussed in the mammography and breast ultrasound

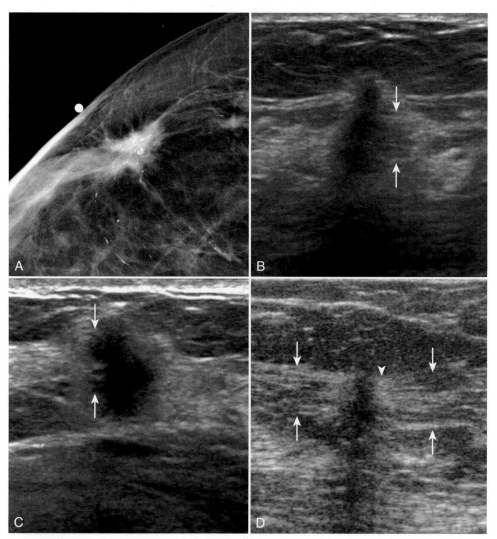

FIGURE 20-23. Spiculation. A, Spiculation is a "hard" mammographic finding that indicates invasion. **B,** Coarse spiculations *(between arrows)* present as alternating hypoechoic and hypoechoic lines radiating from the nodule on ultrasound. The hypoechoic parts represent fingers of invasive tumor or ductal carcinoma in situ, and the hyperechoic lines represent the interface between the tumor and surrounding tissue. Most spicules are fine rather than coarse and present with only a single echogenicity opposite that from the background tissues. **C,** The spiculated lesions surrounded by hyperechoic fibrous tissues are hypoechoic *(between arrows).* **D,** Fine spicules in lesions surrounded by fat appear hyperechoic *(between arrows).* Note that spiculations are most prominent within the coronal plane along the sides of the nodule.

literature. Angular margins are a subcategory of the ACR BIRADS "irregular shape." Angular margin represents a hard sonographic finding indicative of invasion as well as a mammographic finding that has been applied directly to sonography. The angles of the lesion margins can be acute, right angle, or obtuse. A single angle of any type on the surface of the lesion should be considered suspicious and should exclude the lesion from the "probably benign" BIRADS 3 category. Angles on the surface of the nodule occur in regions of low resistance to invasion. In lesions surrounded by fat, angulations can occur on any surface of the nodule (Fig. 20-27, *A*). In fibrous-surrounded lesions, angular margins tend to occur on the edges of the lesion, within loose periductal stromal tissues, and between tissue planes within the

fibrous tissue (Fig. 20-27, *B*). In the approximately two thirds of malignant nodules that arise within anteriorly located TDLUs abutting the anterior mammary fascia, angulations tend to occur at points where Cooper's ligaments intersect the surface of the nodule (Fig. 20-27, *C*). Angular margins have the second best sensitivity of all the suspicious findings (90%) but have the best combination of sensitivity and positive predictive value of any of the findings.

Microlobulations

Microlobulations are 1-mm to 2-mm lobulations that vary in number and distribution along the surface and within the substance of a nodule. They may occur

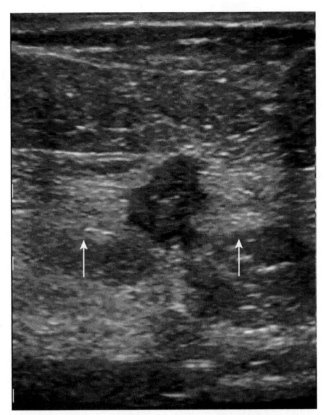

FIGURE 20-24. Echogenic halo with hyperechoic spicules. The thick, poorly defined echogenic halo that can be seen around some invasive malignant lesions surrounded by fat represents hyperechoic spicules too small to be resolved individually. The halo is more often seen and is thicker along the sides of the nodule within the coronal plane *(arrows)* because spicules are more common in the coronal plane and because the spicules that lie within the coronal plane are perpendicular to the ultrasound beam, where they make strong spicular reflectors.

over only a small percentage of the surface of a nodule. Microlobulation is a mixed finding that can be seen with both invasive and DCIS components of tumor, but more often represents in situ components of tumor. It is a mammographic finding that applies directly to sonography. When microlobulations are angular and are associated with a thick echogenic halo, they usually represent fingers of invasive carcinoma (Fig. 20-28, *A*). When the microlobulations are rounded and associated with a thin echogenic capsule, they usually represent DCIS components of tumors. DCIS components can create microlobulations in two ways: ductules or ducts that are distended with tumor and necrosis (Fig. 20-28, *B*), or cancerized lobules (Fig. 20-28, *C*). The size of microlobulations correlates with the histologic grade of the tumor. High-grade lesions tend to have large microlobulations, whereas low-grade lesions tend to have very small microlobulations, and intermediate-grade lesions tend to have intermediate-sized microlobulations.

Taller-than-Wide Shape

Lesions that are larger in the AP dimension than in any horizontal dimension are suspicious for malignancy. This is a mixed finding that can be seen with both invasive and DCIS lesions (Fig. 20-29). Taller-than-wide shape is unique to sonography and is not seen on mammography. Originally described in the Japanese literature, taller than wide (termed "not parallel" in ACR BIRADS ultrasound lexicon) is primarily a feature of small, solid malignant nodules that have a volume of 1 cc (1 mL) or less. Our data confirm this. As lesions enlarge, they tend to become wider than tall (termed

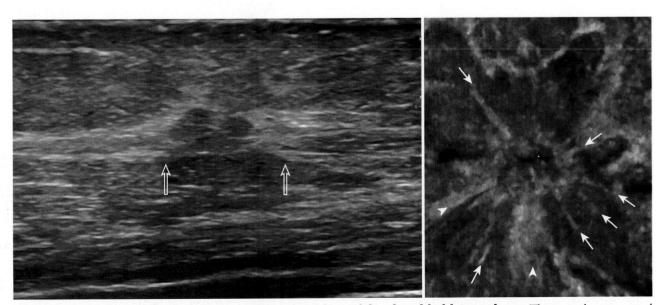

FIGURE 20-25. Three-dimensional or volume imaging with a hand-held transducer. The coronal reconstructed plane can be especially useful in assessing for spiculations. What appears to be a poorly defined, thick, echogenic halo in radial or antiradial planes *(left, arrows)*, can often be resolved as individual hyperechoic spicules in the reconstructed coronal plane *(right, arrows)*. The coronal plane can also better demonstrate other architectural distortions, such as thickened Cooper's ligaments *(right, arrowhead)*.

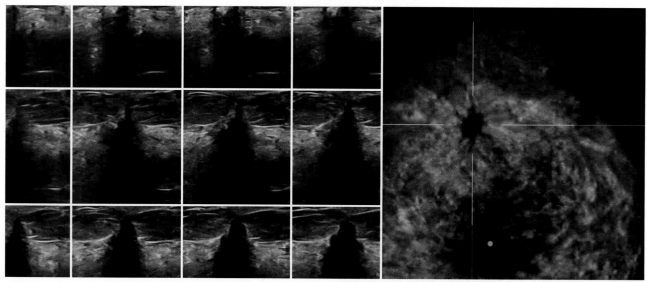

FIGURE 20-26. Three-dimensional or volume imaging with automated breast scanner. Spiculations are better demonstrated on the reconstructed coronal plane *(right)* than on the serial native (original) plane images.

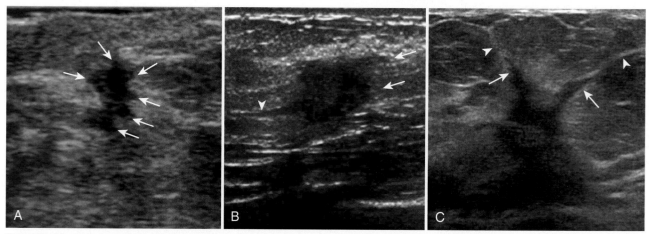

FIGURE 20-27. Angular margins represent invasion of carcinoma into low-resistance pathways. A, Fat offers little resistance to invasion, so malignant nodules surrounded by fat can develop angles along any surface *(arrows)*. **B,** In lesions surrounded by hyperechoic fibrous tissues, paths of low resistance are along the periductal tissues *(arrowhead)* and horizontally along the tissue planes within the fibrous tissue *(arrows)*. **C,** Following Cooper's ligaments *(arrowheads)* down to their base, where they intersect the surface of the nodule, is the best way to detect angles *(arrows)* on the surface of malignant solid nodules.

"parallel" in BIRADS lexicon). The best of several explanations for this finding is that the shape of small carcinomas merely reflects the shape of the TDLUs within which the carcinoma arose. Most TDLUs lie in the anterior aspect of the mammary zone and are oriented in a taller-than-wide axis. As malignant lesions expand into the lobar ductal system, which is oriented horizontally within the breast, they tend rapidly to become wider than tall (Fig. 20-30). About 70% of malignant nodules with maximum diameters less than 10 mm are taller than wide. Only 20% of malignant nodules over 2.0 cm in maximum diameter are taller than wide.

Duct Extension and Branch Pattern

Duct extension and branch pattern are "soft" shape findings that correlate with the presence of DCIS components of tumor. Duct extension and branch pattern are mammographic calcification patterns that have been applied to components of solid nodules. Duct extension and branch pattern fall under the category of "effect on surrounding tissues" in the ACR BIRADS ultrasound lexicon. Duct extension and branch pattern can best be demonstrated when the scan plane is oriented parallel to the long axis of the mammary ducts in the region of the

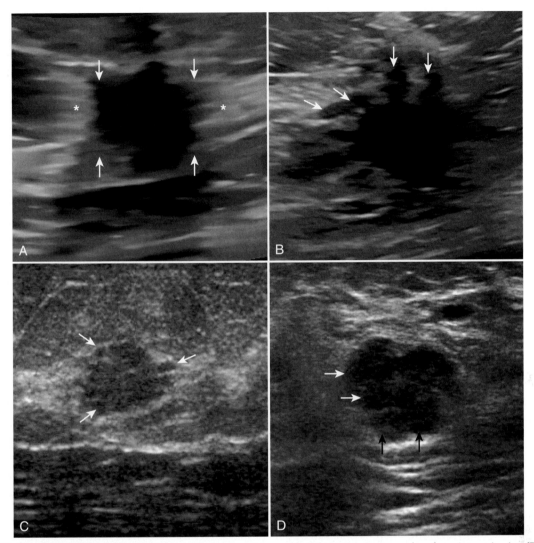

FIGURE 20-28. Microlobulations. These can represent either angles of invasive tumor or ductal carcinoma in situ (DCIS) components of the lesion. **A,** When microlobulations are pointed or angular *(arrows)* and associated with spiculations or thick, echogenic halo *(asterisks)*, they represent fingers of invasive tumor. **B,** When microlobulations appear as small "tennis rackets" *(arrows)* projecting from the surface of the nodule, they represent surrounding lobules distended with DCIS or cancerous lobules. Microlobulations that are round or oval shaped with thin, echogenic capsules represent tumor-distended ducts. The thin capsule represents the intact duct wall. **C,** Small microlobulations *(arrows)* correspond to minimally distended ducts that are filled with low-nuclear-grade DCIS. **D,** Large microlobulations *(arrows)* correspond to grossly distended ducts that contain high–nuclear-grade DCIS.

nodule. Duct extension usually manifests as a single projection of solid growth toward the nipple from the main nodule (Fig. 20-31). Because the duct extension often involves the highly distensible lactiferous sinus portion of the major lobar duct, it can be quite large, up to 5 mm in diameter. Branch pattern manifests as a projection of the solid nodule into multiple small ducts peripherally (Fig. 20-32). Because these are small ducts, branch-pattern involvement is generally smaller than duct extension.

The size of the branch pattern correlates with the histologic grade of the lesion. High-grade lesions tend to have large branch patterns; low-grade lesions tend to

have small branch patterns; and intermediate-grade lesions tend to have intermediate-sized branches. The presence of duct extension or branch pattern is not a specific sign of malignancy, but rather suggests an intraductal growth pattern. Benign intraductal lesions such as papillomas and chronic periductal mastitis and fibrosis can also demonstrate duct extension or branch pattern. In fact, when only duct extension or branch pattern is present, the lesion is a benign papilloma in 87% of cases. However, 6% of such lesions represent DCIS, and another 7% represent papillomas that have atypia in the surface epithelium. Even in the absence of other suspicious findings, the risk of malignancy in nodules that

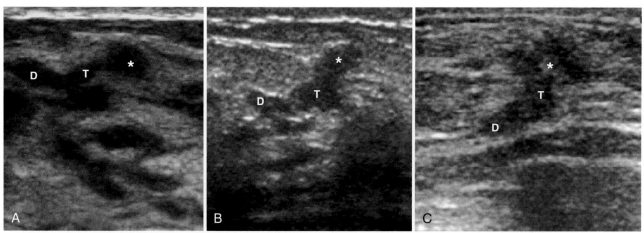

FIGURE 20-29. Terminal ductolobular unit (TDLU) carcinoma. Taller-than-wide orientation corresponds to a small, in situ or invasive carcinoma involving a single TDLU. **A,** Normal lobule *(asterisk)*, its extralobular terminal duct *(t)*, and part of the segmental duct *(d)*. The TDLU orientation is taller than wide. **B,** Small, intermediate-nuclear-grade DCIS grossly distends the lobule *(asterisk)* and its extralobular terminal duct, remaining oriented in the taller-than-wide axis of the lobule from which it arose. **C,** Small, low-nuclear-grade invasive ductal carcinoma more grossly distends and distorts the lobule *(asterisk)* and extralobular terminal duct from which it arose, but remains oriented taller than wide. Note the angles that indicate invasion into the surrounding tissues.

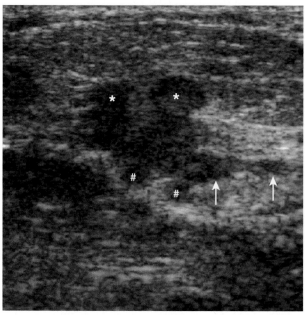

FIGURE 23-30. Ductal carcinoma in situ (DCIS). Growth of DCIS changes shape to wider than tall. As malignant solid nodules enlarge, DCIS components grow down the lobar duct toward the nipple and develop cancerized adjacent lobules, changing from taller-than-wide to wider-than-tall shape. Tumor-distended anterior lobules (*); tumor-distended but smaller posterior lobules (#); and tumor-distended lobar duct *(arrows)*.

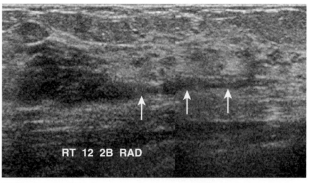

FIGURE 20-31. Duct extension of ductal carcinoma in situ. DCIS growing within the lobar duct toward nipple. Most invasive duct carcinomas contain DCIS components. In some cases the DCIS growing away from the tumor toward the nipple within the lobar duct may grossly distend the duct enough to allow recognition of duct extension sonographically *(arrows)*. If such duct extensions are not recognized on ultrasound, they might be transected at surgery, leading to positive margins, local recurrence, and the need for re-resection.

have duct extension or branch pattern as their only suspicious finding is greater than 2% for lesions, and such lesions must be excluded from the BIRADS 3 category. It is important to recognize duct extension and branch pattern for two reasons: (1) to minimize false-negative characterization of pure DCIS and (2) to identify exten-sive intraductal components of tumor. Solid nodules that have long duct extensions or extensive branch patterns tend to have extensive intraductal (DCIS) components (EIC) that increase the likelihood of local recurrence.

Acoustic Shadowing

Acoustic shadowing is a "hard" suspicious internal characteristic finding that suggests the presence of invasive malignancy. Acoustic shadowing tends to occur in solid nodules that lie on the spiculated end of the malignant

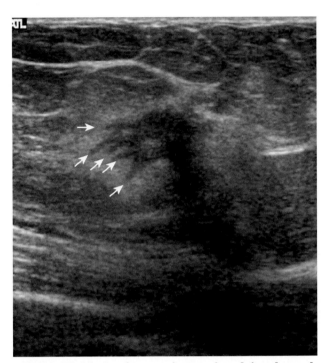

FIGURE 20-32. In situ carcinoma involving branch ducts. Growth of DCIS into small ducts that lie peripherally can distend the ducts enough to permit recognition of the involvement as branch pattern *(arrows)*. Branch pattern ducts are multiple and are usually smaller and shorter than duct extensions, but their width is proportionate to the nuclear grade of the DCIS within them.

spectrum and represent about one third of all solid malignant nodules. The desmoplastic components of the tumor substance and spiculations cause the shadowing (Fig. 20-33, *A*). Because breast carcinomas can be internally heterogeneous, only part of a solid malignant nodule might give rise to acoustic shadowing (Fig. 20-33, *B*). Other parts of the lesion might be associated with **normal** or **enhanced sound transmission.** High-grade invasive ductal carcinomas, the most common circumscribed malignant nodules, do not usually cause shadowing. In fact, they most often have associated enhanced sound transmission (Fig. 20-34, *A*), and many intermediate-grade lesions demonstrate normal sound transmission (Fig. 20-34, *B*). Even pure DCIS that is high nuclear grade may be associated with enhanced through-transmission. Special-type tumors and invasive lobular carcinomas also tend to cause either acoustic shadowing or enhanced sound transmission. Most invasive lobular carcinomas and tubulolobular carcinomas cause acoustic shadowing. Some tubular carcinomas less than 1.5 cm in diameter and most 1.5 cm or larger in maximum diameter cause acoustic shadowing. The differential diagnosis for malignant nodules that cause acoustic shadowing, in order of frequency, is (1) low-grade to intermediate-grade invasive ductal carcinoma, (2) invasive lobular carcinoma, (3) tubulolobular carcinoma, and (4) tubular carcinoma. The differential diag-

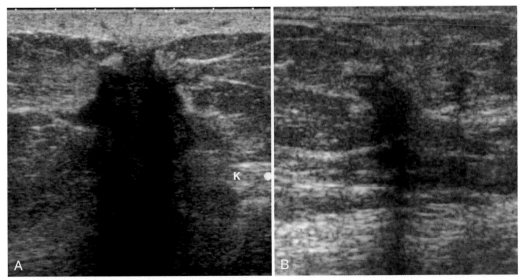

FIGURE 20-33. Cancer causing acoustic shadowing. Acoustic shadowing is a "hard" finding that suggests the presence of desmoplastic invasive tumor. Any acoustic shadowing should be considered suspicious—whether **A,** complete, or **B,** partial. Tumors that are becoming progressively more de-differentiated and that are polyclonal or that contain mixtures of low-grade and intermediate-grade or high-grade components tend to create partial shadows.

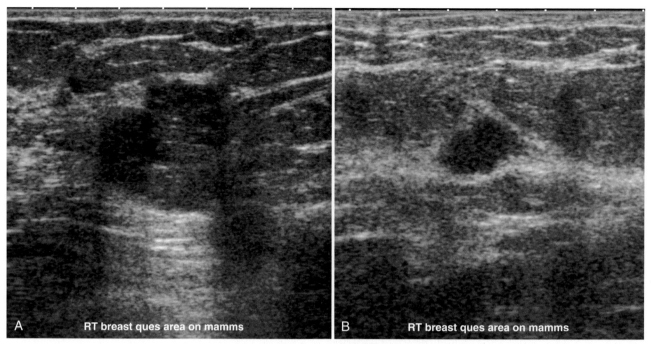

FIGURE 20-34. Variable sound transmission deep to carcinomas. About one third of malignant nodules cause acoustic shadowing, the other two-thirds have either normal sound transmission or enhanced sound transmission. **A,** High-grade invasive ductal carcinomas tend to be associated with enhanced sound transmission. **B,** Intermediate-grade invasive duct carcinomas tend to be associated with normal or mixed sound transmission.

nosis for malignant nodules associated with enhanced sound transmission, in order of frequency, includes (1) high-grade invasive ductal carcinoma; (2) high-nuclear-grade DCIS; (3) colloid carcinoma, usually when 1.5 cm in diameter or larger; (4) medullary carcinoma; and (5) invasive papillary carcinoma.

Calcifications

Calcifications are mammographic suspicious findings that have been applied directly to sonography. Calcifications within solid nodules are soft suspicious sonographic findings that suggest the presence of DCIS components. In the ACR BIRADS ultrasound lexicon, calcifications can be classified as macrocalcifications or microcalcifications. Microcalcifications can occur within or outside a mass. The calcifications develop within necrotic debris within the center of the lumen of DCIS-distended ductules or ducts. Because microlobulations, duct extensions, and branch patterns represent DCIS components of the tumor distending ducts, malignant calcifications can often be found within the other soft findings that represent DCIS. Thus, many malignant calcifications can be found within the center of microlobulations, duct extensions, or branch patterns (Fig. 20-35). The calcifications that are shown on sonography are smaller than the beam width and therefore subject to volume averaging. They are usually in the 200 to 500–micron size range. Calcifications that

are narrower than the beam width do not cast acoustic shadows, appear larger than their true size, and appear less echogenic than their true echogenicity. Most **benign calcifications** lie within a fairly echogenic background, so that when volume is averaged with the surrounding echogenic tissues, they are no longer bright enough to be identified sonographically. **Malignant calcifications** lie within rather homogeneously hypoechoic tumor substance and remain visible even though they are subject to volume averaging with surrounding tissues. Thus, sonography can generally demonstrate a higher percentage of malignant than benign microcalcifications.

Hypoechogenicity

Marked hypoechogenicity of the substance of a solid nodule (compared to fat) is a mixed suspicious internal characteristic sonographic finding of malignancy. It can be the result of several different tumor characteristics. High-grade invasive ductal carcinomas that are highly cellular and contain abundant hyaluronic acid in the ECM may appear hypoechoic because of the high water content. Pure DCIS may appear hypoechoic because of either necrosis or secretions within the lumina of tumor-distended ducts. Low-grade invasive ductal carcinomas can appear "markedly hypoechoic" because of acoustic shadowing (Fig. 20-36). In recent years, as we have pushed the transducer frequency, bandwidth, and

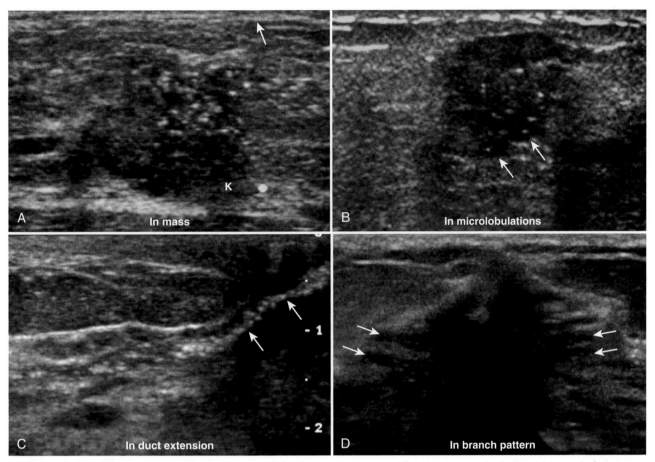

FIGURE 20-35. Microcalcifications. These appear as bright echoes too small to create acoustic shadows. Microcalcifications are "soft" findings that suggest the presence of DCIS elements. **A,** Microcalcifications can occur amorphously within a mass. However, most malignant breast calcifications occur within the necrotic debris in the center of the lumen of tumor-distended ducts. **B to D,** Other soft findings can each represent tumor-filled ducts, and calcifications often occur inside other soft findings, such as **B,** within microlobulations *(arrows);* **C,** within duct extensions *(arrows);* or **D,** within branch patterns *(arrows).*

system dynamic range to their limits, the percentage of malignant nodules that appears markedly hypoechoic has decreased from about 70% to 50%. However, digitally encoded harmonic ultrasound can make a larger percentage of solid nodules appear markedly hypoechoic compared with the surrounding fat (Fig. 20-37).

Multiple Findings

None of the individual findings achieves a sensitivity of 98% or greater because breast carcinoma is too heterogeneous to be detected with high sensitivity using a single finding. Remember that single findings can detect only cases at one end of the malignant spectrum and some mixed cases, but not cases at the other end of the spectrum. However, because the average breast carcinoma has five or six of the suspicious findings, the overall sensitivity for breast cancer of the algorithm using multiple findings easily exceeds our goal of 98% or greater.

Benign Findings

Only if no suspicious findings are present should one of three benign findings be sought. The benign findings are (1) **pure and total hyperechogenicity,** which represents interlobular stromal fibrous tissue; (2) an **elliptical shape with wider-than-tall orientation,** with the lesion completely encompassed by a thin, echogenic capsule; and (3) a **gently lobulated shape with wider-than-tall orientation with three or fewer lobulations,** with the lesion completely encompassed by a thin, echogenic capsule. If a nodule fits into one of these three categories, it can be characterized as BIRADS 3, "probably benign."

Hyperechoic Tissue

Purely hyperechoic tissue is normal interlobular stromal fibrous tissue, which can cause either palpable or mammographic abnormalities (Fig. 20-38). To be considered

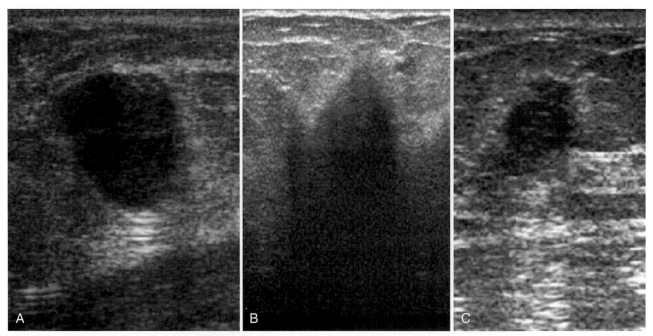

FIGURE 20-36. Hypoechoic carcinomas. Malignant nodules are often markedly hypoechoic in comparison to fat. Hypoechogenicity can be the result of **A,** high cellularity and high content of hyaluronic acid within the extracellular matrix, or **B,** from intense acoustic shadowing associated with invasive carcinomas. **C,** Necrosis within the lumen of tumor containing ductules can cause marked hypoechogenicity in lesions composed of pure DCIS.

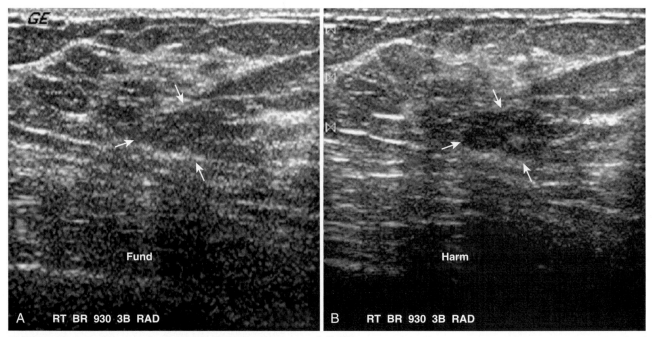

FIGURE 20-37. Harmonic imaging improves mass visibility. A, Nodules that are isoechoic with surrounding tissues and difficult to identify with fundamental imaging *(arrows)* often appear **B,** markedly hypoechoic and more conspicuous *(arrows)* when viewed with harmonics.

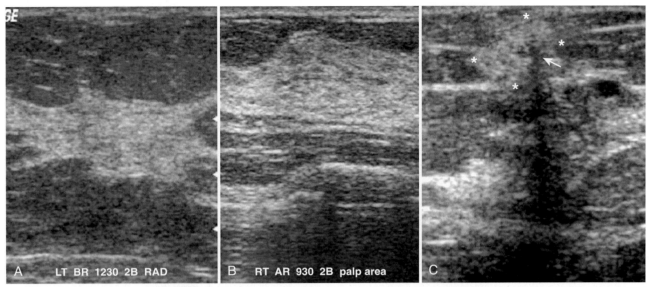

FIGURE 20-38. Hyperechoic fibrous tissue collections. Normal isolated collections of hyperechoic interlobular stromal fibrous tissue can cause **A,** mammographic nodules and masses, or **B,** palpable ridges. The negative predictive value of purely and intensely hyperechoic tissue is essentially 100%. However, collections of hyperechoic tissue should not contain any hypoechoic or isoechoic areas that are larger than normal ducts or TDLUs. **C,** Certain small, invasive carcinomas can present with tiny hypoechoic central foci *(arrow)* surrounded by very thick, echogenic halos (*). Near-field volume averaging or tangential imaging through the thick, echogenic halo of such lesions can make them falsely appear to be purely hyperechoic.

benign, the hyperechoic tissue can contain normal-sized ducts or TDLUs, but it should contain no isoechoic or hypoechoic structures larger than normal ducts or lobules. Purely hyperechoic carcinomas are exceedingly rare, but occasionally a carcinoma may have a very small, hypoechoic central nidus and a very thick, echogenic halo, and technical errors such as volume averaging or tangential imaging through the halo can make the lesion falsely appear to be purely hyperechoic (Fig. 20-38, *C*).

Wider-than-Tall Shape

An **elliptical, wider-than-tall shape** is the classic shape of fibroadenomas. However, we require that this shape also be encompassed completely by a thin, echogenic capsule to meet strict criteria for BIRADS 3 classification (Fig. 20-39, *A*).

A **gently lobulated, wider-than-tall shape** that contains three or fewer lobulations is the second most common shape of fibroadenomas. As for elliptical lesions, there must be a demonstrable thin, echogenic capsule surrounding the entire lesion before it can be classified as BIRADS 3 (Fig. 20-39, *B*).

Nodules that appear to be elliptical in one view and gently lobulated in the orthogonal view are common. The negative predictive value of the elliptical shape is 97%, and the negative predictive value of the gently lobulated shape is 99%, in a population of nodules with 33% malignant nodules.

Thin Echogenic Capsule

It is important to combine the elliptical or gently lobulated shapes with the presence of a complete, thin, echogenic capsule in order to minimize false-negative results in circumscribed carcinomas (which may be surrounded by a thin echogenic pseudocapsule) and in pure DCIS (surrounded by the intact thin echogenic duct wall) because they are almost never elliptical or gently lobulated in shape. They are usually associated with other suspicious findings, such as angular margins, taller-than-wide shape, microlobulations, duct extension, or branch pattern. The thin echogenic pseudocapsule that can be seen around circumscribed carcinomas is often absent along part of the surface of the nodule. By combining the presence of a **complete, thin, echogenic capsule with the elliptical or gently lobulated shape,** we can achieve a negative predictive value of greater than 99%.

Rocking the transducer in its short axis and heeling and toeing the transducer along its long axis are often necessary to demonstrate the presence of a thin, echogenic capsule along the edges of the nodule. Using less compression often helps to demonstrate the thin echogenic capsule in benign nodules that are surrounded by hyperechoic fibrous tissue.

The sensitivity for carcinoma in the entire population of solid nodules and the negative predictive value for nodules meeting strict criteria for BIRADS 3 both exceed 98%. Thus, by using multiple findings in a strict

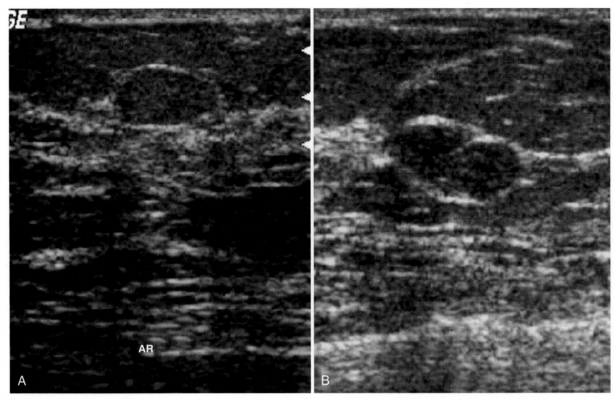

FIGURE 20-39. Fibroadenoma. A, Classic shape of benign fibroadenomas is elliptical. Such lesions are wider than tall and completely encompassed by a thin, echogenic capsule. **B,** Second most common shape of benign fibroadenomas is gently lobulated. Classic lobulated fibroadenomas have three or fewer lobulations, are wider than tall, and are completely encompassed by a thin, echogenic capsule.

TABLE 20-3. CHARACTERIZATION OF SOLID BREAST NODULES

	BENIGN HISTOLOGY	MALIGNANT HISTOLOGY	TOTALS
Negative sonogram (BIRADS 2 and 3)	287 (TN)	1 (FN)	288
Positive sonogram (BIRADS 4 and 5)	610 (FP)	477 (TP)	1087
TOTALS	897	478	1375

BIRADS, Breast Imaging Reporting and Data System; *TN,* true negative; *FN,* false negative; *FP,* false positive; *TP,* true positive.
 Sensitivity: 406/407 = 99.8%.
 Negative predictive value: 245/246 = 99.6%.
 Specificity: 245/804 = 30.5%.
 Positive predictive value: 406/965 = 42.1%.
 Accuracy: (245 + 406)/1211 = 53.8%.

algorithmic approach, we are able to identify a subgroup of solid nodules that meets the mammographic definition for BIRADS 3: a 2% or lower risk of being malignant (Table 20-3). Table 20-4 shows the results of sonographic characterization into BIRADS categories. Note that the actual percentage of malignant nodules within each BIRADS category falls within the predicted risk for that specific category.

Complex and Complicated Cysts

Simple cysts are anechoic and surrounded completely by a thin, echogenic wall or capsule with enhanced sound transmission and thin-edge shadows (Fig. 20-40). Cysts that meet strict criteria for being simple are "definitively benign" and do not require further diagnosis. Biopsy, aspiration, and even follow-up are not necessary. Aspiration of simple cysts is generally reserved for relief of pain and tenderness in very tense simple cysts.

In the ACR BIRADS ultrasound lexicon, a distinction is made between complex and complicated cysts. Any cyst that is not simple is either complicated or complex. **Complex cysts** have thick and irregular walls, mural nodules, thick septations, and internal blood flow. Cysts that are complex are at increased risk of containing papillomas or carcinomas. **Complicated cysts,** on the other hand, contain echogenic fluid, fluid-debris levels, or fat-fluid levels. They are generally benign, at low risk of

TABLE 20-4. CHARACTERIZATION OF 1375 SOLID NODULES INTO BIRADS CATEGORIES*

BIRADS CATEGORY	NO. OF NODULES BIOPSIED	NO. OF MALIGNANT NODULES	EXPECTED RISK OF CANCER	ACTUAL RISK OF CANCER
2	17	0	0%	0%
3	271	1	<2%	0.7%
4a	558	64	3%-49%	12%
4b	217	133	50%-89%	61%
5	312	280	>90%	91%
TOTALS	1375	478	20%-50%	35%

*All 1375 nodules have undergone biopsy.

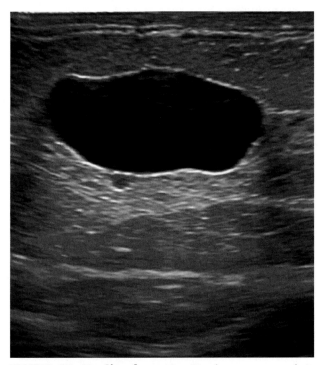

FIGURE 20-40. Simple cysts. Simple cysts are anechoic and have enhanced sound transmission, well-circumscribed borders, thin-edge shadows, and thin, echogenic walls. They are benign (BIRADS 2) and require no aspiration or follow-up.

containing papillomas or carcinomas, and are part of the broad spectrum of benign **fibrocystic change** (FCC). Cysts that have both complex and complicated features should be classified as the more suspicious of the two, complex.

In general, clinicians are too concerned about cysts that are not simple. A good general rule is that most nonsimple cysts fall within the benign FCC spectrum, and malignant cysts are relatively uncommon. However, general rules are never comforting to an individual patient, who is usually quite sure she is the exception to the rule. The greatest difficulty in developing a systematic algorithm for evaluating nonsimple breast cysts is that the "gold standard" for diagnosing cysts (aspiration

with fluid cytology or follow-up) is much less reliable than the histologic gold standard used for solid nodules. It takes many more cases over a much longer period to develop an algorithm for nonsimple cysts than it does for developing a solid nodule algorithm. The algorithm used for evaluation of nonsimple cysts has been derived from the mammographic and solid nodule algorithms. It contains multiple suspicious and benign findings, requires looking for suspicious findings first, and looking for benign findings only in cases with no suspicious findings. The presence of even a single suspicious finding requires exclusion from BIRADS 2 category, and in most cases, exclusion from the BIRADS 3 category as well.

Every effort should be made to characterize as many nonsimple cysts as BIRADS 2 as possible. There are simply too many nonsimple cysts to biopsy, aspirate, or even follow. However, cysts that are not simple must meet strict criteria before they can be characterized as BIRADS 2 or even BIRADS 3, and any cyst characterized as BIRADS 3 lesions should undergo short-interval follow-up. If strict criteria for BIRADS 2 or 3 cannot be met, the lesion should be characterized as BIRADS 4a by default. We believe strongly that complex cysts classified as BIRADS 4a should not be assessed with fluid cytology, but should be evaluated histologically, preferably by ultrasound-guided directional vacuum-assisted biopsy (DVAB). A marker should always be deployed in cases undergoing ultrasound-guided DVAB. If the histology reveals atypia or malignancy, the marker will be necessary to help localize the biopsy site for surgical excision.

Intracystic Papillary Lesions

Cysts that are not simple may involve an intracystic papillary lesion or inflammation and infection. Sonography does not distinguish benign intracystic papilloma from carcinoma as effectively as it characterizes solid nodules because of the direction of invasion. Invasion arising from solid nodules is *outwardly* directed, greatly affecting the shape and the surface characteristics of the lesion. However, invasion arising from intracystic lesions

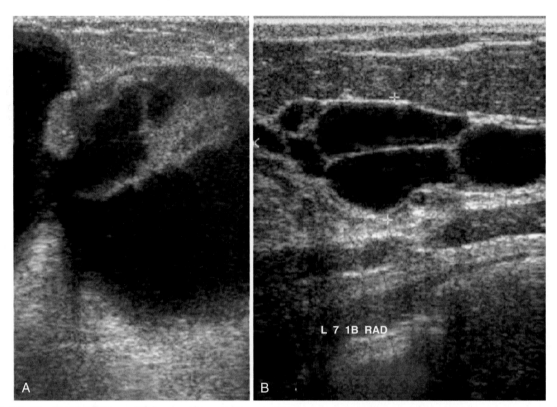

FIGURE 20-41. Septations within cystic masses. A, Thick, isoechoic septations within complex cysts are suspicious for intracystic papilloma or intracystic papillary carcinoma. **B,** Thin, echogenic septations within complex cysts are not suspicious. Such septations represent residual walls of cystically dilated acini within a single TDLU and can be thought of as clusters of simple cysts.

is *inwardly* directed, into the fibrovascular stalk of the lesion. It does not affect the surface characteristics and shape necessary for sonographic characterization of solid nodules, making the findings used for solid nodules less effective for cysts. Any intracystic papillary lesion should be characterized as BIRADS 4a or higher and undergo histologic evaluation. Acutely inflamed or infected cysts can be characterized as BIRADS 3 and can undergo ultrasound-guided aspiration. The aspirated fluid should be sent for Gram stain and culture, but generally not for cytology.

Findings that are suspicious for true intracystic papillary lesions include thick isoechoic septations, certain mural nodules, a Doppler-demonstrable vascular stalk within a thick septation, and clustered complex microcysts. Thick, isoechoic septations are suspicious for **intracystic papilloma** or **intracystic carcinoma** (Fig. 20-41, *A*), whereas thin echogenic septations merely represent **fibrocystic change** and the intact walls between multiple ductules with severe cystic dilation within an individual TDLU (Fig. 20-41, *B*). Most **mural nodules** are caused by **papillary apocrine metaplasia** (PAM), which is part of the benign FCC spectrum, or they are pseudonodules caused by tumefactive sludge or lipid layers rather than papillomas or intracystic papillary carcinomas. Suspicious mural nodules demonstrate loss of the thin echogenic outer cyst wall along their points of attachment, extension beyond the circular or oval

shape of the cyst into surrounding ducts (Fig. 20-42, *A*), or angular margins at the point of attachment. Mural nodules that are caused by PAM remain confined within the circular or round shape of the cyst in which they lie and do not disrupt the thin, echogenic outer cyst wall (Fig. 20-42, *B*).

Papillomas and intracystic carcinomas are generally vascular and tend to develop easily demonstrable and prominent vascular stalks (Fig. 20-43, *A*), whereas mural nodules and thick internal septations caused by florid PAM rarely develop vascular stalks (Fig. 20-43, *B*). Papillomas and intracystic carcinomas frequently undergo hemorrhagic infarction that can obscure vascularity. Most benign intracystic papillomas have a single feeding vessel, whereas malignant intracystic papillary lesions tend to incite the formation of multiple feeding vessels (Fig. 20-43, *B*). Clustered complex microcysts most frequently merely represent FCC and apocrine metaplasia (Fig. 20-44, *A*), but high-nuclear-grade micropapillary DCIS can also appear as complex clustered microcysts (Fig. 20-44, *B*). The gray-scale appearances of microcysts caused by apocrine metaplasia and micropapillary DCIS, unfortunately, are virtually indistinguishable. However, clustered microcysts caused by micropapillary DCIS are usually vascular on color Doppler sonography, whereas microcysts caused by apocrine metaplasia, like mural nodules caused by apocrine metaplasia, are usually avascular on color Doppler ultrasound assessment. A positive

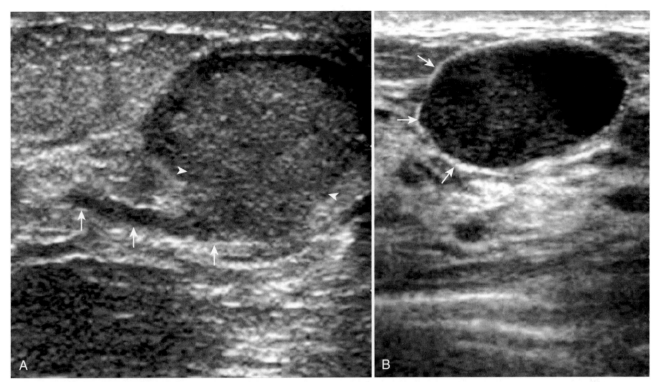

FIGURE 20-42. Complex cysts with mural nodules. A, Mural nodules that protrude beyond a circular or elliptical shape *(arrowheads),* lack a thin echogenic capsule at the point of attachment to the cyst wall, are angular at the point of attachment, or extend into surrounding ducts *(arrows)* are suspicious for intracystic papilloma or intracystic papillary carcinoma. **B,** Mural nodules that are caused by papillary apocrine metaplasia (PAM) remain confined within the circular or elliptical shape of the cyst. The thin, echogenic outer wall of the cyst is intact all along the attached surface of the mural nodule *(arrows).*

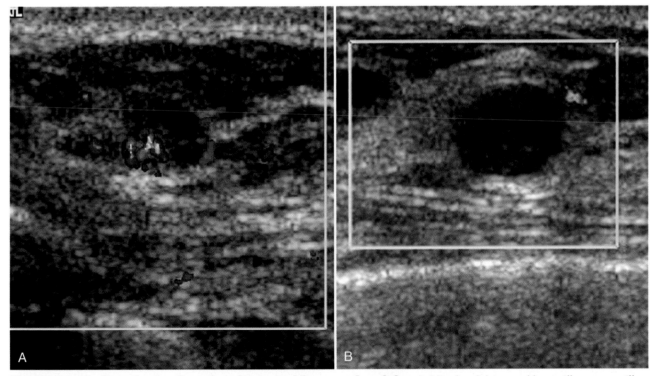

FIGURE 20-43. Use of color Doppler ultrasound for mural nodules. A, Mural nodules caused by papilloma or papillary carcinoma frequently have very prominent vascular stalks. Mural nodules caused by intracystic carcinoma, as in this case, tend to be fed by multiple vessels, whereas benign papillomas tend to be fed by a single vessel. **B,** Mural nodules caused by PAM rarely develop a fibrovascular stalk with demonstrable flow on color Doppler ultrasound.

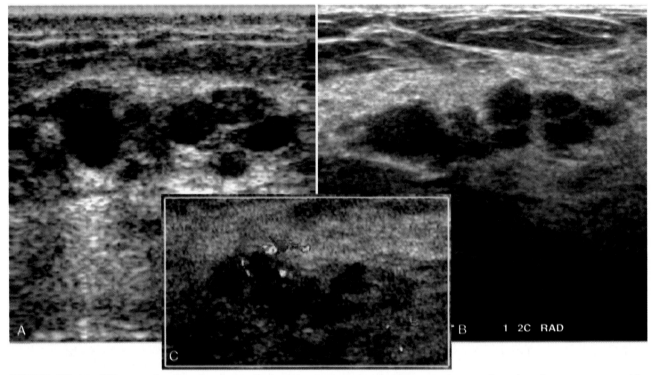

FIGURE 20-44. Microcysts. Complex clustered microcysts can represent **A,** fibrocystic change, where the microcysts are caused by PAM, or **B,** neoplasm, where the microcysts represent ducts distended with secretions and micropapillary DCIS. Unfortunately, the grayscale appearances of fibrocystic change (FCC) and DCIS may be indistinguishable. **C,** However, complex clustered microcysts caused by micropapillary DCIS frequently show internal blood flow on color or power Doppler ultrasound, whereas clustered microcysts caused by PAM, as with mural nodules caused by PAM, rarely have demonstrable internal flow.

Doppler ultrasound assessment is always a better positive predictor than a negative Doppler ultrasound assessment is a negative predictor. If even one of these suspicious findings is present, the cystic lesion should be characterized as BIRADS 4a or higher and should be evaluated histologically (Fig. 20-45).

Inflammation and Infection

The findings that are suspicious for acute inflammation or infection are (1) uniform isoechoic thickening of the cyst wall, (2) fluid-debris levels (tumefactive sludge or layered pus), and (3) inflammatory hyperemia of cyst wall and surrounding tissues. Usually, all three findings coexist (Fig. 20-46, *A*). Uniform isoechoic thickening is typical of inflammation, not tumor, so this finding does not raise much concern about malignancy. Debris levels can be shown to shift to the dependent portion of the complex cyst when the patient is placed in lateral decubitus or upright positions (Fig. 20-46, *B* and *C*). However, tumefactive sludge may be so viscous that it requires 5 minutes or more to shift to the new dependent position. The hyperemic vessels in the wall of inflamed cysts course in a direction parallel to the cyst wall, in contrast to vessels that feed intracystic malignancies, which tend to course perpendicular to the cyst wall. Uniform wall thickening may be seen in cysts with fibrotic walls, but in such cases, there is no hyperemia

or tenderness of the thickened wall because cysts with fibrotic walls represent the healed phase of acute inflammation.

These findings indicate acute inflammation, which is common in FCC, but do not necessarily indicate infection. Even after aspirating pus under ultrasound guidance, the clinician cannot determine whether the cyst is infected or merely inflamed. This requires Gram stain and culture.

The fluid and debris within acutely inflamed cysts usually can be completely aspirated, but the residually thickened cyst wall will persist. If the cyst was not infected, usually the fluid and debris do not reaccumulate, and the residually thickened wall gradually resolves over a few days. A short-interval follow-up in 10 to 14 days may be done to document resolution.

Because the sonographic appearances of acute inflammation are so characteristic and do not raise questions about neoplasm, we usually do not perform cytologic evaluation of the aspirated cyst fluid. Rather, we obtain Gram stain and culture and for most patients provide a 72-hour antibiotic coverage for *Staphylococcus* while awaiting culture results.

Benign (BIRADS 2) Cysts

Only when there are no findings suspicious for true intracystic papillary lesions or acute inflammation do we

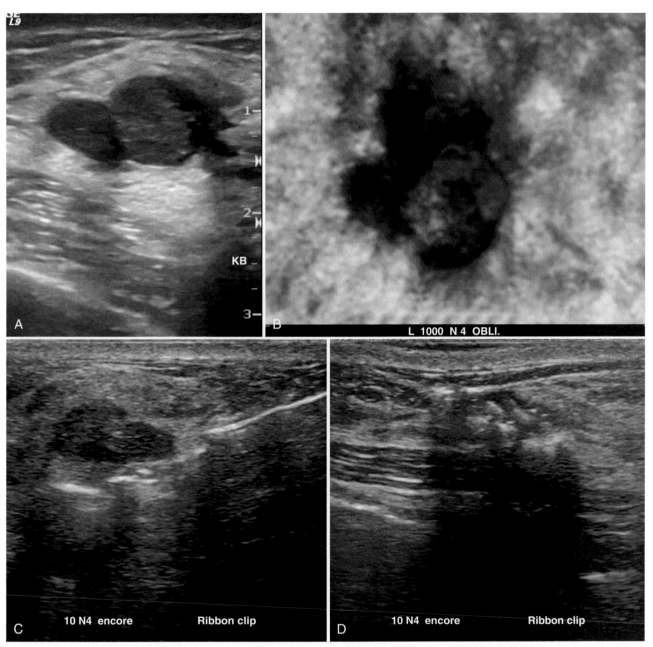

FIGURE 20-45. Ultrasound-guided vacuum-assisted needle biopsy of suspicious complex cyst. Fluid cytology is inadequate for evaluating complex cysts, so histology is necessary. Ultrasound-guided, vacuum-assisted biopsy with marker deployment is our preferred method. **A,** Standard radial view of a complex cyst nearly filled by a bilobed mural nodule. **B,** Three-dimensional maximum-intensity projection (MIP) image of the complex cyst. **C,** Aperture of the vacuum needle is positioned under the lesion. **D,** The lesion has been removed, and echogenic air-impregnated pellets that contain a metallic clip have been placed. Histology showed an intracystic papilloma with atypical duct hyperplasia.

look for "definitively benign" (BIRADS 2) findings. Many types of nonsimple cysts can be characterized as BIRADS 2, and these generally would be classified as complicated cysts rather than complex cysts in the ACR BIRADS ultrasound lexicon. Cysts that can be characterized as BIRADS 2 include (1) cysts with mobile cholesterol crystals, (2) cysts with milk of calcium, (3) cysts with fat-fluid levels, (4) lipid cysts, (5) cysts with calcified walls, (6) cysts with thin echogenic septations, and (7) cysts of skin origin.

Cysts can contain particles suspended in fluid that are so light that they can be moved by the energy of the B-mode imaging or color or power Doppler ultrasound beam. Such particles are subcellular in size and are often seen with uncomplicated FCC. Generally, high-transmit power settings are necessary to cause such particles to move during real-time B-mode imaging. However, the energy of the color or power Doppler ultrasound beam is high enough to cause these particles to move at even default low-power settings, creating what has been

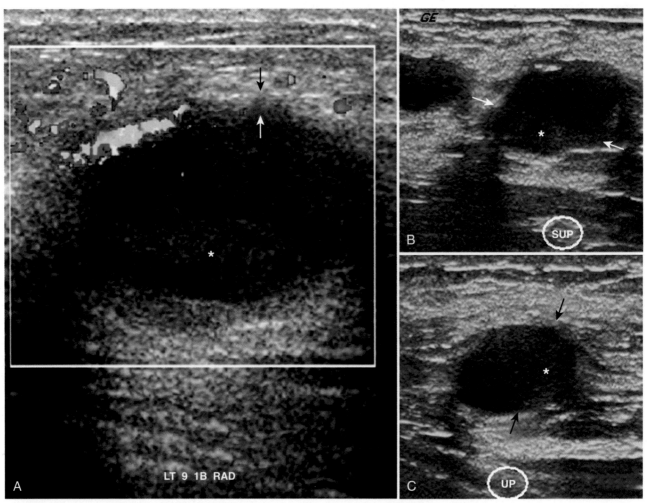

FIGURE 20-46. Inflamed or infected cyst. A, Acutely inflamed or infected cysts demonstrate three findings: (1) abnormal uniform isoechoic wall thickening *(between arrows),* (2) dependent debris *(asterisk),* and (3) hyperemia of the thickened wall. **B,** Supine, and **C,** upright, images show the debris *(asterisk),* resembling sludge within a gallbladder, shifting to the dependent part of the cyst when the position of the patient is changed from supine to upright or lateral decubitus positions. Note the change in the position of the interface between the nondependent fluid and the dependent debris or pus *(between arrows).*

termed "color streaking." Particles are forced posteriorly by the energy of the Doppler ultrasound beam, creating vertically oriented color streaks within the cyst as they move (Fig. 20-47). The particles that cause color streaking appear to be cholesterol crystals, which can be seen on cytologic evaluation as birefractive crystals when viewed with polarized light.

Milk of calcium is a BIRADS 2 mammographic finding that has been directly applied to sonography. Milk of calcium is a collection of tiny calculi within the lumen of a cyst. Such calculi are very common in benign FCC and can be demonstrated definitively on horizontal beam mammographic films. Sonography can prove the presence of milk of calcium by demonstrating that the calcifications move within the cyst to new dependent positions created by lateral decubitus or upright positioning of the patient (Fig. 20-48). Although mammography can generally show smaller and more numerous calcifications, sonography has one advantage over mam-

mography in demonstrating milk of calcium. Mammography requires dozens of small calcifications before the classic "teacup" appearance can be shown on horizontal beam films, whereas sonography can definitively demonstrate milk of calcium even with only a single mobile calculus in a cyst (Fig. 20-49). Thus, although less sensitive than mammography for calcifications, sonography can be more specific than mammography for milk of calcium. This is particularly true in cases where mammography shows a nonspecific cluster of punctate microcalcifications that might require biopsy, but sonography shows benign clustered microcysts, each containing one or more tiny calculi (Fig. 20-50).

Fat-fluid levels within cysts are definitively benign mammographic findings that have been directly applied to ultrasound. Fat-fluid levels are rarely demonstrated on mammography, and usually only within classic galactoceles, but are much more frequently demonstrated by sonography. The lipid layer appears echogenic compared

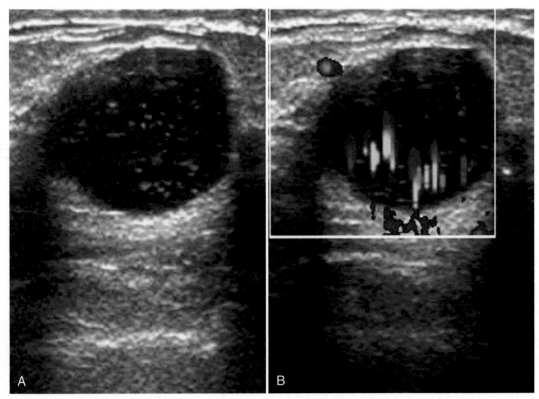

FIGURE 20-47. Cyst with scintillating echoes and color streaking. A, This complicated cyst contains floating punctate echoes that move posteriorly while being scanned, creating a scintillating appearance on gray-scale sonography. **B,** Power Doppler ultrasound pushes the echoes posteriorly faster and with more energy than does the gray-scale beam. The echoes move fast enough that color persistence creates the appearance of "color streaking," an artifact that should not be confused with blood flow.

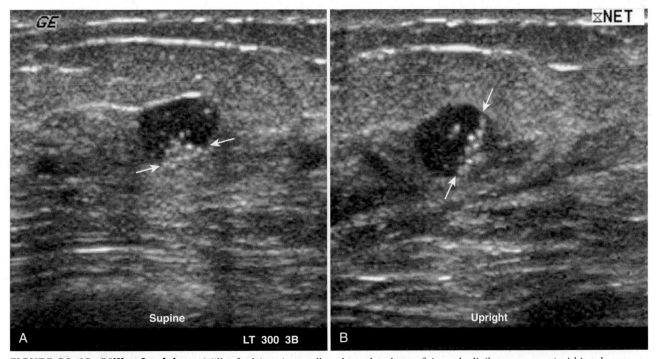

FIGURE 20-48. Milk of calcium. Milk of calcium is actually a dependent layer of tiny calculi *(between arrows)* within a breast cyst that moves when the patient changes position. **A,** The calculi lie along the dependent posterior wall in the supine position. **B,** The calculi fall to the dependent inferior position when the patient is in the upright position and scanned in the longitudinal plane.

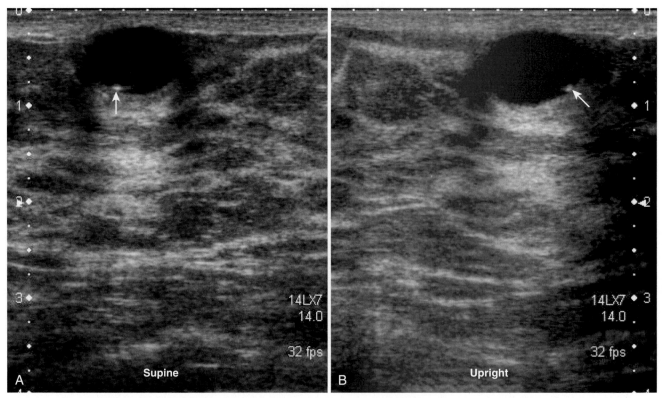

FIGURE 20-49. Milk of calcium presenting as single calculus within cyst. A, Sonogram shows a single stone *(arrow)* lying on the posterior wall of cyst in the supine position. **B,** Stone falls to the dependent inferior wall of the cyst *(arrow)* when the patient is upright and the cyst is scanned in the longitudinal plane.

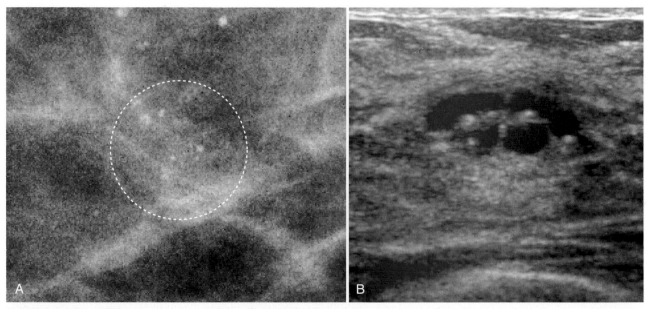

FIGURE 20-50. Milk of calcium within clustered microcysts. A, Mammogram shows a nonspecific cluster of punctate and granular calcifications. **B,** Sonography shows a cluster of microcysts (avascular on color Doppler), many of which contain single dependent calculi, that is definitively benign.

to cyst fluid and floats on the fluid in the nondependent portion of the cyst. The lipid layer can be forced to move within the cyst to a new nondependent position by changing the patient's position from supine to lateral decubitus or upright (Fig. 20-51). As with tumefactive

sludge, lipid layers tend to shift very slowly within a cyst when the patient's position is changed, requiring up to 5 minutes to document the shift of a fat-fluid level. During the shift in position, the shape of the interface between the lipid and fluid layers changes and is usually

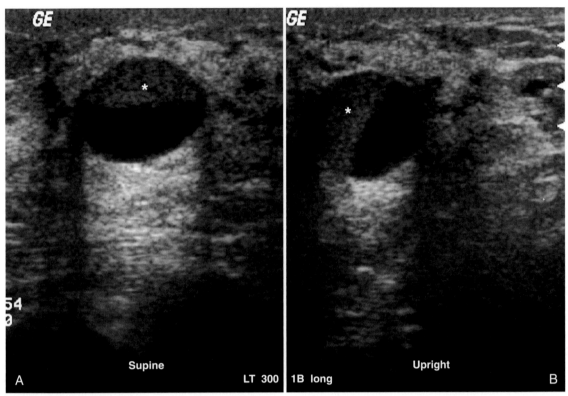

FIGURE 20-51. Fat-fluid level. The lipid layer is echogenic compared with cyst fluid and moves within the cyst to its nondependent part when the patient changes position. **A,** The echogenic lipid layer *(asterisk)* floats to the nondependent anterior wall of the cyst, and the interface is oriented horizontally when the patient is scanned in the supine position. **B,** The echogenic lipid layer *(asterisk)* has floated to the new nondependent superior wall, and the interface is oriented vertically when the patient is in the supine position and the cyst is scanned longitudinally.

obliquely oriented with respect to the tabletop and has a sigmoid shape. The oblique orientation of the interface in combination with the sigmoid shape is characteristic of a fat-fluid level in the process of equilibrating to a new position and may represent a shortcut to waiting 5 minutes for the fat-fluid level to shift. Power Doppler ultrasound **fremitus** can also be used to distinguish a mural nodule from a fat-fluid level. The lipid layer is not attached to the cyst wall, so the fremitus artifact will not pass through it. On the other hand, true papillary lesions that are attached to the cyst wall will vibrate and transmit the fremitus artifact on power Doppler; having the patient hum in a deep voice creates an orange artifact on power Doppler ultrasound (Fig. 20-52).

Lipid cysts or oil cysts are definitively benign mammographic findings that can be applied directly to ultrasound. Unfortunately, lipid cysts usually appear more definitively benign on mammography than sonography. Most lipid cysts lack enhanced sound transmission, and most have some suspicious features on sonography, such as (1) mural nodules; (2) thick septations; (3) thick walls; and (4) fluid debris levels (Fig. 20-53). This should not be surprising because most lipid cysts originate in chronic seromas/hematomas, which often manifest such findings. The suspicious sonographic findings in lipid cysts, unlike those in cysts containing true papillary lesions,

are avascular. Nevertheless, lipid cysts frequently appear more worrisome sonographically than on spot compression mammograms. Thus, when sonographic and mammographic findings are discordant, we rely more on the mammographic findings in this subset of patients, unless color Doppler ultrasound shows internal vascularity.

Eggshell calcifications are benign findings that have been applied directly to sonography. In general, eggshell calcifications are so definitively benign on mammography that they do not require sonographic assessment (Fig. 20-54, *A* and *B*). Occasionally they will be seen on sonography in a patient who has not had mammography or for whom the mammograms are not available. Punctate calcifications that occur within the normal thin, echogenic cyst wall represent incomplete eggshell calcifications and therefore can also be considered to be BIRADS 2 sonographic findings (Fig. 20-54, *C*). In such cases the sonographic findings are more definitively benign than the mammographic findings. Calcifications that are suspended within the lumen of a cyst cannot be characterized as BIRADS 2. In most cases they occur with PAM) but can also occur in DCIS (Fig. 20-54, *D*).

Clustered macrocysts are identical to thinly septated cysts (see Fig. 20-41, *B*). The septations actually represent the residual walls of individual, cystically dilated ductules within an individual TDLU. Each cystically

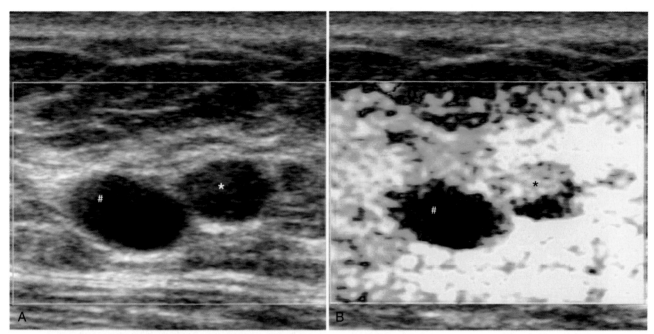

FIGURE 20-52. Acorn cysts of two different types. A, Sonogram shows two cysts that have crescentic echogenic thickening along the anterior wall, resembling the caps on acorns. The echogenic material in the left acorn cyst (#) is **floating lipid debris,** whereas the echogenic material along the anterior wall of the right acorn cyst (*asterisk*) is **papillary apocrine metaplasia** (PAM). Unfortunately, the distinction cannot be made from a single image obtained in the supine position. Changing position can help but often takes 5 minutes; with power Doppler vocal fremitus, the distinction can be made virtually instantly. Having the patient hum in a deep voice creates an **orange artifact** on power Doppler in normal breast tissues and within any mural nodules or thick septations that are attached to the wall of the cyst, but not within unattached debris. **B,** Power Doppler ultrasound image shows that the **vocal fremitus artifact** does not fill the echoes caused by the unattached debris level in the left acorn cyst (#) but does fill the attached echogenic PAM (*asterisk*) within the right acorn cyst.

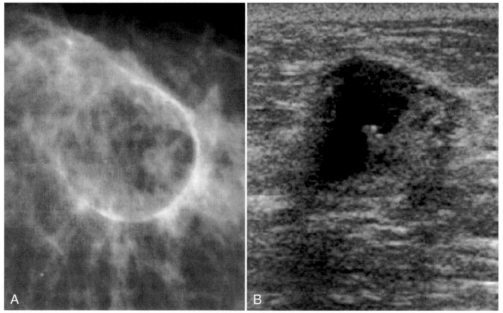

FIGURE 20-53. Lipid cyst. Mammographic spot compression views can more accurately characterize lipid cysts than sonography. On ultrasound images, **A,** lesions that appear to be classic benign lipid cysts on mammography often have suspicious features, such as **B,** thick irregular wall, thick isoechoic septations, and mural nodules. These sonographically suspicious features are typical of chronic hematomas, from which most lipid cysts arise.

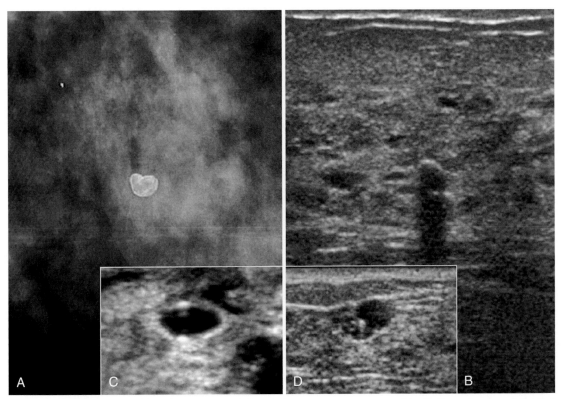

FIGURE 20-54. Eggshell calcification. A, Eggshell calcifications are mammographic findings that are definitively benign. **B,** Dense eggshell calcifications cause acoustic shadowing on ultrasound. **C,** Punctate calcifications confined to the thin echogenic cysts walls can be thought of as incomplete eggshell calcifications and therefore are benign. **D,** Nondependent and nonmobile punctate calcifications within the interior of the cyst are nonspecific and can be associated with PAM or DCIS.

dilated ductule can be thought of as a simple cyst; a thinly septated cyst is actually a cluster of simple cysts, each having BIRADS 2 characteristics.

Cysts of skin origin are benign and usually represent **sebaceous cysts** or **epidermal inclusion cysts.** Sebaceous cysts have three typical appearances: (1) a complex or solid-appearing lesion that lies entirely within the skin (Fig. 20-55, *A*); (2) a complex cyst that lies mainly within the subcutaneous tissues but has clawlike hyperechoic skin wrapped around it (Fig. 20-55, *B*); and (3) a lesion that lies entirely within the subcutaneous fat but has an associated, abnormally hypoechoic, thickened inflamed gland neck that courses through the skin (Fig. 20-55, *C*). The gland neck is obliquely oriented and is often better demonstrated by heeling or toeing the transducer to change the angle of incidence. Because cysts of skin origin are so superficial in location that they are subject to severe volume-averaging artifact, optimal demonstration of one of these three patterns usually requires that an acoustic standoff be used.

Foam and Acorn Cysts

If BIRADS 2 findings cannot be demonstrated, one of two BIRADS 3 appearances can be sought: (1) the "foam cyst" appearance or (2) the "acorn cyst" appearance. **Foam cysts** are cysts whose lumens are completely

filled with low-level echoes (Fig. 20-56, *A*). Other names include gel cysts and inspissated cysts. In fact, the sonographic foam cyst appearance can actually represent a spectrum of lesions, from those completely filled with PAM to those that contain only echogenic proteinaceous debris or lipid material. Other foam cysts may contain mixtures of PAM and proteinaceous or fatty debris. Such lesions have sonographic features that overlap with those of fibroadenomas, and in about 3% of cases, determining with certainty whether the lesion is cystic or solid may not be possible. In these patients, the clinician either must assume that the lesion is a solid nodule and characterize it or must attempt to aspirate it. When assumed to be solid nodules, these lesions usually have characteristics that allow them to be characterized as BIRADS 3. Aspiration may be attempted, but it cannot be determined in advance whether the cyst can be aspirated. When the internal echoes are all caused by PAM, the lesion cannot be aspirated. When the lesion is filled with proteinaceous or fatty debris, it can be completely aspirated. If partially filled with PAM, the lesion will be only partially aspirated. Cytologic evaluation of aspirate of such lesions often shows clusters of apocrine cells diagnostic of benign FCC.

Acorn cysts have either a mural nodule or a crescentic, eccentrically thickened wall caused by PAM that does not completely fill the cyst (Fig. 20-56, *B*). Unlike

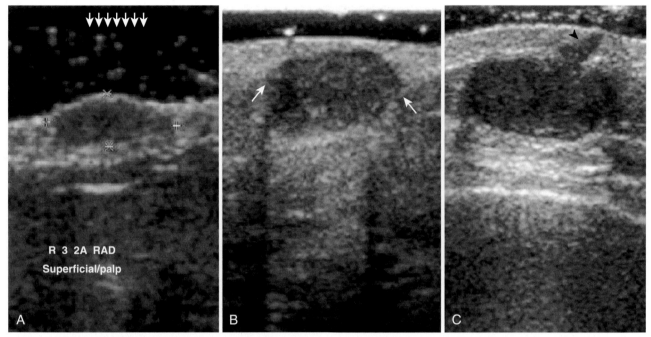

FIGURE 20-55. Benign sebaceous skin cysts. A, Sebaceous cyst is entirely within the skin *(caliper markers).* **B,** Cyst is primarily within the subcutaneous fat, but a thin "claw sign" of echogenic skin *(arrows)* can be shown to wrap around the cyst, confirming that it originates within the skin. **C,** Cyst is entirely within the subcutaneous fat, but a dilated and obstructed gland neck can be seen coursing obliquely through the skin *(arrowhead).* A standoff of acoustic gel is necessary to see these lesions. To show the obliquely oriented hair follicle, heeling or toeing of the transducer may be necessary.

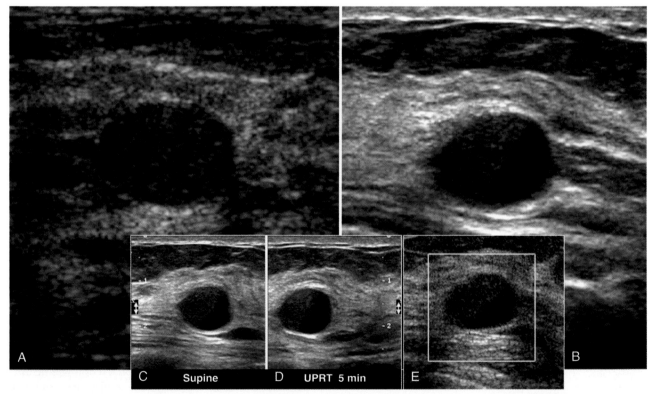

FIGURE 20-56. Foam and acorn cysts. A, Foam cysts are filled with diffuse low-level echoes and can be difficult to distinguish from solid nodules. Foam cysts have also been called **inspissated cysts, gel cysts,** and **mucoceles. B,** Acorn cysts have an echogenic concave rim of papillary apocrine metaplasia (PAM) that appears similar to the cap on an acorn. Unlike similar-appearing lipid layers within cysts that have fat-fluid levels, the position of the PAM does not change from the supine **(C)** to the upright **(D)** or left lateral decubitus positions. **E,** Color Doppler ultrasound image shows that, unlike intracystic papillomas or carcinomas, PAM rarely has a demonstrable vascular stalk.

the echogenic crescent within cysts that contain fat-fluid levels, the echogenic crescent caused by PAM does not shift within the cyst when the patient changes position, regardless of duration (Fig. 20-56, *C* and *D*). In these cases the normal, thin, echogenic outer cyst wall is preserved along the entire thickened wall, and there is no vascular stalk (Fig. 20-56, *E*).

Acorn cysts and foam cysts that are characterized as BIRADS 3 should undergo short-interval follow-up. If it cannot be determined whether a lesion is cystic or solid, and if it can be characterized as BIRADS 3, the patient should be offered the options of attempted aspiration, biopsy, or short-interval follow-up. Unfortunately, if one of these lesions cannot be completely aspirated, one should proceed with DVAB and deployment of a marker. If a complex cyst cannot be characterized as BIRADS 2 or 3, it must be characterized as BIRADS 4a and evaluated histologically. The algorithm for complex cysts is necessarily elaborate because of their wide histopathologic variability.

NICHE APPLICATIONS FOR BREAST ULTRASOUND

There are several niche indications for breast ultrasound that occur much less frequently than palpable and mammographic abnormalities. These include assessment of nipple discharge, mastitis, implants, and regional lymph nodes, as well as correlation with contrast-enhanced breast magnetic resonance imaging (MRI), so-called second-look ultrasound after MRI. Assessment of regional lymph nodes and MRI correlation are the newest and fastest-growing niche applications.

Nipple Discharge

Nipple discharge is an important niche application for breast ultrasound. Nipple discharge can be caused by large duct papillomas, carcinoma, duct ectasia, benign fibrocystic change with communicating cysts, and hyperprolactinemia. In some cases the discharge is idiopathic.

Galactography is still considered the procedure of choice for evaluating nipple discharge, but the role of ultrasound has expanded, primarily because ultrasound-guided DVAB is such an effective way to diagnose and remove papillomas. Sonography is used when galactography fails technically or the patient's intermittent discharge has stopped. Ultrasound can also be used with galactography and in some cases can obviate both diagnostic and localizing galactography and surgery. Even when an intraductal papillary lesion is demonstrated by galactography, ultrasound is required because it is much more practical to perform ultrasound-guided DVAB of an intraductal papillary lesion than stereotactic biopsy with galactographic demonstration of the affected duct and lesion. Additionally, sonography can be justified

for evaluation of low-risk nipple discharge, whereas galactography should be reserved for high-risk discharge. **High-risk discharge** is unilateral, spontaneous, from a single duct orifice, and clear, serous, serosanguineous, or frankly bloody. Discharge is considered high risk because it is often caused by papillomas or carcinoma. Galactography is practical because only a single duct system needs to be evaluated. **Low-risk discharge** is bilateral, from multiple duct orifices, is expressible rather than spontaneous, and is milky or greenish in color. It is considered low risk because it is usually caused by fibrocystic change or duct ectasia. It is not practical to perform galactography on multiple duct systems in the same side, which would be necessary for many cases of low-risk-secretions; however, it is possible to evaluate all the ductal systems in a breast with ultrasound. Furthermore, in my experience, even low-risk secretions can also be caused by intraductal papillary lesions, which sonography can readily demonstrate.

Most **intraductal papillary lesions** that cause nipple discharge lie within the large mammary ducts under or near the areola. Such ducts are readily demonstrated on sonography if appropriate scan planes and maneuvers are used, especially when the ducts are distended with secretions. The central ducts are generally radially oriented, so radial scans are essential to demonstrate the ducts optimally in their long axis. Warm room temperature, warm acoustic gel, and special maneuvers, such as the two-handed compression maneuver and the rolled nipple technique, help minimize shadowing that can arise in the nipple and areola.

Large **duct papillomas** appear to be isoechoic nodules (less echogenic than the duct wall) within ectatic fluid-filled ducts. The appearance of papillomas varies with the degree and distribution of duct dilation, with the diameter and length of the lesion, and with involvement of branch ducts and TDLUs. Small, ovoid lesions less than 1 cm in length that do not expand the duct lumen are benign in more than 98% of cases and qualify for BIRADS 3 characterization (Fig. 20-57). However, because they cause an offensive discharge, papillomas are usually removed at the patient's request, even when classified as probably benign. Intraductal papillary lesions that expand the duct to a greater degree than the associated duct ectasia, that are longer than 1.5 cm, or that involve branch ducts have a greater than 2% risk of being malignant and should be characterized as BIRADS 4a or higher (Fig. 20-58). Papillary lesions that affect TDLUs are, by definition, **peripheral papillomas,** regardless of their distance from the nipple. Peripheral papillomas are at much higher risk than large duct papillomas. Any papillary lesion that arises from or involves a TDLU must be considered at least "mildly suspicious" and should be characterized as BIRADS 4a or higher and biopsied.

Sonography can show causes of nipple discharge other than large duct papilloma, such as **carcinoma, duct ectasia, communicating cysts,** and **hyperprolactinemia**

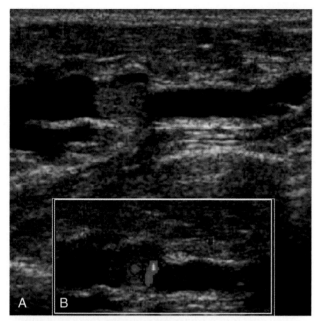

FIGURE 20-57. Intraductal papillary lesion. A, Small, ovoid intraductal papillary lesions that do not expand the duct represent benign large duct papillomas in more than 98% of cases. **B,** Even small intraductal papillomas typically have a readily demonstrable vascular stalk.

(Fig. 20-59). Galactography is probably superior to sonography for demonstrating causes of nipple discharge other than papilloma. Our current practice is to schedule patients who present with nipple discharge for both sonography and galactography.

When ultrasound-guided DVAB is used to biopsy intraductal papillary lesions, a marker is deployed to facilitate image-guided excisional biopsy should the histology be atypical or malignant. In 90% of patients in whom all imaging evidence of the lesion is removed, the nipple discharge stops for at least 2 years.

Infection

The main uses of sonography in patients who present with mastitis is to determine whether there is an abscess, to determine its maturity and whether or not it is multiloculated, and to guide aspiration of, or drain placement into, the abscess in appropriate cases. The appearance of abscesses varies, depending on whether the mastitis is puerperal or nonpuerperal and whether it is centrally or peripherally located. **Peripheral abscesses** in puerperal mastitis usually arise in preexisting galactoceles (Fig. 20-60) whereas peripheral abscesses in nonpuer-

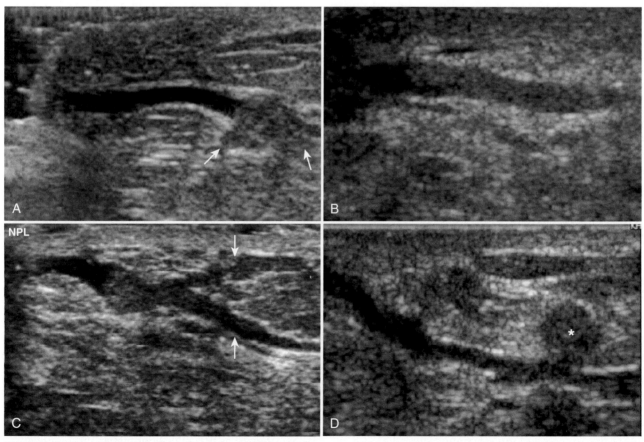

FIGURE 20-58. High-risk intraductal papillary lesions. Intraductal papillary lesions that have greater than a 2% risk of being malignant and that should be characterized as BIRADS 4 and undergo biopsy include **A,** lesions that expand the duct or breach *(arrows)* its wall; **B,** lesions that are longer than 1.5 cm; **C,** lesions that involve multiple peripheral branch ducts *(arrows),* or **D,** lesions that involve TDLUs *(asterisk)* (peripheral papillomas).

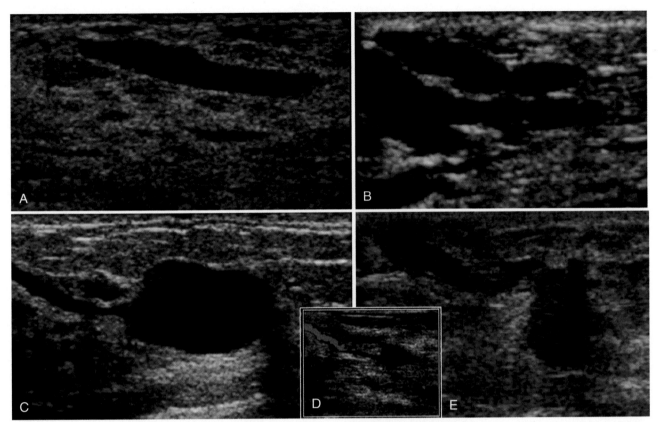

FIGURE 20-59. Lesions other than papillomas that cause nipple discharge. Duct ectasia usually involves one lobar ductal system at a time. **A,** Early in its course, only a single duct might be involved. **B,** Over time, additional lobar ducts can become involved, leading to multiple dilated ducts. When all the ducts are severely involved, one must consider hyperprolactinemia as an underlying factor. **C,** Communicating cysts. **D,** Confirmation that the cyst truly communicates with the ductal system can be made by showing a "color-swoosh" with the communicating duct when the cyst undergoes ballottement with the transducer. **E,** Pure ductal carcinoma in situ (DCIS) and invasive duct carcinomas that have DCIS components can also give rise to nipple discharge.

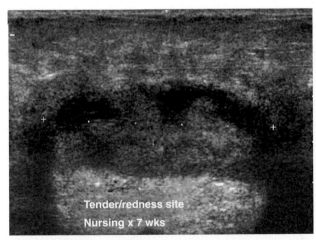

FIGURE 20-60. Peripheral puerperal abscess. Often arising within preexisting galactoceles, peripheral puerperal abscesses *(caliper markers)* have very irregular walls and mixtures of fluid and echogenic debris.

peral mastitis often arise within inflamed cysts. **Central abscesses**, whether arising from puerperal or nonpuerperal mastitis (Fig. 20-61), usually result from rupture of an inflamed or infected duct and tend to be elongated in a plane that is parallel to the inflamed duct. Unilocular

abscesses can be treated with ultrasound-guided aspirations as needed. Loculated abscesses may require placement of a drain or surgical drainage. In some cases, sonography may be used to determine if there is an underlying inflammatory carcinoma.

Implants

Magnetic resonance imaging is generally considered the modality of choice for evaluating mammary implants. However, most patients with implants at risk for **rupture** are within the mammographic screening cohort. Patients with implants present with palpable lumps and mammographic densities that require sonographic evaluation much more often than they present for MR evaluation of their implants. Thus, sonographers must understand the wide variations of normal in implants and must be able to identify intracapsular and extracapsular rupture, silicone granulomas, herniation, and capsular infection.

Sonography allows identification of the type of implant, its implantation site, and many associated complications. The **capsule** that surrounds the implant is fibrous and is a normal foreign body reaction to the implant. The capsule is abnormal only when (1) it becomes too thick and causes capsular contracture, (2) it develops a tear through which the implant can herniate, or (3) it becomes inflamed or infected. The implant is filled with saline or silicone gel and is surrounded by a silicone elastomer shell. The **shell**, a part of the implant, must be distinguished from the capsule, which is living tissue formed by the patient in response to the implant.

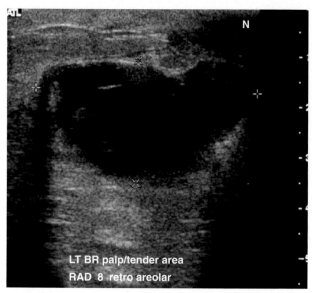

FIGURE 20-61. Central periareolar abscess. Whether puerperal or nonpuerperal, central periareolar abscesses *(caliper markers)* usually arise when an inflamed or infected duct ruptures, spilling its contents into the periductal tissues; *n,* nipple.

Normal implants can give rise to palpable abnormalities in certain cases. **Radial folds** may be palpable when the patient is in certain positions. It is important to scan the patient when she is in the position where she feels the lump, because radial folds are dynamic and frequently present only in certain positions, usually upright. Only anteriorly located radial folds will be palpable (Fig. 20-62, *A*). Radial folds on the posterior surface of the implant are almost never palpable. In patients with saline implants, the **fill valve** can cause palpable abnormalities. Fill valves are generally placed behind the nipple. In certain cases, however, the valve may not be placed directly behind the nipple, or the implant may have rotated after placement. In such cases the valve may be palpable if overlying breast tissue is minimal. In other cases, valves become palpable years after the implant is placed because of eversion of the valve (Fig. 20-62, *B*). **Eversion** is most likely to occur in implants that are under chronic pressure resulting from capsular contracture.

In **intracapsular rupture** the shell develops a tear through which silicone gel extravasates into the space between the shell and the capsule; the capsule remains intact. The classic findings of intracapsular rupture are the **stepladder sign** ("linguini" sign in MRI literature) and abnormally increased echogenicity in the extravasated gel that lies within the intracapsular extrashell space (Fig. 20-63). Unfortunately, these signs have low sensitivity for intracapsular rupture because they are only present in cases where nearly all the silicone gel has extravasated from the shell and the shell is completely

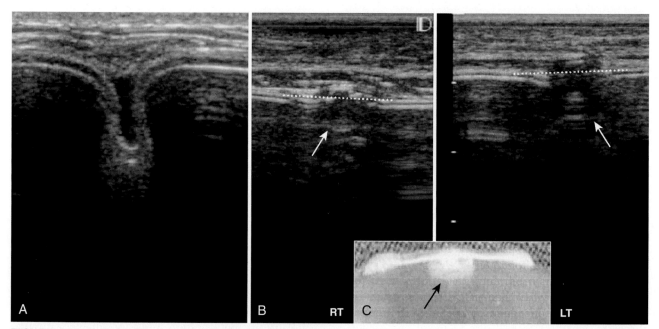

FIGURE 20-62. Palpable implant components. A, Anterior radial folds can cause palpable abnormalities; these folds often feel "crinkly." **B,** Single-lumen saline implants have fill valves. In some cases, particularly with capsular contracture, increased pressure within the implant may cause the valve, which is normally flush with the outer surface of the implant shell *(RT, dotted line),* to evert and become palpable *(LT).*

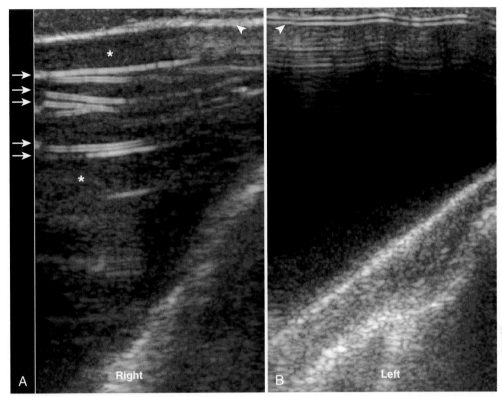

FIGURE 20-63. Breast implant rupture. A, Classic findings of intracapsular rupture of a single-lumen silicone gel implant are the "stepladder sign" *(arrows)* and hyperechoic silicone gel *(asterisk)* in the right breast. Several linear, horizontally oriented echoes represent folds in a collapsed shell. Several of these are double echogenic lines that represent the inner and outer surfaces of each fold of the shell *(arrows)*. The extravasated gel that lies outside the implant shell has become hyperechoic *(asterisk)*. Note that only a single echogenic line that represents the peri-implant capsule can be seen on the right *(arrowhead)*. **B, Normal left breast implant.** Note that the superficial aspect of the unruptured left implant shows the double echogenic line *(white arrowhead)* of the shell at the anterior aspect of the silicone gel.

collapsed. In cases of intracapsular rupture, lesser degrees of collapse merely lead to abnormal, sheetlike separation of the shell inwardly away from the capsule (Fig. 20-64, *A*). There is a continuous spectrum of intracapsular collapse from involvement of a single radial fold to complete collapse. Radial folds are quite dynamic, forming when the patient is in one position, then disappearing when the patient assumes another position; the apex of radial folds therefore is prone to fatigue fractures. Because radial folds normally contain anechoic peri-implant effusion that is identical to silicone gel in echogenicity, for any individual radial fold, it is impossible to know whether the fluid within the fold is normal effusion or extravasated silicone gel from a fatigue fracture at the apex of the fold, unless the extravasated gel within the fold becomes hyperechoic (Fig. 20-64, *B*). Radial folds should be considered normal unless they contain hyperechoic contents (snowstorm appearance). Intracapsular ruptures with only minimal collapse can be distinguished from radial folds by shape that can be evaluated with orthogonal views that are oriented parallel and perpendicular to the long axis of the fold. Radial folds are one-dimensional (1-D), showing a long separation between the capsule and shell parallel to the long axis of the fold,

but a very short separation when the fold is imaged perpendicular to the long axis (Fig. 20-64, *B*). Intracapsular ruptures are 2-D, showing long, capsular-shell separations in both views (Fig. 20-64, *A*).

In **extracapsular rupture** there is a tear in the capsule as well as in the shell, and silicone gel extravasates into the breast tissues outside the capsule. By definition, all cases of extracapsular rupture must be preceded by intracapsular rupture, although in many cases the intracapsular component is difficult to demonstrate sonographically. Extracapsular rupture indicates that silicone gel has extravasated not only from the implant shell, but also through the capsule into surrounding tissues. The classic finding is the **silicone granuloma** with a "snowstorm" appearance. Such granulomas are markedly hyperechoic and well circumscribed anteriorly but have an incoherent, "dirty" shadow posteriorly. Silicone granulomas can occur superficial to implants (Fig. 20-65, *A*), but they most often occur at the edges of the implant, where the shell is thinnest and where fatigue fractures are more likely to occur (Fig. 20-65, *B*). In certain cases, extravasated silicone gel forms a thin sheet over the outer surface of the implant rather than a discrete mass (Fig. 20-65, *C*). In other cases, extravasated silicone gel can migrate

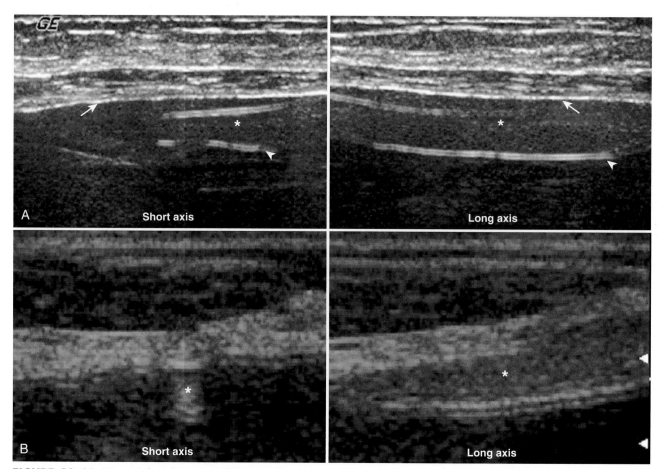

FIGURE 20-64. Breast implant partial rupture. In cases of intracapsular rupture, where collapse is incomplete, the classic stepladder sign may be absent. **A,** In partial collapse, there will be abnormal sheetlike separation between the capsule *(arrow)* and the shell *(arrowhead).* The extravasated gel that has extruded into the abnormal space between the capsule and the shell tends to become hyperechoic over time *(asterisk).* **B,** In many cases the earliest leakage of silicone gel arises from the apex of radial folds, where fatigue fractures of the shell are common. Radial folds are U shaped when viewed in short axis. Only if the fluid within the radial fold becomes hyperechoic *(asterisk)* can one be sure that the fold is the site of intracapsular rupture and not merely a variation of normal.

away from the edge of the implant to the axilla, chest wall, back, or abdominal wall (Fig. 20-65, *D*). Extravasated silicone gel can be picked up and carried by lymphatic vessels into the axillary lymph nodes, where it accumulates from the medullary sinuses within the mediastinum of the lymph node outwardly. Early **accumulation of silicone gel within lymph nodes** can be difficult to detect because the hyperechoic silicone gel has similar hyperechogenicity to the lymph node mediastinum, although gel in the lymph node hilum will cause a subtle, dirty-appearing shadow that will help to detect the silicone gel. As more silicone gel accumulates, the diagnosis of silicone gel accumulation within the lymph node becomes more obvious. When silicone gel fills the cortical sinusoids as well as the medullary sinusoids, the cortex of the lymph node becomes hyperechoic, and dirty shadowing arises from the entire lymph node (Fig. 20-65, *E*).

Silicone granulomas have a spectrum of appearances. Not all present with the classic snowstorm appearance. Large, acute accumulations of extracapsular silicone gel can appear complex and cystic (Fig. 20-66, *A*). Over time, these may become solid appearing and isoechoic (Fig. 20-66, *B*). The classic snowstorm appearance develops late, after the solid, isoechoic phase. Very late in the history of a silicone granuloma, so much foreign body granuloma may develop that the lesion can become hypoechoic, causing architectural distortion and developing more intense acoustic shadowing—findings that simulate those of stellate breast malignant lesions (Fig. 20-66, *C*). The sensitivity of ultrasound for extracapsular rupture will be enhanced if the sonographer can recognize the entire spectrum of its sonographic appearances.

The presence of implants should not discourage necessary ultrasound-guided procedures. With ultrasound guidance, an angle of approach that is almost parallel to the surface of the implant can be used. A large amount of local anesthetic can be injected between the lesion and the implant to "hydrodissect" the lesion away from the implant and create a safe working space.

It is important to remember that patients with implants are subject to the same disease processes as

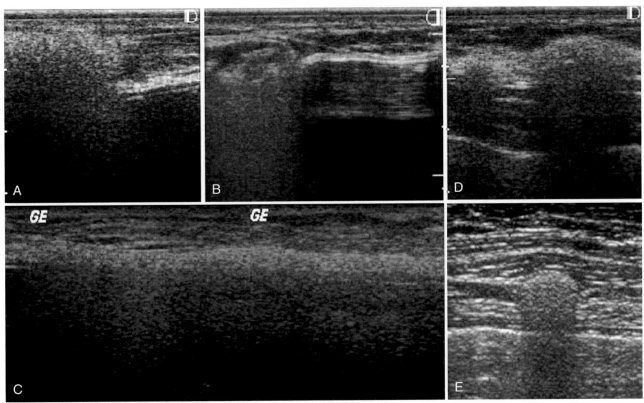

FIGURE 20-65. Silicone granulomas: typical "snowstorm" appearance of extracapsular rupture. Silicone granulomas that manifest the snowstorm sign are hyperechoic and have a well-circumscribed superficial border and a posterior border obscured by "dirty" incoherent shadowing. **A,** Silicone granulomas can occur anterior to the implant. **B,** However, most occur along the edges of the implant, where the shell is thinner. **C,** Silicone granulomas can spread over the surface of the implant in a thin sheet rather than forming a discrete mass. **D,** Silicone granulomas can migrate away from the edge of the implant to lie on the chest or abdominal wall or in the axilla. **E,** Extravasated silicone can be carried by lymphatics to regional lymph nodes, where it fills the lymph nodes with hyperechoic gel, giving a snowstorm appearance, from the medulla outward, as with this Rotter node that lies between the pectoralis major and pectoralis minor muscles.

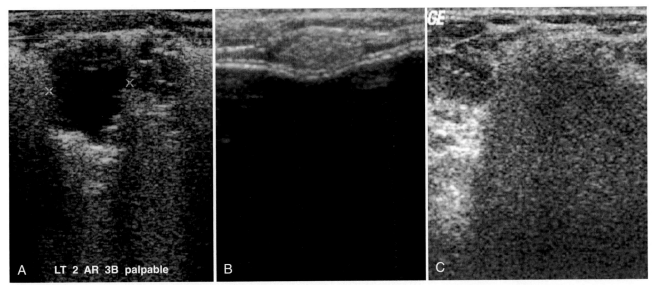

FIGURE 20-66. Silicone granulomas: less common appearances of extracapsular rupture. **A,** Large collections of acutely extravasated silicone gel can have a complex cystic appearance. **B,** Silicone granulomas of a few weeks to a few months' duration can appear to be isoechoic solid nodules. These usually progress to the snowstorm appearance within months. **C,** Silicone granulomas that are many years old can develop so much foreign body reaction that they become intensely shadowing masses that simulate malignancy. Note also that, although most silicone granulomas result from extracapsular rupture, they can form between the capsule and the shell in certain patients, as in image **B.**

patients without implants. Most patients are satisfied with their implants and experience no implant-related problems. The major problem for the sonographer is that the implants are distracting. One may spend so much time and effort assessing implants that one misses the real reason for presentation, a breast cancer. To reduce the risk of missing a breast carcinoma, it is important to evaluate breast tissues *overlying* the implant before turning attention to the implants.

Regional Lymph Node Assessment

The status of lymph nodes and the maximum diameter of breast carcinomas are two of the most important prognostic indicators for invasive breast carcinoma. The sentinel lymph node procedure has evolved into the method of choice for assessing lymph node status. However, ultrasound and ultrasound-guided biopsy can be very useful to assess regional lymph nodes in patients with suspicious breast nodules who are about to undergo ultrasound-guided biopsy of the breast lesion. This can be performed before lumpectomy to help determine whether to perform a sentinel lymph node procedure or to proceed straight to axillary dissection.

Normal lymph nodes have a sonographic appearance similar to miniature kidneys. They are oval shaped in the long axis, C shaped in the short axis, and flat in the AP dimension (Fig. 20-67, *A*). The **cortex** is hypoechoic; the **medulla**, which lies just deep to the cortex, is hyperechoic; and the fat within the **mediastinum** of the lymph node is isoechoic. In younger patients the

entire mediastinum usually appears hyperechoic, but in older patients the hyperechoic mediastinum fills with fat and is compressed into a thin band just deep to the hypoechoic cortex (Fig. 20-67, *B*). The flow of lymph passes through afferent lymphatic channels, which enter the lymph node from the periphery. The lymph then passes, in order, through the subcapsular sinusoids, cortical sinusoids, medullary sinusoids, and then out the efferent lymphatics, which exit through the hilum.

Many gray-scale criteria have evolved for evaluating lymph nodes; including size, shape, and echogenicity. Minimum diameters greater than 1 cm are considered abnormal. However, we have often seen morphologically abnormal metastatic lymph nodes with minimum diameters less than 1 cm and normal atrophic lymph nodes with minimum diameters well over 1 cm. Thus, **size** is a poor criterion for metastasis. Metastatic lymph nodes tend to become **abnormally round** in shape, but unfortunately this is a late finding. The morphologic finding of **eccentric cortical thickening** is much more sensitive than "rounding" of the lymph node. The cortex in some (not all) metastatic lymph nodes becomes **abnormally hypoechoic.** However, the lymph node cortex always appears hypoechoic when scanned with harmonics. We use harmonics in all cases because it makes the lymph node cortex more conspicuous and makes the lymph nodes easier to find and characterize. Thus, harmonics minimizes the usefulness of marked hypoechogenicity as a suspicious finding. Morphologic assessment of the lymph node is more effective than evaluating its size, shape, and echogenicity. Eccentric cortical thickening has

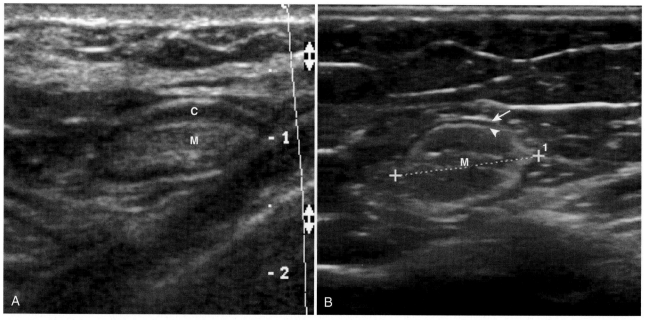

FIGURE 20-67. Lymph node: spectrum of normal appearances. A, In young patients the mediastinum of the lymph node tends to be uniformly hyperechoic because the medullary cords and sinuses fill the entire mediastinum *(m)*. **B,** In older patients who have had repeated episodes of inflammation, the center of the mediastinum *(m)* becomes infiltrated with isoechoic fat, and the medulla *(arrowhead)* becomes compressed into a thin band just deep to the hypoechoic cortex *(c)*.

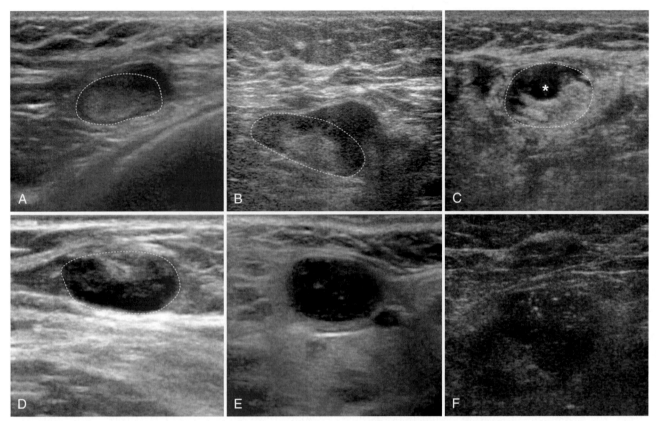

FIGURE 20-68. Hallmark of lymph node metastasis: spectrum of cortical thickening. A, Metastases that implant near the midcortical sinusoids tend to thicken the cortex focally and equally in inward and outward directions. **B,** Metastases that implant within the subcapsular sinusoids tend to cause focal, outwardly bulging cortical thickening ("mouse ear"). **C,** Metastases that implant toward the inner part of the cortical sinusoids cause focal cortical thickenings that bulge inwardly into the lymph node mediastinum ("rat bite" defect). **D,** Metastases that implant extensively throughout the cortical sinusoids can cause symmetrical cortical thickening indistinguishable from the cortical thickening caused by inflammation. **E,** Cortical thickening so severe that the hilum is obliterated is usually caused by metastasis and is strongly against the node being benign and reactive. **F,** Microcalcifications within a lymph node indicate metastasis until proved otherwise, especially if the primary breast lesion presents with microcalcifications.

a high positive predictive value. Lymph nodes that demonstrate eccentric cortical thickening should be considered positive for metastasis. The biopsy should specifically target the area of the cortex that is focally thickened.

Metastases tend initially to implant within the subcapsular or cortical sinusoids and grow there, causing focal cortical thickening. Thus, the hallmark of lymph node metastases is cortical thickening. The pattern of thickening depends on where the metastases first implant. Metastases that implant near the center of the cortical sinusoids tend to widen the cortex focally and equally in inward and outward directions (Fig. 20-68, *A*). Metastases that implant in the subcapsular sinusoids tend to bulge outwardly, creating a "mouse ear" configuration (Fig. 20-68, *B*). Metastases that implant toward the inner side of the cortical sinusoids tend to bulge into the lymph node mediastinum, creating "rat bite" defects in the hilum (Fig. 20-68, *C*). When metastasis fills cortical sinusoids throughout the entire lymph node, the cortical thickening becomes uniform, an appearance that can be simulated by benign reactive lymph nodes (Fig. 20-68, *D*). Metastases cause severe enough cortical thickening

to obliterate the hilum much more frequently than inflammation (Fig. 20-68, *E*). Lymph nodes that contain microcalcifications are metastatic, especially when the primary breast lesion presents with microcalcifications (Fig. 20-68, *F*).

Lymph nodes that demonstrate mild to moderate, symmetrical cortical thickening of 3 mm or greater have a lower positive predictive value for metastasis and are more nonspecific than lymph nodes with clear-cut eccentric cortical thickening. These nodes can be reactive or metastatic; comparing to adjacent lymph nodes is the best way to determine whether a lymph node with symmetrical cortical thickening is a benign reactive node or a metastatic node. Unless there is obvious evidence of inflammation in the ipsilateral breast or upper extremity, reactive lymph nodes are usually reacting to a systemic stimulus; thus all the lymph nodes will be reactive. Usually, more than one axillary lymph node can be seen in the same field of view simply by rotating the transducer. If adjacent lymph nodes show both mild to moderate, symmetrical cortical thickening of near-equal degrees, the nodes are more likely reactive than meta-

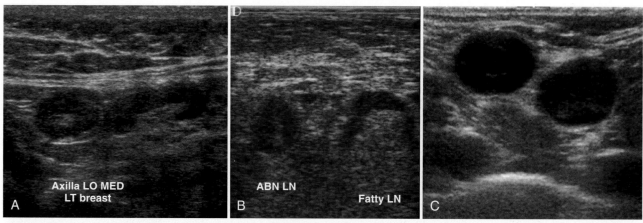

FIGURE 20-69. Comparison with adjacent lymph nodes to assess significance of symmetrical cortical thickening. A, When adjacent lymph nodes within the axilla show similar degrees of symmetrical cortical thickening, the lymph nodes are more likely reactive than metastatic. If contralateral axillary lymph nodes show similar degrees of thickening, the risk of metastasis is reduced even further. **B,** If the adjacent lymph node shows normal cortical thickness, the risk of metastasis in the node with symmetrical cortical thickening is increased. **C,** When the cortical thickening is so severe that the mediastinum of the lymph node is obliterated, the etiology should be assumed to be metastatic, even when adjacent lymph nodes are involved to a similar degree.

static (Fig. 20-69, *A*). However, if the adjacent node is sonographically normal, the node with symmetrical cortical thickening is more likely to be metastatic (Fig. 20-69, *B*). Assessment of adjacent lymph nodes is not necessary when cortical thickening is so severe that the hilum is completely obliterated, because this occurs much more frequently in metastatic than reactive nodes (Fig. 20-69, *C*). Although Doppler sonography can also be used to help determine whether a node with symmetrical cortical thickening is reactive or metastatic, gray-scale imaging of adjacent lymph nodes usually makes this unnecessary.

We now routinely scan the axillary lymph nodes in any patient in whom we find a BIRADS 4 or BIRADS 5 breast lesion. If an abnormal lymph node that is suspicious for metastatic disease is identified, we perform ultrasound-guided core biopsy on the lymph node at the same time the breast lesion is biopsied. If cortical thickening is localized, the part of the node with thickened cortex should be targeted for biopsy (Fig. 20-70). We now place a marker in every lymph node that is biopsied and obtain specimen radiographs of removed lymph nodes to confirm that positive lymph nodes are removed at axillary dissection.

If abnormal lymph nodes are identified within level 1 of the axilla, the next highest level of nodes should be assessed with sonography. As discussed earlier, the pectoralis minor muscle determines the level of the lymph nodes. Nodes that lie lateral and inferior to the lateral edge of the pectoralis muscle are level 1 lymph nodes. These are the first nodes involved by metastases, except in rare cases where the sentinel lymph node is a level 2 node. Lymph nodes behind the pectoralis minor muscle are level 2, and those that lie superior and medial to the medial edge of the pectoralis muscle are level 3, or infra-

clavicular, lymph nodes (Fig. 20-71). Rotter lymph nodes lie between the pectoralis major and minor muscles and lie anterior to and at the same level as level 2 lymph nodes (Fig. 20-72). If undetected and untreated, they can give rise to chest wall invasion. If level 3 nodes are positive, supraclavicular and jugular lymph nodes should be assessed. Internal mammary lymph nodes should be evaluated in all cases, but especially when the primary lesion is medial and deep, and when bulky axillary adenopathy may cause **tumor damming** and collateral flow medially (Fig. 20-73). Presence of metastasis to internal mammary lymph nodes is especially important to patients and radiation oncologists. Internal mammary lymph nodes chains are no longer routinely treated with radiation because of potential long-term cardiac complications. However, if there are known internal mammary nodal metastases, the radiation oncologist will add an internal mammary field to the treatment. Internal mammary lymph node metastasis is most common in the first three interspaces just lateral to the sternum.

If both the breast lesion and the lymph node are positive, a sentinel lymph node procedure becomes unnecessary. However, if the lymph nodes appear normal on sonography, or if nodes appear abnormal and the biopsy is negative, the patient will still need a sentinel lymph node procedure, as originally planned. The value added is in an **abnormal lymph node sonogram with a positive biopsy.** There is no value in a negative lymph node biopsy, and it creates one extra procedure. Thus, we believe that ultrasound-guided lymph node biopsies should be reserved for cases where both the breast lesion and lymph node are highly likely to be malignant. We do not believe that core biopsy of a lymph node with benign cytology adversely affects the sentinel node procedure that is still necessary. Tumor damming within the

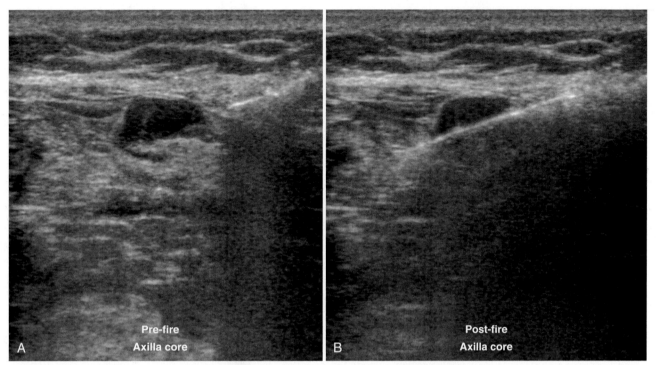

FIGURE 20-70. Ultrasound-guided biopsy of abnormal axillary lymph nodes. Ultrasound-guided biopsy confirming lymph node metastasis obviates a sentinel lymph node procedure and allows the surgeon to proceed directly to axillary dissection. In patients with BIRADS 4 or 5 breast lesions undergoing biopsy, abnormal lymph nodes should be biopsied at the same time. **A,** Prefire image of an abnormal level 1 axillary lymph nodes with eccentric cortical thickening. The needle is specifically targeting the part of the lymph node where the cortex is thickened. **B,** Postfire image shows that the core needle has passes through the abnormally thickened part of the cortex.

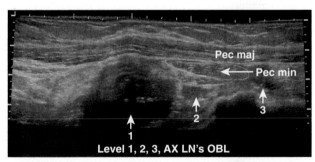

FIGURE 20-71. Metastases to three lymph node levels. Extended-FOV, obliquely oriented sonogram shows metastasis to all three levels of axillary lymph nodes. Massive adenopathy and microcalcifications are seen in a level 1 lymph node that lies lateral and inferior to the pectoralis minor muscle *(dotted oval)*. A mildly enlarged level 2 lymph node lies posterior to the pectoralis muscle. A moderately enlarged level 3 lymph node with a microcalcification lies superior and medial to the pectoralis muscle.

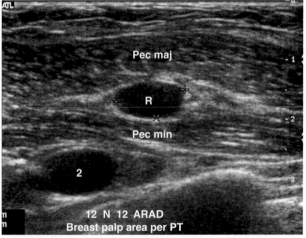

FIGURE 20-72. Metastasis to level 2 and Rotter lymph nodes. Rotter lymph nodes *(R)* lie between the pectoralis minor and major muscles at the same level as level 2 lymph nodes *(2)* and, if unrecognized, can be a source for chest wall invasion. This patient has gross metastasis that obliterates the mediastinum of level 2 and Rotter lymph nodes.

sentinel node that forces collateral flow around the node is the main cause of false-negative sentinel lymph node procedures. These are exactly the nodes that are identified and proved to be positive with sonography. Removing these patients from the sentinel lymph node cohort actually reduces false-negative sentinel lymph node procedures.

Finally, in patients in whom sonography cannot obviate the sentinel lymph node procedure, ultrasound can be used to aid in the injection of technetium sulfur colloid. With the aid of a gamma detector, ultrasound can be used to identify the sentinel node and guide

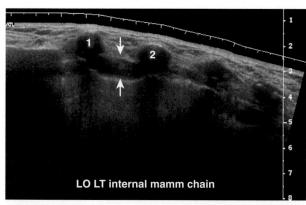

FIGURE 20-73. Metastasis to internal mammary lymph nodes. Long-axis extended-FOV image shows a gross internal mammary lymph node metastasis (between arrows) lying between the first (1) and second (2) costal cartilages.

needle localization of both the primary and the sentinel lymph node.

New contrast agents being developed that specifically enhance lymphatics and lymph node sinusoids will help in identifying lymph node metastases and targeting abnormal areas of lymph node cortex for biopsy.

Sonographic–Magnetic Resonance Correlation

The role of contrast-enhanced MRI in local and regional staging of breast cancer has expanded greatly in recent years, along with the role of ultrasound correlation after MRI. Breast MRI shows the true extent of breast cancer preoperatively better than any other imaging modality, allowing the most appropriate treatment planning. It minimizes positive margins, number of surgeries necessary to obtain clear margins, and true recurrences and so-called recurrences that result from unrecognized and unresected additional foci of carcinoma present before surgery. MRI also shows the size of invasive breast cancers and the associated DCIS components better than other imaging tests. Breast MRI allows detection of ipsilateral multifocal and multicentric and synchronous contralateral malignancy with much higher sensitivity than other modalities. In our patient population, MRI demonstrates multifocal or multicentric disease in 30% of patients and synchronous contralateral breast cancer in 6% of patients.

Although the most sensitive modality for invasive breast cancer, MRI does have problems. First, because of the high rate of false-positive results with contrast-enhanced breast MRI, treatment decisions require histologic confirmation of the cause of abnormal enhancement. Thus, image-guided biopsy of abnormal areas of enhancement is necessary, but MRI-guided biopsy ties up a valuable resource. We believe that MRI-guided biopsies are not as accurate as ultrasound (as long as we are sure that we have accurately identified an area

of abnormal enhancement on MRI) and less accurate than widely believed precisely because MR biopsies are not true real-time biopsies. Further, sensitivity of MRI for DCIS has not been completely established. We believe that MRI is very sensitive for high-nuclear-grade (HNG) DCIS, is moderately sensitive for intermediate-nuclear-grade (ING) DCIS, and has lower sensitivity for low-nuclear-grade (LNG) DCIS, but exact sensitivity is unknown.

Breast ultrasound performed after breast MRI to evaluate areas of abnormal contrast enhancement on MRI (so-called second-look ultrasound, even when a "first look" ultrasound was never performed) can be helpful in overcoming some, but not all, of the limitations of breast MRI. Ultrasound can be very useful in assessing abnormal enhancement shown on MRI and in decreasing false-positive breast MRI results caused by ANDIs. Additionally, ultrasound guidance of interventional procedures is less costly and more efficient than MRI guidance and is truly real-time. Finally, unless Combidex contrast enhancement is used with MRI, sonography is better at characterizing regional lymph nodes and at guiding biopsy of abnormal nodes.

"Second look" breast ultrasound is very effective at confirming the presence of additional ipsilateral or contralateral foci of invasive breast cancer identified on MRI, guiding "mapping" biopsies and localizing the foci for surgery. Invasive breast cancers present primarily with "hard" findings that overlap little with the findings of normal anatomy and benign ANDIs (Fig. 20-74). In most cases with enhancing foci of invasive carcinoma, ultrasound virtually ensures identification of the same invasive lesion identified on MRI. However, sonographic identification of additional foci of DCIS is more difficult. Sonography is not as sensitive for DCIS as it is for invasive breast cancer. DCIS presents with "soft" findings that overlap greatly with the findings of normal anatomy and benign ANDIs. How heavily we weight soft findings sonographically depends on the indication for breast ultrasound. We must keep in mind that "post-test" probability depends on "pretest" probability. In breast ultrasound, we deal with three different patient groups, each with a different prevalence of breast cancer (pretest probability): the screening group, the diagnostic group, and the MRI correlation group. Different sets of rules are needed for interpreting studies in these patients. In the screening group the risk of cancer will be about 3 to 6 per 1000 patients. In the diagnostic group the risk will be about 3% to 8%, and in the MRI correlation group, a group with biopsy-proven cancer and one or more additional foci of abnormal enhancement on MRI, the risk is 30% to 40% (Fig. 20-75). In the screening group, we must deemphasize soft findings, because these will almost always represent benign ANDIs. In the diagnostic group, we weight soft and hard findings almost equally, and in the MRI correlation group, we weight soft findings heavily, especially when the MRI

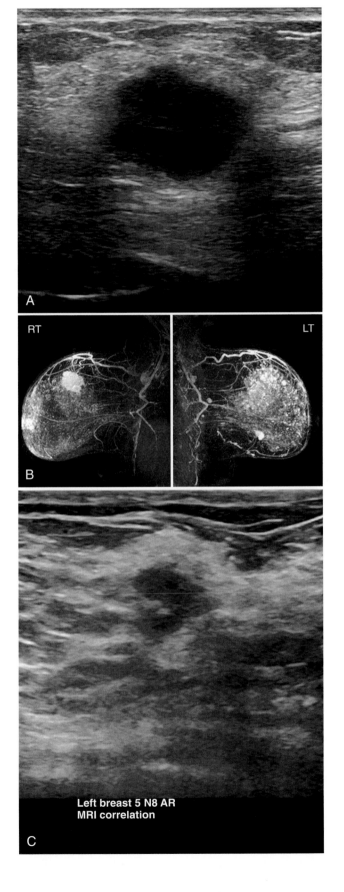

A

RT   LT

B

Left breast 5 N8 AR
MRI correlation

C

FIGURE 20-74. Contralateral invasive carcinoma detected on MRI and verified on "second look" ultrasound. A, Targeted diagnostic sonogram of a high-grade invasive carcinoma in upper right breast that presented as a palpable lump. Ultrasound-guided biopsy showed high-grade invasive carcinoma. **B,** Staging MRI showed right breast carcinoma and an enhancing mass inferiorly in the contralateral left breast. **C,** Second-look ultrasound showed irregular mass corresponding to the left breast lesion on MRI. Ultrasound-guided biopsy showed synchronous high-grade invasive duct carcinoma.

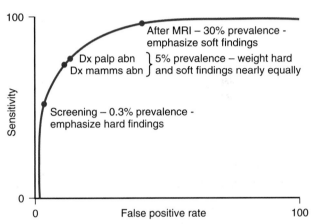

ROC CURVE FOR BREAST ULTRASOUND
RULES OF INTERPRETATION CHANGE WITH INDICATION

After MRI – 30% prevalence - emphasize soft findings

Dx palp abn } 5% prevalence – weight hard
Dx mamms abn } and soft findings nearly equally

Screening – 0.3% prevalence - emphasize hard findings

Sensitivity

False positive rate

FIGURE 20-75. Second-look ultrasound should be interpreted differently from screening or targeted diagnostic breast sonography. In patients undergoing screening breast ultrasound, the risk of malignancy is only about 3 per 1000 patients. The vast majority of lesions that present with only "soft" suspicious findings will be benign lesions, so soft findings should be weighted less heavily in characterizing lesions. In diagnostic patients, the risk of malignancy is about 5%, so we weight soft and hard findings almost equally in palpable lesions and lesions that present on mammography. In patients with proven breast carcinoma who have additional suspicious masslike or non-masslike enhancement, the risk of malignancy exceeds 30%. "Soft" findings must be emphasized on second-look ultrasound because they often represent in situ carcinoma.

enhancement pattern is "non-mass-like," clumped, or ductal (Fig. 20-76).

Doppler Sonography

Once a breast malignancy exceeds about 3 mm in size, it must stimulate neovascularity to continue to grow. To accomplish this, tumors elaborate a variety of angiogenesis factors. A net of peripheral neovessels forms to nourish the rapidly proliferating periphery of the tumor. Much attention has focused on detecting this neovascularity with Doppler ultrasound, with and without

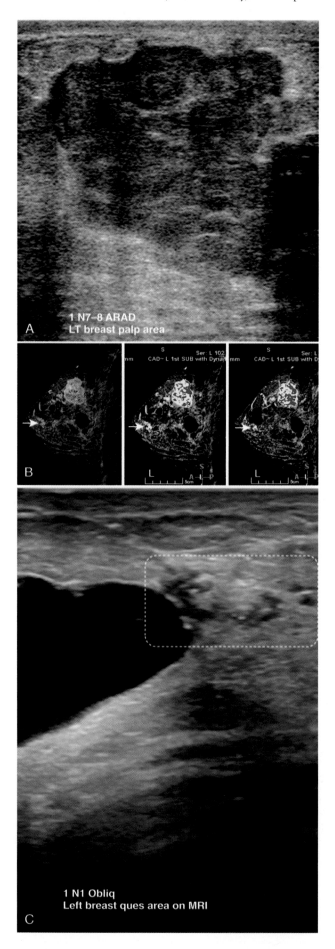

FIGURE 20-76. High-grade invasive duct carcinoma with second in situ lesion presenting only with "soft" findings. A, Targeted diagnostic ultrasound shows an irregularly shaped mass that presented as a palpable lump. Ultrasound-guided biopsy showed high-grade invasive ductal carcinoma. **B,** MRI shows an ipsilateral non-masslike area *(arrow)* of clumped enhancement farther inferiorly that lies just inferior to a large cyst. **C,** Second-look ultrasound shows no mass. Only the soft findings of branching ducts and microcalcifications *(within dotted box)* next to a large, simple cyst correspond to clumped enhancement on MRI. Ultrasound-guided vacuum biopsy showed intermediate-nuclear-grade in situ carcinoma.

contrast agents. Subjective findings, such as presence or absence of flow, and the distribution and pattern of vessels have been evaluated. Semiquantitative criteria such as vessel density, peak systolic velocity (PSV), pulsatility indices, resistive index (RI), and systolic-to-diastolic velocities have been evaluated. However, all these subjective and semiquantitative criteria can easily be altered by using too much compression pressure during scanning. Only a few authors have appropriately emphasized how critical it is to use exceedingly light compression when assessing blood flow in the breast. Tumor vessels have no muscle or elastic to prop them open and are very soft. The transducer is hard, the chest wall is firm, and even the weight of the sonographer's arm on the transducer can compress a lesion between the probe and chest wall enough to decrease or even completely ablate flow within breast lesions (Fig. 20-77). Not only can the presence or absence of flow be affected, but semiquantitative criteria (e.g., PSV, RI) can also be altered. When used for characterizing breast lesions, Doppler sonography must be performed with such light scan pressure that the transducer barely contacts the skin. In some cases, using a standoff of acoustic gel may be necessary so that Doppler ultrasound–detectable blood flow will not be affected.

We have found that the most useful Doppler ultrasound feature in characterizing breast nodules is comparing the pulsed Doppler spectral waveform in the periphery of the lesion with that in the center of the lesion. In **benign lesions** the waveforms obtained from the center and from the periphery of the lesions are similar to each other—low impedance flow with relatively low systolic velocities and rounded systolic peaks. In **malignant lesions** the waveforms obtained from the periphery are similar to those obtained from benign lesions—low impedance with rounded systolic peaks. The waveforms obtained from the center of malignant lesions, however, demonstrate higher impedance, higher systolic velocities, and sharp systolic peaks (Fig. 20-78). These intratumoral waveforms are probably a manifestation of increased pressures within the ECM of tumors that extrinsically compresses the thin-walled sinusoidal vessels within the center of the tumor.

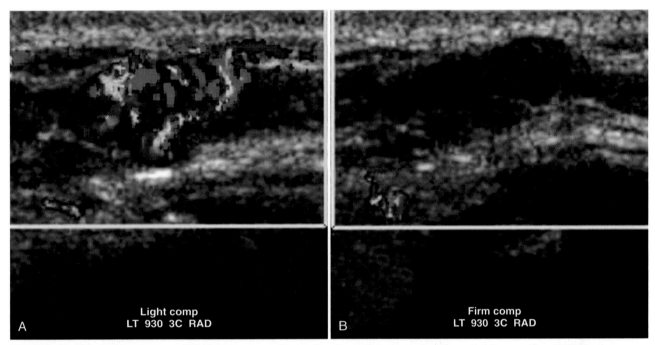

FIGURE 20-77. Importance of light pressure for color Doppler examination. A, Micropapillary DCIS lesion appears exceedingly hypervascular when scanned with light pressure. **B,** Lesion appears avascular when just the weight of the scanning arm is allowed to rest on the transducer while scanning.

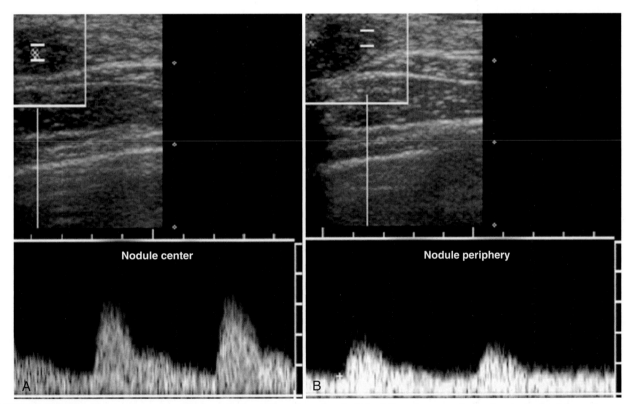

FIGURE 20-78. Central and peripheral Doppler signals. A, Pulsed Doppler spectral waveforms obtained from the center of malignant solid nodule tend to have high peak systolic velocity (PSV) and relatively high resistive index (RI). **B,** Waveforms obtained from the periphery of a malignant solid breast nodule tend to have lower PSV, more rounded systolic peaks, and lower RI. Benign solid nodules differ in that they tend to have low PSV, rounded systolic peaks, and relatively low RI in both the interior and the periphery of the nodule.

We have found the gray-scale image characteristics much more powerful and accurate than Doppler sonography in characterizing most solid nodules. In only a small percentage of cases has Doppler sonography added useful information to the gray-scale imaging in characterizing solid breast nodules. In our experience, Doppler sonography is most helpful in small, high-grade invasive carcinomas 6 or 7 mm in diameter or smaller. Such lesions are typically circumscribed, have not developed numerous suspicious gray-scale findings, and are the lesions most likely to be mischaracterized as BIRADS 3 by imaging alone. Despite their small size, such lesions are frequently quite vascular compared with benign lesions of the same size. We believe the gray-scale image will continue to be better for characterizing breast lesions than Doppler sonography in most cases, even with the use of contrast agents.

Doppler sonography can be useful in assessing the aggressiveness of breast solid nodules. Increased vascularity on Doppler ultrasound is a manifestation of biologically aggressive (high histologic grade) lesions that are most likely to spread distantly hematogenously. Patients with such lesions are those most likely to benefit from aggressive adjuvant chemotherapy, particularly antiangiogenesis drugs.

In niche applications, Doppler sonography is useful for assessing internal echoes within cysts and ectatic ducts, diagnosing acute inflammation or infection, and avoiding large vessels, particularly arteries, during interventional procedures. Doppler ultrasound is essential in diagnosing vascular conditions such as **arteriovenous malformations, arteriovenous fistulas, venous malformations,** and **superficial venous thrombosis (Mondor's disease)**. Doppler ultrasound is valuable in distinguishing between reactive or inflamed lymph nodes and metastasis-bearing nodes in certain cases.

Real, rather than artifactual, internal echoes frequently complicate breast cysts. Such echoes can result from a variety of cellular and acellular particles within the cyst. It can be difficult with static gray-scale images alone to distinguish between the different causes of internal echoes. Additionally, some markedly hypoechoic solid nodules can have a pseudocystic appearance. Demonstrating an internal vessel on color Doppler ultrasound indicates that the lesion is either solid or a cyst completely filled by a papillary lesion (Fig. 20-79). As always the case with Doppler sonography, a positive study is more valuable than a negative study because in certain solid nodules, a central vessel will not be demonstrable. In other cases, the energy of the Doppler beam will

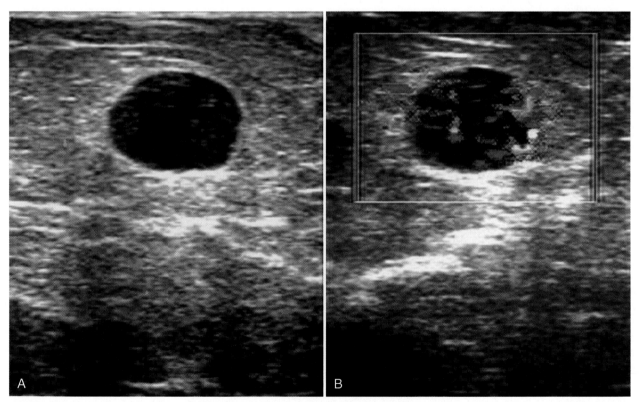

FIGURE 20-79. Pseudocystic solid nodule versus complicated cyst. Color Doppler ultrasound can be helpful in distinguishing between complex cysts and solid nodules when the distinction is uncertain based on the image alone. **A,** Metastatic leiomyosarcoma of the breast shows a pseudocystic appearance on the sonogram. **B,** Color Doppler sonography shows abundant internal flow, indicating that the lesion is solid.

displace particles within the cyst to move posteriorly—so-called color streaking. Particles that can be moved solely by the energy of the Doppler beam are tiny, subcellular in size, and are usually cholesterol crystals that are part of the benign FCC spectrum. Color Doppler sonography can be useful in distinguishing between an echogenic lipid layer or tumefactive sludge within a cyst and a true intracystic papillary lesion. Intracystic papillary lesions, whether benign or malignant, are among the most vascular lesions of the breast and usually have a prominent vascular stalk that is demonstrable with color or power Doppler sonography (Fig. 20-80, *A*). Demonstration of a vessel within such an intracystic area of increased echogenicity indicates the presence of an intracystic papilloma or carcinoma. Benign intracystic papillomas tend to have a single, large, feeding vessel within the vascular stalk, whereas malignant intracystic papillary lesions tend to be fed by multiple feeding vessels.

Ectatic ducts, like cysts, often contain echogenic secretions or blood that can be difficult to distinguish from intraductal papillomas or DCIS by gray-scale imaging alone. Ballottement of ectatic ducts that contain diffuse low-level echoes can cause the echoes to slosh back and forth within the duct. This can be appreciated on the gray-scale image in certain cases and can be documented on a single hard-copy image by using color Doppler sonography. The secretions are echogenic enough to create a color signal when moving within the duct. They tend to move posteriorly during compression and anteriorly during compression release, creating color signals of opposite color. Demonstrating such a "color swoosh" documents that the internal echoes are caused by inspissated echogenic secretions or blood rather than tumor. It is important that the color signal fills the duct, because in some cases, echogenic blood resulting from an intraductal papillary lesion can lead to a color swoosh, but the underlying papillary lesion will cause a defect in the color signal. As with intracystic papillary lesions, intraductal papillary lesions are often vascular enough to have a demonstrable vascular stalk on color Doppler sonography (Fig. 20-80, *B*). This helps to identify intraductal papillary lesions and to distinguish them from echogenic lipid or debris layers within the duct.

Acute breast pain is a frequent indication for breast ultrasound. In most patients the cause for pain is unclear. In some, however, sonography with Doppler may show an acute inflammatory etiology for pain. Acutely inflamed cysts and acute periductal mastitis are the most common causes for this pain. The normally thin, echogenic wall of acutely inflamed cyst or duct becomes thick and isoechoic and also becomes hyperemic (Fig. 20-81). The walls of noninflamed cysts and ducts have no demonstrable flow on color Doppler sonography. Inflammatory hyperemia with the thickened walls of acutely inflamed cysts and ducts can be easily demonstrated by color or power Doppler ultrasound. Interestingly, the direction in which the vessels course within the walls of inflamed cysts and ducts differs from the orientation of vessels that feed intracystic or intraductal papillary lesions. Vessels that lie within the walls of inflamed ducts or within the periductal tissues course *parallel* to the duct wall, because they are feeding and draining the duct wall and periductal tissues. Vessels that feed intraductal papillary lesions are oriented *perpendicular* to the axis of the duct wall, because the vessels are merely passing through the wall to feed a lesion inside the duct. Doppler ultrasound and other imaging findings in acutely inflamed or infected peri-implant capsules are similar to those in acutely inflamed cysts or ducts.

Acute superficial venous thrombosis of the breast (Mondor's disease) can also be a cause of acute pain. Compression gray-scale sonography and color Doppler sonography are essential in making the diagnosis as in lower-extremity deep vein thrombosis.

Doppler sonography can be helpful in assessing **lymph nodes** that are not normal but have nonspecific imaging findings that prevent determination of whether the node is merely inflamed or contains metastasis. The histologic and biologic behavior of lymph node metastases is usually identical to that of the primary lesion. A vascular primary tumor will tend to have a vascular lymph node metastasis. If the spectral waveforms obtained from the center of the primary are high impedance and have high and sharp systolic peaks, the waveforms obtained from lymph node metastases from that primary will have similar waveforms. Conversely, inflamed or reactive lymph nodes will usually have low-impedance waveforms with low, rounded systolic peaks. The pattern of blood vessels within lymph nodes can also be helpful. Inflamed or reactive lymph nodes tend to be fed by a single hilar artery that arborizes to various degrees within the mediastinum of the lymph nodes (Fig. 20-82, *A*). Well-differentiated and low-grade lymphomas can have a similar pattern. Metastases to lymph nodes can stimulate development of transcapsular tumor neovascularity (Fig. 20-82, *B*). Metastases tend to implant in the subcapsular and cortical sinusoids and the neovessels that they generate penetrate through the lymph node capsule. With Doppler ultrasound, the presence of transcapsular feeding arteries is a better positive predictor of metastasis than the absence of transcapsular vessels is an indicator of inflammation. Not all lymph node metastases stimulate formation of transcapsular neovessels.

ULTRASOUND-GUIDED INTERVENTION

The use of sonography for guiding interventional procedures is almost unlimited. Any type of interventional procedure for a lesion that is visible by sonography can be guided by sonography. Sonographic guidance is usually quicker, more precise, and less expensive than mammographic, stereotaxic, or MR guidance.

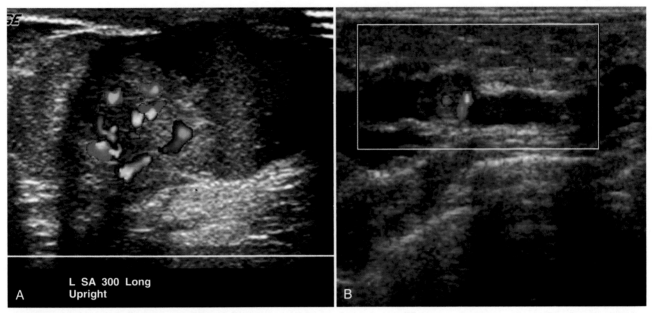

FIGURE 20-80. Intracystic papillary lesions and intraductal papillomas. A, Intracystic papillary lesions, whether benign or malignant, are among the most vascular lesions in the breast. One or more vascular stalks and internal vascularity are usually readily demonstrable on color or power Doppler ultrasound. Malignant lesions tend to be fed by multiple vessels, whereas benign intracystic papillomas usually have a single feeding vessel. **B,** Even very small intraductal papillomas usually have a vascular stalk demonstrable on color or power Doppler ultrasound.

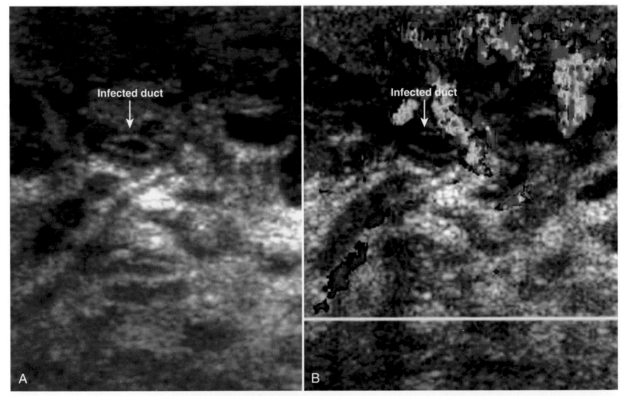

FIGURE 20-81. Duct wall hyperemia in acute periductal mastitis. A, Gray-scale image shows uniform isoechoic wall thickening in the inflamed or infected duct *(arrow)*. The noninflamed ectatic duct just to the right has a normal, thin, echogenic wall. **B,** Color Doppler sonogram shows marked hyperemia of the wall and tissues around the inflamed duct. The vessel is oriented parallel to the wall.

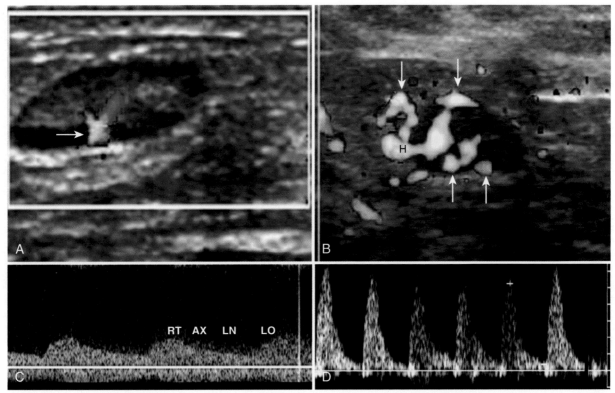

FIGURE 20-82. Color Doppler flow patterns and special waveforms help distinguish between metastatic and inflammatory etiologies of mild lymphadenopathy. A, Benign reactive lymph node is usually fed by a single hilar artery *(arrow).* **B,** Lymph nodes that bear metastasis often develops transcapsular feeding vessels *(arrows)* in addition to having a normal hilar artery *(h).* C, Pulsed Doppler spectral waveforms obtained from benign reactive nodes tend to have low RI and low PSV with rounded systolic peaks. **D,** Waveforms obtained from metastasis-bearing lymph nodes tend to have high RI, high PSV, and sharp systolic peaks.

Ultrasound guidance is truly real time, whereas stereotaxic and MRI guidance are not.

Our strong preference is to place the **needle along the long axis of the transducer,** enabling the needle to be visualized along its entire course in real time throughout the entire procedure. A short-axis approach allows visualization of the needle only when it is within the short axis of the ultrasound beam and requires a much steeper approach. This is especially problematic for deeply located lesions and in patients with implants. The main difficulty encountered during a long-axis approach is in keeping the needle and the long axis of the transducer exactly parallel to each other. Watching the ultrasound monitor before the needle has passed far enough into the breast to be within the ultrasound beam is the main cause of misalignment. It is best to watch one's hands until the needle is deep enough within the breast to be within the ultrasound beam before moving the eyes to the ultrasound monitor. Once the needle is within the beam, it is relatively easy to keep it precisely parallel to the beam.

Ultrasound can be used to guide cyst aspiration (Fig. 20-83), needle localization for surgical biopsy with specimen sonography (Fig. 20-84), sentinel node injection, sentinel node localization, abscess drainage, percutaneous ductography, foreign body removal (broken localization wires), and biopsy using fine needles, large Tru-Cut needles (Fig. 20-85), vacuum-assisted biopsy (Fig. 20-86), and en bloc removal. Sonography can be used to locate and orient the lumpectomy cavity for booster doses of external radiation, to guide placement of brachytherapy needles, and for placement of partial-breast irradiation balloons. It can also be used to guide lesion ablation using laser, radiofrequency, and cryotherapy.

We place a marker after every core needle biopsy and after every vacuum-assisted biopsy for several reasons. First, if the biopsy reveals malignant or atypical histology, a needle localization excisional biopsy will frequently be necessary. Second, if the lesion is malignant, the patient may receive chemotherapy before surgery. After chemotherapy, all imaging evidence of the lesion may disappear, but a needle localization of the marker will still be necessary. Finally, the presence of markers placed in a benign lesion helps immensely in interpreting follow-up mammograms.

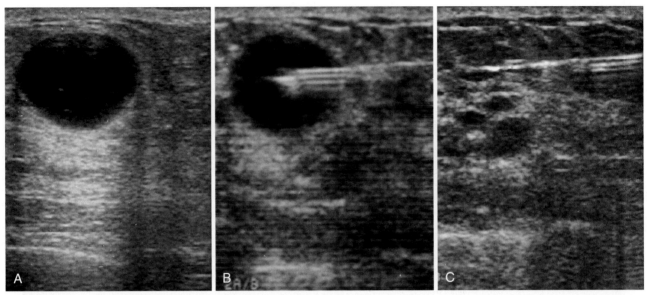

FIGURE 20-83. Technique of needle aspiration and biopsy. Ultrasound images show tender, simple tension cyst **A,** before aspiration; **B,** during aspiration; and **C,** after aspiration. Ultrasound-guided interventional procedures of the breast are performed with the needle oriented along the long axis of the transducer, with angulation of the needle and appropriate heeling or toeing of the transducer to place the needle almost parallel to the transducer face and perpendicular to the ultrasound beam.

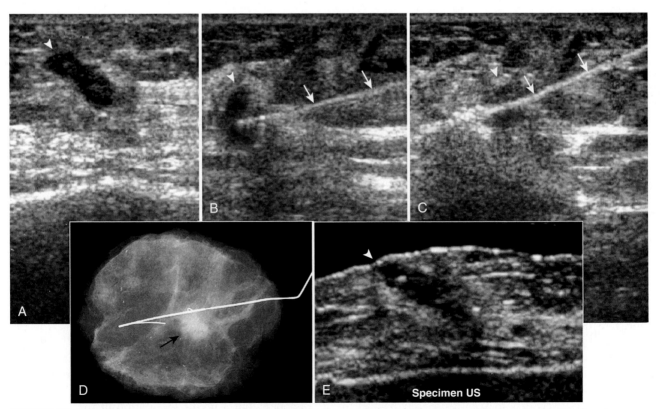

FIGURE 20-84. Ultrasound-guided wire localization for excisional biopsy. A, Nodule *(arrowhead)* before the procedure. **B,** Nodule *(arrowhead)* with the localization needle *(arrows)* in place. **C,** Localization wire *(arrows)* in place after the needle is removed *(arrowhead,* nodule). **D,** Specimen radiograph shows the nodule *(arrow)* in center of specimen. **E,** Specimen sonogram, however, shows the nodule extending to superficial margin of specimen *(arrowhead)*.

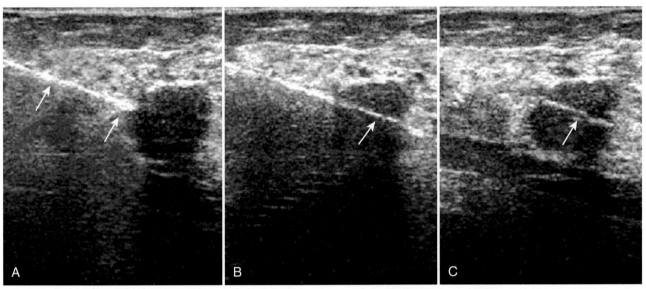

FIGURE 20-85. Ultrasound-guided needle biopsy with a 14-gauge Tru-Cut needle. A, Needle *(arrows)* has been advanced to the edge of the nodule in the prefire position. **B,** Needle *(arrow)* has been fired through the nodule and now is in the postfire position. **C,** Needle has been withdrawn, but a vapor trail of microbubbles *(arrow)* can still be seen within the needle tract, which documents that the needle did pass through the target nodule.

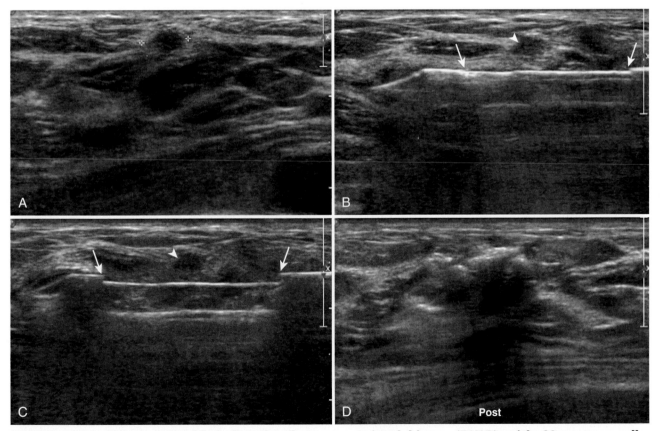

FIGURE 20-86. Ultrasound-guided directional vacuum-assisted biopsy (DVAB) with 10-gauge needle. A, High-grade 5-mm invasive ductal carcinoma. **B,** Vacuum probe has been placed just deep to the lesion, with the closed aperture *(arrows)* just deep to the nodule. **C,** Aperture has been opened *(arrows)*. There is ringdown artifact deep to the aperture created by the vacuum holes. **D,** Lesion has been removed and a marker placed, consisting of air-impregnated pellets, one of which contains a metallic clip.

References

1. Kolb TM, Lichy J, Newhouse JH. Occult cancer in women with dense breasts: detection with screening ultrasound—diagnostic yield and tumor characteristics. Radiology 1998;207:191-199.
2. Kolb TM, Lichy J, Newhouse JH. Comparison of the performance of screening mammography, physical examination, and breast ultrasound and evaluation of factors that influence them: an analysis of 27,825 patient evaluations. Radiology 2002;225:165-175.
3. Buchberger W, DeKoekkoek-Doll P, et al. Incidental findings on sonography of the breast: clinical significance and diagnostic workup. AJR Am J Roentgenol 1999;173:921-927.
4. Kaplan SS. Clinical utility of bilateral whole-breast ultrasound in the evaluation of women with dense breast tissue. Radiology 2001; 221:641-649.

Bibliography

General

Berg WA, Campassi C, Langenberg P, Sexton MJ. Breast Imaging Reporting and Data System: inter- and intraobserver variability in feature analysis and final assessment. AJR Am J Roentgenol 2000;174:1769-1777.

Farria DM, Mund DF, Bassett LW. Evaluation of missed cancers using screening mammography (abstract). AJR Am J Roentgenol 1995; 126:1645.

Ma L, Fishell E, Wright B, et al. Case-control study of factors associated with failure to detect breast cancer by mammography. J Natl Cancer Inst 1992;84:781-785.

Equipment and Physics

Kremkau FW. Multiple-element transducers. Radiographics 1993;13: 1163-1176.

Ritchie WGM. Axial resolution. Ultrasound Q 1992;10:80-100.

Smith SW, Trahey GE, von Ramm OT. Two-dimensional arrays for medical ultrasound. Ultrason Imaging 1992;14:213-233.

Breast Anatomy and Technique

Blend R, Rideout DF, Kaizer L, et al. Parenchymal patterns of the breast defined by real-time ultrasound. Eur J Cancer Prev 1995;4:293-298.

Moy L, Slanetz PJ, Moore R, et al. Specificity of mammography and ultrasound in the evaluation of a palpable abnormality: retrospective review. Radiology 2002;225:176-181.

Richter K. Technique for detecting and evaluating breast lesions. J Ultrasound Med 1994;13:797-802.

Stavros AT. An introduction to breast ultrasound. In: Parker SH, Jobe WE, editors. Percutaneous breast biopsy. New York, Raven Press; 1993. pp. 95-110.

Teboul M, Halliwell M. Atlas of ultrasound of ductal echography of the breast. Cambridge, Mass: Blackwell Science; 1995.

Yang WT, Ahuja A, Tang A, et al. Ultrasonographic demonstration of normal axillary lymph nodes: a learning curve. J Ultrasound Med 1995;14:823-827.

Targeted Indications

Dennis MA, Parker SH, Klaus AJ, et al. Breast biopsy avoidance: the value of normal mammograms and normal sonograms in the setting of a palpable lump. Radiology 2001;219:186-191.

Langer TG, Shaw de Paredes E. Evaluation of nonpalpable mammographic nodules. Appl Rad 1991;4:19-28.

Leung JW, Kornguth PJ, Gotway MB. Utility of targeted sonography in the evaluation of focal breast pain. J Ultrasound Med 2002;21:521-526; quiz 528-529.

Lunt LG, Peakman DJ, Young JR. Mammographically guided ultrasound: a new technique for assessment of impalpable breast lesions. Clin Radiol 1991;44:85-88.

McNicholas MM, Mercer PM, Miller JC, et al. Color Doppler sonography in the evaluation of palpable breast masses. AJR Am J Roentgenol 1993;161:765-771.

Perre CI, Koot VC, de Hooge P, Leguit P. The value of ultrasound in the evaluation of palpable breast tumours: a prospective study of 400 cases. Eur J Surg Oncol 1994;20:637-640.

Weinstein SP, Conant EF, Orel SG, et al. Retrospective review of palpable breast lesions after negative mammography and sonography. J Women Imaging 2000;2:15-18.

Solid Nodules

Baker JA, Kornguth PJ, Soo MS, et al. Sonography of solid breast lesions: observer variability of lesion description and assessment. AJR Am J Roentgenol 1999;172:1621-1625.

Butler RS, Venta LA, Wiley EL, et al. Sonographic evaluation of infiltrating lobular carcinoma. AJR Am J Roentgenol 1999;172: 325-330.

Chao TC, Lo YF, Chen SC, Chen MF. Prospective sonographic study of 3093 breast tumors. J Ultrasound Med 1999;18:363-370; quiz 371-372.

Cohen MA, Sferlazza SJ. Role of sonography in evaluation of radial scars of the breast. AJR Am J Roentgenol 2000;174:1075-1078.

Conant EF, Dillon RL, Palazzo J, et al. Imaging findings in mucin-containing carcinomas of the breast: correlation with pathologic features. AJR Am J Roentgenol 1994;163:821-824.

Ellis RL. Differentiation of benign versus malignant breast disease. Radiology 1999;210:878-880.

Finlay ME, Liston JE, Lunt LG, Young JR. Assessment of the role of ultrasound in the differentiation of radial scars and stellate carcinomas of the breast. Clin Radiol 1994;49:52-55.

Fornage BD, Lorigan JG, Andry E. Fibroadenoma of the breast: sonographic appearance. Radiology 1989;172:671-675.

Fornage BD, Sneige N, Faroux MJ, Andry E. Sonographic appearance and ultrasound-guided fine-needle aspiration biopsy of breast carcinomas smaller than 1 cm³. J Ultrasound Med 1990;9:559-568.

Franquet T, De Miguel C, Cozcolluela R, Donoso L. Spiculated lesions of the breast: mammographic-pathologic correlation. Radiographics 1993;13:841-852.

Hall FM. Sonography of the breast: controversies and opinions. AJR Am J Roentgenol 1997;169:1635-1636.

Jackson VP. Management of solid breast nodules: what is the role of sonography? Radiology 1995;196:14-15.

Kobayashi T, Shinozaki H, Yomon M, et al. Hyperechoic pattern in breast cancer: its bio-acoustical genesis and tissue characterization. J UOEH 1989;11:181-187.

Kornguth PJ, Bentley RC. Mammographic-pathologic correlation. Part 1. Benign breast lesions. J Women Imaging 2001;3:29-37.

Kossoff G. Causes of shadowing in breast sonography. Ultrasound Med Biol 1988;14(Suppl):211-215.

Leucht WJ, Rabe DR, Humbert KD. Diagnostic value of different interpretative criteria in real-time sonography of the breast. Ultrasound Med Biol 1988;14(Suppl 1):59-73.

Liberman L, Bonaccio E, Hamele-Bena D, et al. Benign and malignant phylloides tumors: mammographic and sonographic findings. Radiology 1996;198:121-124.

Meyer JE, Amin E, Lindfors KK, et al. Medullary carcinoma of the breast: mammographic and ultrasound appearance. Radiology 1989;170: 79-82.

Moon WK, Im JG, Koh YH, et al. Ultrasound of mammographically detected clustered microcalcifications. Radiology 2000;217:849-854.

Moss HA, Britton PD, Flower CD, et al. How reliable is modern breast imaging in differentiating benign from malignant breast lesions in the symptomatic population? Clin Radiol 1999;54:676-682.

Rahbar G, Sie AC, Hansen GC, et al. Benign versus malignant solid breast masses: ultrasound differentiation. Radiology 1999;213:889-894.

Richter K, Willrodt RG, Opri F, et al. Differentiation of breast lesions by measurements under craniocaudal and lateromedial compression using a new sonographic method. Invest Radiol 1996;31:401-414.

Rizzatto G, Chersevani R, Abbona M, et al. High-resolution sonography of breast carcinoma. Eur J Radiol 1997;24:11-19.

Rubin E. Cutting-edge sonography obviates breast biopsy. Diagn Imaging (San Francisco) 1996;(Suppl):AU14-AU16, AU32.

Schepps B, Scola FH, Frates RE. Benign circumscribed breast masses: mammographic and sonographic appearance. Obstet Gynecol Clin North Am 1994;21:519-537.

Schoonjans JM, Brem RF. Sonographic appearance of ductal carcinoma in situ diagnosed with ultrasonographically guided large-core needle biopsy: correlation with mammographic and pathologic findings. J Ultrasound Med 2000;19:449-457.

Shimato SH, Sawaki A, Niimi R, et al. Role of ultrasonography in the detection of intraductal spread of breast cancer: correlation with pathologic findings, mammography and MR imaging. Eur Radiol 2000; 10:1726-1732.

Skaane P, Engedal K. Analysis of sonographic features in the differentiation of fibroadenoma and invasive ductal carcinoma. AJR Am J Roentgenol 1998;170:109-114.

Skaane P, Skjorten F. Ultrasonographic evaluation of invasive lobular carcinoma. Acta Radiol 1999;40:369-375.

Stavros AT. Ultrasound of breast pathology. In: Parker SH, editor. Percutaneous breast biopsy. New York: Raven Press; 1993. pp. 111-127.

Stavros AT. Ultrasound of DCIS. In: Silverstein JM, editor. Ductal carcinoma in situ: a diagnostic and therapeutic dilemma. Baltimore: Williams & Wilkins; 1997. pp. 135-177.

Stavros AT. Ultrasound of DCIS. In: Silverstein JM, editor. Ductal carcinoma in situ: a diagnostic and therapeutic dilemma. 2nd ed. Baltimore: Williams & Wilkins; 2002. pp. 128-167.

Stavros AT, Thickman D, Rapp CL, et al. Solid breast nodules: use of sonography to distinguish between benign and malignant lesions. Radiology 1995;196:123-134.

Teboul M, Halliwell M. Atlas of ultrasound and ductal echography of the breast: the introduction of anatomic intelligence into breast imaging. London: Blackwell Science; 1995.

Vignal P, Meslet MR, Romeo JM, Feuilhade F. Sonographic morphology of infiltrating breast carcinoma: relationship with the shape of the hyaluronan extracellular matrix. J Ultrasound Med 2002;21:532-538.

Williams JC. Ultrasound of solid breast nodules. Radiology 1996;198:123-134.

Cystic Lesions

Bargum K, Nielsen SM. Case report: fat necrosis of the breast appearing as oil cysts with fat-fluid levels. Br J Radiol 1993;66:718-720.

Chatterton BE, Spyropoulos P. Colour Doppler induced streaming: an indicator of the liquid nature of lesions. Br J Radiol 1998;71:1310-1312.

Karstrup S, Solvig J, Nolsoe CP, et al. Acute puerperal breast abscesses: ultrasound-guided drainage. Radiology 1993;188:807-809.

Liberman L, Feng TL, Susnik B. Case 35: intracystic papillary carcinoma with invasion. Radiology 2001;219:781-784.

Loyer EM, Kaur H, David CL, et al. Importance of dynamic assessment of the soft tissues in the sonographic diagnosis of echogenic superficial abscesses. J Ultrasound Med 1995;14:669-671.

Maier WP, Au FC, Tang CK. Nonlactational breast infection. Am Surg 1994;60:247-250.

Nightingale KR, Kornguth PJ, Walker WF, et al. A novel ultrasonic technique for differentiating cysts from solid lesions: preliminary results in the breast. Ultrasound Med Biol 1995;21:745-751.

Stavros AT. Ultrasound of breast pathology. In: Parker SH, editor. Percutaneous breast biopsy. New York: Raven Press; 1993. pp. 111-127.

Nipple Discharge and Intraductal Papillary Lesions

Cilotti A, Bagnolesi P, Napoli V, et al. [Solitary intraductal papilloma of the breast: an echographic study of 12 cases]. Radiol Med 1991;82:617-620.

Dennis MA, Parker S, Kaske TI, et al. Incidental treatment of nipple discharge caused by benign intraductal papilloma through diagnostic Mammotome biopsy. AJR Am J Roentgenol 2000;174:1263-1268.

Rissanen T, Typpo T, Tikkakoski T, et al. Ultrasound-guided percutaneous galactography. J Clin Ultrasound 1993;21:497-502.

Mammary Implants

Ahn CY, DeBruhl ND, Gorczyca DP, et al. Comparative silicone breast implant evaluation using mammography, sonography, and magnetic resonance imaging: experience with 59 implants. Plast Reconstr Surg 1994;94:620-627.

Berg WA, Caskey CI, Hamper UM, et al. Diagnosing breast implant rupture with MR imaging, ultrasound, and mammography. Radiographics 1993;13:1323-1336.

Caskey CI, Berg WA, Anderson ND, et al. Breast implant rupture: diagnosis with ultrasound. Radiology 1994;190:819-823.

Chung KC, Wilkins EG, Beil Jr RJ, et al. Diagnosis of silicone gel breast implant rupture by ultrasonography. Plast Reconstr Surg 1996;97:104-109.

DeBruhl ND, Gorczyca DP, Ahn CY, et al. Silicone breast implants: ultrasound evaluation. Radiology 1993;189:95-98.

Everson LI, Parantainen H, Detlie T, et al. Diagnosis of breast implant rupture: imaging findings and relative efficacies of imaging techniques. AJR Am J Roentgenol 1994;163:57-60.

Harris KM, Ganott MA, Shestak KC, et al. Silicone implant rupture: detection with ultrasound. Radiology 1993;187:761-768.

Leibman AJ. Imaging of the breast after cosmetic surgery. Appl Rad 1993;4:45-48.

Leibman AJ. Imaging of complications of augmentation mammaplasty. Plast Reconstr Surg 1994;93:1134-1140.

Leibman AJ, Kruse B. Breast cancer: mammographic and sonographic findings after augmentation mammoplasty. Radiology 1990;174:195-198.

Leibman AJ, Sybers R. Mammographic and sonographic findings after silicone injection. Ann Plast Surg 1994;33:412-414.

Levine RA, Collins TL. Definitive diagnosis of breast implant rupture by ultrasonography. Plast Reconstr Surg 1991;87:1126-1128.

Peters W, Pugash R. Ultrasound analysis of 150 patients with silicone gel breast implants. Ann Plast Surg 1993;31:7-9.

Petro JA, Klein SA, Niazi Z, et al. Evaluation of ultrasound as a tool in the follow-up of patients with breast implants: a preliminary, prospective study. Ann Plast Surg 1994;32:580-587.

Reynolds HE, Buckwalter KA, Jackson VP, et al. Comparison of mammography, sonography, and magnetic resonance imaging in the detection of silicone-gel breast implant rupture. Ann Plast Surg 1994;33:247-255; discussion 256-257.

Rivero MA, Schwartz DS, Mies C. Silicone lymphadenopathy involving intramammary lymph nodes: a new complication of silicone mammaplasty. AJR Am J Roentgenol 1994;162:1089-1090.

Rosculet KA, Ikeda DM, Forrest ME, et al. Ruptured gel-filled silicone breast implants: sonographic findings in 19 cases. AJR Am J Roentgenol 1992;159:711-716.

Shestak KC, Ganott MA, Harris KM, Losken HW. Breast masses in the augmentation mammaplasty patient: the role of ultrasound. Plast Reconstr Surg 1993;92:209-216.

Inflammation/Infection of the Breast

Crowe DJ, Helvie MA, Wilson TE. Breast infection: mammographic and sonographic findings with clinical correlation. Invest Radiol 1995;30:582-587.

Hayes R, Michell M, Nunnerley HB. Acute inflammation of the breast: the role of breast ultrasound in diagnosis and management. Clin Radiol 1991;44:253-256.

Hughes LE. The duct ectasia/periductal mastitis complex. In: Hughes LE, Mansel RE, Webster DJT, editors. Benign disorders and diseases of the breast: concepts and clinical management. 2nd ed. Philadelphia: Saunders; 2000. pp. 143-165.

Doppler Ultrasound of the Breast

Cosgrove DO, Kedar RP, Bamber JC, et al. Breast diseases: color Doppler ultrasound in differential diagnosis. Radiology 1993;189:99-104.

Dock W. Duplex sonography of mammary tumors: a prospective study of 75 patients. J Ultrasound Med 1993;12:79-82.

Fornage BD. Role of color Doppler imaging in differentiating between pseudocystic malignant tumors and fluid collections. J Ultrasound Med 1995;14:125-128.

Hayes R, Michell M, Nunnerley HB. Acute inflammation of the breast: the role of breast ultrasound in diagnosis and management. Clin Radiol 1991;44:253-256.

Kubek KA, Chan L, Frazier TG. Color Doppler flow as an indicator of nodal metastasis in solid breast masses. J Ultrasound Med 1996;15:835-841.

Madjar H, Prompeler HJ, Sauerbrei W, et al. Color Doppler flow criteria of breast lesions. Ultrasound Med Biol 1994;20:849-858.

Mehta TS, Raza S. Power Doppler sonography of breast cancer: does vascularity correlate with node status or lymphatic vascular invasion? AJR Am J Roentgenol 1999;173:303-307.

Ozdemir A, Ozdemir H, Maral I, et al. Differential diagnosis of solid breast lesions: contribution of Doppler studies to mammography and gray scale imaging. J Ultrasound Med 2001;20:1091-1101; quiz 1102.

Walsh JS, Dixon JM, Chetty U, Paterson D. Colour Doppler studies of axillary node metastases in breast carcinoma. Clin Radiol 1994;49:189-191.

Yang WT, Metreweli C. Colour Doppler flow in normal axillary lymph nodes. Br J Radiol 1998;71:381-383.

The Scrotum

Brian Gorman

Chapter Outline

$\mathcal{D}$iagnostic ultrasound is the most common imaging technique used to supplement the physical examination of the scrotum and is an accurate means of evaluating many scrotal diseases. Technical advancements in high-resolution real-time and color flow Doppler sonography have led to an increase in the clinical applications of scrotal sonography.

SONOGRAPHIC TECHNIQUE

It is helpful if the patient can localize a palpable nodule within the scrotum, which the sonographer can then palpate during the examination. The patient is examined in the supine position. The scrotum is elevated with a towel draped over the thighs, and the penis is placed on the patient's abdomen and covered with a towel. Alternatively, the scrotal sac may be supported by the examiner's hand. A high-frequency (7.5-15 MHz) linear array transducer is typically used because it provides increased resolution of the scrotal contents. If greater penetration is needed because of scrotal swelling, a 6-MHz or lower-frequency transducer may be used. A direct-contact scan is most often performed using acoustic coupling gel. Images of both testes are obtained in transverse and sagittal planes. If possible, a transverse scan showing both testes for comparison is obtained using a dual-imaging technique, a larger-footprint transducer, or extended–field of view imaging. Additional views may be obtained

in the coronal or oblique planes, with the patient upright or performing the Valsalva maneuver when necessary. Color flow and power mode Doppler sonography are also performed to evaluate testicular blood flow in normal and pathologic states.

ANATOMY

The adult testes are ovoid glands measuring 3 to 5 cm in length, 2 to 4 cm in width, and 3 cm in anteroposterior dimension. Each testis weighs 12.5 to 19 g. Testicular size and weight decrease with age.[1,2] The testes are surrounded by a dense white fibrous capsule, the **tunica albuginea.** Multiple thin septations (septula) arise from the innermost aspect of the tunica albuginea and converge posteriorly to form the **mediastinum testis** (Fig. 21-1).

The mediastinum testis forms the support for the entering and exiting testicular vessels and ducts. As the septula proceed posteriorly from the tunica albuginea, they form 250 to 400 wedge-shaped lobuli that contain the **seminiferous tubules.** There are approximately 840 tubules per testis. As the tubules course centrally, they join other seminiferous tubules to form 20 to 30 larger ducts, known as the **tubuli recti.** The tubuli recti enter the mediastinum testis, forming a network of channels within the testicular stroma, called the **rete testis.** The rete terminate in 10 to 15 efferent ductules at the supe-

SCROTAL SONOGRAPHY: CURRENT USES

Evaluation of location and characteristics of scrotal masses.

Detection of occult primary tumor in patients with known metastatic disease.

Follow-up of patients with testicular microlithiasis.

Follow-up of patients with previous testicular neoplasms, leukemia, or lymphoma.

Evaluation of extratesticular pathologic lesions.

Evaluation of acute scrotal pain.

Evaluation of scrotal trauma.

Localization of the undescended testis.

Detection of varicoceles in infertile men.

Evaluation of testicular ischemia with color and power Doppler sonography.

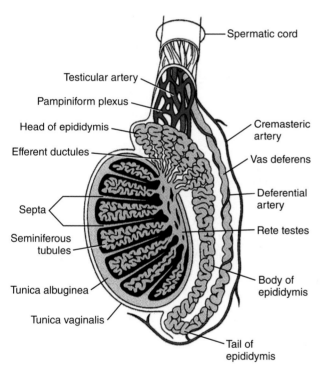

FIGURE 21-1. Normal intrascrotal anatomy. *(From Sudakoff GS, Quiroz F, Karcaaltincaba M, Foley WD. Scrotal ultrasonography with emphasis on the extratesticular space: anatomy, embryology, and pathology. Ultrasound Q 2002;18:255-273.)*

rior portion of the mediastinum, which carry the seminal fluid from the testis to the epididymis.

Sonographically the **normal testis** has a homogeneous echotexture composed of uniformly distributed medium-level echoes, similar to that of the thyroid (Fig. 21-2, *A*). The **septula testis** may be seen as linear echogenic or hypoechoic structures (Fig. 21-2, *B*). The **mediastinum testis** is sometimes seen as a linear echogenic band extending craniocaudally within the testis (Fig. 21-2, *C*). Its appearance varies according to the amount of fibrous and fatty tissue present. It is best visualized between the ages of 15 and 60 years.

The **epididymis** is a curved structure measuring 6 to 7 cm in length and lying posterolateral to the testis. It is composed of a head, a body, and a tail. The **head** of the epididymis, also known as the **globus major**, is located adjacent to the superior pole of the testis and is the largest portion of the epididymis. It is formed by 10 to 15 efferent ductules from the rete testis joining together to form a single convoluted duct, the **ductus epididymis**. This duct forms the body and the majority of the tail of the epididymis. It measures approximately 600 cm in length and follows a convoluted course from the head to the tail of the epididymis. The **body** or **corpus** of the epididymis lies adjacent to the posterolateral margin of the testis. The **tail** or **globus minor** is loosely attached to the lower pole of the testis by areolar tissue. The ductus epididymis forms an acute angle at the inferior aspect of the globus minor and courses cephalad on the medial aspect of the epididymis to the spermatic cord. Sonographically, the epididymis is normally isoechogenic or slightly more echogenic than the testis, and its echotexture may be coarser. The globus major normally measures 10 to 12 mm in diameter and lies lateral to the superior pole of the testis (Fig. 21-2, *D*). The body tends to be isoechoic or slightly less echogenic than the globus major and testis. The normal body measures less than 4 mm in diameter, averaging 1 to 2 mm.

The **appendix testis**, a remnant of the upper end of the paramesonephric (müllerian) duct, is a small ovoid structure usually located on the superior pole of the testis or in the groove between the testis and the head of the epididymis. The appendix testis is identified sonographically in 80% of testes and is more readily visible when a hydrocele is present[3] (Fig. 21-2, *E*). The appendix testis may appear stalk-like and pedunculated, cystic, or even calcified.[4] The **appendices of the head and tail** of the epididymis are blind-ending tubules (vasa aberrantia) derived from the mesonephric (wolffian) duct; they form small stalks, which may be duplicated, and project from the epididymis[5] (Fig. 21-2, *F*). Rarely, other appendages, the paradidymis (organ of Giraldés) and the superior and inferior vas aberrans of Haller, may be seen.[6] The appendages of the epididymis are most often identified sonographically as separate structures when a hydrocele is present.

Knowledge of the arterial supply of the testis is important for interpretation of color flow Doppler sonography of the testis. Testicular blood flow is supplied primarily by the deferential, cremasteric (external spermatic), and testicular arteries. The **deferential artery** originates from the inferior vesical artery and courses to the tail of the epididymis, where it divides and forms a capillary network. The **cremasteric artery** arises from the inferior epigastric artery. It courses with the remainder of the structures of the spermatic cord through the inguinal ring, continuing to the surface of the tunica vaginalis, where it anastomoses with capillaries of the testicular and deferential arteries. The **testicular arteries** arise from the

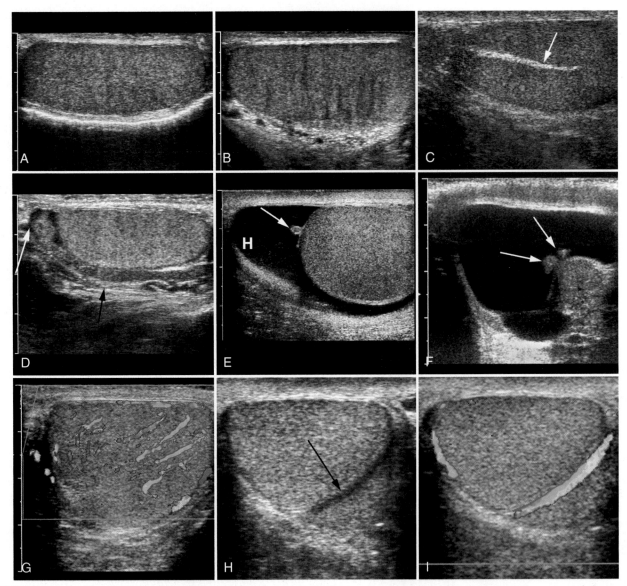

FIGURE 21-2. Normal intrascrotal anatomy. Longitudinal scans show **A,** normal homogeneous echotexture of the testis; **B,** striated appearance of the septula testis; **C,** mediastinum testis *(arrow)* as a linear echogenic band of fibrofatty tissue; **D,** head *(white arrow)* and body *(black arrow)* of epididymis; **E,** hydrocele *(H)* and appendix testis *(arrow);* and **F,** appendages of epididymis *(arrows).* **G,** Color Doppler scan shows normal testicular arteries. **H,** Transverse scan shows hypoechoic band of transmediastinal artery *(arrow).* **I,** Color Doppler scan shows transmediastinal artery.

anterior aspect of the aorta immediately below the origin of the renal arteries. They course through the inguinal canal with the spermatic cord to the posterosuperior aspect of the testis. On reaching the testis, the testicular artery divides into branches that pierce the tunica albuginea and arborize over the surface of the testis in a layer known as the **tunica vasculosa.** Centripetal branches arise from these capsular arteries; these branches course along the septula to converge on the mediastinum. From the mediastinum, these branches form recurrent rami that course centrifugally within the testicular parenchyma, where they branch into arterioles and capillaries[7] (Fig. 21-2, *G*). In about half of normal testes a **transmediastinal artery** supplies the testis, entering

through the mediastinum and coursing toward the periphery of the gland. These arteries may be unilateral or bilateral and single or multiple, and they are frequently seen as a hypoechoic band in the midtestis[7,8] (Fig. 21-2, *H* and *I*). The transmediastinal artery may be associated with acoustic shadowing obscuring the distal aspect of the testis and giving rise to the "two-tone" testis appearance.[9]

The velocity waveforms of the **normal capsular** and **intratesticular arteries** show high levels of antegrade diastolic flow throughout the cardiac cycle, reflecting the low vascular resistance of the testis (Fig. 21-3, *A*). Supratesticular arterial waveforms vary in appearance. Two main types of waveforms exist: a low-resistance wave-

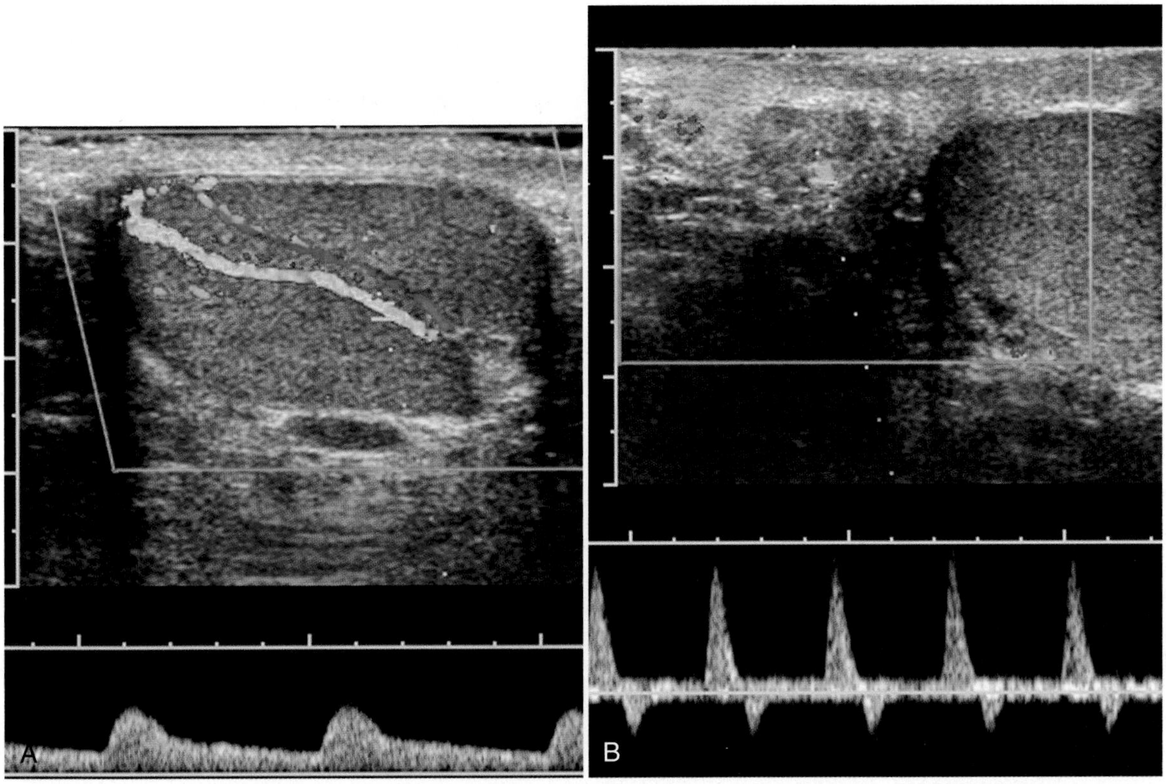

FIGURE 21-3. Spectral Doppler of normal intratesticular and extratesticular arterial flow. A, Intratesticular artery has a low-impedance waveform with large amount of end diastolic flow. **B,** Extratesticular scrotal arterial supply (cremasteric and deferential arteries) has high-impedance waveform with reversed flow in diastole.

form such as the capsular and intratesticular arteries and a high-resistance waveform with sharp, narrow systolic peaks and little or no diastolic flow[10] (Fig. 21-3, *B*). This high-resistance waveform is believed to reflect the high vascular resistance of the extratesticular tissues. The deferential and cremasteric arteries within the **spermatic cord** primarily supply the epididymis and extratesticular tissues, but they also supply the testis through anastomoses with the testicular artery.

The spermatic cord consists of the vas deferens; the cremasteric, deferential, and testicular arteries; a pampiniform plexus of veins; the lymphatics; and the nerves of the testis. Sonographically, the normal spermatic cord lies just beneath the skin and is difficult to distinguish from the adjacent soft tissues of the inguinal canal.[11] It may be visualized within the scrotum when a hydrocele is present or with the use of color flow Doppler sonography.

The **dartos,** a layer of muscle fibers lying beneath the scrotal skin, is continuous with the scrotal septum, which divides the scrotum into two chambers. The walls of the chambers are formed by the fusion of the three fascial layers.

The **tunica vaginalis** is the space between these scrotal fascial layers and the tunica albuginea of the testis. During embryologic development, the tunica vaginalis arises from the **processus vaginalis,** an outpouching of fetal peritoneum that accompanies the testis in its descent

into the scrotum. The upper portion of the processus vaginalis, extending from the internal inguinal ring to the upper pole of the testis, is normally obliterated. The lower portion, the tunica vaginalis, remains as a closed pouch folded around the testis. Only the posterior aspect of the testis, the site of attachment of the testis and epididymis, is not in continuity with the tunica vaginalis. The inner or visceral layer of the tunica vaginalis covers the testis, epididymis, and lower portion of the spermatic cord. The outer or parietal layer of the tunica vaginalis lines the walls of the scrotal pouch and is attached to the fascial coverings of the testis. A small amount of fluid is normally present between these two layers, especially in the polar regions and between the testicle and epididymis.

The scrotal covering layers are normally indistinguishable by sonography and are visualized as a single echogenic stripe. If any type of fluid is present in the scrotal wall, the tunica vaginalis may be identified as a separate structure.[1]

SCROTAL MASSES

With ultrasonographic examination, intrascrotal masses can be detected with a sensitivity of almost 100%. Sonography is important in the evaluation of scrotal masses because its accuracy is 98% to 100% in distinguishing intratesticular and extratesticular pathologic features.[12] This distinction is important in disease management because most extratesticular masses are benign, but the majority of intratesticular lesions are malignant.[13]

Most malignant testicular neoplasms are more hypoechoic than normal testicular parenchyma; however, hemorrhage, necrosis, calcification, or fatty changes can produce areas of increased echogenicity within tumors.

Testicular neoplasms account for 1% to 2% of all malignant neoplasms in men.[14] Approximately 65% to 94% of patients with testicular neoplasms present with painless unilateral testicular masses or diffuse testicular enlargement, and 4% to 14% present with symptoms of metastatic disease.[1,15,16] Most primary testicular tumors are of germ cell origin and are generally malignant. Only 60% of testicular germ cell tumors are of one histologic subtype; the others are of two or more histologic subtypes. Although several histologic subtypes of germ cell tumor may be present, clinically it is important to recognize only two basic tumor types: **seminomas** and **nonseminomatous germ cell tumors** (NSGCTs). Seminomas and NSGCTs behave differently biologically and therefore have different therapeutic and prognostic implications.[17] Seminomas are more radiosensitive and usually have a better prognosis.

Gonadal stromal tumors, arising from Sertoli or Leydig cells, account for 3% to 6% of testicular masses,[1,16] and the majority of these mesenchymal neoplasms are benign.

Malignant Tumors

Germ Cell Tumors

Seminomas. Seminoma is the most common single-cell type of testicular tumor in adults, accounting for 40% to 50% of all germ cell neoplasms. It is also a common component of mixed germ cell tumors, occurring in 30% of these tumors. Seminomas tend to occur in slightly older patients than do other testicular neoplasms, with a peak incidence in the fourth and fifth decades.[1,18,19] Although seminomas may occur at older or younger ages, they rarely occur before puberty. They are less aggressive than other testicular tumors and are usually confined within the tunica albuginea at presentation, with only 25% of patients having metastases at diagnosis. As a result of the radiosensitivity and chemosensitivity of the primary tumor and its metastases, seminomas have the most favorable prognosis of the malignant testicular tumors. A **second primary synchronous or metachronous germ cell tumor** occurs in 1% to 2.5% of patients with seminomas (Fig. 21-4; see also Fig. 21-5, *D*).

Seminoma is the most common tumor type in **cryptorchid testes.** Between 8% and 30% of patients with seminoma have a history of undescended testes.[16,19] The risk of a seminoma developing is substantially increased in an undescended testis, even after orchiopexy. There is

---

PATHOLOGIC CLASSIFICATION OF TESTICULAR TUMORS

GERM CELL TUMORS
Seminoma
Classic
Spermatocytic
Nonseminomatous germ cell tumors
Mixed malignant germ cell
Embryonal cell carcinoma
Yolk sac tumor (endodermal sinus tumor)
Teratoma
Choriocarcinoma

STROMAL TUMORS
Leydig cell (interstitial)
Sertoli cell
Granulosa cell
Mixed undifferentiated sex cord

MIXED GERM CELL–STROMAL TUMORS
Gonadoblastoma
Germ cell–stromal–sex cord

METASTATIC NEOPLASMS
Lymphoma
Leukemia
Myeloma
Carcinoma

OTHER*
Adrenal rests
Epidermoid cyst
Malacoplakia
Carcinoid tumor
Mesenchymal tumor

Data from Mostofi FK, Sobin LH. Histological typing of testis tumours. In *International histological classification of tumors of the testes.* Geneva, 1977, World Health Organization.
*Rare tumors and nonneoplastic tumorous conditions.

---

also an increased risk of malignancy developing in the contralateral, normally located testis. Sonography is often used to screen for an occult tumor in both testes after orchiopexy. In patients who have had an orchiectomy for germ cell tumor, sonography is also used to screen the remaining testis because of increased risk of tumor. Patients with a normally located, but atrophic testis have an increased risk of germ cell tumor, especially seminoma **(Video 21-1).**

Macroscopically, seminoma is a homogeneously solid, firm, round or oval tumor that varies in size from a small nodule in a normal-size testis to a large mass causing diffuse testicular enlargement.[14] The sonographic features of pure seminoma parallel this homogeneous macroscopic appearance (Fig. 21-5). Pure seminomas

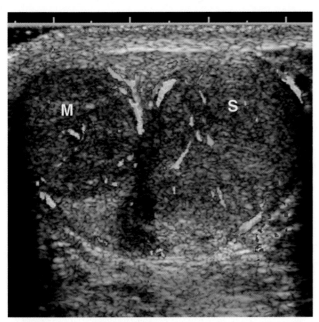

FIGURE 21-4. Mixed tumor. Transverse scan of coexistent mixed germ cell tumor *(M)* and seminoma *(S).*

usually have predominantly uniform, low-level echoes without calcification, and they appear hypoechoic compared with normally echogenic testicular parenchyma.[20] With high-resolution sonography, some seminomas may have a more heterogeneous echotexture (Fig. 21-5, *E*). Rarely, seminomas become necrotic and appear partly cystic on sonography (Fig. 21-5, *I*).

Nonseminomatous Germ Cell Tumors. NSGCTs include **embryonal carcinomas, teratomas, yolk sac tumors, choriocarcinomas**, and **mixed germ cell tumors.** These tumors occur more often in younger patients than do seminomas, with a peak incidence during the latter part of the second decade and the third decade. They are uncommon before puberty and after age 50. These malignancies are more aggressive than seminomas, frequently invading the tunica albuginea and resulting in distortion of the testicular contour (Fig. 21-6). They frequently cause visceral metastases.[1] The sonographic appearance of NSGCTs reflects the histologic features. Typically, these tumors are more heterogeneous than seminoma and may have both solid and cystic components. Coarse calcifications are common. It is not possible to distinguish the various subtypes of NSGCTs on sonography.

Mixed germ cell tumors are the most common NSGCTs and are the second most common primary testicular malignancy after seminoma, constituting 40% of all germ cell tumors. They contain nonseminomatous germ cell elements in various combinations. Seminomatous elements may also be present but do not influence prognosis.[17] The most common combination, previously called "teratocarcinoma," is teratoma and embryonal cell carcinoma.

Pure **embryonal cell carcinoma** is a rare tumor accounting for only 2% to 3% of testicular germ cell neoplasms.[21] It often occurs in combination with other neoplastic germ cell elements, particularly yolk sac tumor and teratoma. As with other NSGCTs, embryonal cell tumors occur in younger patients than seminomas do, with a peak incidence during the latter part of the second and third decades. The infantile form, **endodermal sinus tumor** or **yolk sac tumor,** is the most common germ cell tumor in infants younger than 2 years, accounting for 60% of testicular neoplasms in this age group. Yolk sac tumor is associated with elevated levels of α-fetoprotein in 95% of infants. Both embryonal cell carcinoma and yolk sac tumor are less radiosensitive and chemosensitive than seminomas. The sonographic features of pure embryonal cell carcinoma are similar to those of mixed NSGCTs (Fig. 21-6, *A-C*). Cystic areas are present in one third of tumors, and echogenic foci, with or without acoustic shadowing, may also be seen.

Teratomas constitute approximately 5% to 10% of primary testicular neoplasms. They are defined according to the World Health Organization (WHO) classification on the basis of the presence of derivatives of the different germinal layers (endoderm, mesoderm, and ectoderm). The three WHO categories of teratoma are (1) mature, (2) immature, and (3) teratoma with malignant transformation.[16] One third of teratomas metastasize, usually by a lymphatic route, within 5 years.[1] The peak incidence is in infancy and early childhood, with another peak in the third decade of life. In infants and young children, teratomas are the second most common testicular tumor and usually are mature and well differentiated. Occasional cases may contain immature elements, but metastases are rare.[19] After puberty, teratomas typically contain immature and mature elements admixed with other germ cell types. Teratomas in adults are usually malignant. Elevated levels of α-fetoprotein or human chorionic gonadotropin may be found and are suggestive of malignancy.[17] Sonographically, the teratoma is usually a well-defined, markedly inhomogeneous mass containing cystic and solid areas of various sizes and appears similar to other NSGCTs. Dense echogenic foci causing acoustic shadowing are common, resulting from focal calcification, cartilage, immature bone, fibrosis, and noncalcific scarring[20] (Fig. 21-6, *D* and *E*).

Pure **choriocarcinoma** is the rarest type of germ cell tumor, accounting for less than 0.5% of malignant primary testicular tumors.[21] Only 18 cases were encountered among more than 6000 testicular tumors registered at the Armed Forces Institute of Pathology.[22] Approximately 23% of mixed germ cell tumors contain a component of choriocarcinoma.[19] The peak incidence is in the second and third decades. These tumors are highly malignant and metastasize early by hematogenous and lymphatic routes. Patients may have symptoms resulting from hemorrhagic metastases: hemoptysis, hematemesis, and central nervous system (CNS)–related symptoms.

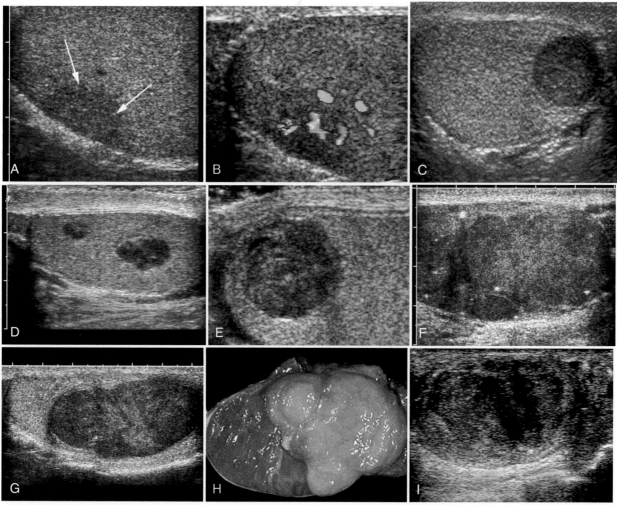

FIGURE 21-5. Seminoma: spectrum of appearances. Longitudinal scans. **A** and **B,** Subtle hypoechoic seminoma *(arrows)* with increased flow. **C,** Typical homogeneous hypoechoic seminoma. **D,** Two small foci of seminoma. **E,** Slightly heterogeneous seminoma. **F,** Seminoma associated with microlithiasis and coarser calcifications. **G,** Seminoma occupying most of testis. Typical homogeneous hypoechoic sonographic appearance. **H,** Gross specimen of seminoma in **G. I,** Necrotic seminoma replacing testicle.

Gynecomastia is common because of the high levels of circulating chorionic gonadotropins produced by all these tumors.[23] Metastases may be present without any evidence of choriocarcinoma in the testicle. Hemorrhage with focal necrosis of tumor is an almost invariable feature, and calcification may be present, giving a sonographic appearance similar to the other NSGCTs (Fig. 21-6, *F*).

Gonadal Stromal Tumors

Gonadal stromal tumors account for 3% to 6% of all testicular neoplasms. Approximately 20% of these tumors occur in children.[20] The term *gonadal stromal tumor* refers to a neoplasm containing Leydig, Sertoli, thecal, granulosa, or lutein cells and fibroblasts in various degrees of differentiation. These tumors may contain single or multiple cell types because of the totipotentiality of the gonadal stroma.[16] Gonadal stromal tumors in

conjunction with germ cell tumors are called **gonadoblastomas.** The majority of gonadoblastomas occur in male patients with cryptorchidism, hypospadias, and female internal secondary sex organs.[19]

The majority of stromal tumors are **Leydig cell tumors.** They account for 1% to 3% of all testicular neoplasms and occur predominantly in patients age 20 to 50 years.[18,19,23] Patients most often present with painless testicular enlargement or a palpable mass. Approximately 15% to 30% of patients present with gynecomastia resulting from the secretion of androgens or estrogens or both. Impotence, loss of libido, or precocious virilization may also occur in young men. The tumor is bilateral in 3% of cases. From 10% to 15% of the tumors are malignant, having invaded the tunica at diagnosis. Leydig cell tumors are homogeneous, but foci of hemorrhage and necrosis are present in 25% of tumors.[18,23] These gonadal tumors are usually small, solid, and hypoechoic on sonography and may show mainly peripheral flow on

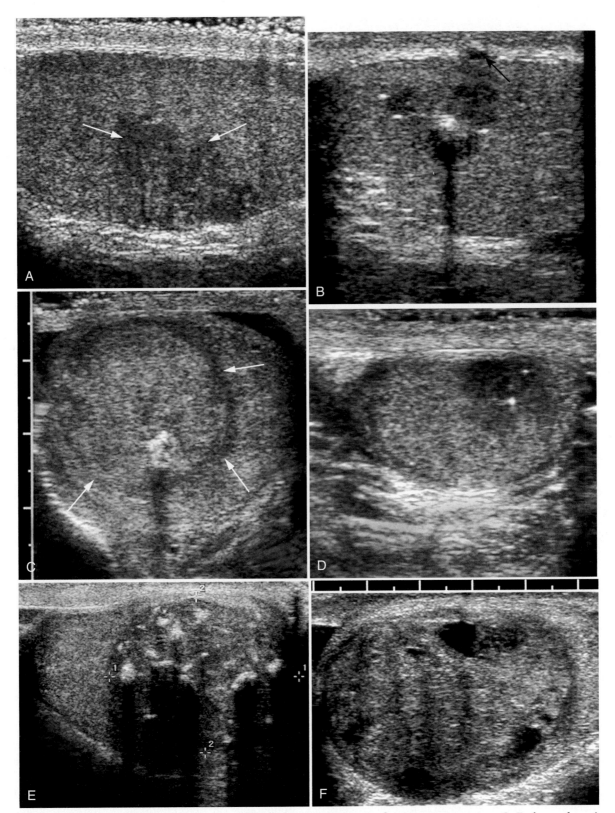

FIGURE 21-6. Nonseminomatous germ cell tumors: spectrum of appearances. A to **C, Embryonal carcinoma. A,** Longitudinal scan shows relatively homogeneous tumor *(arrows)*. **B,** Longitudinal scan shows partly cystic calcified mass invading the tunica *(arrow)*. **C,** Transverse scan shows tumor *(arrows)* with coarse calcification. **D** and **E, Teratoma.** Longitudinal scans show **D,** cystic change and calcification, and **E,** extensive calcification. **F, Mixed germ cell tumor.** Longitudinal scan shows a large tumor with cystic change occupying most of the testis.

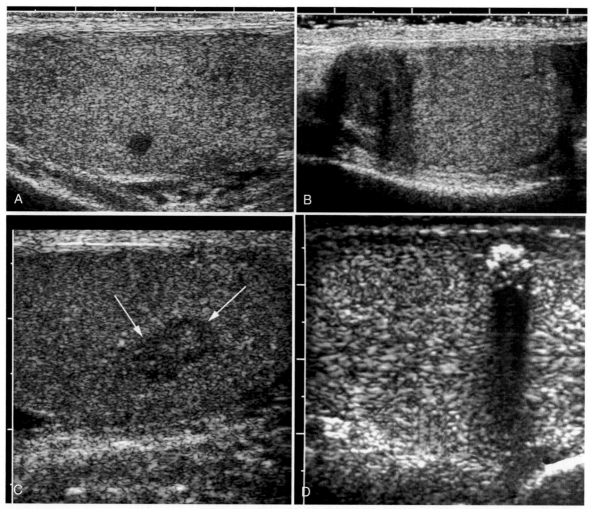

FIGURE 21-7. Stromal tumors: spectrum of appearances. A to C, Leydig cell tumor. Longitudinal scans show **A,** small, hypoechoic solid mass in the midtestis; **B,** hypoechoic solid mass at the upper pole of the testis; and **C,** subtle hypoechoic mass *(arrows)* in the midtestis. The patient had bilateral stromal tumors. **D,** Transverse scan of large-cell calcifying **Sertoli cell tumor.**

color Doppler imaging[24] (Fig. 21-7, *A-C*). Cystic spaces resulting from hemorrhage and necrosis are occasionally seen in larger lesions.

Sertoli cell tumors are rare and account for less than 1% of all testicular tumors; they occur with equal frequency in all age groups.[25] The most common presentation is with a painless testicular mass. Feminization with gynecomastia may occur, especially with malignant Sertoli cell tumors or with the large-cell calcifying variant. Sertoli cell tumors may occur in undescended testes, in patients with testicular feminization, Klinefelter's syndrome, and Peutz-Jeghers syndrome.[26] Sertoli cell tumors are usually small and homogeneous, as reflected in the sonographic appearance, which shows a small, hypoechoic mass similar to a Leydig cell tumor. Occasionally, hemorrhage or necrosis may occur, giving a more heterogeneous appearance on sonography. The large-cell calcifying Sertoli cell tumor is a subtype with distinctive clinical, histologic, and sonographic features.[26] These tumors are often bilateral

and multifocal and may be almost completely calcified (Fig. 21-7, *D*).

Occult Primary Tumors

Sonography is an important diagnostic tool for patients who present with mediastinal, retroperitoneal, or supraclavicular metastases from metastatic testicular carcinoma but have a normal physical examination of the testes (Fig. 21-8). The detection of the **occult primary tumor** is important in disease management because if the tumor is not removed, metastasis will continue. Sonography can detect nonpalpable testicular neoplasms. Unlike mediastinal and CNS extragonadal tumors, which are often primary lesions, retroperitoneal germ cell tumors are usually metastases from primary testicular germ cell tumors.[27,28] The primary testicular tumor may regress, despite widespread advancing metastatic disease, resulting in an echogenic fibrous and possibly calcific scar. Hypothetically, regression is caused by the high

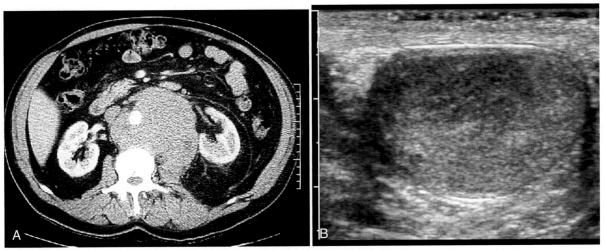

FIGURE 21-8. Occult testicular seminoma with retroperitoneal metastases. A, Contrast-enhanced CT scan showing extensive retroperitoneal adenopathy from seminoma. **B,** Longitudinal sonographic scan shows occult homogeneous hypoechoic seminoma. The physical examination of the testis was negative.

metabolic rate of the tumor and vascular compromise from the tumor outgrowing its blood supply. Usually, no viable tumor cells are identifiable on histologic section in these cases, although intratubular malignant germ cells may be present.[14,15,27] The size of the affected testis is often normal or small. The sonographic finding of an echogenic focus with or without posterior acoustic shadowing is not specific for a "burned-out" tumor, but it strongly suggests this diagnosis in the context of histologically proven testicular metastases[29] (Fig. 21-9).

Approximately 95% of primary testicular neoplasms larger than 1.6 cm in diameter show increased vascularity on color flow Doppler examination. However, color Doppler findings do not appear to be important in the evaluation of adult testicular tumors.[30] Color flow may help to identify tumors that are relatively isoechoic with testicular parenchyma,[31] but focal or diffuse inflammatory lesions cannot be distinguished from neoplasms on the basis of color flow Doppler or pulsed Doppler findings.

Nonpalpable testicular tumors have also been detected with sonography in patients presenting for scrotal discomfort or infertility.[32-35] Incidentally discovered nonpalpable lesions are often benign, but approximately 20% to 30% are malignant.[33,34,36] Management of these patients is controversial. Many believe that if tumor markers and the chest radiograph are normal, patients can undergo an excisional testicular biopsy using an inguinal, organ-sparing approach. In these patients, intraoperative sonography may facilitate resection of the testicular mass. If the frozen section shows a benign lesion, the testis can usually be spared.[33] Sonographic follow-up rather than excision of an incidentally detected lesion ("incidentaloma") is only recommended if there is a strong clinical suggestion that the lesion is nonneoplastic (i.e., recent history of trauma or infection).

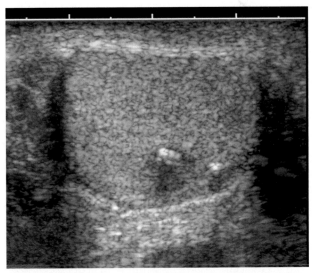

FIGURE 21-9. "Burned-out" germ cell tumor. Longitudinal scan shows a partly calcified nonviable germ cell tumor in a patient with retroperitoneal metastases. Notice the hypoechoic mass around the focus of calcification.

Testicular Metastases

Metastases, Lymphoma, and Leukemia

Malignant lymphoma is the most common secondary testicular neoplasm. Lymphoma accounts for 1% to 8% of all testicular tumors and is the most common testicular tumor in men older than 60 years. However, testicular involvement occurs in only 0.3% of patients with lymphoma.[16] The peak age at diagnosis of lymphoma is 60 to 70 years; 80% of the patients are older than 50 at diagnosis. Malignant lymphoma is the most common bilateral testicular tumor, occurring bilaterally either in a synchronous or more often in a metachronous manner

TESTICULAR METASTASES

LYMPHOMA
Mostly non-Hodgkin's lymphoma

LEUKEMIA
Second most common
Acute leukemia: 64%
"Sanctuary" site

NONLYMPHOMA METASTASES
Lung and prostate most common
Kidney, stomach, colon, pancreas, melanoma

in 6% to 38% of cases. One half of bilateral testicular neoplasms are malignant lymphomas.[16,18] Most malignant lymphomas of the testicle are of the non-Hodgkin's type. Hodgkin's lymphoma of the testis is extremely rare.

Testicular lymphoma most frequently occurs in association with disseminated disease or as the initial manifestation of occult nodal disease. Approximately 10% of the patients with lymphoma present with a testicular mass and appear to have a relatively good prognosis, although meticulous examination usually reveals lymph node involvement.[16] True primary lymphoma of the testis has not been conclusively documented.[17] Most patients with malignant lymphoma of the testis have a painless testicular mass or diffuse testicular enlargement. Approximately 25% of the patients have constitutional symptoms of lymphoma, such as fever, weakness, anorexia, or weight loss.

Lymphoma of the testis is often large at diagnosis. The tunica vaginalis is usually intact, but unlike germ cell tumors, extension into the epididymis and spermatic cord is common, occurring in up to 50% of cases.[37] The scrotal skin is rarely involved. Grossly, the tumor is not encapsulated but compresses the parenchyma to the periphery. The sonographic appearance of lymphoma is nonspecific and similar to that of seminoma. Most malignant lymphomas are homogeneous and hypoechoic, and they diffusely replace the testis;[16] however, focal hypoechoic lesions can occur (Fig. 21-10). Hemorrhage and necrosis are rare.

Color flow Doppler imaging shows increased vascularity in testicular lymphoma, and the appearance may resemble diffuse inflammation[38] (Fig. 21-10, C). Unlike inflammation, lymphoma is usually painless, and the testes are not tender to palpation.

Leukemia is the second most common metastatic testicular neoplasm. Primary testicular leukemia is rare, but leukemic infiltration of the testicle during bone marrow remission is common in children.[16,39] The testis appears to act as a "sanctuary" site for leukemic cells during chemotherapy because of the **blood-testis barrier,** which inhibits concentration of chemotherapeutic agents.[39] The highest frequency of testicular involvement is found in patients with acute leukemia (64%). Approximately 25% of patients with chronic leukemia have testicular involvement. Most cases of testicular involvement occur within 1 year of the discontinuation of long-term remission maintenance chemotherapy.

The sonographic appearance of leukemia is nonspecific and similar to lymphoma. Patients most frequently present with diffuse infiltration, which produces diffusely enlarged, hypoechoic testes (Fig. 21-10, E).

Myeloma

Involvement of the testis is usually a manifestation of diffuse myeloma, although rarely the testis may be the site of primary focal myeloma (plasmacytoma).[40] The testis may have single or multiple nodules that appear hypoechoic and homogeneous on sonographic examination. Bilateral involvement occurs in approximately 20% of cases.[17]

Other Metastases

Nonlymphomatous metastases to the testes are uncommon, representing 0.02% to 5% of all testicular neoplasms.[41] The most frequent primary sites are the **lung** and **prostate.**[18] Other frequent primary sites for metastatic neoplasms include melanoma, kidney, colon, stomach, and pancreas.[42] Most metastases are clinically silent, being discovered incidentally at autopsy or after orchiectomy for prostatic carcinoma. Testicular metastases are most common in patients during the sixth and seventh decades.[1] They are usually multiple and are bilateral in 15% of cases.[18] Because primary germ cell tumors may also be multicentric and bilateral, these features are not helpful in distinguishing primary from metastatic testicular neoplasms. Widespread systemic metastases are usually present in patients with testicular metastases. Possible routes of metastases to the testis include retrograde venous, hematogenous, retrograde lymphatic, and direct tumor invasion. Metastases from sites remote from the testis, such as the lung and skin, most likely spread hematogenously. Retrograde venous extension through the spermatic vein occurs in renal cell carcinoma and may also occur in bladder and prostate tumors.[43] Neoplasms with metastases to the periaortic lymph nodes may involve the testis through retrograde lymphatic extension. Colorectal carcinoma may directly invade the testes. Sonographic features of nonlymphomatous testicular metastases vary. The appearance is often hypoechoic but may be echogenic or complex (Fig. 21-10, F).[1]

Other rare tumors of the testis include hamartoma (Fig. 21-11), dermoid, hemangioma, intratesticular adenomatoid tumor, carcinoid, carcinoma of the

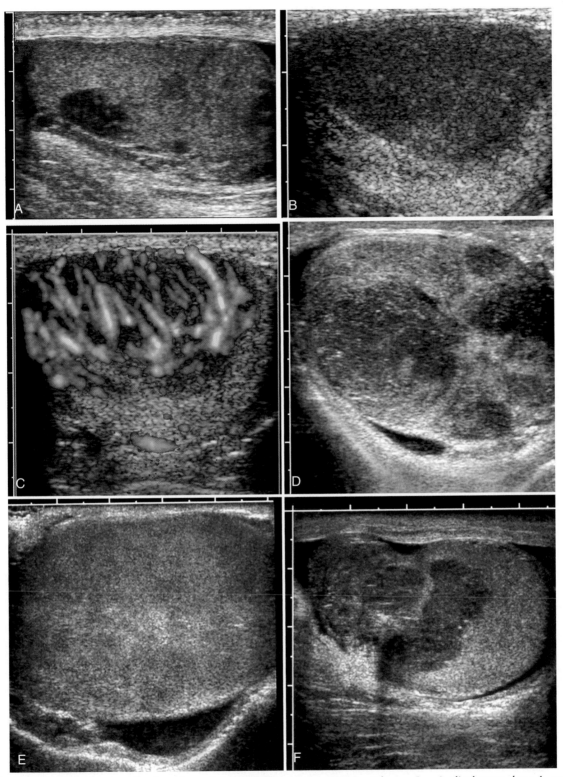

FIGURE 21-10. Lymphoma, leukemia, and metastases. A to **D, Lymphoma.** Longitudinal scans show **A,** two subtle hypoechoic foci of lymphoma, and **B,** diffuse, homogeneous hypoechoic involvement of the testis. **C,** Longitudinal power Doppler image of **B** shows marked vascularity of lymphoma, with **D,** corresponding longitudinal scan. **E, Leukemia.** Longitudinal scan shows diffuse hypoechoic involvement. **F, Melanoma metastasis.** Longitudinal scan shows a hypoechoic mass in the upper pole of the testis and epididymis.

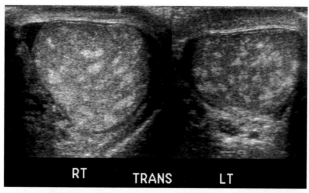

FIGURE 21-11. Dual transverse image shows multiple bilateral hamartomas. The patient had Cowden disease, an inherited autosomal dominant disorder, which causes multiple hamartomas in the gastrointestinal tract.

TESTICULAR CYSTIC LESIONS

BENIGN
Tunica albuginea cysts
Tunica vaginalis cysts
Intratesticular cysts
Tubular ectasia of rete testis
Cystic dysplasia
Epidermoid cysts
Abscess

MALIGNANT
Nonseminomatous germ cell tumor
Necrosis or hemorrhage in tumor
Tubular obstruction by tumor
Lymphoma

mediastinum testis, neuroectodermal tumor, Brenner tumor, fibroma, fibrosarcoma, osteosarcoma, chondrosarcoma, and undifferentiated sarcoma.

Benign Intratesticular Lesions

Cysts

Testicular cysts are discovered incidentally on sonography in 8% to 10% of the male population.[44] Cystic testicular lesions are not always benign because testicular tumors (especially NSGCTs) may undergo cystic degeneration from hemorrhage or necrosis. The distinction between a benign cyst and a cystic neoplasm is of utmost clinical importance. Simple intratesticular cysts can be managed conservatively without the need for surgical intervention.[45] Of the 34 cystic testicular masses discovered with sonography by Hamm et al.,[44] 16 were neoplastic, and all of these had sonographic features of complicated cysts. NCGCTs, especially those with tera-

toma elements, are the most common tumors to contain both cystic and solid components.

Cysts of the tunica albuginea are located within the tunica, which surrounds the testis. They vary in size from 2 to 30 mm and are well defined. They are usually solitary and unilocular but may be multiple or multilocular[44,46] (Fig. 21-12, *A*). The mean age at presentation is 40 years, but cysts also occur in the fifth and sixth decades.[47] The cysts may be asymptomatic, but patients frequently present with cysts that are clinically palpable, firm scrotal nodules. Histologically, they are simple cysts lined with cuboid or low columnar cells and filled with serous fluid.[48] Complex tunica albuginea cysts may simulate a testicular neoplasm.[49] Careful scanning in multiple planes may help identify the benign nature of a tunica albuginea cyst.

Cysts of the tunica vaginalis are rare and arise from the visceral or parietal layer of the tunica vaginalis. They may be single or multiple. Sonographically, they usually appear anechoic but may have septations or may contain echoes caused by hemorrhage.[50]

Intratesticular cysts are simple cysts filled with clear serous fluid; they vary in size from 2 to 18 mm.[51] Sonographically, they are well-defined, anechoic lesions with thin, smooth walls and posterior acoustic enhancement. Hamm et al.[44] reported that in all 13 of their cases, the cysts were located near the mediastinum testis, supporting the theory that they originate from the rete testis, possibly secondary to posttraumatic or postinflammatory stricture formation (Fig. 21-12. *D-F*).

Tubular Ectasia of Rete Testis

Tubular ectasia of the rete testis can be mistaken for a testicular neoplasm.[52-55] This tubular ectasia is usually associated with epididymal obstruction caused by inflammation or trauma. Variably sized cystic lesions are seen in the region of the mediastinum testis with no associated soft tissue abnormality, and no flow on color flow Doppler imaging is seen (Fig. 21-12, *B-D*). Most of these lesions are bilateral and asymmetrical. There is frequently an associated spermatocele. The characteristic sonographic appearance and location should allow distinguishing this benign condition from a malignancy, thus avoiding an orchiectomy. Characteristic findings on magnetic resonance imaging (MRI) include intratesticular abnormal signal intensity similar to that of water in the region of the mediastinum testis.[52]

Cystic Dysplasia

Cystic dysplasia is a rare congenital malformation, usually occurring in infants and young children, although one case was reported in a 30-year-old man.[56,57] This lesion is thought to result from an embryologic defect that prevents connection of the tubules of the rete testis and the efferent ductules. Pathologically, the lesion con-

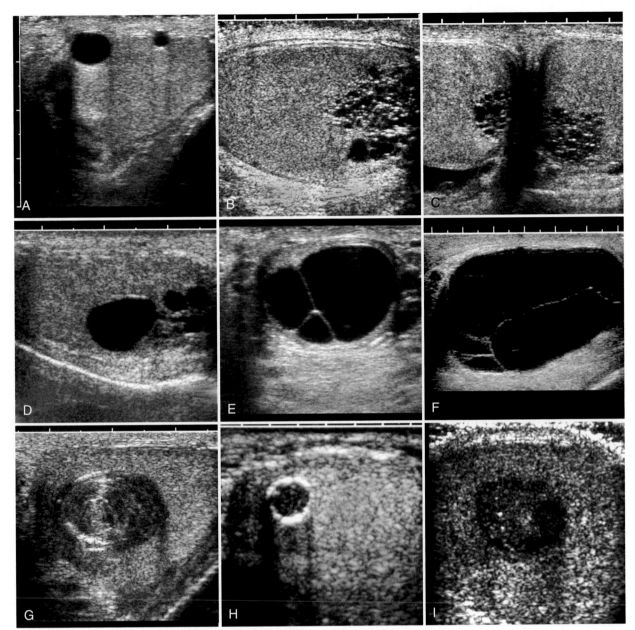

FIGURE 21-12. Benign cystic lesions of the testis. A, Tunica albuginea cysts. Longitudinal scan shows two cysts arising from the tunica. These cysts are usually palpable. **B and C, Cystic dilation in rete testis.** Longitudinal and transverse scans show dilated tubules of the rete testis in both testes. **D,** Benign intratesticular cyst associated with dilated rete testis on longitudinal scan. **E and F,** Benign intratesticular cyst with multiple septations. **G to I, Epidermoid cyst** (benign). **G,** Typical whorled appearance; **H,** typical peripheral calcification. **I,** Transverse scan shows hypoechoic mass with central calcifications similar to other tumors on gray scale, but avascular on Doppler examination. (**H** *courtesy Ben Hollenberg, MD, Presbyterian Hospital, Charlotte, NC.*)

sists of multiple, interconnecting cysts of various sizes and shapes, separated by fibrous septae. This lesion originates in the rete testis and extends into the adjacent parenchyma, resulting in pressure atrophy of the adjacent testicular parenchyma. The cysts are lined by a single layer of flat or cuboidal epithelium. Sonographically, the appearance is similar to acquired cystic dilation of the rete testis. Renal agenesis or dysplasia frequently coexists with testicular cystic dysplasia.[57]

Epidermoid Cysts

The epidermoid cyst is a benign, generally well-circumscribed tumor of germ cell origin, representing approximately 1% of all testicular tumors. These tumors occur at any age but are most common during the second to fourth decades.[18] Usually, patients present with a painless testicular nodule; one-third the tumors are discovered incidentally on physical examination. Diffuse, painless testicular enlargement occurs in 10% of patients. Pathologically, the tumor wall is composed of fibrous tissue with an inner lining of squamous epithelium. The cyst is filled with flaky, cheesy, white keratin. Although the histogenesis of epidermoid cysts is controversial, current opinion is that most are derived from epithelial rests or inclusions and have no malignant potential.[58] Also, epidermoid cysts may represent monomorphic or monodermal development of a teratoma along the line of ectodermal cell differentiation. These benign lesions can be differentiated from premalignant teratomas only through histologic examination.

Sonographically variable, epidermoid cysts are generally well-defined, avascular masses and may be multiple or bilateral.[58] A characteristic whorled appearance, like the layers of an onion skin, corresponds to the alternating layers of compacted keratin and desquamated squamous cells seen histologically[59-61] (Fig. 21-12, G; **Video 21-2**). This appearance, however, may not be pathognomonic because it may rarely be seen with teratoma.[62] Another typical appearance of epidermoid cyst is a well-defined hypoechoic mass with an echogenic capsule that may be calcified (Fig. 21-12, H). There may be central calcification giving a "bull's eye" or target appearance[58] (Fig. 21-12, I). Epidermoid cysts may also have the nonspecific appearance of a hypoechoic mass with or without calcifications and may resemble germ cell tumors. Avascularity is a clue to the diagnosis.[61] When the sonographic appearance is characteristic, histologic confirmation is still obtained by a conservative testicle-sparing approach with local excision (enucleation).[63] MRI has been used to support the sonographic diagnosis of epidermoid cysts if further confirmation is desired before testis-sparing surgery.[64,65] Distinguishing an epidermoid cyst from a teratoma requires careful pathologic examination of the cyst wall and adjacent testis.

Abscess

Testicular abscesses are usually a complication of epididymo-orchitis; they may also result from an undiagnosed testicular torsion, a gangrenous or infected tumor, or a primary pyogenic orchitis. Infectious causes of abscess formation are **mumps, smallpox, scarlet fever, influenza, typhoid, sinusitis, osteomyelitis,** and **appendicitis.**[66] A testicular abscess may rupture through the tunica vaginalis, resulting in formation of a pyocele or a fistula to the skin.

Most often, sonography shows an enlarged testicle containing a predominantly fluid-filled mass with hypoechoic or mixed echogenic areas (Fig. 21-13, A). In one atypical appearance, the testicular architecture was disrupted with hyperechoic striations separating hypoechoic spaces[67] (Fig. 21-13, B and C). The striations were thought to be fibrous septa in the hypoechoic, necrotic testicular parenchyma. Testicular abscesses have no diagnostic sonographic features but can often be

distinguished from tumors on the basis of clinical symptoms.

In patients with acquired immunodeficiency syndrome (AIDS), distinguishing an abscess from a neoplastic process may be difficult on sonographic examination. Clinical findings may be helpful; however, orchiectomy is frequently necessary to obtain a histologic diagnosis.[68,69]

Segmental Infarction

Segmental testicular infarction may occur after **torsion, trauma, bacterial endocarditis, vasculitis, leukemia,** and **hypercoagulable states.**[70] Spontaneous infarction of the testis is rare. The sonographic appearance depends on the age of the infarction. Initially, a typical segmental infarct is seen as a focal, wedge-shaped or round hypoechoic mass.[71] The focal hypoechoic mass cannot be distinguished from a neoplasm on the basis of its gray-scale sonographic appearance.[72,73] These lesions should have reduced or absent blood flow, depending on the age of the infarction.[71] If a well-circumscribed, nonpalpable, relatively peripheral, hypoechoic mass shows a complete lack of vascularity on power Doppler imaging or after the administration of sonographic contrast agent, it may be possible to distinguish such benign infarctions from neoplasm[74,75] (Fig. 21-14). With time, the hypoechoic mass or the entire testicle often decreases in size and develops areas of increased echogenicity because of fibrosis or dystrophic calcification.[67] The early sonographic appearance may be difficult to distinguish from a testicular neoplasm, but infarcts decrease substantially in size, whereas tumors characteristically enlarge with time.[1,73]

Sarcoidosis

Sarcoidosis may involve the epididymis or the testis.[76-78] Genital involvement occurs in less than 1% of patients with systemic sarcoidosis.[1] The clinical presentation is acute or recurrent epididymitis or painless enlargement of the testis or epididymis. Sonographically, sarcoid lesions are irregular, hypoechoic solid masses in the testis or epididymis (Fig. 21-15). Occasionally, hyperechoic, calcific foci with acoustic shadowing may be seen.[10] Distinguishing sarcoidosis from an inflammatory process or a neoplasm is difficult on sonography alone. Resection or orchiectomy may be necessary for definitive diagnosis.

Adrenal Rests

Congenital adrenal hyperplasia (CAH) is an autosomal recessive disease involving an adrenocortical enzyme defect. This disease may become clinically obvious early in life or in early adulthood. Patients often present with a testicular mass or enlargement, and with precocious puberty, with or without salt-depletion syndrome. **Adrenal rests** arise from aberrant adrenocortical cells

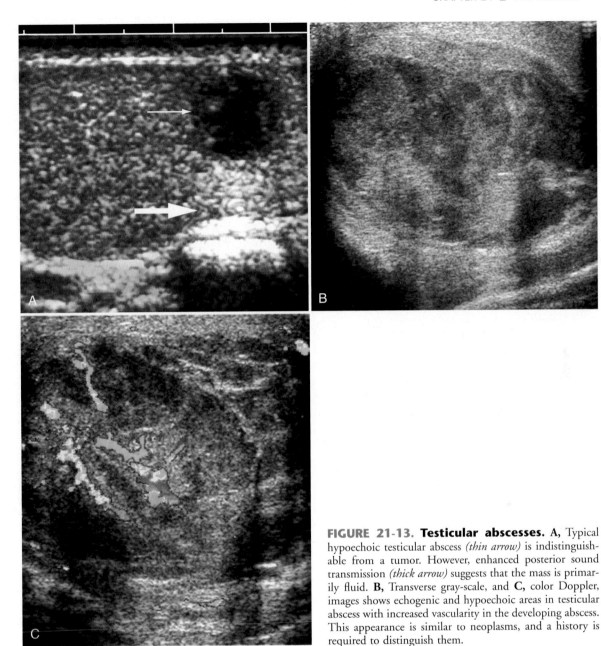

FIGURE 21-13. Testicular abscesses. A, Typical hypoechoic testicular abscess *(thin arrow)* is indistinguishable from a tumor. However, enhanced posterior sound transmission *(thick arrow)* suggests that the mass is primarily fluid. **B,** Transverse gray-scale, and **C,** color Doppler, images shows echogenic and hypoechoic areas in testicular abscess with increased vascularity in the developing abscess. This appearance is similar to neoplasms, and a history is required to distinguish them.

that migrate with gonadal tissues in the fetus. They can form **tumorlike masses** in response to elevated levels of circulating corticotropin in CAH and Cushing's syndrome and rarely may undergo malignant transformation. On sonography, these lesions are multifocal hypoechoic lesions (Fig. 21-16). Occasionally, posterior acoustic shadowing has been described. Many adrenal rests demonstrate spokelike vascularity with multiple peripheral vessels radiating toward a central point within the mass. Usually, if the patient has the appropriate hormonal abnormalities associated with CAH and if sonography shows the appropriate findings, no further work-up is necessary.[79,80] If confirmation of the diagnosis is required, a biopsy under ultrasound guidance may be obtained intraoperatively when the testis is exposed.

Splenogonadal Fusion

Splenogonadal fusion is a rare congenital anomaly in which there is fusion of the spleen and gonad. It usually occurs on the left side and is most often associated with cryptorchidism.[81] There are two types of splenogonadal fusion: continuous and discontinuous. In the more common **continuous** form, the gonad is linked to the spleen by a fibrous cord of splenic tissue. In the **discontinuous** form, ectopic splenic tissue is attached to the testis. Rarely, ectopic splenic tissue may occur on the epididymis or spermatic cord. Splenogonadal fusion may mimic testicular malignancy. The diagnosis may be established by documenting uptake on a technetium-99m sulfur colloid scan.

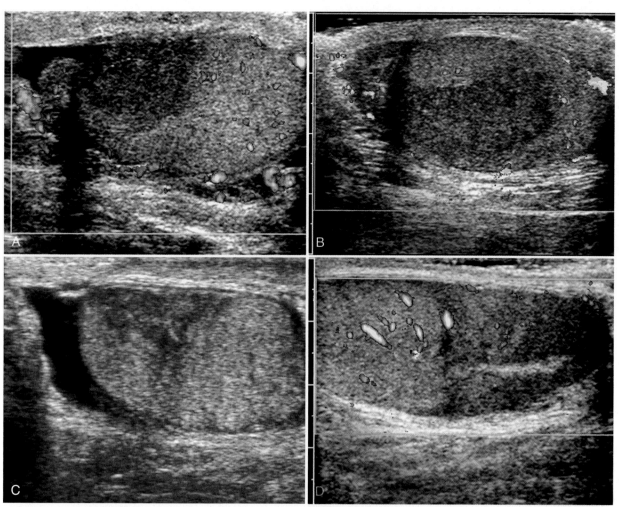

FIGURE 21-14. Testicular infarcts: spectrum of appearances. A and **B, Acute infarct. A,** Longitudinal power Doppler scan shows an avascular area at the upper pole from partial torsion. **B,** Longitudinal color Doppler scan shows an avascular area in the midtestis caused by vasculitis. **C** and **D, Chronic infarct. C,** Longitudinal scan shows a peripheral wedge-shaped hypoechoic area caused by prior mumps orchitis. **D,** Longitudinal power Doppler scan shows lack of vascularity in the lower pole.

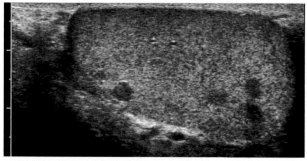

FIGURE 21-15. Testicular sarcoid. Longitudinal scan of the testis shows multiple, small, hypoechoic, solid masses resulting from sarcoid.

Scrotal Calcifications

Scrotal calcifications may be seen within the parenchyma of the testicle, on the surface of the testicle, or freely located in the fluid between the layers of the tunica vaginalis. Large, smooth, curvilinear calcifications without

an associated soft tissue mass are characteristic of a large-cell calcifying **Sertoli cell tumor**, although occasionally, **burned-out germ cell tumors** may have a similar appearance.[82] Scattered calcifications may be found in **tuberculosis, filariasis,** and **scarring** from regressed germ cell tumor or trauma.

Testicular microlithiasis is a condition in which calcifications are present within the seminiferous tubules of the testis either unilaterally or bilaterally. It is postulated that microlithiasis is caused by defective Sertoli cell phagocytosis of degenerating tubular cells, which then calcify within the seminiferous tubules.[83,84] Microlithiasis has been classified as diffuse and limited.[85] In the **diffuse** form, innumerable small, hyperechoic foci are diffusely scattered throughout the testicular parenchyma. These tiny (1-3 mm) foci rarely show a shadow and occasionally show a comet-tail appearance (Fig. 21-17). In the **limited** form, previously thought to be insignificant, less than five hyperechoic foci are seen per image of the testis (Fig. 21-17, *B*).

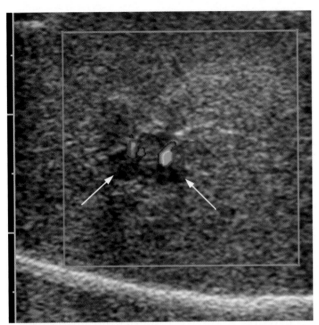

FIGURE 21-16. Adrenal rest. Intraoperative color Doppler image shows an intratesticular mass *(arrows)* with blood flow present near the mediastinum testis.

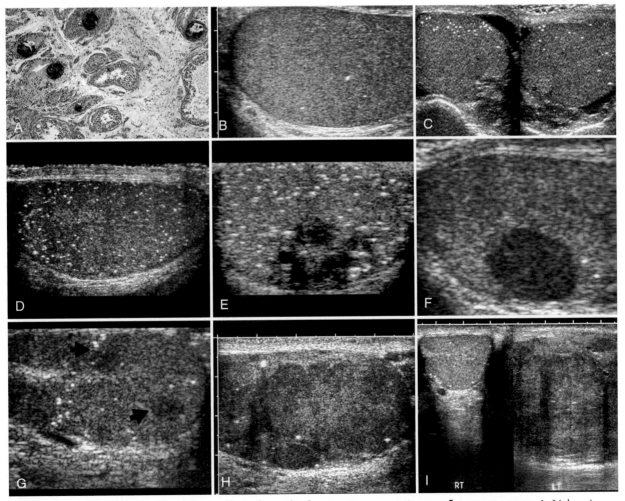

FIGURE 21-17. Microlithiasis and associated testicular tumors: spectrum of appearances. A, Light microscopy examination shows multiple intratubular calcifications *(dark areas)* characteristic of microlithiasis. **B,** Longitudinal scan shows a few tiny calcifications of limited microlithiasis. **C** and **D,** Diffuse microlithiasis. **E,** Transverse scan of testis shows microlithiasis and partially cystic mass caused by **mixed germ cell tumor. F,** Limited microlithiasis with **seminoma.** Longitudinal scan shows a few tiny calcifications and a homogeneous hypoechoic mass. **G,** Microlithiasis and two foci of seminoma. Longitudinal scan shows multiple tiny calcifications and two hypoechoic homogeneous masses *(arrows).* **H** and **I,** Microlithiasis and seminoma. **H,** Longitudinal scan shows large hypoechoic mass with multiple small and coarser calcifications. **I,** Dual transverse image shows large hypoechoic left testicular mass and microcalcifications in the right testis.

Microlithiasis is seen in 1% to 2% of the patients referred for testicular sonography and has a reported prevalence in the general population of 0.6% to 0.9%.[86] Microlithiasis has been associated with cryptorchidism, Klinefelter's syndrome, Down syndrome, pulmonary alveolar microlithiasis, AIDS, neurofibromatosis, previous radiotherapy, and subfertility.[83,86-88] Most importantly, many reports associate microlithiasis with **testicular germ cell neoplasms** (seminoma or nonseminoma), **intratubular germ cell neoplasia,** and **extratesticular germ cell tumor**[85,89-98] (Fig. 21-17). There is general agreement that an association with malignancy exists, but controversy surrounds the strength of this association and the significance of limited microlithiasis.[99-104] Prospective data show that coexisting testicular tumors occur more frequently in patients who have both diffuse and limited microlithiasis, occurring in 5% to 10% of patients.[85] Despite case reports, it is not yet clear, however, whether the incidence of de novo testicular tumors is significantly increased in patients with preexisting microlithiasis.[97] Therefore, no consensus exists on the appropriate follow-up (clinical or radiologic) for patients with testicular microlithiasis. Annual sonography is usually recommended if there are additional risk factors such as infertility, testicular atrophy, or contralateral testicular malignancy. Annual physical examination and periodic self-examination are suggested for those who have no additional risk factors.[85,86,99,100]

Extratesticular scrotal calculi arise from the surface of the tunica vaginalis and may break loose to migrate between the two layers of the tunica (Fig. 21-18). These fibrinoid loose bodies have been called **scrotal pearls** because of their macroscopic appearance, which is usually round, pearly white, and rubbery. Histologically, they consist of fibrinoid material deposited around a central nucleus of hydroxyapatite.[105] They may result from inflammation of the tunica vaginalis or torsion of the appendix testis or epididymis. Hydroceles facilitate the sonographic diagnosis of scrotal calculi.

Extratesticular Pathologic Lesions

Hydrocele, Hematocele, and Pyocele

Serous fluid, blood, pus, or urine may accumulate in the space between the parietal and visceral layers of the tunica vaginalis lining the scrotum. These fluid collections are confined to the anterolateral portions of the scrotum because of the attachment of the testis to the epididymis and scrotal wall posteriorly (the bare area)[5] (Fig. 21-19). The normal scrotum contains a few milliliters of serous fluid between the layers of the tunica vaginalis, and this is usually visible on sonographic examination.

Hydrocele is an abnormal accumulation of serous fluid between the layers of the tunica vaginalis. Rarely, hydrocele may be loculated around the spermatic cord

EXTRATESTICULAR TUMORS

BENIGN
Adenomatoid tumor
Fibroma
Lipoma
Hemangioma
Leiomyoma
Neurofibroma
Cholesterol granuloma
Adrenal rest
Papillary cystadenoma

MALIGNANT
Fibrosarcoma
Liposarcoma
Rhabdosarcoma
Histiocytoma
Lymphoma
Metastases

above the testis and epididymis[106] (Fig. 21-19, *A-C*). Hydrocele is the most common cause of painless scrotal swelling[10] and may be congenital or acquired. The **congenital type** results from incomplete closure of the processus vaginalis, with persistent open communication between the scrotal sac and the peritoneum, usually resolving by 18 months of age. **Acquired hydroceles** may be idiopathic or caused by epididymitis, epididymo-orchitis, torsion, and rarely tumors. Hydroceles associated with testicular tumors are usually small.[1,107,108] Sonography is useful in detecting a potential cause of the hydrocele by allowing evaluation of the testicle when a large hydrocele hampers palpation. Hydroceles are characteristically anechoic collections with good sound transmission surrounding the anterolateral aspects of the testis. Low-level to medium-level echoes from fibrin bodies or cholesterol crystals may occasionally be visualized moving freely within a hydrocele.[109] Rarely, a large hydrocele may impede testicular venous drainage and cause absence of antegrade arterial diastolic flow.[107]

Hematoceles and **pyoceles** are less common than simple hydroceles. Hematoceles result from trauma, surgery, neoplasms, or torsion.[110] Pyoceles result from rupture of an abscess into an existing hydrocele or directly into the space between the layers of the tunica vaginalis. Both hematoceles and pyoceles contain internal septations and loculations (Fig. 21-19, *D-F*). Thickening of the scrotal skin and calcifications may be seen in chronic cases.

Varicocele

A varicocele is a collection of abnormally dilated, tortuous, and elongated veins of the pampiniform plexus

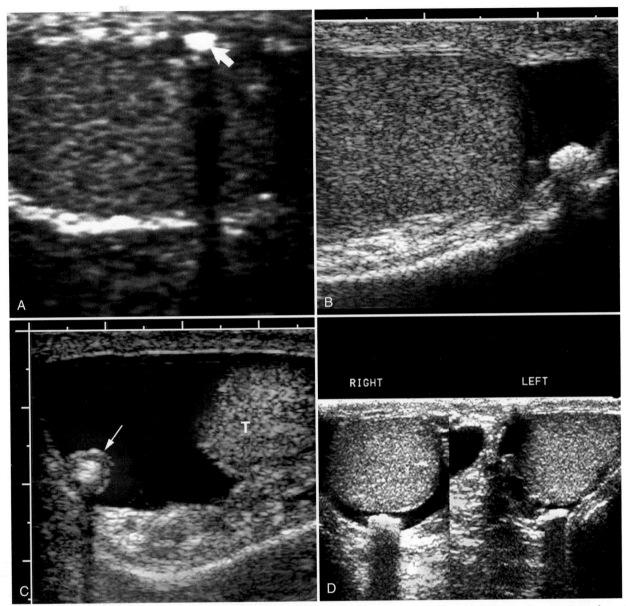

FIGURE 21-18. Benign intrascrotal calcification. A, Calcified tunica plaque on the tunica vaginalis. **B** to **D, Scrotal pearls. B,** Mobile scrotal calcification in a small hydrocele. **C,** Longitudinal scan shows a mostly calcified scrotal pearl *(arrow)* in a hydrocele; *T,* testis. **D,** Bilateral scrotal pearls.

located posterior to the testis, accompanying the epididymis and vas deferens within the spermatic cord[10] (Fig. 21-20). The veins of the pampiniform plexus normally range from 0.5 to 1.5 mm in diameter, with a main draining vein up to 2 mm in diameter.

There are two types of varicoceles: primary (idiopathic) and secondary. The **idiopathic varicocele** is caused by incompetent valves in the internal spermatic vein, which permit retrograde passage of blood through the spermatic cord into the pampiniform plexus. Varicocele affects approximately 15% of men, but occurs in up to 40% of men attending infertility clinics.[111,112] Varicocele is the most common correctable cause of male infertility.[113] Idiopathic varicoceles occur on the left side

in 98% of cases and are most common in men age 15 to 25 years. The left-sided predominance probably occurs because the venous drainage on the left side is into the renal vein, as opposed to the right spermatic vein, which drains directly into the vena cava. Idiopathic varices normally distend when the patient is upright or performs the Valsalva maneuver and may decompress when the patient is supine. Primary varicoceles are bilateral in up to 70% of cases.

Secondary varicoceles result from increased pressure on the spermatic vein or its tributaries by marked hydronephrosis, an enlarged liver, abdominal neoplasms, or venous compression by a retroperitoneal mass.[19] Secondary varicocele may also occur in the **nutcracker**

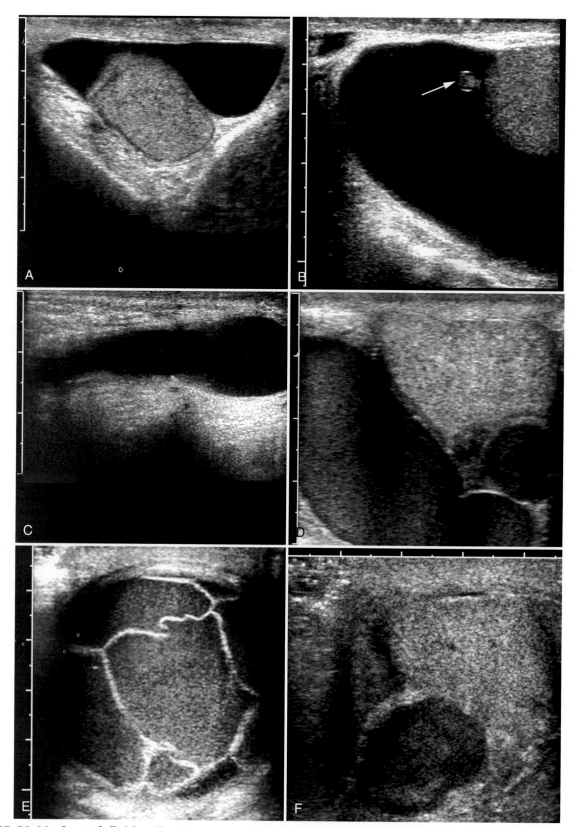

FIGURE 21-19. Scrotal fluid collections: spectrum of appearances. A, Hydrocele. Transverse scan shows hydrocele anterolaterally with attachment of testis to tunica vaginalis posteriorly. **B, Hydrocele.** Fluid outlines appendix testis *(arrow).* **C, Hydrocele of cord**. Longitudinal scan of inguinal region shows elongated fluid collection above the level of the testis and epididymis. **D, Hematocele.** Transverse scan shows loculated fluid with internal echoes. **E, Hematocele.** Transverse scan shows fluid with internal echoes and linear membranes. **F, Pyocele.** Transverse scan shows fluid collection with internal echoes.

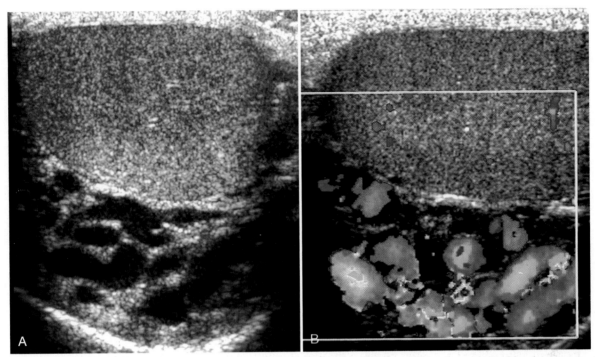

FIGURE 21-20. Varicocele. A, Longitudinal, and **B,** color Doppler, images show serpentine, hypoechoic, dilated veins posterior to the testis. The blood flow in a varicocele is slow and may be detected only with low-flow Doppler settings or the Valsalva maneuver.

syndrome (nutcracker phenomenon), in which the superior mesenteric artery compresses the left renal vein.[114] A search for neoplastic obstruction of gonadal venous return must be undertaken in cases of a right-sided, nondecompressible, or newly discovered varicocele in a patient older than 40 years because these cases are rarely idiopathic[10] (Fig. 21-21). The appearance of secondary varicoceles is not affected by patient position.

In infertile men, sonography aids in the diagnosis of clinically palpable and subclinical varicoceles. Sonography is also of value in assessing testicular size before and after treatment, because varicocele may be associated with a decreased testicular volume.[112] There is poor correlation between the size of the varicocele and the degree of testicular tissue damage leading to infertility.

Sonographically, the varicocele consists of multiple, serpentine, anechoic structures more than 2 mm in diameter, creating a tortuous, multicystic collection located adjacent or proximal to the upper pole of the testis and head of the epididymis. A high-frequency transducer in conjunction with low-flow Doppler settings should be used to optimize slow-flow detection within varices. Slowly moving red blood cells may be visualized with high-frequency transducers, even when flow is too slow to be detected by Doppler imaging. Venous flow can be augmented with the patient in the upright position or during Valsalva maneuver **(Video 21-3).** Varicoceles follow the course of the spermatic cord into the inguinal canal and are easily compressed by the transducer.[1] Rarely, varicoceles may be intrates-

ticular, either in a subcapsular location or around the mediastinum testis[115,116] (Fig. 21-22).

Scrotal Hernia

A scrotal hernia is another common paratesticular mass. Although scrotal hernias are usually diagnosed on the basis of clinical history and physical examination, sonography is useful in the evaluation of atypical cases. The hernia may contain small bowel or colon, with or without omentum. The presence of bowel loops within the hernia may be confirmed by the visualization of valvulae conniventes or haustrations and detection of peristalsis on real-time examination. If these features are absent, distinguishing a hernia from other extratesticular multicystic masses, such as hematoceles and pyoceles, may be difficult. The presence of highly echogenic material within the scrotum may result from a hernia-containing omentum or other fatty masses such as lipomas (Fig. 21-23). Hernias occur anteromedial to the spermatic cord, whereas lipomas are lateral or inferior to the cord.[117] Sonographic examination of the inguinal canal may identify the extension of omentum or bowel loops from the inguinal canal into the scrotum.

Tumors

Extratesticular scrotal neoplasms are rare and usually involve the epididymis. Most extratesticular neoplasms in adults are benign, but extratesticular neoplasms in children are frequently malignant.[118] The most common

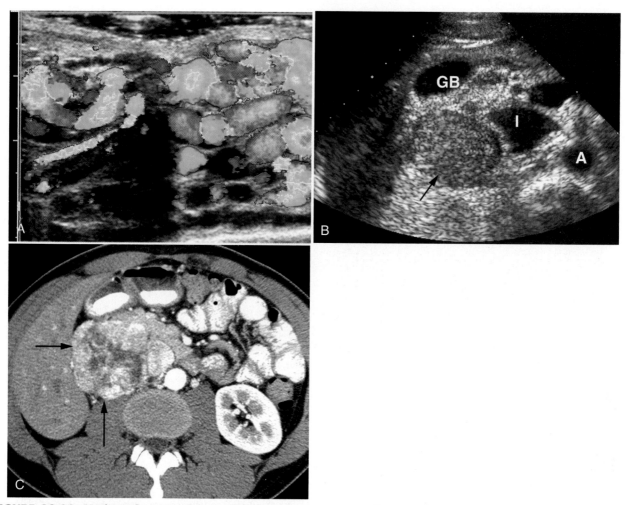

FIGURE 21-21. Varicocele caused by retroperitoneal paraganglioneuroma. A, Longitudinal scan shows extremely dilated veins of large, right varicocele. **B,** Transverse abdominal sonogram shows paraganglioneuroma *(arrow)* adjacent to the inferior vena cava *(I); A,* aorta; *GB,* gallbladder. **C,** Axial CT scan shows the vascular mass *(arrows)* adjacent to inferior vena cava.

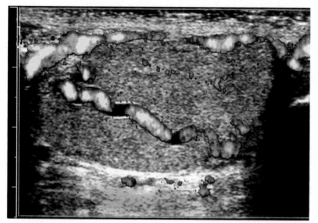

FIGURE 21-22. Intratesticular varicocele. Longitudinal scan shows the dilated vein.

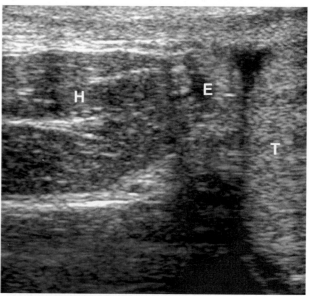

FIGURE 21-23. Herniated mesenteric fat. Longitudinal scan shows herniated fat *(H)* above testis *(T)* and epididymis *(E).*

extratesticular neoplasm in adults is the **benign adenomatoid tumor.**[15] It is most frequently located in the epididymis, especially in the tail, but may also arise in the spermatic cord or testicular tunica (Fig. 21-24, *D* and *E*). This neoplasm occasionally invades adjacent testicular parenchyma. It may occur at any age but most often affects patients age 20 to 50 years.[1,119] Adenomatoid tumors are generally unilateral, solitary, well defined, and round or oval, rarely measuring more than 5 cm in diameter. Occasionally, they may appear plaquelike and poorly defined. Sonography usually shows a solid, well-circumscribed mass with echogenicity that is at least as great as the testis.[1] It may also be hypoechoic.

Other benign extratesticular tumors are rare and include **fibromas, hemangiomas, lipomas** (Fig. 21-24, *F*), **leiomyomas** (Fig. 21-24, *G*), **neurofibromas,** and **cholesterol granulomas. Adrenal rests** may also be encountered in the spermatic cord, testis, epididymis, rete testis, and tunica albuginea in approximately 10% of infants.

Papillary cystadenomas of the epididymis may be seen in patients with Hippel-Lindau disease. These

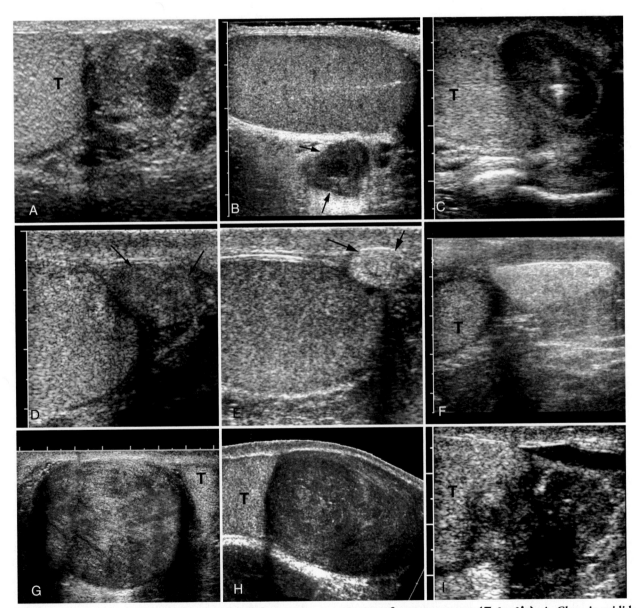

FIGURE 21-24. Extratesticular scrotal solid masses: spectrum of appearances (*T,* testis). A, Chronic epididymitis. Longitudinal scan of the scrotum shows mass in the tail of the epididymis. **B, Sperm granuloma.** Longitudinal scan shows hypoechoic solid mass *(arrows)* posterior to the testis in a patient with vasectomy. **C, Fibrous pseudotumor.** Longitudinal scan shows a mass of mixed echogenicity inferior to the testis. **D, Benign adenomatoid tumor of epididymis.** Longitudinal scan shows a hypoechoic mass *(arrows)* in the tail. **E, Benign adenomatoid tumor of the tunica.** Longitudinal scan shows a hyperechoic mass *(arrows).* **F, Intrascrotal lipoma.** Longitudinal scan shows a hyperechoic mass inferior to the testis. **G, Leiomyoma of cord.** Longitudinal scan shows a solid mass superior to the testis. **H, Rhabdomyosarcoma.** Longitudinal extended–field of view scan in a 12-year-old shows a large, paratesticular mass inferior to the testis. **I, Metastasis from lung carcinoma.** Longitudinal scan shows a mass in the tail of the epididymis.

tumors are considered **hamartomas** and are usually found in the epididymal head.[50] Primary extratesticular scrotal malignant neoplasms include **fibrosarcoma, liposarcoma, histiocytoma,** and **lymphoma** in adults and **rhabdomyosarcoma** in children (Fig. 21-24, *H*). Size of the lesion and the presence of color flow may be helpful in the diagnosis of extratesticular scrotal masses.[120,121] Larger masses (>1.5 cm) with prominent color flow that present without clinical symptoms of inflammation are more likely to be malignant.

Metastatic tumors to the epididymis are also rare. The most common primary sites include the testicle, stomach, kidney, prostate, colon, and less often the pancreas[122,123] (Fig. 21-24, *I*).

Epididymal Lesions

Sperm Granuloma

Sperm granulomas are thought to arise from extravasation of spermatozoa into the soft tissues surrounding the epididymis, producing a necrotizing granulomatous response.[1] These lesions may be painful or asymptomatic, and they are most often found in patients after vasectomy. Sperm granulomas may also be associated with prior epididymal infection or trauma. The typical sonographic appearance is that of a solid, hypoechoic or heterogeneous mass, usually located in the epididymis, although it may simulate an intratesticular lesion (Fig. 21-24, *B*). Chronic sperm granuloma may contain calcification.[124]

Fibrous Pseudotumor

Fibrous pseudotumor is a rare, nonneoplastic mass of reactive fibrous tissue that may involve the tunica vaginalis or epididymis. On sonography, fibrous pseudotumors may appear as hypoechoic, hyperechoic, or heterogeneous paratesticular masses[125-127] (Fig. 21-24, *C*).

Cystic Lesions

Spermatoceles are more common than **epididymal cysts.** Both were seen in 20% to 40% of all asymptomatic patients studied by Leung et al.,[128] and 30% were multiple cysts. Both epididymal cysts and spermatoceles are thought to result from dilation of the epididymal tubules, but the contents of these masses differ.[10] Cysts contain clear serous fluid, whereas spermatoceles are filled with spermatozoa and sediment containing lymphocytes, fat globules, and cellular debris, giving the fluid a thick, milky appearance.[1] Both lesions may result from prior episodes of epididymitis or trauma. Spermatoceles and epididymal cysts appear identical on sonography: anechoic, circumscribed masses with no or few internal echoes; loculations and septations are often seen (Fig. 21-25). Rarely, a spermatocele may be hyper-

echoic.[5] Differentiation between a spermatocele and an epididymal cyst is rarely important clinically. Spermatoceles almost always occur in the head of the epididymis, whereas epididymal cysts arise throughout the length of the epididymis.

Postvasectomy Changes in Epididymis

Sonographic changes in the epididymis are very common in patients after vasectomy.[129,130] These findings include epididymal enlargement with tubular ectasia and the development of sperm granulomas and cysts (Fig. 21-26; **Video 21-4**). It is assumed that vasectomy produces increased pressure in the epididymal tubules, causing tubular rupture with subsequent formation of sperm granulomas. The dilated vas deferens may be seen in addition to the dilated epididymis. An unusual appearance described as "dancing megasperm" is occasionally seen in patients with vasectomy **(Video 21-5).** High reflective echoes within the dilated epididymis appear to move independently, shown histologically to be aggregations of spermatozoa and macrophages.[131]

Chronic Epididymitis

Patients with incompletely treated acute **bacterial epididymitis** usually present with a chronically painful scrotal mass (Fig. 21-24, *A*). Patients with chronic granulomatous epididymitis caused by spread of **tuberculosis** from the genitourinary tract complain of a hard, nontender scrotal mass.[10] Sonography most often shows a thickened tunica albuginea and a thickened, irregular epididymis (Fig. 21-27). Calcification may be identified within the tunica albuginea or epididymis.[1] Untreated granulomatous epididymitis will spread to the testes in 60% to 80% of cases. Focal testicular involvement may simulate the appearance of a testicular neoplasm on sonography.

ACUTE SCROTAL PAIN

The differential diagnosis of an acutely painful and swollen scrotum includes torsion of the spermatic cord and testis, torsion of a testicular appendage, epididymitis or orchitis, acute hydrocele, strangulated hernia, idiopathic scrotal edema, Henoch-Schönlein purpura, abscess, traumatic hemorrhage, hemorrhage into a testicular neoplasm, and scrotal fat necrosis. **Torsion of the spermatic cord** and acute **epididymitis** or **epididymo-orchitis** are the most common causes of acute scrotal pain. These entities cannot be distinguished by physical examination or laboratory tests in up to 50% of patients.[132] Immediate surgical exploration has been advised in boys and young men with acute scrotal pain, unless a definitive diagnosis of epididymitis or orchitis can be made. This aggressive approach has resulted in an

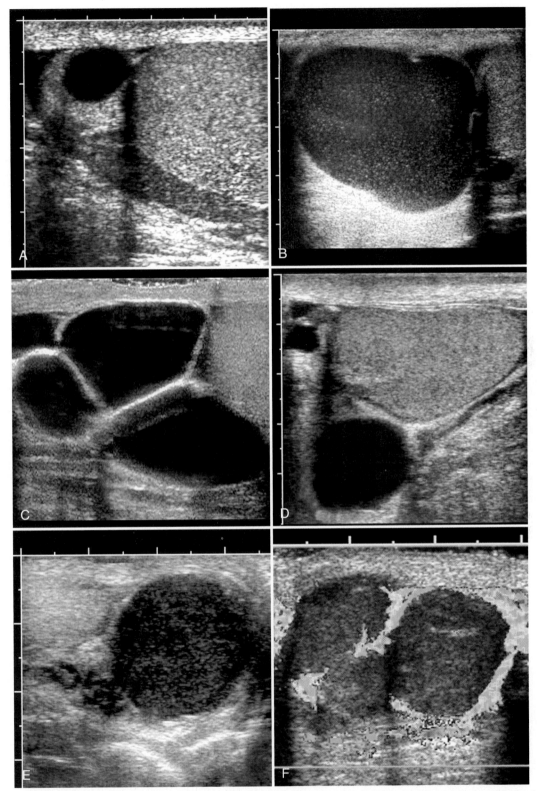

FIGURE 21-25. Extratesticular scrotal cysts: spectrum of appearances. A, Spermatocele. Longitudinal scan shows an anechoic cyst in head of the epididymis. **B, Spermatocele.** Longitudinal scan shows a large cyst containing internal echoes in head of the epididymis. **C, Septate spermatocele.** Longitudinal scan shows a septate cyst in head of the epididymis. **D, Epididymal cyst.** Longitudinal scan shows a cyst in body of the epididymis. **E, Cyst of vas deferens remnant.** Longitudinal scan shows a cyst with internal echoes inferior to the testis (surgically proven). **F, Epidermoid inclusion cyst of epididymis.** Longitudinal color Doppler scan shows bilobed cystic mass in head of the epididymis surrounded by vessels.

CAUSES OF ACUTE SCROTAL PAIN

Torsion of the testis
Epididymo-orchitis
Testicular appendage torsion
Strangulated hernia
Idiopathic scrotal edema
Trauma
Henoch-Schönlein purpura

increased testicular salvage rate from torsion, but also an increase in unnecessary surgical procedures. Testicular radionuclide scintigraphy, MRI, real-time sonography, and Doppler sonography have been used to increase the accuracy of distinguishing between infection and torsion.[133] Currently, sonography using color flow or power Doppler is the imaging study of choice to diagnose the cause of acute scrotal pain.

Torsion

Torsion is more common in boys than in men, and it represents only 20% of the acute scrotal pathologic phenomena in postpubertal males.[1] However, prompt diagnosis is necessary because torsion requires immediate surgery to preserve the testis. The testicular salvage rate is 80% to 100% if surgery is performed within 5 to 6 hours of the onset of pain, 70% if surgery is performed within 6 to 12 hours, and only 20% if surgery is delayed for more than 12 hours.[134]

There are two types of testicular torsion: intravaginal and extravaginal. **Intravaginal torsion** is the more common type, occurring most frequently at puberty. It results from anomalous suspension of the testis by a long stalk of spermatic cord, resulting in complete investment of the testis and epididymis by the tunica vaginalis. This anomaly has been likened to a bell-clapper (Fig. 21-28). Anomalous testicular suspension is bilateral in 50% to 80% of patients. There is a tenfold greater incidence of torsion in undescended testes after orchiopexy. **Extravaginal torsion** most often occurs in newborns without the "bell clapper" deformity. It is thought to result from a poor or absent attachment of the testis to the scrotal wall, allowing rotation of the testis, epididymis, and tunica vaginalis as a unit and causing torsion of the cord at the level of the external ring[135,136] (Fig. 21-28, *D*). The more compliant veins are obstructed before the arteries in both forms of torsion, resulting in early vascular engorgement and edema of the testicle.

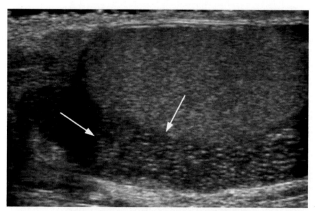

FIGURE 21-26. Postvasectomy change in epididymis. Longitudinal image of the scrotum shows tubular ectasia of the epididymis in a patient who had a vasectomy.

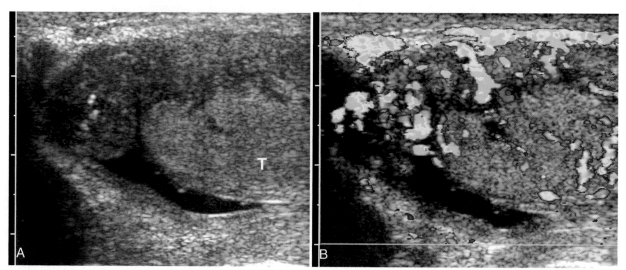

FIGURE 21-27. Tuberculous epididymo-orchitis. A, Longitudinal scan shows a heterogeneous mass with calcification involving the head and body of the epididymis and the adjacent testis *(T)*. **B,** Longitudinal color Doppler image shows increased vascularity in the epididymis and adjacent testis.

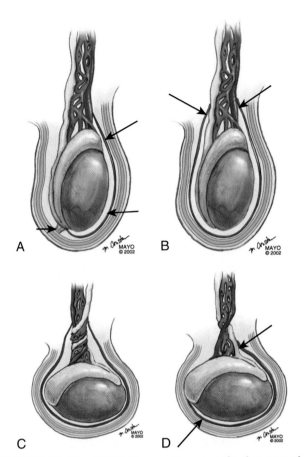

FIGURE 21-28. "Bell clapper" anomaly, intravaginal torsion, and extravaginal torsion. A, Normal anatomy. The tunica vaginalis *(arrows)* does not completely surround the testis and epididymis, which are attached to the posterior scrotal wall *(short arrow)*. **B, Bell-clapper anomaly.** The tunica vaginalis *(arrows)* completely surrounds the testis, epididymis, and part of the spermatic cord, predisposing to torsion. **C, Intravaginal torsion.** Bell-clapper anomaly with complete torsion of the spermatic cord, compromising the blood supply to the testis. **D, Extravaginal torsion in a neonate.** Tunica vaginalis *(arrows)* is in normal position, but abnormal motility allows rotation of the testis, epididymis, and spermatic cord.

Several gray-scale sonographic changes occur in the acute phase of torsion, within 1 to 6 hours.[132,137,138] Initially the testis becomes enlarged, with a normal echogenicity, and later it becomes heterogeneous and hypoechoic compared with the contralateral normal testis[139-141] (Fig. 21-29). A hypoechoic or heterogeneous echogenicity may indicate nonviability.[142] Generalized testicular hyperechogenicity has been reported in the absence of histologic changes of testicular hemorrhage or infarction.[140]

Torsion may change the position of the long axis of the testis (Fig. 21-29, *B*). Extratesticular sonographic findings typically occur in torsion and are important to recognize. The spermatic cord immediately cranial to the testis and epididymis is twisted, causing a characteristic **torsion knot** or "whirlpool pattern" of concentric layers

seen on sonography or MRI[137,143,144] (Fig. 21-29, *G* and *H*). The epididymis may be enlarged and heterogeneous because of hemorrhage and may be difficult to separate from the torsion knot of the spermatic cord. This spherical epididymis-cord complex can be mistaken for epididymitis.[137] A reactive hydrocele and scrotal skin thickening are often seen with torsion. Large, echogenic or complex extratesticular masses caused by hemorrhage in the tunica vaginalis or epididymis may be seen in patients with undiagnosed torsion.[145] The gray-scale findings of acute and subacute torsion are not specific and may be seen in testicular infarction caused by epididymitis, epididymo-orchitis, and traumatic testicular rupture or infarction.

Color Doppler sonography is the most useful and most rapid technique to establish the diagnosis of testicular torsion and to help distinguish torsion from epididymo-orchitis[132,139,146] (Fig. 21-29). In torsion, blood flow is absent in the affected testicle or significantly less than in the normal, contralateral testicle. Meticulous scanning of the testicular parenchyma with the use of low-flow detection Doppler settings (low pulse repetition frequency, low wall filter, high Doppler gain) is important because testicular vessels are small and have low flow velocities, especially in prepubertal boys. Color flow Doppler sonography is more sensitive for showing decreased testicular flow in incomplete torsion than is nuclear scintigraphy.[147] Power Doppler and frequency shift color Doppler sonography are used, although the techniques appear to have equivalent sensitivity in the diagnosis of torsion.[148-153] In testicular torsion, color Doppler sonography has a sensitivity of 80% to 98%, a specificity of 97% to 100%, and an accuracy rate of 97%.[137,146,154] The use of intravascular contrast agents in sonography may improve the sensitivity of detecting blood flow in the scrotum, but this has not yet been proved in a large series.[150] In pediatric patients, it may be difficult to document flow in a normal testis.[155] In practice, many surgeons elect to explore the testis surgically if clinical symptoms and signs are suggestive and results of the sonographic examination are equivocal.

Potential pitfalls in using sonography in the diagnosis of torsion are **partial torsion, torsion/detorsion,** and **ischemia from orchitis.** Torsion of at least 540 degrees is necessary for complete arterial occlusion.[146,156] With partial torsion of 360 degrees, or less, arterial flow may still occur, but venous outflow is often obstructed, causing diminished diastolic arterial flow on spectral Doppler examination[157,158] (Fig. 21-29). If spontaneous detorsion occurs, flow within the affected testis may be normal, or it may be increased and mimic orchitis.[159] Spontaneous detorsion rarely occurs and leaves a segmental testicular infarction.[74,75] Segmental testicular infarction may also occur with Henoch-Schönlein purpura or with orchitis (see Fig. 21-14). Orchitis may also cause global ischemia of the testis and mimic torsion.[159]

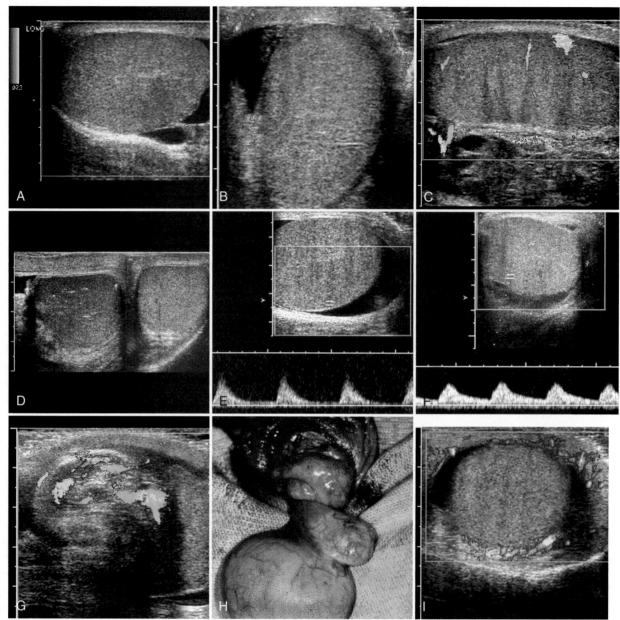

FIGURE 21-29. Torsion of spermatic cord and testis: spectrum of appearances. A to D, Acute torsion. Longitudinal power Doppler scans show **A,** no flow in the testis, and **B,** abnormal, transverse, and vertical orientation of the testis with no flow. **C,** After manual detorsion of case in **B,** longitudinal color Doppler scan shows the normal orientation of the testis with blood flow present. The testis has a striated appearance caused by the previous ischemia. **D,** Dual transverse gray-scale scan shows enlarged hypoechoic right testis resulting from torsion and skin thickening in the right hemiscrotum. **E, Partial torsion.** Longitudinal scan with spectral Doppler shows a high-resistance testicular arterial waveform with little diastolic flow because of venous occlusion; small, reactive hydrocele was found. **F,** After spontaneous detorsion of case in **E,** longitudinal scan with spectral Doppler shows return of diastolic flow. **G, Torsion knot.** Longitudinal scan with acute spermatic cord torsion shows the "torsion knot" complex of epididymis and spermatic cord. **H, Acute torsion.** Intraoperative photograph shows the twisted spermatic cord that gives the torsion knot appearance on sonograph. **I, Subacute torsion** (3 days of pain). Transverse power Doppler scan shows absent flow within the testis with surrounding hyperemia. *(H from Winter T.C. Ultrasonography of the scrotum. Appl Radiol 2002;31(3). H courtesy Drs. R.E. Berger, University of Washington, Seattle, and T.C. Winter, University of Wisconsin, Madison.)*

In subacute or chronic torsion, color Doppler shows no flow in the testis and increased flow in the paratesticular tissues, including the epididymis-cord complex and dartos fascia (Fig. 21-29).

Torsion of the testicular appendage is a common cause of acute scrotal pain and may mimic testicular torsion clinically. Patients are rarely referred for imaging because the pain is usually not severe, and the twisted appendage may be evident clinically as the "blue dot" sign.[160] The sonographic appearance of the twisted testicular appendage has been described as an avascular hypoechoic mass adjacent to a normally perfused testis and surrounded by an area of increased color Doppler perfusion.[146] However, the twisted appendage may appear as an echogenic extratesticular mass situated between the head of the epididymis and the upper pole of the testis.[161]

Epididymitis and Epididymo-orchitis

Epididymitis is the most common cause of acute scrotal pain in postpubertal men, causing 75% of all acute intrascrotal inflammatory processes. It usually results from a lower urinary tract infection and is less often hematogenous or traumatic in origin. The common causative organisms are *Escherichia coli, Pseudomonas,* and *Klebsiella.* Sexually transmitted organisms causing urethritis, such as gonococci and chlamydiae, are common causes of epididymitis in young men. Less frequently, epididymitis may be caused by tuberculosis, mumps, or syphilitic orchitis.[162,163] The age of peak incidence is 40 to 50 years. Typically, patients present with the insidious onset of pain, which increases over 1 to 2 days. Fever, dysuria, and urethral discharge may also be present.

In **acute epididymitis**, sonography characteristically shows thickening and enlargement of the epididymis, involving the tail initially and frequently spreading to the entire epididymis[164] (Fig. 21-30, *A* and *B*). The echogenicity of the epididymis is usually decreased, and its echotexture is often coarse and heterogeneous, probably because of edema or hemorrhage, or both. Reactive hydrocele formation is common, and associated skin thickening may be seen. Color flow Doppler sonography usually shows increased blood flow in the epididymis or testis, or both, compared with the asymptomatic side[165] (Fig. 21-30, *C*).

Direct extension of epididymal inflammation to the testicle, called **epididymo-orchitis,** occurs in up to 20% of patients with acute epididymitis. Isolated orchitis may also occur. In such cases, increased blood flow is localized to the testis (Fig. 21-30, *D* and *E;* **Video 21-6**). Testicular involvement may be focal or diffuse. Characteristically, **focal orchitis** produces a hypoechoic area adjacent to an enlarged portion of the epididymis. Color Doppler shows increased flow in the hypoechoic area of the testis; increased flow in the tunica vasculosa may be visible as lines of color signal radiating from the mediastinum testis.[166] These lines of color correspond to septal accentuation that is visible as hypoechoic bands on gray-scale sonography (Fig. 21-30, *H* and *I*). Spectral Doppler shows increased diastolic flow in uncomplicated orchitis (Fig. 21-31, *A*). If left untreated, the entire testicle may become involved, appearing hypoechoic and enlarged. As pressure in the testis increases from edema, venous infarction with hemorrhage may occur, appearing hyperechoic initially and hypoechoic later (Fig. 21-30).[166] Ischemia and subsequent infarction may occur when the vascularity of the testis is compromised by venous occlu-

sion in the epididymis and cord.[167] When vascular disruption is severe, resulting in complete testicular infarction, the changes are indistinguishable from those seen in testicular torsion. Color Doppler sonography may show focal areas of reactive hyperemia and increased blood flow associated with relatively avascular areas of infarction in both the testis and the epididymis in patients with severe epididymo-orchitis. Diastolic flow reversal in the arterial waveforms of the testis is an ominous finding, associated with testicular infarction in severe epididymo-orchitis[168] (Fig. 21-31, *B*).

In addition to infarction, other complications of acute epididymo-orchitis include abscess and pyocele (see Figs. 21-13 and 21-19, *F*). Chronic changes may be seen in the epididymis or testis from clinically resolved epididymo-orchitis. Swelling of the epididymis may persist and appear as a heterogeneous mass on sonography (see Fig. 21-24, *A*). The testis may have a persistent, striated appearance of septal accentuation from fibrosis (Figs. 21-32 and 21-33). This striated appearance of the testis is nonspecific and may also be seen after ischemia from torsion or during a hernia repair.[166,169] A similar heterogeneous appearance in the testis may be seen in elderly patients because of **seminiferous tubule atrophy and sclerosis.**[170] Focal areas of infarction in the testis may persist as wedge-shaped or cone-shaped hypoechoic areas or may appear as hyperechoic scars.[166] If complete infarction of the testis has occurred because of epididymo-orchitis, the testis may become small, with a hypoechoic or heterogeneous echotexture.

Fournier Gangrene

Fournier gangrene is a **necrotizing fasciitis of the perineum** occurring most frequently in men age 50 to 70 years who are debilitated or who have diabetes mellitus.[131] Multiple organisms are usually involved, including *Klebsiella, Streptococcus, Proteus,* and *Staphylococcus.* Surgical debridement of devitalized tissue is usually required, and morbidity and mortality are high without prompt treatment. Ultrasound may be helpful in diagnosis by showing scrotal wall thickening containing gas.

TRAUMA

Prompt diagnosis of a ruptured testis is crucial because of the direct relationship between early surgical intervention and testicular salvageability. Approximately 90% of ruptured testicles can be saved if surgery is performed within the first 72 hours, whereas only 45% may be salvaged after 72 hours.[171]

Clinical diagnosis is often impossible because of marked scrotal pain and swelling, and sonography can be valuable in the assessment of tunica albuginea integrity and the extent of testicular hematoma.[81,171-173] Sonographic features include focal areas of altered testicular

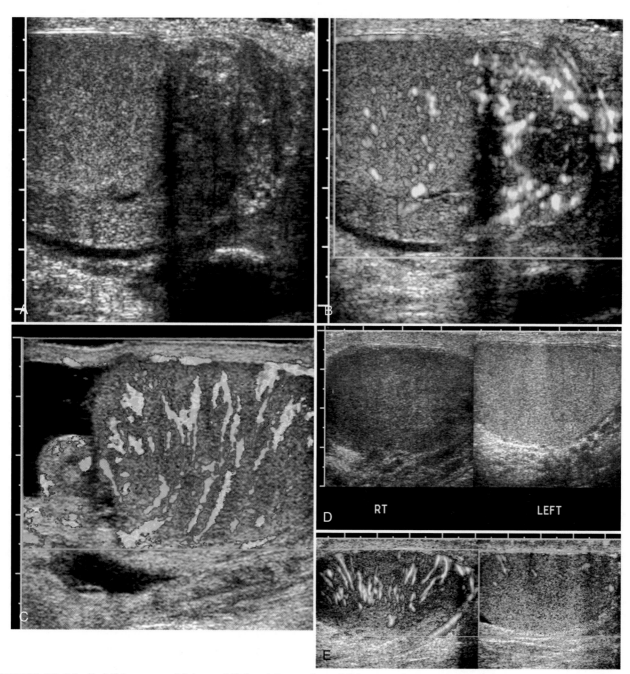

FIGURE 21-30. Epididymo-orchitis, epididymitis, and orchitis: spectrum of appearances. A and **B, Acute epididymitis.** Longitudinal gray-scale and color Doppler images show enlargement and a heterogeneous echotexture of tail of the epididymis, with greatly increased flow in tail of the epididymis and minimally increased flow in the adjacent testis. **C, Acute epididymo-orchitis.** Longitudinal color Doppler scan shows increased flow in the epididymis and testis. **D** and **E, Acute orchitis.** Longitudinal dual-image gray-scale and color Doppler images show that right testis is hypoechoic and has greatly increased flow.

echogenicity, corresponding to areas of hemorrhage or infarction, and hematocele formation in 33% of patients. A discrete **fracture plane** is rarely identified (Fig. 21-34, *B*). A visibly intact tunica albuginea should exclude rupture, but testicular hematoma may obscure the tunica[81] (Fig. 21-34, *A*). Tunical disruption associated with extrusion of the seminiferous tubules is specific for rupture (Fig. 21-34, *E*; **Video 21-7**). However, the sensitivity of the diagnosis of rupture based on tunical dis-

ruption alone is only 50%. Heterogeneity of the testis with associated testicular contour irregularity may be helpful in making the diagnosis of rupture.[81,172,173]

Although not specific for a ruptured testicle, these features may suggest the diagnosis in the appropriate clinical setting, prompting immediate surgical exploration. Color Doppler imaging can be helpful because rupture of the tunica albuginea is almost always associated with disruption of the tunica vasculosa and loss of

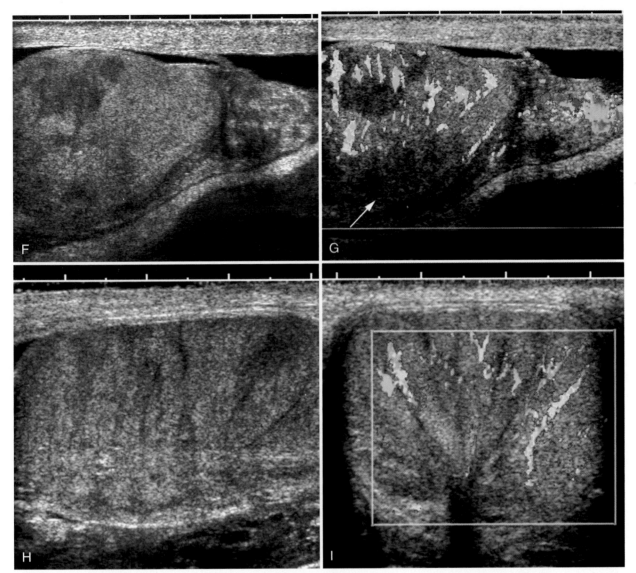

FIGURE 21-30, cont'd. F, Longitudinal gray-scale scan with 3 weeks of epididymo-orchitis unresolved with antibiotic therapy shows hypoechoic areas in the testis and an enlarged heterogeneous tail of the epididymis. **G,** Color Doppler image shows increased flow in the testis and epididymis with an area of decreased flow due to ischemia *(arrow).* **H** and **I, Acute orchitis.** Longitudinal gray-scale and color Doppler images show hypoechoic bands caused by septal accentuation from edema and increased vascularity of the testis.

blood supply to part or all of the testis[81] (Fig. 21-34, *C*). A complex intrascrotal hematoma may be difficult to distinguish from testicular rupture.[174] Patients with large, intrascrotal hematomas or hematoceles will often undergo surgical exploration because it is difficult to exclude rupture sonographically in the presence of surrounding complex fluid.[81] Sonography can also be used to discern the severity of scrotal trauma resulting from bullet wounds, and foreign bodies can be localized.[175] A careful gray-scale and color flow Doppler evaluation of the epididymis should be performed in all examinations done for blunt trauma. Traumatic epididymitis may be an isolated finding that should not be confused with an infectious process.[176]

CRYPTORCHIDISM

The testes normally begin their descent through the inguinal canal into the scrotal sac at about 36 weeks of gestation. The gubernaculum testis is a fibromuscular structure that extends from the inferior pole of the testis to the scrotum and guides the testis in its descent, which normally has been completed at birth. **Undescended testis** is one of the most common genitourinary anomalies in male infants. At birth, 3.5% of male infants weighing more than 2500 g have an undescended testis; 10% to 25% of these cases are bilateral. This figure decreases to 0.8% by age 1 year because the testes descend spontaneously in most infants. The incidence of

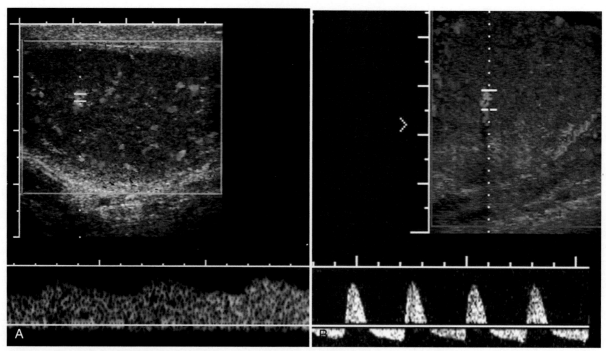

FIGURE 21-31. Spectral Doppler changes in orchitis. A, Uncomplicated orchitis. Longitudinal scan with spectral Doppler tracing shows increased diastolic flow in the testis. **B, Orchitis with venous compromise.** Longitudinal scan with spectral Doppler tracing in more severe orchitis shows reversal of flow in diastole caused by edema impeding venous flow.

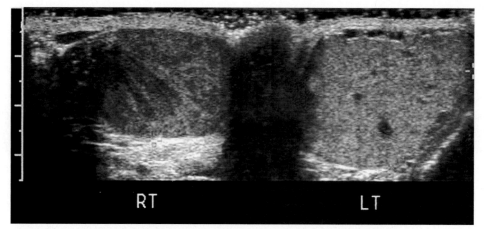

FIGURE 21-32. Heterogeneous "striped" testis. Transverse dual image shows heterogeneity in the right testis with marked septal accentuation from previous orchitis. This appearance may also be seen after ischemia.

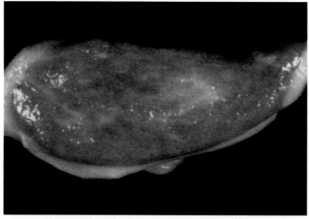

FIGURE 21-33. Fibrosis of testis after orchitis. Pathologic specimen of testis shows linear bands of fibrosis *(white areas)* caused by previous severe orchitis. A similar "end stage" testis could have this appearance due to ischemia.

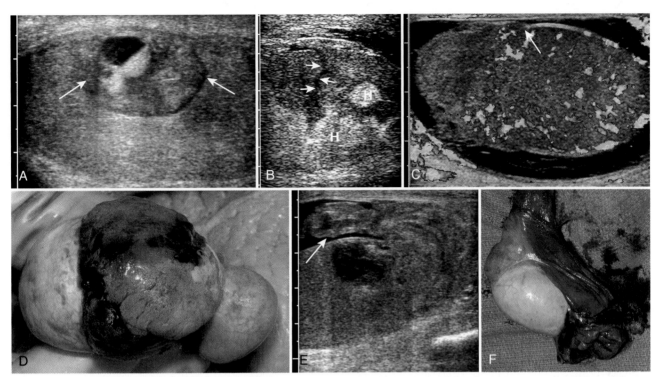

FIGURE 21-34. Testicular trauma: spectrum of appearances. A, Hematoma. Longitudinal image shows hematoma *(arrows)* on the anterior surface of the testis. Tunica intact at surgery. **B, Fracture of testis.** Transverse scan shows a heterogeneous testicle with a linear band *(arrows)* indicating a fracture. *H,* Testicular hematoma. **C, Tunical tear.** Longitudinal color Doppler image shows contour irregularity of the testis with disruption of the tunica *(arrow).* Extruded testis parenchyma shows no color flow. **D,** Same case as **C.** Photograph during surgery shows tunical tear in the exposed right testis. **E, Rupture of testis.** Longitudinal image shows rupture of the testis with extrusion of seminiferous tubules *(arrow).* **F,** In same case as **E,** photograph during surgery shows a tear in the tunica inferiorly with extrusion of seminiferous tubules.

undescended testes increases to 30% in premature infants, approaching 100% in neonates who weigh less than 1 kg at birth. Complete descent is necessary for full testicular maturation.[177,178]

Malpositioned testes may be located anywhere along the pathway of descent from the retroperitoneum to the scrotum. Most (80%) undescended testes are palpable, lying at or below the level of the inguinal canal. **Anorchia** occurs in 4% of the remaining patients with impalpable testes.[178]

Localization of the undescended testis is important for the prevention of two potential complications of cryptorchidism: **infertility** and **cancer.** The undescended testis is more likely to undergo malignant change than the normally descended testis.[1] The most common malignancy is seminoma. The risk of malignancy is increased in both the undescended testis after orchiopexy and the normally descended testis. Therefore, careful serial examinations of both testes are essential.

Sonographically, the **undescended testis** is often smaller and slightly less echogenic than the contralateral, normally descended testis (Fig. 21-35). A large lymph node or the pars infravaginalis gubernaculi (PIG), which is the distal bulbous segment of the gubernaculum testis, can be mistaken for the testis. After completion of testicular descent, the PIG and the gubernaculum normally

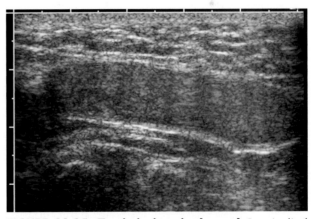

FIGURE 21-35. Testis in inguinal canal. Longitudinal scan shows an elongated, ovoid, undescended testis.

atrophy. If the testis remains undescended, both structures persist. The PIG is located distal to the undescended testis, usually in the scrotum, but it may be found in the inguinal cord. Sonographically, the PIG is a hypoechoic, cordlike structure of echogenicity similar to the testis, with the gubernaculum leading to it.[179]

Sonography is often used in the initial evaluation of cryptorchidism, although the value of this has been questioned because it is insensitive in detecting high intra-abdominal testes.[180] MRI has also been used in cryptorchidism because it is more sensitive than ultrasound in detecting undescended testes in the retroperitoneum.[181,182] Nonvisualization of an undescended testis on sonography or MRI does not exclude its presence, and therefore laparoscopy or surgical exploration should be performed if clinically indicated.

Acknowledgment

Frank Thornton, MD, assisted in gathering images.

References

Anatomy

1. Krone KD, Carroll BA. Scrotal ultrasound. Radiol Clin North Am 1985;23:121-139.
2. Trainer TD. Histology of the normal testis. Am J Surg Pathol 1987;11:797-809.
3. Johnson KA, Dewbury KC. Ultrasound imaging of the appendix testis and appendix epididymis. Clin Radiol 1996;51:335-337.
4. Sellars ME, Sidhu PS. Ultrasound appearances of the testicular appendages: pictorial review. Eur Radiol 2003;13:127-135.
5. Black JA, Patel A. Sonography of the normal extratesticular space. AJR Am J Roentgenol 1996;167:503-506.
6. Allen TD. Disorders of the male external genitalia. In: Kelalis PP, King LR, editors. Clinical pediatric urology. Philadelphia: Saunders; 1976. p. 636-668.
7. Middleton WD, Bell MW. Analysis of intratesticular arterial anatomy with emphasis on transmediastinal arteries. Radiology 1993;189:157-160.
8. Fakhry J, Khoury A, Barakat K. The hypoechoic band: a normal finding on testicular sonography. AJR Am J Roentgenol 1989;153:321-323.
9. Bushby LH, Sellars ME, Sidhu PS. The "two-tone" testis: spectrum of ultrasound appearances. Clin Radiol 2007;62:1119-1123.
10. Middleton WD, Thorne DA, Melson GL. Color Doppler ultrasound of the normal testis. AJR Am J Roentgenol 1989;152:293-297.
11. Gooding GA. Sonography of the spermatic cord. AJR Am J Roentgenol 1988;151:721-724.

Scrotal Masses

12. Rifkin MD, Kurtz AB, Pasto ME, Goldberg BB. Diagnostic capabilities of high-resolution scrotal ultrasonography: prospective evaluation. J Ultrasound Med 1985;4:13-19.
13. Carroll BA, Gross DM. High-frequency scrotal sonography. AJR Am J Roentgenol 1983;140:511-515.
14. Grantham JG, Charboneau JW, James EM, et al. Testicular neoplasms: 29 tumors studied by high-resolution ultrasound. Radiology 1985;157:775-780.
15. Kirschling RJ, Kvols LK, Charboneau JW, et al. High-resolution ultrasonographic and pathologic abnormalities of germ cell tumors in patients with clinically normal testes. Mayo Clin Proc 1983;58:648-653.
16. Javadpour N. Principles and management of testicular cancer. New York, Thieme; 1986.
17. Damjanov I. Tumors of the testis and epididymis. In: Murphy WM, editor. Urological pathology. 2nd ed. Philadelphia: Saunders; 1997. p. 342-400.
18. Talerman A, Roth LM. Pathology of the testis and its adnexa. In: Talerman A, Roth LM, editors. Germ cell tumors. New York: Churchill Livingstone; 1986.
19. Jacobsen GK, Talerman A. Atlas of germ cell tumors. J Pathol 1989;160:86-87.
20. Schwerk WB, Schwerk WN, Rodeck G. Testicular tumors: prospective analysis of real-time ultrasound patterns and abdominal staging. Radiology 1987;164:369-374.
21. Ulbright TM. Germ cell neoplasms of the testis. Am J Surg Pathol 1993;17:1075-1091.

22. Mostofi FK, Price EB. Tumors of the male genital system. In: Atlas of tumor pathology. Washington, DC: Armed Forces Institute of Pathology; 1973.
23. Emory TH, Charboneau JW, Randall RV, et al. Occult testicular interstitial-cell tumor in a patient with gynecomastia: ultrasonic detection. Radiology 1984;151:474.
24. Maizlin ZV, Belenky A, Kunichezky M, et al. Leydig cell tumors of the testis: gray scale and color Doppler sonographic appearance. J Ultrasound Med 2004;23:959-964.
25. Gabrilove JL, Freiberg EK, Leiter E, Nicolis GL. Feminizing and non-feminizing Sertoli cell tumors. J Urol 1980;124:757-767.
26. Young S, Gooneratne S, Straus Jr FH, et al. Feminizing Sertoli cell tumors in boys with Peutz-Jeghers syndrome. Am J Surg Pathol 1995;19:50-58.
27. Tasu JP, Faye N, Eschwege P, et al. Imaging of burned-out testis tumor: five new cases and review of the literature. J Ultrasound Med 2003;22:515-521.
28. Mindrup SR, Konety BR. Testicular recurrence from "primary" retroperitoneal germ cell tumor. Urology 2004;64:1031.
29. Shawker TH, Javadpour N, O'Leary T, et al. Ultrasonographic detection of "burned-out" primary testicular germ cell tumors in clinically normal testes. J Ultrasound Med 1983;2:477-479.
30. Horstman WG, Melson GL, Middleton WD, Andriole GL. Testicular tumors: findings with color Doppler ultrasound. Radiology 1992;185:733-737.
31. Luker GD, Siegel MJ. Pediatric testicular tumors: evaluation with gray-scale and color Doppler ultrasound. Radiology 1994;191:561-564.
32. Hindley RG, Chandra A, Saunders A, O'Brien TS. Impalpable testis cancer. BJU Int 2003;92:572-574.
33. Powell TM, Tarter TH. Management of nonpalpable incidental testicular masses. J Urol 2006;176:96-98; discussion 99.
34. Carmignani L, Gadda F, Gazzano G, et al. High incidence of benign testicular neoplasms diagnosed by ultrasound. J Urol 2003;170:1783-1786.
35. Carmignani L, Morabito A, Gadda F, et al. Prognostic parameters in adult impalpable ultrasonographic lesions of the testicle. J Urol 2005;174:1035-1038.
36. Horstman WG, Haluszka MM, Burkhard TK. Management of testicular masses incidentally discovered by ultrasound. J Urol 1994;151:1263-1265.
37. Mostofi FK, Sobin LH. Histological typing of testis tumours. In: International histological classification of tumors of the testes. Geneva: World Health Organization; 1977.
38. Mazzu D, Jeffrey Jr RB, Ralls PW. Lymphoma and leukemia involving the testicles: findings on gray-scale and color Doppler sonography. AJR Am J Roentgenol 1995;164:645-647.
39. Rayor RA, Scheible W, Brock WA, Leopold GR. High-resolution ultrasonography in the diagnosis of testicular relapse in patients with acute lymphoblastic leukemia. J Urol 1982;128:602-603.
40. Iizumi T, Shinohara S, Amemiya H, et al. Plasmacytoma of the testis. Urol Int 1995;55:218-221.
41. Grignon DJ, Shum DT, Hayman WP. Metastatic tumours of the testes. Can J Surg 1986;29:359-361.
42. Werth V, Yu G, Marshall FF. Nonlymphomatous metastatic tumor to the testis. J Urol 1982;127:142-144.
43. Hanash KA, Carney JA, Kelalis PP. Metastatic tumors to testicles: routes of metastasis. J Urol 1969;102:465-468.
44. Hamm B, Fobbe F, Loy V. Testicular cysts: differentiation with ultrasound and clinical findings. Radiology 1988;168:19-23.
45. Shergill IS, Thwaini A, Kapasi F, et al. Management of simple intratesticular cysts: a single-institution 11-year experience. Urology 2006;67:1266-1268.
46. Martinez-Berganza MT, Sarria L, Cozcolluela R, et al. Cysts of the tunica albuginea: sonographic appearance. AJR Am J Roentgenol 1998;170:183-185.
47. Dogra VS, Gottlieb RH, Rubens DJ, Liao L. Benign intratesticular cystic lesions: ultrasound features. Radiographics 2001;21 Spec No:273-281.
48. Warner KE, Noyes DT, Ross JS. Cysts of the tunica albuginea testis: a report of 3 cases with a review of the literature. J Urol 1984;132:131-132.
49. Poster RB, Spirt BA, Tamsen A, Surya BV. Complex tunica albuginea cyst simulating an intratesticular lesion. Urol Radiol 1991;13:129-132.

50. Sudakoff GS, Quiroz F, Karcaaltincaba M, Foley WD. Scrotal ultrasonography with emphasis on the extratesticular space: anatomy, embryology, and pathology. Ultrasound Q 2002;18:255-273.

51. Takihara H, Valvo JR, Tokuhara M, Cockett AT. Intratesticular cysts. Urology 1982;20:80-82.

52. Tartar VM, Trambert MA, Balsara ZN, Mattrey RF. Tubular ectasia of the testicle: sonographic and MR imaging appearance. AJR Am J Roentgenol 1993;160:539-542.

53. Brown DL, Benson CB, Doherty FJ, et al. Cystic testicular mass caused by dilated rete testis: sonographic findings in 31 cases. AJR Am J Roentgenol 1992;158:1257-1259.

54. Weingarten BJ, Kellman GM, Middleton WD, Gross ML. Tubular ectasia within the mediastinum testis. J Ultrasound Med 1992;11: 349-353.

55. Older RA, Watson LR. Tubular ectasia of the rete testis: a benign condition with a sonographic appearance that may be misinterpreted as malignant. J Urol 1994;152:477-478.

56. Cho CS, Kosek J. Cystic dysplasia of the testis: sonographic and pathologic findings. Radiology 1985;156:777-778.

57. Keetch DW, McAlister WH, Manley CB, Dehner LP. Cystic dysplasia of the testis: sonographic features with pathologic correlation. Pediatr Radiol 1991;21:501-503.

58. Atchley JT, Dewbury KC. Ultrasound appearances of testicular epidermoid cysts. Clin Radiol 2000;55:493-502.

59. Sanderson AJ, Birch BR, Dewbury KC. Case report: multiple epidermoid cysts of the testes–the ultrasound appearances. Clin Radiol 1995;50:414-415.

60. Malvica RP. Epidermoid cyst of the testicle: an unusual sonographic finding. AJR Am J Roentgenol 1993;160:1047-1048.

61. Stein MM, Stein MW, Cohen BC, et al. Unusual sonographic appearance of an epidermoid cyst of the testis. J Ultrasound Med 1999;18:723-726.

62. Maizlin ZV, Belenky A, Baniel J, et al. Epidermoid cyst and teratoma of the testis: sonographic and histologic similarities. J Ultrasound Med 2005;24:1403-1409; quiz 1410-1411.

63. Eisenmenger M, Lang S, Donner G, et al. Epidermoid cysts of the testis: organ-preserving surgery following diagnosis by ultrasonography. Br J Urol 1993;72:955-957.

64. Cho JH, Chang JC, Park BH, et al. Sonographic and MR imaging findings of testicular epidermoid cysts [see comment]. AJR Am J Bennett 2002;178:743-748.

65. Langer JE, Ramchandani P, Siegelman ES, Banner MP. Epidermoid cysts of the testicle: sonographic and MR imaging features. AJR Am J Roentgenol 1999;173:1295-1299.

66. Hermansen MC, Chusid MJ, Sty JR. Bacterial epididymo-orchitis in children and adolescents. Clin Pediatr 1980;19:812-815.

67. Mevorach RA, Lerner RM, Dvoretsky PM, Rabinowitz R. Testicular abscess: diagnosis by ultrasonography. J Urol 1986;136:1213-1216.

68. Korn RL, Langer JE, Nisenbaum HL, Miller Jr WT, Cheung LP. Non-Hodgkin's lymphoma mimicking a scrotal abscess in a patient with AIDS. Journal of Ultrasound in Medicine 1994;13:715-718.

69. Smith FJ, Bilbey JH, Filipenko JD, Goldenberg SL. Testicular pseudotumor in the acquired immunodeficiency syndrome. Urology 1995;45:535-537.

70. Wu VH, Dangman BC, Kaufman Jr RP. Sonographic appearance of acute testicular venous infarction in a patient with a hypercoagulable state. J Ultrasound Med 1995;14:57-59.

71. Bilagi P, Sriprasad S, Clarke JL, et al. Clinical and ultrasound features of segmental testicular infarction: six-year experience from a single centre. Eur Radiol 2007;17:2810-2818.

72. Flanagan JJ, Fowler RC. Testicular infarction mimicking tumour on scrotal ultrasound: a potential pitfall. Clin Radiol 1995;50:49-50.

73. Einstein DM, Paushter DM, Singer AA, et al. Fibrotic lesions of the testicle: sonographic patterns mimicking malignancy. Urol Radiol 1992;14:205-210.

74. Ledwidge ME, Lee DK, Winter 3rd TC, et al. Sonographic diagnosis of superior hemispheric testicular infarction.[see comment]. AJR Am J Roentgenol 2002;179:775-776.

75. Sriprasad S, Kooiman GG, Muir GH, Sidhu PS. Acute segmental testicular infarction: differentiation from tumour using high-frequency colour Doppler ultrasound. Br J Radiol 2001;74:965-967.

76. Carmody JP, Sharma OP. Intrascrotal sarcoidosis: case reports and review. Sarcoidosis Vasc Diffuse Lung Dis 1996;13:129-134.

77. Winter 3rd TC, Keener TS, Mack LA. Sonographic appearance of testicular sarcoid. J Ultrasound Med 1995;14:153-156.

78. Eraso CE, Vrachliotis TG, Cunningham JJ. Sonographic findings in testicular sarcoidosis simulating malignant nodule. J Clin Ultrasound 1999;27:81-83.

79. Avila NA, Premkumar A, Shawker TH, et al. Testicular adrenal rest tissue in congenital adrenal hyperplasia: findings at Gray-scale and color Doppler ultrasound. Radiology 1996;198:99-104.

80. Vanzulli A, DelMaschio A, Paesano P, et al. Testicular masses in association with adrenogenital syndrome: ultrasound findings. Radiology 1992;183:425-429.

81. Bhatt S, Dogra VS. Role of ultrasound in testicular and scrotal trauma. Radiographics 2008;28:1617-1629.

82. Gierke CL, King BF, Bostwick DG, et al. Large-cell calcifying Sertoli cell tumor of the testis: appearance at sonography. AJR Am J Roentgenol 1994;163:373-375.

83. Vegni-Talluri M, Bigliardi E, Vanni MG, Tota G. Testicular microliths: their origin and structure. J Urol 1980;124:105-107.

84. Breger RC, Passarge E, McAdams AJ. Testicular intratubular bodies. J Clin Endocrinol Metab 1965;25:1340-1346.

85. Middleton WD, Teefey SA, Santillan CS. Testicular microlithiasis: prospective analysis of prevalence and associated tumor. Radiology 2002;224:425-428.

86. Kim B, Winter 3rd TC, Ryu JA. Testicular microlithiasis: clinical significance and review of the literature. Eur Radiol 2003;13: 2567-2576.

87. Nistal M, Paniagua R, Diez-Pardo JA. Testicular microlithiasis in 2 children with bilateral cryptorchidism. J Urol 1979;121:535-537.

88. Janzen DL, Mathieson JR, Marsh JI, et al. Testicular microlithiasis: sonographic and clinical features [see comment]. AJR Am J Roentgenol 1992;158:1057-1060.

89. Backus ML, Mack LA, Middleton WD, et al. Testicular microlithiasis: imaging appearances and pathologic correlation. Radiology 1994;192:781-785.

90. Patel MD, Olcott EW, Kerschmann RL, et al. Sonographically detected testicular microlithiasis and testicular carcinoma. J Clin Ultrasound 1993;21:447-452.

91. Cast JE, Nelson WM, Early AS, et al. Testicular microlithiasis: prevalence and tumor risk in a population referred for scrotal sonography. AJR Am J Roentgenol 2000;175:1703-1706.

92. Bennett HF, Middleton WD, Bullock AD, Teefey SA. Testicular microlithiasis: ultrasound follow-up. Radiology 2001;218:359-363.

93. Bach AM, Hann LE, Hadar O, et al. Testicular microlithiasis: what is its association with testicular cancer [see comment]? Radiology 2001;220:70-75.

94. Frush DP, Kliewer MA, Madden JF. Testicular microlithiasis and subsequent development of metastatic germ cell tumor. AJR Am J Roentgenol 1996;167:889-890.

95. Smith WS, Brammer HM, Henry M, Frazier H. Testicular microlithiasis: sonographic features with pathologic correlation. AJR Am J Roentgenol 1991;157:1003-1004.

96. McEniff N, Doherty F, Katz J, Schrager CA, Klauber G. Yolk sac tumor of the testis discovered on a routine annual sonogram in a boy with testicular microlithiasis. AJR Am J Roentgenol 1995;164: 971-972.

97. Miller FN, Sidhu PS. Does testicular microlithiasis matter? A review [see comment]. Clin Radiol 2002;57:883-890.

98. Quane LK, Kidney DD. Testicular microlithiasis in a patient with a mediastinal germ cell tumour [see comment]. Clin Radiol 2000; 55:642-644.

99. Dagash H, Mackinnon EA. Testicular microlithiasis: what does it mean clinically? BJU Int 2007;99:157-160.

100. Lam DL, Gerscovich EO, Kuo MC, McGahan JP. Testicular microlithiasis: our experience of 10 years. J Ultrasound Med 2007;26: 867-873.

101. Ringdhal E, Claybrook K, Teague JL, et al. Testicular microlithiasis and its relation to testicular cancer on ultrasound findings of symptomatic men. J Urol 2004;172:1904-1906.

102. Sakamoto H, Shichizyou T, Saito K, et al. Testicular microlithiasis identified ultrasonographically in Japanese adult patients: prevalence and associated conditions. Urology 2006;68:636-641.

103. Konstantinos S, Alevizos A, Anargiros M, et al. Association between testicular microlithiasis, testicular cancer, cryptorchidism and history of ascending testis. Int Braz J Urol 2006;32:434-438; discussion 439.

104. Serter S, Gumos B, Unlu M, et al. Prevalence of testicular microlithiasis in an asymptomatic population. Scand J Urol Nephrol 2006; 40:212-214.

105. Linkowski GD, Avellone A, Gooding GA. Scrotal calculi: sonographic detection. Radiology 1985;156:484.

106. Rathaus V, Konen O, Shapiro M, et al. Ultrasound features of spermatic cord hydrocele in children. Br J Radiol 2001;74:818-820.

107. Nye PJ, Prati Jr RC. Idiopathic hydrocele and absent testicular diastolic flow. J Clin Ultrasound 1997;25:43-46.

108. Worthy L, Miller EI, Chinn DH. Evaluation of extratesticular findings in scrotal neoplasms. J Ultrasound Med 1986;5:261-263.

109. Gooding GA, Leonhardt WC, Marshall G, et al. Cholesterol crystals in hydroceles: sonographic detection and possible significance. AJR Am J Roentgenol 1997;169:527-529.

110. Cunningham JJ. Sonographic findings in clinically unsuspected acute and chronic scrotal hematoceles. AJR Am J Roentgenol 1983; 140:749-752.

111. Beddy P, Geoghegan T, Browne RF, Torreggiani WC. Testicular varicoceles. Clin Radiol 2005;60:1248-1255.

112. Zucchi A, Mearini L, Mearini E, et al. Varicocele and fertility: relationship between testicular volume and seminal parameters before and after treatment. J Androl 2006;27:548-551.

113. Gonda RL Jr, Karo JJ, Forte RA, O'Donnell KT. Diagnosis of subclinical varicocele in infertility. AJR Am J Roentgenol 1987; 148:71-75.

114. Graif M, Hauser R, Hirshebein A, et al. Varicocele and the testicular-renal venous route: hemodynamic Doppler sonographic investigation. J Ultrasound Med 2000;19:627-631.

115. Tetreau R, Julian P, Lyonnet D, Rouviere O. Intratesticular varicocele: an easy diagnosis but unclear physiopathologic characteristics. J Ultrasound Med 2007;26:1767-1773.

116. Atasoy C, Fitoz S. Gray-scale and color Doppler sonographic findings in intratesticular varicocele. J Clin Ultrasound 2001;29: 369-373.

117. Bhosale PR, Patnana M, Viswanathan C, Szklaruk J. The inguinal canal: anatomy and imaging features of common and uncommon masses. Radiographics 2008;28:819-835; quiz 913.

118. Sung T, Riedlinger WF, Diamond DA, Chow JS. Solid extratesticular masses in children: radiographic and pathologic correlation. AJR Am J Roentgenol 2006;186:483-490.

119. Pavone-MacAluso M, Smith PH, Bagshaw MA. Testicular cancer and other tumors of the genitourinary tract. New York: Plenum Press; 1985.

120. Alleman WG, Gorman B, King BF, et al. Benign and malignant epididymal masses evaluated with scrotal sonography: clinical and pathologic review of 85 patients. J Ultrasound Med 2008;27: 1195-1202.

121. Yang DM, Kim SH, Kim HN, et al. Differential diagnosis of focal epididymal lesions with gray scale sonographic, color Doppler sonographic, and clinical features. J Ultrasound Med 2003;22:135-142; quiz 143-144.

122. Smallman LA, Odedra JK. Primary carcinoma of sigmoid colon metastasizing to epididymis. Urology 1984;23:598-599.

123. Wachtel TL, Mehan DJ. Metastatic tumors of the epididymis. J Urol 1970;103:624-627.

124. Oh C, Nisenbaum HL, Langer J, et al. Sonographic demonstration, including color Doppler imaging, of recurrent sperm granuloma. J Ultrasound Med 2000;19:333-335.

125. Krainik A, Sarrazin JL, Camparo P, et al. Fibrous pseudotumor of the epididymis: imaging and pathologic correlation. Eur Radiol 2000;10:1636-1638.

126. Al-Otaibi L, Whitman GJ, Chew FS. Fibrous pseudotumor of the epididymis. AJR Am J Roentgenol 1997;168:1586.

127. Oliva E, Young RH. Paratesticular tumor-like lesions. Semin Diagn Pathol 2000;17:340-358.

128. Leung ML, Gooding GA, Williams RD. High-resolution sonography of scrotal contents in asymptomatic subjects. AJR Am J Roentgenol 1984;143:161-164.

129. Reddy NM, Gerscovich EO, Jain KA, et al. Vasectomy-related changes on sonographic examination of the scrotum. J Clin Ultrasound 2004;32:394-398.

130. Ishigami K, Abu-Yousef MM, El-Zein Y. Tubular ectasia of the epididymis: a sign of postvasectomy status. J Clin Ultrasound 2005; 33:447-451.

131. Stewart VR, Sidhu PS. The testis: the unusual, the rare and the bizarre. Clin Radiol 2007;62:289-302.

Acute Scrotal Pain

132. Mueller DL, Amundson GM, Rubin SZ, Wesenberg RL. Acute scrotal abnormalities in children: diagnosis by combined sonography and scintigraphy. AJR Am J Roentgenol 1988;150:643-646.

133. Watanabe Y, Dohke M, Ohkubo K, et al. Scrotal disorders: evaluation of testicular enhancement patterns at dynamic contrast-enhanced subtraction MR imaging [see comment]. Radiology 2000;217:219-227.

134. Hricak H, Lue T, Filly RA, et al. Experimental study of the sonographic diagnosis of testicular torsion. J Ultrasound Med 1983;2:349-356.

135. Pillai SB, Besner GE. Pediatric testicular problems. Pediatr Clin North Am 1998;45:813-830.

136. Paltiel HJ. Sonography of pediatric scrotal emergencies. Ultrasound Q 2000;16:53-71.

137. Prando D. Torsion of the spermatic cord: sonographic diagnosis. Ultrasound Q 2002;18:41-57.

138. Sidhu PS. Clinical and imaging features of testicular torsion: role of ultrasound. Clin Radiol 1999;54:343-352.

139. Middleton WD, Melson GL. Testicular ischemia: color Doppler sonographic findings in five patients. AJR Am J Roentgenol 1989; 152:1237-1239.

140. Chinn DH, Miller EI. Generalized testicular hyperechogenicity in acute testicular torsion. J Ultrasound Med 1985;4:495-496.

141. Winter TC 3rd. Ultrasonography of the scrotum. App Radiol 2002;31.

142. Middleton WD, Middleton MA, Dierks M, et al. Sonographic prediction of viability in testicular torsion: preliminary observations. J Ultrasound Med 1997;16:23-27; quiz 29-30.

143. Vijayaraghavan SB. Sonographic differential diagnosis of acute scrotum: real-time whirlpool sign, a key sign of torsion. J Ultrasound Med 2006;25:563-574.

144. Trambert MA, Mattrey RF, Levine D, Berthoty DP. Subacute scrotal pain: evaluation of torsion versus epididymitis with MR imaging. Radiology 1990;175:53-56.

145. Vick CW, Bird K, Rosenfield AT, et al. Extratesticular hemorrhage associated with torsion of the spermatic cord: sonographic demonstration. Radiology 1986;158:401-404.

146. Lerner RM, Mevorach RA, Hulbert WC, Rabinowitz R. Color Doppler ultrasound in the evaluation of acute scrotal disease. Radiology 1990;176:355-358.

147. Fitzgerald SW, Erickson S, DeWire DM, et al. Color Doppler sonography in the evaluation of the adult acute scrotum [see comment]. J Ultrasound Med 1992;11:543-548.

148. Barth RA, Shortliffe LD. Normal pediatric testis: comparison of power Doppler and color Doppler ultrasound in the detection of blood flow. Radiology 1997;204:389-393.

149. Bader TR, Kammerhuber F, Herneth AM. Testicular blood flow in boys as assessed at color Doppler and power Doppler sonography. Radiology 1997;202:559-564; erratum 203:580.

150. Oley BD, Frush DP, Babcock DS, et al. Acute testicular torsion: comparison of unenhanced and contrast-enhanced power Doppler ultrasound, color Doppler ultrasound, and radionuclide imaging. Radiology 1996;199:441-446.

151. Luker GD, Siegel MJ. Scrotal US in pediatric patients: comparison of power and standard color Doppler ultrasound. Radiology 1996; 198:381-385.

152. Albrecht T, Lotzof K, Hussain HK, Shedden D, Cosgrove DO, de Bruyn R. Power Doppler US of the normal prepubertal testis: does it live up to its promises? Radiology 1997;203:227-231.

153. Lee Jr FT, Winter DB, Madsen FA, et al. Conventional color Doppler velocity sonography versus color Doppler energy sonography for the diagnosis of acute experimental torsion of the spermatic cord. AJR Am J Roentgenol 1996;167:785-790.

154. Burks DD, Markey BJ, Burkhard TK, et al. Suspected testicular torsion and ischemia: evaluation with color Doppler sonography. Radiology 1990;175:815-821.

155. Atkinson Jr GO, Patrick LE, Ball Jr TI, et al. The normal and abnormal scrotum in children: evaluation with color Doppler sonography. AJR Am J Roentgenol 1992;158:613-617.

156. Bude RO, Kennelly MJ, Adler RS, Rubin JM. Nonpulsatile arterial waveforms: observations during graded testicular torsion in rats. Acad Radiol 1995;2:879-882.

157. Dogra VS, Rubens DJ, Gottlieb RH, Bhatt S. Torsion and beyond: new twists in spectral Doppler evaluation of the scrotum. J Ultrasound Med 2004;23:1077-1085.

158. Sanelli PC, Burke BJ, Lee L. Color and spectral Doppler sonography of partial torsion of the spermatic cord. AJR Am J Roentgenol 1999;172:49-51.

159. Alcantara AL, Sethi Y. Imaging of testicular torsion and epididymitis/orchitis: diagnosis and pitfalls. Emerg Radiol 1998;5:394-402.

160. Dresner ML. Torsed appendage: diagnosis and management—blue dot sign. Urology 1973;1:63-66.

161. Hesser U, Rosenborg M, Gierup J, et al. Gray-scale sonography in torsion of the testicular appendages. Pediatr Radiol 1993;23:529-532.

162. Chung JJ, Kim MJ, Lee T, et al. Sonographic findings in tuberculous epididymitis and epididymo-orchitis. J Clin Ultrasound 1997;25:390-394.

163. Basekim CC, Kizilkaya E, Pekkafali Z, et al. Mumps epididymo-orchitis: sonography and color Doppler sonographic findings. Abdom Imaging 2000;25:322-325.

164. Gondos B, Wong TW. Non-neoplastic diseases of the testis and epididymis. In: Murphy WM, editor. Urological pathology. 2nd ed. Philadelphia: Saunders; 1997. p. 277-341.

165. Horstman WG, Middleton WD, Melson GL. Scrotal inflammatory disease: color Doppler ultrasound findings. Radiology 1991;179:55-59.

166. Cook JL, Dewbury K. The changes seen on high-resolution ultrasound in orchitis. Clin Radiol 2000;55:13-18.

167. Hourihane DO. Infected infarcts of the testis: a study of 18 cases preceded by pyogenic epididymoorchitis. J Clin Pathol 1970;23:668-675.

168. Sanders LM, Haber S, Dembner A, Aquino A. Significance of reversal of diastolic flow in the acute scrotum. J Ultrasound Med 1994;13:137-139.

169. Casalino DD, Kim R. Clinical importance of a unilateral striated pattern seen on sonography of the testicle. AJR Am J Roentgenol 2002;178:927-930.

170. Harris RD, Chouteau C, Partrick M, Schned A. Prevalence and significance of heterogeneous testes revealed on sonography: ex vivo sonographic-pathologic correlation. AJR Am J Roentgenol 2000;175:347-352.

Trauma

171. Jeffrey RB, Laing FC, Hricak H, McAninch JW. Sonography of testicular trauma. AJR Am J Roentgenol 1983;141:993-995.

172. Kim SH, Park S, Choi SH, et al. Significant predictors for determination of testicular rupture on sonography: a prospective study. J Ultrasound Med 2007;26:1649-1655.

173. Buckley JC, McAninch JW. Use of ultrasonography for the diagnosis of testicular injuries in blunt scrotal trauma. J Urol 2006;175:175-178.

174. Cohen HL, Shapiro ML, Haller JO, Glassberg K. Sonography of intrascrotal hematomas simulating testicular rupture in adolescents. Pediatr Radiol 1992;22:296-297.

175. Learch TJ, Hansch LP, Ralls PW. Sonography in patients with gunshot wounds of the scrotum: imaging findings and their value. AJR Am J Roentgenol 1995;165:879-883.

176. Gordon LM, Stein SM, Ralls PW. Traumatic epididymitis: evaluation with color Doppler sonography. AJR Am J Roentgenol 1996;166:1323-1325.

Cryptorchidism

177. Elder JS. Cryptorchidism: isolated and associated with other genitourinary defects. Pediatr Clin North Am 1987;34:1033-1053.

178. Harrison JH, Gittes RF, Stamey TA, et al. Campbell's urology. 4th ed. Philadelphia: Saunders; 1979.

179. Rosenfield AT, Blair DN, McCarthy S, et al. The pars infravaginalis gubernaculi: importance in the identification of the undescended testis. Society of Uroradiology Award paper. AJR Am J Roentgenol 1989;153:775-778.

180. Friedland GW, Chang P. The role of imaging in the management of the impalpable undescended testis. AJR Am J Roentgenol 1988;151:1107-1111.

181. Fritzsche PJ, Hricak H, Kogan BA, et al. Undescended testis: value of MR imaging. Radiology 1987;164:169-173.

182. Kier R, McCarthy S, Rosenfield AT, et al. Nonpalpable testes in young boys: evaluation with MR imaging. Radiology 1988;169:429-433.

CHAPTER 22

The Rotator Cuff

Marnix T. van Holsbeeck, Dzung Vu, and J. Antonio Bouffard

Chapter Outline

Shoulder pain has many causes. Tendinitis, rotator cuff strain, and partial-thickness or full-thickness tear may cause pain and weakness on elevation of the arm.[1] The pain in rotator cuff disease is often worse at night and may keep the patient awake. Underlying these symptoms in many patients over 40 years of age is failure of the rotator cuff fibers.[2] The supraspinatus tendon fibers typically fail first. The subscapularis and infraspinatus tendons, two other tendons of the rotator cuff, fail when the tear extends. The teres minor, the fourth component of the rotator cuff, is rarely affected. Calcific tendinitis, cervical radiculopathy, and acromioclavicular arthritis may mimic rotator cuff pathology. Contrast arthrography has long been the premier radiologic examination used to diagnose full-thickness tears of the rotator cuff.[3] Two competing noninvasive imaging techniques, ultrasound and magnetic resonance imaging (MRI), are taking over the role of arthrography. High-resolution real-time ultrasound has been shown to be a cost-effective means of examining the rotator cuff.[4-9] Ultrasound is the modality of choice in our institution. In the last 15 years, we performed more than 40,000 shoulder ultrasound studies.

CLINICAL CONSIDERATIONS

Rotator cuff fiber failure is the most common cause of shoulder pain and dysfunction in patients older than 40.[1] Epidemiologic studies by Codman, DePalma, and others have demonstrated that the frequency of rotator cuff fiber failure increases with age.[10-12] This aging of tendons

has been shown in imaging studies as well.[13-16] The earliest changes are often located in the substance of the tendon, resulting in so-called delamination of the cuff. Fiber failure is a step-by-step process from partial-thickness tear, almost always first in the supraspinatus, to massive tears involving multiple cuff tendons.

Rotator cuff tear may occur insidiously and, in fact, may be unnoticed by the patient, a process termed by some as **creeping tendon ruptures.**[17] Asymptomatic tears affect up to 30% of the population over age 60.[13] When a larger group of fibers fails at once, the shoulder demonstrates pain at rest and accentuation of pain on use of the rotator cuff (e.g., extension, abduction, or external rotation). When even greater numbers of fibers fail at one time, a process known as **acute extension of the shoulder** may demonstrate sudden onset of substantial weakness in flexion, abduction, and external rotation.

As persons age, the rotator cuff becomes increasingly susceptible to tearing with less severe amounts of applied force. Thus, although a major force is required to tear the usual rotator cuff of a 40-year-old person, a relatively trivial force may result in tear of the rotator cuff of the average 60-year-old individual. This is analogous to the predisposition of older women to femoral neck fractures. Although differences of the acromial shape, abnormalities of the acromial-clavicular joint, and other factors may also affect the susceptibility of the rotator cuff to fiber failure, age-related deterioration and loading of the rotator cuff seem to be the dominant factors in determining the failure patterns of the cuff tendons. In a retrospective study of siblings of patients with rotator cuff tears, the relative risk of developing symptomatic full-thickness tears in the siblings compared to controls was 4.65. The authors concluded that genetic factors may also play a role in the development of tendon tears in shoulders.[18]

Symptoms of rotator cuff fiber failure in the acute phase usually include pain at rest and on motion. Later, subacromial crepitance occurs when the arm is rotated in the partially flexed position, and finally, arm weakness occurs. When the rotator cuff fails, shoulder instability can result, and so-called impingement may then manifest. The humeral head is no longer stabilized and may impinge on the tissues between the head and the acromion (acromial process) or between the head and the posterior glenoid in cases of subacromial impingement, the process will lead to osteosclerosis and remodeling of the acromion, and it may result in a traction spur along the coracoacromial ligament.[19]

TECHNICAL CONSIDERATIONS

Mechanical sector scanners with frequencies between 5 and 10 MHz used in the early 1980s provided adequate detail in detecting full-thickness tears.[20] The utility of these transducers was limited by several factors: near-field artifact, narrow superficial image field, and tendon **anisotropy.** This last artifact is caused by the anisotropic structure of tendons and still affects the scanning of tendons significantly. Parallelism of collagenous structures within the cuff results in peculiar imaging characteristics; the echogenicity of the tendon depends on the angle of the transducer relative to the tendon during tendon interrogation. Oblique insonation of the tissues will result in heterogeneous appearance of the tendons. With optimal perpendicular technique, the center of the image will appear hyperechoic, whereas the side lobes will often be hypoechoic if one scans over the round surface of the proximal humerus. This hypoechogenicity can be mistaken for pathology by the inexperienced ultrasound reader.

State-of-the-art imaging of the cuff should be done with a high-resolution linear array transducer with a broad-bandwidth frequency capability, typically 5 to 13 MHz.[20] These transducers demonstrate marked improvement in near resolution compared with the older devices. The broad superficial field of view is helpful to improve the near-field image. Tissue harmonics has been shown to improve tendon surface visibility over conventional ultrasound.[21] In recent years the ultrasound machines have changed from heavy, space occupying ultrasound equipment to lightweight, laptop ultrasound systems with ergonomic ultrasound probes. Parallel with this trend, the high-expense equipment can often be replaced with more affordable pieces that are marketed for focused use in clinics,[20,22] in the operating room, and at the point of injury.[23,24] Several manufacturers now make ultrasound units that weigh less than 5 kg (11 1b); prices of equipment applicable for use in musculoskeletal ultrasound have decreased by more than 80% compared with prices in the 1990s.[20]

ANATOMY AND SONOGRAPHIC TECHNIQUE

Understanding the complex three-dimensional (3-D) rotator cuff anatomy during sonography is crucial to successful rotator cuff sonography. Bone often limits the examination done by the inexperienced operator. For those starting in shoulder ultrasound, but who have experience in MRI arthrography, we recommend performing a quick ultrasound examination before and after each arthrogram. This allows examiners to test their diagnostic abilities instantaneously. Those who have no experience with arthrography can scan in the operating room or anatomy laboratory. Surgical exploration or dissection may teach the most valuable lessons. Those initial steps are necessary to improve knowledge of the anatomy, which is essential in mastering the technique and accelerating the learning curve. Some investigators have been combining arthrographic technique with the sonographic examination, called **arthrosonography,** which may be more sensitive in assessing synovial proliferation and estimating the size of rotator cuff tears.[25] Future applications may also include the diagnosis of labral abnormalities.[26-29] As with MRI, ultrasound's display of anatomy improves when enhanced by injection of intra-articular fluid. Saline used as a contrast agent in arthrosonography is much less expensive than gadolinium, the contrast agent universally used for MR arthrography.

The bony landmarks guide the shoulder ultrasound examination (Fig. 22-1). The fingers of the examiner can palpate the acromion, the scapular spine, the coracoid, and the acromioclavicular joint. Transducer orientation relative to those landmarks will be essential in making corrections to the technique in viewing complex shoulder pathology. External bony landmarks are important in shoulder imaging when scanning a patient with significant pathology and loss of normal soft tissue landmarks.

The patient is scanned while seated on a rotating stool without armrests. The examiner sits comfortably on a stool adjusted so that the examiner rises above the shoulder level of the patient. Both shoulders, starting with the less symptomatic one, should be examined if the examiner is a beginner. The following technique is used at our institution.[8]

Transverse images through the long biceps are obtained with the arm and forearm on the patient's thigh, the palm supinated (Fig. 22-2). **The bicipital groove** serves as the anatomic landmark to differentiate the subscapularis tendon from the supraspinatus tendon.

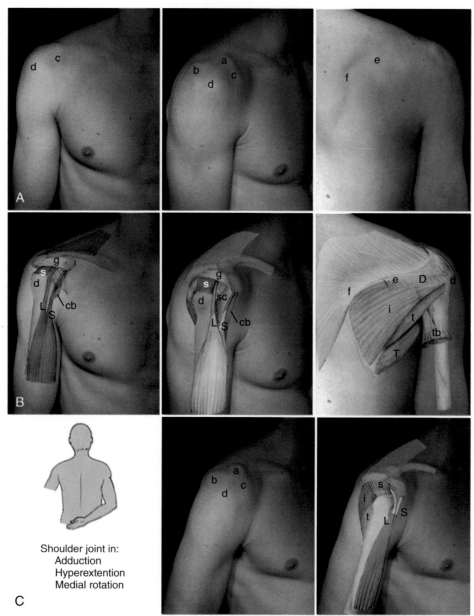

FIGURE 22-1. Right shoulder joint with surface anatomy and underlying musculoskeletal structures. **A,** Neutral position of the shoulder: frontal view *(left image)*, side view *(middle image)*, and posterior view *(right image)* of superficial anatomy. The bony prominences formed by the clavicle *(a)*, acromion *(b)*, and coracoid process *(c)* that limit the acoustic window for shoulder ultrasound are visible subcutaneously. Other visible contours represent the greater tuberosity *(d)* and spine of the scapula *(e)*, which ends at the medial flat surface *(f)*, over which slides the aponeurosis of the trapezius muscle. **B,** Anatomy in neutral position. Frontal view *(left image)* shows coracoacromial ligament *(g)*, supraspinatus tendon attachment *(s)*, and biceps brachii, with the short head *(S)* originating from the coracoid medially and the long head *(L)* extending into the joint deep to the coracoacromial ligament. The coraco-brachial tendon *(cb)* is another tendon that originates from the coracoid. Side view *(middle image)* shows how the subscapularis *(sc)* is a separate tendon at the anterior aspect of the shoulder. This tendon is divided from the supraspinatus *(S)* by the long head of biceps tendon and by the rotator cuff interval. Posterior view *(right image)* with trapezius *(t)*, infraspinatus *(i)*, teres minor *(t)*, triceps brachii *(tb)*, and teres major *(T)*. The deltoid *(D)* has been cut, and its edge is seen around the acromion. On all anatomic drawings that follow, the deltoid has been removed. On ultrasound, we look through the deltoid to see the rotator cuff. **C,** By using adduction, hyperextension and internal (medial) rotation, one can free more supraspinatus tendon for visualization. The most vulnerable zone of the supraspinatus *(S)* is anterior to the acromion and lateral to the intracapsular long *(L)* biceps tendon. The zone of the rotator cuff where most tears occur **(critical zone)** can be found in the trapezoidal space between the bony prominences of the lateral clavicle *(a)*, anterior acromion *(b)*, coracoid *(c)*, and anterior greater tuberosity. The subscapularis tendon in this position hides under the coracoid and medial to the short head of biceps *(S)*.

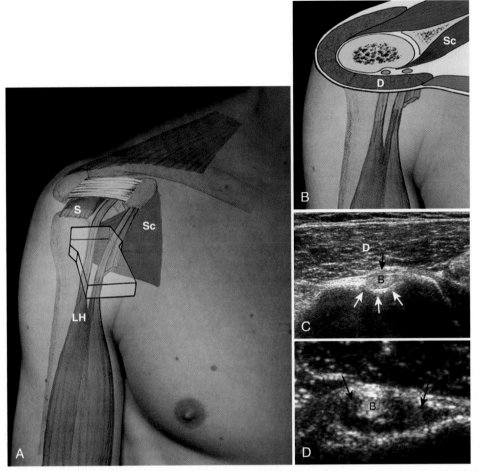

FIGURE 22-2. Short-axis or transverse scan of the long biceps tendon. A, View of the long head *(LH)* and the short head of biceps tendon. Transducer position is indicated by a transparent symbol. For this scan, the patient rests the dorsum of the hand comfortably on the thigh with elbow flexed. *S,* Supraspinatus tendon; *Sc,* subscapularis tendon. **B,** Cross section through the biceps groove at the level of the subscapularis *(Sc).* The deltoid *(D)* is hoof shaped and covers the two biceps tendons and the subscapularis tendon in the front of the shoulder. This is the anatomic view of the shoulder in neutral position and with the transducer placed transversely over the bicipital groove. The cross sections of the long and short heads of biceps are seen close together. **C,** Deep to the deltoid *(D),* the proximal long biceps *(B)* rests in the bicipital groove *(arrows).* The transverse ligament *(black arrow)* represents the lateral extension of the subscapularis and covers the long biceps. A small segment of the subscapularis is noted between the bone surface of the humerus and the short head of the biceps at the right edge of the image. **D,** Transverse scan over the lower part of the bicipital groove in a patient with rotator cuff disease. The long biceps tendon *(B)* appears enveloped in a distended hypoechoic sheath *(arrows).* The hypoechogenicity of the tendon sheath may represent fluid, synovial hypertrophy, or both. It is important to scan the lowest recess of the biceps synovial sheath. In a patient who sits for the examination, fluid will precipitate to the most dependent portion of the synovium.

The groove is concave; bright echoes reflect off the bony surface of the humerus. The tendon of the long head of the biceps is visualized as a hyperechoic oval structure within the bicipital groove on the transverse images. The tendon courses through the rotator cuff interval and divides the subscapularis from the supraspinatus tendon. Scanning should begin with the proximal long biceps tendon above the biceps tendon groove. The intracapsular biceps shows more obliquely in the shoulder capsule. The capsular biceps is located in a space typically referred to as the **rotator cuff interval.** The space varies between 1 and 3 cm in width.[30] In this interval between the superior subscapular and the anterior supraspinatus, a **sling** of connective tissue surrounds the proximal long biceps tendon. Deep to the biceps, inserting on the

bicipital groove, the sling consists of fibers of the superior glenohumeral ligament. Superficial to the biceps are fibers of the **coracohumeral ligament,**[31] which courses from the coracoid medially, covers the biceps in the rotator cuff interval, and attaches on the humerus laterally. At its lateral insertion, the coracohumeral ligament forks around the anterior supraspinatus. The deep layer appears more distinct and has been called the **rotator cuff cable,**[32] a structure at the articular margin of the supraspinatus. The superficial coracohumeral ligament is thinner and less distinctly visible. The sonographers may occasionally recognize the rotator cuff cable because of its unique anisotropic characteristics oriented perpendicular to the longitudinal fibers of the critical zone of the supraspinatus. After scanning the biceps in the capsule, the long biceps is followed throughout its course in the bicipital groove; the scan should extend as far down as the musculotendinous junction. This allows detection of the smallest fluid collections in the medial triangular recess at the distal end of the tendon sheath.[33] Such small biceps sheath collections are a very sensitive indicator of joint fluid. A 90-degree rotation of the transducer into a longitudinal view will ascertain the intactness of the biceps tendon.[34] The transducer must be carefully aligned along the biceps groove (Fig. 22-3). Gentle pressure on the distal aspect of the transducer is necessary to align the transducer parallel to the tendon to avoid artifact due to anisotropy (Fig. 22-4).

The transducer position is then returned to the transverse plane and moved proximally along the humerus to visualize the **subscapularis tendon,** which appears as a band of medium-level echoes deep to the subdeltoid fat and bursa. The subscapularis tendon is viewed parallel to its axis (Fig. 22-5) for its long-axis view; scanning during passive and external rotation may be helpful in assessing the integrity of the subscapularis tendon, which may be disrupted in patients with chronic anterior shoulder dislocation. External rotation is also necessary to diagnose subluxation of the long biceps tendon, especially if only present intermittently.[35] The short-axis view of the subscapularis is best evaluated over the ledge of the lesser tuberosity as close as possible to the bicipital groove (Fig. 22-6).

The normal **subdeltoid bursa** is recognized as a thin, hypoechoic layer between the deltoid muscle on one side and the rotator cuff tendons and biceps tendon on the deep side. Hyperechoic peribursal fat surrounds the outer aspect of the synovial layer.[36]

The **supraspinatus tendon** is scanned perpendicular to its axis (transversely) by moving the transducer laterally posteriorly. The sonographic window is very narrow, and careful transducer positioning is essential (Fig. 22-7). The supraspinatus tendon is visualized as a band of medium-level echoes deep to the subdeltoid bursa and superficial to the bright echoes originating from the bone surface of the greater tuberosity.

The rest of the examination is done with the arm adducted and hyperextended and the shoulder in moderate internal rotation[5,7,37] (Fig. 22-8). This position can best be explained to patients by asking them to reach to the opposite back pocket. This placement of the hand is often alternated with the hand position over the back pocket on the side of the affected shoulder with maximum elbow adduction. The latter position puts more tension on the tendon. It may make a lesion of the cuff stand out more clearly; however, the position may also mislead the examiner to overestimate the size of tears.[38] Both longitudinal sections along the course of the supraspinatus tendon and images transverse to the tendon insertion and perpendicular to the humeral head are obtained. Correct orientation is achieved when an imaging plane

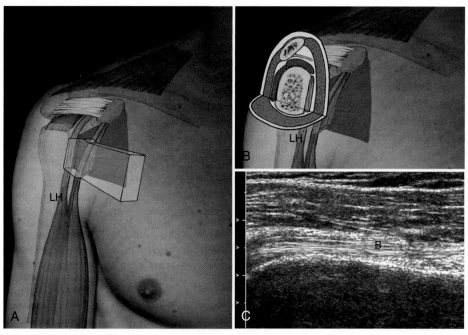

FIGURE 22-3. Long-axis or longitudinal scan of the long biceps tendon. A, In the neutral position, the long biceps is found in the bicipital groove, about midline over the anterior humerus. Transducer position is indicated by the transparent symbol. **B,** Longitudinal cross section through the biceps. The deltoid is also hoof shaped in the sagittal plane. This is the anatomic view of the shoulder in neutral position and with the transducer placed longitudinally over the bicipital groove. The long head of the biceps *(LH)* appears as a tubular structure. **C,** Longitudinal scan shows the biceps tendon *(B)* with distinct fibrillar architecture deep to the deltoid. Note the distinct longitudinal linear reflections in the tubular structure of a normal long biceps. When the layered structure is absent, the clinician should consider the possibility of scar tissue replacing a torn tendon.

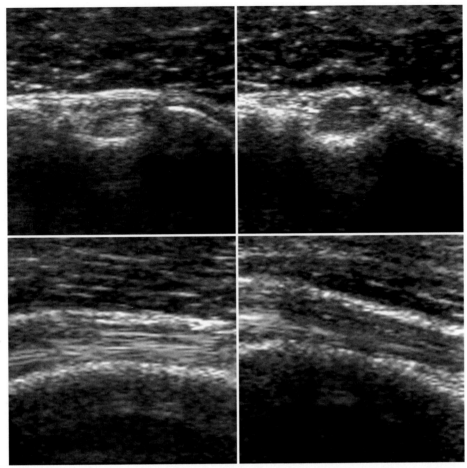

FIGURE 22-4. Composite of images through proximal long biceps showing tendon anisotropy. The predominant longitudinal orientation of the collagen in tendons such as the biceps make them strong anisotropic reflectors. *Top images,* Transverse imaging approach; *bottom images,* sagittal scanning through the middle of the bicipital groove. The column on the left shows correct scanning technique. Normal tendons appear hyperechoic only when scanned perpendicularly. The column on the right demonstrates how tendons appear hypoechoic as the angle of the transducer diverges from 90 degrees. Visualization of this transition of tendon echogenicity from hyperechoic to hypoechoic may be used at times to improve tissue contrast; it is also a useful technique to distinguish tendon from scar.

shows crisp bone surface definition and sharp outline of the cartilage of the humeral head. During longitudinal scanning, the transducer overlays the acromion medially and the lateral aspect of the greater tuberosity laterally (Fig. 22-8, *B* and *C*). The transducer sweeps around the humeral head circumferentially, and the transducer should be held perpendicular to the humeral head surface at all times. This sweeping motion through the supraspinatus tendon starts anteriorly next to the long biceps tendon. We cover an area of approximately 2.5 cm lateral to the long biceps tendon. Infraspinatus tendon is scanned beyond this point. The musculotendinous junction shows as hypoechoic muscle surrounding hyperechoic infraspinatus tendon. The transverse scan starts just lateral to the acromion and translates downward over the supraspinatus tendon and the greater tuberosity. The critical zone is that portion of the tendon that begins approximately 1 cm posterolateral to the biceps tendon. Failure to adequately visualize this area may cause a false-negative result.[5]

Scanning of the supraspinatus tendon is followed by the visualization of the infraspinatus and teres minor tendons by moving the transducer posteriorly and in the plane parallel to the scapular spine. The **infraspinatus tendon** appears as a beak-shaped soft tissue structure as it attaches to the posterior aspect of the greater tuberosity[6] (Fig. 22-9). Internal and external shoulder rotation may be helpful in the examination of the infraspinatus tendon. This maneuver relaxes and contracts the infraspinatus tendon in alternating fashion. At this level, a portion of the posterior glenoid labrum is seen as a hyperechoic triangular structure. The fluid of the infraspinatus recess surrounds the labrum. Optimal image contrast for detection of intra-articular fluid will be obtained by bringing the arm in external rotation (Fig. 22-10). In this position the normal labrum will be covered by infraspinatus tendon. Both structures appear hyperechoic and become almost indistinguishable in a joint without effusion. In contrast, hypoechoic fluid or synovium may considerably separate these tissues in the

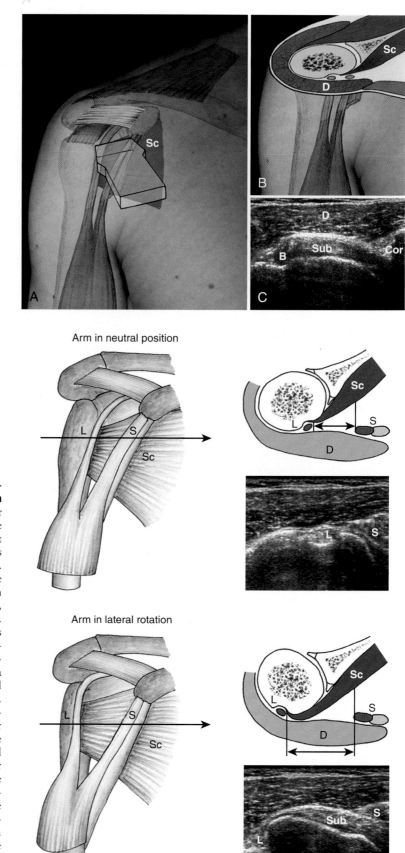

FIGURE 22-5. Long-axis view of subscapularis tendon, or transverse scan through anterior shoulder. A, Transducer position for the examination of the long axis of the subscapularis *(Sc)* is indicated by the transparent transducer. **B,** Cross section of the subscapularis *(Sc)* and the two tendons of the proximal biceps. The subscapularis tendon can be seen over the humerus and between the two biceps tendons. In neutral position or in internal (medial) rotation, there is little separation of the two biceps tendons. In extreme rotation, the long head may actually pass under the short head. **C,** Long-axis sonogram visualized with external rotation shows the subscapularis tendon *(Sub)* parallel to its axis, viewed as a band of medium-level echoes deep to the deltoid muscle *(D)*; *B,* biceps tendon; *Cor,* coracoid. **D,** Dual images illustrate the use of external rotation in bringing out the subscapularis from under the coracoid and short head of biceps *(S)*. In the neutral position, long head *(L)* of the biceps will show over the middle of the proximal anterior humerus. In external rotation, long head of the biceps separates from the short head. The subscapularis tendon *(Sub)* shows in its full length over the anterior humeral head; *D,* deltoid. Anatomic diagrams on the left show the long biceps position in frontal view. Arrows indicate what happens to the cross-sectional anatomy with internal rotation *(top)* and external rotation *(bottom)*.

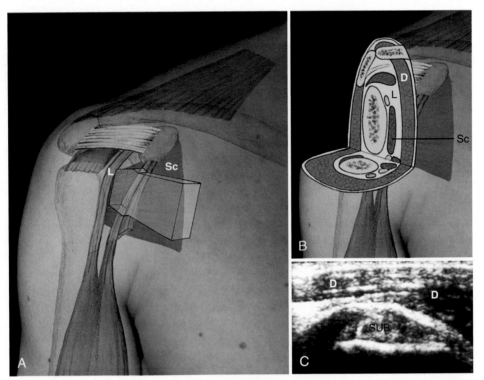

FIGURE 22-6. Short-axis view of subscapularis, or sagittal scan through anterior shoulder. A, The transparent transducer indicates the placement of the transducer. **B,** The subscapularis tendon *(Sc)* covers the humeral head and the humeral head cartilage of the anterior shoulder. The tendon is visualized through the deltoid *(D)*. The space superior to the subscapularis, the **rotator cuff interval,** is a space with loose mesenchymal tissue surrounding the intracapsular biceps *(L)*. **C,** Deep to the deltoid *(D)*, the subscapularis *(SUB)* tapers in thickness from its superior to inferior border.

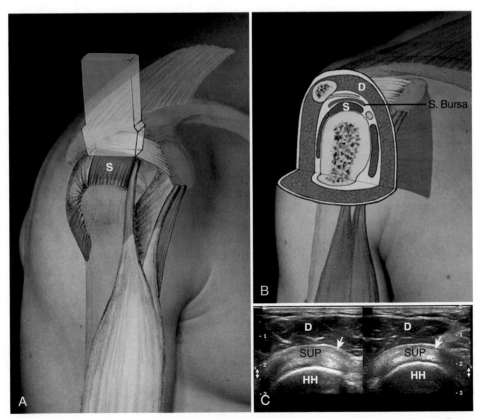

FIGURE 22-7. Short-axis scan of supraspinatus tendon. A, With the arm in extension and internal rotation, the transducer is placed between the anterior acromion and the coracoid. The transducer is swept from the edge of the acromion down to the level of the lateral greater tuberosity. **B,** This section in the plane of the transducer shows how the supraspinatus is covered most immediately by the subdeltoid bursa *(S. Bursa)* deep to the deltoid *(D)*. **C,** The supraspinatus tendon *(SUP)* shows as a band of medium-level echoes deep to the subdeltoid bursa *(arrows)* and draped over the cartilage of the humeral head *(HH)*. The swollen symptomatic tendon shows on the left side of the split-screen image; the patient's normal shoulder shows on the right. *D,* Deltoid muscle. Compare the thickness of the hypoechoic bursa with the thickness of the hyaline cartilage covering the humeral head. A normal bursa does not exceed the thickness of normal cartilage.

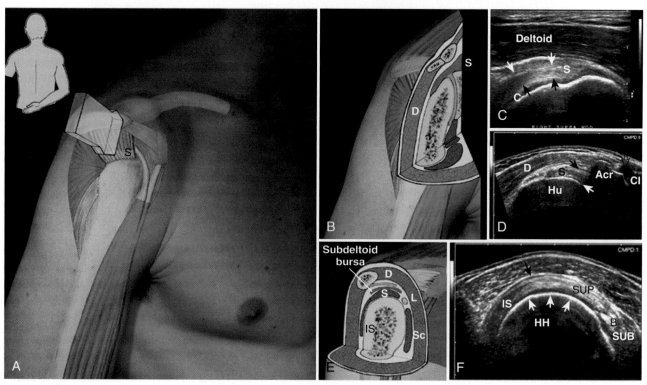

FIGURE 22-8. Long-axis scan of supraspinatus tendon. A, With the arm in extension and internal rotation, the transducer is placed perpendicular to the curvature of the acromial process for the view along the bulk of the largest number of fibers of the supraspinatus. We refer to this view as the long-axis view. **B,** This section demonstrates the challenge posed by the acromioclavicular joint and the lateral acromion that cover part of the supraspinatus *(S).* The positioning of the patient (as seen in **A,** *inset)* frees the critical zone and moves it into the acoustic window deep to the acromioclavicular ligament. **C,** Longitudinal image through a left supraspinatus. More tendon will stretch beyond the lateral and anterior aspect of the acromion than in the neutral position. Echogenicity changes within the rotator cuff are related to tendon anisotropy. The propagation of ultrasound through supraspinatus tendon *(S)* appears uneven. This feature stands out more clearly in one sublayer of the supraspinatus tendon *(arrows).* The fibers in this layer have a longitudinal orientation along the long axis of the tendon; *C,* hyaline cartilage over the humeral head. **D,** Panoramic overview through a right supraspinatus demonstrates the anatomic relationship of the longitudinal supraspinatus tendon *(S)* with the acromion *(Acr)* and acromioclavicular joint *(open arrow).* This image can best be viewed side by side with **B.** Deltoid *(D)* originates from the acromion; *Cl,* lateral clavicle; *Hu,* proximal humerus. The shape of the tendon has often been compared to a parrot's beak. Hypoechoic tissue covers the tendon on either side. Hypoechogenicity between tendon and bone represents hyaline cartilage *(white arrow),* and the thin, hypoechoic layer between tendon and deltoid corresponds to subdeltoid bursa *(black arrow).* **E,** Sagittal section shows relationship of supraspinatus joining the infraspinatus, which is located more posteriorly. Also noted is the separation of the anterior supraspinatus from the subscapularis *(Sc)* by the intracapsular long biceps *(L).* **F,** Panoramic overview of the transverse anatomy of supraspinatus *(SUP)* relative to the subscapularis *(SUB)* and the intracapsular biceps *(B)* in the front and the infraspinatus *(IS)* in the back. Again, the tendon appears sandwiched between two hypoechoic layers. Note that the normal subdeltoid bursa *(black arrow)* remains slightly thinner than the hyaline cartilage *(white arrows)* over the humeral head *(HH).* The supraspinatus and infraspinatus form a conjoined tendon, whereas the biceps tendon separates supraspinatus and subscapularis. The image has been made by making a circular sweep over the tendons in a movement following the hoof shape of the deltoid in the sagittal plane, as illustrated in **E.**

joint with arthritis. The hypoechoic articular cartilage of the humeral head, which shows lateral to the labrum, contrasts significantly with the hyperechogenicity of the fibrocartilage. Scanning is extended medially to encompass the spinoglenoid notch and the suprascapular vessels and nerve. Visualization of the notch may be improved by bringing the transducer in the transverse plane, but with the medial end of the transducer slightly more cephalad than the lateral end. Using the external-internal rotation dynamic during visualization of the neurovascular bundle that wraps around the spinoglenoid notch will show distention of the suprascapular vein during external rotation. The transversely oriented transducer is moved distally, and the teres minor is then visualized.

The **teres minor tendon** is a trapezoidal structure[39] (Fig. 22-11), differentiated from the infraspinatus tendon by its broader and more muscular attachment. Tears of the teres minor are rare. In cases of **quadrilateral space syndrome** with entrapment of the axillary nerve, the teres minor can be unilaterally smaller and appear hyperechoic.[40] Small joint effusions will also be imaged in this location.[41] Demonstration of this effusion helps distinguish articular processes, such as rheumatoid arthritis and septic arthritis, which will cause effusion. In rotator cuff disease, it is rare to find fluid in this location.

Coronal images through the **acromioclavicular joints** are obtained at the end of the examination. Right-left comparison can show degenerative or traumatic pathol-

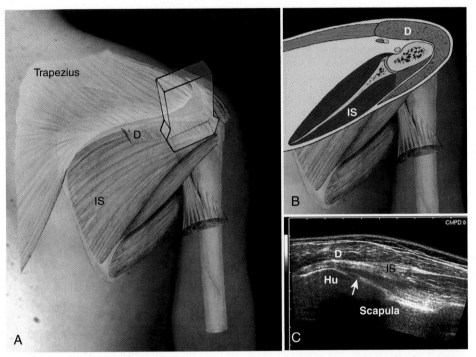

FIGURE 22-9. Long-axis view of the infraspinatus. A, With the arm at the patient's side, the operator can scan the infraspinatus *(IS)* from its origin on the scapula to its insertion on the posterior greater tuberosity; *D,* deltoid. The transducer is placed over the posterior joint (on the left of the transducer) and oriented toward the tuberosity insertion. **B,** Oblique anatomic section along the infraspinatus *(IS)* long axis; *D,* deltoid. **C,** Panoramic view along the plane shown in **B.** The infraspinatus *(IS)* thins out toward its humeral insertion *(Hu)* and appears sandwiched between the deltoid *(D)* and the humerus. Arrow indicates the location of the joint.

ogy that can mimic or cause impingement-like symptoms. The superior glenoid labrum can be shown with the transducer aligned posterior to the acromioclavicular joint and oriented perpendicular to the superior glenoid. A curved, linear array transducer will be necessary if diagnosis of **superior labral detachment** (SLAP lesions) is sought.

THE NORMAL CUFF

The Adolescent Cuff

The rotator cuff tendons and the intracapsular biceps are hyperechoic relative to the deltoid muscle bellies (Fig. 22-12). The cuff tendons are enveloped in a thin synovial layer that is normally thinner than 1.5 mm and appears hypoechoic relative to the tendons. The thickness of this bursal layer does not change. The **subacromial-subdeltoid bursa** is as thick over the long biceps tendon as it is over the subscapularis, supraspinatus, and infraspinatus tendons. A correctly performed examination will show a neatly defined bursa that shows as a hypoechoic stripe thinner than the thickness of the hypoechoic hyaline cartilage over the humeral head. This extra-articular bursa is a virtual space, because it contains lubricant synovial fluid; this fluid cannot be distinguished on a routine shoulder ultrasound study. The

bursa is hoof shaped in cross section, and it often extends from the coracoid anteriorly around the lateral shoulder and posteriorly past the glenoid. If the subdeltoid bursa extends that far anteriorly, it is in direct continuity with the **coracobrachial bursa.** The pleural space and the bursal synovial space have a number of similarities, including the virtual space (which can become distended in effusions), the thin lubricating layer of fluid in their lumen, and the extensive network of capillary vessels and lymph vessels in their walls. Those vessels are not visible with color flow Doppler sonogram in patients with normal rotator cuff anatomy, but distended vessels have been shown in the power and color flow Doppler sonograms of patients with inflamed cuffs.[42] The boundary between the bursa and the deltoid muscle consists of the so-called peribursal fat. This layer appears hyperechoic, and its thickness is remarkably uniform; body habitus seems to have little influence on the thickness of this fat layer.

Rotator cuff pathology is rare in young patients, although bursal and labral pathology can occur. Some of these conditions can mimic tendon tears. It is important to know that the adolescent cuff consists of more muscle than the aging cuff. The relative length of tendon to muscle increases with age.[43] Hypoechoic areas in the cuff in patients under age 20 may simply represent muscle, and the finding should not easily be attributed to a tear. Meticulous right-left comparison of the thickness of the

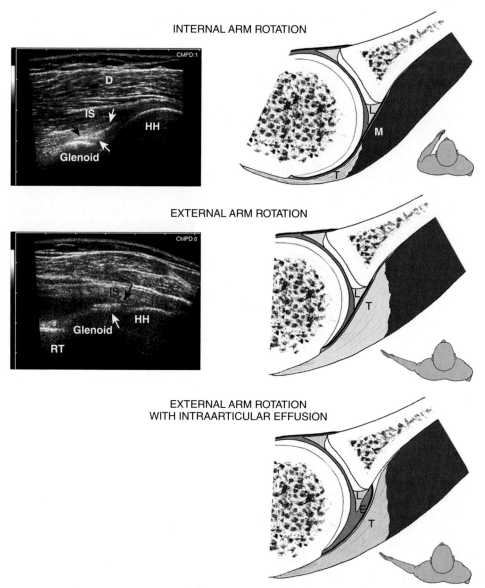

FIGURE 22-10. Relationship of infraspinatus tendon and muscle relative to glenoid labrum. With the arm in medial (internal) and lateral (external) rotation. *Top diagram,* Fibrous glenoid labrum *(L)* appears as a hyperechoic triangle deep to the infraspinatus muscle *(M).* Look at the corresponding ultrasound image on the left. With the arm in internal rotation, the contrast between the hypoechoic muscle *(IS)* and the labrum *(arrows)* is accentuated. *Middle diagram,* When the arm is in external rotation, the hyperechoic tendon *(T)* is in direct proximity to the hyperechoic labrum. Look at the ultrasound inset on the left. The separating interface, which is barely perceptible *(black arrow),* represents the actual location of the synovium. *Bottom diagram,* External rotation is the preferred position to detect effusion. If there is effusion *(E),* hypoechoic fluid distends the synovium between the posterior labrum and the deep surface of the infraspinatus. *HH,* Humeral head.

subscapular tendons in adolescents may demonstrate tears of the anterior rotator cuff resulting from athletic injuries. In our experience, the subscapular insertion appears the weaker link of the rotator cuff in the growing shoulder. Ultrasound has proved its usefulness in detecting subscapularis tendon tears.[44]

Age-Related Changes

The rotator cuff in individuals under age 30 years is watertight. Arthrographic studies show that no commu-

nication should exist between the glenohumeral joint and the subacromial-subdeltoid bursa.[25] Postmortem and cadaver studies have shown a high prevalence of rotator cuff tears in aging shoulders. Keyes[45] examined 73 unselected cadavers and found full-thickness tears of the supraspinatus in 13.4% of shoulders. Full-thickness tears were not recorded for those younger than age 50 years; the prevalence over age 50 was 31%. Wilson and Duff[46] examined an unselected series of 74 bodies at postmortem and 34 dissecting-room cadavers over age 30 years. They found full-thickness tears of the supra-

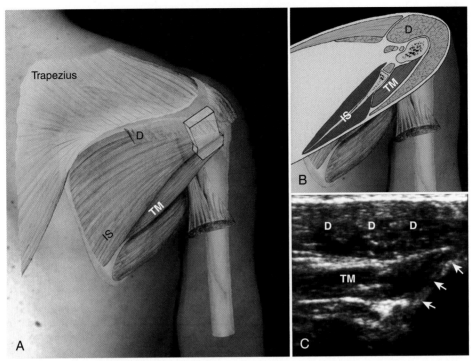

FIGURE 22-11. Long-axis view of the teres minor. A, The probe placed parallel to the spine of the scapula and just proximal to the prominence caused by the muscle belly of the teres major (look at the surface landmarks in Fig. 22-1) can show the short tendinous insertion of the teres minor *(TM); IS,* infraspinatus; *D,* deltoid, severed proximally. **B,** Obliquely along the teres minor insertion, diagram shows the "muscular" (fleshy) insertion of the teres minor tendon; *TM,* teres minor; *IS,* infraspinatus. **C,** Teres minor *(TM)* is seen as a trapezoidal structure deep to the inferior deltoid *(D);* humerus *(arrows).* The insertion appears hypoechoic, as opposed to other rotator cuff tendon insertions that have more fibrinous and therefore more hyperechoic insertions.

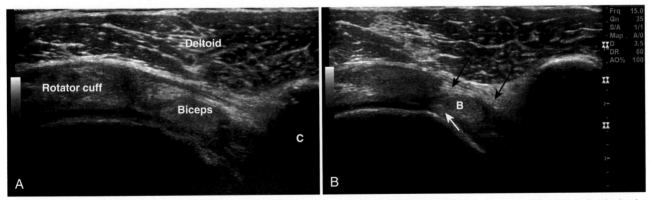

FIGURE 22-12. Short-axis view of supraspinatus and rotator cuff interval. A, In young and healthy individuals, the rotator cuff contrasts significantly in echogenicity with the deltoid. The cuff tendons appear hyperechoic relative to the deltoid. *C,* Coracoid process. **B,** In the rotator cuff interval, a hyperechoic "sling" surrounds the biceps. Fibers of the superior glenohumeral ligament *(white arrow)* are seen deep to the intracapsular biceps *(B),* and fibers of the coracohumeral ligament *(black arrows)* course superficially.

spinatus tendon in 11% and partial-thickness tears in 10% of the shoulders. Fukuda et al.[47] reported a 7% prevalence of complete tears and a 13% prevalence of incomplete tears in a study of cadavers that included no details on age. With such high percentages of rotator cuff tears in cadaver studies, how many of these tears would have been asymptomatic? A study we conducted showed that ultrasound can detect asymptomatic tears.

Ninety volunteer subjects (47 women and 43 men) in a population who had never sought medical attention for shoulder disease underwent shoulder sonography; 77% (69 of 90) were white, 13% (12 of 90) were black, 9% (8 of 90) were Asian, and 1% (1 of 90) was Hispanic. Eighteen subjects were between ages 30 and 39 years; 18 were 40 to 49 years old; 18 were 50 to 59; 13 were 60 to 69; 13 were 70 to 79; and 10 were 80 to 99 years old. The proportion of women to men was almost equal for each decade.

No statistically significant differences were found in the prevalence of rotator cuff lesions in each gender for

ROTATOR-CUFF CHANGES IN ASYMPTOMATIC ADULTS
DOMINANT VERSUS NON-DOMINANT

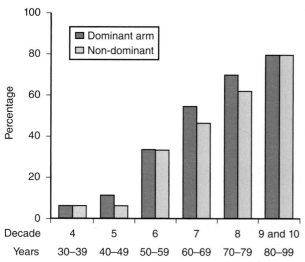

FIGURE 22-13. Asymptomatic rotator cuff tears. Percentage of shoulders with rotator cuff tears in asymptomatic adults in different age groups. Chart shows comparison between dominant and nondominant arms.

ROTATOR-CUFF CHANGES IN ASYMPTOMATIC ADULTS
IMPINGEMENT GRADES

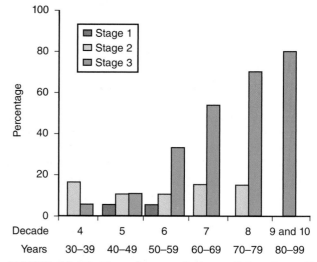

FIGURE 22-14. Prevalence of stage 1 to stage 3 impingement for dominant arm in different age groups. Abnormalities in the subacromial space were staged sonographically as follows: **stage 1** if bursal thickness 1.5 to 2 mm; **stage 2** if bursal thickness over 2 mm; **stage 3** if partial-thickness or full-thickness rotator cuff tear.

either the dominant or the nondominant arm (Fig. 22-13). We found no statistically significant differences in the incidence of rotator lesions related to gender or reported level of exertional activities. However, the prevalence of rotator cuff tears in dominant and nondominant arms showed a linear increase after the fifth decade of life. This difference was statistically significant among patients in the third, fourth, and fifth decades and older.[13] The cumulative percentage of partial-thickness and full-thickness tears was approximately 33% between ages 50 and 59 years, 55% between 60 and 69 years, 70% between 70 and 79 years, and as high as 78% above age 80 (Fig. 22-14). A total of 25 full-thickness and 15 partial-thickness tears were found. Sixteen individuals or 64% of the people with tears had bilateral rotator cuff tears. The youngest subject with a partial-thickness tear was 35 years old. The youngest subject with a full-thickness tear was 54 years old. The age range for partial-thickness tears was 35 to 80. The age range of full-thickness tears was 54 to 92. The average age in the partial-thickness group was 56 years. The average age in the full-thickness group was 63 years.

In 19 cases (46%) the rotator cuff tears had associated intrasynovial fluid. In 15 of these patients the fluid was located in the biceps tendon sheath, and in the remaining four cases it was located in the subacromial-subdeltoid bursa. There were two individuals with tears and fluid in the biceps tendon sheath and in the bursa simultaneously. The infraspinatus recess appeared normal in all our patients. Eleven effusions were noted in the long biceps tendon sheath in subjects who did not have tears of the cuff. There was never excess fluid in the subacromial-subdeltoid bursa in the absence of rotator cuff tear.

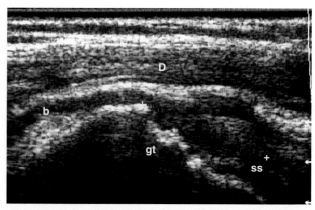

FIGURE 22-15. Bone change in asymptomatic full-thickness rotator cuff tear. Longitudinal scan through the supraspinatus tendon *(ss)* shows retraction of tissue (calipers). The bone surface of the uncovered greater tuberosity *(gt)* is irregular. The subdeltoid bursa *(b)* is filled with fluid. *D,* Deltoid muscle.

Shallow erosion or irregularity of the bone surface under the tear was noted in 90% of tears; bone changes were present in all but four partial-thickness tears. Greater tuberosity irregularity was noted in 37 shoulders or in 21% of shoulders in this study. Twelve shoulders showed irregular greater tuberosities and no rotator cuff tear. A statistically significant correlation between asymptomatic rotator cuff tears and irregularity of the greater tuberosity was found (Fig. 22-15).

Twenty of the full-thickness tears were considered large and involved more than one tendon. Three tears were massive and greater than 4 cm in diameter, and three tears were small and less than 2 cm in width when measured over the base of the greater tuberosity. Ten partial-thickness tears were mixed echogenicity, and five were hypoechoic. Nine mixed-echogenicity lesions and two hypoechoic tears exhibited bone change in the greater tuberosity.

Our results indicate that the finding of a rotator cuff abnormality or an effusion in the biceps tendon sheath can be compatible with normal and pain-free mobility of the shoulder. Rotator cuff findings should be interpreted with care in patients over age 50. A rotator cuff tear is not necessarily the cause of the pain in an aging shoulder and can be an incidental finding. **Degenerative rotator cuff changes** may be regarded as a natural correlate of aging, with a statistically significant linear increase after the fifth decade of life. On the one hand, clinical judgment must be used to distinguish asymptomatic from symptomatic rotator cuff tears. On the other hand, finding a rotator cuff tear should not stop the clinician from searching for other causes of shoulder pain. Our shoulder ultrasound reading is done in conjunction with the reading of the initial shoulder radiographic evaluation. We have found missed primary or secondary neoplasms of bone, myeloma, and Pancoast tumors using this careful approach. Limited and painful shoulder elevation can result from a number of diseases, of which rotator cuff disease is the most common. Simultaneous occurrence of a full-thickness tear with a tumor in or around the shoulder is not rare in our experience.

Yamaguchi et al.[48] studied the contralateral asymptomatic arm of patients with symptomatic tears in one arm. In a follow-up averaging 2.8 years, 51% of asymptomatic shoulders became symptomatic. In 23 patients the tears were reevaluated with ultrasound. None of the tears had healed, and none had become smaller. In 9 of the 23 patients the tears had increased in size. In patients with tears that were first asymptomatic and then symptomatic, the ability of performing daily activities decreased significantly.

In a study of middle-aged tennis players, Brasseur et al.[49] showed that tears of the rotator cuff were more than twice as common in the dominant arm. The tears discovered by ultrasound had been symptomatic at one time or other in 90% of the players. However, there was no relationship between the presence of a tear or calcification at the time of the study and the presence or absence of pain.[4]

PREOPERATIVE APPEARANCES

Criteria of Rotator Cuff Tears

Rotator cuff ultrasound has become more popular partly because the imaging of the rotator cuff has been per-

fected with a high degree of sophistication. In addition, patients and clinicians have contributed to the recent surge in interest in shoulder ultrasound. Patients who have undergone both ultrasound and MRI of the shoulder prefer ultrasound over MRI.[50,51] Clinicians who have thorough knowledge of shoulder anatomy and pathology now have access to compact ultrasound technology. These physicians see the advantages with in-office ultrasound; the technique is low cost and provides the opportunity for patient education during the visit.[20,22]

With respect to the **reproducibility** of the study of the rotator cuff, several radiologists have tested agreement between experienced radiologist readers and have found good to excellent interobserver agreement for full-thickness rotator cuff tear evaluation (kappa values between 0.6 and 0.81). In cases of partial-thickness tears and for intratendinous changes, the interobserver variability was higher.[52-54] O'Connor et al.[54] noted poor agreement between an experienced operator and a less experienced operator with only 6 months of training in shoulder ultrasound. This study concluded that rigorous training with measurement of competency will be required if the medical community wants to keep this technique at its current degree of diagnostic credibility.

Previously published sonographic criteria for rotator cuff pathology can be categorized into four groups: nonvisualization of the cuff, localized absence or focal nonvisualization, discontinuity, and focal abnormal echogenicity.[55]

Nonvisualization of the Cuff

Direct contact of the humeral head with the acromion is an indication of massive cuff tear. In this situation the ultrasound image shows deltoid muscle directly on top of the humeral head (Fig. 22-16). In some cases, thickened bursa and fat will be noted between the deltoid muscle and the surface of the humeral head. This tissue layer is more hypoechoic and patchy in texture. The thickness of this layer will depend on the location of the tear, but generally it will be thinner and more irregular than the normal cuff layer. Some bursae have been noted to be up to 5 mm thick. This synovial layer has been mistaken for normal cuff by the inexperienced sonographer. With massive tears, exceeding 4 cm, the humeral head may ascend through the defect because of pulling of the deltoid muscle. The supraspinatus tendon is retracted under the acromion, and as a rule, surgical reattachment will be challenging at this stage (Fig. 22-17). The extent of tear should be reported because multiple tendons are often involved. The diagnosis of these tears can be predicted on shoulder radiographs. Some centers use radiographs with comparison views during active shoulder abduction or anteroposterior supine views of the subacromial space to counteract the gravitational pull on the humerus.[56] The subacromial space should not be smaller than 5 mm.

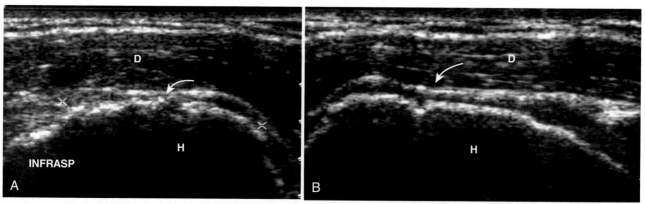

FIGURE 22-16. Nonvisualization of cuff. A, Transverse view shows the deltoid muscle *(D)* in direct contact with the humeral head *(H)*. Hyperechoic layer *(curved arrow)* of fat lies deep to the deltoid; this layer is interposed between deltoid and humerus. **B,** Longitudinal view through the expected location of the supraspinatus tendon; supraspinatus is absent. Hyperechoic layer of fat *(curved arrow)* is noted deep to the deltoid *(D)*. *H,* Humeral head.

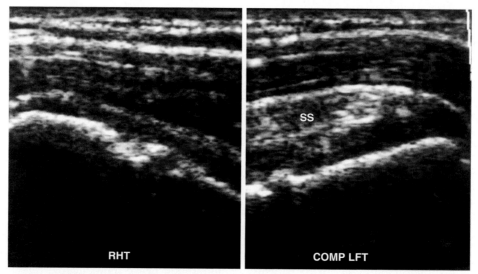

FIGURE 22-17. Irreparable rotator cuff tear. Longitudinal right-left comparison shows a significant discrepancy in the thickness of the soft tissues. The supraspinatus tendon *(SS)* appears normal in the asymptomatic left shoulder *(LFT)*. The supraspinatus tendon in the right *(RHT)* shoulder is retracted out of sight. The deltoid and the subdeltoid fascial layer cover the humeral head directly. Arthroscopy showed the torn edge of the supraspinatus tendon withdrawn beyond the glenoid cavity. The rotator cuff defect was deemed irreparable.

Focal Nonvisualization of the Cuff

Smaller tears will appear as localized absence of supraspinatus tendon or, in rare cases, local absence of subscapularis or infraspinatus tendon. The most common tear pattern is caused by disease at the tendon-bone junction. The tendon will retract from the bone surface, leaving a bare area of bone (Fig. 22-18). This finding has been reported in the past as the "naked tuberosity" sign.[57] The bone surface of the greater tuberosity and anatomic neck of the humerus are irregular in approximately 79% of this type of tears; anatomic study confirmed these bone changes.[58] This pathologic process affects not only the surface of the bone, but also the internal structure of the greater tuberosity. The exterior changes consist of pitting of the cortex, erosion of bone,

sclerosis, fragmentation of the tuberosity, and crystal deposition beyond the tidemark.[58] The changes of the architecture of the tuberosity manifest as fewer trabeculae and fewer connections between trabeculae. The vast majority of such tears will occur anteriorly in the supraspinatus tendon and in the critical zone. Characteristically, a small amount of tissue will be preserved surrounding the biceps tendon. Ideally, such tears can be confirmed in two perpendicular scan planes. Sometimes this will not be possible because the tear may show full thickness in one plane but may not be identified as such in the orthogonal plane. This phenomenon has been attributed to partial-volume averaging in tears that are smaller than the footprint of the transducers. Small **horizontal tears** typically appear on longitudinal images but can be missed on transverse images.[57] A helpful finding is the "infolding" of bursal and peribursal fat tissue into the focal defect. With few exceptions, this infolding is a sign of a full-thickness tear. If the tear is larger, bursal and peribursal tissue will approximate the bone surface (Fig. 22-18). Large bursal surface tears can occasionally show this pattern of infolding.[50]

Focal nonvisualization should not be confused with segmental thinning of cuff after rotator cuff surgery. This thinning is normal after most tendon-bone reimplantations. In these patients a bony trough is detected as a rounded or V-shaped defect in the humeral contour. The tendon is brought down into this narrow slit. The

tendon is not repaired onto the tuberosity anatomically with a broad insertion but with a tapered end. It is well known that a number of these reconstructions fail to be watertight even after successful surgery. The rents in the capsule cause additional focal thinning. In a patient with a negative baseline study, re-tears can be identified by visualizing anechoic fluid leaking through a tear.

Discontinuity in the Cuff

The term **discontinuity** has been used for tears located more proximally in the tendon. These tears tend to be of the **vertical type** and are more often traumatic.[57,59] The patient may have a history of prior shoulder dislocation. Discontinuity is observed when the small defects fill with joint fluid or hypoechoic reactive tissue[60] (Fig. 22-19). Such defects are often accentuated by placing the arm in extension and internal rotation (Fig. 22-20). Often, a small amount of bursal fluid is also present. The sonographer can use this fluid as a natural contrast medium to show the tear in more detail. Manual compression of the subdeltoid bursa can move the fluid through the tear into the joint. This maneuver will show the tear more clearly. A focally bright interface around a segment of hyaline cartilage and deep to hypoechoic tendon is considered a sign of a full-thickness tear (see Fig. 22-19). This sign has been named the **cartilage-interface sign** in an earlier report.[57]

Focal Abnormal Echogenicity

Cuff echogenicity may be diffusely or focally abnormal. Diffuse abnormalities of cuff echogenicity have proved to be unreliable sonographic signs for cuff tear, especially

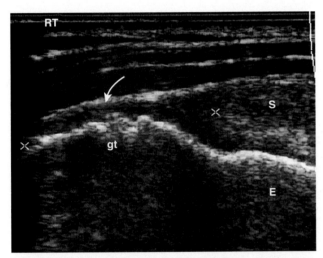

FIGURE 22-18. Horizontal full-thickness tear. Longitudinal image through the supraspinatus tendon *(S)* shows 2-cm retraction of the torn tendon (distance between calipers). Bursa and peribursal fat *(curved arrow)* rest directly on the irregular bone surface of the greater tuberosity *(gt)*. *E,* Humeral epiphysis.

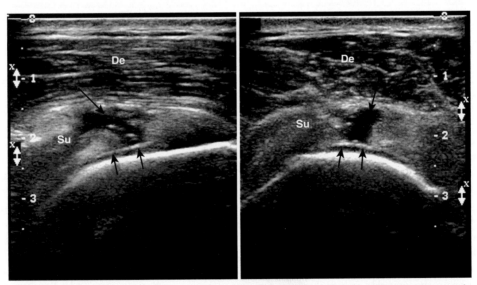

FIGURE 22-19. Vertical full-thickness tear. *Left,* Longitudinal, and *right,* transverse, split-screen images through the supraspinatus tendon *(Su)* show an anechoic area of discontinuity *(large arrows)* within the rotator cuff layer. The cartilage of the humeral head is surrounded by a bright interface *(small arrows). De,* Deltoid muscle.

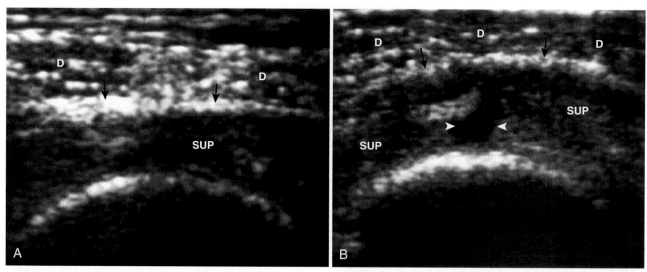

FIGURE 22-20. Discontinuity of the cuff. A, Transverse scans of the supraspinatus tendon *(SUP)* in neutral position. **B,** Transverse scans of the supraspinatus tendon with the arm in extension and internal rotation show a small tear filled with fluid *(arrowheads).* Note the tear is more distinctly visible with the arm in extension. *D,* Deltoid muscle; *arrows,* subdeltoid bursa.

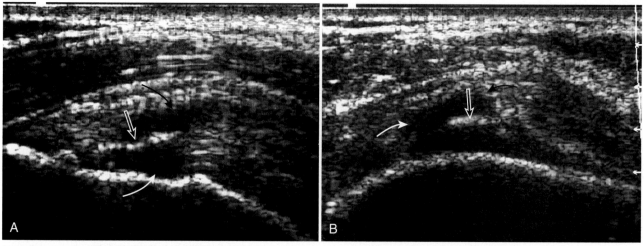

FIGURE 22-21. Focal abnormal echogenicity. A, Longitudinal supraspinatus tendon view of an articular side partial-thickness tear, the so-called rim rent. A linear hyperechoic lesion in the supraspinatus tendon *(open arrow)* is surrounded by hypoechoic edema *(curved arrows).* **B,** Transverse supraspinatus tendon view of same partial-thickness defect. The same hyperechoic lesion is noted.

when there is no associated bone surface change.[61] Focal abnormal echogenicity has been associated with small full-thickness and partial-thickness tears. An area of increased echogenicity might represent a new interface within the tendon at the site of fiber failure, as observed in some partial-thickness tears.[8] The small, linear or comma-shaped hyperechoic lesion is often surrounded by edema or fluid and appears as a hypoechoic halo (Fig. 22-21). The partial-thickness tears are similar to the **rim rents** first observed pathologically by Codman.[10] A slightly different type of partial-thickness tear can appear as an anechoic spot on the articular or bursal side of the tendon.[8] Careful inspection of the synovial surfaces of the tendon is necessary. Only those focal hypoechoic

defects that violate the surface may be considered tears by the arthroscopist (Fig. 22-22). **Intrasubstance lesions** are the most common type of partial lesions and account for almost 50% of the defects. We do not call them "tears" because they are not considered tears by the surgeons who cannot observe them by direct tendon inspection. This poses a diagnostic problem similar to that of intrasubstance lesions of the menisci seen on MRI studies. Associated bone or synovial findings may be helpful if the ultrasound findings are equivocal.[61] Tissue harmonics makes the intratendinous cleavage or delamination stand out more visibly. Because of this new technology, diagnostic accuracy for partial-thickness tear has recently improved.[62]

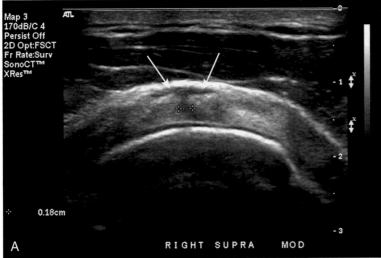

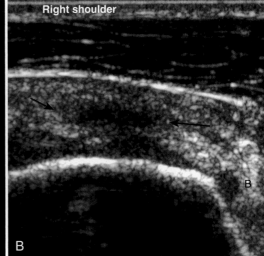

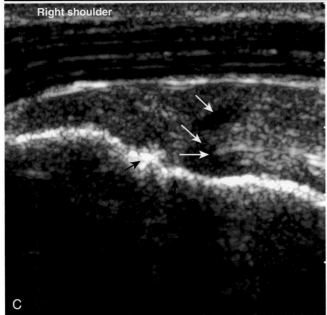

FIGURE 22-22. Focal abnormal echogenicity. A, Transverse supraspinatus tendon view of a bursal-side partial-thickness tear. The hypoechoic change violates the bursal surface *(arrows).* **B,** Transverse supraspinatus tendon view of hypoechoic change within the substance of the tendon. **C,** Longitudinal view through the same abnormality as in **B.** The hypoechoic disruption appears intrasubstance *(arrows);* intact tendon fibers *(large arrow),* which are seen curving toward the bone, still cover the articular surface of the tendon. The greater tuberosity surface is irregular *(small black arrows).* Such lesions cannot be seen on arthroscopy.

Associated Findings

Subdeltoid Bursal Effusion

Visualization of subdeltoid bursal effusion is the most reliable associated finding of rotator cuff tear (Fig. 22-23). It is found in both full-thickness and partial-thickness tears. Anechoic fluid differs from hypoechoic edema of the bursal synovium. Edema is a common finding in shoulder impingement but is only rarely associated with a tear. Edema and fluid can be distinguished from each other using the transducer compression test. A synovial recess filled with fluid will be emptied by compression; a recess with synovial edema changes little in shape. Other causes for fluid in the bursa include calcium milk with synovitis and septic bursitis. Hollister et al.[63] found that the sonographic appearance of bursal fluid had a specificity of 96% for the diagnosis of rotator cuff tears. Similar results were found by Farin et al.[64] In our prospective study of rotator cuff disease, all patients with fluid in the bursa had a rotator cuff tear.[13]

Joint Effusion

Joint fluid can be found in the joint recesses, including the infraspinatus, subcoracoid, and axillary recesses. In a patient who sits in the upright position, most fluid will accumulate in the dependent portion of the biceps tendon sheath. Approximately half of these effusions are associated with rotator cuff tears.[6] The other half result from a variety of articular causes of shoulder disease. When a large fluid collection is found in the infraspinatus recess without fluid in the subdeltoid bursa, inflammatory or infectious causes of joint disease should always be excluded.[41]

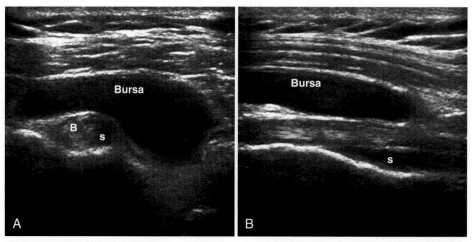

FIGURE 22-23. Subdeltoid bursal effusion. A, Transverse view over the anterior shoulder demonstrates fluid in two different synovial compartments. Synovial effusion *(s)* surrounds the long biceps tendon *(B)*. This fluid does not extend beyond the biceps groove. The larger collection of fluid noted deep to the deltoid fills the subdeltoid bursa and extends both medial and lateral to the confines of the groove. **B,** Longitudinal scan of the long biceps tendon shows joint effusion *(s)* extending deep to the tendon. The subdeltoid bursa extends as a large sac over the anterior aspect of the shoulder. Fluid in joint and bursa signifies rotator cuff tear in most patients.

Concave Subdeltoid Fat Contour

In the normal shoulder, the bright linear echoes from the subdeltoid bursal fat are convex. Concavity of the subdeltoid contour may be noted in medium and large tears, reflecting the absence of cuff tendon. It may be possible to approximate the deltoid and the humeral surface even in smaller tears using transducer compression at the site of the tear.

Bone Surface Irregularity

Only recently has bone irregularity been cited in imaging literature as an important and common associated finding in rotator cuff tears.[8,10,58,65] The majority of partial-thickness and full-thickness tears of the distal 1 cm of the rotator cuff are associated with small bone spurs and pits in the bone surface of the greater tuberosity. Use of higher-frequency transducers for rotator cuff imaging may have made these findings more evident. The tuberosity abnormality matches the tendon abnormality in location, size, and shape. The cause of the abnormality is unknown. Trauma from an impaction of the tuberosity on the acromion during shoulder elevation has been considered.

Tear Size and Muscle Atrophy

Several studies have attempted to quantify rotator cuff tears. Ultrasound is capable of measuring tears as accurately as MRI if the tears are relatively small. However, both MRI and ultrasound tend to underestimate the size of tears compared with measurement at surgery. If the diameter of the tear exceeds 3 cm, ultrasound assessment is more limited.[66,67] New emphasis has been placed on quantifying the muscle loss that accompanies chronic tears of the rotator cuff. Sofka et al.[68] demonstrated that fatty atrophy shows as increased echogenicity in muscles with torn tendons. The teres minor tendon was mentioned as the only muscle that occasionally atrophies without being torn. Newer methods of estimating atrophy have used criteria that assess the surface of the tendon and visibility of the pennate structure and central aponeurosis.[69,70] The most reproducible measurement thus far has been the "occupation ratio," which can be assessed on sagittal images at the level of the suprascapular notch medial to the acromial process.[70]

Pathology of Rotator Cuff Interval

The subscapularis, superior glenohumeral, and coracohumeral ligaments can be distinguished from the conjoint tendons of the rotator cuff. High-frequency transducer technology currently available allows the diagnosis of hyperemia and fibrosis, seen as a mass within the interval of patients with adhesive capsulitis.[71] In diabetic patients in particular, the differential diagnosis occasionally must be made between rotator cuff tears and adhesive capsulitis. Tears of the rotator cuff interval and abnormalities of the subscapularis have also been diagnosed with more confidence recently. Detection of these tears is important because these defects require an open approach different from the arthroscopic surgical approach of the more common tears of the supraspinatus and infraspinatus tendons.[72,73]

POSTOPERATIVE APPEARANCES

The literature suggests that sonography can play an important role in the postoperative follow-up after rotator cuff repair.[74,75] Because surgery may distort sonographic landmarks, sonography in the postoperative patient is more difficult than in the preoperative patient. It is therefore important to understand the surgical procedures used in acromioplasty and cuff repair.

In **acromioplasty** the anterior inferior aspect of the acromion is surgically removed. Sonographically, this appears as disruption of the normal, rounded, smooth acromial contour. After surgery, the acromion appears pointed (Fig. 22-24). Because the inferior aspect of the acromion is removed, a greater extent of the supraspinatus tendon may be visualized.

Repair of a cuff tear creates unique sonographic landmarks. The cuff tendons are reimplanted into a trough made perpendicular to the axis of the supraspinatus tendon. The reimplantation trough is placed in the humerus at a site that provides optimal tendon tension. The trough appears sonographically as a defect in the humeral contour, which is best viewed with the transducer longitudinal to the supraspinatus tendon (Fig. 22-25, *A*), with the shoulder in extension. Suture material may be seen deep in the trough as specular echoes. Scanning the arm in extension and internal rotation may be necessary to visualize this site of tendon reimplantation, especially when it is medially placed (Fig. 22-25, *B*). Failure to scan in this position may lead to a false-positive diagnosis. Such a maneuver, however, should be used with care, especially in the immediate postoperative period, to avoid reinjury of the friable, newly reimplanted tendons.

Recent improvements in arthroscopic repair have culminated in a more anatomic tendon reconstruction. The two-row repair shows as two reflective surfaces at the placement of the anchors, best seen on longitudinal images. One anchor is typically placed close to the articular margin (medial anchor) and one more laterally in the tuberosity.[76] The number of anchors is proportionate to the size of the original defect in the cuff.

Sonographic appearances of the cuff tendons never return to normal in the postoperative patient. Tendons, especially the supraspinatus, are often echogenic and thinned when compared with the contralateral shoulder. Joint effusions are common and best visualized along the biceps tendon. Because resection of the subdeltoid bursa removes an important landmark, dynamic scanning is especially important in distinguishing a thin, hyperechoic cuff from adjacent deltoid muscle.

In patients with shoulder arthroplasty, ultrasound can be used to demonstrate tears that develop postoperatively.[77] These tears can explain postoperative shoulder pain in some patients. The subscapularis tears in particular are important lesions to detect because they can lead to further deterioration of the shoulder function through anterior instability.[78]

Recurrent Tear

Sonographically, recurrent tears most often appear as absence of the cuff. Fluid filling a defect in a rotator cuff repair and loose sutures or screws are other indications of recurrent tear (Fig. 22-26). Unless baseline scans are available in the postoperative period, it may be difficult to differentiate small, recurrent tears from the appearances created when only a small amount of cuff tendon remains to be reattached. Thinning of the tendon is useless as a criterion, and bone irregularity is the rule in the postoperative patient. Recurrent tears are common, occurring in up to 40% of patients with repair of a small defect and 80% of patients with large tears preoperatively.

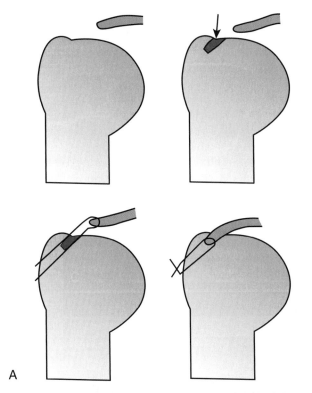

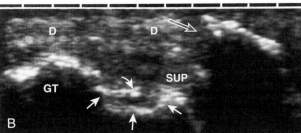

FIGURE 22-24. Rotator cuff repair. A, Drawing demonstrates the surgical technique for cuff reimplantation, with creation of trough *(arrow)* in the humeral head, reimplantation of the residual tendon within that trough, and characteristic method of suture placement. **B,** Longitudinal supraspinatus tendon *(SUP)* image shows characteristic appearances of reimplantation trough *(arrows)*. Acromioplasty defect *(open arrow)* is also visualized. *D,* Deltoid muscle; *GT,* greater tuberosity; *curved arrow,* reimplantation suture. *(From Mack LA, Nyberg DA, Matsen FA 3rd, et al. Sonography of the postoperative shoulder. AJR Am J Roentgenol 1988;150:1089-1093.)*

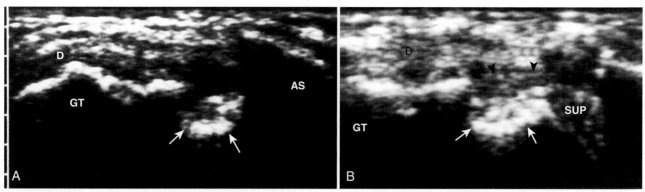

FIGURE 22-25. Postoperative rotator cuff: importance of examination during extension. A, Longitudinal supraspinatus tendon view in neutral position of a patient after repair of full-thickness rotator cuff tear demonstrates the reimplantation trough, but fails to reveal evidence of the supraspinatus tendon, thus suggesting recurrent injury. **B,** Scan with the arm in extension and internal rotation demonstrates that the repair is intact. The residual supraspinatus tendon *(SUP)* is thinned. Note absence of characteristic echoes of the subdeltoid bursa *(arrowheads). AS,* Acromial shadow; *D,* deltoid muscle; *GT,* greater tuberosity; *arrows,* reimplantation trough. *(From Mack LA, Nyberg DA, Matsen FA. Sonographic evaluation of rotator cuff. Radiol Clin North Am 1988;25:161-177.)*

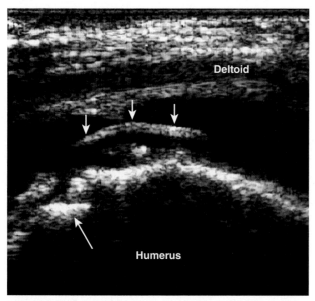

FIGURE 22-26. Recurrent tear: postoperative ultrasound examination. Longitudinal scan along the deltoid muscle in the region of the reimplantation trough *(arrow).* A loose suture *(small arrows)* is noted within the subdeltoid bursal effusion. The supraspinatus has left this subdeltoid space. The proximal humerus has an abnormal, round appearance. The anatomic neck has disappeared through the process of bone remodeling.

PITFALLS IN INTERPRETATION

Inadequate transducer positioning is the most common error in scanning the rotator cuff. False-positive and false-negative results may be produced in this manner. For example, scanning the supraspinatus tendon transversely with the transducer placed laterally may artifactually mimic a rotator cuff tear. An oblique transverse scan of the supraspinatus tendon can be falsely reported as

thinning of the cuff. The examiner must therefore view the cuff in two orthogonal planes. Visualization of neatly depicted bony contour will help in avoiding these pitfalls.

A cause of tendon heterogeneity is the geometric relationship of the tendon to the transducer. As demonstrated by Crass et al.[79] and Fornage,[80] failure to orient the transducer parallel to the fibers of the tendon may result in artifactual areas of decreased echogenicity (Fig. 22-27). When only a small area of the tendon is parallel to the transducer, a focal area of increased echogenicity may be produced, mimicking a small, partial-thickness or full-thickness tear. This artifact is especially pronounced with sector transducers.

ROTATOR CUFF CALCIFICATIONS

Calcifications can affect any of the four tendons of the rotator cuff. Subscapular tendon calcifications can be particularly difficult to diagnose without the aid of ultrasound. The calcium can burst out from the tendon into the subacromial-subdeltoid bursa and cause an acute and very painful inflammatory synovitis.[81] Standard texts on calcific tendinitis have distinguished a chronic phase of formation and an acute phase of resorption.[82] Ultrasound appears incapable of staging calcium according to these phases. However, increases in color Doppler signal have been noted in more painful calcifications.[83] Ultrasound has also shown great potential in demonstrating the physical form of the crystal deposition.[84] Aggregates of calcium can be solid, pastelike, or liquid (Fig. 22-28). The liquid deposits appear hyperechoic without shadow; the calcium paste casts a vague shadow; and hard deposits show with distinct acoustic shadow. This unique capability of ultrasound aids in the treatment when ultrasound is used to localize and aspirate calcium.[85,86]

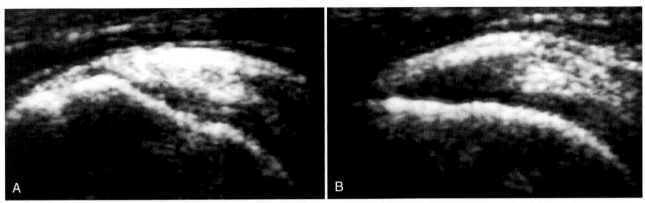

FIGURE 22-27. Artifactual areas of decreased tendon echogenicity. A and **B,** Two views of the same supraspinatus tendon demonstrate considerable changes in echogenicity that may be artifactually created by transducer position and orientation.

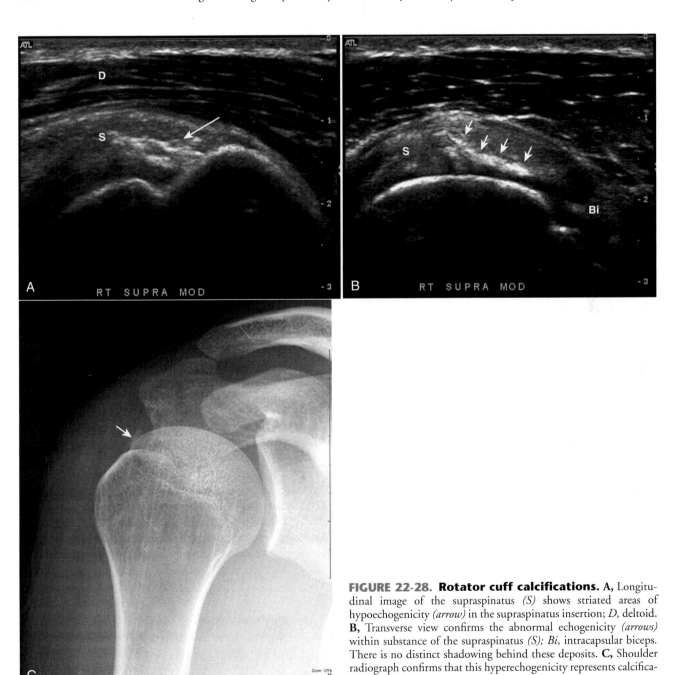

FIGURE 22-28. Rotator cuff calcifications. A, Longitudinal image of the supraspinatus *(S)* shows striated areas of hypoechogenicity *(arrow)* in the supraspinatus insertion; *D,* deltoid. **B,** Transverse view confirms the abnormal echogenicity *(arrows)* within substance of the supraspinatus *(S); Bi,* intracapsular biceps. There is no distinct shadowing behind these deposits. **C,** Shoulder radiograph confirms that this hyperechogenicity represents calcification *(arrow).*

Before the procedure, the clinician will decide on the size and number of needles necessary for treatment. Expectations for complete recovery are lower if the pain is caused by rock-type calcifications. A small amount of corticosteroid is then often added after multiple passes have been made through the calcium, using 16- to 18-gauge needles. In a retrospective study of 44 patients at a minimum of 8 months' follow-up, 75% of patients noted statistically significant improvement after the lavage of calcium under ultrasound guidance.[87] The authors noted the need for randomized clinical trials on this subject, in part because the natural history of calcific tendinitis can result in spontaneous healing. When all other treatment of calcifications fails, calcium deposits can be marked under ultrasound guidance to add precision to the surgical evacuation of the lesions.[88]

References

1. Matsen FA, Arntz CT. Subacromial impingement. In Matsen FA, editor. The shoulder. Philadelphia: Saunders; 1990.
2. Neviaser RJ, Neviaser TJ. Observations on impingement. Clin Orthop Relat Res 1990:60-63.
3. Resnick D. Shoulder arthrography. Radiol Clin North Am 1981;19: 243-253.
4. Mack LA, Matsen 3rd FA, et al. Ultrasound evaluation of the rotator cuff. Radiology 1985;157:205-209.
5. Mack LA, Gannon MK, Kilcoyne RF, Matsen 3rd RA. Sonographic evaluation of the rotator cuff: accuracy in patients without prior surgery. Clin Orthop Relat Res 1988:21-27.
6. Middleton WD, Reinus WR, Totty WG, et al. Ultrasonographic evaluation of the rotator cuff and biceps tendon. J Bone Joint Surg Am 1986;68:440-450.
7. Crass JR, Craig EV, Feinberg SB. Ultrasonography of rotator cuff tears: a review of 500 diagnostic studies. J Clin Ultrasound 1988; 16:313-337.
8. van Holsbeeck MT, Kolowich PA, Eyler WR, et al. Ultrasound depiction of partial-thickness tear of the rotator cuff. Radiology 1995;197:443-446.
9. Dinnes J, Loveman E, McIntyre L, Waugh N. The effectiveness of diagnostic tests for the assessment of shoulder pain due to soft tissue disorders: a systematic review. Health Technol Assess 2003;7:iii, 1-166.

Clinical Considerations
10. Codman EA. The shoulder. 2nd ed. Boston: Thomas Todd; 1934.
11. DePalma AF. Surgery of the shoulder. 2nd ed. Philadelphia: Lippincott; 1973.
12. Refior HJ, Krodel A, Melzer C. Examinations of the pathology of the rotator cuff. Arch Orthop Trauma Surg 1987;106:301-308.
13. Milgrom C, Schaffler M, Gilbert S, van Holsbeeck M. Rotator cuff changes in asymptomatic adults: the effect of age, hand dominance and gender. J Bone Joint Surg Br 1995;77:296-298.
14. Sher JS, Uribe JW, Posada A, et al. Abnormal findings on magnetic resonance images of asymptomatic shoulders. J Bone Joint Surg Am 1995;77:10-15.
15. Raven PB. Asymptomatic tears of the rotator cuff are commonplace. Sports Med Diagn 1995;17:11-12.
16. Miniaci A, Dowdy PA, Willits KR, Vellet AD. Magnetic resonance imaging evaluation of the rotator cuff tendons in the asymptomatic shoulder. Am J Sports Med 1995;23:142-145.
17. Petterson G. Rupture of the tendon aponeurosis of the shoulder joint in antero-inferior dislocation. Acta Chir Scand Suppl 1942;77:1-187.
18. Harvie P, Ostlere SJ, Teh J, et al. Genetic influences in the aetiology of tears of the rotator cuff: sibling risk of a full-thickness tear. J Bone Joint Surg Br 2004;86:696-700.
19. Neer Jr CS. Anterior acromioplasty for the chronic impingement syndrome in the shoulder: a preliminary report. J Bone Joint Surg Am 1972;54:41-50.

Technical Considerations
20. Churchill RS, Fehringer EV, Dubinsky TJ, Matsen FA 3rd. Rotator cuff ultrasonography: diagnostic capabilities. J Am Acad Orthop Surg 2004;12:6-11.
21. Strobel K, Zanetti M, Nagy L, Hodler J. Suspected rotator cuff lesions: tissue harmonic imaging versus conventional ultrasound of the shoulder. Radiology 2004;230:243-249.
22. Al-Shawi A, Badge R, Bunker T. The detection of full-thickness rotator cuff tears using ultrasound. J Bone Joint Surg Br 2008;90: 889-892.
23. Kwon D, Bouffard JA, van Holsbeeck M, et al. Battling fire and ice: remote guidance ultrasound to diagnose injury on the International Space Station and the ice rink. Am J Surg 2007;193:417-420.
24. Fincke EM, Padalka G, Lee D, et al. Evaluation of shoulder integrity in space: first report of musculoskeletal ultrasound on the International Space Station. Radiology 2005;234:319-322.

Anatomy and Sonographic Technique
25. Lee HS, Joo KB, Park CK, et al. Sonography of the shoulder after arthrography (arthrosonography): preliminary results. J Clin Ultrasound 2002;30:23-32.
26. Taljanovic MS, Carlson KL, Kuhn JE, et al. Sonography of the glenoid labrum: a cadaveric study with arthroscopic correlation. AJR Am J Roentgenol 2000;174:1717-1722.
27. Schydlowsky P, Strandberg C, Galatius S, Gam A. Ultrasonographic examination of the glenoid labrum of healthy volunteers. Eur J Ultrasound 1998;8:85-89.
28. Schydlowsky P, Strandberg C, Tranum-Jensen J, et al. Post-mortem ultrasonographic assessment of the anterior glenoid labrum. Eur J Ultrasound 1998;8:129-133.
29. Schydlowsky P, Strandberg C, Galbo H, et al. The value of ultrasonography in the diagnosis of labral lesions in patients with anterior shoulder dislocation. Eur J Ultrasound 1998;8:107-113.
30. Cole BJ, Rodeo SA, O'Brien SJ, et al. The anatomy and histology of the rotator interval capsule of the shoulder. Clin Orthop Relat Res 2001:129-137.
31. Le Corroller T, Cohen M, Aswad R, Champsaur P. [The rotator interval: hidden lesions?]. J Radiol 2007;88:1669-1677.
32. Morag Y, Jacobson JA, Lucas D, et al. Ultrasound appearance of the rotator cable with histologic correlation: preliminary results. Radiology 2006;241:485-491.
33. Rakofsky M. Fractional arthrography of the shoulder. Stuttgart: Gustav Fischer; 1987.
34. Ptasznik R, Hennessy O. Abnormalities of the biceps tendon of the shoulder: sonographic findings. AJR Am J Roentgenol 1995;164: 409-414.
35. Farin PU, Jaroma H, Harju A, Soimakallio S. Medial displacement of the biceps brachii tendon: evaluation with dynamic sonography during maximal external shoulder rotation. Radiology 1995;195: 845-848.
36. van Holsbeeck M, Strouse PJ. Sonography of the shoulder: evaluation of the subacromial-subdeltoid bursa. AJR Am J Roentgenol 1993; 160:561-564.
37. Crass JR, Craig EV, Feinberg SB. The hyperextended internal rotation view in rotator cuff ultrasonography. J Clin Ultrasound 1987; 15:416-420.
38. Ferri M, Finlay K, Popowich T, et al. Sonography of full-thickness supraspinatus tears: comparison of patient positioning technique with surgical correlation. AJR Am J Roentgenol 2005;184:180-184.
39. Mack LA, Nyberg DA, Matsen FA 3rd. Sonographic evaluation of the rotator cuff. Radiol Clin North Am 1988;26:161-177.
40. Brestas PS, Tsouroulas M, Nikolakopoulou Z, et al. Ultrasound findings of teres minor denervation in suspected quadrilateral space syndrome. J Clin Ultrasound 2006;34:343-347.
41. van Holsbeeck M, Introcaso J, Hoogmartens M. Sonographic detection and evaluation of shoulder joint effusion. Radiology 1990;15: 416-420.

The Normal Cuff
42. Newman JS, Adler RS, Bude RO, Rubin JM. Detection of soft tissue hyperemia: value of power Doppler sonography. AJR Am J Roentgenol 1994;163:385-389.
43. Petersson CJ. Ruptures of the supraspinatus tendon: cadaver dissection. Acta Orthop Scand 1984;55:52-56.

44. Farin P, Jaroma H. Sonographic detection of tears of the anterior portion of the rotator cuff (subscapularis tendon tears). J Ultrasound Med 1996;15:221-225.
45. Keyes EL. Observations on rupture of the supraspinatus tendon: based upon a study of seventy-three cadavers. Ann Surg 1933;97: 849-856.
46. Wilson CL, Duff G. Pathologic study of degeneration and rupture of the supraspinatus tendon. Arch Surg 1943;47:121-135.
47. Fukuda H, Mikasa M, Yamanaka K. Incomplete thickness rotator cuff tears diagnosed by subacromial bursography. Clin Orthop Relat Res 1987:51-58.
48. Yamaguchi K, Tetro AM, Blam O, et al. Natural history of asymptomatic rotator cuff tears: a longitudinal analysis of asymptomatic tears detected sonographically. J Shoulder Elbow Surg 2001;10: 199-203.
49. Brasseur JL, Lucidarme O, Tardieu M, et al. Ultrasonographic rotator cuff changes in veteran tennis players: the effect of hand dominance and comparison with clinical findings. Eur Radiol 2004;14:857-864.

Preoperative Appearances
50. Teefey SA, Middleton WD, Payne WT, Yamaguchi K. Detection and measurement of rotator cuff tears with sonography: analysis of diagnostic errors. AJR Am J Roentgenol 2005;184:1768-1773.
51. Middleton WD, Payne WT, Teefey SA, et al. Sonography and MRI of the shoulder: comparison of patient satisfaction. AJR Am J Roentgenol 2004;183:1449-1452.
52. Le Corroller T, Cohen M, Aswad R, et al. Sonography of the painful shoulder: role of the operator's experience. Skeletal Radiol 2008;37: 979-986.
53. Middleton WD, Teefey SA, Yamaguchi K. Sonography of the rotator cuff: analysis of interobserver variability. AJR Am J Roentgenol 2004;183:1465-1468.
54. O'Connor PJ, Rankine J, Gibbon WW, et al. Interobserver variation in sonography of the painful shoulder. J Clin Ultrasound 2005;33: 53-56.
55. Middleton WD. Status of rotator cuff sonography. Radiology 1989; 173:307-309.
56. Bloom RA. The active abduction view: a new maneuver in the diagnosis of rotator cuff tears. Skeletal Radiol 1991;20:255-258.
57. van Holsbeeck M, Introcaso JH, Kolowich PA. Sonography of tendons: patterns of disease. Instr Course Lect 1994;43:475-481.
58. Jiang Y, Zhao J, van Holsbeeck MT, et al. Trabecular microstructure and surface changes in the greater tuberosity in rotator cuff tears. Skeletal Radiol 2002;31:522-528.
59. Teefey SA, Middleton WD, Bauer GS, et al. Sonographic differences in the appearance of acute and chronic full-thickness rotator cuff tears. J Ultrasound Med 2000;19:377-378; quiz 383.
60. Sorensen AK, Bak K, Krarup AL, et al. Acute rotator cuff tear: do we miss the early diagnosis? A prospective study showing a high incidence of rotator cuff tears after shoulder trauma. J Shoulder Elbow Surg 2007;16:174-180.
61. Jacobson JA, Lancaster S, Prasad A, et al. Full-thickness and partial-thickness supraspinatus tendon tears: value of ultrasound signs in diagnosis. Radiology 2004;230:234-242.
62. Guerini H, Feydy A, Campagna R, et al. [Harmonic sonography of rotator cuff tendons: are cleavage tears visible at last?]. J Radiol 2008; 89:333-338.
63. Hollister MS, Mack LA, Patten RM, et al. Association of sonographically detected subacromial/subdeltoid bursal effusion and intraarticular fluid with rotator cuff tear. AJR Am J Roentgenol 1995;165:605-608.
64. Farin PU, Jaroma H, Harju A, Soimakallio S. Shoulder impingement syndrome: sonographic evaluation. Radiology 1990;176:845-849.
65. Wohlwend JR, van Holsbeeck M, Craig J, et al. The association between irregular greater tuberosities and rotator cuff tears: a sonographic study. AJR Am J Roentgenol 1998;171:229-233.
66. Bryant L, Shnier R, Bryant C, Murrell GA. A comparison of clinical estimation, ultrasonography, magnetic resonance imaging,

and arthroscopy in determining the size of rotator cuff tears. J Shoulder Elbow Surg 2002;11:219-224.
67. Kluger R, Mayrhofer R, Kroner A, et al. Sonographic versus magnetic resonance arthrographic evaluation of full-thickness rotator cuff tears in millimeters. J Shoulder Elbow Surg 2003;12:110-116.
68. Sofka CM, Haddad ZK, Adler RS. Detection of muscle atrophy on routine sonography of the shoulder. J Ultrasound Med 2004;23:1031-1034.
69. Strobel K, Hodler J, Meyer DC, et al. Fatty atrophy of supraspinatus and infraspinatus muscles: accuracy of ultrasound. Radiology 2005; 237:584-589.
70. Khoury V, Cardinal E, Brassard P. Atrophy and fatty infiltration of the supraspinatus muscle: sonography versus MRI. AJR Am J Roentgenol 2008;190:1105-1111.
71. Lee JC, Sykes C, Saifuddin A, Connell D. Adhesive capsulitis: sonographic changes in the rotator cuff interval with arthroscopic correlation. Skeletal Radiol 2005;34:522-527.
72. Flury MP, John M, Goldhahn J, et al. Rupture of the subscapularis tendon (isolated or in combination with supraspinatus tear): when is a repair indicated? J Shoulder Elbow Surg 2006;15:659-664.
73. Lyons RP, Green A. Subscapularis tendon tears. J Am Acad Orthop Surg 2005;13:353-363.

Postoperative Appearances
74. Mack LA, Nyberg DA, Matsen 3rd FR, et al. Sonography of the postoperative shoulder. AJR Am J Roentgenol 1988;150:1089-1093.
75. Crass JR, Craig EV, Feinberg SB. Sonography of the postoperative rotator cuff. AJR 1988;148:561-564.
76. Anderson K, Boothby M, Aschenbrener D, van Holsbeeck M. Outcome and structural integrity after arthroscopic rotator cuff repair using 2 rows of fixation: minimum 2-year follow-up. Am J Sports Med 2006;34:1899-1905.
77. Westhoff B, Wild A, Werner A, et al. The value of ultrasound after shoulder arthroplasty. Skeletal Radiol 2002;31:695-701.
78. Sofka CM, Adler RS. Sonographic evaluation of shoulder arthroplasty (original report). AJR Am J Roentgenol 2003;180:1117-1120.

Pitfalls in Interpretation
79. Crass JR, van de Vegte GL, Harkavy LA. Tendon echogenicity: ex vivo study. Radiology 1988;167:499-501.
80. Fornage BD. The hypoechoic normal tendon: a pitfall. J Ultrasound Med 1987;6:19-22.

Rotator Cuff Calcifications
81. Resnick D, Niwayama G. Diagnosis of bone and joint disorders. 2nd ed. Philadelphia: Saunders; 1988.
82. Gartner J, Simons B. Analysis of calcific deposits in calcifying tendinitis. Clin Orthop Relat Res 1990:111-120.
83. Chiou HJ, Chou YH, Wu JJ, et al. Evaluation of calcific tendonitis of the rotator cuff: role of color Doppler ultrasonography. J Ultrasound Med 2002;21:289-295; quiz 296-297.
84. Farin PU. Consistency of rotator cuff calcifications: observations on plain radiography, sonography, computed tomography, and at needle treatment. Invest Radiol 1996;31:300-304.
85. Farin PU, Jaroma H, Soimakallio S. Rotator cuff calcifications: treatment with ultrasound-guided technique. Radiology 1995;195:841-843.
86. Chiou HJ, Chou YH, Wu JJ, et al. The role of high-resolution ultrasonography in management of calcific tendinitis of the rotator cuff. Ultrasound Med Biol 2001;27:735-743.
87. Lin JT, Adler RS, Bracilovic A, et al. Clinical outcomes of ultrasound-guided aspiration and lavage in calcific tendinosis of the shoulder. HSS J 2007;3:99-105.
88. Kayser R, Hampf S, Seeber E, Heyde CE. Value of preoperative ultrasound marking of calcium deposits in patients who require surgical treatment of calcific tendinitis of the shoulder. Arthroscopy 2007;23:43-50.

CHAPTER 23

The Tendons

Bruno D. Fornage, Didier H. Touche, and
Beth S. Edeiken-Monroe

Chapter Outline

The tendons of the extremities are particularly well suited for sonographic examination using high-frequency transducers (up to 20 MHz) because of their superficial location. Also, tendons are best evaluated dynamically during their gliding motion, for which the unique real-time capability of sonography is invaluable. Sonography of the musculoskeletal system in general and of the tendons of the extremities in particular continues to grow in popularity, with tendon sonography now extensively performed by rheumatologists, orthopedic surgeons, physiatrists, and sports medicine physicians. This has led to the replication of many early studies performed by radiologists.

Sonography has become the first-line imaging modality in many centers specializing in musculoskeletal imaging and sports medicine worldwide, even where magnetic resonance imaging (MRI) is available. Indeed, in expert hands, high-frequency sonography, combined with physical examination and plain radiography, can solve many diagnostic challenges, making MRI unnecessary. The vast majority of tendon disorders are related to trauma and inflammation and are associated with athletic or occupational activities that result in overuse of the tendon, mostly through excessive tension or repetitive microtrauma.

ANATOMY

Tendons are made of dense connective tissue and are extremely resistant to traction forces.[1] The densely packed collagen fibers are separated by a small amount of ground substance with a few elongated fibroblasts and are arranged in parallel bundles. The **peritenon** is a layer of loose connective tissue that wraps around the tendon and sends intratendinous septa between the bundles of collagen fibers. In large tendons, blood and lymphatic vessels course with nerve endings in these septa, whereas small tendons are almost avascular. At the musculotendinous junction, muscle fibers interdigitate with collagen fibrils. The bony insertion of tendons is usually calcified and characterized by cartilaginous tissue. Tendons usually attach to tuberosities, spinae, trochanters, processes, or ridges. Blood supply to tendons is poor, and nutritional exchange occurs mostly through the ground substance. With aging, the ground substance and fibroblasts decrease, whereas the fibers and fat in the tendon increase.

In certain areas of mechanical constraint, tendons are associated with additional structures that provide mechanical support, protection, or both. **Fibrous sheaths** keep certain tendons close to the bones and prevent them from "bowstringing"; examples include the flexor and extensor retinacula in the wrist, the fibrous sheaths ("pulleys") of the flexor tendons in the fingers, and the peroneal and flexor retinacula in the foot. The sesamoid bones are intended to reinforce tendons' strength. **Synovial sheaths** are double-walled tubular structures that surround some tendons; the inner wall of these sheaths is in intimate contact with the tendon, and the two layers are in continuity with each other at both ends and also occasionally through a **mesotenon.** A minimal amount of synovial fluid allows the tendon to glide smoothly within its sheath. Large tendons (e.g., patellar, Achilles) lack a synovial sheath and are surrounded instead by a sheath of loose areolar and adipose tissue known as **paratenon. Synovial bursae** are small, fluid-filled pouches found in particular locations that act as bolsters to facilitate the motion (play) of tendons.

INSTRUMENTATION AND SONOGRAPHIC TECHNIQUE

Because of their wider field of view and their better resolution in the near field relative to those of other types of transducers, linear array electronic transducers are the best choice for tendon sonography. Images of exquisite resolution are obtained with the broad-bandwidth (e.g., 5-12 MHz, 7-15 MHz) linear array transducers that are available on current state-of-the-art scanners (Fig. 23-1). Some mechanical transducers of up to 20 MHz are also found on some commercially available scanners.

The width of the field of view (FOV) of most high-frequency broadband linear array transducers is limited to about 4 cm. Although most scanners allow splitting of the screen on the monitor to obtain a montage of two contiguous scans, thereby doubling the width of the field of view, the measurements of lesions that straddle the two half screens are inaccurate if the two contiguous views overlap. The image processing technique known as extended–field of view or **panoramic** imaging allows stretching the FOV width up to 50 to 60 cm. With the accurate measurement of the structures visualized on those extended sonograms, this technique removed a long-standing limitation of real-time sonography and has been particularly effective in musculoskeletal sonography, in which long anatomic segments or lesions are often scanned[2,3] (Figs. 23-2 and 23-3).

Real-time spatial compound scanning involves the acquisition of echoes at a given point in an image using multiple different apertures generated by computed beam-steering technology. The images obtained from the multiple lines of sight are compounded in real time. Real-time compound scanning has shown some success in reducing the amount of speckle in the image, making uniform tissue appear more uniform and boundaries more continuous (Fig. 23-4). This may appear beneficial in imaging the fibrillar texture of tendons and reducing the anisotropy artifact. These potential benefits must be carefully weighed against the risks; the unavoidable blurring associated with this technique obscures minute lesions, and the reduction or disappearance of subtle useful artifacts, such as fine trails of shadowing or comet-tail artifacts, may prevent the detection of tiny reflectors, such as foreign bodies or microcalcifications.

Electronic beam steering is available on some high-end scanners. This may be useful when the beam from the linear array transducer is not perpendicular to the tendon and needs to be corrected slightly to hit the tendon fibers at a 90-degree angle.[4] This technique helps reduce the anisotropy artifact related to the obliquity or concavity of tendons without the blurring associated with real-time spatial compound scanning (Fig. 23-5). In addition, beam steering changes the image format of linear array transducers from rectangular to trapezoidal and thus widens the FOV.

Tissue harmonic imaging (THI) is available with high-frequency linear array transducers. Because THI boosts both spatial and contrast resolutions, it can help in confirming the anechoic appearance of minute and deep-seated fluid collections, such as small joint effusions, ganglia, or early acute tenosynovitis, which would otherwise display spurious echoes on fundamental imaging.

Color Doppler imaging is now available not only on high-end but also on midrange and even laptop-type

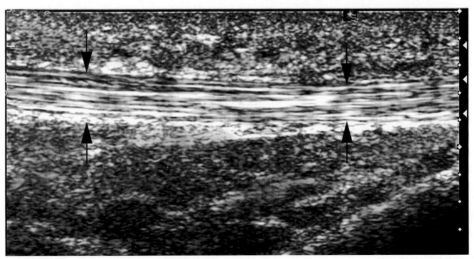

FIGURE 23-1. Normal patellar tendon. Longitudinal sonogram of the midportion of the patellar tendon using a 5 to 13–MHz linear array transducer shows the fibrillar echotexture of the tendon *(arrows).*

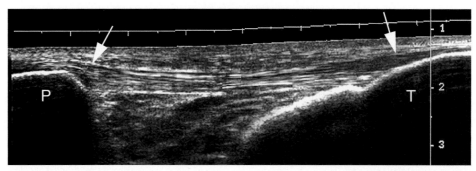

FIGURE 23-2. Normal patellar tendon. Longitudinal extended–field of view sonogram shows both insertions *(arrows)* of the patellar tendon; *P,* patella; *T,* tibia.

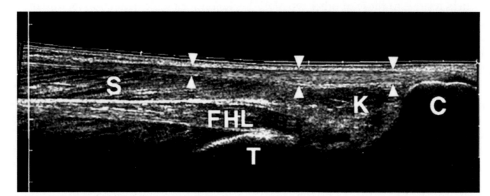

FIGURE 23-3. Normal Achilles tendon. Longitudinal extended-field-of-view sonogram shows the entire length of the Achilles tendon *(arrowheads)* from its origin to its insertion into the calcaneus *(C); K,* Kager's fatty triangle; *FHL,* flexor hallucis longus muscle; *S,* termination of soleus muscle; *T,* tibia.

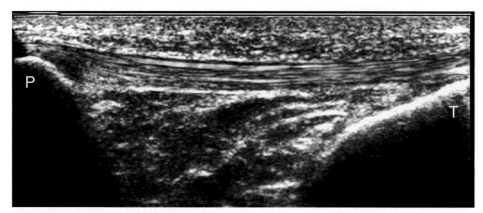

FIGURE 23-4. Real-time spatial compounding. Real-time spatial compound longitudinal sonogram of the patellar tendon shows the tendon margins well. Note the associated blur. *P,* Patella; *T,* tibia.

portable scanners, and it is always good practice to use it when evaluating inflammatory or tumoral conditions. **Power Doppler imaging** is preferred because of its greater sensitivity in flow detection, especially in light of the low baseline vascularity of tendons. It is important to keep in mind that the color Doppler signals associated with inflammatory conditions of tendons are easily obliterated by even modest pressure exerted with the transducer, or when the tendon is stretched, such as by flexion of the knee for the patellar tendon or dorsiflexion of the foot for the Achilles tendon[5] (Figs. 23-6 and 23-7).

Color Doppler imaging has been used to evaluate and quantitate the excursion velocity and gliding characteristics of some tendons in the hand.[6-8] Anecdotal reports on the use of ultrasound contrast agents to enhance the visibility of the blood supply to the largest tendons[9-11] are of academic interest and probably not clinically significant.

Elastography (or elasticity imaging) is the mapping of elasticity of tissues. This can be achieved with MRI or with sonography. Although manufacturers recently commercialized software providing elastograms, thus far

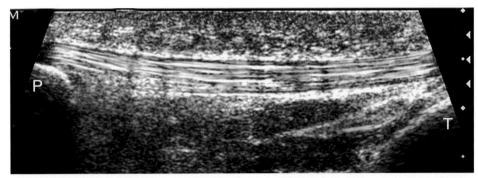

FIGURE 23-5. Electronic beam steering. Longitudinal sonogram of the patellar tendon using electronic beam steering to achieve a trapezoidal format. This allows the beam to remain perpendicular to the tendon fibers even at the patellar insertion, thus avoiding areas of false hypoechogenicity. *P,* Patella; *T,* tibia.

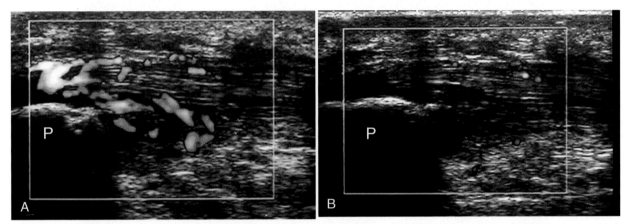

FIGURE 23-6. Effect of examination technique on power Doppler findings: patellar tendinitis. A, Longitudinal sonogram obtained without pressure exerted on the tendon with the transducer shows significant hypervascularity; *P,* patella. **B,** Longitudinal sonogram obtained with the usual pressure applied with the transducer shows the nearly complete disappearance of hypervascularity on the power Doppler vascular signals; *P,* patella.

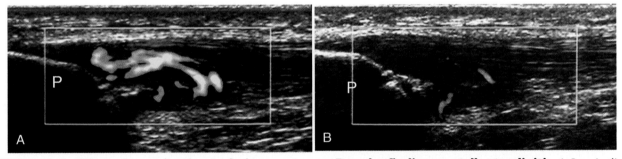

FIGURE 23-7. Effect of examination technique on power Doppler findings: patellar tendinitis. A, Longitudinal sonogram obtained with the knee extended shows substantial hypervascularity; *P,* patella. **B,** Longitudinal sonogram obtained with the knee flexed shows the nearly complete disappearance of vascularity seen by the power Doppler signals; *P,* patella.

these images remain crude, difficult to obtain, and of questionable clinical value.

A combination of longitudinal and transverse scans provides a **three-dimensional** (3-D) approach to tendon examination. Ultrasound scanners capable of 3-D reconstruction of sonograms are commercially available, but no direct benefit of the use of 3-D sonography in the evaluation of superficial tendons has been reported to date (Fig. 23-8).

Once mandatory with the use of 7.5-MHz probes, standoff pads are no longer needed with the use of high–frequency transducers, whose focal zone can be adjusted to the very first millimeters of the scan. However, a thin **standoff pad** remains useful for evaluating very superficial tendons, such as the extensor tendons of the fingers at the dorsum of the hand, or tendons coursing in regions with an uneven surface, such as the flexor tendons in the fingers[12] (Fig. 23-9). A standoff pad is also used to cor-

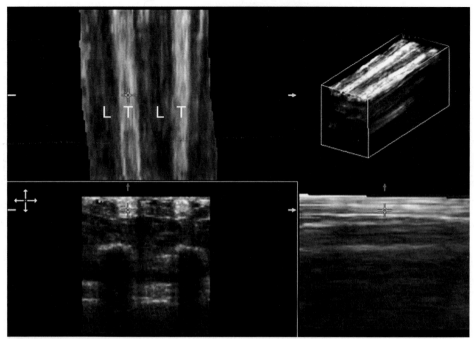

FIGURE 23-8. Three-dimensional sonographic examination of flexor tendons of fingers in palm. *Top left,* Reconstructed coronal sonogram shows the flexor tendons *(T)* of the third and fourth fingers and the companion lumbrical muscles *(L).* *Top right,* Volume rendering; *bottom left,* transverse sonogram; *bottom right,* longitudinal sonogram.

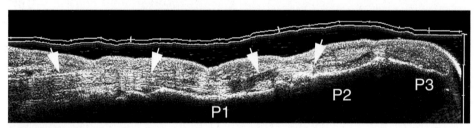

FIGURE 23-9. Normal finger. Longitudinal extended-field-of-view sonogram obtained with a thin standoff pad shows the normal superficial and deep flexor tendons *(arrows)* coursing along the phalanges; *P1,* first phalanx; *P2,* second phalanx; *P3,* third phalanx. Note that the tendons exhibit normal echogenicity only in the segments that are parallel to the linear array transducer; the tendons are falsely hypoechoic in the segments that lie oblique to the beam.

relate the sonographic findings with the palpation findings. This is accomplished by sliding one or two fingers of one hand between the pad and the skin while keeping the transducer in place over the region of interest with the other hand. This palpation under "sonoscopy" allows the clinician to focus during real-time observation with sonography on the region of palpable concern and, conversely, to appreciate the firmness of the sonographic abnormality. When a standoff pad is used, care should be taken to maintain the ultrasound beam strictly perpendicular to the region being examined and avoid artifacts.[13]

When examining tendons with sonography, the operator should take full advantage of the real-time capability by examining the tendon at rest and during active and passive mobilization through **flexion and extension maneuvers.**[13] A valuable reference for the normal anatomy of the region being examined is obtained by scanning the corresponding area in the contralateral

> ### TENDON SONOGRAPHY: EXAMINATION TECHNIQUE
>
> Use linear array transducer.
> Use highest frequency available.
> Identify and correct anisotropy-related artifacts (false hypoechogenicity) caused by improper angle of insonation of the tendon.
> Always combine longitudinal and transverse scans.
> Check contralateral tendon for reference.
> Perform dynamic examination during flexion and extension maneuvers.
> Use power Doppler sonographic imaging.

extremity or region, although the clinician should always consider the possibility of bilateral tendon disorders.

Another advantage of real-time sonography is the accurate guidance during **interventional procedures.** Aspiration of fluid from or injection of drugs or contrast agent into the fluid-distended synovial sheath of a tendon or an adjacent bursa can be performed safely under ultrasound guidance.[14,15]

NORMAL SONOGRAPHIC APPEARANCE

All normal tendons are echogenic and display a characteristic **fibrillar echotexture** on longitudinal scans[13] (Fig. 23-10). The higher the frequency, the greater the number of visible fibrils. The fine echogenic lines have been shown to correspond to the interfaces between the collagen bundles and the endotenon.[16] No specific sonographic appearance seems to correlate with areas of tendon fragility, the so-called vulnerable zones, where ruptures occur most frequently, such as the area of the Achilles tendon located 2.5 to 6 cm from its insertion into the calcaneus. Although easily seen when surrounded by hypoechoic muscles, tendons are less well demarcated when they are surrounded by echogenic fat. A key step in the identification of tendons is their mobilization under real-time sonographic monitoring on longitudinal scans.

On transverse sonograms, the reflective bundles of fibers give rise to a **finely punctate echogenic pattern** (Fig. 23-11). Transverse scans provide the most accurate measurements of tendon thickness.[13] However, because of the small size of the structures measured, meticulous care in the measurement technique must be taken; substantial interobserver variability has been reported.[17]

Like tendons, **nerves** are echogenic with a fibrillar echotexture. However, the hypoechoic bundles of axons are thicker than the bundles of fibrils, and at high frequencies, fewer interfaces are seen within a nerve than within a tendon of the same caliber. On transverse sonograms, this results in a honeycomb pattern for nerves and slightly decreased overall echogenicity compared with tendons (Fig. 23-12).

Sesamoid bones appear as hyperreflective structures associated with acoustic shadowing (Fig. 23-13). At high frequencies, **synovial sheaths** appear as thin, hypoechoic underlining of the tendon (Fig. 23-14). The largest synovial bursae (e.g., deep infrapatellar, retrocalcaneal) can be seen on sonograms as flat, hypoechoic structures that contain only a sliver of fluid and are only a few millimeters thick[18] (Fig. 23-15).

Optimal display of the echogenic fibrillar texture of a tendon requires that the ultrasound beam be strictly perpendicular to the tendon's axis. The slightest obliquity causes scattering of the beam, which results in an **artifactual hypoechogenicity**[19] referred to as the **anisotropic property** of tendons (Fig. 23-16). Early erroneous descriptions of hypoechoic normal tendons were caused by this **anisotropy artifact.** When a linear array transducer is used, the artifact occurs wherever the tendon or a tendon segment is not parallel to the transducer's footprint. Rocking the transducer by pressing more firmly on one end usually suffices to bring the footprint of the probe back in a direction parallel to the tendon's axis. When the anisotropy artifact is caused by a tendon's curved (concave or convex) course, straightening the tendon through muscle contraction usually clears the artifact (Fig. 23-16). If this is not possible, the alternative is to examine the tendon segment by segment, changing the position of the probe so its footprint is parallel to the segment of the tendon being examined. Transverse scans are equally affected by the tendon anisotropy artifact, with falsely hypoechoic sections being displayed whenever the transverse scan plane is not perpendicular to the tendon's axis (Fig. 23-16, *G* and *H*).

Shoulder

Sonography of the rotator cuff and the rest of the shoulder is discussed in Chapter 22.

Elbow

The anterior and lateral aspects of the elbow are best examined with the elbow extended. The common **extensor** tendon, which includes tendons from the extensor digitorum, extensor digiti minimi, extensor carpi ulnaris, and extensor carpi radialis brevis muscles, inserts into the lateral aspect of the lateral epicondyle (Fig. 23-17). Similarly, a common tendon of origin for the superficial **flexor** muscles, which include the pronator teres, flexor carpi radialis, palmaris longus, flexor carpi ulnaris, and flexor digitorum superficialis muscles, inserts into the medial epicondyle. At the anterior aspect of the extended elbow, the tendon of the **biceps** brachii muscle can be visualized as it inserts into the radial tuberosity. Because of the oblique direction of that tendon, it usually appears slightly hypoechoic (Fig. 23-18). The cubital bursa, which is located between the tendon and the radial tuberosity to facilitate the tendon's gliding, is normally not seen.

With the elbow flexed at a 90-degree angle, the tendon of the **triceps** brachii muscle is readily identifiable on both longitudinal and transverse scans as it inserts onto the olecranon (Fig. 23-19).

Hand and Wrist

In the **carpal tunnel** the echogenic tendons of the **flexor digitorum profundus** (FDP) and **flexor digitorum superficialis** (FDS) muscles are surrounded by the hypoechoic ulnar bursa and are best seen when the wrist is moderately flexed. The **median nerve** courses outside the ulnar bursa and anterior to the flexor tendons of the second finger[20] (Fig. 23-20, *A*). On transverse scans, the flexor tendons are seen to move during contraction of the fist. The median nerve is also subject to marked

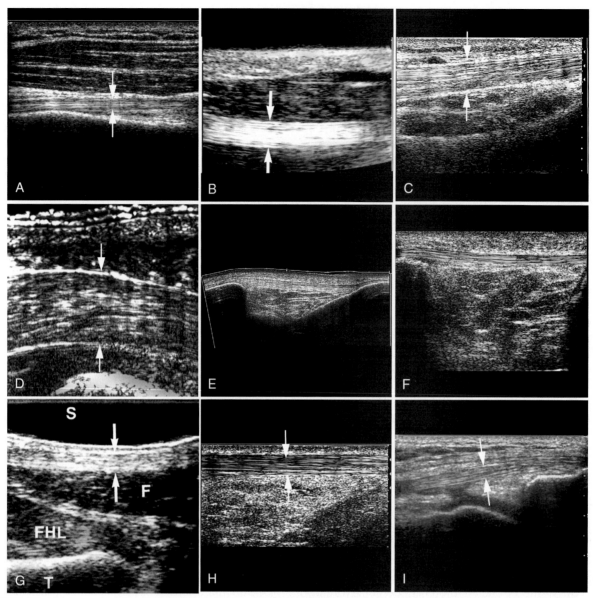

FIGURE 23-10. Longitudinal sonograms of normal tendons. All tendons exhibit a fibrillar echotexture, with more interfaces being visualized with higher-frequency transducers. **A,** Tendon of the long biceps *(arrows)* at the anterior aspect of the shoulder. **B,** Tendon of the flexor pollicis longus *(arrows)* in the thenar area. **C,** Pair of superficial and deep flexor tendons *(arrows)* of the third finger in the palm. **D,** Pair of superficial and deep flexor tendons *(arrows)* of the third finger at the metacarpophalangeal joint obtained with a 20-MHz transducer. Note the higher number of interfaces depicted within the tendons compared with image **C,** which was obtained at 13 MHz. **E,** Patellar tendon scanned at 7.5 MHz. **F,** Patellar tendon scanned at 13 MHz shows more internal interfaces than in image **E. G,** Longitudinal scan of Achilles tendon using a 5-MHz transducer shows the echogenic tendon *(arrows)* with few internal interfaces; *F,* Kager's fatty triangle; *FHL,* flexor hallucis longus muscle; *S,* standoff pad; *T,* tibia. **H,** Achilles tendon scanned at 13 MHz. The fibrillar echotexture of the tendon *(arrows)* is much better depicted than in image **G. I,** Tendon of the flexor hallucis longus muscle *(arrows)* in the distal sole of the foot.

changes in shape at various degrees of flexion of the wrist and fingers as it is deformed and displaced by the moving flexor tendons. The median nerve is slightly less echogenic than the tendons and, as with other major peripheral nerve trunks, appears to comprise multiple hypoechoic tubules, with their interfaces responsible for the median nerve's overall low echogenicity[21] (Fig. 23-20, *B*).

In the **palm** the pairs of FDP and FDS tendons are clearly identified. On longitudinal scans, the play of the tendons of a given finger is appreciated in real time during flexion and extension of that finger. On transverse scans, the pairs of FDP and FDS tendons appear as rounded echogenic structures adjacent to the corresponding hypoechoic lumbrical muscles (Fig. 23-21).

In the **fingers** the flexor tendons follow the concavity of the phalanges and therefore are affected by the anisotropy artifact on longitudinal scans along most of their course, except for the segments strictly perpendicular to

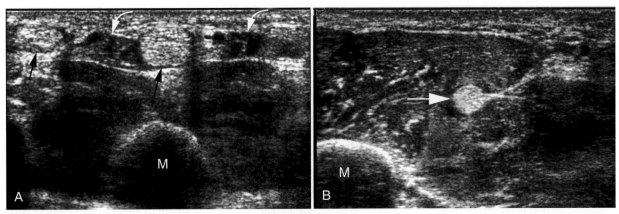

FIGURE 23-11. Transverse sonograms of normal tendons. A, Transverse scan of the palm of the hand shows the normal echogenic, rounded superficial and deep flexor tendons of the second and third fingers *(arrows)* adjacent to the hypoechoic lumbrical muscles *(curved arrows); M,* metacarpal bone. **B,** Transverse sonogram of the thenar region shows the echogenic round cross section of the tendon of the flexor pollicis longus muscle *(arrow)* surrounded by the hypoechoic muscles; *M,* metacarpal bone.

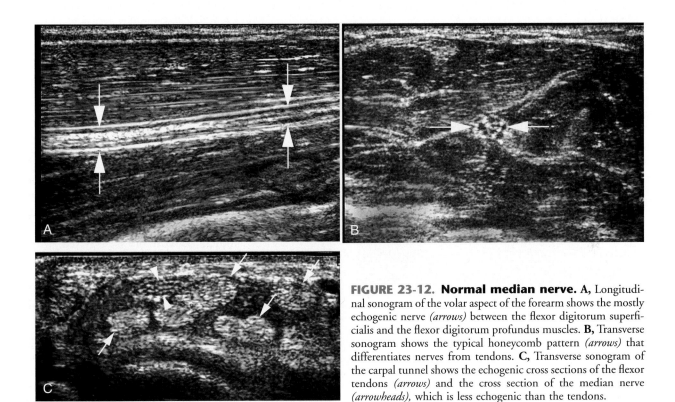

FIGURE 23-12. Normal median nerve. A, Longitudinal sonogram of the volar aspect of the forearm shows the mostly echogenic nerve *(arrows)* between the flexor digitorum superficialis and the flexor digitorum profundus muscles. **B,** Transverse sonogram shows the typical honeycomb pattern *(arrows)* that differentiates nerves from tendons. **C,** Transverse sonogram of the carpal tunnel shows the echogenic cross sections of the flexor tendons *(arrows)* and the cross section of the median nerve *(arrowheads),* which is less echogenic than the tendons.

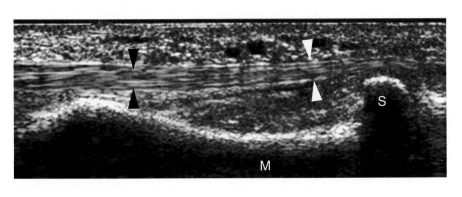

FIGURE 23-13. Tendons of the foot. Longitudinal sonogram of the medial aspect of the sole of the foot shows the tendon of the flexor hallucis longus muscle *(arrowheads)* and a sesamoid bone *(S); M,* first metatarsal bone.

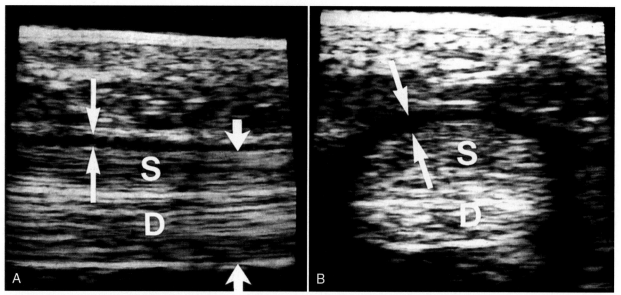

FIGURE 23-14. Synovial sheath of flexor tendons of third finger in palm (15-MHz transducer). A, Longitudinal sonogram shows the echogenic superficial *(S)* and deep *(D)* flexor tendons *(short arrows)* with a typical fibrillar texture; long arrows indicate synovial sheath. **B,** Transverse scan shows the echogenic cross section of the superficial *(S)* and deep *(D)* tendons; arrows indicate synovial sheath.

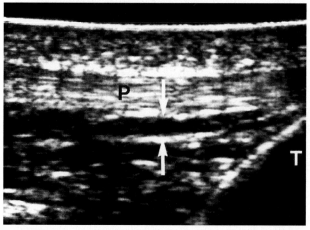

FIGURE 23-15. Normal infrapatellar bursa. Longitudinal scan of the knee shows the deep infrapatellar bursa *(arrows)* posterior to the distal patellar tendon *(P); T,* tibia.

the ultrasound beam[22,23] (see Figs. 23-9 and 23-16, *E* and *F*).

Some of the fibrous sheaths (pulleys) that maintain the flexor tendons in place and prevent them from bowstringing during flexion of the finger can be visualized on sagittal sonograms as a barely visible, hypoechoic focal thickening of the anterior margin of the flexor tendons (Fig. 23-22). In a cadaver study, sonography demonstrated the A2 (proximal phalanx) pulley in 100% of cases, with a mean length of 16 mm, and the A4 (middle phalanx) pulley in 67% of cases, with a mean length of 6 mm.[24] Transverse sonograms of the fingers at the level of the first phalanx can demonstrate the passage of the rounded FDP tendon, which inserts onto the base of the distal phalanx, through the splitting of

the FDS tendon, which inserts onto the middle phalanx[25] (Fig. 23-23).

Knee

Sonography is an excellent technique for visualizing the extensor tendons of the knee.[26,27] Because both the quadriceps and the patellar tendons may be slightly concave anteriorly when the knee is extended and the quadriceps relaxed, scans should be obtained during contraction of the quadriceps muscle or with the knee flexed, which straightens the tendons and eliminates the anisotropy-related artifacts (see Fig. 23-16).

The **quadriceps tendon** comprises the tendons of the rectus femoris, vastus lateralis, vastus medialis, and vastus intermedius muscles, which usually are not distinguished sonographically as separate structures. The quadriceps tendon lies underneath the subcutaneous fat and anterior to a fat pad and the collapsed suprapatellar bursa (Fig. 23-24). On transverse scans, the quadriceps tendon's cross section is oval.

The **patellar tendon** extends from the patella to the tibial tuberosity over a length of 5 to 6 cm (Fig. 23-25, *A*). On transverse sections, the patellar tendon has a convex anterior and a flat posterior surface (Fig. 23-25, *B*). At its midportion, the tendon is about 4 to 5 mm thick and 20 to 25 mm wide.[26] The subcutaneous prepatellar and infrapatellar bursae are not normally visible, but the deep infrapatellar bursa may appear as a flattened anechoic structure 2 to 3 mm thick (see Fig. 23-15).

Sonography has been used in the evaluation of **collateral ligaments** of the knee and of the iliotibial band.[28,29] Normal ligaments are not always easily

Text continued on p. 916.

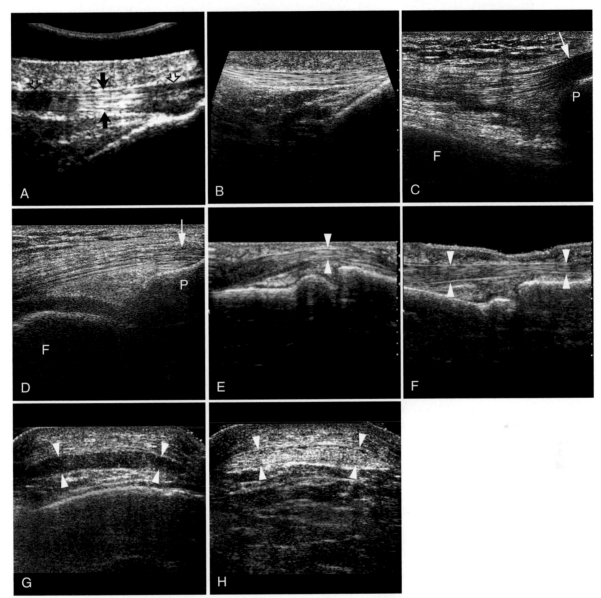

FIGURE 23-16. False hypoechogenicity caused by anisotropic property of tendons. A to **E,** Longitudinal sonograms. **A,** Sonogram of the distal patellar tendon obtained with a 10-MHz curved array sector transducer. The tendon exhibits normal echogenicity *(arrows)* only in the narrow midportion of the scan, where the beam is perpendicular to the tendon. On either side, obliquity of the beam is responsible for the tendon's artifactual hypoechogenicity *(open arrows)*. **B,** Sonogram of the patellar tendon obtained using the trapezoidal format (electronic beam steering) of a linear array transducer. The beam is perpendicular to the tendon fibers along the entire tendon, resulting in the correct display of the tendon's echogenicity. **C,** Sonogram of the quadriceps tendon with knee extended and quadriceps relaxed shows the false hypoechogenicity of the patellar insertion *(arrow)*. **D,** Sonogram obtained with the knee flexed and quadriceps tendon straightened shows normal echogenicity at the patellar insertion *(arrow)*. **E,** With the finger fully extended, the flexor tendons are curved and exhibit their normal echogenicity *(arrowheads)*. only in the midportion of the scan. **F,** Moderate flexion of the joint straightens the tendons, which now display their normal echogenicity along their entire course *(arrowheads)*. **G** and **H,** Transverse sonograms. **G,** Patellar tendon with the scan plane not strictly perpendicular to the tendon's axis, which results in artifactual hypoechogenicity *(arrowheads)*. **H,** Patellar tendon with scan plane strictly perpendicular to the tendon; normal echogenicity is displayed *(arrowheads)*.

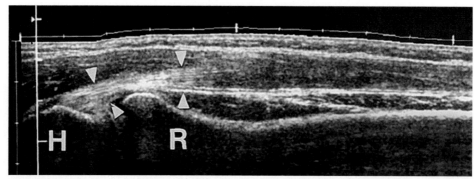

FIGURE 23-17. Normal extensor tendon at elbow. Coronal extended-field-of-view sonogram of the lateral aspect of the elbow shows normal common tendon of the extensor muscles of the forearm at the elbow, with the normal, echogenic tendon *(arrowheads)* inserting into the lateral epicondyle; *H,* humerus; *R,* radius.

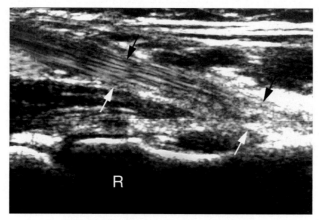

FIGURE 23-18. Anterior aspect of extended elbow. Longitudinal sonogram shows the oblique biceps tendon *(arrows)* inserting into the radial tuberosity; *R,* radial head.

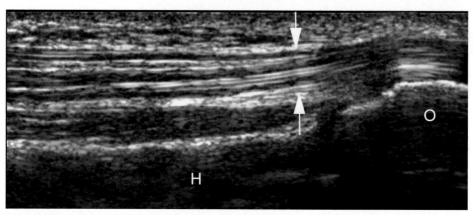

FIGURE 23-19. Posterior aspect of flexed elbow. Longitudinal sonogram of the tendon of the triceps *(arrows); H,* humerus; *O,* olecranon.

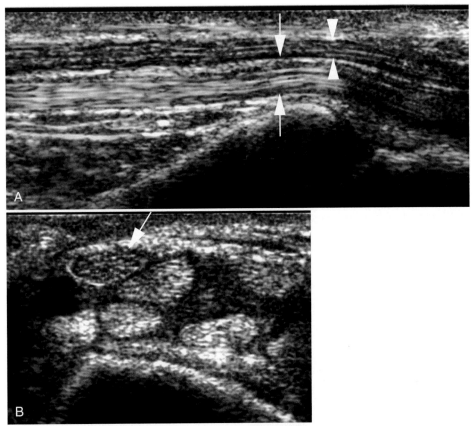

FIGURE 23-20. Flexor tendons of fingers in wrist. A, Longitudinal sonogram of the volar aspect of the wrist shows the median nerve *(arrowheads)* coursing anterior to the flexor tendons of the index finger *(arrows)*. Note the higher echogenicity of the tendons compared with that of the nerve. **B,** Transverse sonogram of the wrist in moderate flexion shows the echogenic cross sections of the superficial and deep flexor tendons of the fingers in the hypoechoic ulnar bursa. The arrow points to the oval section of the median nerve.

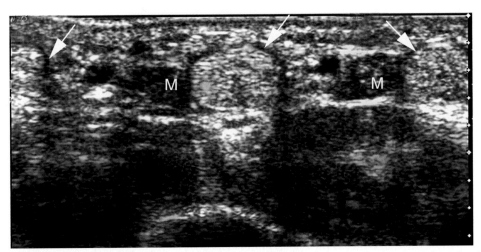

FIGURE 23-21. Superficial and deep flexor tendons of fingers. Transverse sonogram of the palm shows the normal, echogenic, rounded pairs of superficial and deep flexor tendons of the second, third, and fourth fingers *(arrows)* adjacent to the hypoechoic lumbrical muscles *(M)*.

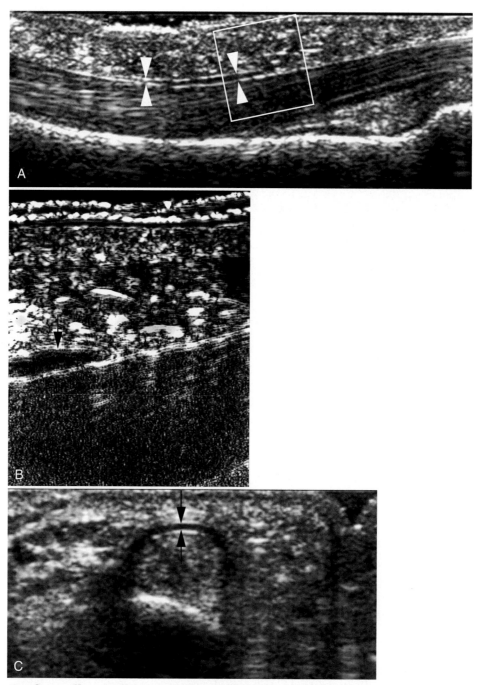

FIGURE 23-22. Tendon pulleys in first and second phalanges of third finger. A, Longitudinal sonogram of the first phalanx of the third finger shows the pulley as a very thin (inframillimetric) hypoechoic band of tissue anterior to the flexor tendons *(arrowheads).* **B,** Longitudinal sonogram obtained at 20 MHz of the region indicated with a box on image **A** shows the distal end of the pulley *(arrows).* **C,** Transverse sonogram shows the hypoechoic pulley *(arrow).*

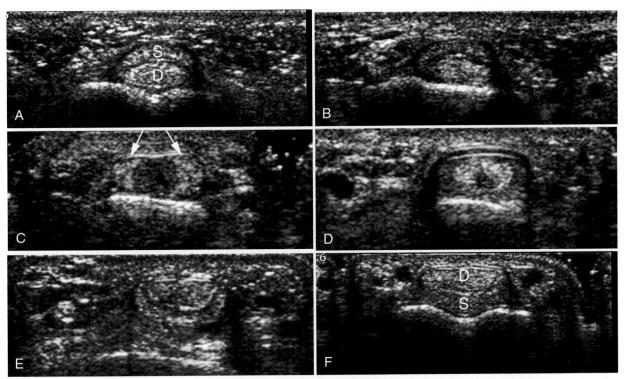

FIGURE 23-23. Relationship between superficial and deep flexor tendons. Transverse sonograms at different levels of the first phalanx of the third finger from the base to the proximal interphalangeal joint. **A,** Transverse sonogram at the base of the first phalanx shows the superficial tendon *(S)* above the deep tendon *(D)*. **B,** The superficial tendon becomes thinner and spreads laterally. **C,** The superficial tendon has split in two halves *(arrows),* seen on each side of the round deep tendon, which appears hypoechoic on this scan because of anisotropy. **D,** The two halves of the superficial tendon have reunited behind the deep tendon. **E,** The superficial tendon now has the shape of a cup containing the deep tendon, which is now superficial. **F,** Transverse sonogram obtained at the level of the base of the middle phalanx shows the deep tendon *(D)* lying anterior to the superficial tendon *(S)*.

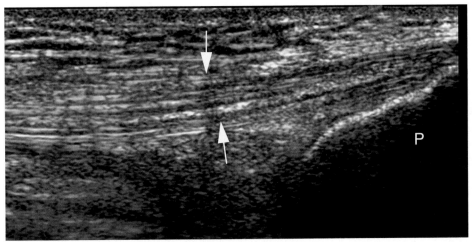

FIGURE 23-24. Normal quadriceps tendon. Longitudinal scan shows the echogenic tendon *(arrows)* surrounded by fat; *P,* patella.

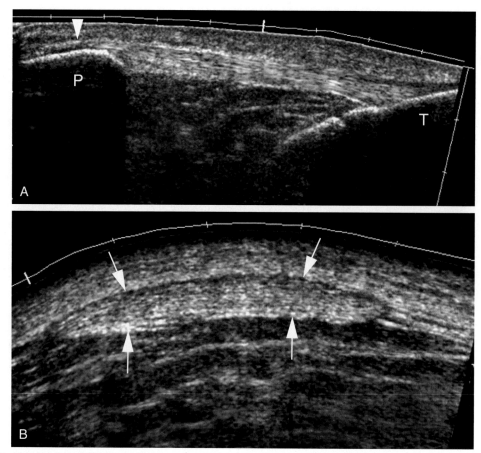

FIGURE 23-25. Normal patellar tendon. A, Longitudinal extended-field-of-view sonogram shows the tendon from its insertion into the patella *(P)* to its termination into the anterior tibial tuberosity. Note the prepatellar fibers *(arrowhead)*. *T,* tibia. **B,** Transverse sonogram shows the convex anterior and flat posterior surfaces *(arrows)*.

delineated from the articular capsule and the surrounding subcutaneous fatty tissues. In chronic injuries of the medial collateral ligament, sonography can demonstrate calcifications within a thickened hypoechoic ligament; this is known as Pellegrini-Stieda disease.[30] A few early reports have claimed good results in the evaluation of the **cruciate ligaments.**[31,32] However, sonographic examination of these tendons is limited because it is virtually impossible to scan them other than obliquely, which results in an artifactual hypoechoic appearance.[33] It is therefore difficult to evaluate cruciate tendons other than for gross rupture. As a rule, the cruciate ligaments should be assessed with MRI.

Foot and Ankle

The **Achilles tendon** is formed by the fusion of the aponeuroses of the soleus and gastrocnemius muscles, and it inserts onto the posterior surface of the calcaneus. The Achilles tendon is echogenic and exhibits a characteristic fibrillar texture on longitudinal sonograms.[34] The termination of the hypoechoic soleus muscle is easily identified anterior to the origin of the Achilles tendon (Fig. 23-26). The fatty Kager's triangle, which lies ante-

rior to the distal half of the tendon (see Fig. 23-3), is usually echogenic but may show some individual variation in echogenicity. More anteriorly lie the hypoechoic flexor hallucis longus muscle and the echogenic posterior surface of the tibia. The small, flattened, hypoechoic retrocalcaneal bursa is sometimes seen in the angle formed by the tendon and the calcaneus. The tendon fibers at the bony insertion have a short oblique course, which explains their artifactual hypoechogenicity (Fig. 23-26, *C*); this appearance should not be mistaken for the subcutaneous calcaneal bursa, which is not normally seen. A sonographic study of the Achilles tendon revealed two tendinous portions of different echogenicity representing the portions arising from the soleus and gastrocnemius muscles.[35]

On transverse sonograms, the cross section of the Achilles tendon is grossly elliptical and tapers medially. The tendon plane is remarkable in that instead of being strictly coronal, it is slanted anteriorly and medially (Fig. 23-27). Because of this configuration, there is a risk of overestimating the thickness of the tendon on strictly sagittal scans, and measurements should therefore be taken from transverse scans. At 2 to 3 cm superior to its insertion, the Achilles tendon is 5 to 7 mm thick and 12

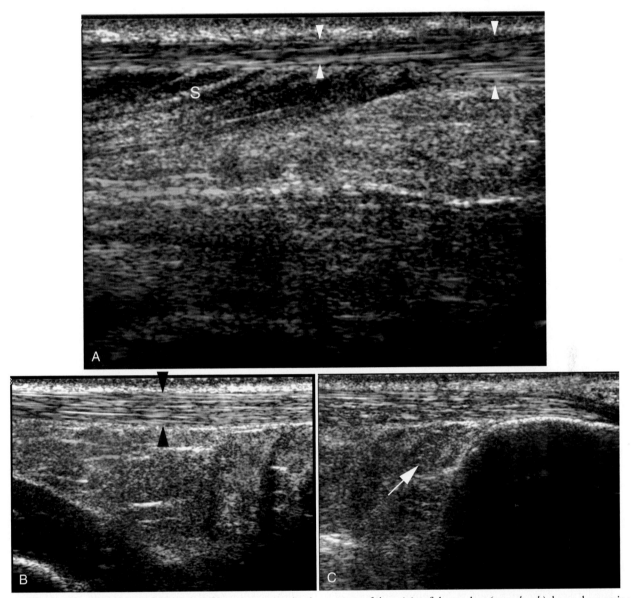

FIGURE 23-26. Normal Achilles tendon. A, Longitudinal sonogram of the origin of the tendon *(arrowheads)* shows the termination of the muscular fibers of the soleus muscle *(S)* that connect to the tendon. **B,** Longitudinal sonogram of the midportion of the tendon *(arrowheads)* shows its typical fibrillar echotexture. **C,** Longitudinal sonogram of the termination of the tendon shows the small retrocalcaneal bursa *(arrow)* with no fluid.

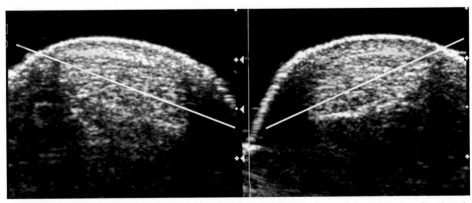

FIGURE 23-27. Oblique orientation of normal Achilles tendons. Transverse sonograms of both Achilles tendons of the same subject show the oblique orientation *(white lines)* of the planes of the tendons, *Left,* left tendon; *right,* right tendon.

to 15 mm wide.[34] A weak positive correlation has been found between the tendon's thickness and the subject's height.[36,37]

In the **ankle,** sonography demonstrates the tendons of the peroneus longus and brevis muscles laterally and those of the tibialis posterior muscle medially. The tendons of the flexor digitorum longus and flexor hallucis longus muscles can also be identified posterior to the medial malleolus, whereas the tendons of the tibialis anterior, extensor hallucis longus, and extensor digitorum longus muscles are seen at the anterior aspect of the ankle joint.[38] Dynamic examination during specific flexion and extension maneuvers of the ankle and foot help identify individual tendons. The ankle tendons are enveloped in synovial sheaths. In a study of ankles of asymptomatic volunteers, a small amount of fluid was found in the posterior tibial and common peroneal tendon sheaths in 71% and 12%, respectively.[39]

In the **foot** the examination technique and normal sonographic appearance of the flexor and extensor tendons of the toes do not differ significantly from those of the tendons of the fingers.[23]

PATHOLOGY

Tendon disorders result most often from trauma (tears), noninflammatory degenerative conditions (grouped under the term **tendinosis**), and inflammatory conditions (tendinitis, peritendinitis).

Tears

It is currently acknowledged that most tendon ruptures represent the final stage of progressive destruction of the fibrils. Tears usually occur in tendons that have been rendered fragile by such factors as aging, presence of calcifications, general or local corticosteroid therapy, and underlying systemic diseases (e.g., rheumatoid arthritis, seronegative spondyloarthropathies, lupus erythematosus, diabetes mellitus, gout).[40-43]

Complete Tears

Tears resulting from direct trauma to the tendons (e.g., lacerations) are rare. The vast majority of complete tears result from excessive tension applied to the tendon or from normal tension applied in a movement performed in abnormal conditions. Recent complete tendon tears are often diagnosed clinically. If physical examination is delayed, however, the diagnosis may be indeterminate because of inflammatory changes. Sonography can show the full-thickness discontinuity of the tendon. The gap between the torn tendon fragments is filled with hypoechoic hemorrhagic fluid (or clot) or granulomatous tissue, depending on the age of the lesion (Fig. 23-28). The gap varies in length, and when the torn

---

SONOGRAPHIC SIGNS OF TENDON TEARS

Discontinuity of fibers (partial or complete)
Focal thinning of the tendon
Hematoma of variable size, usually small
Bone fragment (in bone avulsion)
Nonvisualization of retracted tendon (in complete tear)

---

fragments are separated by a long distance, the tendon may not be visualized at all. **Nonvisualization** of the tendon may occur in complete ruptures of the rotator cuff, biceps brachii tendon, and flexor tendons of the fingers. Excluding ruptures of the Achilles tendon, in which a hematoma can develop around the whole tendon, ruptures are usually associated with minimal focal hemorrhage. With avulsion of the tendon from the bone, one or more bone fragments may appear as bright, echogenic foci with acoustic shadowing.[44]

Incomplete Tears

Accurate sonographic diagnosis of an incomplete tear is important because early diagnosis and treatment will prevent a subsequent complete rupture. However, partial tears are difficult to diagnose clinically and to differentiate from focal areas of tendinosis or tendinitis.

Sonographically, recent partial ruptures appear as focal hypoechoic defects with discontinuity of the fibrillar pattern either within the tendon or at its attachment[18,45] (Fig. 23-29). A focal irregularity at the tendon's surface may be the only sign of a small partial tear. A partial rupture may also present as only a focal thinning of the tendon, such as in the rotator cuff. Special mention must be made of **intrasubstance tears** or splits, which often occur in the ankle tendons and appear as longitudinal hypoechoic clefts[46] (Fig. 23-29, *B*). Subtle sonographic findings may become more apparent on dynamic examination of the tendon during active or passive flexion-extension movements of the associated muscle(s). Three-dimensional evaluation of partial ruptures requires a combination of longitudinal and transverse scans. Indirect signs of tendon rupture include effusion in the tendon sheath or thickening of an adjacent bursa.

A sensitivity of 94% has been reported for sonography in the diagnosis of partial tears of the Achilles tendon.[45] Other studies have reported the superiority of MRI over sonography in the diagnosis of incomplete Achilles tendon tears.[47] Although sonography is an acceptable method for diagnosing complete tears of the Achilles tendon, it is limited in differentiating partial ruptures or even microruptures from focal areas of tendinosis.[48,49] In the knee, when the patellar tendon is partially detached from the patellar apex, longitudinal scans show the

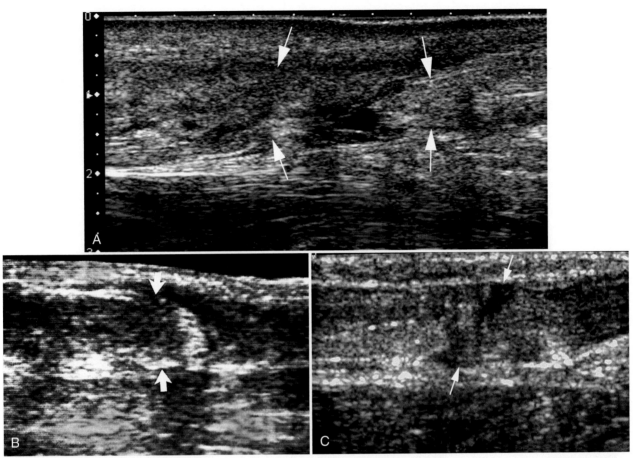

FIGURE 23-28. Complete ruptures involving middle third of Achilles tendon. A, Longitudinal sonogram shows the gap between the two ends *(arrows)* of the torn tendon, which is filled with echogenic tissue and a minimal amount of fluid. **B,** Longitudinal sonogram shows the retracted, swollen upper fragment *(arrows)* surrounded by organizing hematoma. **C,** Longitudinal sonogram shows the discontinuity of the tendon fibers *(arrows).*

discontinuity of the tendon fibers, whereas transverse scans obtained inferior to the patellar apex demonstrate the round defect in the midline of the tendon (Fig. 23-29, *C*). This may be indistinguishable from classic lesions of tendinosis seen at the upper insertion of the tendon.

Tendinosis

The term **tendinosis** is used to describe degenerative changes in a tendon without clinical or histopathologic signs of inflammation within the tendon or paratenon. Most often, it is associated with painful focal or diffuse nodular thickening of the tendon. Tendinosis has been mainly described in the patellar tendon ("jumper's knee") and the Achilles tendon (achillodynia). A strong relationship exists between tendinosis and the repetitive microtrauma of overuse injuries. The normal age-related degeneration is probably accelerated with increased stress or decreased resistance of the tendon; this is particularly obvious in sports-related injuries.

A wide range of histopathologic changes have been described, including degenerative changes (myxoid and hyaline degeneration, fibrinoid necrosis, microcysts), regeneration (neovascularization and granulation tissue), and microtears. A constant finding, however, is the absence of inflammatory cells. The clinical distinction between tendinosis and tendinitis is not always straightforward.

Sonographically, the lesions of tendinosis appear as focal or diffuse areas of greatly decreased echogenicity and tendon enlargement. In the Achilles tendon the lesions involve preferentially the middle third of the tendon, whereas in the patellar tendon the lesions are most often located at the upper insertion of the tendon. In both locations, however, the tendon can be diffusely swollen with focal or diffuse hypoechoic areas.[50] Color and power Doppler ultrasound show increased vascularity, usually from the deep surface of the upper patellar tendon and from the deep surface of the distal Achilles tendon[51-53] (Fig. 23-30). Sonography of the patellar tendon showed hypoechoic focal lesions consistent with tendinosis in 14% of asymptomatic athletes with no previous history of jumper's knee.[54] However, the significance of these abnormalities in asymptomatic athletes remains unclear. It was shown in basketball players that

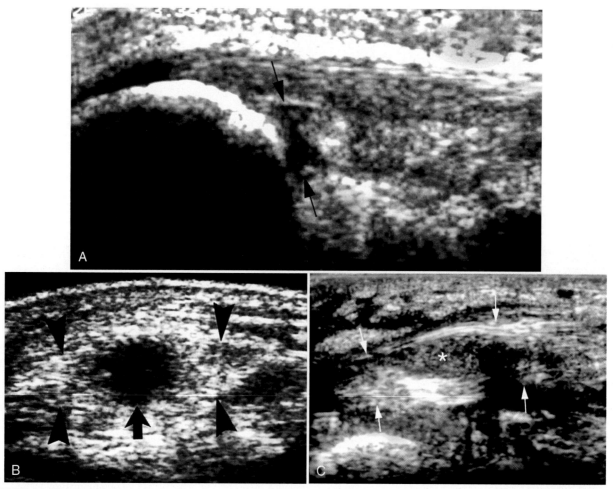

FIGURE 23-29. Partial tendon tears. A, Partial rupture of patellar tendon at its insertion into patella. Longitudinal sonogram shows the partial detachment from the patella of the deep fibers of the tendon with a small anechoic hematoma *(arrows)*. **B, Partial detachment of superior portion of patellar tendon.** Transverse scan shows a well-defined, round, hypoechoic midline hematoma *(arrow)*. The arrowheads indicate the tendon's margins. **C, Posterior tibial tendon split.** Coronal sonogram of the ankle shows the central split (*) separating the tendon's fibers *(arrows)*.

hypoechoic areas in the patellar tendon can resolve, remain unchanged, or increase without predicting symptoms of jumper's knee.[55] In contrast, a study of asymptomatic elite soccer players revealed sonographic abnormalities in 18% of the patellar tendons and 11% of the Achilles tendons; players with abnormal patellar tendons had a 17% risk of developing symptomatic jumper's knee during the 12-month season, whereas those with abnormal Achilles tendons had a 45% risk of developing Achilles tendinosis.[56] Early detection of occult tendinosis should prompt adequate treatment to prevent chronic, therapy-resistant symptoms and subsequent tendon ruptures.

Color Doppler sonographic examination of Achilles tendinosis can demonstrate the presence of vessels not only outside but also inside the thickened Achilles tendon, mostly in the ventral portion of the tendon. Ultrasound-guided sclerosis of these vessels has been attempted in the treatment of painful chronic Achilles tendinosis.[5,57] Reports that the presence of hypervascu-

larity on color Doppler sonographic imaging is associated with pain[58,59] have not been confirmed.[60]

Inflammation

Edema associated with inflammation is responsible for the thickening and decreased echogenicity of the tendons, synovial sheath, or paratenon involved. The increased vascularity associated with inflammation can be depicted with power Doppler sonography,[61,62] which can also be used to document response to therapy of patients with inflammatory lesions.[63]

Tendinitis

As with tendinosis, tendinitis may be associated with athletic or occupational activities, but on pathologic examination, there is evidence of acute inflammation, often in addition to preexisting degenerative changes of tendinosis. Tendinitis may affect the whole tendon or

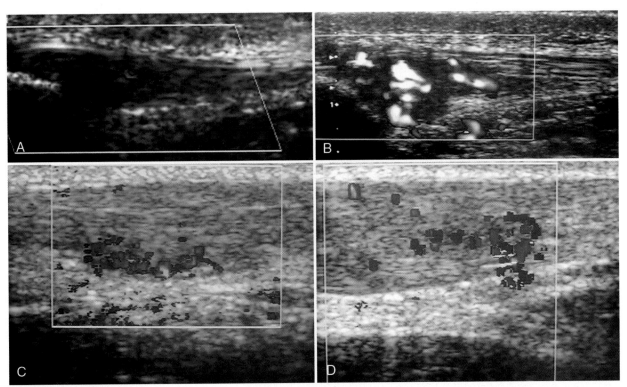

FIGURE 23-30. Tendinosis. A and **B,** "Jumper's knee." Longitudinal color and power Doppler sonograms show the hypoechoic thickening of the upper third of the patellar tendon with substantial associated hypervascularity. **C** and **D, Achillodynia.** Longitudinal sonograms of the Achilles tendon show thickening and decreased echogenicity of the tendon with a minimal but unequivocal increase in vascularity at the deep surface of the tendon.

SONOGRAPHIC SIGNS OF TENDINITIS

Thickening of the tendon
Decreased echogenicity
Blurred margins
Increased vascularity on color flow Doppler
Calcifications in chronic tendinitis

only part of it. For example, in the patellar tendon, focal tendinitis, like tendinosis, often involves the upper insertion of the tendon, whereas focal involvement of the distal insertion typically occurs after surgical transposition of the tibial tuberosity.

Sonographically, in **acute tendinitis** the tendon is thickened, and the margins are often poorly defined. There is also a diffuse decrease in echogenicity.[26,34] Because improper scanning may result in a falsely hypoechoic tendon, the examination technique must be flawless. Power Doppler ultrasound is used to document the focal or diffuse increase in vascularity (Fig. 23-31). Comparison with sonograms of the unaffected contralateral tendons is often useful. The presence of flow in a focal area of decreased echogenicity confirms the diagnosis of focal tendinitis and rules out an acute partial tear, because blood flow is not expected to be present

in the blood-filled cavity resulting from the tear. Power Doppler sonography can also be used to monitor a patient's response to anti-inflammatory therapy. A decrease in size of the tendon and a return to a normal level of echogenicity and very low vascularity indicate healing.

In **chronic tendinitis** the margins of the tendon may be deformed and bumpy. Sonography can detect minute intratendinous calcifications, which appear as bright foci with or without acoustic shadowing, occasionally with a comet-tail artifact. As a rule, the size and shape of these calcifications are better appreciated on low-kilovoltage radiographs, easily obtained with the use of a mammographic unit[64] (Fig. 23-32).

Peritendinitis

In peritendinitis the inflammation takes place in the paratenon, the layer of connective tissue that wraps around the tendon in the absence of a synovial sheath. This condition is frequently found in the Achilles tendon. Sonographically, peritendinitis is characterized by a hypoechoic thickening of the peritenon, with the tendon remaining grossly unaffected. Because gray-scale sonography is often unable to diagnose mild peritendinitis with sufficient reliability,[48] power Doppler imaging is very helpful in documenting the increased vascularity associated with this condition[61] (Fig. 23-33).

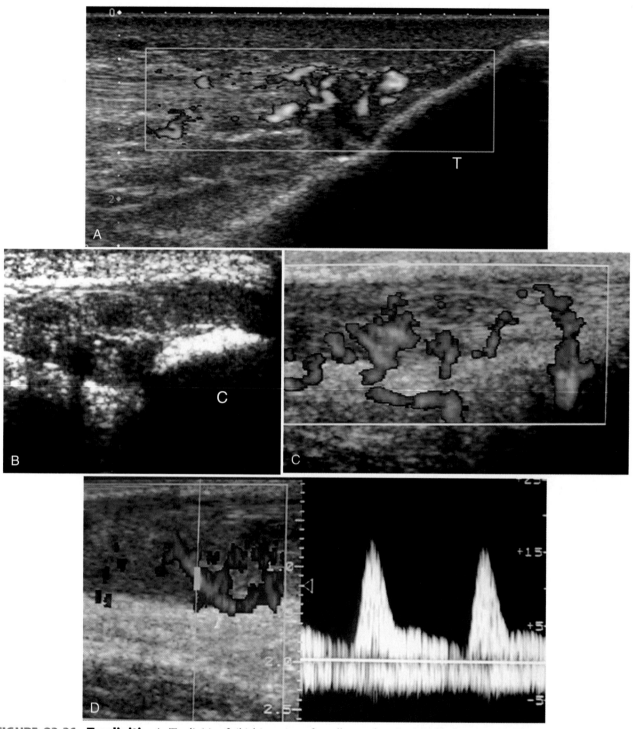

FIGURE 23-31. Tendinitis. A, Tendinitis of tibial insertion of patellar tendon. Longitudinal power Doppler sonogram shows the focal area of decreased echogenicity and hypervascularity; *T,* tibia. **B,** Tendinitis of distal Achilles tendon. Longitudinal sonogram shows the swelling and decreased echogenicity of the tendon; *C,* calcaneus. **C** and **D,** Achilles tendinitis. Longitudinal power and spectral Doppler sonograms show the hypervascularity of the diffusely swollen and hypoechoic tendons.

Tenosynovitis

Tenosynovitis is defined as the inflammation of a tendon sheath. Any tendon surrounded by a synovial sheath—especially tendons in the hand, wrist, and ankle—can be affected. Trauma, including repetitive microtrauma, and pyogenic infection are most often responsible for acute tenosynovitis. Cases of tenosynovitis caused by a foreign body retained within a tendon sheath in the hand have been reported.[65] Sonographically, the diagnosis of acute tenosynovitis is made when fluid, even a minimal quantity, is identified in the sheath[66-68] (Fig. 23-34). Internal

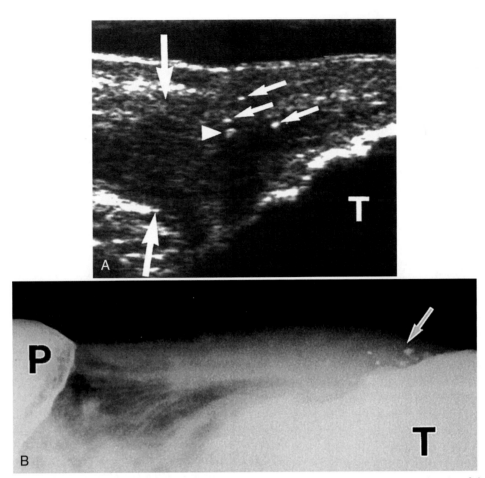

FIGURE 23-32. Chronic calcified patellar tendinitis. A, Longitudinal scan of the lower attachment of the tendon shows a markedly thickened, hypoechoic tendon *(long arrows)* with blurred contours and tiny hyperechoic calcifications *(short arrows)*, one with a comet-tail artifact *(arrowhead)*. **B,** Lateral low-kilovoltage radiograph obtained with a mammographic unit shows the swollen patellar tendon and the small calcifications *(arrow); T,* tibia; *P,* patella.

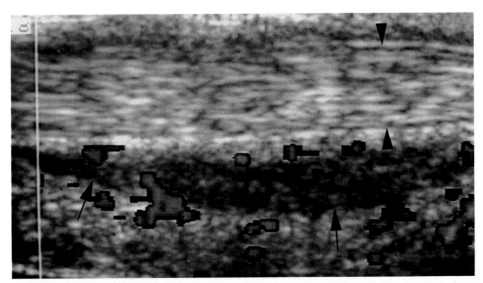

FIGURE 23-33. Achilles peritendinitis. Longitudinal power Doppler sonogram shows the hypoechoic thickening of the paratenon *(arrows)* anterior to the tendon *(arrowheads)* and the associated increased vascularity.

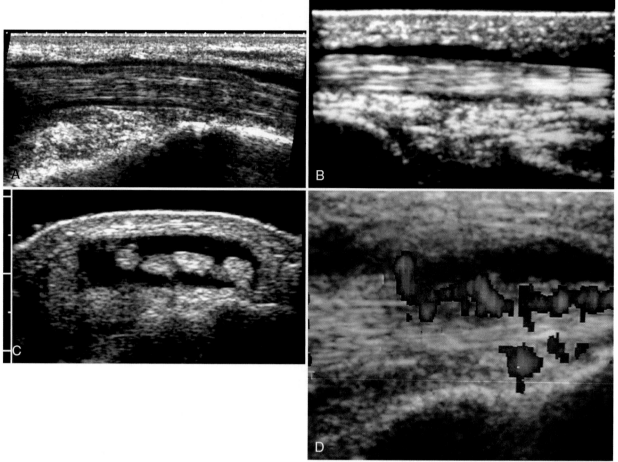

FIGURE 23-34. Tenosynovitis. A, Mild tenosynovitis of posterior tibial tendon at ankle. Coronal sonogram shows a minimal amount of fluid in the tendon sheath. **B, Acute tenosynovitis** of flexor digitorum tendon in hand. **C,** Transverse sonogram of the wrist demonstrates fluid surrounding the flexor tendons. **D,** Tenosynovitis of peronei tendons. Coronal power Doppler sonogram shows fluid in the synovial sheath and hypervascularity around the tendons.

echoes representing debris can be seen in suppurative tenosynovitis, a serious condition that, if left untreated, can lead to the rapid destruction of the tendon.[69]

Chronic tenosynovitis is characterized by a hypoechoic thickening of the synovial sheath, most often with little or no fluid (Fig. 23-35). The thickening of the sheath may impair the movement of tendons in narrow passages. In **de Quervain's tenosynovitis** the tendons of the abductor pollicis longus and extensor pollicis brevis muscles are constricted by the thickened sheath in the pulley over the radial styloid process. Sonography can demonstrate the hypoechoic thickening of the tendon sheath[23,70] (Fig. 23-35, *B*), and power Doppler sonography may demonstrate increased vascularity in the tissues involved. Sonography can be used to guide the injection of contrast medium into the sheath for **tenography,** a study that silhouettes the sheath wall but cannot demonstrate its thickness. Sonography has also been used to guide injection of steroids into the synovial sheath of the posterior tibial tendon in patients with chronic inflammatory arthropathy.[71]

Rheumatoid arthritis has a predilection for synovial tissues, including tendon sheaths in the distal extremities. Sonography has proved effective in the diagnosis of **rheumatoid tenosynovitis** in the hand.[72,73] The tendon sheath involved by the pannus is extremely hypoechoic, and occasionally, fluid is also present in the sheath, which enhances the visibility of the **pannus** (Fig. 23-36). Power Doppler ultrasound shows significant hypervascularity of the pannus. Sonographic findings of tendon involvement include thickening and nonhomogeneity of the tendon, with margins that appear jagged.[74] At a later stage, sonography can demonstrate a marked thinning of the tendon or a partial or complete rupture.[75]

Bursitis

Bursitis most often involves the subdeltoid, olecranal, radiohumeral, patellar, and calcaneal bursae. Trauma and, more importantly, repetitive microtrauma play a major role in bursitis, although in many cases, no initiating factor can be found. **Prepatellar bursitis,** also known

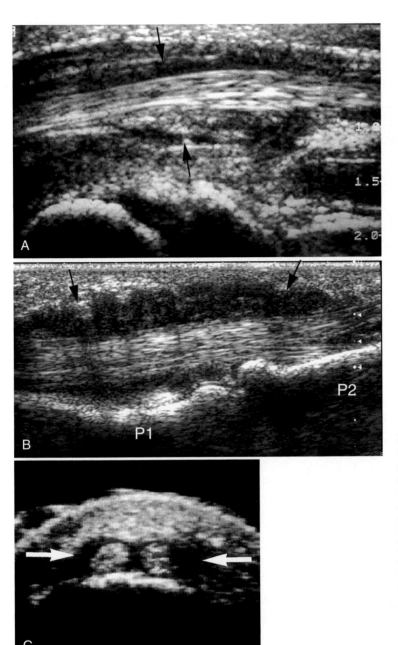

FIGURE 23-35. Chronic tenosynovitis. A, Chronic tenosynovitis of flexor digitorum tendons after surgical treatment of carpal tunnel syndrome. Longitudinal sonogram of the volar aspect of the wrist shows the thickened hypoechoic bursa *(arrows)* and the absence of any substantial amount of fluid. **B,** Chronic posttraumatic tenosynovitis of flexor digitorum tendons of index finger. Longitudinal sonogram shows the hypoechoic thickened synovial sheath *(arrows)*, which contains no fluid. Note the grossly intact flexor tendons, with the superficial tendon inserting into the base of the second phalanx. *P1,* first phalanx; *P2,* second phalanx. **C, De Quervain's tenosynovitis.** Transverse sonogram of the wrist shows the thickened, hypoechoic synovial sheath *(arrows)* surrounding the tendons of the abductor pollicis longus and extensor pollicis brevis muscles.

as "housemaid's knee," is a common finding in subjects who spend extended periods kneeling, such as carpet layers.[76] Transient accumulation of fluid in the subacromial bursa has been demonstrated on sonograms of the shoulder for as long as 16 to 20 hours after handball training.[77] In the early acute stage of bursitis, when the bursa is filled with fluid, sonograms demonstrate a sonolucent, fluid-filled collection with poorly defined margins. In the chronic stage, a complex sonographic appearance with internal echogenic debris results from the presence of granulomatous tissue, precipitated fibrin, and occasionally calcification. Power Doppler imaging often shows increased vascularity in the thickened wall of the bursa and around it[78,79] (Fig. 23-37). Because the bursa and the adjacent tendon may be involved in the same pathologic process, careful examination of the adjacent tendon is recommended; in 82% of patients with distal third Achilles tendon tendinosis, retrocalcaneal bursitis was also present.[79]

Enthesopathy

Inflammatory enthesopathy, or **enthesitis,** is defined as an inflammation of the insertion of tendons into the bones. This is usually seen in seronegative spondyloarthropathies, but it can also be occupational, metabolic, drug induced, infective, or degenerative. Tendons usually involved include the patellar and Achilles, as well as the

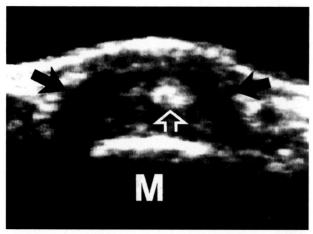

FIGURE 23-36. Rheumatoid tenosynovitis of extensor tendon of finger at dorsum of hand. Transverse scan shows the hypoechoic pannus *(arrows)* surrounding the tendon *(open arrow); M,* metacarpal bone.

plantar fascia. Sonographically, the tendon insertion appears swollen and hypoechoic, with calcifications developing in chronic lesions, ranging from fine calcifications to bony spurs.[80-82] Often, there is coexisting bursitis.

Nonarticular Osteochondroses

Osgood-Schlatter and Sinding-Larsen-Johansson diseases are both nonarticular osteochondroses of the knee that occur in ossification centers subjected to traction stress. Both conditions occur in adolescents, typically in boys involved in athletic activities. Although the diagnosis is strongly suggested by the clinical history, radiographic studies are often performed to confirm the diagnosis. High-resolution sonography has been used in the evaluation of these two conditions.[83-86] **Osgood-Schlatter disease** is osteochondrosis of the tibial tuber-

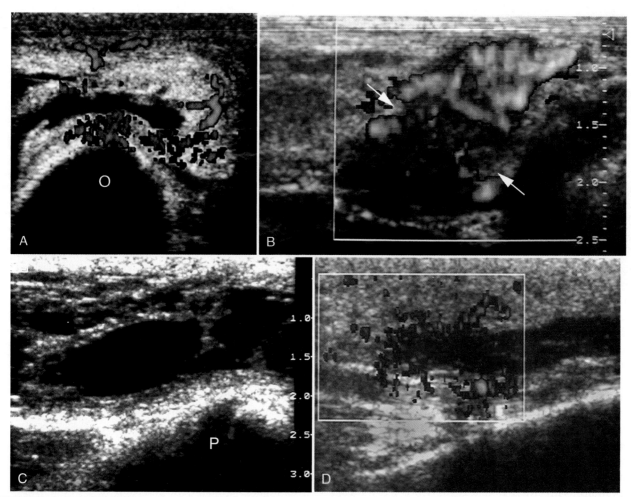

FIGURE 23-37. Bursitis. A, Transverse power Doppler sonogram of the posterior aspect of the elbow shows the thick-walled, fluid-containing olecranal bursa and the bursa's hypervascularity. *O,* olecranon. **B,** Longitudinal sonogram of the distal arm with the elbow flexed shows the enlarged, hypervascular subtendinous bursa of the triceps brachii muscle. **C, Prepatellar bursitis.** Longitudinal sonogram shows the fluid-filled subcutaneous prepatellar bursa; *P,* patella; **D,** Infrapatellar bursitis. Longitudinal power Doppler sonogram shows the hypervascularity around the distended subcutaneous infrapatellar bursa.

osity. In one study of 70 cases, sonography revealed swelling of the anechoic cartilage in 100%, fragmentation of the echogenic ossification center of the anterior tibial tuberosity in 75%, diffuse thickening of the patellar tendon in 22%, and deep infrapatellar bursitis in 17% of cases[85] (Fig. 23-38). **Sinding-Larsen-Johansson disease** is osteochondrosis of the accessory ossification center at the lower pole of the patella. In this rare disease, sonography can demonstrate the fragmented echogenic ossification center and the swollen hypoechoic cartilage and surrounding soft tissues, including the origin of the patellar tendon.[86]

Impaired Tendon Motion and Entrapment

Sonography has the advantage of showing in real-time the normal and abnormal motion of tendons. The gliding of the extensor pollicis longus tendon has been studied in the wrist.[87] In patients with a "snapping" iliopsoas tendon, sonography showed that the snapping was provoked by the sudden flipping of the iliopsoas tendon around the iliac muscle, allowing abrupt contact of the tendon against the pubic bone and producing an audible snap.[88] Sonography can confirm in real time the subluxation of the long head of the biceps tendon[89] and the peroneal tendons.[90] Ultrasound has also shown the entrapment of the flexor tendons of a finger complicating a fracture.[91]

Postoperative Patterns

After surgical repair, tendons remain enlarged, hypoechoic, and heterogeneous with blurred, irregular margins[18,92,93] (Fig. 23-39). The internal linear echoes that constitute the tendon's echotexture are thinner and shorter than in normal tendons. Sonography cannot reliably differentiate recurrent tears and tendinitis from postoperative changes. On postoperative transverse scans, the tendon usually has a rounded cross section. The postoperative pattern may last for several months or even years. Occasionally, sonography can detect bright, echogenic foci caused by residual synthetic suture material or calcification. Postoperative Doppler sonographic studies may demonstrate residual hypervascularization in tendons (Fig. 23-39, C). A long-term follow-up study of ruptured Achilles tendons, most repaired surgically, showed that their average thickness was 12 mm (range, 7-20 mm), compared with 5 mm for the controls, and that 14% of the healed tendons contained calcifications.[94] A study comparing the sonographic appearance after surgical repair of Achilles tendon rupture with that after nonsurgical treatment found no difference except for more limited gliding function of the tendon after surgery. In addition, there was a weak correlation between the sonographic findings and the clinical outcome.[92]

Tumors and Pseudotumors

Benign tumors of tendons or their sheaths include **giant cell tumors** and **osteochondromas**. The giant cell tumor of tendon sheaths is considered a circumscribed form of pigmented villonodular synovitis. It preferentially involves the flexor surface of the fingers and is usually found in young and middle-aged women. Local recurrences are possible after incomplete excision. Sonographically, giant cell tumors appear as hypoechoic masses, sometimes with lobulated contours.[23,95] Power Doppler imaging reveals substantial internal vascularity in 71% of lesions.[96]

Malignant tumors are rare. **Synovial sarcomas** may arise from a tendon sheath, appearing as an irregular or lobulated hypoechoic mass, which may contain calcifications.

In 95% of patients with **familial hypercholesterolemia,** sonography demonstrates multiple hypoechoic **xanthomas** in the Achilles tendon and can detect early focal xanthomas in tendons that are not yet enlarged.[97] In 30 adults with familial hypercholesterolemia the mean thickness of the Achilles tendon was 11.1 mm, compared with 4.5 mm in normal subjects and 4.9 mm in a group with nonfamilial hypercholesterolemia.[98] The use of a cutoff value of 5.8 mm for the thickness of the Achilles tendon has been reported to yield a sensitivity of 75% and a specificity of 85% for sonography in the diagnosis of familial hypercholesterolemia.[99] In familial hypercholesterolemia mutation carriers, sonography increased the clinical diagnosis of xanthomas from 43% to 68%.[100] Sonography has also been shown to detect hypoechoic infiltration of the Achilles tendon in 38% of children with familial hypercholesterolemia.[101] Sonography can be used to monitor the effect of therapy on the Achilles tendon's thickness and echotexture.

Intratendinous rheumatoid nodules appear on sonograms as hypoechoic nodules.[72] In contrast, various appearances have been reported for **gouty tophi** within or adjacent to tendons. An early report mentioned highly echogenic foci with acoustic shadowing, thus claiming easy differentiation from intratendinous rheumatoid nodules.[102] However, another study showed the tophi to be hypoechoic with a peripheral increase in vascularity on color Doppler imaging.[103] The sonographic appearances of gouty tophi likely parallel the degree of their calcification and associated inflammation.

In dialysis-related **amyloidosis,** joint synovial membranes and capsules as well as tendons (e.g., supraspinatus) may be thickened, with the amount of thickening increasing with the duration of dialysis.[104]

Ganglion cysts most often occur in the hand but can develop from any joint or tendon sheath. Sonography demonstrates the oval fluid collection adjacent to the joint space or tendon (Fig. 23-40). Occasionally, chronic cysts have internal echoes, causing the cyst to mimic a hypoechoic solid tumor.

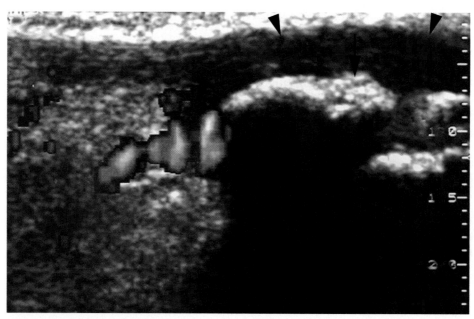

FIGURE 23-38. Osgood-Schlatter disease. Longitudinal power Doppler sonogram shows swelling of the cartilage, fragmentation of the echogenic ossification center of the anterior tibial tuberosity, and deep infrapatellar bursitis.

Baker's cyst is another type of cyst that often occurs adjacent to a joint. Baker's cysts are caused by an abnormal distention of the gastrocnemiosemimembranous bursa, which frequently communicates with the knee joint through a slit-shaped opening at the posteromedial aspect of the joint capsule. Baker's cysts are frequently associated with pathologic conditions that increase the intra-articular pressure through overproduction of synovial fluid, capsular sclerosis, or synovial hypertrophy, most often rheumatoid arthritis. Baker's cysts present clinically as popliteal masses that can be asymptomatic or symptomatic. Ruptured cysts or large cysts dissecting into the calf produce a swollen, painful limb that mimics thrombophlebitis. A Baker's cyst typically appears sonographically as a fluid-filled collection.[105-107] Occasionally, longitudinal scans demonstrate a second anechoic area anterior to the tendon of the gastrocnemius muscle. Transverse scans confirm that both areas represent sections of the same cyst, which surrounds the tendon of the muscle[108] (Fig. 23-41). Internal echoes representing fibrinous strands or debris and synovial thickening can be seen in inflamed or infected cysts. In patients with rheumatoid arthritis, a Baker's cyst may be completely filled with pannus, thus mimicking a solid mass. Power Doppler sonography demonstrates the hypervascularity of the pannus and differentiates it from debris. Osteochondromatosis can also develop in a Baker's cyst, giving rise to hyperechoic loose bodies, which cast acoustic shadows when calcified.[109] In a recently ruptured cyst, sonography can demonstrate the leak as a subcutaneous fluid collection that extends distally into the lower calf down to the ankle. However, when examination is deferred, the sonographic diagnosis may be more prob-lematic because the leaking fluid has been resorbed, and only an ill-defined residual hypoechoic area remains (Fig. 23-42).

OTHER IMAGING MODALITIES

Although it can silhouette the tendons, particularly when the tendons are surrounded by fat, **low-kilovoltage radiography** cannot demonstrate their structure. However, plain radiography remains the best modality for unequivocally documenting the presence of fine calcifications in tendons or bursae.

Tenography is performed by injecting contrast medium into the tendon's synovial sheath. This imaging technique provides detailed global views of the inner wall of the sheath but cannot appreciate the thickness of the wall as sonography.[110,111] Similarly, **bursography** consists of direct opacification of a bursa. These two techniques have been replaced by cross-sectional imaging in daily practice. MRI after **ultrasound-guided bursography** has been used recently to better evaluate the deep and superficial infrapatellar bursae and the radial and ulnar bursae of the wrist.[112,113]

Computed tomography (CT) has rarely been used in the evaluation of tendons.[114,115] MRI, on the other hand, because of its excellent contrast and spatial resolution and multiplanar-imaging capability, has become the modality of choice for soft tissue imaging and the "gold standard" for imaging tendons in the United States.[116] However, its cost is about 10 times that of sonography, often for obtaining similar diagnostic information.

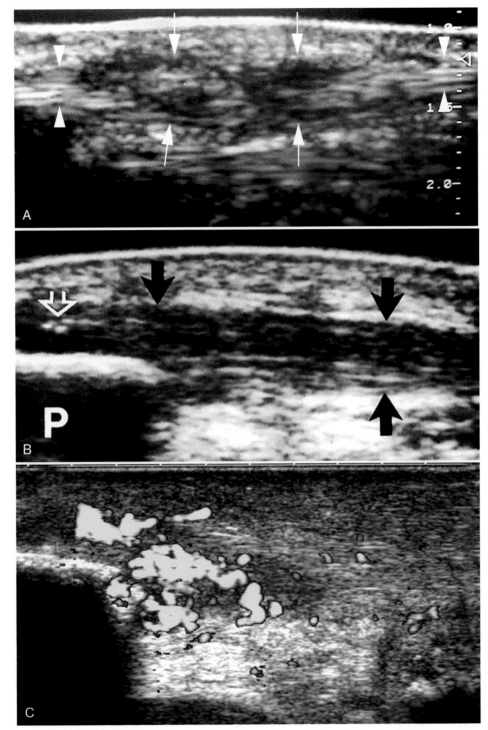

FIGURE 23-39. Postoperative patterns. A, Longitudinal scan shows tendon of the palmaris longus muscle after surgical repair of a complete rupture, with focal hypoechoic thickening of the tendon *(arrows)*. The arrowheads indicate normal tendon. **B,** Longitudinal scan shows patellar tendon 15 months after surgery for tendinitis, with diffusely thickened, heterogeneous, hypoechoic tendon *(arrows)* with poorly defined margins and minute calcifications *(open arrow); P,* patella. **C,** Longitudinal power Doppler sonogram shows the residual thickening and hypervascularity of the upper portion of the patellar tendon. Residual chronic postoperative inflammatory changes in the patellar tendon followed percutaneous fixation of a fracture of the tibial shaft that involved inserting an intramedullary rod through the tendon.

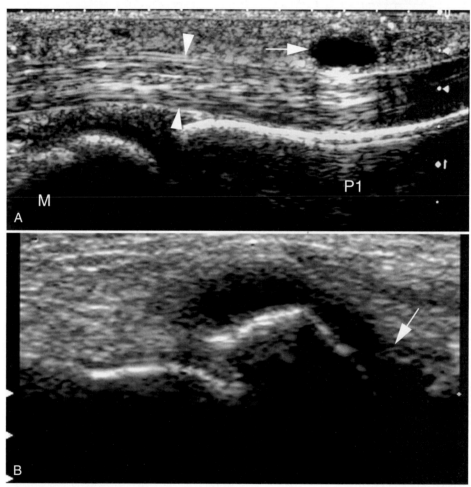

FIGURE 23-40. Ganglion cyst. A, Longitudinal sonogram of the first phalanx of the third finger shows a well-defined, 0.4 × 0.2–cm cyst *(arrow)* anterior to the flexor tendons of the finger *(arrowheads).* Note the distal acoustic enhancement. *M,* metacarpal bone; *P1,* first phalanx. **B,** Longitudinal view of the wrist demonstrates a small ganglion cyst dorsal to the wrist bones. Note the small neck *(arrow)* connecting the cyst to the joint.

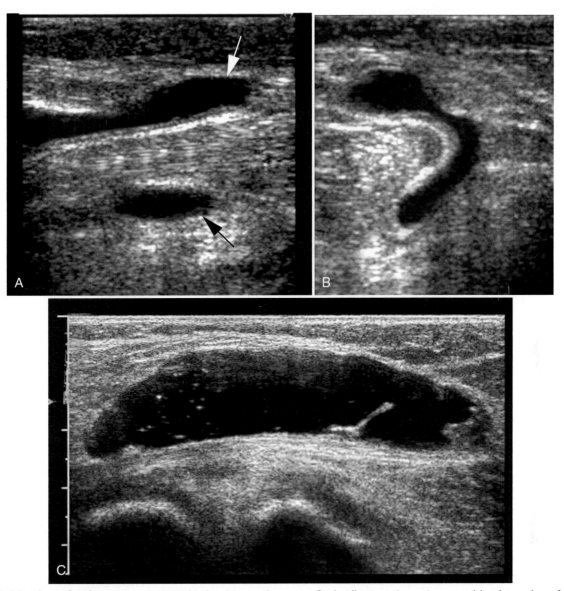

FIGURE 23-41. Baker's cyst. A, Longitudinal sonogram shows two fluid collections *(arrows)* separated by the tendon of the gastrocnemius medialis muscle. **B,** Transverse sonogram shows that the two collections are parts of the same cyst, which wraps around the tendon of the gastrocnemius medialis muscle. **C,** Longitudinal sonogram shows a large popliteal cyst.

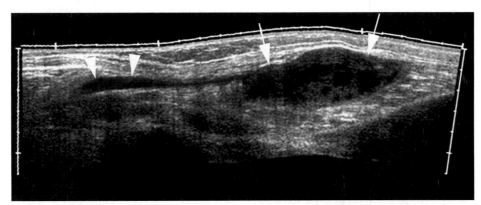

FIGURE 23-42. Ruptured Baker's cyst. Longitudinal extended-field-of-view sonogram of the calf shows a complex mass *(arrows)* that is connected to a small amount of residual fluid in the popliteal fossa *(arrowheads)* representing the ruptured cyst.

High-frequency sonography is currently the only real-time cross-sectional imaging technique, and it provides unique dynamic information. Sonograms can be quickly obtained along virtually any orientation, and very-high-frequency transducers now provide exquisite spatial and contrast resolution. In experienced hands, in specific anatomic locations, and for specific pathologic conditions (e.g., ankle tendon tears, patellar tendinopathy, epicondylitis), high-resolution sonography has been reported to be almost as accurate as or even more accurate than MRI.[117-120] However, because of the small size of the structures being examined and the possibility of significant technique-related artifacts, **tendon sonography is operator dependent,** requiring skill, adequate training, and sufficient experience to achieve the best results.[17,121]

References

Anatomy

1. McMaster PE. Tendon and muscle ruptures: clinical and experimental studies on the causes and location of subcutaneous ruptures. J Bone Joint Surg 1933;15:705-722.

Instrumentation and Sonographic Technique

2. Lin EC, Middleton WD, Teefey SA. Extended field of view sonography in musculoskeletal imaging. J Ultrasound Med 1999;18: 147-152.
3. Fornage BD, Atkinson EN, Nock LF, Jones PH. Ultrasound with extended field of view: phantom-tested accuracy of distance measurements. Radiology 2000;214:579-584.
4. Connolly DJ, Berman L, McNally EG. The use of beam angulation to overcome anisotropy when viewing human tendon with high frequency linear array ultrasound. Br J Radiol 2001;74:183-185.
5. Ohberg L, Lorentzon R, Alfredson H. Neovascularisation in Achilles tendons with painful tendinosis but not in normal tendons: an ultrasonographic investigation. Knee Surg Sports Traumatol Arthrosc 2001;9:233-238.
6. Cigali BS, Buyruk HM, Snijders CJ, et al. Measurement of tendon excursion velocity with colour Doppler imaging: a preliminary study on flexor pollicis longus muscle. Eur J Radiol 1996;23:217-221.
7. Soeters JN, Roebroeck ME, Holland WP, et al. Non-invasive measurement of tendon excursion with a colour Doppler imaging system: a reliability study in healthy subjects. Scand J Plast Reconstr Surg Hand Surg 2004;38:356-360.
8. Oh S, Belohlavek M, Zhao C, et al. Detection of differential gliding characteristics of the flexor digitorum superficialis tendon and subsynovial connective tissue using color Doppler sonographic imaging. J Ultrasound Med 2007;26:149-155.
9. Rudzki JR, Adler RS, Warren RF, et al. Contrast-enhanced ultrasound characterization of the vascularity of the rotator cuff tendon: age- and activity-related changes in the intact asymptomatic rotator cuff. J Shoulder Elbow Surg 2008;17(Suppl):96-100.
10. Zardi EM, Rizzello G, Afeltra A. Color and power Doppler sonography of Achilles tendons before and after contrast medium: what is their role? Ultraschall Med 2007;28:52-56.
11. Koenig MJ, Torp-Pedersen S, Holmich P, et al. Ultrasound Doppler of the Achilles tendon before and after injection of an ultrasound contrast agent: findings in asymptomatic subjects. Ultraschall Med 2007;28:52-56.
12. Fornage BD, Touche DH, Rifkin MD. Small parts real-time sonography: a new "water-path." J Ultrasound Med 1984;3:355-357.
13. Fornage BD. Ultrasonography of muscles and tendons. Examination technique and atlas of normal anatomy of the extremities. New York: Springer-Verlag; 1988.
14. Sofka CM, Adler RS. Ultrasound-guided interventions in the foot and ankle. Semin Musculoskelet Radiol 2002;6:163-168.
15. Mehdizade A, Adler RS. Sonographically guided flexor hallucis longus tendon sheath injection. J Ultrasound Med 2007;26:233-237.

Normal Sonographic Appearance

16. Martinoli C, Derchi LE, Pastorino C, et al. Analysis of echotexture of tendons with ultrasound. Radiology 1993;186:839-843.
17. Brushøj C, Henriksen BM, Albrecht-Beste E, et al. Reproducibility of ultrasound and magnetic resonance imaging measurements of tendon size. Acta Radiol 2006;47:954-959.
18. Fornage BD, Rifkin MD. Ultrasound examination of tendons. Radiol Clin North Am 1988;26:87-107.
19. Fornage BD. The hypoechoic normal tendon: a pitfall. J Ultrasound Med 1987;6:19-22.
20. Jacob D, Cohen M, Bianchi S. Ultrasound imaging of non-traumatic lesions of wrist and hand tendons. Eur Radiol 2007;17: 2237-2247.
21. Silvestri E, Martinoli C, Derchi LE, et al. Echotexture of peripheral nerves: correlation between ultrasound and histologic findings and criteria to differentiate tendons. Radiology 1995;197:291-296.
22. Fornage BD, Rifkin MD. Ultrasound examination of the hand. Radiology 1986;160:853-854.
23. Fornage BD, Rifkin MD. Ultrasonic examination of the hand and foot. Radiol Clin North Am 1988;26:109-129.
24. Hauger O, Chung CB, Lektrakul N, et al. Pulley system in the fingers: normal anatomy and simulated lesions in cadavers at MR imaging, CT, and ultrasound with and without contrast material distention of the tendon sheath. Radiology 2000;217:201-212.
25. McNally EG. Ultrasound of the small joints of the hands and feet: current status. Skeletal Radiol 2008;37:99-113.
26. Fornage BD, Rifkin MD, Touche DH, Segal P. Sonography of the patellar tendon: preliminary observations. AJR Am J Roentgenol 1984;143:179-182.
27. Lee MJ, Chow K. Ultrasound of the knee. Semin Musculoskelet Radiol 2007;11:137-148.
28. De Flaviis L, Nessi R, Leonardi M, Ulivi M. Dynamic ultrasonography of capsulo-ligamentous knee joint traumas. J Clin Ultrasound 1988;16:487-492.
29. Goh LA, Chhem RK, Wang SC, Chee T. Iliotibial band thickness: sonographic measurements in asymptomatic volunteers. J Clin Ultrasound 2003;31:239-244.
30. Brys P, Velghe B, Geusens E, et al. Ultrasonography of the knee. J Belge Radiol 1996;79:155-159.
31. Röhr E. Die sonographische Darstellung des hinteren Kreuzbandes. Röntgenblatter 1985;38:377-379.
32. Scherer MA, Kraus M, Gerngross H, Lehner K. [Importance of ultrasound in postoperative follow-up after reconstruction of the anterior cruciate ligament]. Unfallchirurg 1993;96:47-54.
33. Hsu CC, Tsai WC, Chen CP, et al. Ultrasonographic examination of the normal and injured posterior cruciate ligament. J Clin Ultrasound 2005;33:277-282.
34. Fornage BD. Achilles tendon: ultrasound examination. Radiology 1986;159:759-764.
35. Bertolotto M, Perrone R, Martinoli C, et al. High-resolution ultrasound anatomy of normal Achilles tendon. Br J Radiol 1995;68: 986-991.
36. Koivunen-Niemela T, Parkkola K. Anatomy of the Achilles tendon (tendo calcaneus) with respect to tendon thickness measurements. Surg Radiol Anat 1995;17:263-268.
37. Pang BS, Ying M. Sonographic measurement of Achilles tendons in asymptomatic subjects: variation with age, body height, and dominance of ankle. J Ultrasound Med 2006;25:1291-1296.
38. De Maeseneer M, Marcelis S, Jager T, et al. Sonography of the normal ankle: a target approach using skeletal reference points. AJR Am J Roentgenol 2009;192:487-495.
39. Nazarian LN, Rawool NM, Martin CE, Schweitzer ME. Synovial fluid in the hindfoot and ankle: detection of amount and distribution with ultrasound. Radiology 1995;197:275-278.

Pathology

40. Downey DJ, Simkin PA, Mack LA, et al. Tibialis posterior tendon rupture: a cause of rheumatoid flat foot. Arthritis Rheum 1988;31: 441-446.
41. Ismail AM, Balakrishnan R, Rajakumar MK. Rupture of patellar ligament after steroid infiltration: report of a case. J Bone Joint Surg 1969;51B:503-505.
42. Kricun R, Kricun ME, Arangio GA, et al. Patellar tendon rupture with underlying systemic disease. AJR Am J Roentgenol 1980;135: 803-807.

43. Morgan J, McCarty DJ. Tendon ruptures in patients with systemic lupus erythematosus treated with corticosteroids. Arthritis Rheum 1974;17:1033-1036.
44. Kaempffe FA, Lerner RM. Ultrasound diagnosis of triceps tendon rupture: a report of 2 cases. Clin Orthop 1996;332:138-142.
45. Kalebo P, Allenmark C, Peterson L, Sward L. Diagnostic value of ultrasonography in partial ruptures of the Achilles tendon. Am J Sports Med 1992;20:378-381.
46. Waitches GM, Rockett M, Brage M, Sudakoff G. Ultrasonographic-surgical correlation of ankle tendon tears. J Ultrasound Med 1998; 17:249-256.
47. Neuhold A, Stiskal M, Kainberger F, Schwaighofer B. Degenerative Achilles tendon disease: assessment by magnetic resonance and ultrasonography. Eur J Radiol 1992;14:213-220.
48. Paavola M, Paakkala T, Kannus P, Jarvinen M. Ultrasonography in the differential diagnosis of Achilles tendon injuries and related disorders: a comparison between pre-operative ultrasonography and surgical findings. Acta Radiol 1998;39:612-619.
49. Kayser R, Mahlfeld K, Heyde CE. Partial rupture of the proximal Achilles tendon: a differential diagnostic problem in ultrasound imaging. Br J Sports Med 2005;39:838-842.
50. Nicol AM, McCurdie I, Etherington J. Use of ultrasound to identify chronic Achilles tendinosis in an active asymptomatic population. J R Army Med Corps 2006;152:212-216.
51. Hoksrud A, Ohberg L, Alfredson H, Bahr R. Color Doppler ultrasound findings in patellar tendinopathy (jumper's knee). Am J Sports Med 2008;36:1813-1820.
52. Tan SC, Chan O. Achilles and patellar tendinopathy: current understanding of pathophysiology and management. Disabil Rehabil 2008;30:1608-1615.
53. Leung JL, Griffith JF. Sonography of chronic Achilles tendinopathy: a case-control study. J Clin Ultrasound 2008;36:27-32.
54. Cook JL, Khan KM, Harcourt PR, et al. Patellar tendon ultrasonography in asymptomatic active athletes reveals hypoechoic regions: a study of 320 tendons. Victorian Institute of Sport Tendon Study Group. Clin J Sport Med 1998;8:73-77.
55. Khan KM, Cook JL, Kiss ZS, et al. Patellar tendon ultrasonography and jumper's knee in female basketball players: a longitudinal study. Clin J Sport Med 1997;7:199-206.
56. Fredberg U, Bolvig L. Significance of ultrasonographically detected asymptomatic tendinosis in the patellar and Achilles tendons of elite soccer players: a longitudinal study. Am J Sports Med 2002;30:488-491.
57. Ohberg L, Alfredson H. Ultrasound-guided sclerosis of neovessels in painful chronic Achilles tendinosis: pilot study of a new treatment. Br J Sports Med 2002;36:173-175.
58. Cook JL, Kiss ZS, Ptasznik R, Malliaras P. Is vascularity more evident after exercise? Implications for tendon imaging. AJR Am J Roentgenol 2005;185:1138-1140.
59. Reiter M, Ulreich N, Dirisamer A, et al. Colour and power Doppler sonography in symptomatic Achilles tendon disease. Int J Sports Med 2004;25:301-305.
60. Van Snellenberg W, Wiley JP, Brunet G. Achilles tendon pain intensity and level of neovascularization in athletes as determined by color Doppler ultrasound. Scand J Med Sci Sports 2007;17:530-534.
61. Premkumar A, Perry MB, Dwyer AJ, et al. Sonography and MR imaging of posterior tibial tendinopathy. AJR Am J Roentgenol 2002;178:223-232.
62. Richards PJ, Dheer AK, McCall IM. Achilles tendon (TA) size and power Doppler ultrasound (PD) changes compared to MRI: a preliminary observational study. Clin Radiol 2001;56:843-850.
63. Newman JS, Laing TJ, McCarthy CJ, et al. Power Doppler sonography of synovitis: assessment of therapeutic response: preliminary observations. Radiology 1996;198:582-584.
64. Fornage B, Touche D, Deshayes JL, et al. Diagnostic des calcifications du tendon rotulien: comparaison échoradiographique. J Radiol 1984;65:355-359.
65. Howden MD. Foreign bodies within finger tendon sheaths demonstrated by ultrasound: two cases. Clin Radiol 1994;49:419-420.
66. Middleton WD, Reinus WR, Totty WG, et al. Ultrasound of the biceps tendon apparatus. Radiology 1985;157:211-215.
67. Gooding GAW. Tenosynovitis of the wrist: a sonographic demonstration. J Ultrasound Med 1988;7:225-226.
68. García Triana M, Fernández Echevarria MA, Alvaro RL, et al. *Pasteurella multocida* tenosynovitis of the hand: sonographic findings. J Clin Ultrasound 2003;31:159-162.
69. Jeffrey Jr RB, Laing FC, Schechter WP, et al. Acute suppurative tenosynovitis of the hand: diagnosis with ultrasound. Radiology 1987;162:741-742.
70. Giovagnorio F, Andreoli C, De Cicco ML. Ultrasonographic evaluation of de Quervain disease. J Ultrasound Med 1997;16:685-689.
71. Brophy DP, Cunnane G, Fitzgerald O, et al. Technical report: ultrasound guidance for injection of soft tissue lesions around the heel in chronic inflammatory arthritis. Clin Radiol 1995;50:120-122.
72. Fornage BD. Soft tissue changes in the hand in rheumatoid arthritis: evaluation with ultrasound. Radiology 1989;173:735-737.
73. Kotob H, Kamel M. Identification and prevalence of rheumatoid nodules in the finger tendons using high-frequency ultrasonography. J Rheumatol 1999;26:1264-1268.
74. Grassi W, Tittarelli E, Blasetti P, et al. Finger tendon involvement in rheumatoid arthritis: evaluation with high-frequency sonography. Arthritis Rheum 1995;38:786-794.
75. Coakley FV, Samanta AK, Finlay DB. Ultrasonography of the tibialis posterior tendon in rheumatoid arthritis. Br J Rheumatol 1994; 33:273-277.
76. Myllymaki T, Tikkakoski T, Typpo T, et al. Carpet-layer's knee: an ultrasonographic study. Acta Radiol 1993;34:496-499.
77. Kruger-Franke M, Fischer S, Kugler A, et al. [Stress-related clinical and ultrasound changes in shoulder joints of handball players]. Sportverletz Sportschaden 1994;8:166-169.
78. Balint PV, Sturrock RD. Inflamed retrocalcaneal bursa and Achilles tendonitis in psoriatic arthritis demonstrated by ultrasonography. Ann Rheum Dis 2000;59:931-933.
79. Gibbon WW, Cooper JR, Radcliffe GS. Distribution of sonographically detected tendon abnormalities in patients with a clinical diagnosis of chronic Achilles tendinosis. J Clin Ultrasound 2000;28:61-66.
80. Balint PV, Kane D, Wilson H, et al. Ultrasonography of entheseal insertions in the lower limb in spondyloarthropathy. Ann Rheum Dis 2002;61:905-910.
81. Falsetti P, Acciai C, Lenzi L, et al. Ultrasound of enthesopathy in rheumatic diseases. Mod Rheumatol 2009;19:103-113.
82. Filippou G, Frediani B, Selvi E, et al. Tendon involvement in patients with ochronosis: an ultrasonographic study. Ann Rheum Dis 2008;67:1785.
83. De Flaviis L, Nessi R, Scaglione P, et al. Ultrasonic diagnosis of Osgood-Schlatter and Sinding-Larsen-Johansson diseases of the knee. Skeletal Radiol 1989;18:193-197.
84. Blankstein A, Cohen I, Heim M, et al. Ultrasonography as a diagnostic modality in Osgood-Schlatter disease: a clinical study and review of the literature. Arch Orthop Trauma Surg 2001;121:536-539.
85. Bergami G, Barbuti D, Pezzoli F. [Ultrasonographic findings in Osgood-Schlatter disease]. Radiol Med (Torino) 1994;88:368-372.
86. Barbuti D, Bergami G, Testa F. [Ultrasonographic aspects of Sinding-Larsen-Johansson disease]. Pediatr Med Chir 1995;17:61-63.
87. Chen M, Tsubota S, Aoki M, et al. Gliding distance of the extensor pollicis longus tendon with respect to wrist positioning: observation in the hands of healthy volunteers using high-resolution ultrasonography. J Hand Ther 2009;22:44-48.
88. Deslandes M, Guillin R, Cardinal E, et al. The snapping iliopsoas tendon: new mechanisms using dynamic sonography. AJR Am J Roentgenol 190:576, 2008.
89. Armstrong A, Teefey SA, Wu T, et al. The efficacy of ultrasound in the diagnosis of long head of the biceps tendon pathology. J Shoulder Elbow Surg 2006;15:7-11.
90. Neustadter J, Raikin SM, Nazarian LN. Dynamic sonographic evaluation of peroneal tendon subluxation. AJR Am J Roentgenol 2004;183:985-988.
91. Pandey T, Al Kandari SA, Al Shammari SA. Sonographic diagnosis of the entrapment of the flexor digitorum profundus tendon complicating a fracture of the index finger. J Clin Ultrasound 2008; 36:371-373.
92. Moller M, Kalebo P, Tidebrant G, et al. The ultrasonographic appearance of the ruptured Achilles tendon during healing: a longitudinal evaluation of surgical and nonsurgical treatment, with comparisons to MRI appearance. Knee Surg Sports Traumatol Arthrosc 2002;10:49-56.

93. Alfredson H, Zeisig E, Fahlström M. No normalisation of the tendon structure and thickness after intratendinous surgery for chronic painful midportion Achilles tendinosis. Br J Sports Med 2009;43:948-949.

94. Bleakney RR, Tallon C, Wong JK, et al. Long-term ultrasonographic features of the Achilles tendon after rupture. Clin J Sport Med 2002;12:273-278.

95. Middleton WD, Patel V, Teefey SA, Boyer MI. Giant cell tumors of the tendon sheath: analysis of sonographic findings. AJR Am J Roentgenol 2004;183:337-339.

96. Wang Y, Tang J, Luo Y. The value of sonography in diagnosing giant cell tumors of the tendon sheath. J Ultrasound Med 2007;26: 1333.

97. Bude RO, Adler RS, Bassett DR, et al. Heterozygous familial hypercholesterolemia: detection of xanthomas in the Achilles tendon with ultrasound. Radiology 1993;188:567-571.

98. Ebeling T, Farin P, Pyorala K. Ultrasonography in the detection of Achilles tendon xanthomata in heterozygous familial hypercholesterolemia. Atherosclerosis 1992;97:217-228.

99. Descamps OS, Leysen X, Van Leuven F, Heller FR. The use of Achilles tendon ultrasonography for the diagnosis of familial hypercholesterolemia. Atherosclerosis 2001;157:514-518.

100. Junyent M, Gilabert R, Zambón D, et al. The use of Achilles tendon sonography to distinguish familial hypercholesterolemia from other genetic dyslipidemias. Arterioscler Thromb Vasc Biol 2005;25: 2203-2208.

101. Koivunen-Niemela T, Viikari J, Niinikoski H, et al. Sonography in the detection of Achilles tendon xanthomata in children with familial hypercholesterolaemia. Acta Paediatr 1994;83:1178-1181.

102. Tiliakos N, Morales AR, Wilson Jr CH. Use of ultrasound in identifying tophaceous versus rheumatoid nodules [letter]. Arthritis Rheum 1982;25:478-479.

103. Gerster JC, Landry M, Dufresne L, Meuwly JY. Imaging of tophaceous gout: computed tomography provides specific images compared with magnetic resonance imaging and ultrasonography. Ann Rheum Dis 2002;61:52-54.

104. Jadoul M, Malghem J, van de Berg B, et al. Ultrasonographic detection of thickened joint capsules and tendons as marker of dialysis-related amyloidosis: a cross-sectional and longitudinal study. Nephrol Dial Transplant 1993;8:1104-1109.

105. McDonald DG, Leopold GR. Ultrasound B-scanning in the differentiation of Baker's cyst and thrombophlebitis. Br J Radiol 1972;45:729-732.

106. Gompels BM, Darlington LG. Evaluation of popliteal cysts and painful calves with ultrasonography: comparison with arthrography. Ann Rheum Dis 1982;41:355-359.

107. Strome GM, Bouffard JA, van Holsbeeck M. The knee. In Fornage BD, editor. Musculoskeletal ultrasound. New York: Churchill Livingstone; 1995. p. 201-219.

108. Helbich TH, Breitenseher M, Trattnig S, et al. Sonomorphologic variants of popliteal cysts. J Clin Ultrasound 1998;26:171-176.

109. Moss GD, Dishuk W. Ultrasound diagnosis of osteochondromatosis of the popliteal fossa. J Clin Ultrasound 1984;12:232-233.

Other Imaging Modalities

110. Engel J, Luboshitz S, Israeli A, Ganel A. Tenography in de Quervain's disease. Hand 1981;13:142-146.

111. Gilula LA, Oloff L, Caputi R, et al. Ankle tenography: a key to unexplained symptomatology. Part II. Diagnosis of chronic tendon disabilities. Radiology 1984;151:581-587.

112. Viegas FC, Aguiar RO, Gasparetto E, et al. Deep and superficial infrapatellar bursae: cadaveric investigation of regional anatomy using magnetic resonance after ultrasound-guided bursography. Skeletal Radiol 2007;36:41-46.,

113. Aguiar RO, Gasparetto EL, Escuissato DL, et al. Radial and ulnar bursae of the wrist: cadaveric investigation of regional anatomy with ultrasonographic-guided tenography and MR imaging. Skeletal Radiol 2006;35:828-832.

114. Mourad K, King J, Guggiana P. Computed tomography and ultrasound imaging of jumper's knee: patellar tendinitis. Clin Radiol 1988;39:162-165.

115. Rosenberg ZS, Feldman F, Singson RD, et al. Ankle tendons: evaluation with computed tomography. Radiology 1988;166:221-226.

116. Beltran J, Mosure JC. Magnetic resonance imaging of tendons. Crit Rev Diagn Imaging 1990;30:111-182.

117. Rockett MS, Waitches G, Sudakoff G, Brage M. Use of ultrasonography versus magnetic resonance imaging for tendon abnormalities around the ankle. Foot Ankle Int 1998;19:604-612.

118. Nallamshetty L, Nazarian LN, Schweitzer ME, et al. Evaluation of posterior tibial pathology: comparison of sonography and MR imaging. Skeletal Radiol 2005;34:375-380.

119. Warden SJ, Kiss ZS, Malara FA, et al. Comparative accuracy of magnetic resonance imaging and ultrasonography in confirming clinically diagnosed patellar tendinopathy. Am J Sports Med 2007;35:427-436..

120. Miller TT, Shapiro MA, Schultz E, Kalish PE. Comparison of sonography and MRI for diagnosing epicondylitis. J Clin Ultrasound 2002;30:193-202.

121. O'Connor PJ, Grainger AJ, Morgan SR, et al. Ultrasound assessment of tendons in asymptomatic volunteers: a study of reproducibility. Eur Radiol 2004;14:1968-1973.

CHAPTER 24

Musculoskeletal Interventions

Ronald S. Adler

Chapter Outline

The real-time nature of ultrasound makes it ideally suited to provide guidance for a variety of musculoskeletal interventional procedures.[1-10] Continuous observation of needle position ensures proper placement and allows continuous monitoring of the distribution of injected and aspirated material. The adverse effects of improper needle placement during corticosteroid administration are well documented.[11-16] Likewise, decompression of fluid-filled lesions and fragmentation of calcific deposits may be performed.

The current generation of high-frequency transducers for small parts sonography allows excellent depiction of soft tissue detail and articular surfaces, particularly in the hand, wrist, foot, and ankle.[17] This allows needle placement in non-fluid-distended structures, such as a non-distended joint, tendon sheath, or bursa. The injected agent also produces a **contrast** effect, which can improve delineation of surrounding structures (e.g., labral morphology) and provide additional information regarding the agent's distribution.[18,19] Ultrasound guidance has broad appeal because it does not involve ionizing radiation; this feature is particularly advantageous in the pediatric population and during pregnancy.

Ultrasound-guided injections in the musculoskeletal system include injection of joints, tendon sheaths, bursae, and ganglion cysts. The chapter emphasizes the most common injections performed at my institution, an orthopedic and rheumatology specialty hospital. The most common clinical indication for ultrasound-guided injections generally relates to **pain** that does not respond to other conservative measures, regardless of the anatomic site. The pain may result from a chronic repetitive injury in the work environment, a sports-related injury, or an underlying inflammatory disorder, such as rheumatoid arthritis.

TECHNICAL CONSIDERATIONS

Diagnostic and subsequent interventional examinations are often performed using either linear or curved, phased array transducers, based on depth and local geometry. Needle selection is based on specific anatomic conditions (i.e., depth and size of region of interest). We employ a freehand technique in which the basic principle is to ensure needle visualization as a specular reflector.[7] This relies on orienting the needle so that it is perpendicular (or nearly so) to the insonating beam (Fig. 24-1). The needle then becomes a specular reflector, often having a strong ringdown artifact. Although needle guides are available and may be of value, a freehand technique allows greater flexibility in adjusting needle position during a procedure. Further, needle visualization can be enhanced by injecting a small amount of anesthetic and observing the corresponding moving echoes in either gray-scale or color flow sonographic imaging.[1]

Patient positioning should be assessed first to ensure comfort and optimal visualization of the anatomy. It is important to keep in mind that tendons display inherent **anisotropy;** they will look hypoechoic if the transducer footprint is not parallel to the tendon.[17] Therefore the transducer must be oriented to maximize tendon echogenicity to avoid false interpretation of the tendon as being complex fluid or synovium. An offset may be required at the skin entry point of the needle relative to the transducer to allow for the appropriate needle orientation. Deep structures, such as tendons about the hip, are often better imaged using a curved linear or sector transducer, operating at center frequencies of about 3.5 to 7.5 MHz. Superficial, linearly oriented structures, such as in the wrist or ankle, are best approached using a linear array transducer with higher center frequencies (>10 MHz). Transducers with a small footprint ("hockey stick") are particularly well suited to superficial injections. These factors should be assessed before skin preparation.

The immiscible nature of the steroid anesthetic mixture may likewise produce temporary contrast effect (Fig. 24-2). In vitro experiments suggest that this prop-

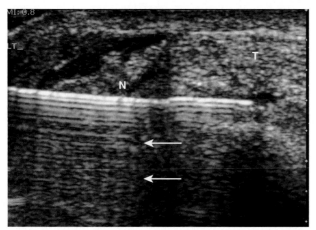

FIGURE 24-1. Needle as specular reflector with reverberation artifact. A 25-gauge needle (N) has been positioned into the retrocalcaneal bursa deep to the Achilles tendon (T). Note that the needle is a specular reflector with a characteristic reverberation artifact (arrows).

erty is caused by alterations in acoustic impedance by the scattering material, formed by the suspension of steroid in an aqueous background; this results in an increase in echo intensity of about 20 dB.[19] This contrast effect has the advantage of increasing the conspicuity of the delivered agent during real time, enabling the operator to better define the distribution of delivered agent during ultrasound-guided therapy (**Video 24-1**).

INJECTION TECHNIQUE

We employ a sterile technique; the area in question is cleaned with iodine-based solution and draped with a sterile drape (Fig. 24-3). The transducer is immersed into iodine-based solution and surrounded by a sterile drape. A drape is also placed over portions of the ultrasound unit. A sonographer or radiologist positions the transducer; a radiologist positions the needle and performs the procedure. We use 1% lidocaine and bupivacaine (0.25%-0.75%) for local anesthesia. Once the needle is in position, the procedure is undertaken while imaging in real time. Depending on anatomic location, a 1.5-inch or spinal needle with stylet is used to administer the anesthetic-corticosteroid mixture, generally consisting of local long-acting anesthetic and one of the standard injectable corticosteroid derivatives (e.g., triamcinolone).

Two approaches to performing injections are long axis and short axis, which relate needle orientation to the structure being injected.[9] The **long-axis approach** refers to needle placement in the plane parallel to the structure

BASELINE   EARLY   LATE

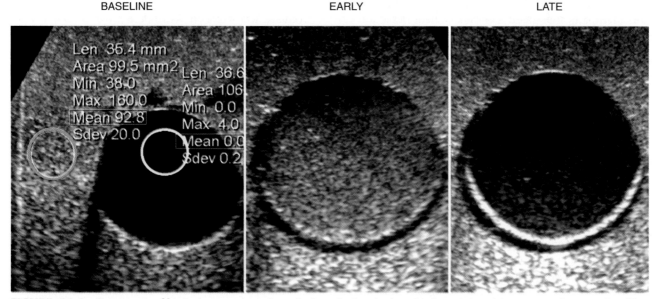

Len 35.4 mm
Area 99.5 mm2
Min 38.0   Len 36.6
Max 160.0   Area 106
Mean 92.8   Min 0.0
Sdev 20.0   Max 4.0
              Mean 0.0
              Sdev 0.2

FIGURE 24-2. Contrast effect. A suspension of anesthetic and triamcinolone has been injected into a cyst phantom. **Baseline:** Before injection, anechoic "cyst" is shown in a scattering medium, with baseline pixel intensities listed. **Early:** The early mixing phase is obtained immediately after injection. A contrast effect is evident, in which the cyst becomes almost isoechoic to the background. **Late:** 20 minutes after injection. In the late phase, apparent gravitational effect results in settling of the suspension toward the dependent portions of the cyst phantom and development of a contrast gradient.

of interest (Fig. 24-4). For example, longitudinal imaging of the hip to display a hip effusion might be used as the plane to direct the needle for ultrasound-guided aspiration. Alternatively, the **short-axis approach** refers to needle entry in the plane perpendicular to the long axis of a structure (Fig. 24-5). For example, injection of the retrocalcaneal bursa or metatarsophalangeal joint might use a lateral approach. In our experience, the short-axis approach works well when performing injections or aspirations in small joints and tendon sheaths of the hand and foot. The long-axis approach appears better suited for deep joint injections, such as in the hip or shoulder. It is important to recognize, however, that

such approaches serve merely as guidelines, and that no single method necessarily applies to any specific injection.

INJECTION MATERIALS

Most injections involve use of a long-acting corticosteroid in combination with a local anesthetic in relatively small volumes. **Injectable steroids** usually come in either **crystalline** form, associated with a slower rate of absorption, or a **soluble** form, characterized by rapid absorption.[20-22] Crystalline agents include triamcinolone and methylprednisolone acetate (Depo-Medrol). A common soluble agent is Celestone, which includes a rapidly absorbed betamethasone salt. A reactive inflammatory response or flushing response may occur with crystalline steroids, but typically not with soluble agents.[13]

The most significant complications associated with injectable steroid use in the musculoskeletal system relate to **chondrolysis** (when used in weight-bearing joints), **depigmentation, fat necrosis,** and **impaired healing response** (when used in soft tissues).[11-14] Impaired healing has been associated with tendon, ligament, and plantar fascia rupture. The most frequently used mixtures contain insoluble particles, so a systemic injection could theoretically result in an "embolic phenomenon," which has been implicated as a mechanism for neurologic complications associated with transforaminal injections. We have not encountered this as a complication when performing injections in the appendicular skeletal system.

The most common **anesthetics** are lidocaine (Xylocaine) and bupivacaine (Marcaine).[22,23] Both are characterized as "local injectable anesthetics" but differ in the

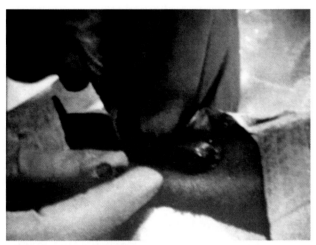

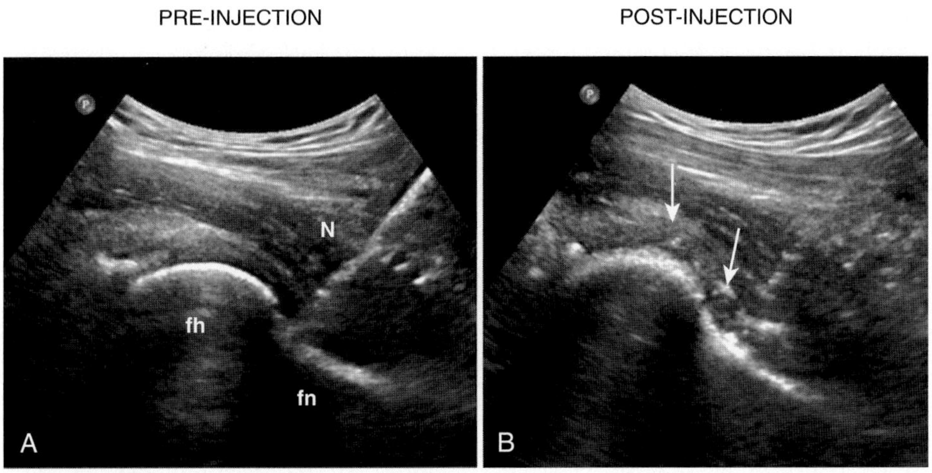

FIGURE 24-3. Sterile technique used for ultrasound-guided interventions. The current setup illustrates a dorsal approach for injection of the first metatarsophalangeal joint. A linear high-frequency transducer with a hockey stick configuration is convenient for injection of small joints, as illustrated here. In this case the needle is in the plane perpendicular to the transducer; the transducer parallels the joint so that the needle is imaged in cross section (short-axis approach).

PRE-INJECTION   POST-INJECTION

FIGURE 24-4. Long-axis approach: injection of left hip. The long-axis approach is suitable for deep joint injections, such as the hip or shoulder. **A,** Before injection, 22-gauge spinal needle *(N)* has been positioned at the femoral head-neck junction in a 50 year-old woman with a labral tear demonstrated on MRI (not shown), to assess relief after therapeutic injection. **B,** After injection, confirmation of intra-articular deposition of injected material is obtained by the presence of micro-bubbles *(arrows)* deep to the joint capsule; *fh,* femoral head; *fn,* femoral neck.

PRE-INJECTION   POST-INJECTION

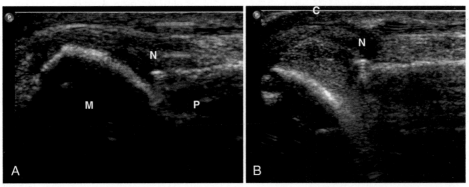

FIGURE 24-5. Short-axis approach for injection of first metatarsophalangeal (MTP) joint. A, Long-axis view shows 25-gauge needle positioned in MTP joint of 53-year-old woman with plantar plate injury; needle *(N)* is seen in cross section; *M,* metatarsal head; *P,* proximal phalanx. **B,** While monitoring the injection in real time, the joint capsule distends and fills with echogenic material; *C,* capsule.

onset of effect and duration. Lidocaine is characterized by early onset (seconds) and short duration (1-2 hours). Bupivacaine becomes effective in 5 to 10 minutes and generally last 4 to 6 hours. In addition to allergic reactions, potential adverse effects include neurotoxicity and cardiotoxicity; these are generally rare when small doses are used under image guidance, taking care to avoid an intravascular injection. Bupivacaine has also been associated with chondrolysis when used for intra-articular applications, but only with constant infusions during arthroscopy and in vitro.[24] Chondrolysis is probably not an issue with the small, fixed volumes of bupivacaine typically employed during injections in the musculoskeletal system.

INJECTION OF JOINTS

A high-frequency linear transducer is used for hand, wrist, elbow, foot and ankle injections. A short-axis approach is often technically easier for small joint injections. The needle should enter the skin parallel to the plane of the joint space. Superficial joints usually appear as separations between the normally continuous specular echoes produced by cortical surfaces. As in other fluid-containing structures, the presence of an effusion is a helpful feature in visualizing the needle as it enters the joint, because it provides a fluid standoff.

The short-axis approach entails scanning across the joint and looking for the transition from one cortical surface to the next, marking the skin (with a surgical marker) and then placing a needle into the joint using ultrasound guidance. When imaging the joint in long axis, the needle will be seen in cross section (Fig. 24-5). Needle placement is confirmed by injecting a small amount of 1% lidocaine, which should display distention of the joint, as well as echoes filling the joint. Small joint injections generally require 0.5 to 1 mL of the therapeutic mixture. In our experience, this approach

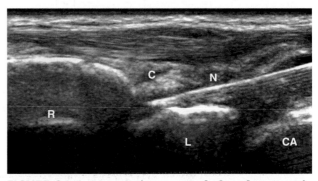

FIGURE 24-6. Long-axis approach for therapeutic radiocarpal joint injection. A 25-gauge needle *(N)* has been positioned deep to the dorsal capsule *(C)* and above the lunate bone *(L)* of 19-year-old female patient with chronic wrist pain, to assess relief; *R,* radius; *CA,* capitate.

works well in the **metatarsophalangeal** or **metacarpophalangeal** (MTP/MCP) and **interphalangeal** (IP) joints, midfoot, ankle, and elbow. Occasionally, a long-axis approach may be efficacious, as in the radiocarpal joint and lateral gutter of the ankle (Fig. 24-6). Ultrasound guidance allows the clinician to negotiate osteophytes and joint bodies. It allows identification of capsular outpouching, thereby affording a more convenient, indirect approach into a joint than slipping a needle into a small joint space.

A long-axis approach and a spinal needle are used when performing injections of large joints such as the shoulder or hip (Fig. 24-7). A greater volume is usually injected, typically 5 mL of the steroid-anesthetic mixture. In the case of adhesive capsulitis, significantly larger volumes of local anesthetic (5-10 mL) may be added to provide additional joint distention. We generally approach the glenohumeral joint using a posterior approach, with the patient in a decubitus position and the arm placed in cross-adduction. An intermediate-frequency, linear or curvilinear transducer will suffice in most cases. A linear transducer often results in better

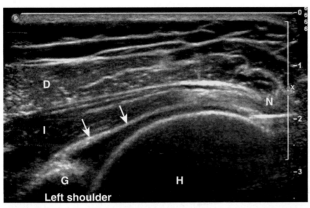

FIGURE 24-7. Long-axis approach for glenohumeral joint injection. A 22-gauge needle *(N)* has been positioned deep to the posterior capsule *(arrows)* during a glenohumeral joint injection in 42-year-old woman with adhesive capsulitis. Mild fluid distension of the posterior recess of the joint is evident. *H,* Humeral head; *G,* glenoid; *I,* infraspinatus muscle; *D,* deltoid muscle.

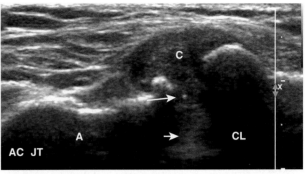

FIGURE 24-8. Short-axis approach to injection of acromioclavicular (AC) joint. A 25-gauge needle *(long thin arrow)* is seen in cross section in a distended hypertrophic AC joint during therapeutic injection in 73-year-old woman with pain centered over AC joint. The joint appears widened, containing echogenic material caused by the contrast effect *(short thick arrow)* of the therapeutic agent. *A,* Acromion; *CL,* clavicle; *C,* distended capsule.

anatomic detail than curved arrays. The interface of the glenohumeral joint is usually seen with the patient in the decubitus position, as well as the hypoechoic articular cartilage overlying the humeral head. We perform this injection using a long-axis approach, with the needle directed toward the joint along the articular cartilage and deep to the posterior capsule. A test injection with 1% lidocaine should show bright echoes filling the posterior recess or distributed along the articular cartilage **(Video 24-1).**

The hip is approached similarly in long axis, with the transducer placed over the proximal anterior thigh at the level of the joint[25] (see Fig. 24-4). The approach is similar to that used in evaluating the joint for an effusion. Ideally, the anterior capsule is imaged at the head-neck junction of the femur. In this approach the scan plane is lateral to the neurovascular bundle. The needle may be directed into the joint while maintaining its position in the scan plane of the transducer. A test injection of 1% lidocaine confirms the intra-articular needle position, and the therapeutic injection follows.

Fibrous joints, such as the **acromioclavicular** (AC) joint, can likewise be injected using ultrasound guidance (Fig. 24-8). A short-axis technique is employed similar to that used in the foot. The majority of these injections can be performed using a 1.5-inch needle with a small volume (0.5-1.0 mL) of therapeutic mixture. In addition to the AC joint, this approach is useful in the sternoclavicular joint and pubic symphysis.

SUPERFICIAL PERITENDINOUS AND PERIARTICULAR INJECTIONS

Peritendinous injection of anesthetic and long-acting corticosteroid is an effective means to treat tenosynovitis, bursitis, and ganglion cysts in the hand, foot, and ankle.

These structures are superficially located and well delineated on sonography. Ultrasound-guided injections are an effective means to ensure correct localization of therapeutic agents.

Foot and Ankle

In my experience, peritendinous injections in the foot and ankle are most often requested for patients with chronic **achillodynia** or those with medial or lateral ankle pain caused by posterior tibial or peroneal **tendinosis** or **tenosynovitis.** Less often, patients are referred to help differentiate pain from posterior impingement and stenosing tenosynovitis of the flexor hallucis longus tendon.[26] This distinction can be difficult, sometimes requiring diagnostic and therapeutic injection of the corresponding tendon sheath. Patients with plantar foot pain caused by plantar fasciitis and forefoot pain resulting from painful neuromas are also frequently referred for ultrasound-guided injections.[27,28]

The large majority of patients with achillodynia have pain referable to the enthesis, with associated retrocalcaneal bursitis and Achilles tendinosis. **Enthesis** is the site of attachment of a muscle or ligament to bone where the collagen fibers are mineralized and integrated into bone. A retrocalcaneal bursal injection may help alleviate local pain and inflammation (Fig. 24-9). We scan the patient in a prone position with the ankle in mild dorsiflexion, using a linear transducer of 10 MHz or higher frequency. A 1.5-inch needle usually suffices in these patients, with placement using a short-axis approach. The deep retrocalcaneal bursa is usually well seen. A small amount of anesthetic will help confirm position by active distention of the bursa in real time.

We similarly approach posterior **tibial** or **peroneal** tendons in short axis (Fig. 24-10). Patients with pain in this distribution have been shown to benefit from local

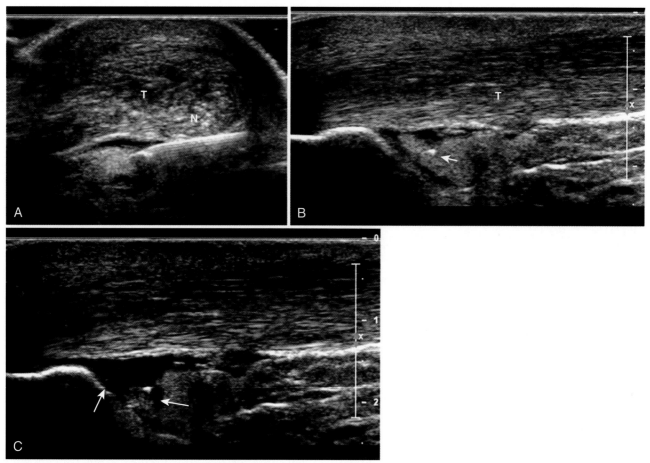

FIGURE 24-9. Retrocalcaneal bursa injection. A, Short-axis view shows Achilles tendon *(T)* in 59-year-old man with retrocalcaneal pain and history of Haglund's deformity. A 25-gauge needle *(N)* enters perpendicular to the tendon's long axis and terminates in a small, retrocalcaneal bursal effusion. **B,** Rotating transducer 90 degrees results in the more typical short-axis view, with the needle *(arrow)* seen in cross section. **C,** While observing in real time, the bursa distends *(arrows)* and fills with echogenic material (contrast effect). The needle is still evident within the distended bursa.

PRE-INJECTION   POST-INJECTION

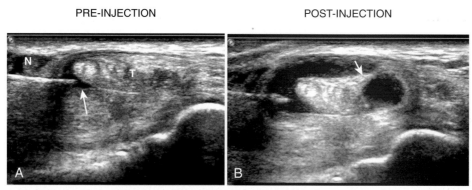

FIGURE 24-10. Tendon sheath injection using short-axis approach. A 17-year-old female patient with medial ankle pain was referred for ultrasound-guided injection of posterior tibial tendon sheath. **A,** Preinjection view shows 25-gauge needle *(N)* within a small, tendon sheath effusion *(long arrow)* in the inframalleolar portion of the tendon *(T)*. The tendon, which is inhomogeneous, is seen in cross section. **B,** Postinjection view shows that the tendon sheath is distended, confirming appropriate deposition of the injected material. Note that the tendon margins are better delineated because of a tenosonographic effect of the injected fluid. The vascular pedicle *(short arrow)* of the tendon is evident.

tendon sheath injections. The presence of preexisting tendon sheath fluid can facilitate needle visualization. However, careful scanning should be done before the procedure to assess the needle trajectory relative to adjacent neurovascular structures. Use of color or power Doppler sonographic imaging can facilitate visualization of the neurovascular bundle. The posterior tibial nerve is closely related to adjacent vascular structures and is usually well seen before bifurcating into medial and lateral plantar branches. Fluid frequently is seen in relation to the posterior tibial tendon, in the submalleolar region. The peroneal tendons are less predictable. Use of power Doppler sonography in conjunction with real-time guidance can help localize areas of inflammation for guided injection. In **stenosing tenosynovitis** the tendons may be surrounded only by a thickened retinaculum, proliferative synovium, or scar tissue. In this case, use of a test injection of local anesthesia can be invaluable to confirm the distribution of the therapeutic agent within the tendon sheath in real time.

The **flexor hallucis longus** (FHL) tendon poses a more challenging problem because of its close relation to the neurovascular bundle of the posterior medial ankle. One helpful feature in performing FHL tendon sheath injections is that tendon sheath effusions tend to localize at the posterior recess of the tibiotalar joint. The neurovascular bundle is easily circumvented by placing the needle lateral to the Achilles tendon while scanning medially (Fig. 24-11). This approach allows flexibility in needle placement while maintaining the needle perpendicular to the insonating beam.

Ultrasound diagnosis of **plantar fasciitis** includes thickening of the medial band of the plantar fascia and fat pad edema. One treatment option for severe plantar fasciitis is regional corticosteroid injection, typically performed using anatomic landmarks. However, "blind" injections into the heel have been associated with rupture of the plantar fascia and failure of the longitudinal arch.[13] Ultrasound can be used to guide a needle along the plantar margin of the fascia, thus avoiding direct intra-fascial injection.[26] The plantar fascia is imaged with the patient prone and the foot mildly dorsiflexed, using a long-axis approach. The transducer is centered over the medial band, which is most often implicated in these patients. A mark is placed over the posterior aspect of the heel and the needle advanced superficial to the plantar fascia, approximately to the margin of the medial tubercle (Fig. 24-12). We perform a perifascial injection using this approach, monitoring the distribution of injected material in real time.

Interdigital (Morton's) neuromas, a common cause of forefoot pain especially in women, have been described at sonography as hypoechoic masses replacing the normal hyperechoic fat in the interdigital web spaces. Occasionally, a dilated hypoechoic tubular structure can be seen associated with the neuroma, reflecting the enlarged feeding interdigital nerve. The second and third web spaces are most often involved. We generally inject Morton's neuromas using a dorsal approach while imaging the neuroma in long axis[28] (Fig. 24-13). This approach is well tolerated by the majority of patients. In certain patients, however, a plantar approach to injecting the nodule is preferred, such as those with severe subluxation at the MTP joint. In either case, the needle is positioned directly within the neuroma and/or adjacent intermetatarsal bursa (if present) and a small volume of therapeutic mixture injected, similar to that used for a small joint injection (0.5 mL).

Hand and Wrist

In the hand and wrist, **de Quervain's tendinosis** is a frequently encountered tendinopathy involving the abductor pollicis longus and extensor pollicis brevis tendons that responds to local administration of anti-inflammatory agents (Fig. 24-14). Injections are also frequently requested for patients with **rheumatoid arthritis** or **psoriatic arthritis.** These patients typically

PRE-INJECTION   POST-INJECTION

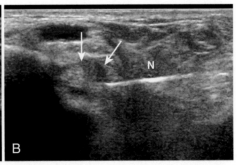

FIGURE 24-11. Flexor hallucis longus (FHL) tendon sheath injection. Short-axis approach with ultrasound guidance in 31-year-old professional dancer with posteromedial ankle pain during plantar flexion. **A,** Preinjection image depicts the tendon *(T)* at the level of the posterior sulcus of the talus *(TA).* The arrows show relationship of the tendon to the neurovascular structures. **B,** Postinjection image depicts 25-gauge needle *(N)* situated within the distended tendon sheath *(arrows)* below the neurovascular structures.

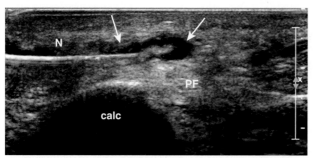

FIGURE 24-12. Plantar fascia injection. The proximal medial band of the plantar fascia *(PF)* is thickened and inhomogeneous *(arrows)* in a 36-year-old man with hindfoot pain; *calc,* calcaneus. A 25-gauge needle *(N)* has been positioned superficial to this plantar fascia and a perifascial injection performed. The injected material *(arrows)* loculates along the superficial margin of the medial band.

experience severe tenosynovitis, which can lead to secondary tendon rupture and deformity. The approach is similar to that used for superficial structures in the foot and ankle. A short-axis approach avoids the surrounding neurovascular structures, and the corresponding tendon sheaths are injected.

INJECTION OF DEEP TENDONS

Frequently requested deep tendon injections include those for the bicipital tendon sheath, iliopsoas tendon, gluteal tendon insertion onto the greater trochanter, and hamstring tendon origin.

PRE-INJECTION   POST-INJECTION

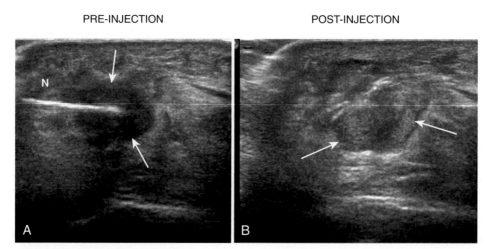

FIGURE 24-13. Morton's neuroma injection. A, Preinjection image shows 25-gauge needle *(N)* positioned in a third web space neuroma using a dorsal approach in 45-year-old woman with forefoot pain. Neuroma appears as a heterogeneous hypoechoic nodule *(arrows)* within the normal echogenic fat. **B,** After injection and needle removal, the nodule appears expanded and echogenic *(arrows).* The injected material often decompresses into an adjacent adventitial bursa, which frequently accompanies these nodules.

PRE-INJECTION   POST-INJECTION

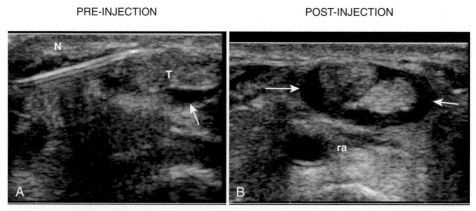

FIGURE 24-14. Injection of first dorsal compartment of wrist. This 70-year-old woman with de Quervain's tendinosis had clinical symptoms of wrist pain radiating along the extensor surface of the forearm. **A,** Preinjection image shows 25-gauge needle *(N)* positioned in the first dorsal compartment tendon sheath under ultrasound guidance. The tendons *(T)* are inhomogeneous, with a small effusion evident *(arrows)* in the dependent part of the tendon sheath. **B,** After injection and needle removal, the injected material distends the sheath *(arrows),* producing a tenosonographic effect; the intrinsic tendon abnormalities become more conspicuous; *ra,* radial artery.

PRE-INJECTION   POST-INJECTION

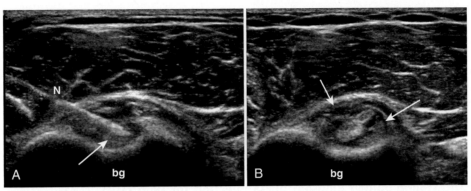

FIGURE 24-15. Biceps tendon sheath injection. Biceps tendinosis is clinically suspected and a biceps tendon sheath injection requested for this 41-year-old man with development of anterior shoulder pain after arthroscopic surgery for labral tear. **A,** Preinjection image shows 25-gauge needle *(N)* placed superficial to the long head of the biceps tendon *(arrow); bg,* bicipital groove. **B,** After injection and needle removal, there is distension of the tendon sheath by fluid *(arrows)* containing low-level echoes caused by contrast effect.

Biceps Tendon

Anterior shoulder pain with radiation into the arm may be secondary to bicipital tendinitis or tenosynovitis.[29] The biceps tendon can be palpated, but if nondistended, the sheath may offer less than 2 mm of clearance to place a needle. This is complicated by the caudal extension of the subacromial subdeltoid bursa, which may overlie the bicipital tendon sheath. A non-image-guided injection could therefore result in delivery into an extratendinous synovial space, or possibly result in an intratendinous injection. We have found that ultrasound guidance enables localization of therapeutic agent to the biceps tendon sheath.[10]

The patient is placed recumbent with the forearm supinated and the shoulder mildly elevated. The bicipital groove is oriented anteriorly. A linear transducer, typically 7.5 MHz, is used with a lateral approach and 25- or 22-gauge needle (Fig. 24-15). The long head of the biceps tendon is scanned in short axis. When fluid distends the bicipital tendon sheath, the tip is directed into the fluid. Otherwise, the needle is directed along the superficial margin of the tendon, and a test injection of local anesthetic is used to confirm local distention of the sheath, which is then followed by administration of the long-acting corticosteroid. The presence of fluid distention of the sheath with superficially located microbubbles helps to confirm a successful injection.

Iliopsoas Tendon

The iliopsoas tendon lies superficial to and along the medial margin of the anterior capsule of the hip. The tendon inserts onto the lesser trochanter. A bursa that frequently communicates with the hip is seen in this location and may be distended because of underling joint pathology or a primary iliopsoas bursitis. Alternatively, iliopsoas tendinosis may occur in the absence of a pre-existing bursitis for which a peritendinous injection

is requested.[30] A lateral approach to the tendon often requires use of a lower-frequency transducer and curved linear or sector geometry. The neurovascular bundle lies medial and superficial to the tendon, so it is advantageous to approach from the lateral margin of the tendon and perform a small test injection to confirm needle position. A successful injection will show the appearance of fluid or microbubbles distending a bursa that follows the course of the long axis of the tendon (Fig. 24-16).

BURSAL AND GANGLION CYST INJECTIONS

Distended bursae around tendinous insertions provide anatomic localization for therapeutic agents. Injection of these areas is often requested for the patient with localized **bursitis** and abnormality of the adjacent tendon. Examples include the retrocalcaneal, iliopsoas, greater trochanteric, and ischial bursae (Fig. 24-17). Alternatively, the presence of a bursitis, distended synovial cyst, or ganglion cyst may cause mechanical impingement of adjacent tendons. The decompression of these cysts with subsequent administration of a therapeutic agent may alleviate these symptoms[31,32] (Fig. 24-18). Ultrasound guidance allows the clinician to avoid intratendinous injections as well as adjacent neurovascular structures. Furthermore, the needle may be redirected as necessary in the presence of a multiloculated cyst (Fig. 24-19).

Calcific Tendinitis

The presence of symptomatic intratendinous calcification involves the deposition of **calcium hydroxyapatite.** This often appears as a nodular echogenic mass within the tendon, which may or may not display posterior acoustic shadowing.[33] Although most often affecting the shoulder, this may occur elsewhere in the musculo-

PRE-INJECTION   POST-INJECTION

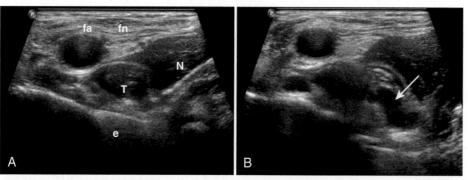

FIGURE 24-16. Ultrasound-guided iliopsoas bursa injection for pain relief. This 66-year-old woman with a total hip arthroplasty had developed pain with hip flexion. **A,** Preinjection image shows 22-gauge spinal needle *(N)* positioned deep to the tendon *(T)* at the level of the iliopectineal eminence *(e),* using a short-axis approach; *fa,* femoral artery; *fn,* femoral nerve. **B,** After injection and needle removal, fluid surrounds the tendon within the distended iliopsoas bursa *(arrow).*

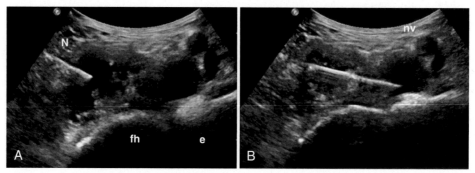

FIGURE 24-17. Ultrasound-guided aspiration and injection of multiloculated iliopsoas bursa. A, Image shows 22-gauge spinal needle *(N)* positioned into the lateral component of the bursa in 65-year-old woman with groin pain; *fh,* femoral head; *e,* iliopectineal eminence. **B,** After aspiration of the lateral component, the needle has been advanced into the medial component for aspiration and subsequent injection with therapeutic mixture; *nv,* neurovascular structures.

PRE-INJECTION   POST-INJECTION

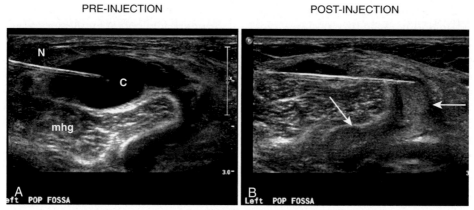

FIGURE 24-18. Ultrasound-guided aspiration and injection of clinically suspected Baker's cyst. A, Preinjection image shows 22-gauge needle *(N)* positioned in the cyst *(C)* under ultrasound guidance in 59-year-old woman with posterior knee pain and swelling; *mhg,* medial head of gastrocnemius muscle. **B,** After cyst aspiration and injection of the therapeutic mixture, the anechoic fluid is replaced by echogenic fluid resulting from contrast effect *(arrows).*

skeletal system. Ultrasound-guided fragmentation and lavage have been described as an excellent method to reduce the level of calcification and to deposit therapeutic agents.[34-37] We currently employ a single-needle technique, with the needle acting as inflow for anesthetic/ sterile saline and as an outflow for the calcium solution (Fig. 24-20). The elasticity of the pseudocapsule encasing the calcification is sufficient to decompress the calcific mass in the majority of cases **(Video 24-2).** After multiple lavages, the needle is used to inject anesthetic

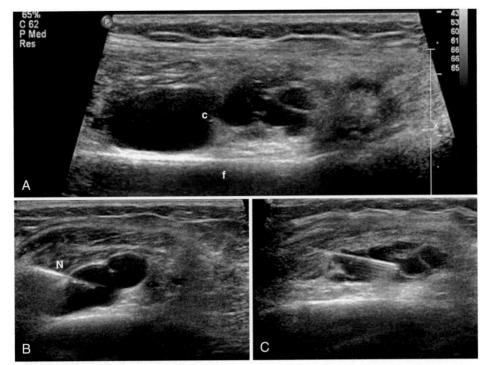

FIGURE 24-19. Ultrasound-guided aspiration and injection of multiloculated ganglion cyst. A, Baseline sonogram shows a multiloculated cyst *(c)* within the vastus lateralis muscle of the left knee and superficial to the lateral margin of the femur *(f)* in 41-year-old woman. **B,** 20-gauge spinal needle *(N)* was initially positioned into the proximal component of the cyst; **C,** Subsequently, the needle was redirected into the distal component. Multiple lavages and aspiration enabled complete decompression of the cyst (not shown).

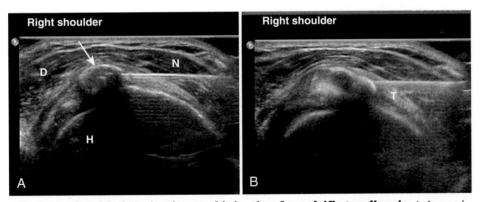

FIGURE 24-20. Ultrasound-guided aspiration and injection for calcific tendinosis. A, Image shows 20-gauge spinal needle *(N)* positioned into the calcification *(arrow)* under ultrasound guidance in 42-year-old man with shoulder pain; *H,* humeral head; *D,* deltoid. **B,** Series of repeat lavage and aspirations of the calcification are performed with the calcification eventually largely replaced by fluid contents within the surrounding pseudocapsule of the calcific mass; *T,* rotator cuff tendons. Notice that the degree of posterior acoustic shadowing has diminished, and that the center of the calcification *(arrow on* **A***)* is partially replaced by fluid. After numerous lavages, the calcification is typically fenestrated, and a therapeutic mixture is injected and often decompresses into the subdeltoid bursa (not shown).

and anti-inflammatory mixture. The injected mixture is distributed within the calcification and adjacent subdeltoid bursa in most cases. If the calcification is too small or fragmented, precluding lavage and decompression, the single needle is used to fenestrate the calcium deposit, and a peritendinous therapeutic injection has been shown to be effective.

INTRATENDINOUS INJECTIONS: PERCUTANEOUS TENOTOMY

Recent literature suggests that image guidance can be useful for performing percutaneous tenotomy and intratendinous injections with either autologous blood or platelet-rich plasma (PRP).[38-42] All these methods are

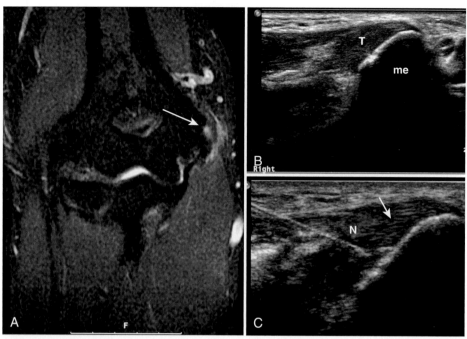

FIGURE 24-21. Ultrasound-guided injection of autologous blood to induce healing response. A, Coronal inversion-recovery MR scan of the affected elbow in 43-year-old man with medial epicondylitis shows increased signal intensity *(arrow)* of the common flexor tendon mass and adjacent collateral ligament. **B,** Long-axis ultrasound image of the tendon *(T)* and adjacent medial epicondyle *(me)* shows that tendon is predominantly hypoechoic, reflecting underlying tendinosis. **C,** Image shows 22-gauge needle *(N)* placed within the common flexor tendon mass, for purposes of mechanical fenestration, and injection of 5 mL of autologous blood, obtained from an antecubital vein. Tendon echogenicity *(small arrow)* is increased by microbubbles within the injected blood.

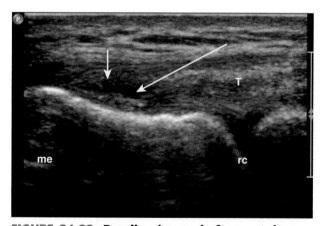

FIGURE 24-22. Baseline image before autologous blood injection. Common extensor tendon mass *(T)* in 50-year-old woman with partial tear of the deep portion of the tendon *(short arrow, extensor carpi radialis brevis)* as it inserts on the medial epicondyle *(me); rc,* radiocapitellar joint; *long arrow,* plane of needle entry for percutaneous tenotomy and autologous blood injection. (Same patient is shown in Video 24-3.)

associated with secondary release of local growth factors, such as platelet-derived growth factor (PDGF), which in turn may produce a direct healing response.[41] Preliminary data show significant promise in promoting ultrasound-guided tendon repair. "Dry needling" techniques have been employed successfully in patients with lateral epicondylitis refractory to other conservative measures.[38] Likewise, autologous blood injections and PRP injec-

tions have been successfully used in both the elbow and the knee[39-41] (Figs. 24-21 and 24-22; **Video 24-3**). The advantage of performing these injections under ultrasound guidance becomes evident when the clinician wants to generalize such techniques to include tendons close to neurovascular structures, such as the hamstring tendon origin.

CONCLUSION

Ultrasound offers distinct advantages in providing guidance for delivery of therapeutic injections. Most importantly, ultrasound allows the operator to visualize the needle and make adjustments in real time, to ensure that medication is delivered to the appropriate location. The current generation of ultrasound scanners provides excellent depiction of relevant musculoskeletal anatomy. The needle has a unique sonographic appearance and can be monitored with real-time imaging, as can the steroid-anesthetic mixture. Given these advantages, ultrasound guidance should become the method of choice to perform a large variety of guided musculoskeletal interventions.

References

1. Christensen RA, Van Sonnenberg E, Casola G, Wittich GR. Interventional ultrasound in the musculoskeletal system. Radiol Clin North Am 1988;26:145-156.

2. Cunnane G, Brophy DP, Gibney RG, FitzGerald O. Diagnosis and treatment of heel pain in chronic inflammatory arthritis using ultrasound. Semin Arthritis Rheum 1996;25:383-389.

3. Brophy DP, Cunnane G, Fitzgerald O, Gibney RG. Technical report: ultrasound guidance for injection of soft tissue lesions around the heel in chronic inflammatory arthritis. Clin Radiol 1995;50:120-122.

4. Cardinal E, Chhem RK, Beauregard CG. Ultrasound-guided interventional procedures in the musculoskeletal system. Radiol Clin North Am 1998;36:597-604.

5. Koski JM. Ultrasound-guided injections in rheumatology. J Rheumatol 2000;27:2131-2138.

6. Grassi W, Farina A, Filippucci E, Cervini C. Sonographically guided procedures in rheumatology. Semin Arthritis Rheum 2001;30:347-353.

7. Sofka CM, Collins AJ, Adler RS. Use of ultrasonographic guidance in interventional musculoskeletal procedures: a review from a single institution. J Ultrasound Med 2001;20:21-26.

8. Sofka CM, Adler RS. Ultrasound-guided interventions in the foot and ankle. Semin Musculoskelet Radiol 2002;6:163-168.

9. Adler RS, Sofka CM. Percutaneous ultrasound-guided injections in the musculoskeletal system. Ultrasound Q 2003;19:3-12.

10. Adler RS, Allen A. Percutaneous ultrasound-guided injections in the shoulder. Tech Shoulder Elbow Surg 2004;5(2):122-133.

11. Unverferth LJ, Olix ML. The effect of local steroid injections on tendon. J Sports Med 1973;1:31-37.

12. Ford LT, DeBender J. Tendon rupture after local steroid injection. South Med J 1979;72:827-830.

13. Gottlieb NL, Riskin WG. Complications of local corticosteroid injections. JAMA 1980;243:1547-1548.

14. Oxlund H, Manthorpe R. The biochemical properties of tendon and skin as influenced by long-term glucocorticoid treatment and food restriction. Biorheology 1982;19:631-646.

15. Stapczynski JS. Localized depigmentation after steroid injection of a ganglion cyst on the hand. Ann Emerg Med 1991;20:807-809.

16. Shrier I, Matheson GO, Kohl 3rd HW. Achilles tendonitis: are corticosteroid injections useful or harmful? Clin J Sport Med 1996;6:245-250.

17. Bouffard JA, Eyler WR, Introcaso JH, van Holsbeeck M. Sonography of tendons. Ultrasound Q 1993;11:259-286.

18. Koski JM, Saarakkala SJ, Heikkinen JO, Hermunen HS. Use of air-steroid-saline mixture as contrast medium in greyscale ultrasound imaging: experimental study and practical applications in rheumatology. Clin Exp Rheumatol 2005;23:373-378.

19. Luchs JS, Sofka CM, Adler RS. Sonographic contrast effect of combined steroid and anesthetic injections: in vitro analysis. J Ultrasound Med 2007;26:227-231.

Injection Materials

20. Curatolo M, Bogduk N. Pharmacologic pain treatment of musculoskeletal disorders: current perspectives and future prospects. Clin J Pain 2001;17:25-32.

21. Caldwell JR. Intra-articular corticosteroids: guide to selection and indications for use. Drugs 1996;52:507-514.

22. Kannus P, Jarvinen M, Niittymaki S. Long- or short-acting anesthetic with corticosteroid in local injections of overuse injuries? A prospective, randomized, double-blind study. Int J Sports Med 1990;11:397-400.

23. Cox B, Durieux ME, Marcus MA. Toxicity of local anaesthetics. Best Pract Res Clin Anaesthesiol 2003;17:111-136.

24. Gomoll AH, Kang RW, Williams JM, et al. Chondrolysis after continuous intra-articular bupivacaine infusion: an experimental model investigating chondrotoxicity in the rabbit shoulder. Arthroscopy 2006;22:813-819.

Injection of Joints

25. Sofka CM, Saboeiro G, Adler RS. Ultrasound-guided adult hip injections. J Vasc Interv Radiol 2005;16:1121-1123.

Superficial Peritendinous and Periarticular Injections

26. Mehdizade A, Adler RS. Sonographically guided flexor hallucis longus tendon sheath injection. J Ultrasound Med 2007;26:233-237.

27. Tsai WC, Wang CL, Tang FT, et al. Treatment of proximal plantar fasciitis with ultrasound-guided steroid injection. Arch Phys Med Rehabil 2000;81:1416-1421.

28. Sofka CM, Adler RS, Ciavarra GA, Pavlov H. Ultrasound-guided interdigital neuroma injections: short-term clinical outcomes after a single percutaneous injection—preliminary results. HSS J 2007;3:44-49.

Injection of Deep Tendons

29. Middleton WD, Reinus WR, Totty WG, et al. Ultrasound of the biceps tendon apparatus. Radiology 1985;157:211-215.

30. Adler RS, Buly R, Ambrose R, Sculco T. Diagnostic and therapeutic use of sonography-guided iliopsoas peritendinous injections. AJR Am J Roentgenol 2005;185:940-943.

Bursal and Ganglion Cyst Injections

31. Breidahl WH, Adler RS. Ultrasound-guided injection of ganglia with corticosteroids. Skeletal Radiol 1996;25:635-638.

32. Chiou HJ, Chou YH, Wu JJ, et al. Alternative and effective treatment of shoulder ganglion cyst: ultrasonographically guided aspiration. J Ultrasound Med 1999;18:531-535.

33. Farin PU, Jaroma H. Sonographic findings of rotator cuff calcifications. J Ultrasound Med 1995;14:7-14.

34. Farin PU, Jaroma H, Soimakallio S. Rotator cuff calcifications: treatment with ultrasound-guided technique. Radiology 1995;195:841-843.

35. Farin PU, Rasanen H, Jaroma H, Harju A. Rotator cuff calcifications: treatment with ultrasound-guided percutaneous needle aspiration and lavage. Skeletal Radiol 1996;25:551-554.

36. Aina R, Cardinal E, Bureau NJ, et al. Calcific shoulder tendinitis: treatment with modified ultrasound-guided fine-needle technique. Radiology 2001;221:455-461.

37. Lin JT, Adler RS, Bracilovic A, et al. Clinical outcomes of ultrasound-guided aspiration and lavage in calcific tendinosis of the shoulder. HSS J 2007;3:99-105.

Intratendinous Injections: Percutaneous Tenotomy

38. McShane JM, Nazarian LN, Harwood MI. Sonographically guided percutaneous needle tenotomy for treatment of common extensor tendinosis in the elbow. J Ultrasound Med 2006;25:1281-1289.

39. James SL, Ali K, Pocock C, et al. Ultrasound-guided dry needling and autologous blood injection for patellar tendinosis. Br J Sports Med 2007;41:518-521; discussion 522.

40. Connell DA, Ali KE, Ahmad M, et al. Ultrasound-guided autologous blood injection for tennis elbow. Skeletal Radiol 2006;35:371-377.

41. Mishra A, Pavelko T. Treatment of chronic elbow tendinosis with buffered platelet-rich plasma. Am J Sports Med 2006;34:1774-1778.

42. Gamradt SC, Rodeo SC, Warren RF. Platelet-rich plasma in rotator cuff repair. Tech Orthop 2007;22:26-33.

CHAPTER 25

The Extracranial Cerebral Vessels

Edward I. Bluth and Barbara A. Carroll

Chapter Outline

$\mathcal{S}$troke secondary to atherosclerotic disease is the third leading cause of death in the United States. Many stroke victims survive the catastrophic event with some degree of neurologic impairment.[1] More than 500,000 new cases of cerebrovascular accident (CVA, stroke) are reported annually.[2] Ischemia from severe, flow-limiting stenosis caused by atherosclerotic disease involving the extracranial carotid arteries is implicated in 20% to 30% of strokes.[2] An estimated 80% of CVAs are thromboembolic in origin, often with carotid plaque as the embolic source.[3]

Carotid atherosclerotic plaque with resultant stenosis usually involves the **internal carotid artery** (ICA) within 2 cm of the carotid bifurcation. This location is readily amenable to examination by sonography as well as surgical intervention. **Carotid endarterectomy** (CEA) initially proved to be more beneficial than medical therapy in symptomatic patients with carotid stenoses of more than 70%, as reported in the **North American Symptomatic Carotid Endarterectomy Trial** (NASCET) and the **European Carotid Surgery Trial** (ECST).[4,5]

Subsequent NASCET results for moderate stenoses have shown a net benefit for surgical intervention with carotid narrowing between 50% and 69% of vessel diameter. A 15.7% reduction in the 5-year ipsilateral stroke rate was seen in patients treated surgically, versus 22.2% stroke reduction in those treated medically. These results are not as compelling as those for the higher

degree of stenosis seen in the earlier NASCET trial. The benefit from surgery was greatest in men, patients with recent stroke, and those with hemispheric symptoms. In addition, the NASCET trials dealing with moderate carotid stenoses required rigorous surgical expertise, such that the risks for disabling stroke or death should not exceed 2% to achieve the statistical surgical benefit.[6] The **Asymptomatic Carotid Atherosclerosis Study** (ACAS) trials published in 1995 reported a reduction in ipsilateral stroke in asymptomatic patients with greater than 60% ICA stenoses who undergo CEA.[2] However, these results were less clear-cut than the NASCET trials.

Accurate diagnosis of carotid stenosis clearly is critical to identify patients who would benefit from surgical treatment. In addition, ultrasound can assess plaque morphology, such as determining heterogeneous or homogeneous plaque, known to be an independent risk factor for stroke and **transient ischemic attack** (TIA).

Over the past two decades, carotid sonography has largely replaced angiography as the principal screening method for suspected extracranial carotid atherosclerotic disease. Gray-scale examination, color Doppler, power Doppler, and pulsed Doppler imaging techniques are routinely employed in the evaluation of patients with neurologic symptoms and suspected extracranial cerebral disease.[7]

Ultrasound is an inexpensive, noninvasive, and highly accurate method of diagnosing carotid stenosis.

INDICATIONS FOR CAROTID ULTRASOUND

Evaluation of patients with hemispheric neurologic symptoms, including stroke, transient ischemic attack, and amaurosis fugax.
Evaluation of patients with a carotid bruit.
Evaluation of pulsatile neck masses.
Preoperative evaluation of patients scheduled for major cardiovascular surgical procedures.
Evaluation of nonhemispheric or unexplained neurologic symptoms.
Follow-up of patients with proven carotid disease.
Evaluation of patients after carotid revascularization, including stenting.
Intraoperative monitoring of vascular surgery.
Evaluation of suspected subclavian steal syndrome.
Evaluation of a potential source of retinal emboli.
Follow-up of carotid dissection.
Follow-up of radiation therapy to the neck in select patients.

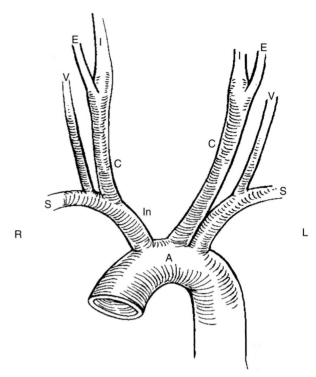

FIGURE 25-1. Branches of aortic arch and extracranial cerebral arteries. *R,* Right side; *L,* left side; *A,* aortic arch; *C,* common carotid artery; *E,* external carotid artery; *In,* innominate artery; *I,* internal carotid artery; *S,* subclavian artery; *V,* vertebral artery.

Angiography is an expensive, invasive test with potential morbidity, which is why reliance on carotid sonography without preoperative angiography is becoming increasingly common. **Magnetic resonance angiography** (MRA) and computed tomography (CT) are additional noninvasive screening tools for the identification of carotid bifurcation disease as well as for clarification of ultrasound findings. Angiography is often now reserved for those patients for whom the ultrasound or MRA was equivocal or inadequate.

Other carotid ultrasound applications include the evaluation of carotid bruits, monitoring the progression of known atherosclerotic disease,[7-9] assessment during or after CEA or stent placement,[10] preoperative screening prior to major vascular surgery, and evaluation after the detection of retinal cholesterol emboli.[7] Also, **nonatherosclerotic carotid diseases** can be evaluated, including follow-up of carotid dissection,[11-15] examination of fibromuscular dysplasia or Takayasu's arteritis, assessment of malignant carotid artery invasion,[16,17] and workup of pulsatile neck masses and carotid body tumors.[18,19]

CAROTID ARTERY ANATOMY

The first major branch of the aortic arch is the innominate or brachiocephalic artery, which divides into the right subclavian artery and right **common carotid artery** (CCA). The second major branch is the left CCA, which is generally separate from the third major branch, the left subclavian artery (Fig. 25-1).

The right and left CCAs ascend into the neck posterolateral to the thyroid gland and lie deep to the jugular vein and sternocleidomastoid muscle. The CCAs have different proximal configurations, with the right originating at the bifurcation of the innominate (brachiocephalic) artery into the common carotid and subclavian arteries. The left CCA usually originates directly from the aortic arch but often arises with the brachiocephalic trunk. This is known as a "bovine arch" configuration. The CCA usually has no branches in its cervical region. Occasionally, however, it may give off the superior thyroid artery, vertebral artery, ascending pharyngeal artery, and occipital or inferior thyroid artery. At the carotid bifurcation, the CCA divides into the **external carotid artery** (ECA) and the **internal carotid artery** (ICA). The ICA usually has no branching vessels in the neck. The ECA, which supplies the facial musculature, has multiple branches in the neck. The ICA may demonstrate an ampullary region of mild dilation just beyond its origin.

CAROTID ULTRASOUND EXAMINATION

Carotid artery ultrasound examinations are performed with the patient supine, the neck slightly extended, and the head turned away from the side being examined. Some operators prefer to perform the examination at the patient's side, whereas others prefer to sit at the patient's head. The examination sequence also varies

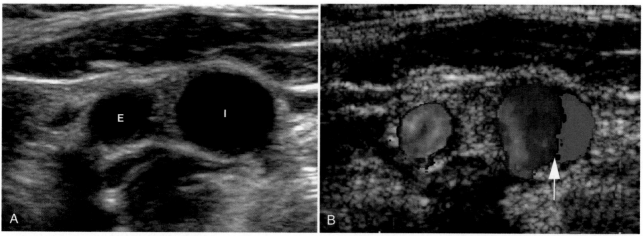

FIGURE 25-2. Carotid sonographic anatomy. A, Transverse image of the left carotid bifurcation. The larger, more lateral vessel is the internal carotid artery *(I); E,* external carotid artery. **B,** Color Doppler shows normal flow separation *(arrow)* in the proximal internal carotid artery.

with operator preference. This sequence includes the gray-scale examination, Doppler spectral analysis, and color Doppler blood flow interrogations. Power Doppler sonography may or may not be employed. A 5 to 12–MHz transducer is used for gray-scale imaging and a 3 to 7–MHz transducer for Doppler sonography; the choice depends on the patient's body habitus and technical characteristics of the ultrasound machine. Color Doppler flow imaging and power Doppler imaging may be performed with 5 to 10–MHz transducers. In cases of critical stenosis, the Doppler parameters should be optimized to detect extremely slow flow.

Gray-scale sonographic examination begins in the transverse projection. Scans are obtained along the entire course of the cervical carotid artery, from the supraclavicular notch cephalad to the angle of the mandible (Fig. 25-2). Inferior angulation of the transducer in the supraclavicular area images the CCA origin. The left CCA origin is deeper and more difficult to image consistently than the right. The **carotid bulb** is identified as a mild widening of the CCA near the bifurcation. Transverse views of the **carotid bifurcation** establish the orientation of the external and internal carotid arteries and help define the optimal longitudinal plane in which to perform Doppler spectral analysis. When the transverse ultrasound images demonstrate occlusive atherosclerotic disease, the percentage of "diameter stenosis" or "area stenosis" can be calculated directly using electronic calipers and software analytic algorithms available on most duplex equipment.

After transverse imaging, longitudinal scans of the carotid artery are obtained. The examination plane necessary for optimal longitudinal scans is determined by the course of the vessels demonstrated on the transverse study. In some patients the optimal longitudinal orientation will be nearly coronal, whereas in others it will be almost sagittal. In most cases the optimal longitudinal scan plane will be oblique, between sagittal and coronal.

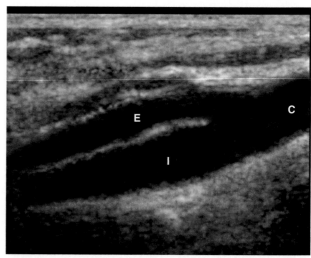

FIGURE 25-3. Carotid bifurcation. Longitudinal image demonstrates common carotid artery *(C);* external carotid artery *(E);* and large, posterior internal carotid artery *(I).*

In approximately 60% of patients, both vessels above the carotid bifurcation and the CCA can be imaged in the same plane (Fig. 25-3); in the remainder, only a single vessel will be imaged in the same plane as the CCA. Images are obtained to display the relationship of both branches of the carotid bifurcation to the visualized plaque disease, and the cephalocaudal extent of the plaque is measured. Several anatomic features differentiate the ICA from the ECA. In about 95% of patients, the ICA is posterior and lateral to the ECA. This may vary considerably, however,[10] and the ICA may be medial to the ECA in 3% to 9% of people. The ICA frequently has an ampullary region of dilation just beyond its origin and is usually larger than the ECA. One reliable distinguishing feature of the ECA is its **branching vessels** (Fig. 25-4, *A*).

The **superior thyroid artery** is often seen as the first branch of the ECA after the bifurcation of the CCA.

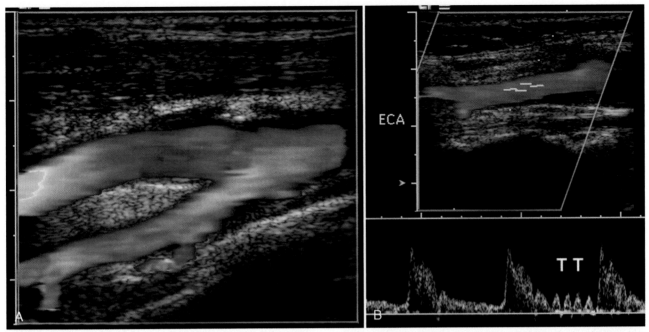

FIGURE 25-4. Normal external carotid artery (ECA). A, Color Doppler ultrasound of bifurcation demonstrates two small arteries originating from the ECA. **B,** ECA spectral Doppler shows the anticipated serrated (sawtooth) flow disturbance from the temporal artery tap *(TT)*.

Occasionally, an aberrant superior thyroid artery branch will arise from the distal CCA. The ICA usually has no branches in the neck, although rarely the ICA gives rise to the ascending pharyngeal, occipital, facial, laryngeal, or meningeal arteries. In some patients, a considerable amount of the ICA will be visible, but in others, only the immediate origin of the vessel will be accessible. Very rarely, the bifurcation may not be visible at all.[19] Rarely, the ICA may be hypoplastic or congenitally absent.[20] A useful method to identify the ECA is the tapping of the superficial temporal artery in the preauricular area, the **temporal tap** (TT). The pulsations are transmitted back to the ECA, where they cause a **sawtooth** appearance on the spectral waveform (Fig. 25-4, *B*). Although the tap helps identify the ECA, this tap deflection may be transmitted into the CCA and even the ICA in certain rare situations.

CAROTID ULTRASOUND INTERPRETATION

Each facet of the carotid sonographic examination is valuable in the final determination of the presence and extent of disease. In most cases the gray-scale, color Doppler, and power Doppler sonographic images and assessments will agree. However, when there are discrepancies between Doppler ultrasound and information, every attempt should be made to discover the source of the disagreement. The more closely the image and Doppler findings correlate, the higher the degree of confidence in the diagnosis. Generally, gray-scale and color

or power Doppler images better demonstrate and quantify low-grade stenoses, whereas high-grade occlusive disease is more accurately defined by Doppler spectral analysis. For **plaque** characterization, assessment must be made in gray scale only, without color or power Doppler ultrasound.

Visual Inspection of Gray-Scale Images

Vessel Wall Thickness and Intima-Media Thickening

Longitudinal views of the layers of the normal carotid wall demonstrate **two nearly parallel echogenic lines,** separated by a hypoechoic to anechoic region (Fig. 25-5). The first echo, bordering the vessel lumen, represents the lumen-intima interface; the second echo is caused by the media-adventitia interface. The media is the anechoic/hypoechoic zone between the echogenic lines. The distance between these lines represents the combined thickness of the **intima and media (I-M complex).** The far wall of the CCA is measured. Many consider measurement of **intima-media thickness** (IMT) to be a surrogate marker for atherosclerotic disease in the *whole* arterial system, not only the cerebrovascular system. Some believe that thickening of the I-M complex greater than 0.8 mm is abnormal and may represent the earliest changes of atherosclerotic disease. However, because thickness of the I-M increases with age, absolute measurements of IMT for any given person may not be a reliable indicator of atherosclerotic risk factors[21] (Fig. 25-6).

Numerous studies support the relationship between IMT and increased risk for myocardial infarction or stroke in asymptomatic patient populations.[14,22-29] IMT may be superior to the coronary artery calcification score for identifying patients at high risk for these cardiovascular events.[14] Assessment of IMT has been advocated as a means of assessing effectiveness of medical interventions to reduce the progression of I-M thickening or even reverse carotid wall thickening. Whether these measurements have validity for assessment of an individual patient versus large groups of patients remains controversial. Studies demonstrating the accuracy of interobserver variability, reproducibility, and precision are needed before IMT assessment can be advocated for individual patient management.

Plaque Characterization

Atheromatous carotid plaques should be carefully evaluated to determine plaque extent, location, surface contour, and texture, as well as to assess luminal stenosis.[30] The plaque should be scanned and evaluated in both the sagittal and the transverse projections.[31] The most common cause of TIAs is **embolism,** not flow-limiting stenosis; less than half of patients with documented TIA have hemodynamically significant stenosis. It is important to identify low-grade atherosclerotic lesions that may contain hemorrhage or ulceration, which can serve as a nidus for emboli that cause both TIAs and stroke.[1] Polak et al.[32] showed that plaque is an independent risk factor for developing a stroke.[32] Of patients with hemispheric stroke symptoms, 50% to 70% demonstrate hemorrhagic or ulcerated plaque. Plaque analysis of CEA specimens has implicated intraplaque hemorrhage as an important factor in the development of neurologic symptoms.[33-39] However, the relationship between sonographic plaque morphology and the onset of symptoms is controversial.

Plaque texture is generally classified as homogeneous or heterogeneous.* The accurate evaluation of plaque can only be made with gray-scale ultrasound, without the use of color or power Doppler. The plaque must be evaluated in both sagittal and transverse planes.[31]

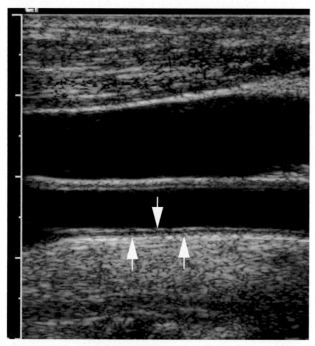

FIGURE 25-5. Normal intima-media (I-M) complex of common carotid artery. The I-M complex *(arrows)* is seen in a left common carotid artery.

---

*References 9, 24, 27, 30, 31, 33-35, 40-44.

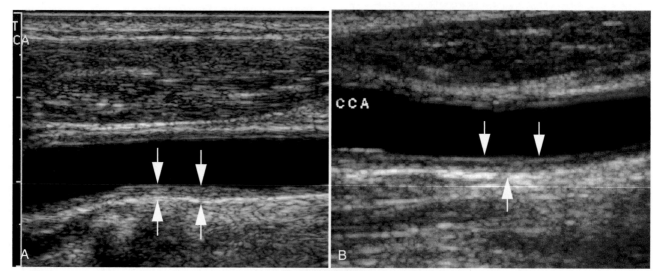

FIGURE 25-6. Abnormal intima-media complex of common carotid artery (CCA). A, Early I-M hyperplasia with loss of the hypoechoic component of the I-M complex and thickening *(arrows).* **B,** Thickening of the I-M complex with hyperplasia *(arrows).*

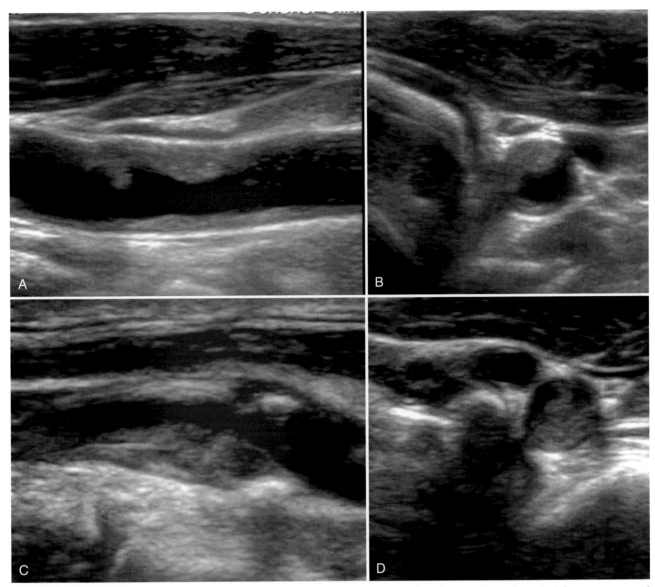

FIGURE 25-7. Homogeneous plaque. A, Sagittal, and **B,** transverse, images show homogeneous plaque in left common carotid artery (type 4). Note the uniform echo texture. **C,** Sagittal, and **D,** transverse, images show homogeneous plaque in proximal left internal carotid artery (type 3). Note the focal hypoechoic area within the plaque, estimated at less than 50% of plaque volume.

Homogeneous plaque has a generally uniform echo pattern and a smooth surface (Fig. 25-7). Sonolucent areas may be seen, but the amount of sonolucency is less than 50% of the plaque volume. The uniform acoustic texture corresponds pathologically to **dense fibrous connective tissue**. **Calcified plaque** produces posterior acoustic shadowing and is common in asymptomatic individuals (Fig. 25-8). **Heterogeneous plaque** has a more complex echo pattern and contains one or more focal sonolucent areas corresponding to more than 50% of the plaque volume (Fig. 25-9). Heterogeneous plaque is characterized pathologically by containing **intraplaque hemorrhage** and deposits of lipid, cholesterol, and proteinaceous material.[10,42] Homogeneous plaque is identified much more often than heterogeneous plaque, occurring in 80% to 85% of patients examined.[32] Sonography accurately determines the presence or absence of

intraplaque hemorrhage (sensitivity, 90%-94%; specificity, 75%-88%).[33,39,42,45-47]

Some sources suggest classifying plaque according to four types. Plaque **types 1 and 2,** similar to heterogeneous plaque and much more likely to be associated

---

ULTRASOUND TYPES OF PLAQUE MORPHOLOGY

Type 1: Predominantly echolucent, with a thin echogenic cap
Type 2: Substantially echolucent with small areas of echogenicity (>50% sonolucent)
Type 3: Predominantly echogenic with small areas of echolucency (<50% sonolucent)
Type 4: Uniformly echogenic

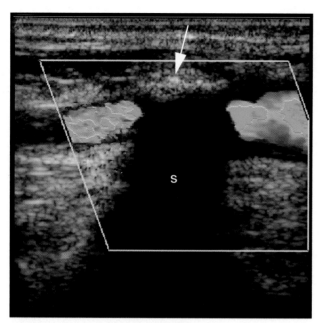

FIGURE 25-8. Calcified plaque. Calcific plaque *(arrow)* produces a shadow *(S)*, which obscures a portion of the left carotid bulb.

with intraplaque hemorrhage and ulceration, are considered unstable and subject to abrupt increases in plaque size after hemorrhage or embolization.[9,31,43,48,49] Types 1 and 2 plaque are typically found in symptomatic patients with stenoses greater than 70% of diameter. Plaque **types 3 and 4** are generally composed of fibrous tissue and calcification. These plaque types are similar to homogeneous plaque. These are generally more benign, stable plaques typically seen in asymptomatic individuals (see Fig. 25-8).

Other methods are being introduced to characterize plaque in a more automated and reproducible manner. Reiter et al.[50] developed a **gray-scale median (GSM) level** for echolucency of plaque after standardizing and adjusting the B-mode images. They obtained standardized GSM levels for asymptomatic patients with greater than 30% stenosis and found that decreasing echolucency of carotid plaques over 6 to 9 months is predictive of major cardiovascular events affecting coronary, peripheral, and cerebrovascular circulation. However, absolute GSM levels were not associated with a specific risk.[50]

Plaque Ulceration

Although ultrasound reportedly detects intraplaque hemorrhage reliably, in general neither angiography nor sonography has proved highly accurate in identifying ulcerated plaque.[48,51] However, virtually all ulcerated plaques that can be accurately identified fit into the heterogeneous pattern.[31,48,51] Sonographic findings that suggest **plaque ulceration** include a focal depression or break in the plaque surface, causing an irregular surface,

or an anechoic area within the plaque that extends to the plaque surface without an intervening echo between the vessel lumen and the anechoic plaque region. Recent studies suggest that color and power Doppler ultrasound may improve sonographic identification of plaque ulceration. Color or power Doppler ultrasound or B-flow imaging (a proprietary non-Doppler imaging technique) may demonstrate slow-moving eddies of color within an anechoic region in plaque, which would suggest ulceration[47] (Fig. 25-10). The demonstration of these flow vortices was 94% accurate in predicting ulcerative plaque at surgery in one study.[52] Preliminary studies suggest that ultrasound contrast agents may further improve the ability to identify plaque surface characteristics.[53]

A potential pitfall in the diagnosis of plaque ulceration may result from a mirror-image artifact producing **pseudoulceration** of the carotid artery. Highly reflective plaque can produce a color Doppler ghost artifact simulating ulceration. However, the region of color within the plaque can be recognized as artifactual because the spectral waveform and color shading within the pseudoulceration are of lower amplitude, but otherwise identical to those within the true carotid lumen.[54] Conversely, pulsed Doppler traces from within **ulcer craters** show low-velocity damped waveforms (Fig. 25-11).

Although the diagnosis of ulceration is controversial, the ability to predict intraplaque hemorrhage reliably, with its associated clinical implications, underscores the importance of ultrasound plaque characterization. The presence of heterogeneous, irregular plaque should be noted because hemorrhagic plaque in a stenosis of less than 50% may be considered a surgical lesion in the appropriate clinical setting. Many now consider heterogeneous plaque to be the "vulnerable," unstable form of plaque that should be treated differently then the more stable homogeneous form of plaque.[55] Plaque characterization should be considered when determining the type of therapy to use in carotid intervention. Angioplasty and subsequent stenting of carotid vessels might be safer if performed in patients with homogeneous plaque than those with heterogeneous plaque.[55]

Gray-Scale Evaluation of Stenosis

Measurements of carotid diameter and area stenosis should be made in the transverse plane, perpendicular to

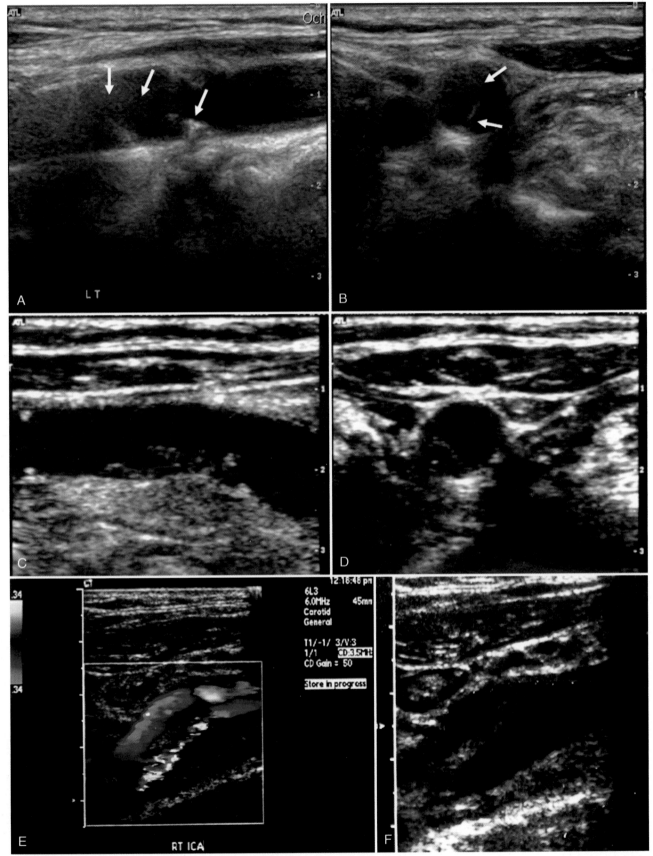

FIGURE 25-9. Heterogeneous plaque in internal carotid artery (ICA). A, Sagittal, and **B,** transverse, images show plaque *(arrows)* virtually completely sonolucent, consistent with heterogeneous plaque (type 1). Note smooth plaque surface. **C,** Sagittal, and **D,** transverse, images show focal sonolucent areas within the plaque greater than 50% of plaque volume, corresponding to heterogeneous plaque (type 2). Note the irregular surface of the plaque. **E,** Sagittal image of the ICA shows heterogeneous sonolucent plaque most evident on color flow duplex imaging by the small, displaced residual lumen. The plaque is completely sonolucent (type 1) and indicative of acute hemorrhage. **F,** On the gray-scale image alone, plaque may be easily overlooked because of the degree of sonolucency.

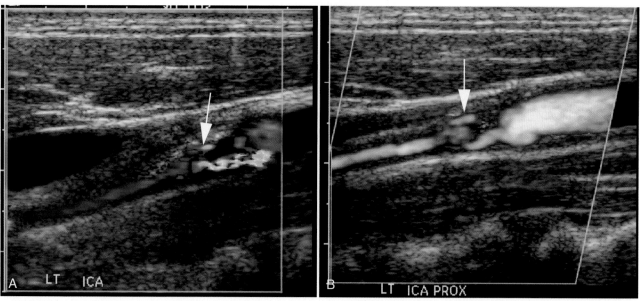

FIGURE 25-10. Plaque ulceration. A, Color Doppler, and **B,** power Doppler, longitudinal images show blood flow *(arrow)* into hypoechoic ulcerated plaque.

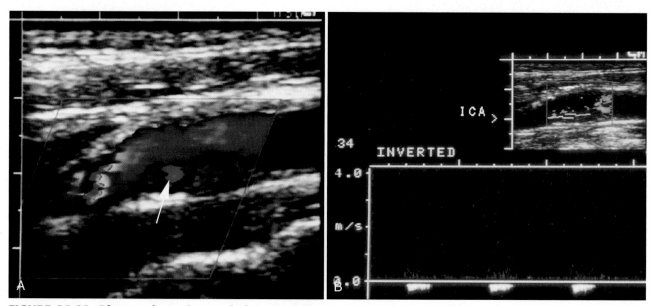

FIGURE 25-11. Plaque ulceration and abnormal flow. A, Longitudinal image of the proximal right internal carotid artery demonstrates heterogeneous plaque with an associated area of reversed low-velocity eddy flow within an ulcer *(arrow).* **B,** Pulsed Doppler waveforms in this ulcer crater demonstrate the extremely damped low-velocity reversed flow, not characteristic of that seen within the main vessel lumen of the ICA.

the long axis of the vessel, using gray-scale, B-flow, or power Doppler sonographic imaging[30] (Fig. 25-12). Measurements made on longitudinal scans may overestimate or underestimate the severity of stenosis by partial "voluming" through an eccentric plaque. The percentage of diameter stenosis and the percentage of area stenosis are not always linearly related. Clinical records should state the type of stenosis measured. Asymmetrical stenoses are most appropriately assessed with "percentage of area stenosis" measurements,[30] although these are often time-consuming and technically difficult. The cephalo-

caudal extent and length of plaques should be noted, along with the presence of **tandem plaques.**

As the severity of a stenosis increases, the quality of the real-time image deteriorates.[54,56] Several factors work against successful image assessment of high-grade stenosis. Plaque calcification and irregularity produce shadowing, which obscures the vessel lumen. Heterogeneous plaque often has acoustic properties similar to flowing blood, producing anechoic plaques or thrombi that are almost invisible on gray-scale images. In the most extreme cases, vessels can show little visible plaque yet

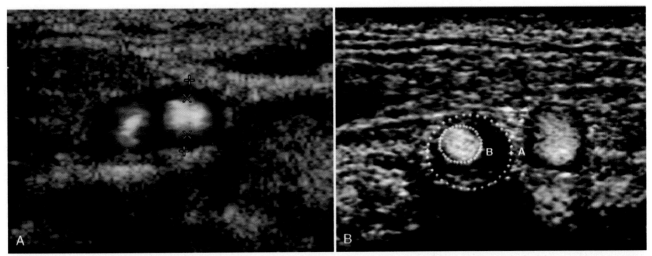

FIGURE 25-12. **Measurement of carotid artery diameter. A,** Power Doppler transverse image shows a less than 50% diameter stenosis *(cursors)*. **B,** Transverse B-mode flow image of the right carotid bifurcation shows measurement of stenosis *(B)* in area of internal carotid artery; *A,* outer ICA area.

be totally occluded (see Fig. 25-9, *E* and *F*). Color Doppler sonography readily identifies such phenomena. For these reasons, real-time gray-scale ultrasound is best suited for the evaluation of non-rate-limiting lesions, and not for quantifying high-grade stenoses, which are more accurately determined by spectral analysis.[57,58] The gray-scale findings and Doppler spectral analysis values must be integrated and correlated for a complete ultrasound assessment of the carotid vessels.

It is probably unnecessary to make a quantitative assessment of the degree of stenosis. Rather, a **qualitative** assessment of the amount of plaque should be made and compared to the Doppler spectral findings to ensure accuracy in grading stenoses. A mismatch between the qualitative assessment of the amount of plaque and the Doppler findings should alert the examiner to a possible technical error. If these cannot be resolved, further assessment with CT angiography or MRA should be considered.

Doppler Spectral Analysis

The **Doppler spectrum** is a quantitative graphic display of the velocities and directions of moving red blood cells (RBCs) present in the Doppler sample volume. Although Doppler assessment of carotid occlusive disease can be performed using frequency data, velocity calculations are preferable. **Velocity** values are potentially more accurate than frequency shift measurements, because **angle theta,** between the transducer line of sight and the blood flow vector, is used to convert a frequency shift to velocity. Frequency shifts vary according to the angle theta and the incident Doppler frequency; velocity measurements take both these factors into account.

The Doppler spectral display represents velocities on the *y* axis and time on the *x* axis. By convention,

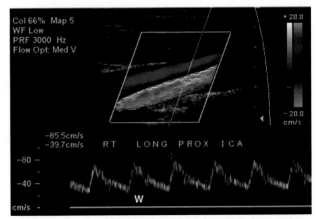

FIGURE 25-13. **Normal internal carotid artery (ICA) waveform.** Normal, low-resistance ICA waveform with clear spectral window *(W)* indicating the absence of spectral broadening.

flow toward the transducer is displayed above the zero-velocity baseline, and flow away from the transducer is below. For ease of analysis, spectra that project below the baseline are often inverted and placed above the baseline, always keeping in mind the true direction of flow within the vessel. The amplitude of each velocity component (number of RBCs with each velocity component) is used to modulate the brightness of the traces. This is also known as a **gray-scale velocity plot.** In the normal carotid artery, the frequency spectrum is narrow in systole and somewhat wider in early and late diastole. There is usually a black zone between the spectral line and the zero-velocity baseline called the **spectral window**[59,60] (Fig. 25-13).

The ICA and ECA branches of the CCA have distinctive spectral waveforms (Fig. 25-14). The **external carotid artery** supplies the high-resistance vascular bed

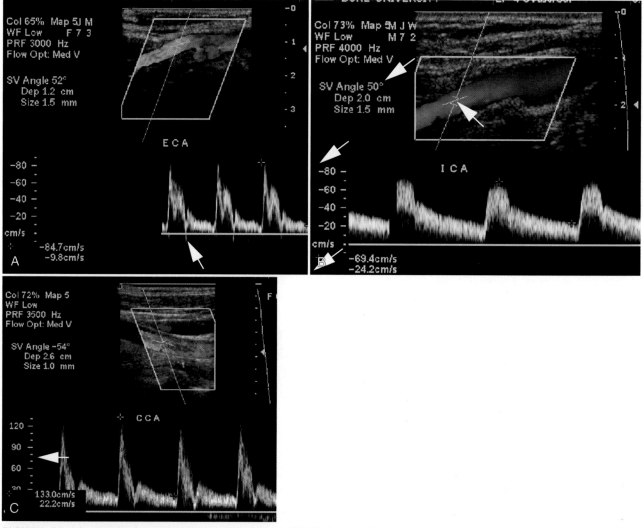

FIGURE 25-14. Normal external carotid artery (ECA), internal carotid artery (ICA), and common carotid artery (CCA) waveforms. A, Right ECA shows a sharp systolic upstroke and relatively low-velocity end diastolic flow *(arrow),* indicating a vessel supplying high-impedance circulation. **B,** ICA shows a larger amount of end diastolic flow consistent with the low-impedance intracerebral circulation. **Angle theta** *(arrow)* is 50 degrees. **C,** Normal distal CCA waveform is a composite of low-resistance ICA and higher-resistance CCA waveforms. Note that flow in **C** is toward the transducer *(arrow)* and the Doppler spectrum is plotted above the baseline. In **A** and **B,** flow is directed away from the transducer. Although these spectra have been inverted, the negative velocity signs *(arrows)* remind the operator of the true flow direction.

of the facial musculature, so its flow resembles that of other peripheral arterial vessels. Flow velocity rises sharply during systole and falls rapidly during diastole, approaching zero or transiently reversing direction. The **internal carotid artery** supplies the low-resistance circulation of the brain and demonstrates flow similar to that in vessels supplying other blood-hungry organs, such as the liver, kidneys, and placenta. The common feature in all low-resistance arterial waveforms is that a large quantity of forward flow continues throughout diastole. The **common carotid artery** waveform is a composite of the internal and external waveforms, but most often the CCA flow pattern more closely resembles that of the ICA, and diastolic flow is generally above the baseline. Approximately 80% of the blood flowing from

the CCA goes through the ICA into the brain, whereas 20% goes through the ECA into the head musculature. The relative decrease in blood flow through the ECA will cause it to have a generally lower-amplitude gray-scale waveform than in either the ICA or the CCA.[10]

Standard Examination

Virtually all state-of-the-art ultrasound equipment offers color and power Doppler, as well as gray-scale capabilities and pulsed Doppler, for the carotid examination. A rapid color Doppler screen allows the detection of abnormal flow patterns, which allows the pulsed Doppler signal volume to be placed in areas that are abnormal, especially those with **high-velocity jets.** These high-velocity jets are located in the region of and immediately distal to a high-grade stenosis (Fig. 25-15). In cases where both gray-scale and color and power Doppler images of an entire carotid artery are normal, only representative spectral tracings from the CCA, ICA, and ECA are necessary to complete the examination.

The standard Doppler spectral examination consists of traces obtained from the proximal and distal CCA, carotid bulb, and proximal ECA; samples in the proximal, middle, and distal ICA; and a representative trace from the vertebral artery. Normal velocities are higher in the proximal CCA and lower in the distal vessel; normal ICA velocities tend to increase from proximal to distal. In addition, blood flow velocities are obtained immediately proximal to, at, and just beyond regions of maximal visible stenosis and at 1-cm intervals distal to the visualized plaque as far cephalad as possible. Positioning the Doppler angle cursor parallel to the vessel walls determines angle theta, used to convert frequency information into velocity values (see Fig. 25-14, *B*). **Doppler angle theta** is defined as the angle between the Doppler transducer line of sight and the direction of blood flow. The ideal angle theta is 0 degrees, as the cosine of this angle is 1, thus resulting in the greatest possible detectable frequency shift. Because this angle is rarely achievable in the clinical setting, a range of angles from 30 to 60 degrees is considered acceptable for carotid spectral analysis.

Certain schools of ultrasound use a technique in which the Doppler angle is set at 60% and the transducer is "heel and toed" to parallel the carotid artery for Doppler spectral analysis. In our experience, it is frequently not possible to optimize cursor placement in the midportion of the vessel using this technique in tortuous vessels. Therefore, our technique involves selecting the site of spectral analysis and paralleling the wall of the vessel at that point, making certain that the Doppler angle does not exceed 60 degrees. Although either technique can be used, results obtained using these different methodologies can result in different velocities. Thus, if the first technique is used, a different set of velocity criteria should be expected than if the second is used. This is one of the factors responsible for the differences in velocity spectral criteria used in different laboratories (Fig. 25-16). When angle theta exceeds 60 to 70 degrees, the accuracy of velocity measurement declines precipitously, to the point that virtually no velocity change is detected at angle theta of 90 degrees (Fig. 25-17). The entire course of the CCA and ICA should be interrogated with a **consistent angle theta** between the transducer and the vessel maintained throughout the examination, when possible. Generally, only the origin of the ECA is evaluated because occlusive plaque is less common here than in the ICA and is rarely clinically significant. A stenosis of the ECA should be noted because it may account for a worrisome cervical bruit when the ICA is normal.[20]

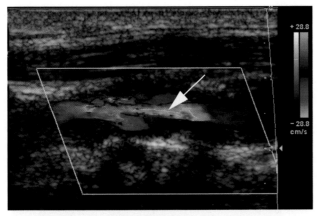

FIGURE 25-15. Color Doppler jet. High-velocity jet *(arrow)* or aliasing color demonstrates the area of highest velocity in the area of stenosis.

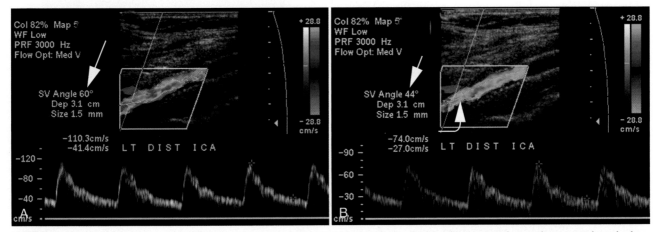

FIGURE 25-16. Doppler angle theta measurement. A, Velocity obtained in the distal internal carotid artery with angle theta of 60 degrees is higher than that obtained at 44 degrees *(arrow).* **B,** However, the sample angle does not parallel the vessel wall at 60 degrees. Note central color aliasing in the region of highest velocity *(curved arrow).*

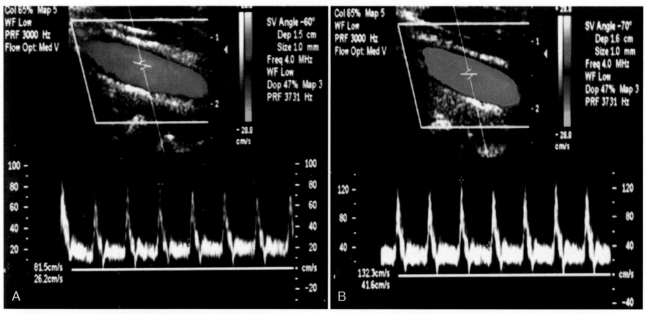

FIGURE 25-17. Incorrect Doppler angle theta. Velocity obtained in the internal carotid artery (ICA) with angle theta of 60 degrees **(A)** is less accurate than the velocity obtained from the same area of the same ICA with an angle theta of 70 degrees **(B)**.

Spectral Broadening

Atheromatous plaque projecting into the arterial lumen disturbs the normal, smooth laminar flow of erythrocytes. The RBCs move with a wider range of velocities, so the spectral line becomes wider, filling in the normally black spectral window. This phenomenon, termed spectral broadening increases in proportion to the severity of carotid artery stenosis[61-63] (Fig. 25-18). Some duplex machines allow the operator to measure the spectral spread between the maximal and minimal velocities (bandwidth) and thus quantitate spectral broadening. The validity of these measurements remains unproved, however, and further correlative studies are needed to document the relationship of quantitative spectral broadening parameters to specific degrees of stenosis.[63] Most tables no longer include a measurement for spectral broadening when grading carotid stenosis. Nevertheless, a visible gestalt of the amount of spectral window obliteration, as well as color Doppler heterogeneity, provides a useful, if not quantitative, predictor of the severity of flow disturbance.

Pitfalls in Interpretation

Pseudospectral broadening can be caused by technical factors, such as too high a gain setting. In such cases the background around the spectral waveform often contains noise. Whenever spectral broadening is suspected, the gain should be lowered to see if the spectral window clears. Similarly, spectral broadening caused by vessel wall motion can occur when the Doppler sample volume is too large or positioned too near the vessel

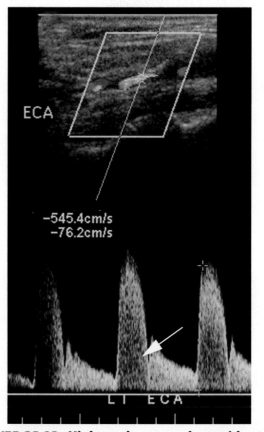

FIGURE 25-18. High-grade external carotid artery (ECA) stenosis. Elevated velocities and visible narrowing. Spectral broadening is present *(arrow)*. Color Doppler spectral broadening is also seen.

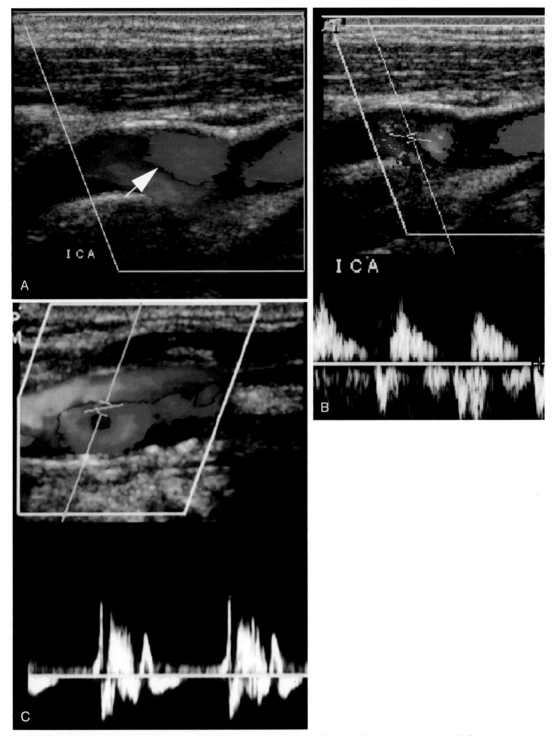

FIGURE 25-19. Disturbed flow pattern is normal at branching of common carotid artery. A, Longitudinal image of left carotid bulb shows color flow separation *(arrow).* **B** and **C,** Two examples of disturbed flow patterns in areas of flow separation between normal carotid bulb and the internal carotid artery *(ICA).*

wall. Decreasing the size of the sample volume and placing it midstream should eliminate this potential pitfall.

Altered flow patterns can normally be found at certain sites in the carotid system. For example, it is normal to find flow separation at the site of branching vessels, such as where the CCA branches into the ECA and ICA.[64] Flow disturbances also occur at sites where there is an abrupt change in the vessel diameter. For example, flow disturbances and bizarre waveforms caused by flow separation may be encountered in a normal carotid bulb where the CCA terminates in a localized area of dilation as it divides into the ECA and ICA[10] (Fig. 25-19).

The tendency for spectral broadening increases in direct proportion to the velocity of blood flow. For example, spectral broadening can be observed in a normal ECA, vertebral arteries, and CCA supplying circulation contralateral to an occluded contralateral ICA. Increased velocity may also account for the disturbed flow that is sometimes observed in the normal extracranial carotid arteries of young athletes with normal cardiac outputs or in patients in pathologically high cardiac output states. It is also seen in arteries supplying **arteriovenous fistulas and malformations.**[10,65] Postoperative spectral broadening may persist for months after CEA in the absence of significant residual or recurrent disease, possibly from changes in wall compliance.

Tortuous carotid vessels can demonstrate spectral broadening and asymmetrical high-velocity flow jets in the absence of plaque disease. Other nonatheromatous causes of disturbed blood flow in the extracranial carotid arteries include **aneurysms, arterial wall dissections,** and **fibromuscular dysplasia.**

High-Velocity Blood Flow Patterns

Carotid stenoses usually begin to cause velocity changes when they exceed 50% diameter (70% cross-sectional area)[1] (Fig. 25-20, *A-C*). Velocity elevations generally increase as the severity of the stenosis increases. At critical stenoses (>95%), the velocity measurements may actually decrease, and the waveform becomes dampened[58,66] (Fig. 25-20, *D* and *E*).

In these cases, correlation with color or power Doppler imaging is essential to diagnose correctly the severity of the stenoses. Velocity increases are focal and most pronounced in and immediately distal to a stenosis, emphasizing the importance of sampling directly in these regions. As one moves further distal from a stenosis, flow begins to reconstitute and assume a more normal pattern, provided a tandem lesion does not exist distal to the initial site of stenosis. Spectral broadening results in the jets of high-velocity flow associated with carotid stenosis; however, correlation with gray-scale and color Doppler images can define other causes of spectral broadening. An awareness of normal flow spectra combined with appropriate Doppler techniques can obviate many potential diagnostic pitfalls.

The degree of carotid stenosis that is considered clinically significant in the symptomatic or asymptomatic patient is in evolution. Initially, it was thought that lesions causing 50% diameter stenosis were significant; this perception changed as more information was gathered from two large clinical trials. As noted earlier, NASCET demonstrated that CEA was more beneficial than medical therapy in symptomatic patients with 70% to 99% ICA stenosis.[4] ECST demonstrated a CEA benefit when the degree of stenosis was greater than 60%.[5] Interestingly, the method used to grade stenoses in the ECST study was significantly different than that used in the NASCET trials. The NASCET trials compared the severity of the ICA stenosis on arteriogram with the residual lumen of a presumably more normal distal ICA. The ECST methodology entailed assessment of the severity of stenosis with a "guesstimation" of the lumen of the carotid artery at the level of the stenosis. The ECST assessment is more comparable to ultrasound's visible assessment of the degree of narrowing, whereas velocity tables currently in use have been derived to correspond to the NASCET angiographic determinations for stenosis. The ECST method for grading carotid artery stenosis tends to give a more severe assessment of narrowing than the NASCET technique (Fig. 25-21).

The initial NASCET trials retrospectively compared velocity data obtained on the Doppler examination with angiographic measurements of stenosis. No standardized ultrasound protocol was employed by the numerous centers involved in the trials. Despite the lack of uniformity, moderate sensitivity and specificity ranging from 65% to 77% were obtained for grading ICA stenoses using Doppler velocities. If ultrasound technique is standardized and criteria are validated in a given laboratory, **peak systolic velocity** (PSV) and peak systolic ratios have proved to be an accurate method for determining carotid stenosis.[67] The ECST group compared three different angiographic measurement techniques: the NASCET, the ECST, and a technique comparing distal CCA measurements with those of ICA stenosis. Researchers concluded that the ECST and NASCET techniques were similar in their prognostic value, whereas the CCA/stenosis measurement was the most reproducible of the three techniques. They also concluded that the CCA method, although reproducible, would be invalidated by the presence of CCA disease.[68] Virtually all investigators advocate using the NASCET angiographic measurement technique.

The results of these trials, as well as the more recent ACAS and moderate NASCET studies, have generated reappraisals of the Doppler velocity criteria that most accurately define 70% or greater stenosis and, more recently, greater than 50% diameter stenoses.[69] Attempts have been made to determine the Doppler parameters or combination of parameters that most reliably identify a certain-diameter stenosis. Most sources agree that the best parameter is the PSV of the ICA in the region of a stenosis.[66] Using multiple parameters can improve diagnostic confidence, particularly when combined with color and power Doppler imaging.

The degree of stenosis is best assessed using the gray-scale and pulsed Doppler parameters, including ICA PSV, ICA **end diastolic velocity** (EDV), CCA PSV, CCA EDV, **peak systolic ICA/CCA ratio** (SVR), and **peak end diastolic ICA/CCA ratio** (EDR).[66,67,70] Peak systolic velocity has proved accurate for quantifying high-grade stenoses.[57,67] The relationship of PSV to the degree of luminal narrowing is well defined and easily measured.[71,72] Although Doppler velocities have proved

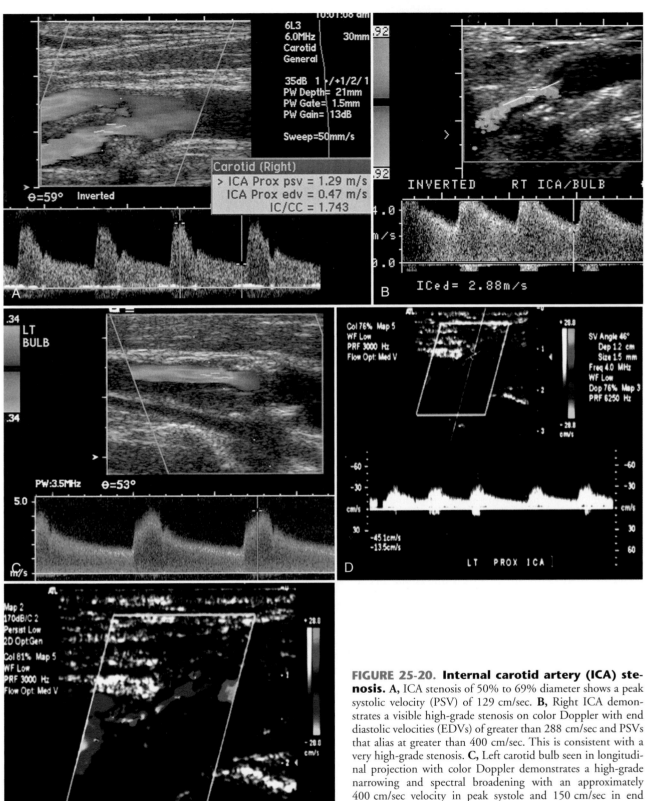

FIGURE 25-20. Internal carotid artery (ICA) stenosis. A, ICA stenosis of 50% to 69% diameter shows a peak systolic velocity (PSV) of 129 cm/sec. **B,** Right ICA demonstrates a visible high-grade stenosis on color Doppler with end diastolic velocities (EDVs) of greater than 288 cm/sec and PSVs that alias at greater than 400 cm/sec. This is consistent with a very high-grade stenosis. **C,** Left carotid bulb seen in longitudinal projection with color Doppler demonstrates a high-grade narrowing and spectral broadening with an approximately 400 cm/sec velocity in peak systole and 150 cm/sec in end diastole, consistent with an 80% to 95% stenosis. **D,** Velocity obtained in the ICA demonstrates low velocities. The PSV is 78 cm/sec, EDV is 22 cm/sec, systolic velocity ratio is 1.7, and diastolic velocity ratio is 2.8. **E,** The color-flow Doppler image demonstrates a markedly narrowed vessel. The degree of stenosis correlates with 95% to 99%.

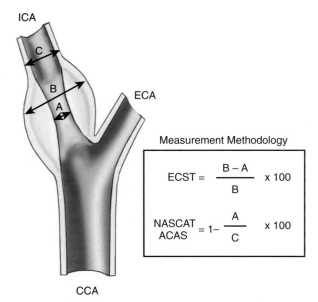

Measurement Methodology

$$ECST = \frac{B - A}{B} \times 100$$

$$\begin{matrix} NASCAT \\ ACAS \end{matrix} = 1 - \frac{A}{C} \times 100$$

FIGURE 25-21. Comparative measurement methodology. Different methodologies for grading internal carotid artery stenoses, from North American Symptomatic Carotid Endarterectomy Trial (NASCET), Asymptomatic Carotid Atherosclerosis Study (ACAS), and European Carotid Surgery Trial (ECST).

reliable for defining 70% or greater stenosis, Grant et al.[67] showed less favorable results for substenosis classification between 50% and 69% using PSV and ICA/CCA PSV ratios. In our experience, however, using all four parameters and determining a correct category for the degree of stenosis is the most efficacious way to ensure accuracy. Agreement for all four parameters for a clinical situation is most common. When there is an outlying parameter, further assessment and careful attention to technique and detail are required. EDV and EDR are particularly useful in distinguishing between high grades of stenosis. Additionally, correlating the visual estimation of the degree of stenosis and the velocity numbers will help in correctly grading stenosis, particularly when the degree of stenosis is "near occlusion" (Figs. 25-22 and 25-23; see also Fig. 25-20, D and E). On rare occasions, alternate imaging methodologies (e.g., MRA, CT angiography) may need to be recommended.

No criteria for grading **external carotid artery stenoses** have been established. A good general rule is that if the ECA velocities do not exceed 200 cm/sec, no significant stenosis is present. However, we usually rely on a visible assessment of the degree of narrowing associated with velocity changes. Occlusive plaque involving the ECA is less common than in the ICA and is rarely clinically significant. Similarly, velocity criteria used to grade **common carotid artery stenoses** have not been well established. However, if one is able to visualize 2 cm proximal and 2 cm distal to a visible CCA stenosis, a PSV ratio obtained 2 cm proximal to the stenosis (vs. in region of greatest visible stenosis) can be used to grade

the "percent diameter stenosis" in a manner similar to that used in peripheral artery studies. A doubling of the PSV across a lesion would correspond to at least a 50% diameter stenosis, and a velocity ratio in excess of 3.5 corresponds to a greater than 75% stenosis. Although duplex ultrasound remains an accurate method of quantifying ICA stenoses, the use of color and power Doppler sonography has significantly improved diagnostic confidence and reproducibility.[73]

One persistent problem with duplex Doppler with gray-scale ultrasound evaluation of the carotids is that different institutions use PSVs ranging from 130 cm/sec[74] to 325 cm/sec[69] to diagnose greater than 70% ICA stenosis. Factors creating these discrepancies include technique and equipment.[75] This wide range of PSVs reinforces the need for individual ultrasound laboratories to determine which Doppler parameters are most reliable in their own institution.[75] Correlation of the velocity ranges obtained by ultrasound with angiographic and surgical results is necessary to achieve accurate, reproducible examinations in a particular ultrasound laboratory.[76]

The Society of Radiologists in Ultrasound, representing multiple medical and surgical specialties, held a consensus conference in 2002 to consider carotid Doppler ultrasound.[77] In addition to guidelines for performing and interpreting carotid ultrasound examinations, panelists devised a set of criteria widely applicable among vascular laboratories (Table 25-1).[77] Although the conference did not recommend all established laboratories with internally validated velocity charts alter their practices, they suggested physicians establishing new laboratories consider using the consensus criteria; those with preexisting charts might consider comparing in-house criteria with those provided by the consensus conference. Velocity criteria corresponding to specific degrees of vascular stenosis are listed in the tables. Our institution uses Table 25-2, which has a category for 80% to 95% stenoses; our surgeons are more inclined to consider surgery for patients with asymptomatic stenoses greater than 80% than for those with less severe stenoses.[30,78]

The ICA values should be obtained at or just distal to the point of maximum visible stenosis and at the point of greatest color Doppler spectral abnormality. Values from the CCA should be obtained 2 cm proximal to the widening in the region of the carotid bulb. Because velocities normally decrease from proximal to distal in the CCA and increase from proximal to distal in the ICA, it is important that standardized levels be used routinely for obtaining the ICA/CCA velocity ratio.

Color Doppler Ultrasound

Color Doppler ultrasound displays blood flow information in real time over the entire image or a selected area. Stationary soft tissue structures, which lack a detectable phase or frequency shift, are assigned an amplitude value

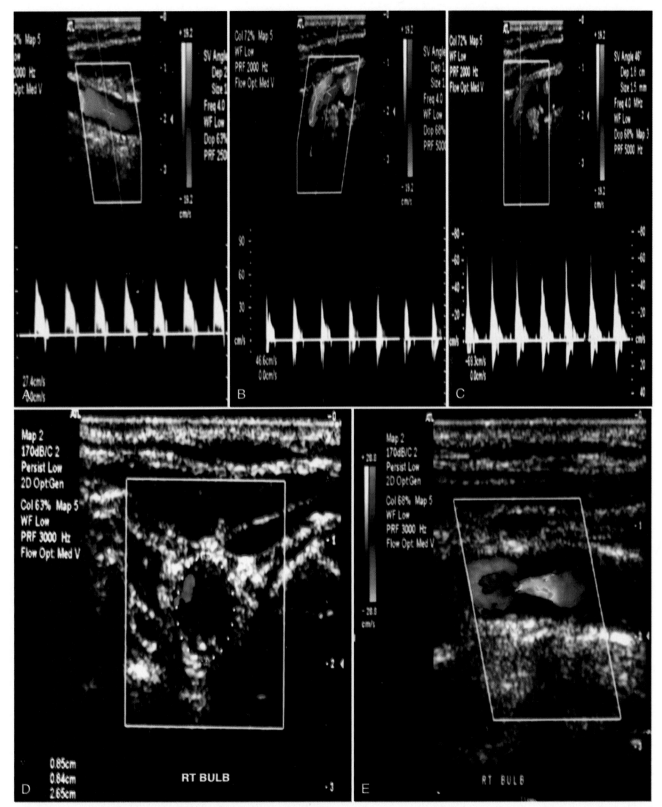

FIGURE 25-22. Abnormal high-resistance waveforms. High-resistance waveforms: **A,** common carotid artery; **B,** proximal internal carotid artery (ICA); and **D,** distal ICA. Color flow Doppler imaging of the carotid bulb in transverse (**D**) and sagittal (**E**) projections demonstrates a significantly narrowed ICA. These findings are consistent with a greater than 95% stenosis of the ICA and a distal tandem stenosis of the intracranial carotid artery.

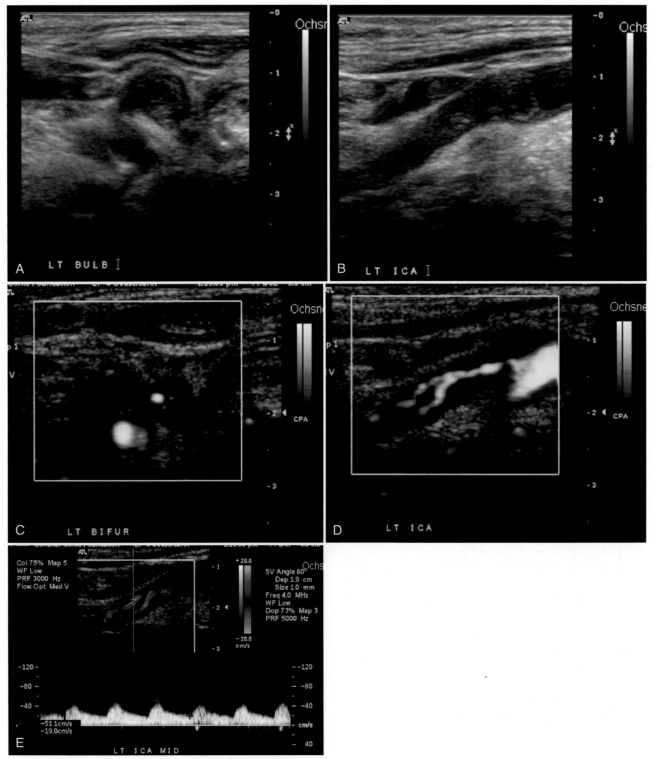

FIGURE 25-23. Near occlusion (95-99% stenosis) with homogeneous plaque. A, Transverse, and **B,** sagittal, gray-scale images of the left internal carotid artery (ICA) demonstrate homogeneous (type 3) plaque. **C,** Transverse, and **D,** sagittal, power Doppler images demonstrate extremely narrowed residual lumen. **E,** Velocity measurements for the ICA were peak systolic velocity, 51 cm/sec; acoustic Doppler velocity, 19 cm/sec; systolic velocity ratio, 51/64 = 0.8; diastolic velocity ratio, 19/12 = 1.5. The combination of visual images and Doppler spectral analysis findings indicate a 95% to 99% stenosis.

TABLE 25-1. DIAGNOSTIC CRITERIA FOR CAROTID ULTRASOUND EXAMINATIONS

	ICA PSV	PLAQUE	ICA/CCA PSV RATIO	ICA EDV
Normal	<125 cm/sec	None	<2.0	<40 cm/sec
<50%	<125 cm/sec	<50% diameter reduction	<2.0	<40 cm/sec
50%-69%	125-230 cm/sec	≥50% diameter reduction	2.0-4.0	40-100 cm/sec
≥70% to near occlusion	>230 cm/sec	≥50% diameter reduction	>4.0	>100 cm/sec
Near occlusion	May be low or undetectable	Visible	Variable	Variable
Total occlusion	Undetectable	Visible, no detectable lumen	Not applicable	Not applicable

From Society of Radiologists in Ultrasound. Consensus Conference on Carotid Ultrasound. October 2002, San Francisco. Radiology 229:340-346, 2003.
ICA, Internal carotid artery; *PSV,* peak systolic velocity; *CCA,* common carotid artery; *EDV,* end diastolic velocity.

TABLE 25-2. ALTERNATIVE DIAGNOSTIC CRITERIA FOR ESTIMATING CAROTID ARTERY DISEASE

DIAMETER STENOSIS	PEAK SYSTOLIC VELOCITY (cm/sec)	PEAK DIASTOLIC VELOCITY (cm/sec)	SYSTOLIC VELOCITY RATIO (VICA/VCCA)	DIASTOLIC VELOCITY RATIO (VICA/VCCA)
0% (normal)	<110	<40	<2.0	<2.6
1%-39% (mild)	<110	<40	<2.0	<2.6
40%-59% (moderate)	<170	<40	<2.0	<2.6
60%-79% (severe)	>170	>40	>2.0	>2.6
80%-95% (critical)	>250	>100	>3.7	>5.5
96%-99%	Velocities demonstrate variability and may be low.			
100% (occlusion)	No flow detected.			

Based on the European Carotid Surgery Trial's methodology of measuring residual lumen to outer vessel margin. Radiographics 8:487-506, 1988; J Vasc Surg 22:697-703, 1995.

and displayed in a gray-scale format with flowing blood in vessels superimposed in color. The mean Doppler frequency shift produced by RBC ensembles pulsing through a selected sample volume is obtained using an autocorrelative method or a time domain processing (speckle motion analysis) method. Color assignments depend on the direction of blood flow relative to the Doppler transducer. Blood flow toward the transducer appears in one color and flow away from the transducer in another. These color assignments are arbitrary and are generally set up so that arterial flow is depicted as red and venous flow as blue. Color saturation displays indicate the variable velocity of blood flow. Deeper shades usually indicate low velocities centered around the zero-velocity color flow baseline. As velocity increases, the shades become lighter or are assigned a different color hue. Some systems allow selected frequency shifts to be displayed in a contrasting color, such as green. This **green-tag feature** provides a real-time estimation of the presence of high-velocity flow.

Setting the color Doppler scale can also be used to create an aliasing artifact corresponding to the highest-velocity flow within a vessel (see Figs. 25-16, *B*; 25-18;

and 25-21). These **high-velocity jets** pinpoint areas for spectral analysis. Color assignments are a function of both the mean frequency shift produced by moving RBC ensembles and the Doppler angle theta. If the vessel is tortuous or diving, angle theta between the transducer and vessel will change along the course of the vessel, resulting in **changing color assignments** that are unrelated to the change in RBC velocity. The color assignments will reverse in tortuous vessels as their course changes relative to the Doppler transducer, even though the absolute direction of flow is unchanged. Portions of a vessel that **parallel the Doppler beam** when angle theta is 90 degrees will have little or no frequency shift detected, and no color will be seen.

Optimal Settings for Low-Flow Vessel Evaluation

Color Doppler flow studies should be performed with optimal flow sensitivity and gain settings. Color flow should fill the entire vessel lumen but not spill over into adjacent soft tissues. The **pulse repetition frequency** (PRF) and frame rates should be set to allow visualiza-

OPTIMIZATION OF COLOR DOPPLER LOW-FLOW VESSEL EVALUATION

- Use low pulse repetition frequency.
- Use Doppler angle of less than 60 degrees.
- Increase gain setting.
- Increase power setting.
- Decrease wall filter.
- Increase persistence.
- Increase dwell time.

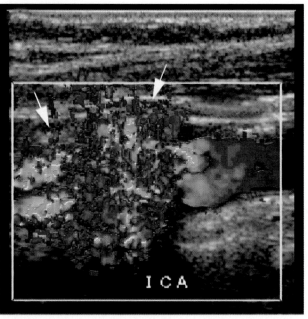

FIGURE 25-24. Color Doppler bruit. Extensive soft-tissue color Doppler bruit (arrows) surrounds the right carotid bifurcation with a 90% right internal carotid artery *(ICA)* stenosis.

tion of flow phenomenon anticipated in a vessel. Frame rates will vary as a function of the width of the area chosen for color Doppler display and for depth of the region of interest. The greater the color image area, the slower the frame rate will be. The deeper the posterior boundary of the color image, the slower the PRF will be. Color Doppler sensitivity should be adjusted to detect anticipated velocities, such that if slow flow in a preocclusive carotid lesion is sought, low-flow settings with decreased sampling rates are employed. However, the system will then alias at lower velocities because of the decrease in PRF. In addition to changes in the PRF, optimization of the Doppler angle, increases in gain and power settings, decrease in the wall filter, increase in persistence, and increase in ensemble or dwell time can be used to optimize low-flow detection.

Flowing blood becomes, in effect, its own contrast medium, with color or power Doppler outlining the patent vessel lumen. This allows determination of the true course of the vessel, facilitating positioning of the Doppler cursor and thus providing more reliable velocity determinations. Furthermore, color Doppler facilitates Doppler spectral analysis by rapidly identifying areas of flow abnormalities. The highest velocities in the region of and immediately distal to a stenosis are seen as **aliasing high-velocity jets of color.** Color Doppler ultrasound facilitates placing the pulsed Doppler range gate in the region of these most striking color abnormalities for pulsed Doppler spectral analysis. The presence of a stenosis can be determined by color Doppler changes in the vessel lumen as well as by visible luminal narrowing. Although color Doppler can be used to determine the presence of hypoechoic plaque, it cannot be used optimally to determine the area of patent lumen in transverse projection because the optimal angle for measuring the area or diameter of narrowing is at 90 degrees to the long axis of the vessel, which is the worst angle for color Doppler imaging. Gray-scale assessment, power Doppler, or B-flow imaging should be used to assess the diameter/area of the patent carotid lumen (see Fig. 25-12). If a stenosis produces a **bruit** or **thrill**, the resultant perivascular tissue vibrations may actually be seen as transient speckles of color in the adjacent soft tissues, more prominent during systole[79] (Fig. 25-24).

Comparisons of color Doppler ultrasound with conventional duplex Doppler sampling techniques and angiography have shown relatively similar accuracy, sensitivity, and specificity.[80] However, color Doppler offers many benefits, including a reduction in examination time by pinpointing areas of color Doppler abnormality for pulsed Doppler spectral analysis. Branches of the ECA are readily detected, facilitating differentiation from the ICA. The real-time flow information over a large cross-sectional area provides a global overview of flow abnormalities and allows ready determination of the course of a vessel. Further, color Doppler improves diagnostic confidence and reproducibility of ultrasound studies, thereby avoiding many potential diagnostic pitfalls.

The laminar blood flow is disrupted in the region of the carotid bifurcation where there is a **normal transient flow reversal** opposite the origin of the ECA (see Fig. 25-19). Color Doppler displays this normal flow separation as an area of flow reversal located along the outer wall of the carotid bulb, which appears either at early systole or in peak systole and persists for a variable period into the diastolic part of the cardiac cycle.[81,82] This flow reversal can produce some strikingly bizarre pulsed Doppler waveforms; however, the color Doppler appearance readily discerns the nature of these waveform changes. Furthermore, the absence of this flow reversal may be abnormal and may represent one of the earliest changes of atherosclerotic disease.[81] The flow reversal seen in the region of the carotid bifurcation is clearly different than that seen with color Doppler aliasing. Contiguous saturated areas of red and blue are seen in this low-velocity flow separation, versus the very different contiguous color hues representing the highest color assignments for forward and reversed flow.

Helical flow in the CCA may be an indirect indication of proximal arterial stenosis but can occur as a normal variant. Color Doppler sonography graphically displays the eccentric spiraling of flow up the CCA.

Advantages and Pitfalls

Color Doppler ultrasound may help avoid potential diagnostic pitfalls. Alterations in cardiovascular physiology, tandem lesions, contralateral carotid disease, arrhythmias, postoperative changes, and tortuous vessels can lead to underestimation or overestimation of the degree of stenosis. In such cases, color Doppler ultrasound can provide direct visualization of the patent lumen in a fashion analogous to angiography.[83] In fact, because angiography images only the vessel lumen and not the vessel wall, color Doppler and power Doppler ultrasound imaging have the potential to evaluate stenoses even more completely than angiography. Because flow patterns are displayed with color Doppler imaging, the local hemodynamic consequences of the lesion are readily discerned. Color and power Doppler ultrasound appear to have particular value in detecting small residual channels of flow in areas of high-grade carotid stenoses[79,80,83-85] (Fig. 25-25). Power Doppler ultrasound offers a comparable advantage and has the theoretical potential to be more sensitive for detecting extremely low-amplitude, low-velocity flow. Finally, color Doppler and power Doppler ultrasound have the potential to clarify image Doppler mismatches, further improving diagnostic accuracy and confidence.

Although color Doppler ultrasound offers many advantages, it is angle dependent and prone to artifacts,

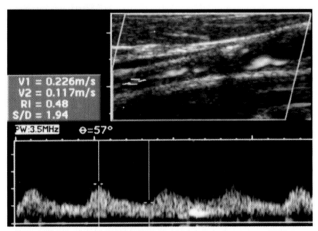

FIGURE 25-25. High-grade "string sign" stenosis of internal carotid artery. Tardus-parvus waveform with low velocity in a long segment.

COLOR DOPPLER EVOLUTION OF CAROTID STENOSIS

ADVANTAGES
Reduction in examination time.
Quick identification of areas of stenosis/high velocity, which facilitates spectral analysis to artifacts.
Improved diagnostic reproducibility and confidence.
Distinguishes occlusion from "string sign."
Simultaneous hemodynamic and anatomic information, velocity, and directional blood flow information.
Improved accuracy in quantitating stenoses.
Clarifies pulsed Doppler/image mismatch.

DISADVANTAGES
Prone to angle dependence.
Resolution less than with gray scale.
Less Doppler spectral than pulsed Doppler.
Slower–frame rates information.
Use cannot characterize plaque.

such as aliasing. The spatial resolution of color Doppler ultrasound is less than that of gray-scale imaging, and the Doppler resolution is inferior to pulsed Doppler spectral analysis. Color saturation cannot be equated with velocity.[75] The color image is corrected for only one angle, so changes in color saturation may simply reflect changes in the vessel course and the relative Doppler angle. Color systems generally compute the mean velocity to produce the color pixel in the image. However, the examiner is usually interested in determining the maximum velocity; therefore pulsed Doppler spectral analysis remains necessary for precise quantification of a hemodynamically significant stenosis.

Power Doppler Ultrasound

The color signal in power Doppler ultrasound is generated from the integrated power Doppler spectrum. The amplitude of the reflected echoes determines the brightness and color tone of the color signal. This amplitude depends on the density of RBCs flowing within the sample volume. Power Doppler ultrasound uses a larger dynamic range with a better signal-to-noise (S/N) ratio than color Doppler ultrasound. Because power Doppler ultrasound does not evaluate frequencies but rather amplitude (or power), artifacts such as aliasing do not occur. Power Doppler sonography, unlike color Doppler ultrasound, is largely angle independent. These features combine to make power Doppler ultrasound exquisitely sensitive to detecting a **residual string of flow** in the region of a suspected carotid occlusion.[84]

It is also hypothesized that power Doppler ultrasound has better edge definition than color Doppler ultra-

POWER DOPPLER EVALUATION OF CAROTID STENOSIS

ADVANTAGES
No aliasing.
Potentially increases accuracy of grading stenoses.
Aids in distinguishing preocclusive from occlusive lesions.
Potentially superior depiction of plaque surface morphology.
Increased sensitivity to detecting low-velocity, low-amplitude blood flow.
Angle independent.

DISADVANTAGES
Does not provide direction or velocity flow information.
Very motion sensitive (poor temporal resolution).

CAUSES OF IMAGE/ DOPPLER MISMATCH

Cardiac arrhythmia
Cardiac valvular disease; cardiomyopathy
Severe aortic stenosis
Hypotension or hypertension
Tandem lesions
Contralateral carotid stenosis
Nonstenotic plaque
Long-segment, concentric high-grade stenosis
Carotid dissection
Preocclusive lesion
Tortuous vessels
Calcified plaque; hypoechoic or anechoic plaque
Anatomic variants

sound. The combination of improved edge definition and relative angle-independent flow imaging offers the potential for better visual assessment of the degree of stenosis using power Doppler.[86] Better edge definition may also allow power Doppler ultrasound to define plaque surface characteristics more clearly[87] (see Fig. 25-10, B).

Despite the many potential benefits of power Doppler ultrasound, it does not provide velocity or directional flow information.[88] Also, power Doppler is very motion sensitive, which may result in a **pseudostring** of flow. If the vibrations of soft tissue at an echogenic interface exceed the clutter filter level, color information may be displayed in areas where there is no blood flow. Pulsed Doppler evaluation of a color or power string should always be performed to confirm the presence of real flow.

Power Doppler screening may produce an accurate and cost-effective method for patients at risk for carotid disease.[89,90] Power Doppler imaging used independent of spectral analysis was effectively performed in 89 of 100 patients. The sensitivity for the detection of 40% or greater stenoses using power Doppler was 91%, with 79% specificity. This would be reasonable for a screening test, allowing patients with greater than 40% stenoses to undergo more expensive spectral analysis. Some believe that using this less expensive power Doppler screening could result in a more cost-effective approach to carotid Doppler screening. In addition, carotid power Doppler imaging, as well as carotid B-flow imaging, is ideally suited to combined use with vascular contrast agents that may be widely available in the future.

Pitfalls and Adjustments

Although absolute velocity determinations are valuable in assessing the degree of vascular stenosis, these measurements are less reliable in certain patients.[1] Variations in cardiovascular physiology may affect carotid velocity measurements[91,92]. For example, velocities produced by a stenosis in a **hypertensive patient** may be higher than those in a normotensive individual with comparable narrowing, especially in the setting of a wide-pulsed pressure. On the other hand, a **reduction in cardiac output** will diminish both systolic and diastolic velocities (Fig. 25-26). **Cardiac arrhythmias, aortic valvular lesions,** and **severe cardiomyopathies** can cause significant aberrations in the shape of carotid flow waveforms and alter systolic and diastolic velocity readings (Fig. 25-27). Use of an **aortic balloon pump** can also distort the Doppler velocity spectrum (Fig. 25-28). These alterations can invalidate the use of standard Doppler parameters to quantify stenoses. **Bradycardia**, for example, produces increased stroke volume, causing systolic velocities to increase, whereas **prolonged diastolic runoff** causes spuriously decreased end diastolic values. Patients with isolated **severe or critical aortic stenosis** may demonstrate duplex waveform abnormalities, including prolonged acceleration time, decreased peak velocity, delayed upstroke, and rounded waveforms.[93] However, **mild or moderate aortic stenosis** usually results in little or no sonographic abnormality. **Tortuous or kinked carotid arteries** represent either congenital or acquired changes in the carotid artery. The clinical significance of these is debatable; however, the **vascular tortuosity** frequently results in eccentric jets of high-velocity flow, which may show elevated velocities in the absence of significant stenosis[94] (Fig. 25-29). Conversely, if the carotid bulb is capacious, a large plaque burden may still fail to produce anticipated velocity increases. The relative difference in area between the distal CCA and the residual patent lumen of the large bulb is not sufficient to produce a greater than 50% velocity change. Some refer to this as **nonstenotic (homogeneous) plaque** (Fig. 25-30). Frequently, an **image/Doppler mismatch** alerts the examiner to potential pitfalls.

Color Doppler can be used to overcome diagnostic dilemmas in these situations, particularly when "cine

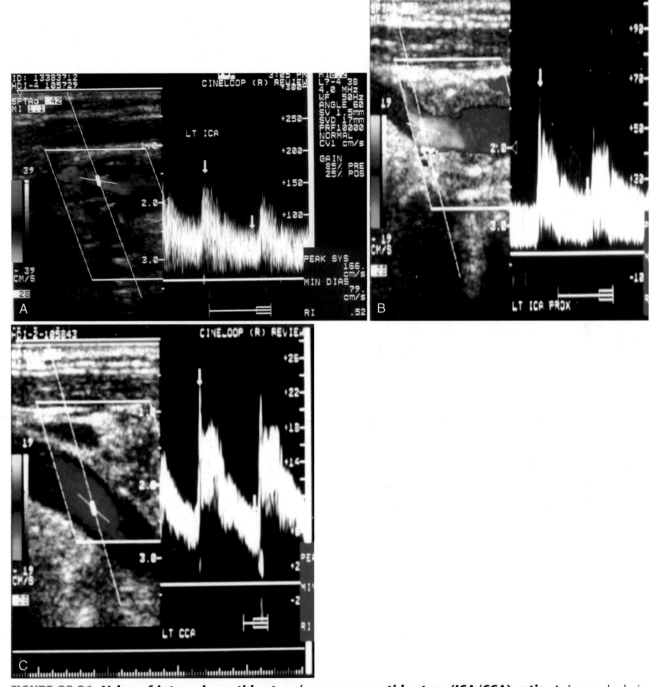

FIGURE 25-26. Value of internal carotid artery/common carotid artery (ICA/CCA) ratio. A, Increased velocity ICA and CCA in a patient with hypertension. ICA peak systolic velocity (PSV) is 166 cm/sec; end diastolic velocity (EDV) is 79 cm/sec. CCA velocities: PSV = 96 cm/sec; EDV = 36 cm/sec. ICA/CCA systolic velocity ratio (SVR) is 1.7, and diastolic velocity ratio (DVR) is 2.2, corresponding to a degree of stenosis less than 50%. **B,** Low velocities in left ICA: PSV = 67 cm/sec, EDV = 23 cm/sec. **C,** In left CCA, PSV = 23 cm/sec; EDV = 8 cm/sec. SVR is 2.9, and DVR is 2.9, corresponding to a 50% to 69% stenosis in patient with cardiomyopathy.

loop" playback capabilities are present. Cine loop allows the computer to store up to 10 seconds of the previous color Doppler flow recording for playback at the real-time rate or frame by frame. This allows the clinician to assess the filling of all parts of the vessel lumen. **Obstructive lesions in one carotid can affect velocities in the contralateral vessel.** For example, severe unilateral ICA stenosis or occlusion may cause shunting of increased flow through the contralateral carotid system. This increased flow artificially increases velocity measurements in the contralateral vessel, particularly in areas of stenosis.[94-97] Conversely, a proximal common carotid or

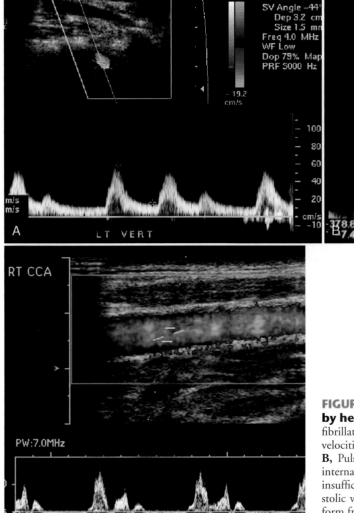

FIGURE 25-27. Abnormal Doppler waveforms caused by heart disease. A, Patient with aortic valvular disease and atrial fibrillation shows irregular pulsed Doppler rhythm with varying velocities and a delayed upstroke consistent with aortic stenosis. **B,** Pulsed Doppler waveforms in a patient with an 80% to 99% internal carotid artery *(ICA)* stenosis and combined aortic stenosis/insufficiency show a striking disparity in peak-systolic and end diastolic velocities due to severe aortic insufficiency. **C,** Doppler waveform from common carotid artery *(CCA)* in patient with aortic valve insufficiency. Note reversal of flow in diastole.

innominate artery stenosis may reduce flow, with consequent reduction of velocity measurements in a stenosis that is distal to the point of obstruction **(tandem lesion)** (see Fig. 25-22).

Velocity ratios that compare velocity values in the ICA to those in the ipsilateral CCA can help avoid some pitfalls.[58] Of particular value are the **peak systolic ratio** (PSV in ICA vs. PSV in CCA)[63,98] and the **end diastolic ratio** (ICA/CCA EDV).[70] Grant et al. have shown that PSV ICA/CCA ratios are comparable in accuracy to PSV values for determining the degree of ICA stenosis.[67] Although the peak systolic velocity and peak systolic ICA/CCA velocity ratio have shown relative comparable sensitivities and specificities, at times the velocity ratio will more correctly identify the degree of stenosis and the absolute velocity. Velocity ratios should always be employed when unusually high or low CCA velocities or significant asymmetry of CCA velocities is detected. Long-segment, high-grade stenoses frequently will not demonstrate the anticipated degree of ICA velocity elevation. In such situations, the velocity ratio coupled

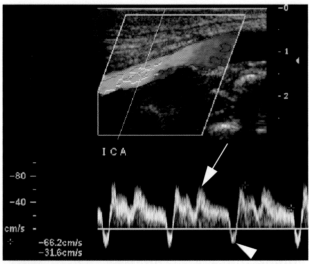

FIGURE 25-28. Abnormal Doppler waveform caused by aortic balloon pump. Internal carotid artery *(ICA)* pulsed Doppler trace shows the effect of an aortic balloon pump on carotid waveforms. Inflation of the device in systole *(arrow)* produces a second systolic peak, whereas deflation produces flow reversal *(arrowhead)* in end diastole.

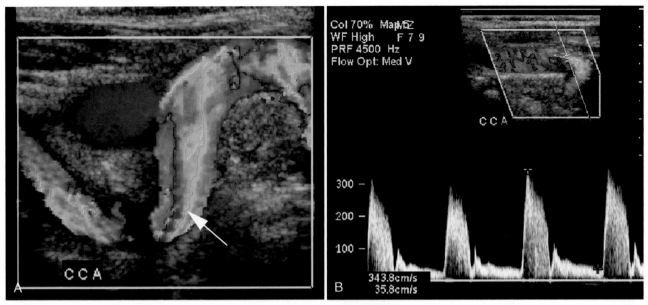

FIGURE 25-29. Abnormal Doppler flow caused by tortuous vessel. A, Tortuous common carotid artery *(CCA)* displays color Doppler eccentric jets of flow *(arrow).* **B,** Spuriously elevated velocity is caused by an eccentric jet in a tortuous proximal left CCA without any visible stenosis.

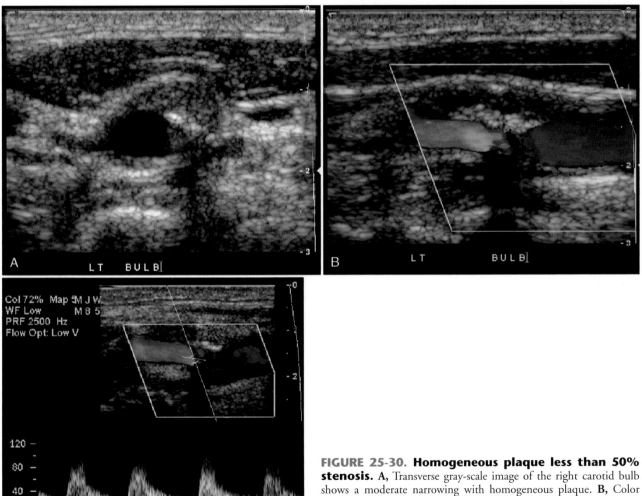

FIGURE 25-30. Homogeneous plaque less than 50% stenosis. A, Transverse gray-scale image of the right carotid bulb shows a moderate narrowing with homogeneous plaque. **B,** Color Doppler flow imaging shows a moderate stenosis. **C,** On Doppler spectral analysis, there is no corresponding increase in systolic velocity in the area of narrowing (88.7 cm/sec). This stenosis is less than 50% in patient with capacious carotid bulb.

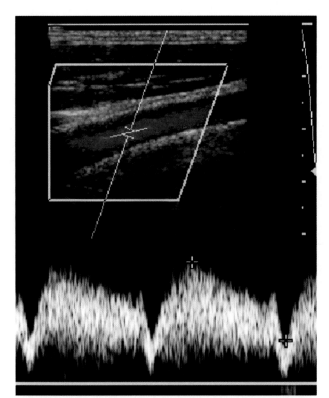

FIGURE 25-31. Abnormal common carotid artery velocity caused by innominate artery stenosis. Low, right CCA velocities with a presteal waveform distal to a severe innominate artery stenosis.

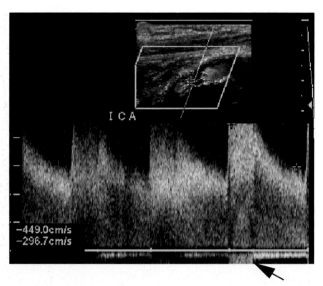

FIGURE 25-32. Aliasing of Doppler waveform in the region of a high-grade (80%-95%) stenosis; *ICA,* internal carotid artery. Highest velocities are wrapped around *(arrow)* and displayed below the zero-velocity baseline.

with the gray-scale/color/power Doppler appearance may provide insight into the actual degree of narrowing. As discussed for spectral broadening, color and power Doppler sonography are invaluable in the avoidance of pitfalls related to spurious Doppler spectral traces.

Although high-grade stenoses usually produce increased velocity in the region of a plaque and distal to it, high-grade intracranial or extracranial occlusive **lesions in tandem may reduce anticipated velocity shifts** and produce an atypical high-resistance ICA waveform (see Fig. 25-22). Vessels should be examined as far cephalad as possible to avoid missing a distal tandem lesion. Flow immediately distal to stenosis of greater than 95% frequently demonstrates very-low-velocity **tardus-parvus waveforms,** versus the anticipated high velocities seen in a high-grade stenosis (see Fig. 25-25). **High-grade vascular narrowings,** particularly those of a circumferential nature that occur over a long segment of a vessel, may also produce damped waveforms without a high-velocity frequency shift. Although no definite velocity elevations are present in such a long, circumferential narrowing, spectral broadening and disturbed flow distal to such a narrowing are usually apparent. In addition, the fusiform narrowings are usually detected with the real-time image, particularly if color Doppler is employed. **Innominate artery occlusions** may result in tardus-parvus waveforms and even carotid steal patterns similar to those noted in the vertebral artery (Fig. 25-31).

Another source of error in pulsed Doppler ultrasound analysis is **aliasing**, which is caused by the inability to detect the true peak velocity because the Doppler sampling rate, the PRF, is too low. A classic visual example of aliasing can be seen in Western films, with the apparent reversal of stagecoach wheel spokes when the wagon wheel rotations exceed the film frame rate. The maximal detectable frequency shift can be no greater than half the PRF. With aliasing, the tips of the time velocity spectrum (representing high velocities) are cut off and wrap around to appear below the baseline (Fig. 25-32). If aliasing occurs, **continuous wave probes** used in conjunction with duplex pulsed Doppler can readily demonstrate the true peak velocity shift. Aliasing can also be overcome or decreased by **increasing the angle theta** (the angle of Doppler insonation), thereby reducing the detected Doppler shift, or by decreasing the insonating sound beam frequency. **Increasing the PRF** increases the detectable frequency shift, but the PRF increase is limited by the depth of the vessel as well as the center frequency of the transducer.[30,60] One can also **shift the zero baseline** and reassign a larger range of velocities to forward flow to overcome aliasing. It is also valid to **add velocity values above and below the baseline** to obtain an accurate velocity value, provided that multiple wraparounds do not occur, as seen in extremely high velocities. Aliasing may sometimes be useful in color Doppler image interpretation, where color-flow Doppler aliasing can accent the severity of flow disturbances as well as define the patent lumen.

Internal Carotid Artery Occlusion

Distinguishing between a **string sign** and a **totally occluded carotid artery** has major clinical significance.

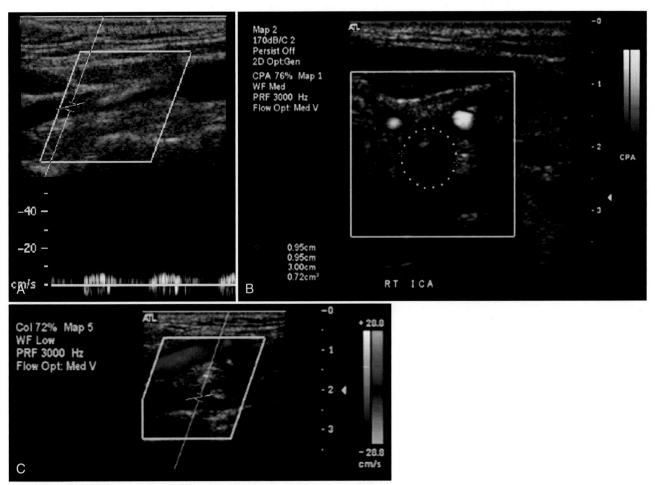

FIGURE 25-33. Near occlusion and total occlusion of internal carotid artery. A, Preocclusive trickle of flow in a left ICA. **B,** Hypoechoic heterogenous plaque completely occluding the lumen of the ICA. In this color Doppler image, no flow is demonstrated in the ICA. **C,** Color Doppler image shows an absence of flow in patient with ICA occlusion.

Grubb et al.[99] showed that untreated preocclusive lesions carry about a 5% per year risk for stroke. Thus, intervention in this patient population is particularly important.

Carotid occlusion is diagnosed when no flow is detected in a vessel. Occasionally, transmitted pulsations into an occluded ICA may mimic abnormal flow in a patent vessel. The pulsed Doppler cursor should be clearly located in the ICA lumen, and arterial pulsatile flow should be identified. Close attention should be paid to the direction of flow and the nature of pulsations. **True center-stream sampling** should be documented by transverse scanning, and the sample volume reduced in size as much as possible. Extraneous pulsations should seldom be transmitted to the center of the thrombus.[61]

As a high-grade stenosis approaches occlusion, the high-velocity jet is reduced to a mere trickle. It may be difficult to locate the small residual string of flow within a largely occluded lumen using gray-scale imaging alone, particularly if the adjacent plaque or thrombus is anechoic, making the residual lumen invisible during real-time examination, or if calcified plaque obscures visualization. In critical high-grade stenoses (>95%),

standard-sensitivity color Doppler settings may fail to demonstrate a string of residual flow. Thus, it is always prudent to employ the **slow-flow sensitivity settings** on color Doppler to discriminate between critical stenoses and occlusions.[80,83] Alternatively, power Doppler ultrasound (with its increased sensitivity to detecting low-amplitude, slow-velocity signals) may be used to visualize a **residual string of blood flow** (Fig. 25-33). Color Doppler is 95% to 98% accurate in distinguishing high-grade stenosis from complete occlusion on angiography when appropriate technical parameters are employed.[100-102]

The presence of a high-grade ICA stenosis or occlusion can often be inferred from inspection of the ipsilateral CCA on a pulsed Doppler waveform or color/power Doppler image (see Fig. 25-31). The pulsed Doppler waveforms in the ipsilateral CCA and ICA proximal to a lesion frequently demonstrate an asymmetrical, high-resistance signal with decreased, absent, or reversed diastolic flow, except when there are **ECA collaterals to the intracranial circulation** (Fig. 25-34). The main intracranial/extracranial collateral pathway exists between the orbital and ophthalmic arteries. Other collateral pathways include the occipital branch of the ECA to the

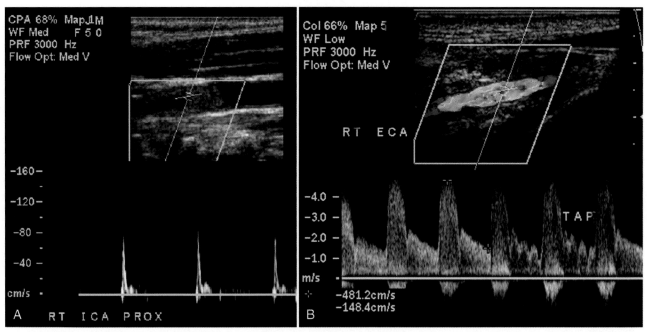

FIGURE 25-34. Internal carotid artery occlusion. A, Complete left ICA occlusion shows a spiked waveform consistent with an occlusion. **B,** Proximal left external carotid artery *(ECA)* trace shows a low-resistance waveform consistent with collaterals to intracranial circulation, as well as increased velocity caused by a stenosis; *TAP,* temporal artery tap.

INTERNAL CAROTID ARTERY OCCLUSION: SONOGRAPHIC FINDINGS

"Internalization" of ipsilateral external carotid artery waveform.

Absence of flow in internal carotid artery (ICA) by color Doppler, power Doppler, or pulsed Doppler ultrasound.

Reversal of flow in segment of ICA or common carotid artery (CCA) proximal to occluded segment.

Thrombus or plaque completely fills lumen of ICA on gray-scale, color Doppler, or power Doppler images.

Dampened high-resistance waveform in ipsilateral CCA or proximal ICA.

Contralateral CCA may demonstrate significantly higher velocities than ipsilateral CCA.

vertebral artery and cervical branches off the arch with the vertebral artery. Similarly, color or power Doppler images may show a flash of color flow in systole but a conspicuous decrease or absence of color flow in diastole, which is asymmetrical compared to the contralateral side. The diagnosis of carotid occlusion versus a string sign is made more accurately with color and power Doppler than with gray-scale duplex scanning and may obviate the need for angiography to confirm a sonographically diagnosed ICA occlusion.[100,101]

Another pitfall in the diagnosis of a totally occluded ICA is **mistaking a patent ECA** (or one of its branches)

for the ICA. The situation is especially confusing when the ECA/ICA collaterals open in response to long-standing ICA disease and the ECA acquires a low-resistance waveform (internalization) (Fig. 25-35). One technique that can aid in identifying the ECA is scanning at the origin of the vessel while simultaneously tapping the temporal artery. Percussion of the superficial temporal artery often results in a serrated distortion of the Doppler waveform in the ECA (80% of ECAs percussed in one study;[102] see Fig. 25-4, *B*). However, this maneuver should be used with caution because the temporal tap can also be seen in the CCA and ICA, although less frequently (54% and 33%, respectively) than in the ECA.[103] Branching vessels are a unique feature of the ECA, which can also be used to differentiate this vessel from the ICA. Color Doppler sonography can facilitate the identification of such branching vessels (see Fig. 25-4, *A*). Usually, the combination of vessel size, position, waveform shape, presence of branches, and the temporal tap response can correctly identify the ECA.

Although distal propagation of the thrombus almost invariably occurs after an ICA occlusion, CCA occlusions are often localized. Flow may be maintained in the ECA and ICA but must be reversed in one of the two vessels. Sonography is the preferred method for evaluating the maintenance of flow around the carotid bifurcation after proximal CCA occlusion. Most often, retrograde flow in the ECA will supply antegrade flow in the ipsilateral ICA. Occasionally, the opposite flow pattern will be encountered[61,104,105] (Fig. 25-36).

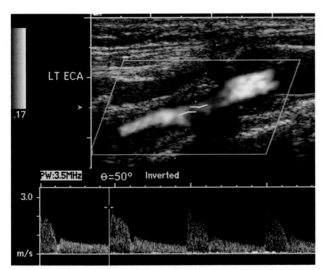

FIGURE 25-35. Chronic occlusion. Long-standing internal carotid artery occlusion results in low-resistance waveform in the external carotid artery.

Preoperative Strategies for Patients with Carotid Artery Disease

The preoperative workup of carotid disease is evolving in response to NASCET, ECST, and ACAS results.[4,5,106] The issue of numbers to be used for a carotid ultrasound examination depends on the intent of the examination. Why are we doing the study? How will we use the results? If the examination is a screening test, are we evaluating all patients, or only symptomatic patients? If we intend to select patients for surgery on the basis of the ultrasound alone, then a different set of variables is likely to produce the desired outcome. The purpose of a carotid examination and the patient population being screened will impact the selection of velocity thresholds. For example, screening of high-risk, asymptomatic patients might best be performed with high-velocity thresholds with increased specificity, whereas symptomatic patients more likely to undergo surgery for optimal treatment would dictate lower thresholds with increased sensitivity.

Although many still consider angiography as the standard, its critics cite significant intraobserver variability and frequent underestimation of the degree of stenosis.[107] Comparisons of angiographic and sonographic estimations of carotid stenosis reveal a closer surgical correlation with the ultrasound measurements.[1] Carotid ultrasound has proved highly accurate in detecting high-grade stenoses, as well as differentiating critical stenoses from occlusion, particularly since the advent of color and power Doppler ultrasound. MRA is currently demonstrating comparable accuracy as ultrasound and angiography for the detection and quantification of carotid stenosis. Like sonography, MRA can depict plaque morphology, but it can also evaluate intracranial circulation. MRA may be helpful in situations where calcified plaque obscures the underlying carotid lumen from insonation.

Many investigators now suggest replacing preoperative angiography with a combination of carotid sonography and MRA. They advocate utilizing angiography only in cases where MRA and carotid ultrasound have discordant results, or they are inadequate.[108-110] Other studies support the use of carotid ultrasound alone before endarterectomy.[109-115] Numerous studies show that more than 90% of surgical candidates can be adequately screened using clinical assessment and ultrasound alone. However, in suspected aortic arch proximal vessel disease or in cases of suspected complete occlusion, some practitioners still advocate preoperative angiography.

Randoux et al.[116] reported strong correlation among CT angiography, gadolinium-enhanced MRA, and conventional angiography for estimating carotid stenoses. When MRA is contraindicated, CT angiography could provide an alternative noninvasive preoperative imaging tool.

Postoperative Ultrasound

The **endarterectomized carotid artery** demonstrates many characteristic features[117,118] (Fig. 25-37). A discrete wedge between the normal I-M complex and the endarterectomized surface is frequently seen, as are periodically spaced echogenic sutures. The absent I-M complex has also been shown to regrow. Although routine post-endarterectomy surveillance is not advocated in asymptomatic patients, one study showed that approximately 6% of CEA patients had carotid flaps, residual moderate to moderately severe stenoses, or occluded ECAs.[119] Two of these patients with postoperative abnormalities on ultrasound sustained perioperative stroke. Patients without defects on the postoperative ultrasound had no perioperative sequelae or need for a repeat of procedures. Patients with preoperative stenoses greater than 75% have a greater risk for residual stenoses. Ultrasound appears useful in the symptomatic postoperative population, but its role in the asymptomatic patient population is debatable.[120]

Carotid Artery Stents and Revascularization

Percutaneous transluminal **carotid artery stenting** (CAS) in association with carotid angioplasty is becoming an increasing popular and common means of carotid revascularization. Between 1998 and 2004, the incidence of CEA decreased 17%, whereas incidence of CAS increased 149%.[121] Studies report that CAS is equivalent in safety and efficacy even in patients at increased surgical risk.[122] However, this is a controversial issue. Careful patient selection is critical if the potential benefits of carotid revascularization are to be realized. Ultrasound may be helpful in (1) assessing the presence and severity of stenosis, (2) characterizing the carotid bifurcation,

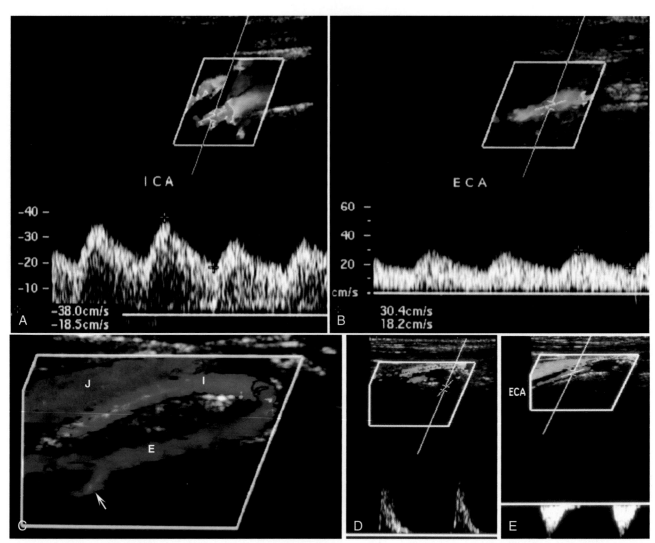

FIGURE 25-36. Common carotid artery (CCA) occlusion causes abnormal internal carotid artery (ICA) waveform. A, Antegrade tardus-parvus waveform is seen in an ICA distal to a CCA occlusion. **B,** Retrograde external carotid artery *(ECA)* flow with a tardus-parvus waveform caused by collateral flow from the contralateral ECA to supply the ipsilateral ICA distal to a CCA occlusion. **C,** Color Doppler image shows antegrade ECA flow *(E)* with an ECA branch *(arrow)* and retrograde ICA flow *(I; J,* internal jugular vein. **D,** Spectral Doppler image shows high-resistance retrograde right ICA flow. **E,** High-resistance antegrade flow in the right ECA distal to a CCA occlusion.

and (3) assessing anatomic variants, vessel tortuosity, and plaque calcification before stent placement (Fig. 25-38).

The role of ultrasound in determining patient selection also remains controversial. Certainly, the accuracy of duplex ultrasound in grading flow-limiting stenosis is well established, with a sensitivity of 94% and a specificity of 92%, and is universally accepted as an important criterion in patient selection.[123] However, although the role of plaque characterization in patient selection remains controversial, it is becoming more important as **vulnerable plaque,** as an etiology of stroke, becomes more appreciated. Vulnerable plaque appears to correlate with heterogeneous or echolucent type 1 or 2 plaque. This type of plaque is associated with intraplaque hemorrhage and is thought to have strong embolic potential. Using **intravascular ultrasound** (IVUS), Diethrich et al.[124] showed a strong correlation between IVUS

plaque characterization and true histologic examination of the plaque after endarterectomy. Considering the accuracy of ultrasound characterization, when intraplaque hemorrhage or vulnerable plaque is identified, CEA rather than CAS might be the preferred method of revascularization to reduce the risk of embolic complications. However, Reiter et al.[125] were unable to use plaque echolucency as a criterion for those at increased risk for post-CAS neurologic events and therefore did not recommend this type of risk stratification. The use of plaque characterization to determine the type of therapeutic intervention needs further assessment.

Grading Carotid Intrastent Restenosis

Sonography allows accurate evaluation of stent placement within the carotid vessels.[126] Carotid **stents** are

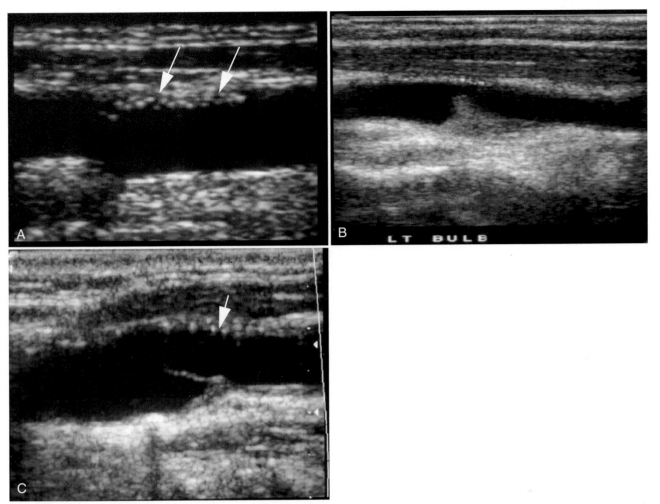

FIGURE 25-37. Post–carotid endarterectomy (CEA) appearances. A, Normal post-CEA changes with a vein patch *(arrows)*. **B,** Abnormal wedge of residual/recurrent plaque/thrombus in newly symptomatic post-CEA patient. **C,** Post-CEA sutures *(arrow)* with a residual intimal flap in lumen.

readily visualized with ultrasound, allowing one to assess disease before, along, and distal to the stent. The rate of post-CAS restenosis has been reported as between 1.9% and 16%.[126-129] Velocity criteria for grading stenoses in a stent may not be the same as for those in the native carotid artery.[130] Some investigators have shown that velocities along the stent are routinely higher than those in a nonstented vessel. Velocity elevations in the range of 125 to 140 cm/sec are fairly common in widely patent stents. In addition, one normally sees an increase in velocity in the distal ICA beyond the deployed stent. At present, slight increases in velocity in a stent that appears widely patent on power or color Doppler are unlikely to indicate significant narrowing or warrant further assessment or intervention.

Fleming et al.[126] and Chahwan et al.[131] showed that normal Doppler ultrasound reliably identifies arteriographically normal carotid arteries after CAS. They also reported that post-CAS carotid velocities did not always correlate with the prestented flow-limiting stenosis tables, and that the velocities appeared to be disproportionately elevated in mild and moderately restenotic

vessels. The disproportionate velocity elevations along the stent may be caused by several factors, including changes in vessel wall compliance and shunting of blood flow away from the ECA. Also, the technique used in many stent trials, which require strict adherence to the 60-degree angle theta technique for Doppler interrogation, may result in systematic velocity increases. As such, it was realized that new tables must be established and validated for the follow-up of patients after CAS. Multiple proposals for grading post-CAS parameters have been suggested[132-136] (Table 25-3).

NONATHEROSCLEROTIC CAROTID DISEASE

Nonatherosclerotic carotid disease is much less common than plaque disease. **Fibromuscular dysplasia** (FMD), a noninflammatory process with hypertrophy of muscular and fibrous arterial walls separated by abnormal zones of fragmentation, involves the middle and distal ICA more frequently than other carotid segments. A

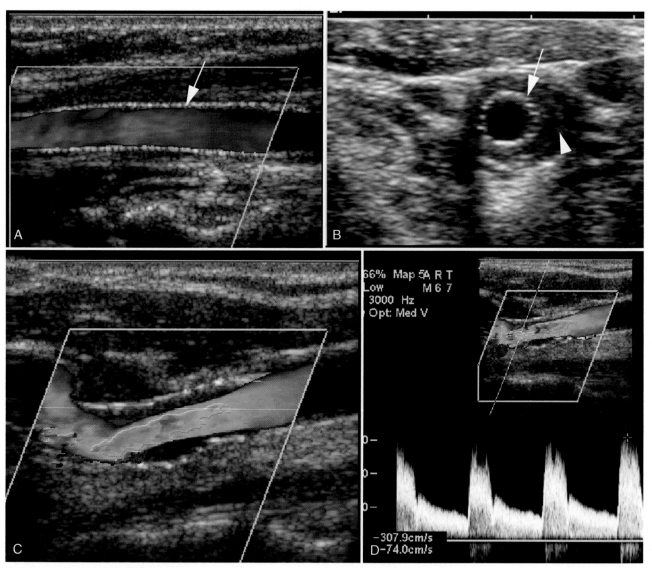

FIGURE 25-38. Carotid stent. A, Normal right carotid stent *(arrow)* shows complete filling on color Doppler examination. **B,** Transverse image of carotid stent *(arrow)* in the carotid bulb shows residual plaque *(arrowhead)* in the lumen. **C** and **D,** Left carotid stent shows visible narrowing on color Doppler **(C)** and elevated velocities **(D)** consistent with a greater than 70% stenosis using standard carotid velocity criteria.

TABLE 25-3. CAROTID ARTERY STENOSIS GRADING

STUDY	DEGREE OF STENOSIS	PSV (cm/sec)	EDV (cm/sec)	ICA/CCA PSV RATIO
Setacci et al.[132]	<30%	≤104		
	30%-50%	105-174		
	50%-70%	175-299		
	≥70%	≥300	≥140	≥3.8
Zhou et al.[133]	>70%	>300	>90	>4
Lal et al.[134]	≥20%	≥150		>2.15
	≥50%	≥220		≥2.7
	≥80%	>340		≥4.15
Armstrong et al.[135]	>50%	>150		>2
	>75%	>300	>125	>4
Chi et al.[136]	≥50%	240		2.45
	≥70%	450		4.3

Modified from Fleming et al.[126] and Chahwan et al.[131]
PSV, Peak systolic velocity; *EDV,* end diastolic velocity; ICA/CCA, internal/common carotids.

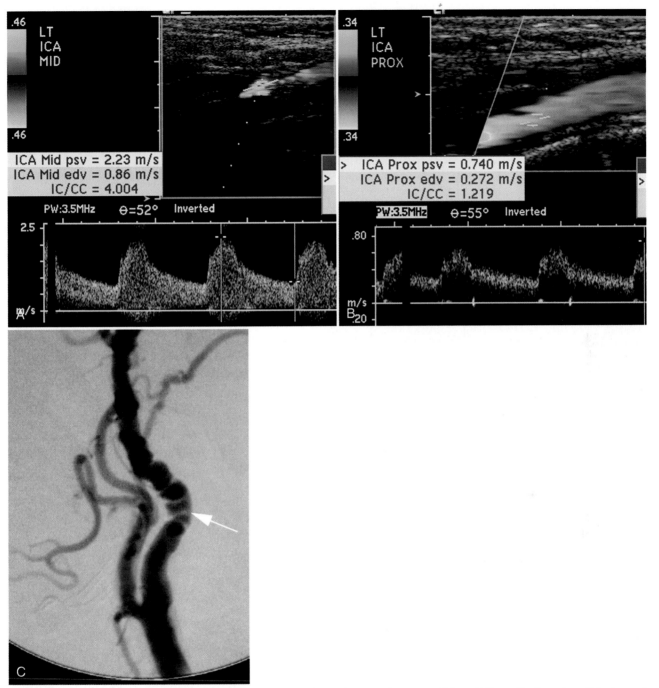

FIGURE 25-39. Fibromuscular dysplasia. A, Longitudinal color Doppler image of the middle to distal portion of the internal carotid artery (ICA) shows velocity elevation and significant stenosis. **B,** Same patient's proximal portion of the ICA shows no stenosis. **C,** Angiogram demonstrates typical appearance of fibromuscular dysplasia in the mid-ICA and distal ICA. Note the beaded appearance resulting from focal bands *(arrow)* of thickened tissue that narrow the lumen.

characteristic "string of beads" appearance has been described on angiography. Only a few reports describe sonographic features of FMD.[137,138] Many patients with FMD demonstrate nonspecific or no obvious abnormalities on ultrasound. FMD may be asymptomatic or can result in carotid dissection or subsequent thromboembolic events (Fig. 25-39). **Arteritis** resulting from autoimmune processes (e.g., Takayasu's arteritis, temporal arteritis) or radiation changes can produce diffuse con-

centric thickening of carotid walls, which most frequently involves the CCA[139] (Fig. 25-40).

Cervical trauma can produce carotid dissections or aneurysms. **Carotid artery dissection** results from a tear in the intima, allowing blood to dissect into the wall of the artery, which produces a false lumen. The false lumen may be blind ended or may reenter the true lumen. The false lumen may occlude or narrow the true lumen, producing symptoms similar to carotid

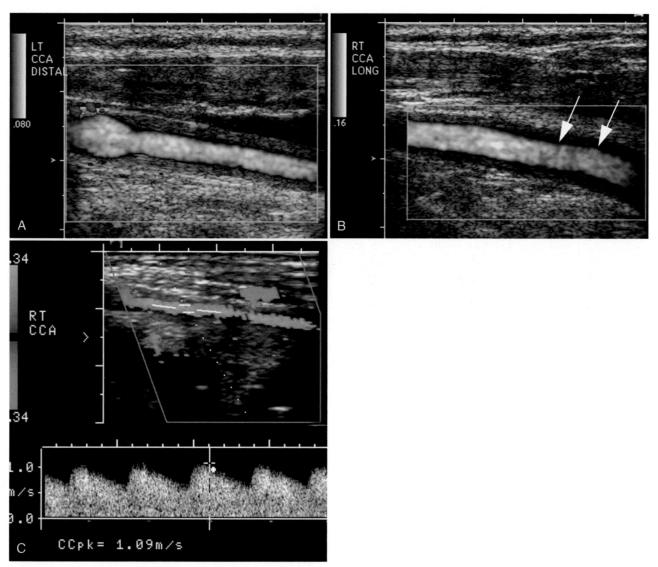

FIGURE 25-40. Long-segment stenosis of common carotid artery (CCA) caused by Takayasu's arteritis.
A, Power Doppler image of left CCA shows long-segment concentric narrowing caused by greatly thickened walls of the artery. **B,** Power Doppler image of right CCA in same patient demonstrates similar concentric narrowing *(arrows)*. **C,** Right spectral Doppler waveform shows a mildly tardus-parvus waveform.

plaque disease. Dissections may arise spontaneously or secondary to trauma or to intrinsic disease with elastic tissue degeneration (e.g., Marfan's syndrome) or may be related to atherosclerotic plaque disease.[15] The ultrasound examination of a carotid dissection may reveal a mobile or fixed **echogenic intimal flap,** with or without thrombus formation. Frequently, there is a striking image/Doppler mismatch with a paucity of gray-scale abnormalities seen in association with marked flow abnormalities (Fig. 25-41).

Color or power Doppler ultrasound may readily clarify the source of this mismatch by demonstrating abrupt tapering of the patent, filled lumen to the point of an ICA occlusion, analogous to angiographic findings. Although the ICA is frequently occluded, demonstrating absent flow with a high-resistance waveform in the proxi-

mal ipsilateral CCA, flow in the ICA may demonstrate high velocities associated with luminal narrowing secondary to hemorrhage and a thrombus in the area of the false lumen. Accordingly, flow velocity waveforms in the CCA may be normal or may demonstrate extremely damped, high-resistance waveforms. MRA, another noninvasive imaging test, readily demonstrates mural hematoma that confirms the diagnosis of ICA dissection. Although angiography is frequently used initially to diagnose a dissection, ultrasound can be used to follow patients to assess the therapeutic response to anticoagulation. Repeat sonographic evaluation of patients with ICA dissection after anticoagulation therapy reveals recanalization of the artery in as many as 70% of cases.[140-142] It is important to consider the diagnosis of dissection as a cause of neurologic symptoms, particu-

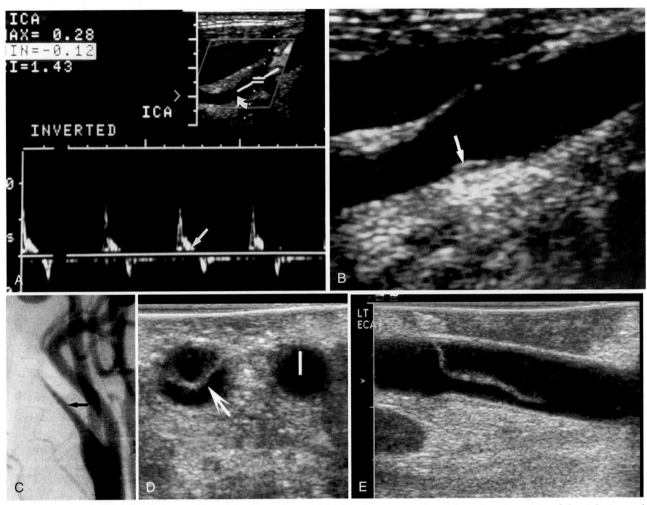

FIGURE 25-41. Carotid artery dissection. A, Abnormal high-resistance waveforms *(arrow)* at the origin of the right internal carotid artery *(ICA)* with no evidence of flow distal to this point *(curved arrow)*. **B,** Gray-scale evaluation of the vessel in the area of the occlusion demonstrates only a small, linear echogenic structure *(arrow)* without evidence of significant atherosclerotic narrowing. **C,** Subsequent angiogram demonstrates the characteristic tapering to the point of occlusion *(arrow)* associated with carotid artery dissection and thrombotic occlusion. **D,** Transverse, and **E,** longitudinal, images of another patient show an intimal flap *(arrow)* in an external carotid artery; *I,* internal carotid artery.

INTERNAL CAROTID ARTERY DISSECTION: SONOGRAPHIC FINDINGS

Internal Carotid Artery
Absent flow or occlusion
Echogenic intimal flap, with or without thrombus
Hypoechoic thrombus, with or without luminal narrowing
Normal appearance

Common Carotid Artery
High-resistance waveform
Damped flow
Normal appearance

---

larly when the clinical presentation, age, and patient history are atypical for that of atherosclerotic disease or hemorrhagic stroke.

The most common **CCA aneurysm** occurs in the region of the carotid bifurcation. These aneurysms may result from atherosclerosis, infection, trauma, surgery, or infectious etiology, such as syphilis. The normal CCA usually measures no more than 1 cm in diameter. **Carotid body tumors,** one of several paragangliomas that involve the head and neck, are usually benign, well-encapsulated masses located at the carotid bifurcation. These tumors may be bilateral, particularly in the familial variant, and are very vascular, often producing an audible bruit. Some of these tumors produce catecholamines, leading to sudden changes in blood pressure during or after surgery. Color Doppler ultrasound demonstrates an extremely vascular soft tissue mass at the carotid bifurcation (Fig. 25-42). Color Doppler

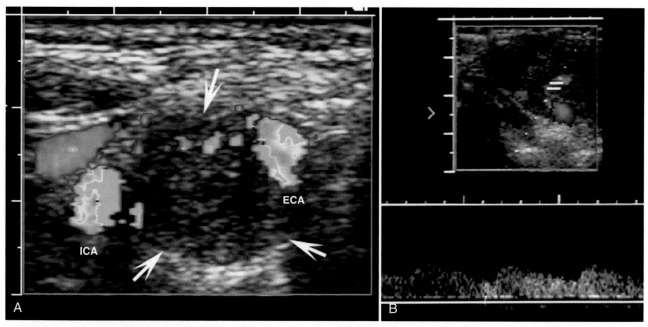

FIGURE 25-42. Carotid body tumor. A, Transverse image of the carotid bifurcation shows a mass *(arrows)* splaying the internal carotid artery *(ICA)* and external carotid artery *(ECA)*. **B,** Pulsed Doppler traces of the carotid body tumor show typical arteriovenous shunt (low-resistance) waveform.

ultrasound can also be used to monitor embolization or surgical resection of carotid body tumors. A classic nonmass is the **ectatic innominate/proximal CCA**, frequently occurring as a pulsatile supraclavicular mass in older women. The request to rule out a carotid aneurysm almost invariably shows the classic normal features of these tortuous vessels (Fig. 25-43).

Extravascular masses (e.g., lymph nodes, hematomas, abscesses) that compress or displace the carotid arteries can be readily distinguished from primary vascular masses, such as aneurysms or pseudoaneurysms (Fig. 25-44). **Posttraumatic pseudoaneurysms** can usually be distinguished from a true carotid aneurysm by demonstrating the characteristic to-and-fro waveforms in the neck of the pseudoaneurysm, as well as the internal variability (yin-yang) characteristic of a pseudoaneurysm (Fig. 25-45).

TRANSCRANIAL DOPPLER SONOGRAPHY

In transcranial Doppler (TCD) ultrasound, a low-frequency 2-MHz transducer is used to evaluate blood flow within the intracranial carotid and vertebrobasilar system and the circle of Willis. Access is achieved through the orbits, foramen magnum, or most often the region of temporal calvarial thinning (**transtemporal window**).[143] However, many patients (up to 55% in one series[144]) may not have access to an interpretable TCD examination. Women, particularly African Americans, have a thick temporal bone through which it is difficult to

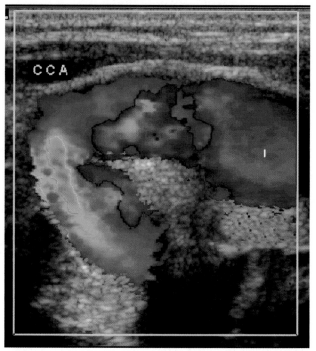

FIGURE 25-43. Ectatic common carotid artery (CCA). Color Doppler image shows ectatic proximal CCA arising from the innominate artery *(I)* and responsible for a pulsatile right supraclavicular mass.

insonate the basal cerebral arteries.[144,145] This difficulty limits the feasibility of TCD imaging as a routine part of the noninvasive cerebrovascular workup.[144]

By using spectral analysis, various parameters are determined, including mean velocity, PSV, EDV, and

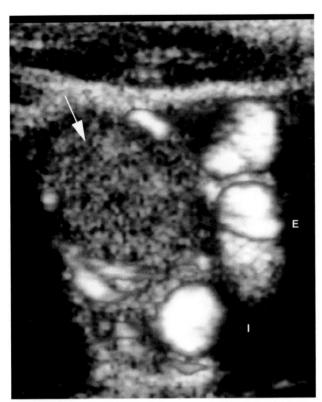

FIGURE 25-44. Pathologic lymph node near carotid bifurcation. Power Doppler image shows a malignant lymph node *(arrow)* lateral to the carotid bifurcation.

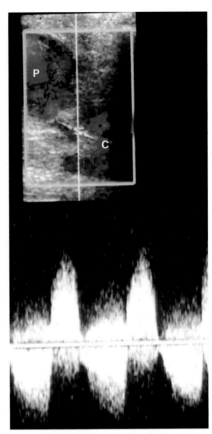

FIGURE 25-45. Pseudoaneurysm of the common carotid artery (CCA). Transverse image of the left distal CCA *(C)* demonstrates a characteristic to-and-fro waveform in the neck of the large pseudoaneurysm *(P)*, which resulted from an attempted central venous line placement.

the pulsatility and resistive indices of the blood vessels. Color or power Doppler ultrasound can improve velocity determination by providing better angle theta determination and localizing the course of vessels.[143] TCD applications include (1) evaluation of intracranial stenoses and collateral circulation, (2) detection and follow-up of vasoconstriction from subarachnoid hemorrhage, (3) determination of brain death, (4) evaluation of patients with sickle cell disease, and (5) identification of arteriovenous malformation.[140-143,146] TCD is most reliable in diagnosing stenoses of the middle cerebral artery (MCA), with sensitivities as high as 91% reported. TCD is less reliable for detecting stenoses of the intracranial vertebrobasilar system, anterior and posterior cerebral arteries, and terminal ICA. However, TCD is helpful in assessing vertebral artery patency and flow direction when no flow is detected in the extracranial vertebral artery (Fig. 25-46). Diagnosis of an intracranial stenosis is based on an increase in the mean velocity of blood flow in the affected vessel compared to that of the contralateral vessel at the same location.[144,145]

Advantages of TCD ultrasound also include its availability to monitor patients in the operating room or angiographic suite for potential cerebrovascular complications.[145] Intraoperative TCD monitoring can be performed with the transducer strapped over the transtemporal window, allowing evaluation of blood flow in the MCA during CEA. The adequacy of cerebral perfusion can be assessed while the carotid artery is clamped.[145,147] TCD is also capable of detecting **intraoperative microembolization** ("HITS"), which produces high-amplitude spikes on the Doppler spectrum.[144,148-150] The technique can be used for the serial evaluation of **vasospasms.** This diagnosis is usually based on serial examinations of the relative increase in blood flow velocity and resistive index changes resulting from a decrease in the lumen of the vessel caused by vasospasms.[145]

VERTEBRAL ARTERY

The vertebral arteries supply the majority of the posterior brain circulation. Through the circle of Willis, the vertebral arteries also provide collateral circulation to other portions of the brain in patients with carotid occlusive disease. Evaluation of the extracranial vertebral artery seems a natural extension of carotid duplex and color Doppler imaging.[151,152] Historically, however, these arteries have not been studied as intensively as the carotids. Symptoms of **vertebrobasilar insufficiency**

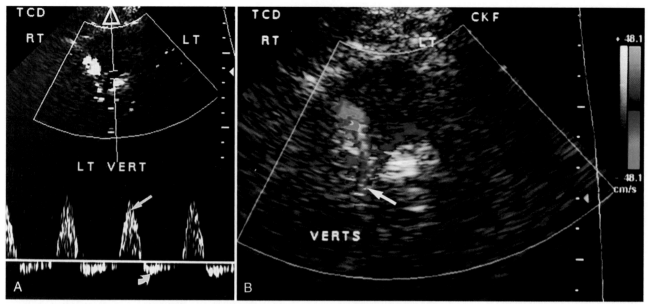

FIGURE 25-46. Transcranial Doppler imaging. A, Transcranial duplex scan of the posterior fossa in a patient with an incomplete left subclavian steal syndrome demonstrates retrograde systolic flow *(arrow)* and antegrade diastolic flow *(curved arrow).* The scan is obtained in a transverse projection from the region of the foramen magnum *(open arrowhead).* **B,** Color Doppler image obtained in the same patient demonstrates that there is retrograde flow not only within the left vertebral artery, but within the basilar artery *(arrow)* as well.

also tend to be rather vague and poorly defined compared with symptoms referable to the carotid circulation. It is often difficult to make an association confidently between a lesion and symptoms. Furthermore, interest in surgical correction of vertebral lesions has been limited. The anatomic variability, small size, deep course, and limited visualization resulting from overlying transverse processes make the vertebral artery more difficult to examine accurately with ultrasound.[151,153,154] The clinical utility of vertebral artery duplex scanning remains under investigation. Its role in diagnosing subclavian steal and presteal phenomena is well established.[155,156] Less clear-cut is the use of vertebral duplex scanning in evaluating vertebral artery stenosis, dissection, or aneurysm.

Anatomy

The vertebral artery is usually the first branch off the subclavian artery (Fig. 25-47). However, variation in the origin of the vertebral arteries is common. In 6% to 8% of people the left vertebral artery arises directly from the aortic arch proximal to the left subclavian artery. In 90% the proximal vertebral artery ascends superomedially, passing anterior to the transverse process of the seventh cervical vertebra (C7), and enters the transverse foramen at the C6 level. The remainder of vertebral arteries enters into the transverse foramen at the C5 or C7 level and, rarely, at the C4 level. The size of vertebral arteries is variable, with the left larger than the right in 42%, the two vertebral arteries equal in size in 26%, and the right

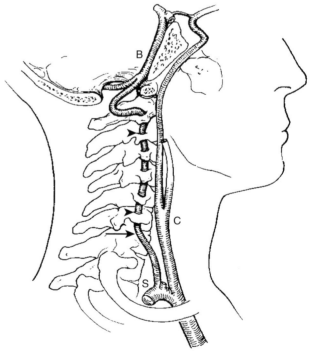

FIGURE 25-47. Vertebral artery course. Lateral diagram of vertebral artery *(arrow)* shows its course through the cervical spine transverse foramina *(arrowheads)* en route to joining the contralateral vertebral artery to form the basilar artery *(B);* *C,* carotid artery; *S,* subclavian artery.

larger than the left in 32% of cases.[157] One vertebral artery may even be congenitally absent. Usually, the vertebral arteries join at their confluence to form the **basilar artery.** Rarely, the vertebral artery may terminate in a posterior inferior cerebellar artery.

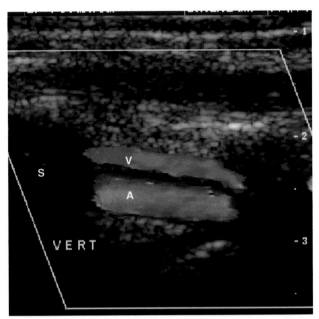

FIGURE 25-48. Normal vertebral artery and vein.
Longitudinal color Doppler image shows a normal vertebral artery *(A)* and vein *(V)* running between the transverse processes of the second to sixth cervical vertebrae (C2-C6), which are identified by their periodic acoustic shadowing *(S)*.

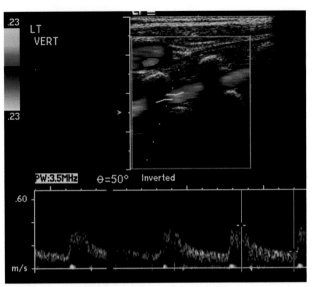

FIGURE 25-49. Normal vertebral artery waveform.
Normal low-resistance waveform of the vertebral artery with filling of the spectral window.

Sonographic Technique and Normal Examination

Vertebral artery visualization with Doppler flow analysis can be obtained in 92% to 98% of vessels[151,158] (Fig. 25-48). Color Doppler facilitates the rapid detection of vertebral arteries but does not significantly improve this detection rate.[154] Vertebral artery duplex examinations are performed by first locating the CCA in the longitudinal plane. The direction of flow in the CCA and jugular vein is determined. A gradual sweep of the transducer laterally demonstrates the vertebral artery and vein running between the transverse processes of C2 to C6, which are identified by their periodic acoustic shadowing. Transverse scanning with color Doppler allows the examiner to visualize the carotid artery and jugular vein at the same time and use them as references to determine the direction of flow in the vertebral artery.[153,155] Angling the transducer caudad allows visualization of the vertebral artery origin in 60% to 70% of the arteries, in 80% on the right-hand side, and in 50% on the left. This discrepancy may relate to the left vertebral artery origin being deeper and arising directly from the aortic arch in 6% to 8% of cases.[153,159]

The presence and direction of flow should be established. Visible plaque disease should be assessed. The vertebral artery supplies blood to the brain and usually has a low-resistance flow pattern similar to that of the CCA, with continuous flow in systole and diastole; however, wide variability in waveform shape has been noted in angiographically normal vessels.[160] Because the vessel is small, flow tends to demonstrate a broader spectrum. The clear spectral window seen in the normal carotid system is often filled in the vertebral artery[61] (Fig. 25-49).

The **vertebral vein** (often a plexus of veins) runs parallel and adjacent to the vertebral artery. Care must be taken not to mistake its flow for that of the adjacent artery, particularly if the venous flow is pulsatile. Comparison with jugular venous flow during respiration should readily distinguish between vertebral artery and vein. At times, the ascending cervical branch of the thyrocervical trunk can be mistaken for the vertebral artery. This can be avoided by looking for landmark transverse processes that accompany the vertebral artery and by paying careful attention to the waveform of the visualized vessel. The ascending cervical branch has a high-impedance waveform pattern similar to that of the ECA.[155]

Transcranial Doppler sonographic examination of the vertebrobasilar artery system can be performed as an adjunct to the extracranial evaluation. The examination is conducted with a 2-MHz transducer with the patient sitting, using a suboccipital midline nuchal approach, or with the patient supine, using a retromastoidal approach. Color or power Doppler facilitates TCD imaging of the vertebrobasilar system.[161]

Subclavian Steal

The **subclavian steal phenomenon** (syndrome) occurs when there is high-grade stenosis or occlusion of the proximal subclavian or innominate arteries with patent vertebral arteries bilaterally. The artery of the ischemic limb "steals" blood from the vertebrobasilar circulation through retrograde vertebral artery flow, which may

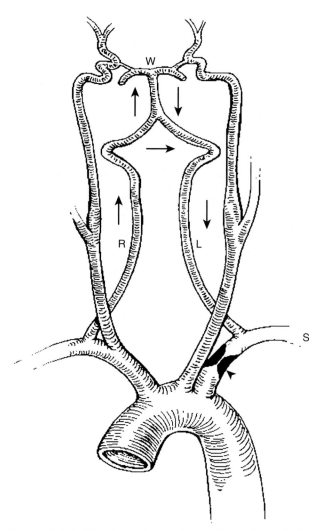

FIGURE 25-50. Hemodynamic pattern in subclavian steal syndrome. Proximal left subclavian artery occlusive lesion *(arrowhead)* decreases flow to the distal subclavian artery *(S)*. This produces retrograde flow *(large arrows)* down the left vertebral artery *(L)* and stealing from the right vertebral artery *(R)* and other intracranial vessels through the circle of Willis *(W)*.

ABNORMAL VERTEBRAL ARTERY WAVEFORMS

Complete Subclavian Steal
Reversal of flow within vertebral artery ipsilateral to stenotic or occluded subclavian or innominate artery.

Incomplete or Partial Subclavian Steal
Transient reversal of vertebral artery flow during systole.
May be converted into a complete steal using provocative maneuvers.
Suggests stenotic, not occlusive, lesion.

Presteal Phenomenon
"Bunny" waveform: systolic deceleration less than diastolic flow.
May be converted into partial steal by provocative maneuvers.
Seen with proximal subclavian stenosis.

Tardus-Parvus or Damped Waveform
Seen with vertebral artery stenosis.

result in symptoms of vertebrobasilar insufficiency (Fig. 25-50). Symptoms are usually most pronounced during exercise of the upper extremity but can be produced by changes in head position. However, there is often poor correlation between vertebrobasilar symptoms and the subclavian steal phenomenon. Usually, flow within the basilar artery is unaffected unless severe stenosis of the vertebral artery supplying the steal exists.[161] Also, surgical or angioplastic restoration of blood flow may not result in relief of symptoms.[162] The subclavian steal syndrome is most often caused by atherosclerotic disease, although traumatic, embolic, surgical, congenital, and neoplastic factors have also been implicated. Although the proximal subclavian stenosis or occlusion may be difficult to image, particularly on the left, the vertebral

artery waveform abnormalities correlate with the severity of the subclavian disease.

Doppler evaluation of the vertebral artery reveals four distinct abnormal waveforms that correlate with subclavian or vertebral artery pathology on angiography. These include the complete subclavian steal, partial or incomplete steal, presteal phenomenon, and tardus-parvus vertebral artery waveforms.[160] In a **complete subclavian steal,** flow within the vertebral artery is completely reversed (Fig. 25-51). **Incomplete steal** or **partial steal** demonstrate transient reversal of vertebral flow during systole[161,163] (Fig. 25-52). Incomplete steal suggests high-grade stenosis of the subclavian or innominate artery rather than occlusion. Provocative maneuvers, such as exercising the arm for 5 minutes or 5-minute inflation of a sphygmomanometer on the arm to induce rebound hyperemia on the side of the subclavian or innominate lesion, can enhance the sonographic findings and convert an incomplete steal to a complete steal.[97,115]

The **presteal** ("bunny") **waveform** shows antegrade flow but with a striking deceleration of velocity in peak systole to a level less than EDV. This is seen in patients with proximal subclavian stenosis, which is usually less severe than in those with partial steal waveform.[163] The bunny waveform can be converted into a partial steal or complete steal waveform by provocative maneuvers, such as the use of a blood pressure cuff (Fig. 25-53). A damped, **tardus-parvus waveform** can be seen in patients with high-grade proximal vertebral stenosis.[156,163]

With a subclavian steal, color Doppler may show two similarly color-encoded vessels between the transverse

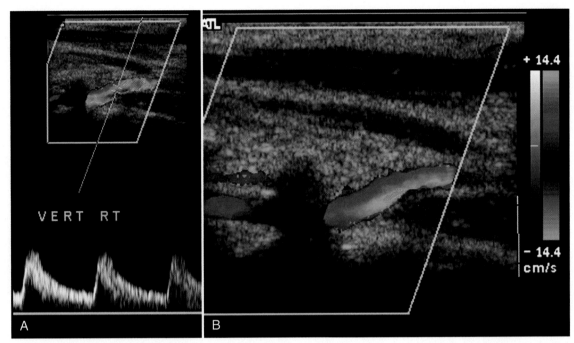

FIGURE 25-51. Vertebral artery flow. A, Subclavian steal causes reversed flow in vertebral artery. Complete vertebral artery flow reversal results from a right subclavian artery occlusion. Flow in this vertebral artery is toward the transducer. **B,** Slightly aberrant vertebral artery with color flow reversal.

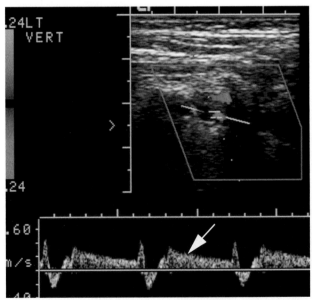

FIGURE 25-52. Incomplete subclavian steal. Flow in early systole is antegrade, flow in peak systole is retrograde, and flow in late systole and diastole *(arrow)* is again antegrade.

processes, representing the vertebral artery and vein.[83] Transverse images of the vertebral artery with color Doppler show reversed flow compared with those of the CCA. A Doppler spectral waveform must be produced in all such cases to avoid mistaking flow reversal within an artery for flow in a pulsatile vertebral vein.[83,155]

Stenosis and Occlusion

Diagnosis of **vertebral artery stenosis** is more difficult than diagnosis of flow reversal. Most hemodynamically significant stenoses occur at the vertebral artery origin, situated deep in the upper thorax and seen in only 60% to 70% of patients.[153,158,159] Even if the vertebral artery origin off the subclavian is visualized, optimal adjustments of the Doppler angle for accurate velocity measurements may be difficult because of the deep location and vessel tortuosity. No accurate reproducible criteria for evaluating vertebral artery stenosis exist. Because flow is normally turbulent within the vertebral artery, spectral broadening cannot be used as an indicator of stenosis. Velocity measurements are not reliable as criteria for stenosis because of the wide normal variation in vertebral artery diameter. Although velocities greater than 100 cm/sec often indicate stenosis, they can occur in angiographically normal vessels. For example, high-flow velocity may be present in a vertebral artery that is serving as a major collateral pathway for cerebral circulation in cases of carotid occlusion[21,119,164] (Fig. 25-54). Thus, only a **focal increase in velocity of at least 50%, visible stenosis on gray-scale or color Doppler, or a striking tardus-parvus vertebral artery waveform** is likely to indicate significant vertebral stenosis. The variability of resistive indices in normal and abnormal vertebral arteries precludes the use of this parameter as an indicator of vertebral disease.[160]

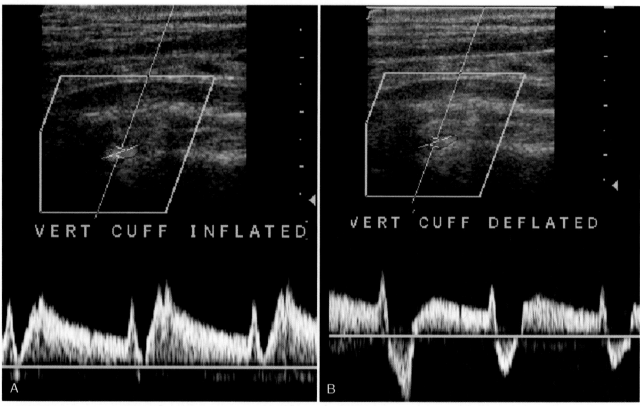

FIGURE 25-53. Incomplete subclavian steal and provocative maneuver. A, Presteal left vertebral artery waveform. Flow decelerates in peak systole but does not reverse. **B,** After provocative maneuver, there is reversal of flow in peak systole in response to a decrease in peripheral arterial pressure.

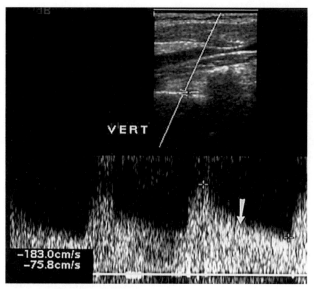

FIGURE 25-54. Increased flow velocity in vertebral artery. Pulsed Doppler spectral trace from a left vertebral artery demonstrates strikingly high velocities and disturbed flow *(arrow)*. Although this degree of velocity elevation and flow disturbance could be associated with a focal stenosis, in this case there was increased velocity throughout the vertebral artery from bilateral internal carotid artery occlusion and increased collateral flow into the vertebral artery.

Diagnosis of **vertebral artery occlusion** is also difficult. Often, the inability to detect arterial flow results from a small or congenitally absent vertebral artery or a technically difficult examination. The differentiation of severe stenosis from occlusion is difficult for the same reasons. Extremely damped blood flow velocity in high-grade stenoses and a decreased number of RBCs traversing the area evaluated may result in a Doppler signal with amplitude too low to be detected.[154] Power Doppler imaging may prove useful in this situation. Visualization of only a vertebral vein may indicate vertebral artery occlusion or congenital absence.

INTERNAL JUGULAR VEINS

The internal jugular veins are the major vessels responsible for the return of venous blood from the brain. The most common clinical indication for duplex and color Doppler flow ultrasound of the internal jugular vein is the evaluation of suspected **jugular venous thrombosis.**[165-172] Thrombus formation may be related to central venous catheter placement. Other indications include a diagnosis of jugular venous ectasia[171-174] and guidance for internal jugular or subclavian vein cannulation,[175-179] particularly in difficult situations where vascular anatomy is distorted.

Sonographic Technique

The normal internal jugular vein is easily visualized. The vein is scanned with the neck extended and the head turned to the contralateral side. Longitudinal and transverse scans are obtained with light transducer pressure on the neck to avoid collapsing the vein. A coronal view from the supraclavicular fossa is used to image the lower segment of the internal jugular vein and the medial segment of the subclavian vein as they join to form the brachiocephalic vein.

The jugular vein lies lateral and anterior to the CCA, lateral to the thyroid gland, and deep to the sternocleidomastoid muscle. The vessel has sharply echogenic walls and a hypoechoic or anechoic lumen. Normally, a valve can be visualized in its distal portion.[168,176,180] The right internal jugular vein is usually larger than the left.[175]

Real-time ultrasound demonstrates **venous pulsations related to right heart contractions,** as well as changes in venous diameter that vary with changes in intrathoracic pressure. Doppler examination graphically depicts these flow patterns (Fig. 25-55). On inspiration, negative intrathoracic pressure causes flow toward the heart and the jugular veins to decrease in diameter. During expiration and during Valsalva maneuver, increased intrathoracic pressure causes a decrease in the blood return, and the veins enlarge, with minimal or no flow noted. The walls of the normal jugular vein collapse

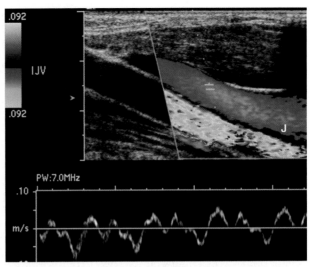

FIGURE 25-55. Normal jugular vein. Complex venous pulsations in a normal jugular vein *(J)* reflect the cycle of events in the right atrium.

completely when moderate transducer pressure is applied. Sudden patient sniffing reduces intrathoracic pressure, causing momentary collapse of the vein on real-time ultrasound, accompanied by a brief increase in venous flow toward the heart as shown by Doppler.[167,169,171]

Thrombosis

Clinical features of jugular venous thrombosis (JVT) include a tender, poorly defined, nonspecific neck mass or swelling. The correct diagnosis may not be immediately obvious.[168] Thrombosis of the internal jugular vein can be completely asymptomatic because of the deep position of the vein and the presence of abundant collateral circulation.[171] This condition was previously diagnosed by **venography,** an invasive procedure prompted only by a high index of suspicion. With the introduction of noninvasive techniques, such as ultrasound, CT,[181] and MRA,[182] JVT is being identified more frequently. Internal jugular thrombosis most often results from complications of **central venous catheterization.**[166,170,171] Other causes include intravenous drug abuse, mediastinal tumor, hypercoagulable states, neck surgery, and local inflammation or adenopathy.[168] Some cases are idiopathic or spontaneous.[168] Possible complications of JVT include suppurative thrombophlebitis, clot propagation, and pulmonary embolism.[168,172]

Real-time examination reveals an enlarged, noncompressible vein, which may contain a visible echogenic intraluminal thrombus. An **acute thrombus** may be anechoic and indistinguishable from flowing blood; however, the characteristic lack of compressibility and absent Doppler or color Doppler flow in the region of a thrombus quickly lead to the correct diagnosis. In addition, there is visible loss of vein response to respiratory maneuvers and venous pulsation. Spectral and color

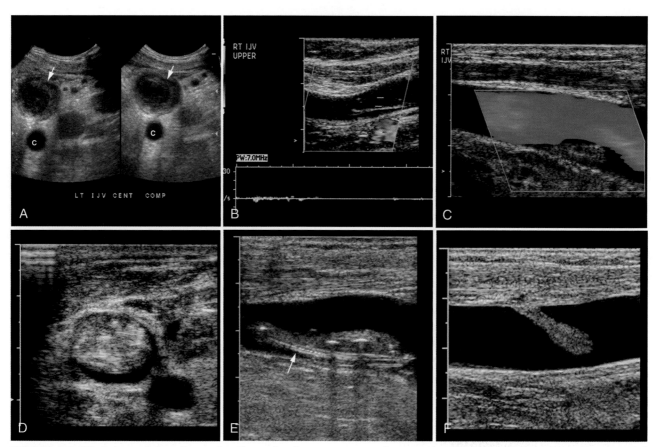

FIGURE 25-56. Internal jugular vein thrombosis: spectrum of appearances. A, Transverse image of an acute left internal jugular vein thrombus *(arrow)*. The vein is distended and noncompressible. *C,* Common carotid artery. **B,** Longitudinal image of a different patient demonstrates a hypoechoic thrombus and no Doppler signal. **C,** Longitudinal color Doppler image shows a small amount of thrombus arising from the posterior wall of the internal jugular vein (IJV). **D,** Transverse image shows an echogenic thrombus, indicating chronic thrombus in IJV. **E,** Longitudinal image demonstrates a thrombus around jugular vein catheter. **F,** Longitudinal images show a thrombus arising from anterior wall. This thrombus probably results from previous catheter placement in this region.

Doppler interrogations reveal absent flow (Fig. 25-56). Collateral veins may be identified, particularly in cases of chronic internal jugular vein thrombosis. Central liquefaction or other heterogeneity of the thrombus also suggests chronicity. **Chronic thrombi** may be difficult to visualize because they tend to organize and are difficult to separate from echogenic perivascular fatty tissue.[176] The absence of cardiorespiratory plasticity in a patent jugular or subclavian vein can indicate a more central, nonocclusive thrombus (Fig. 25-57). The confirmation of bilateral loss of venous pulsations strongly supports a more central thrombus, which can be documented by venography or MRA.

A thrombus that is related to catheter insertion is often demonstrated at the tip of the catheter, although it may be seen anywhere along the course of the vein. The catheter can be visualized as two parallel echogenic lines separated by an anechoic region. Flow is not usually demonstrated in the catheter, even if the catheter itself is patent.

Sonography has proved to be a reliable means of diagnosing jugular and subclavian vein thrombosis and has the advantage over CT and MRI of being inexpensive, portable, and nonionizing and of requiring no intravenous contrast. Sonography has limited access and cannot image all portions of the jugular and subclavian veins, especially those located behind the mandible or below the clavicle, although knowledge of the full extent of a thrombus is not typically a critical factor in treatment planning.[168,172] Serial sonographic examination to evaluate response to therapy after the initial assessment can be performed safely and inexpensively. Sonography can also document venous patency before vascular line placement, facilitating safer and more successful catheter insertion.

Acknowledgment

Thanks to Rita Premo and Barbara Siede for their assistance with manuscript preparation.

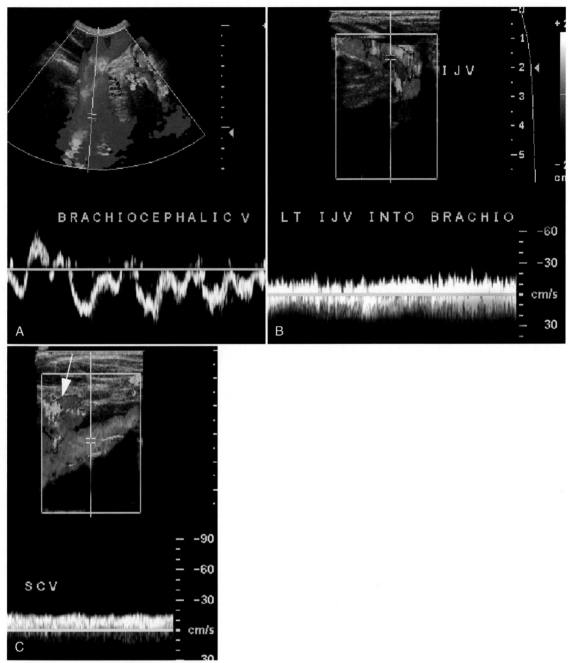

FIGURE 25-57. Normal and abnormal waveforms. A, Brachiocephalic vein has normal cardiorespiratory change in the venous waveforms, implying a patent superior vena cava. **B,** Near-occlusive left central brachiocephalic vein stenosis caused by a prior central venous catheter in another patient. Pulsed Doppler waveform shows reversed nonpulsatile flow in the internal jugular vein *(IJV)*. **C,** Left subclavian vein *(SCV)* shows centrally directed but **monophasic** flow toward an area of central collaterals *(arrow)* in patient with a malfunctioning left arteriovenous dialysis fistula.

References

1. Carroll BA. Carotid sonography. Radiology 1991;178:303-313.
2. Executive Committee, Asymptomatic Carotid Atherosclerosis Study. Endarterectomy for asymptomatic carotid artery stenosis. JAMA 1995;273:1421-1428.
3. Fontenelle LJ, Simper SC, Hanson TL. Carotid duplex scan versus angiography in evaluation of carotid artery disease. Am Surg 1994;60:864-868.
4. North American Symptomatic Carotid Endarterectomy Trial Collaborators. Beneficial effect of carotid endarterectomy in symptomatic patients with high-grade carotid stenosis. N Engl J Med 1991;325:445-453.
5. European Carotid Surgery Trialists' Collaborative Group. Interim results for symptomatic patients with severe (70-99%) or with mild (0-29%) carotid stenosis. MRC European Carotid Surgery Trial. Lancet 1991;337:1235-1243.
6. Barnett HJ, Taylor DW, Eliasziw M, et al. Benefit of carotid endarterectomy in patients with symptomatic moderate or severe stenosis. North American Symptomatic Carotid Endarterectomy Trial Collaborators. N Engl J Med 1998;339:1415-1425.
7. Bluth EI, Bertino RE, Grant EG, et al. ACR guideline for the performance of an ultrasound examination of the extracranial cerebrovascular system. Am Coll Radiol 2007:1037-1040.

8. Derdeyn CP, Powers WJ, Moran CJ, et al. Role of Doppler ultrasound in screening for carotid atherosclerotic disease. Radiology 1995;197:635-643.

9. Merritt CR, Bluth EI. The future of carotid sonography. AJR Am J Roentgenol 1992;158:37-39.

10. Taylor KJW. Clinical applications of carotid Doppler ultrasound. In: Taylor KJW, Burns PN, Wells PNT, editors. Clinical applications of Doppler ultrasound. New York: Raven Press; 1988. p. 120-161.

11. Bluth EI, Shyn PB, Sullivan MA, Merritt CR. Doppler color flow imaging of carotid artery dissection. J Ultrasound Med 1989;8:149-153.

12. Hennerici M, Steinke W, Rautenberg W. High-resistance Doppler flow pattern in extracranial carotid dissection. Arch Neurol 1989;46:670-672.

13. Rothrock JF, Lim V, Press G, Gosink B. Serial magnetic resonance and carotid duplex examinations in the management of carotid dissection. Neurology 1989;39:686-692.

14. O'Leary DH, Polak JF, Kronmal RA, et al. Carotid artery intima and media thickness as a risk factor for myocardial infarction and stroke in older adults. Cardiovascular Health Study Collaborative Research Group. N Engl J Med 1999;340:14-22.

15. Sidhu PS, Jonker ND, Khaw KT, et al. Spontaneous dissections of the internal carotid artery: appearances on colour Doppler ultrasound. Br J Radiol 1997;70:50-57.

16. Gritzmann N, Grasl MC, Helmer M, Steiner E. Invasion of the carotid artery and jugular vein by lymph node metastases: detection with sonography. AJR Am J Roentgenol 1990;154:411-414.

17. Gooding GA, Langman AW, Dillon WP, Kaplan MJ. Malignant carotid artery invasion: sonographic detection. Radiology 1989;171:435-438.

18. Steinke W, Hennerici M, Aulich A. Doppler color flow imaging of carotid body tumors. Stroke 1989;20:1574-1577.

19. Grant EG, Wong W, Tessler F, Perrella R. Cerebrovascular ultrasound imaging. Radiol Clin North Am 1988;26:1111-1130.

Carotid Ultrasound Examination

20. Ide C, De Coene B, Mailleux P, et al. Hypoplasia of the internal carotid artery: a noninvasive diagnosis. Eur Radiol 2000;10:1865-1870.

Carotid Ultrasound Interpretation

21. Polak JF, O'Leary DH, Kronmal RA, et al. Sonographic evaluation of carotid artery atherosclerosis in the elderly: relationship of disease severity to stroke and transient ischemic attack. Radiology 1993;188:363-370.

22. Veller MG, Fisher CM, Nicolaides AN, et al. Measurement of the ultrasonic intima-media complex thickness in normal subjects. J Vasc Surg 1993;17:719-725.

23. Bots ML, Mulder PG, Hofman A, et al. Reproducibility of carotid vessel wall thickness measurements: the Rotterdam Study. J Clin Epidemiol 1994;47:921-930.

24. Csanyi A, Egervari A. Simple clinical method of average intima-media thickness measurement in the common carotid artery. Vasa 1996;25:242-248.

25. Bots ML, Hoes AW, Koudstaal PJ, et al. Common carotid intima-media thickness and risk of stroke and myocardial infarction: the Rotterdam Study. Circulation 1997;96:1432-1437.

26. Kanters SD, Algra A, van Leeuwen MS, Banga JD. Reproducibility of in vivo carotid intima-media thickness measurements: a review. Stroke 1997;28:665-671.

27. Dwyer JH, Sun P, Kwong-Fu H, et al. Automated intima-media thickness: the Los Angeles Atherosclerosis Study. Ultrasound Med Biol 1998;24:981-987.

28. Aminbakhsh A, Frohlich J, Mancini GB. Detection of early atherosclerosis with B mode carotid ultrasonography: assessment of a new quantitative approach. Clin Invest Med 1999;22:265-274.

29. Greenland P, Abrams J, Aurigemma GP, et al. Prevention Conference V. Beyond secondary prevention: identifying the high-risk patient for primary prevention—noninvasive tests of atherosclerotic burden. Writing Group III. Circulation 2000;101:E16-E22.

30. Bluth EI, Stavros AT, Marich KW, et al. Carotid duplex sonography: a multicenter recommendation for standardized imaging and Doppler criteria. Radiographics 1988;8:487-506.

31. Bluth EI. Evaluation and characterization of carotid plaque. Semin Ultrasound CT MR 1997;18:57-65.

32. Polak JF, Shemanski L, O'Leary DH, et al. Hypoechoic plaque at ultrasound of the carotid artery: an independent risk factor for incident stroke in adults aged 65 years or older. Cardiovascular Health Study. Radiology 1998;208:649-654.

33. Langsfeld M, Gray-Weale AC, Lusby RJ. The role of plaque morphology and diameter reduction in the development of new symptoms in asymptomatic carotid arteries. J Vasc Surg 1989;9:548-557.

34. Leahy AL, McCollum PT, Feeley TM, et al. Duplex ultrasonography and selection of patients for carotid endarterectomy: plaque morphology or luminal narrowing? J Vasc Surg 1988;8:558-562.

35. Reilly LM, Lusby RJ, Hughes L, et al. Carotid plaque histology using real-time ultrasonography: clinical and therapeutic implications. Am J Surg 1983;146:188-193.

36. Persson AV, Robichaux WT, Silverman M. The natural history of carotid plaque development. Arch Surg 1983;118:1048-1052.

37. Lusby RJ, Ferrell LD, Ehrenfeld WK, et al. Carotid plaque hemorrhage: its role in production of cerebral ischemia. Arch Surg 1982;117:1479-1488.

38. Edwards JH, Kricheff II, Gorstein F, et al. Atherosclerotic subintimal hematoma of the carotid artery. Radiology 1979;133:123-129.

39. Imparato AM, Riles TS, Gorstein F. The carotid bifurcation plaque: pathologic findings associated with cerebral ischemia. Stroke 1979;10:238-245.

40. Geroulakos G, Ramaswami G, Nicolaides A, et al. Characterization of symptomatic and asymptomatic carotid plaques using high-resolution real-time ultrasonography. Br J Surg 1993;80:1274-1277.

41. Holdsworth RJ, McCollum PT, Bryce JS, Harrison DK. Symptoms, stenosis and carotid plaque morphology: is plaque morphology relevant? Eur J Vasc Endovasc Surg 1995;9:80-85.

42. Bluth EI, Kay D, Merritt CR, et al. Sonographic characterization of carotid plaque: detection of hemorrhage. AJR Am J Roentgenol 1986;146:1061-1065.

43. Merritt CRB, Bluth EI. Ultrasonographic characterization of carotid plaque. In: Labs KH, editor. Diagnostic vascular ultrasound. London: Hodder & Stoughton; 1991.

44. Bluth EI. B-mode evaluation and characterization of carotid plaque. In: Tegler CH, Babikian VL, Gomez CR, editors. Neurosonology. St Louis: Mosby–Year Book; 1991. p. 62-67.

45. Sterpetti AV, Schultz RD, Feldhaus RJ, et al. Ultrasonographic features of carotid plaque and the risk of subsequent neurologic deficits. Surgery 1988;104:652-660.

46. Weinberger J, Marks SJ, Gaul JJ, et al. Atherosclerotic plaque at the carotid artery bifurcation: correlation of ultrasonographic imaging with morphology. J Ultrasound Med 1987;6:363-366.

47. Stahl JA, Middleton WD. Pseudoulceration of the carotid artery. J Ultrasound Med 1992;11:355-358.

48. Bluth EI. Extracranial carotid arteries: intraplaque hemorrhage and surface ulceration. Minerva Cardioangiol 1998;46:81-85.

49. Bluth EI. Plaque morphology as a risk factor for stroke. JAMA 2000;284:177.

50. Reiter M, Effenberger I, Sabeti S, et al. Increasing carotid plaque echolucency is predictive of cardiovascular events in high-risk patients. Radiology 2008;248:1050-1055.

51. Bluth EI, McVay 3rd LV, Merritt CR, Sullivan MA. The identification of ulcerative plaque with high-resolution duplex carotid scanning. J Ultrasound Med 1988;7:73-76.

52. Ballard JL, Deiparine MK, Bergan JJ, et al. Cost-effective evaluation and treatment for carotid disease. Arch Surg 1997;132:268-271.

53. Furst H, Hartl WH, Jansen I, et al. Color-flow Doppler sonography in the identification of ulcerative plaques in patients with high-grade carotid artery stenosis. AJNR Am J Neuroradiol 1992;13:1581-1587.

54. Abildgaard A, Egge TS, Klow NE, Jakobsen JA. Use of sonicated albumin (Infoson) to enhance arterial spectral and color Doppler imaging. Cardiovasc Intervent Radiol 1996;19:265-271.

55. Bluth EI. Value of ultrasound in selecting patients for carotid angioplasty and stent placement. Radiology 2005;237:374-375; author reply 375.

56. Comerota AJ, Cranley JJ, Cook SE. Real-time B-mode carotid imaging in diagnosis of cerebrovascular disease. Surgery 1981;89:718-729.

57. Zwiebel WJ, Austin CW, Sackett JF, Strother CM. Correlation of high-resolution, B-mode and continuous-wave Doppler sonography

with arteriography in the diagnosis of carotid stenosis. Radiology 1983;149:523-532.

58. Jacobs NM, Grant EG, Schellinger D, et al. Duplex carotid sonography: criteria for stenosis, accuracy, and pitfalls. Radiology 1985; 154:385-391.

59. Taylor KJ, Holland S. Doppler ultrasound. Part I. Basic principles, instrumentation, and pitfalls. Radiology 1990;174:297-307.

60. Carroll BA, von Ramm OT. Fundamental of current Doppler technology. Ultrasound Q 1988;6:275-298.

61. Kassam M, Johnston KW, Cobbold RS. Quantitative estimation of spectral broadening for the diagnosis of carotid arterial disease: method and in vitro results. Ultrasound Med Biol 1985;11: 425-433.

62. Douville Y, Johnston KW, Kassam M. Determination of the hemodynamic factors which influence the carotid Doppler spectral broadening. Ultrasound Med Biol 1985;11:417-423.

63. Garth KE, Carroll BA, Sommer FG, Oppenheimer DA. Duplex ultrasound scanning of the carotid arteries with velocity spectrum analysis. Radiology 1983;147:823-827.

64. Phillips DJ, Greene Jr FM, Langlois Y, et al. Flow velocity patterns in the carotid bifurcations of young, presumed normal subjects. Ultrasound Med Biol 1983;9:39-49.

65. Lichtman JB, Kibble MB. Detection of intracranial arteriovenous malformation by Doppler ultrasound of the extracranial carotid circulation. J Ultrasound Med 1987;6:609-612.

66. Robinson ML, Sacks D, Perlmutter GS, Marinelli DL. Diagnostic criteria for carotid duplex sonography. AJR Am J Roentgenol 1988;151:1045-1049.

67. Grant EG, Duerinckx AJ, El Saden SM, et al. Ability to use duplex ultrasound to quantify internal carotid arterial stenoses: fact or fiction? Radiology 2000;214:247-252.

68. Rothwell PM, Gibson RJ, Slattery J, Warlow CP. Prognostic value and reproducibility of measurements of carotid stenosis: a comparison of three methods on 1001 angiograms. European Carotid Surgery Trialists' Collaborative Group. Stroke 1994;25:2440-2444.

69. Moneta GL, Edwards JM, Chitwood RW, et al. Correlation of North American Symptomatic Carotid Endarterectomy Trial (NASCET) angiographic definition of 70% to 99% internal carotid artery stenosis with duplex scanning. J Vasc Surg 1993;17:152-157; discussion 157-159.

70. Friedman SG, Hainline B, Feinberg AW, et al. Use of diastolic velocity ratios to predict significant carotid artery stenosis. Stroke 1988;19:910-912.

71. Kohler TR, Langlois Y, Roederer GO, et al. Variability in measurement of specific parameters for carotid duplex examination. Ultrasound Med Biol 1987;13:637-642.

72. Hunink MG, Polak JF, Barlan MM, O'Leary DH. Detection and quantification of carotid artery stenosis: efficacy of various Doppler velocity parameters. AJR Am J Roentgenol 1993;160:619-625.

73. Horrow MM, Stassi J, Shurman A, et al. The limitations of carotid sonography: interpretive and technology-related errors. AJR Am J Roentgenol 2000;174:189-194.

74. Faught WE, Mattos MA, van Bemmelen PS, et al. Color-flow duplex scanning of carotid arteries: new velocity criteria based on receiver operator characteristic analysis for threshold stenoses used in the symptomatic and asymptomatic carotid trials. J Vasc Surg 1994;19:818-827; discussion 827-828.

75. Kuntz KM, Polak JF, Whittemore AD, et al. Duplex ultrasound criteria for the identification of carotid stenosis should be laboratory specific. Stroke 1997;28:597-602.

76. Alexandrov AV, Vital D, Brodie DS, et al. Grading carotid stenosis with ultrasound: an interlaboratory comparison. Stroke 1997;28: 1208-1210.

77. Society of Radiologists in Ultrasound. Consensus Conference on Carotid Ultrasound. October 2002. Radiology 2003;229:340-346.

78. Carpenter JP, Lexa FJ, Davis JT. Determination of sixty percent or greater carotid artery stenosis by duplex Doppler ultrasonography. J Vasc Surg 1995;22:697-703; discussion 703-705.

79. Middleton WD, Erickson S, Melson GL. Perivascular color artifact: pathologic significance and appearance on color Doppler ultrasound images. Radiology 1989;171:647-652.

80. Erickson SJ, Mewissen MW, Foley WD, et al. Stenosis of the internal carotid artery: assessment using color Doppler imaging compared with angiography. AJR Am J Roentgenol 1989;152: 1299-1305.

81. Middleton WD, Foley WD, Lawson TL. Flow reversal in the normal carotid bifurcation: color Doppler flow imaging analysis. Radiology 1988;167:207-210.

82. Zierler RE, Phillips DJ, Beach KW, et al. Noninvasive assessment of normal carotid bifurcation hemodynamics with color-flow ultrasound imaging. Ultrasound Med Biol 1987;13:471-476.

83. Erickson SJ, Mewissen MW, Foley WD, et al. Color Doppler evaluation of arterial stenoses and occlusions involving the neck and thoracic inlet. Radiographics 1989;9:389-406.

84. Middleton WD, Foley WD, Lawson TL. Color-flow Doppler imaging of carotid artery abnormalities. AJR Am J Roentgenol 1988;150:419-425.

85. Branas CC, Weingarten MS, Czeredarczuk M, Schafer PF. Examination of carotid arteries with quantitative color Doppler flow imaging. J Ultrasound Med 1994;13:121-127.

86. Steinke W, Ries S, Artemis N, et al. Power Doppler imaging of carotid artery stenosis: comparison with color Doppler flow imaging and angiography. Stroke 1997;28:1981-1987.

87. Bluth EI, Althans LE, Sullivan M, et al. Comparison of plaque characterization with grayscale imaging and 3-D power Doppler imaging: can more be learned about intraplaque hemorrhage? JEMU 1999;20:11-15.

88. Griewing B, Morgenstern C, Driesner F, et al. Cerebrovascular disease assessed by color-flow and power Doppler ultrasonography: comparison with digital subtraction angiography in internal carotid artery stenosis. Stroke 1996;27:95-100.

89. Bluth EI, Sunshine JH, Lyons JB, et al. Power Doppler imaging: initial evaluation as a screening examination for carotid artery stenosis. Radiology 2000;215:791-800.

90. Bluth EI. Screening test for carotid disease. Semin Ultrasound CT MR 2003;24:55-61.

91. Zbornikova V, Lassvik C. Duplex scanning in presumably normal persons of different ages. Ultrasound Med Biol 1986;12:371-378.

92. Spencer EB, Sheafor DH, Hertzberg BS, et al. Nonstenotic internal carotid arteries: effects of age and blood pressure at the time of scanning on Doppler ultrasound velocity measurements. Radiology 2001;220:174-178.

93. O'Boyle MK, Vibhakar NI, Chung J, et al. Duplex sonography of the carotid arteries in patients with isolated aortic stenosis: imaging findings and relation to severity of stenosis. AJR Am J Roentgenol 1996;166:197-202.

94. Macchi C, Gulisano M, Giannelli F, et al. Kinking of the human internal carotid artery: a statistical study in 100 healthy subjects by echocolor Doppler. J Cardiovasc Surg (Torino) 1997;38:629-637.

95. Busuttil SJ, Franklin DP, Youkey JR, Elmore JR. Carotid duplex overestimation of stenosis due to severe contralateral disease. Am J Surg 1996;172:144-147; discussion 147-148.

96. AbuRahma AF, Richmond BK, Robinson PA, et al. Effect of contralateral severe stenosis or carotid occlusion on duplex criteria of ipsilateral stenoses: comparative study of various duplex parameters. J Vasc Surg 1995;22:751-761; discussion 761-762.

97. Van Everdingen KJ, van der Grond J, Kappelle LJ. Overestimation of a stenosis in the internal carotid artery by duplex sonography caused by an increase in volume flow. J Vasc Surg 1998;27: 479-485.

98. Blackshear WM, Phillips DJ, Chikos PM, et al. Carotid artery velocity patterns in normal and stenotic vessels. Stroke 1980; 11:67-71.

99. Grubb Jr RL, Derdeyn CP, Fritsch SM, et al. Importance of hemodynamic factors in the prognosis of symptomatic carotid occlusion. JAMA 1998;280:1055-1060.

100. Berman SS, Devine JJ, Erdoes LS, Hunter GC. Distinguishing carotid artery pseudo-occlusion with color-flow Doppler. Stroke 1995;26:434-438.

101. Gortler M, Niethammer R, Widder B. Differentiating subtotal carotid artery stenoses from occlusions by colour-coded duplex sonography. J Neurol 1994;241:301-305.

102. AbuRahma AF, Pollack JA, Robinson PA, Mullins D. The reliability of color duplex ultrasound in diagnosing total carotid artery occlusion. Am J Surg 1997;174:185-187.

103. Kliewer MA, Freed KS, Hertzberg BS, et al. Temporal artery tap: usefulness and limitations in carotid sonography. Radiology 1996; 201:481-484.

104. Bebry AJ, Hines GL. Total occlusion of the common carotid artery with a patent internal carotid artery: identification by duplex ultrasonography—report of a case. J Vasc Surg 1989;10:469-470.

105. Blackshear Jr WM, Phillips DJ, Bodily KC, Strandness Jr DE. Ultrasonic demonstration of external and internal carotid patency with common carotid occlusion: a preliminary report. Stroke 1980; 11:249-252.
106. Lee DH, Gao FQ, Rankin RN, et al. Duplex and color Doppler flow sonography of occlusion and near occlusion of the carotid artery. AJNR Am J Neuroradiol 1996;17:1267-1274.
107. Alexandrov AV, Bladin CF, Maggisano R, Norris JW. Measuring carotid stenosis: time for a reappraisal. Stroke 1993;24:1292-1296.
108. Polak JF, Kalina P, Donaldson MC, et al. Carotid endarterectomy: preoperative evaluation of candidates with combined Doppler sonography and MR angiography—work in progress. Radiology 1993;186:333-338.
109. Johnston DC, Goldstein LB. Clinical carotid endarterectomy decision making: noninvasive vascular imaging versus angiography. Neurology 2001;56:1009-1015.
110. Kuntz KM, Skillman JJ, Whittemore AD, Kent KC. Carotid endarterectomy in asymptomatic patients–is contrast angiography necessary? A morbidity analysis. J Vasc Surg 1995;22:706-714; discussion 714-716.
111. Mattos MA, Hodgson KJ, Faught WE, et al. Carotid endarterectomy without angiography: is color-flow duplex scanning sufficient? Surgery 1994;116:776-782; discussion 782-783.
112. Cartier R, Cartier P, Fontaine A. Carotid endarterectomy without angiography: the reliability of Doppler ultrasonography and duplex scanning in preoperative assessment. Can J Surg 1993;36:411-416.
113. Thusay MM, Khoury M, Greene K. Carotid endarterectomy based on duplex ultrasound in patients with and without hemispheric symptoms. Am Surg 2001;67:1-6.
114. Welch HJ, Murphy MC, Raftery KB, Jewell ER. Carotid duplex with contralateral disease: the influence of vertebral artery blood flow. Ann Vasc Surg 2000;14:82-88.
115. Chen JC, Salvian AJ, Taylor DC, et al. Can duplex ultrasonography select appropriate patients for carotid endarterectomy? Eur J Vasc Endovasc Surg 1997;14:451-456.
116. Randoux B, Marro B, Koskas F, et al. Carotid artery stenosis: prospective comparison of CT, three-dimensional gadolinium-enhanced MR, and conventional angiography. Radiology 2001;220:179-185.
117. Johnson BL, Gupta AK, Bandyk DF, et al. Anatomic patterns of carotid endarterectomy healing. Am J Surg 1996;172:188-190.
118. Kagawa R, Okada Y, Shima T, et al. B-mode ultrasonographic investigations of morphological changes in endarterectomized carotid artery. Surg Neurol 2001;55:50-56; discussion 56-57.
119. Jackson MR, D'Addio VJ, Gillespie DL, O'Donnell SD. The fate of residual defects following carotid endarterectomy detected by early postoperative duplex ultrasound. Am J Surg 1996;172:184-187.
120. Ricotta JJ, DeWeese JA. Is routine carotid ultrasound surveillance after carotid endarterectomy worthwhile? Am J Surg 1996;172:140-142; discussion 143.
121. Goodney PP, Lucas FL, Likosky DS, et al. Changes in the use of carotid revascularization among the Medicare population. Arch Surg 2008;143:170-173.
122. Chaer RA, Derubertis BG, Trocciola SM, et al. Safety and efficacy of carotid angioplasty and stenting in high-risk patients. Am Surg 2006;72:694-698; discussion 698-699.
123. Wolff T, Guirguis-Blake J, Miller T, et al. Screening for carotid artery stenosis: an update of the evidence for the U.S. Preventive Services Task Force. Ann Intern Med 2007;147:860-870.
124. Diethrich EB, Pauliina Margolis M, Reid DB, et al. Virtual histology intravascular ultrasound assessment of carotid artery disease: the Carotid Artery Plaque Virtual Histology Evaluation (CAPITAL) study. J Endovasc Ther 2007;14:676-686.
125. Reiter M, Bucek RA, Effenberger I, et al. Plaque echolucency is not associated with the risk of stroke in carotid stenting. Stroke 2006;37:2378-2380.
126. Fleming SE, Bluth EI, Milburn J. Role of sonography in the evaluation of carotid artery stents. J Clin Ultrasound 2005; 33:321-328.
127. Peterson BG, Longo GM, Kibbe MR, et al. Duplex ultrasound remains a reliable test even after carotid stenting. Ann Vasc Surg 2005;19:793-797.
128. Roffi M, Greutmann M, Eberli FR, et al. Starting a carotid artery stenting program is safe. Catheter Cardiovasc Interv 2008;71: 469-473.
129. Zhou W, Lin PH, Bush RL, et al. Management of in-sent restenosis after carotid artery stenting in high-risk patients. J Vasc Surg 2006;43:305-312.
130. Robbin ML, Lockhart ME, Weber TM, et al. Carotid artery stents: early and intermediate follow-up with Doppler ultrasound. Radiology 1997;205:749-756.
131. Chahwan S, Miller MT, Pigott JP, et al. Carotid artery velocity characteristics after carotid artery angioplasty and stenting. J Vasc Surg 2007;45:523-526.
132. Setacci C, Chisci E, Setacci F, et al. Grading carotid intrastent restenosis: a 6-year follow-up study. Stroke 2008;39:1189-1196.
133. Zhou W, Felkai DD, Evans M, et al. Ultrasound criteria for severe in-stent restenosis following carotid artery stenting. J Vasc Surg 2008;47:74-80.
134. Lal BK, Hobson 2nd RW, Tofighi B, et al. Duplex ultrasound velocity criteria for the stented carotid artery. J Vasc Surg 2008; 47:63-73.
135. Armstrong PA, Bandyk DF, Johnson BL, et al. Duplex scan surveillance after carotid angioplasty and stenting: a rational definition of stent stenosis. J Vasc Surg 2007;46:460-465; discussion 465-466.
136. Chi YW, White CJ, Woods TC, Goldman CK. Ultrasound velocity criteria for carotid in-stent restenosis. Catheter Cardiovasc Interv 2007;69:349-354.

Nonatherosclerotic Carotid Disease
137. Furie DM, Tien RD. Fibromuscular dysplasia of arteries of the head and neck: imaging findings. AJR Am J Roentgenol 1994;162: 1205-1209.
138. Kliewer MA, Carroll BA. Ultrasound case of the day: internal carotid artery web (atypical fibromuscular dysplasia). Radiographics 1991; 11:504-505.
139. Maeda H, Handa N, Matsumoto M, et al. Carotid lesions detected by B-mode ultrasonography in Takayasu's arteritis: "macaroni sign" as an indicator of the disease. Ultrasound Med Biol 1991;17: 695-701.
140. Sturzenegger M. Spontaneous internal carotid artery dissection: early diagnosis and management in 44 patients. J Neurol 1995;242: 231-238.
141. Sturzenegger M, Mattle HP, Rivoir A, Baumgartner RW. Ultrasound findings in carotid artery dissection: analysis of 43 patients. Neurology 1995;45:691-698.
142. Steinke W, Rautenberg W, Schwartz A, Hennerici M. Noninvasive monitoring of internal carotid artery dissection. Stroke 1994;25: 998-1005.

Transcranial Doppler Sonography
143. Lupetin AR, Davis DA, Beckman I, Dash N. Transcranial Doppler sonography. Part 1. Principles, technique, and normal appearances. Radiographics 1995;15:179-191.
144. Comerota AJ, Katz ML, Hosking JD, et al. Is transcranial Doppler a worthwhile addition to screening tests for cerebrovascular disease? J Vasc Surg 1995;21:90-95; discussion 95-97.
145. Rorick MB, Nichols FT, Adams RJ. Transcranial Doppler correlation with angiography in detection of intracranial stenosis. Stroke 1994;25:1931-1934.
146. Ultrasound screening helps prevent stroke in children with sickle cell disease. Science Centric 7 Dec 2008.
147. Lupetin AR, Davis DA, Beckman I, Dash N. Transcranial Doppler sonography. Part 2. Evaluation of intracranial and extracranial abnormalities and procedural monitoring. Radiographics 1995;15: 193-209.
148. Lin SK, Ryu SJ, Chu NS. Carotid duplex and transcranial color-coded sonography in evaluation of carotid-cavernous sinus fistulas. J Ultrasound Med 1994;13:557-564.
149. Mast H, Mohr JP, Thompson JL, et al. Transcranial Doppler ultrasonography in cerebral arteriovenous malformations: diagnostic sensitivity and association of flow velocity with spontaneous hemorrhage and focal neurological deficit. Stroke 1995;26: 1024-1027.
150. Gaunt ME, Martin PJ, Smith JL, et al. Clinical relevance of intraoperative embolization detected by transcranial Doppler ultrasonography during carotid endarterectomy: a prospective study of 100 patients. Br J Surg 1994;81:1435-1439.

Vertebral Artery

151. Bendick PJ, Glover JL. Hemodynamic evaluation of vertebral arteries by duplex ultrasound. Surg Clin North Am 1990;70:235-244.
152. Lewis BD, James EM, Welch TJ. Current applications of duplex and color Doppler ultrasound imaging: carotid and peripheral vascular system. Mayo Clin Proc 1989;64:1147-1157.
153. Visona A, Lusiani L, Castellani V, et al. The echo-Doppler (duplex) system for the detection of vertebral artery occlusive disease: comparison with angiography. J Ultrasound Med 1986;5:247-250.
154. Davis PC, Nilsen B, Braun IF, Hoffman Jr JC. A prospective comparison of duplex sonography vs angiography of the vertebral arteries. AJNR Am J Neuroradiol 1986;7:1059-1064.
155. Bluth EI, Merritt CR, Sullivan MA, et al. Usefulness of duplex ultrasound in evaluating vertebral arteries. J Ultrasound Med 1989;8:229-235.
156. Walker DW, Acker JD, Cole CA. Subclavian steal syndrome detected with duplex pulsed Doppler sonography. AJNR Am J Neuroradiol 1982;3:615-618.
157. Elias DA, Weinberg PE. Angiography of the posterior fossa. In: Taveras JM, Ferrucci JT, editors. Radiology: diagnosis-imaging-intervention. Philadelphia: Lippincott; 1989.
158. Bendick PJ, Jackson VP. Evaluation of the vertebral arteries with duplex sonography. J Vasc Surg 1986;3:523-530.
159. Ackerstaff RG, Grosveld WJ, Eikelboom BC, Ludwig JW. Ultrasonic duplex scanning of the prevertebral segment of the vertebral artery in patients with cerebral atherosclerosis. Eur J Vasc Surg 1988;2:387-393.
160. Carroll BA, Holder CA. Vertebral artery duplex sonography (abstract). J Ultrasound Med 1990;9:S27-S28.
161. De Bray JM, Zenglein JP, Laroche JP, et al. Effect of subclavian syndrome on the basilar artery. Acta Neurol Scand 1994;90:174-178.
162. Thomassen L, Aarli JA. Subclavian steal phenomenon: clinical and hemodynamic aspects. Acta Neurol Scand 1994;90:241-244.
163. Kliewer MA, Hertzberg BS, Kim DH, et al. Vertebral artery Doppler waveform changes indicating subclavian steal physiology. AJR Am J Roentgenol 2000;174:815-819.
164. Nicolau C, Gilabert R, Garcia A, et al. Effect of internal carotid artery occlusion on vertebral artery blood flow: a duplex ultrasonographic evaluation. J Ultrasound Med 2001;20:105-111.

Internal Jugular Veins

165. Williams CE, Lamb GH, Roberts D, Davies J. Venous thrombosis in the neck: the role of real-time ultrasound. Eur J Radiol 1989;9:32-36.
166. Hubsch PJ, Stiglbauer RL, Schwaighofer BW, et al. Internal jugular and subclavian vein thrombosis caused by central venous catheters: evaluation using Doppler blood flow imaging. J Ultrasound Med 1988;7:629-636.
167. Gaitini D, Kaftori JK, Pery M, Engel A. High-resolution real-time ultrasonography: diagnosis and follow-up of jugular and subclavian vein thrombosis. J Ultrasound Med 1988;7:621-627.
168. Albertyn LE, Alcock MK. Diagnosis of internal jugular vein thrombosis. Radiology 1987;162:505-508.
169. Falk RL, Smith DF. Thrombosis of upper extremity thoracic inlet veins: diagnosis with duplex Doppler sonography. AJR Am J Roentgenol 1987;149:677-682.
170. Weissleder R, Elizondo G, Stark DD. Sonographic diagnosis of subclavian and internal jugular vein thrombosis. J Ultrasound Med 1987;6:577-587.
171. De Witte BR, Lameris JS. Real-time ultrasound diagnosis of internal jugular vein thrombosis. J Clin Ultrasound 1986;14:712-717.
172. Wing V, Scheible W. Sonography of jugular vein thrombosis. AJR Am J Roentgenol 1983;140:333-336.
173. Gribbin C, Raghavendra BN, Ginsburg HB. Ultrasound diagnosis of jugular venous ectasia. NY State J Med 1989;89:532-533.
174. Hughes PL, Qureshi SA, Galloway RW. Jugular venous aneurysm in children. Br J Radiol 1988;61:1082-1084.
175. Jasinski RW, Rubin JM. CT and ultrasonographic findings in jugular vein ectasia. J Ultrasound Med 1984;3:417-420.
176. Stevens RK, Fried AM, Hood Jr TR. Ultrasonic diagnosis of jugular venous aneurysm. J Clin Ultrasound 1982;10:85-87.
177. Lee W, Leduc L, Cotton DB. Ultrasonographic guidance for central venous access during pregnancy. Am J Obstet Gynecol 1989;161:1012-1023.
178. Bond DM, Champion LK, Nolan R. Real-time ultrasound imaging aids jugular venipuncture. Anesth Analg 1989;68:700-701.
179. Machi J, Takeda J, Kakegawa T. Safe jugular and subclavian venipuncture under ultrasonographic guidance. Am J Surg 1987;153:321-323.
180. Dresser LP, McKinney WM. Anatomic and pathophysiologic studies of the human internal jugular valve. Am J Surg 1987;154:220-224.
181. Patel S, Brennan J. Diagnosis of internal jugular vein thrombosis by computed tomography. J Comput Assist Tomogr 1981;5:197-200.
182. Braun IF, Hoffman Jr JC, Malko JA, et al. Jugular venous thrombosis: MR imaging. Radiology 1985;157:357-360.

CHAPTER 26

The Peripheral Arteries

Joseph F. Polak and Jean M. Alessi-Chinetti

Chapter Outline

DIAGNOSTIC SCREENING METHODS

The upper and lower extremity arteries are readily evaluated by Doppler ultrasound. Because they are usually located at depths of 6 cm or less, the extremity arteries are more consistently imaged than the abdominal or thoracic arteries. Availability of sufficient imaging windows allows the transducer to be placed over the artery of interest without the presence of overlying attenuating tissues containing bone or gas. Transducers with imaging frequencies greater than 5 MHz can normally be used because the arteries lie close to the skin. Doppler frequencies are typically more than 3 MHz.

Although limited, real-time gray-scale sonography is useful for evaluating the presence of atherosclerotic plaque or confirming the presence of extravascular masses. Color flow Doppler sonographic imaging allows the clinician to survey the area of interest rapidly, determine if vascular structures are present, and if so, characterize their blood flow patterns (Fig. 26-1; **Video 26-1**). The addition of spectral Doppler waveform analysis makes duplex Doppler sonography a powerful diagnostic tool for evaluating the clinical significance of atherosclerotic lesions, differentiating significant arterial stenoses from occlusions and assessing the nature of perivascular masses. Compared with duplex sonography (spectral Doppler and gray-scale sonography) alone, color flow Doppler imaging can more rapidly survey the full length of limb arteries and detect the presence of significant stenoses and occlusions. Color flow imaging decreases the length of the peripheral arterial examination compared with duplex sonography alone,[1] and it improves diagnostic accuracy.[2] As such, peripheral artery imaging is, in fact, color Doppler sonography. Power Doppler sonography, a more sensitive derivative of color Doppler imaging, can further improve the diagnostic performance of Doppler sonography in specific clinical situations.

Compared with angiography, the sonographic approaches discussed in this chapter have the advantage of being **noninvasive, relatively inexpensive, and well suited for serial examinations.** They also permit the **evaluation of soft tissue structures** contiguous to the arteries. **Computed tomography angiography** (CTA) is a more expensive technology than Doppler sonography and requires the administration of contrast material. The use of multidetector CTA has shortened imaging times, improved resolution, and made it competitive with arteriography. **Magnetic resonance angiography** (MRA) is also used to detect the presence of arterial lesions. As with CTA, MRA can also be used to evaluate the soft tissues for nonvascular pathologies. However, MRA requires additional imaging sequences and increases imaging time. CTA and MRA are less operator dependent and, in given clinical situations, more accurate and more reproducible than Doppler sonography. However, the value of Doppler ultrasound is undisputed in patients with poor renal func-

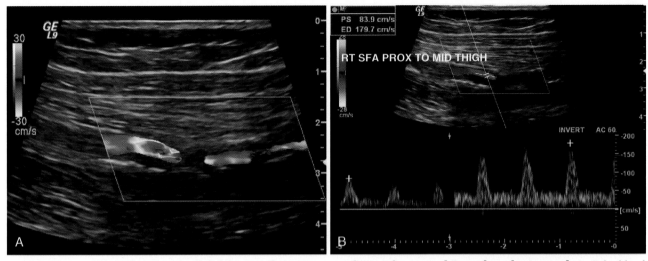

FIGURE 26-1. Stenosis of superficial femoral artery on color and spectral Doppler ultrasound. A, Color blood flow image shows that the site of stenosis causes an alteration in the color signals within the artery. There is aliasing of the color Doppler signals *(blue)* at the site of maximal stenosis. Abnormalities in the color flow signals extend at least 1 cm downstream from the lesion. Calcified plaques cause areas of Doppler signal drop-off distal to the stenosis. **B,** Pulsed Doppler waveforms taken before and at the site of aliasing show a significant increase in velocity (doubling), consistent with a significant stenosis of the superficial femoral artery.

tion. Although MRA and CTA are more cost-effective than sonography in certain clinical scenarios, Doppler ultrasound can often help identify patients requiring direct referral for percutaneous arterial interventions.[3-6]

SONOGRAPHIC TECHNIQUE

Real-Time Gray-Scale Imaging

The diameter of the peripheral arteries that is clinically relevant varies from 1 to 6 mm. Accurate visualization of the arterial wall requires high-resolution transducers, more than 5 MHz, to visualize all the various lesions. A broad frequency range of 5 to 10 MHz is preferred because it offers overall good resolution while permitting good depth penetration, even in the thigh. For detailed visualization of smaller-diameter arteries, higher frequencies of 7 to 12 MHz can be used. At these high frequencies, transducers have poor depth penetration but may be useful for evaluating bypass grafts and the ulnar and radial arteries and smaller arteries of the hand.

The linear phased array transducer is ideal for imaging the extremity arteries. The transducer has sufficient length to permit rapid coverage of long arterial segments by holding it parallel to the artery or graft long axis and by sliding it in a series of nonoverlapping increments. A smaller-footprint, curved array or sector transducer can be useful for imaging the iliac arteries and the more centrally located portions of the subclavian arteries.

Doppler Sonography

Simultaneous display of Doppler spectral waveforms and data and the gray-scale image, **duplex Doppler**

sonography, is the basic requisite for the evaluation of the peripheral arteries and arterial bypass grafts.[7] Careful real-time control is needed to position the Doppler sample gate and accurately detect sites of maximal blood flow velocity in arteries and bypass grafts. The transducer carrier frequencies can vary between 3 to 10 MHz, tending to be best lower than the simultaneously acquired gray-scale image. Selection of a Doppler transducer frequency of approximately 5 MHz sacrifices some sensitivity for detecting slowly moving blood, but decreases the likelihood that the system will alias at sites of rapidly moving blood, such as stenoses or arteriovenous fistulas.

Color Doppler sonography is an essential component of a peripheral arterial sonographic examination. The simultaneous display of moving blood superimposed on a gray-scale image allows a rapid survey of the flow patterns within long sections of the peripheral arteries and bypass grafts.[8] In general, an efficient approach to peripheral vascular sonography relies on color flow Doppler sonography to rapidly identify zones of flow disturbances, then on duplex sonography, including Doppler spectral analysis, to characterize the type of flow abnormality present.[1,9] The color Doppler image displays only the mean frequency shift caused by moving structures. The pixel size (resolution) is also coarser than the corresponding pixel size of gray-scale image. This may cause some ambiguity in alignment of the two separate images and can cause the color Doppler information to overlap beyond the wall of the arteries. Most manufacturers use lower transducer frequencies for the color flow image than for the gray-scale sonographic component of the image. This approach increases the depth penetration of the color flow image without compromising image resolution.

Power Doppler sonography is a variant of color flow Doppler imaging that displays a summation of the Doppler signals caused by moving blood. Advantages of power Doppler over color Doppler flow imaging are (1) the blood flow information does not alias, (2) the signal strengths are much less angle dependent, and (3) slowly moving blood is more easily detected. A disadvantage is the loss of information pertaining to the direction of blood flow, although this information can also be displayed.

DOPPLER FLOW PATTERNS

Normal Arteries

The normal pattern of arterial blood flow in the extremity is different from that seen in the carotid arteries. At rest, the muscles of the extremities cause a high peripheral (distal) resistance and relatively low diastolic blood flow. The typical blood flow profile is a **triphasic pattern** (Fig. 26-2, *top*). First, during systole, there is a strong forward component of blood flow. Second, during early diastole, there is a short reversal of blood flow. Third, during remaining diastole, there is low-amplitude forward blood flow. The magnitude of the forward component of blood flow during diastole varies, disappearing with vasoconstriction caused be cold and increasing with warmth or after exercise (Fig. 26-3).

Stenotic Arteries

The high-resistance pattern seen in normal peripheral arteries at rest is transformed into a low-resistance pattern when an occluded or severely stenotic arterial lesion is located proximal to the artery segment where the Doppler signals are sampled (see Fig. 26-2). This low-resistance pattern resembles that of the internal carotid artery. It is thought to reflect the opening of collateral arterial branches and the loss of normal resting arteriolar tone in response to ischemia. It is typically seen distal to an occluded artery segment but can be seen distal to severe stenotic lesions.

A localized increase in velocity occurs at the site of a stenosis proper. This increase in blood flow velocity causes a shift in the Doppler frequency sampled at the stenosis. The Doppler frequency shift and increase in estimated flow velocity are proportional to the lumen diameter narrowing at the stenosis.[10-12] This can be shown as an increase in color saturation or aliasing on the color Doppler map or as an increase in the peak systolic velocity on the Doppler spectral display (see Fig. 26-1, *A* and *B*). The pattern of blood flow distal to the stenosis is nonlaminar and shows a large variation in both direction and amplitude; this zone of disturbed flow is maintained over a distance of slightly more than 1 cm (see Video 26-1). In certain cases the zone of blood

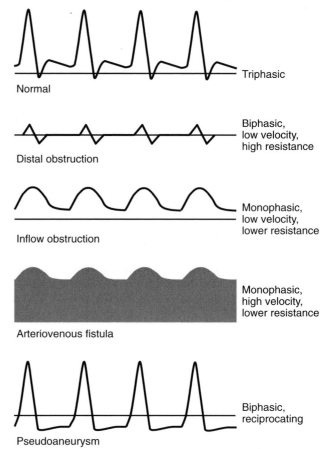

FIGURE 26-2. Diagram of normal and abnormal Doppler arterial waveforms. The normal Doppler spectrum of flowing blood in the lower extremity arteries typically has a **triphasic pattern:** (1) forward flow during systole, (2) a short period of flow reversal in early diastole, and (3) low-velocity flow during the remainder of diastole. Arterial Doppler signals are altered depending on the pathologic change. The four other patterns are examples of common arterial pathologies: distal obstruction, inflow obstruction, arteriovenous fistula, and pseudoaneurysm.

flow disturbance can be very small. This zone of disturbed blood flow is captured by the Doppler waveform as a broadening of the spectral window and by color Doppler imaging as increased variance of the color Doppler signals in the vessel.

Arteriovenous Fistulas

Arteriovenous (AV) fistulas can be either congenital or iatrogenic. **Congenital** AV fistulas present in various forms as abnormal communications between an artery and large, distended venous channels or primary venous anomalies. The abnormalities more easily identified with Doppler ultrasound are usually quite obvious clinically and tend to be located close to the skin surface of the involved extremity.[13] These are normally visualized as distended venous channels into which feed single or multiple arterial branches. Smaller, nondistended veins

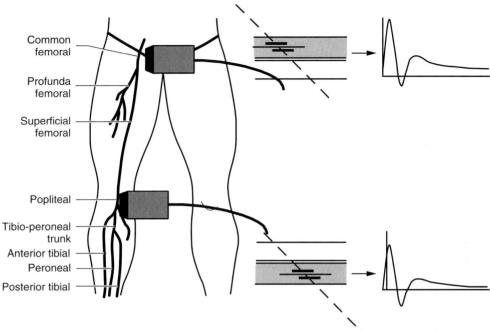

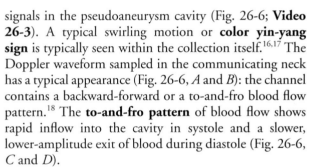

FIGURE 26-3. Normal arterial waveforms. Doppler waveforms at the common femoral and popliteal arteries show triphasic patterns.

that have not dilated may still contain increased blood flow signals caused by the fistula.

Iatrogenic communications often arise after selective arterial or venous catheterization or other forms of penetrating trauma. The communication can be visualized as a "jet of blood" (**Video 26-2**), with the involved vein distended compared to the other side. Blood flow signals in the recipient vein also show an arterial-like appearance, and the feeding artery can have increased diastolic blood flow (Fig. 26-4). The jet of blood has high-velocity signals, and on impact against the opposite vein wall, it can cause a perivascular vibration seen as an artifact on color Doppler imaging.[14] An important differential diagnosis is **compression of a vein by a hematoma.** Venous compression causes a stenosis that increases blood flow velocity signals in the vein and mimics the high-velocity signals of a fistula (Fig. 26-5).

Masses

The differential diagnosis of perivascular masses is facilitated by the use of color Doppler flow imaging, with some diagnostic specificity being offered by Doppler waveform analysis. Blood flow signals within a mass contiguous to an artery suggest the diagnosis of **pseudoaneurysm.** The communication tends to have a wide neck if the aneurysm arises at the anastomosis of a synthetic or autologous vein graft.[15] With an iatrogenic pseudoaneurysm of the native artery, a small-diameter channel communicates to a larger, contained collection of blood. Color Doppler imaging shows blood flow

signals in the pseudoaneurysm cavity (Fig. 26-6; **Video 26-3**). A typical swirling motion or **color yin-yang sign** is typically seen within the collection itself.[16,17] The Doppler waveform sampled in the communicating neck has a typical appearance (Fig. 26-6, *A* and *B*): the channel contains a backward-forward or a to-and-fro blood flow pattern.[18] The **to-and-fro pattern** of blood flow shows rapid inflow into the cavity in systole and a slower, lower-amplitude exit of blood during diastole (Fig. 26-6, *C* and *D*).

Hyperplastic lymph nodes and **malignant lymph nodes** can show both venous and arterial signals radiating from the hilum of the node (Fig. 26-7). These nodes can be mistaken for pseudoaneurysms.[19,20] Points to consider in the differential diagnosis are (1) detection of arterial and venous signals where the communicating channel should be located and (2) absence of a to-and-fro pattern of blood flow.

Tumors can show a "rind" of hypervascularity at their periphery, as in thyroid gland adenomas. **Arterial aneurysms** are easily recognized by their typical location within the confines of the arterial wall. Although fusiform aneurysms follow this rule, it may be quite difficult to differentiate a saccular aneurysm from a pseudoaneurysm.[21]

PERIPHERAL ARTERY DISEASE

Incidence and Clinical Importance

Peripheral vascular disease is at least as prevalent as coronary artery disease or cerebrovascular disease.[22]

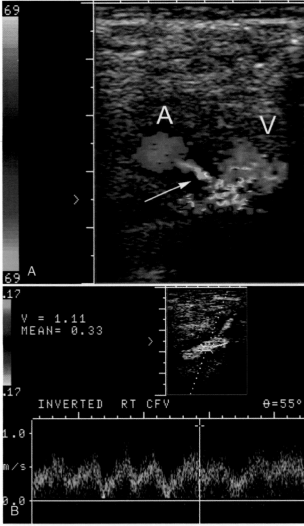

Atherosclerosis is a generalized process in which the clinical presentation and development of symptoms depend on the arterial bed and the target organ. Coronary artery disease and carotid artery disease can present in a catastrophic manner, as myocardial infarction (MI) and cerebrovascular accident (CVA, stroke), respectively. This is very different from peripheral artery disease (PAD). Many patients have PAD for years before seeking medical assistance.[23] This reflects the development of collateral arterial channels bypassing the diseased arterial segment as it progressively narrows. The collaterals are often sufficient to maintain perfusion to the lower extremity. The balance between blood supply and oxygen demand is maintained as long as the patient does not exercise or ambulate too vigorously. In general, patients with PAD can go on for years, decreasing their level of

FIGURE 26-4. Arteriovenous (AV) fistula of femoral vessels after angiogram. A, Color flow Doppler image shows a high-velocity jet *(arrow)* from the common femoral artery *(A)* into the distended common femoral vein *(V).* **B,** The arterial-type signals sampled in the common femoral vein are consistent with a large AV fistula showing an arterialized venous blood flow pattern.

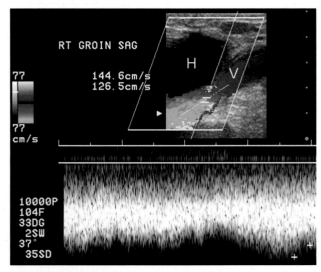

FIGURE 26-5. Extrinsic compression of the common femoral vein *(V)* by a large hematoma *(H)* causes an increase in blood flow velocity. This can mimic the increased velocity seen in veins where an arteriovenous fistula is present.

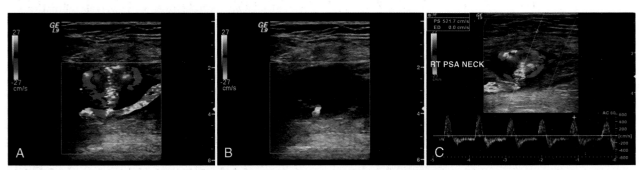

FIGURE 26-6. Systolic and diastolic images of pseudoaneurysm. A, Image during end systole shows filling of the pseudoaneurysm and swirling motion of blood. **B,** Image at end systole shows emptying of the pseudoaneurysm through a small, communicating channel. **C,** Spectral Doppler tracing from the neck channel between the common femoral artery and the perivascular collection shows the classic to-and-fro waveform of a pseudoaneurysm.

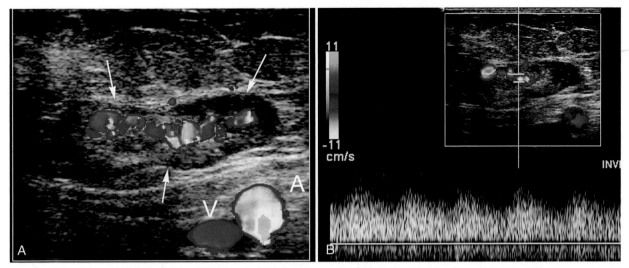

FIGURE 26-7. Groin lymph node with Doppler signal. A, Color Doppler signals in the soft tissues of the groin are complex. Careful examination shows that these signals are from the center of a structure that is a hyperplastic lymph node *(arrows)*. *A,* Femoral artery; *V,* femoral vein. **B,** Spectral Doppler waveform from the center of this mass confirms the presence of a mainly arterial waveform and not the to-and-fro waveform of a pseudoaneurysm.

activity as their disease progresses. Disabling claudication is therefore more likely to be a presenting symptom in the younger patient with high levels of daily activity.

The patient may also seek medical assistance because of the development of chronic changes of arterial insufficiency and poor wound healing. Acute embolic events originating from a more proximal arterial lesion, either from ulcerated plaques or popliteal aneurysms, can cause acute ischemia and extensive tissue loss, leading to amputation unless an intervention is performed. The widespread use of arterial bypass surgery has modified the natural history of PAD. The high patency rates of both arterial bypass surgery and similar patency rates for angioplasty allow patients who previously would have had amputation now to remain asymptomatic[24,25] until other causes of mortality intercede. Acute cardiovascular events (e.g., MI, sudden death) are common causes of mortality in these patients, who already have generalized atherosclerosis.

Sonographic Technique

Duplex Doppler sonography with gray-scale and Doppler spectral analysis is well accepted as the primary noninvasive modality for detecting evidence of lower extremity bypass graft dysfunction. It can also be used to evaluate the success of peripheral angioplasty, atherectomy, and stent placement.[26-31] Doppler imaging of the leg arteries to determine the extent and nature of arterial lesions has become practical with the aid of color Doppler flow imaging. Although duplex Doppler sonography can be used to determine the presence of significant arterial lesions, the task of evaluating the whole leg is labor and time intensive. It takes 30 to 60 minutes to map out the

arterial tree of each leg using Duplex ultrasound.[32] With color Doppler mapping, this task can be accomplished in 15 to 20 minutes.[1] Color Doppler imaging also improves the accuracy of Doppler ultrasound as a diagnostic test for detecting and grading the severity of PAD.[2,29]

Lower Extremity

Normal Anatomy

The deep arteries of the leg travel with an accompanying vein. The **common femoral artery** starts at the level of the inguinal ligament and continues for 4 to 6 cm until it branches into the **superficial and deep femoral arteries** (see Fig. 26-3). The deep femoral artery quickly branches to supply the region of the femoral head and the deep muscles of the thigh. With PAD, collateral pathways often form between this deep femoral artery and the lower portions of the superficial femoral or the popliteal arteries. The superficial femoral artery continues along the medial aspect of the thigh at a depth of 4 to 8 cm until it reaches the adductor canal. At the boundary of the adductor canal, the superficial femoral artery continues as the **popliteal artery.** The popliteal artery crosses posterior to the knee, sending off small geniculate branches, and terminates as two major branches: the **anterior tibial artery** and **tibioperoneal trunk.** The anterior tibial artery courses in the anterior compartment of the lower leg after crossing through the interosseous membrane. It finally crosses the ankle joint as the **dorsalis pedis artery.** The tibioperoneal trunk gives off the **posterior tibial** and the **peroneal** arteries, which supply the calf muscles. The posterior tibial is more superficial than the peroneal artery and can be followed down to its typical location behind the medial malleolus.

The blood flow pattern in all these branches is triphasic (Fig. 26-8; see also Fig. 26-2). There is an early systolic acceleration in velocity, followed by a brief period of low-amplitude flow reversal before returning to antegrade diastolic flow of low velocity. This pattern can be more pulsatile in the profunda femoris artery. **Peak systolic velocity** (PSV) varies with the level of the artery, typically 100 cm/sec at the common femoral, down to 70 cm/sec at the popliteal artery. The tibioperoneal arteries have PSV of 40 to 50 cm/sec. The response to either **exercise** or **transient ischemia** is a loss of the triphasic pattern and the development of a **monophasic pattern** with antegrade blood flow with loss of early diastolic blood flow reversal (Fig. 26-9). Although a monophasic pattern can be seen in lower extremity disease or after exercise, PSV will be decreased in the ischemic limb of a patient with PAD, whereas it is increased in a healthy individual after exercise.

Aneurysms

Diagnostic Criteria. Aneurysms develop as the structural integrity of the arterial wall weakens. **Focal enlargement** of the artery is more likely to occur at the level of the popliteal or distal superficial femoral artery (Fig. 26-10). Aneurysms are often bilateral and can remain asymptomatic for long periods. Ultrasound has become a gold standard in itself for confirming this suspected diagnosis.[33,34] Although ultrasound can visualize the progressive thrombosis that fills in the aneurysm lumen to the level of the dilated wall, the lumen can appear normal at angiography. Ultrasound can be used to follow these aneurysms, as done for abdominal aneurysms. Unfortunately, no strict size criteria can be used to determine surgical suitability. Empirically, a 2-cm cutoff has been adopted.[35] The development of symptoms suggestive of

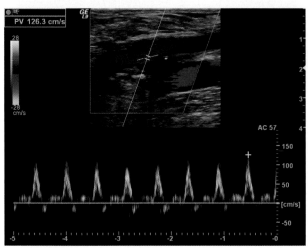

FIGURE 26-8. Normal triphasic waveform of lower extremity arteries.

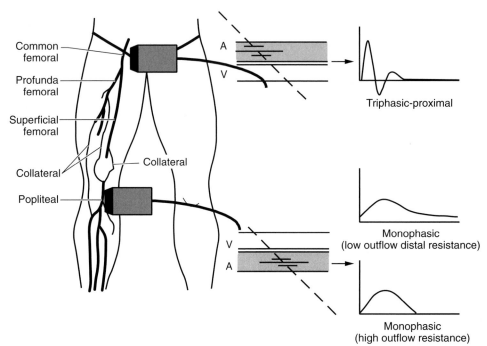

FIGURE 26-9. Significant arterial disease alters Doppler waveform. Sampling occurring distal to an occlusion. Doppler waveform sampled proximal to a high-grade stenosis may be normal or can show loss of the early and then late components of diastolic flow. Distal waveform is monophasic, most often with a relatively strong diastolic component; pattern is called a **tardus-parvus** waveform.

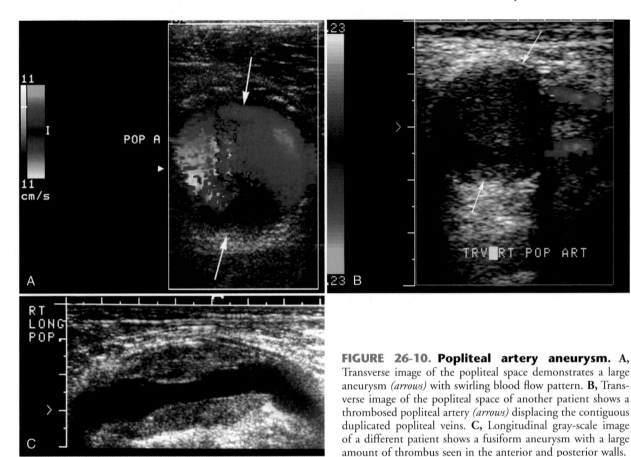

FIGURE 26-10. Popliteal artery aneurysm. A, Transverse image of the popliteal space demonstrates a large aneurysm *(arrows)* with swirling blood flow pattern. **B,** Transverse image of the popliteal space of another patient shows a thrombosed popliteal artery *(arrows)* displacing the contiguous duplicated popliteal veins. **C,** Longitudinal gray-scale image of a different patient shows a fusiform aneurysm with a large amount of thrombus seen in the anterior and posterior walls.

distal embolization by the thrombus accumulating in the lumen is an absolute indication for surgical intervention, regardless of the size of the aneurysm.[35] Aneurysms will typically occlude with time due to accumulating thrombus (Fig. 26-10, *B*). Surgical exclusion (ligation of the aneurysm) is the traditional treatment. Doppler ultrasound can be used to monitor the success of the intervention.[36] Aneurysm exclusion with covered stents is an alternative therapy to surgical intervention (Fig. 26-11). Doppler ultrasound can be used to monitor the patency of the stent and the exclusion of the aneurysm from the circulation[37,38] (**Video 26-4**).

Doppler techniques are useful in confirming the continued patency or occlusion of the lumen within the aneurysm. A bulge or focal enlargement of 20% of the expected vessel diameter constitutes a simple functional definition of an aneurysm. Serial monitoring should be considered in patients with small aneurysms less than 2 cm in size.

Diagnostic Accuracy. Direct pathologic verification of aneurysms diagnosed by ultrasound has shown that the technique is sensitive and specific and also superior to contrast angiography. The accuracy of Doppler techniques for confirming patency or occlusion of the lumen at the level of the aneurysm has yet to be reported, but it is accepted as a gold standard.

Stenoses and Occlusions

Diagnostic Criteria. The effects of peripheral arterial lesions are detectable by a change in the blood flow pattern seen on the arterial Doppler waveform. At the lesion, peak systolic velocity increases (Fig. 26-12; see also Fig. 26-1 and Video 26-1), and early diastolic velocity reversal disappears. Distal to a moderately severe arterial lesion, the early diastolic blood flow reversal decreases and ultimately disappears as the lesion becomes more severe, and peak systolic blood flow velocity will decrease. The diastolic portion of the waveform increases in significance with respect to the decreasing peak systolic blood flow. On occasion, a high-resistance, monophasic pattern with absent diastolic blood flow can be seen, likely caused by peripheral vasoconstriction. The low-resistance pattern distal to the lesion is accentuated as the severity of the lesion increases. With severe lesions, the blood flow pattern is mainly that of forward flow, with end diastolic velocity approaching in amplitude the severely depressed peak systolic velocity.

One explanation for the development of this pattern is progressive dilation of the arterioles within the distant vascular bed due to the release of metabolites caused by local ischemia. Another is the development of many small collateral branches that diminish the effective resistance

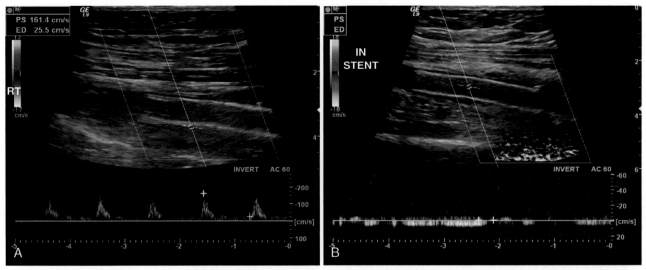

FIGURE 26-11. Occlusion of popliteal artery stent. A, Color Doppler image of the proximal portion of a covered stent used to exclude a popliteal artery aneurysm. Blood flow is seen around the occluded stent, in effect causing a type 1 endoleak. **B,** Spectral Doppler tracing inside the stent confirming occlusion. Some faint venous signals from the contiguous popliteal vein are detected because of the high gain settings.

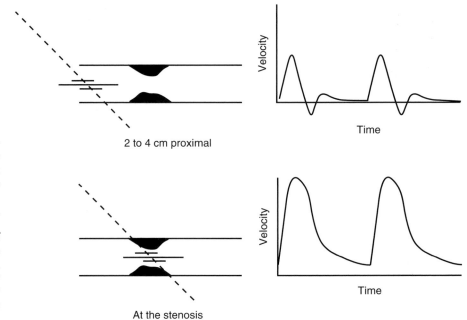

FIGURE 26-12. Blood flow velocity alterations occur with stenosis of at least 50%. Proximal to the lesion, the flow pattern is normal. At the stenosis, the peak systolic velocity increases in proportion to the degree of stenosis. Alterations in the diastolic portion of the Doppler waveform sampled at the lesion depend on the state of the distal arteries and the severity and geometry of the lesion; diastolic flow may increase dramatically or may be almost absent.

of the distal arterial bed. This pattern is present in most cases of sufficiently severe proximal lesions, but it may not be seen when sampling within an artery segment proximal to tandem lesions such as distal high-grade focal lesions or occlusions. Signals in the artery proximal to a high-grade lesion can show a high-resistance pattern (see Fig. 26-9). With absent collaterals, forward blood flow can sometimes only be maintained during systole. The low-resistance pattern, a slow-rise low-amplitude pattern seen distal to segmental occlusions, is called the **tardus-parvus waveform** (see Fig. 26-9). Although seen in most arterial segments distal to occlusions (Fig. 26-13), the

low-resistance blood flow pattern may be absent when there is peripheral vasoconstriction.

Color Doppler imaging can be used to survey the lower extremity arteries and identify likely stenotic lesions, through sites where color Doppler image shows aliasing (see Video 26-1). Focal areas where the measured PSV more than doubles from a contiguous and normal segment have been shown to correspond to lesions of **greater than 50%** narrowing in the lumen diameter of the artery.[39] The velocity measured at the stenosis is divided by the velocity measured proximal to the stenosis. Peak systolic velocity is less sensitive to the

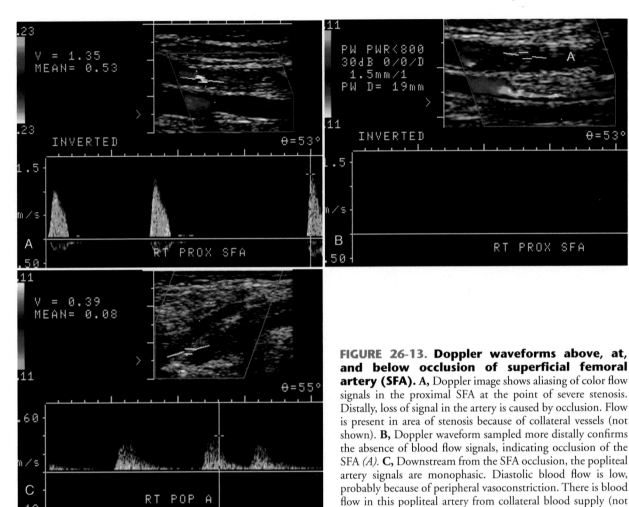

FIGURE 26-13. Doppler waveforms above, at, and below occlusion of superficial femoral artery (SFA). A, Doppler image shows aliasing of color flow signals in the proximal SFA at the point of severe stenosis. Distally, loss of signal in the artery is caused by occlusion. Flow is present in area of stenosis because of collateral vessels (not shown). **B,** Doppler waveform sampled more distally confirms the absence of blood flow signals, indicating occlusion of the SFA *(A)*. **C,** Downstream from the SFA occlusion, the popliteal artery signals are monophasic. Diastolic blood flow is low, probably because of peripheral vasoconstriction. There is blood flow in this popliteal artery from collateral blood supply (not shown).

effects of vasodilation and vasoconstriction, so it is the preferred Doppler velocity parameter used to grade the severity of lower extremity arterial stenoses. Either end diastolic velocities (example EDVs; e.g., ≥80 cm/sec) or PSVs (>200 and >300 cm/sec) can be used as indicators of stenosis severity. However, EDV estimates are more variable than PSV measurements because EDV changes as a function of peripheral vasodilation.

Diagnostic Accuracy and Applications. In their original 1987 paper, Kohler et al.[32] reported that Doppler sonography had a diagnostic sensitivity of 82% and a specificity of 92% for detecting segmental arterial lesions of the femoropopliteal arteries. They emphasized, however, that selective sampling had to be performed along the *full course* of the femoral and popliteal arteries. These segments normally measure 30 to 40 cm, so it is not surprising that such a survey took 1 to 2 hours to perform, especially if the iliac arteries were evaluated.

Color Doppler sonography has been shown to reduce by 40% the time needed to examine the carotid artery for sites of suspected stenosis.[9] A similar effect has been shown when color Doppler imaging is used to detect lower extremity arterial lesions.[1] Diagnostic accuracy is

also improved with color Doppler imaging compared with duplex sonography.[2,40] With color Doppler the examination time is reduced to 30 minutes.[1]

Accuracy of color flow imaging of the peripheral arteries is almost 98% for distinguishing occlusions from nonoccluded segments. Accuracy for the detection of stenoses is greater than 85% for the femoropopliteal arteries,[1,41-43] with some including an evaluation of the iliac arteries[32,40] and runoff arteries.[44] The evaluation of the runoff arteries is not as accurate as for the femoro-popliteal system, especially for the peroneal artery.[3,45,46] However, segments of the tibial arteries might be selected as suitable for the distal anastomosis of bypass grafts.[47-49] Also, other imaging modalities might be unnecessary, relying exclusively on Doppler ultrasound before lower extremity bypass grafting.[50-52] This is more likely for femoropopliteal bypass grafts.[53]

Color Doppler imaging is effective in **triaging** patients with symptoms of lower extremity arterial disease, reducing the need for diagnostic arteriography in more than half of patients presenting for clinical evaluation.[54] Doppler sonography can also be used to triage patients likely to need peripheral angioplasty, therefore with

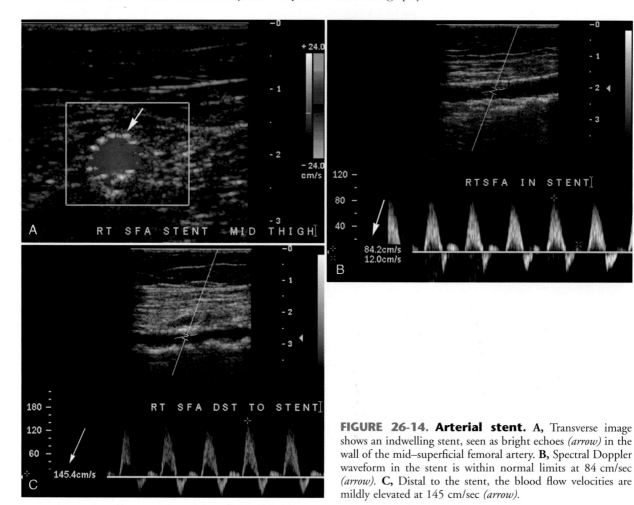

FIGURE 26-14. Arterial stent. A, Transverse image shows an indwelling stent, seen as bright echoes *(arrow)* in the wall of the mid–superficial femoral artery. **B,** Spectral Doppler waveform in the stent is within normal limits at 84 cm/sec *(arrow).* **C,** Distal to the stent, the blood flow velocities are mildly elevated at 145 cm/sec *(arrow).*

better management of more expensive imaging resources such as arteriography.[29,55-57] No large studies have compared the efficacy of color Doppler imaging and CTA. However, cost-effectiveness analysis suggests that either color Doppler imaging or MRA can be used to select patients for interventions as a substitute for contrast arteriography.[6]

Color Doppler imaging and duplex sonography are extremely well suited for the evaluation of sites of percutaneous interventions such as angioplasty, atherectomy, and stent placement (Fig. 26-14). An original 1992 report indicated that one ultrasound measurement made a few days after angioplasty was predictive of lesion recurrence.[58] Subsequent studies have failed to confirm this observation,[59,60] but Doppler sonography can be used to detect recurrence of stenosis or occlusion at the site of a previous intervention. For example, postatherectomy results show a higher incidence of reocclusion than indicated by patients' symptoms; atherectomy was not as efficient as angioplasty, with more lesion recurrences after atherectomy.[61] Questions surround whether repeat imaging at the site of previous intervention is needed, because a repeat intervention might not be done if the patient remains asymptomatic.[62] It does appear,

however, that serial monitoring of sites of angioplasty and stent placement can predict technical success and lesion recurrence.[63,64] No data indicate a benefit of re-intervention at the site of lesions detected by Doppler sonography.[26] In fact, Doppler findings suggest that primary stent deployment is likely superior to stent deployment after angioplasty.[30]

Color Doppler imaging has been used to guide percutaneous interventions, angioplasty, and stent placement, without the use of contrast arteriography or fluoroscopy.[59,65] Success rates have been high, but patient selection is critical to the success of the procedure.

Upper Extremity

Normal Anatomy and Doppler Flow Patterns

The arteries of the upper extremity are accompanied by veins: typically, only one vein at the level of the subclavian vein, occasionally duplicated at the level of the axillary veins, always duplicated at the level of the brachial veins and more distally. The junction of the **subclavian artery** with either the **right brachiocephalic** (innominate) or the **left brachiocephalic** artery can be identified using an imaging window superior to the sternoclavicular joint. The artery is located superficial to the vein when the transducer is placed in the supraclavicular fossa. Near the junction of the middle and proximal thirds of the clavicle, it is necessary to use a window with the transducer placed on the chest, below the clavicle. The artery now lies deep to the subclavian vein. The origin of the **axillary artery** is lateral to the first rib, normally near the junction of the cephalic and the axillary vein. The axillary artery can be followed as it courses medially over the proximal humerus as it becomes the **brachial artery.** In most subjects the artery can be followed to the antecubital fossa, where it trifurcates into the radial, ulnar, and interosseous branches. The **radial** and **ulnar** branches can normally be imaged to the level of the wrist. It is also possible to visualize the smaller **digital** branches. The normal flow pattern is triphasic and similar to the pattern seen in the leg.

Pathophysiology and Diagnostic Accuracy

Most clinical interest in the noninvasive evaluation of the upper extremity arterial branches focuses on the (1) confirmation of pseudoaneurysms, (2) detection of focal stenosis caused by thoracic outlet syndrome (Fig. 26-15), (3) confirmation of native arterial occlusion secondary to emboli or trauma (Fig. 26-16), (4) detection of complications following cardiac catheterization, (5) evaluation of dialysis shunts, and (6) preoperative evaluation of radial artery patency.

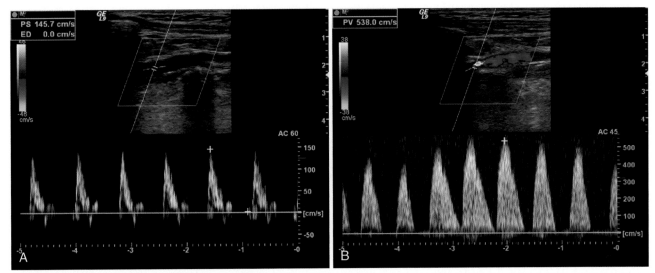

FIGURE 26-15. Thoracic outlet syndrome. A, Normal baseline subclavian artery waveform. **B,** Altered waveform during hyperextension, with compression against the clavicle causing stenosis and thoracic outlet syndrome.

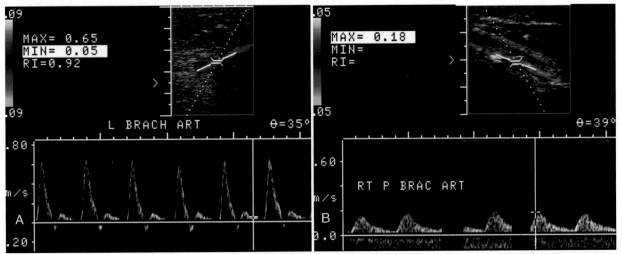

FIGURE 26-16. Normal and abnormal waveforms in brachial arteries. A, Normal waveform pf left side of brachial artery resembles the triphasic waveform seen in lower extremity arteries. **B,** Abnormal waveform of right side of brachial artery is obtained distal to a subclavian artery occlusion. The spectral Doppler waveform shows a low-amplitude (parvus) waveform with a slow systolic rise (tardus). This tardus-parvus waveform is typical distal to an arterial occlusion.

Stenosis can be induced in the artery of patients with **thoracic outlet syndrome** by positioning the arm in the orientation that normally elicits symptoms, most often abducted (Fig. 26-15). Thoracic outlet syndrome is associated with distal arterial embolization, probably through mechanical forces predisposing the artery to develop an aneurysm. Thrombus then forms in the aneurysm and can embolize into the digital arteries. The extent of these acute or chronic occlusions must be mapped to assess the feasibility of bypass surgery before subjecting the patient to angiography. Proximal stenoses and occlusions associated with vasculitis can also be confirmed.[66]

After cardiac catheterization, suspected occlusions can be rapidly confirmed. Large hematomas can be readily evaluated and underlying **pseudoaneurysms** from jeopardized arteriotomy sutures confirmed or excluded. The radial artery is occasionally used as an access site for cardiac catheterization. Pseudoaneurysms can develop following cardiac catheterization[67] (Fig. 26-17).

The radial artery can also be harvested and serve as a donor conduit for coronary bypass surgery. Confirmation of the integrity of the palmar arch of the hand (dominant ulnar artery) is a prerequisite before harvest of the radial artery. This can be tested with Doppler ultrasound, imaging of the distal radial artery, and confirming reversal of blood flow on compression of the more proximal radial artery.[68,69] Ulnar blood flow should increase when the radial artery is compressed and occluded.[69]

VASCULAR AND PERIVASCULAR MASSES

Doppler sonography and color flow Doppler imaging have the ability to document the presence or absence of blood flow within masses located close to vessels or vascular prostheses. Although the presence of blood flow within a perivascular mass can be diagnostic of a pseudoaneurysm, the absence of blood flow makes it easier to justify a more conservative approach. In the case of a suspected hematoma, serial follow-up examinations can be used to document resolution of the process. In the

case of a suspected abscess, a biopsy can be performed without fear of uncontrolled hemorrhage.

Synthetic Vascular Bypass Grafts

The various complications likely to affect the function of synthetic lower extremity bypass grafts[15,70] are a function of the **type of graft** and **time since placement** (Fig. 26-18). In the first and second years after surgery, graft failure can result from technical errors or development of fibrointimal lesions at the anastomoses. Later failures may be caused by the progression of atherosclerotic lesions in the native vessels proximal and distal to the graft. The late complication of an anastomotic pseudoaneurysm occurs on average 5 to 10 years after graft placement and preferentially affects the femoral anastomosis of aortofemoral grafts.[15,71] Infections can occur at any time after graft placement and may be associated with development of anastomotic pseudoaneurysm. With time, atherosclerotic changes and fibrointimal hyperplastic lesions mixed in with areas of chronic thrombus deposition can also develop in the synthetic graft conduit.

Masses: Hematoma versus Pseudoaneurysm

Although the diagnostic accuracy of duplex Doppler sonography is greater than 95% for making the diagnosis of **pseudoaneurysms at the anastomoses of bypass grafts**, no specific waveform patterns have been described.[72,73] The addition of color Doppler imaging can reveal an almost classic appearance of swirling motion of blood in the perivascular mass.[15] This sign is not specific to a pseudoaneurysm because saccular aneurysms share similar flow patterns. The differential diagnosis is normally made when careful real-time imaging confirms that the mass is situated beyond the normal lumen of the vessel. The **to-and-fro sign** seen in native

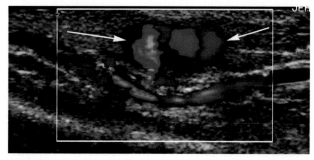

FIGURE 26-17. Radial artery pseudoaneurysm. Pseudoaneurysm *(arrows)* arising in the radial artery after cardiac catheterization.

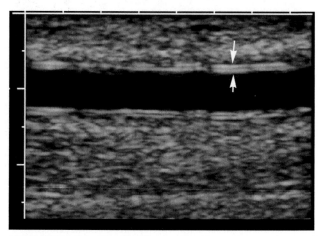

FIGURE 26-18. Synthetic graft. Gray-scale appearance of a synthetic PTFE lower extremity bypass graft *(arrows)*.

pseudoaneurysms is obtained from Doppler spectral analysis of the signal sampled in the communicating channel between the perivascular collection and the native vessel. This neck often does not exist or is very broad, abutting the artery rather than extending as a thin structure for a length of a few centimeters. Typically, anastomotic pseudoaneurysms do not have any distinct communicating channels.

Care must be taken to differentiate perivascular pulsations transmitted within a **hematoma** from flowing blood. Adjustment of the flow sensitivity of the imaging device to minimize this artifact in the normal artery proximal or distal to the site of abnormality can help eliminate this error. Setting the color velocity scale (**peak repetition frequency,** PRF) to a high value can eliminate this artifact while not hindering the detection of the communicating channel.

Occlusions and Anastomotic Stenoses

The absence of Doppler signals within a bypass graft is diagnostic of an **occlusion.** An **anastomotic stenosis** will typically cause a marked increase in the Doppler velocity signals sampled at the anastomosis or beyond. Normally, however, blood flow velocities tend to increase as the graft tapers to the anastomosis. Increases in velocity caused by the geometry of the anastomotic connection are common and can cause up to a 100% increase in velocity without being indicative of a pathologic lesion. No studies have addressed the actual incidence and significance of this finding. Serial monitoring of these sites of disturbed flow may be done on the basis that an increase in velocity over a few months is indicative of a developing stenosis.[74]

AUTOLOGOUS VEIN GRAFTS

Two types of venous bypass grafts are currently used for arterial revascularization: the reversed vein and the "in situ" vein grafts. The **reversed vein** is a segment of native superficial vein that has been harvested from its normal anatomic location, reversed, and then anastomosed to the native artery segments proximal and distal to the diseased segments. The **in situ technique** typically uses the greater saphenous vein, although the lesser saphenous vein can be used for popliteal-to-distal tibioperoneal bypass surgery. The vein is left in its native bed. The valves are lysed and the side branches (perforating veins that normally communicate to deep venous system) are ligated. The proximal and distal portions are mobilized and anastomosed to the selected arterial segments.

Three different mechanisms are responsible for **bypass graft failure.** Early failures are seen within 1 month of surgery and usually result from **technical errors,** including poor suture line placement, opening of unsuspected venous channels in the in situ grafts, poor selection of anastomotic sites, and poorly lysed or disrupted vein valves. For 2 years after surgery, **fibrointimal or fibrotic lesions** tend to develop either at the anastomosis or within the graft conduit, most often at the site of a vein valve. Later failures, after 2 years, are thought to result from the **progressive atherosclerotic process** in the native vessels proximal and distal to the anastomosis.

Stenosis of Venous Bypass Graft

A decreased blood flow velocity within a vein bypass graft indicates a high likelihood of incipient graft occlusion and thrombosis (Fig. 26-19). Bandyk et al.[75,76] have shown that PSV less than 40 or 45 cm/sec can be used to identify such grafts. This diagnostic criterion can appropriately identify only the more severely diseased grafts.[77] It does not identify the site of stenoses likely to progress until they become flow restrictive and finally result in graft thrombosis.[78] The lesions that develop within bypass grafts are most often the result of **fibrointimal hyperplasia,** and their presence must be identified before they can be monitored for possible progression of severity. Color Doppler sonography can be used to survey the 30 to 80 cm–long bypass graft very efficiently. The site of a suspected stenosis can be quickly identified and Doppler spectral analysis used to grade the severity of the stenosis using the PSV ratio (Fig. 26-20). Power Doppler imaging and "B-flow imaging" (a technique that visualizes moving blood) can also be used to better confirm the presence of any stenotic lesions. The PSV ratio is calculated by dividing the peak-systolic velocity measured at the suspected stenosis by that measured in the portion of the graft 2 to 4 cm proximal (Fig. 26-21). Blood flow velocity ratios of 2 or more correspond to **50% diameter stenosis.**[32,57] Blood flow velocity ratios of 3 or more correspond to **75% diameter stenosis.**[27,57] **Critical stenoses** have been empirically identified as those causing a velocity increase by a factor of 3.5, 3.7,

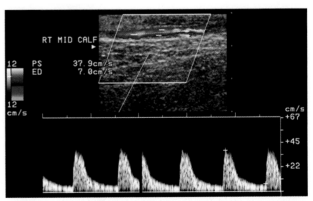

FIGURE 26-19. Abnormal flow velocity of bypass graft. Depressed velocity (<40 cm/sec) in bypass graft in the calf indicates a high likelihood for future occlusion. The diastolic velocity is still preserved.

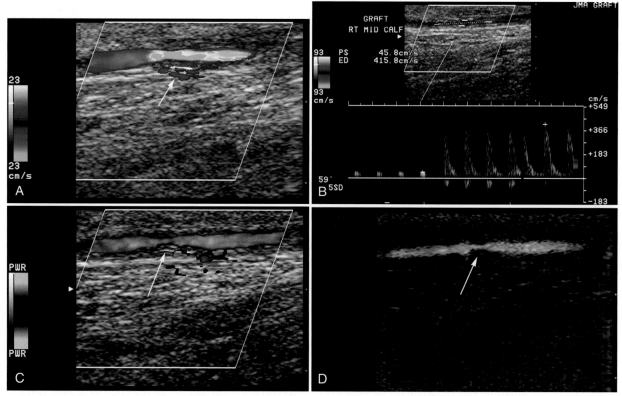

FIGURE 26-20. Focal stenosis of bypass graft in calf. A, Color Doppler sonogram shows a focal site of aliasing with soft tissue bruit *(arrow).* **B,** Color Doppler image shows corresponding segment of the bypass graft was then sampled by displacing the Doppler gate along the graft. A significant increase in peak systolic velocity occurs at the site of aliasing. **C,** Power Doppler image confirms the presence of the lesion *(arrow).* **D,** B-flow image also confirms the severity of the stenosis *(arrow).*

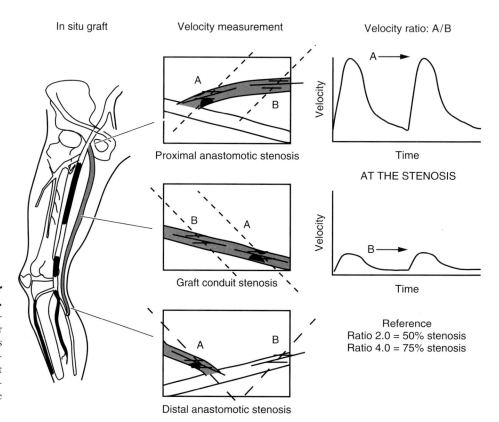

FIGURE 26-21. Doppler flow sampling in graft. Diagram shows the various approaches for sampling the Doppler blood flow velocities in bypass grafts. Sampling of blood flow velocities at the anastomosis must take into account the expected tapering between graft and native artery.

In situ graft

Velocity measurement

Velocity ratio: A/B

Proximal anastomotic stenosis

AT THE STENOSIS

Graft conduit stenosis

Distal anastomotic stenosis

Reference
Ratio 2.0 = 50% stenosis
Ratio 4.0 = 75% stenosis

or even 4.0.[79,80] The blood flow velocity ratio is very accurate for the detection of a stenosis and grading it's severity.[81-83] A potential limitation of Doppler imaging is the presence of tandem lesions, where the flow field of one stenosis overlaps that of another stenosis located more distally.[84]

It is now recognized that the early lesions develop within 3 months of surgery and are detectable by sonography even before the patient develops symptoms,[85] and that an early examination identifies most of the lesions that will ultimately progress and cause graft thrombosis.[86] An intervention, most often a surgical correction of the developing stenosis, is indicated for many of these "early lesions" because, if left alone, they often progress to cause bypass graft occlusion.[85,87] Currently, surveillance is focused more on these early lesions, with intervention once they reach a certain threshold.[88,89] A PSV ratio of 4.0 has been accepted as a threshold defining a critical stenosis requiring treatment.[79] Distal tibial bypass grafts with decreased end diastolic blood flow velocities detected intraoperatively are a high risk for subsequent graft failure.[90] Preoperative measurement of vein diameter also seems to predict different aspects of long-term vein bypass success.[91] As with native arterial disease, ultrasound-guided interventions have shown some therapeutic success, without the need for contrast during endovascular repair or surgical time for direct interventions.[92]

Arteriovenous Fistula

Persistent AV communication through nonligated perforating veins occurs with the in situ technique. AV fistulas can easily be missed during or immediately after surgery because a significant percentage open in the first few postoperative weeks. Color Doppler imaging is a simple and elegant way of documenting the presence of AV fistulas, although findings can mimic those of a stenosis (Fig. 26-22). Intraoperative sonography is used to detect fistulas in need of ligation.[76] Sites of AV communication between the in situ graft and the deeper native veins can be detected postoperatively by Doppler ultrasound alone. Ultrasound is typically used as the only guide for surgical correction, without the need for angiography.[93]

DIALYSIS ACCESS GRAFTS AND FISTULAS

The utility of sonography in the evaluation of dialysis AV fistulas and hemodialysis access grafts has been controversial.[94] However, AV fistulas are the favored approach to long-term dialysis despite the large prevalence of hemodialysis access grafts in the United States (Fig. 26-23).

The native artery-to-vein AV fistula is also preferred to ensure long-term hemodialysis. The AV communication is typically created between the radial artery and a superficial vein such as the distal cephalic (Brescia-Cimino). Its creation requires careful technique, and graft maturation typically takes a month.[95] Ultrasound offers preoperative information on the status of the native arteries and veins, which can increase the technical success rate of fistula creation.[96] Ultrasound measurement of artery diameter can predict failure of the dialysis fistula. Proper fistula maturation is critical to the long-term success of the dialysis fistula. The vein being accessed needs to be close enough to the skin for ease of access. The vein diameter typically increases as the flow rate of the arterialized venous segment increases. Technical errors in fistula formation, such as kinks and stenoses

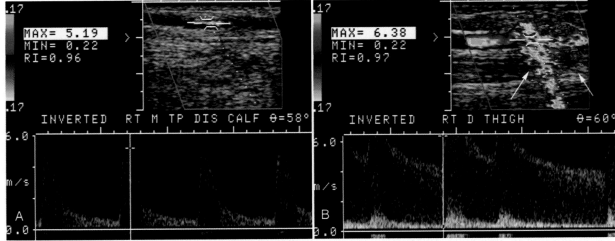

FIGURE 26-22. Bypass graft stenosis and arteriovenous (AV) fistula cause focal elevation of velocity. **A,** Sampling at the site of aliasing of this bypass graft in the calf shows the dramatic increase in blood flow velocity caused by a stenosis. **B,** Sampling of same graft in the thigh shows a dramatically different pattern, with much more flow in diastole and a perigraft tissue bruit *(arrows).* Although this pattern may be seen with a simple stenosis, in this case the elevated blood flow velocity was caused by a patent AV fistula arising from the graft at this location.

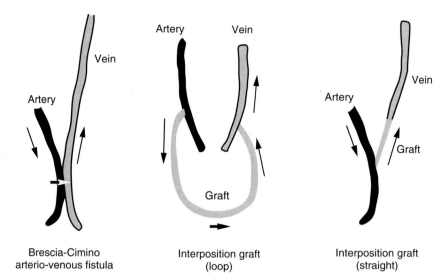

FIGURE 26-23. Dialysis fistula types. Brescia-Cimino arteriovenous fistulas are created by direct suturing (side to side) of an artery to a vein. The interposition grafts are created with synthetic PTFE or biologic analogs for material bridging the artery to a suitable superficial vein.

Brescia-Cimino
arterio-venous fistula

Interposition graft
(loop)

Interposition graft
(straight)

and failure to ligate dominant collateral venous pathways, can lead to failure of vein maturation. Duplex Doppler ultrasound can help identify these fistulas and guide successful corrective interventions.[97]

The alternative type of dialysis access relies on **interposition grafts,** inserted in the forearm, typically synthetic polytetrafluoroethylene (PTFE), and rarely autologous vein. Problems common to interposition access grafts include the development of **microaneurysms, larger aneurysms,** and **stenoses.** Color flow imaging can readily detect perigraft masses or pseudoaneurysm with high accuracy. Color Doppler imaging and duplex sonography can be used to detect stenoses, with an estimated accuracy of 86%, sensitivity of 92%, and specificity of 84%.[98] The loss in specificity is caused by turbulent flow patterns in the tortuous course of the outflow vein and its high baseline velocities. The diagnostic accuracy is improved in straight-segment grafts to the efferent veins, where the sensitivity increases to 95% for a specificity of 97%.[98] The addition of color Doppler does not seem to improve diagnostic accuracy.[99] **Graft thrombosis** ultimately is the source of graft failure and is the ultimate outcome of a dialysis graft. Extension of the effective lifetime of a dialysis access is critical to the dialysis patient because of the limited number of times an AV fistula or dialysis graft can be created. Graft thrombosis is most often seen secondary to low blood flow in the setting of developing stenotic lesions. Duplex Doppler ultrasound can be used to detect these lesions. However, there is controversy as to whether this information extends the lifetime of the access[100] or simply promotes an increased number of interventions without affecting long-term patency.[101]

Few studies provide diagnostic criteria applicable to Doppler ultrasound of **hemodialysis access graft stenosis.**[102-104] PSVs in well-functioning dialysis access grafts are typically 100 to 200 cm/sec (Fig. 26-24), tending to be higher in the first 6 months after graft placement or creation of an AV shunt.[104] Superimposed stenosis can therefore be difficult to detect given the high baseline velocities. A blood flow velocity elevation of 100% (velocity ratios ≥2) is considered to be consistent with the presence of a significant stenosis. Color Doppler, power Doppler, and gray-scale images are also useful for confirming the presence of an anatomic lesion.[102] Stenotic lesions tend to develop on the venous side of the access fistula in more than 80% of cases.[105] Occasionally, the stenosis can be at the level of the subclavian vein, specifically in individuals who have had hemodialysis catheters inserted in the subclavian vein. After percutaneous interventions, Doppler ultrasound can be used to monitor development of recurrent stenosis. Low blood flow states of 50 cm/sec or less are also indicative of a high-grade stenosis in the graft conduit or outflow vein.

COMPLICATIONS OF INVASIVE PROCEDURES

Duplex and color Doppler sonography are useful for evaluating patients who underwent invasive procedures and may have AV fistula or pseudoaneurysm. The number of cases seen has increased in response to the increased use of endovascular procedures. Sonographic findings are usually taken at face value, without the need for angiography or other imaging tests, before a corrective intervention is performed.

Fistulous Communications

Fistulous communications after cardiac catheterization or other angiographic procedures can be quickly detected using color Doppler imaging. An area of **turbulence** is normally seen within either the common femoral or the profunda femoral vein, with arterialized signals shown on the Doppler spectrum (see Fig. 26-4). The actual

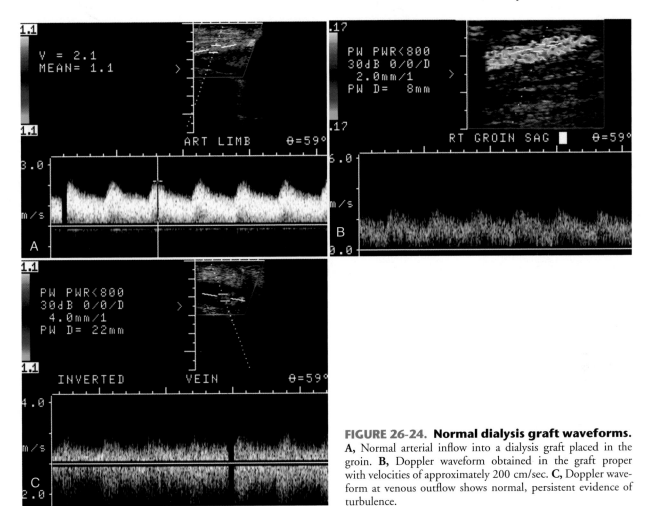

FIGURE 26-24. Normal dialysis graft waveforms.
A, Normal arterial inflow into a dialysis graft placed in the groin. **B,** Doppler waveform obtained in the graft proper with velocities of approximately 200 cm/sec. **C,** Doppler waveform at venous outflow shows normal, persistent evidence of turbulence.

fistulous communication can be seen on the color map, although it may difficult to localize with duplex sonography alone (see Video 26-2). The turbulence associated with the fistula can be confused with turbulent signals caused by extrinsic compression of the vein by a **hematoma** (see Fig. 26-5), another common complication after catheterization. Visualization of the communicating channel should therefore be done with a high–color velocity setting (high-color PRF). An indirect sign of the fistula is dilation of the vein and a poor response to Valsalva maneuver. With small AV communications, the venous velocity signals can easily decrease or disappear during Valsalva (Fig. 26-25). Blood flow signals in a vein recipient of a large AV fistula communication will not decrease during a Valsalva maneuver (Fig. 26-26). Complete abolition of the flow signals during Valsalva suggests that the fistula is small and likely to occlude spontaneously over the next few weeks. **Transcutaneous therapy** to achieve closure of the fistula has been described using ultrasound monitoring and applying pressure over the fistula for 20 to 60 minutes. Success rates of transcutaneous repair attempts are 30% or lower.[106] Another intervention applies a compressive bandage over the site; fistulas resolved in 16 patients

wearing a bandage for 4 to 46 days, with local puncture site ulceration seen in two patients and femoral vein thrombosis in one patient.[107]

Pseudoaneurysms

Pseudoaneurysms can develop after **penetrating trauma** or **arterial catheterization.** The direct communication between the pseudoaneurysm and arterial lumen should be detectable by color flow Doppler imaging. Often, a high-velocity scale (PRF) is needed because blood flow velocities can be very high. The duplex sonographic finding of a "to and fro" sign is typically detected in the communicating channel of the pseudoaneurysm (see Fig. 26-6 and Video 26-3). The "to" component is caused by expansion of the pseudoaneurysm cavity as blood enters during systole. The "fro" component is seen during diastole as the blood stored in the cavity is ejected back into the artery and is more prominent depending on the capacity (size) of the pseudoaneurysm, the compliance of the soft tissues surrounding the pseudoaneurysm, and the pulse pressure between systole and diastole. Pseudoaneurysms can have multiple compartments as well as being solitary.

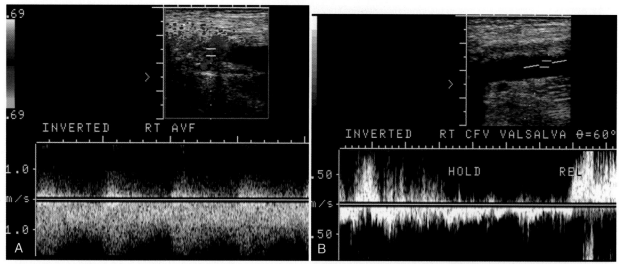

FIGURE 26-25. Waveform in femoral vein suggests small arteriovenous fistula. A, Soft tissue bruit is the only evidence of an AV fistula. **B,** Sampling of the Doppler waveform in the nearby native common femoral vein shows a partial response (decreasing blood flow velocity) during Valsalva maneuver *(HOLD)* and return to normal after maneuver *(REL)*. This suggests that the AV fistula is small.

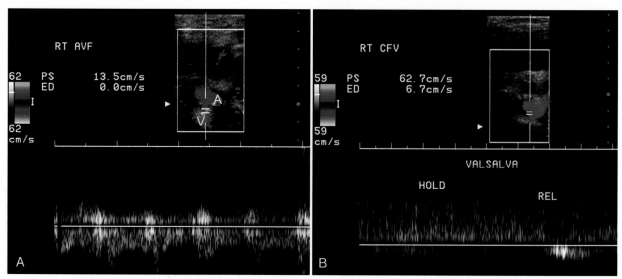

FIGURE 26-26. Waveform in femoral vein suggests large arteriovenous fistula. A, Color Doppler image detects deep-lying AV fistula; *A,* common femoral artery; *V,* common femoral vein. **B,** Poor response (lack of velocity change) to Valsalva maneuver suggests that the AV fistula is relatively large.

Once considered a relative medical emergency, management of pseudoaneurysms has been significantly affected by the wide use of sonography. In a group of patients on bed rest, Kotval et al.[108] found that the natural history of pseudoaneurysms is often benign, documenting spontaneous closure and thrombosis of the patients' pseudoaneurysms. Fellmeth et al.[106] first described the use of **transcutaneous compression therapy** of pseudoaneurysms after catheterization, using a simple protocol of applying pressure with the ultrasound probe over the neck of the pseudoaneurysm. The probe was kept along the long axis of the artery as flow into the cavity was obliterated, using a sequence of up to three transcutaneous pressure applications, each for 20 minutes. Transcutaneous therapy was successful in

more than 80% of cases. These authors emphasized the need for good analgesia, the increased difficulty of repair in anticoagulated patients, and potential complications such as arterial or venous thrombosis. Subsequent reports have confirmed the high success rates of transcutaneous compression,[109,110] even in patients undergoing anticoagulation.[111] Other reports describe greater likelihood of success for smaller pseudoaneurysms and those with longer communicating channels.[112,113] Pseudoaneurysms arising from other arteries (e.g., axillary,[114] brachial[115]) have also been successfully treated with transcutaneous compression therapy.

Ultrasound-guided **thrombin injection** is an alternative therapy that has almost completely replaced ultrasound-guided compression[116-118] (Fig. 26-27; **Videos**

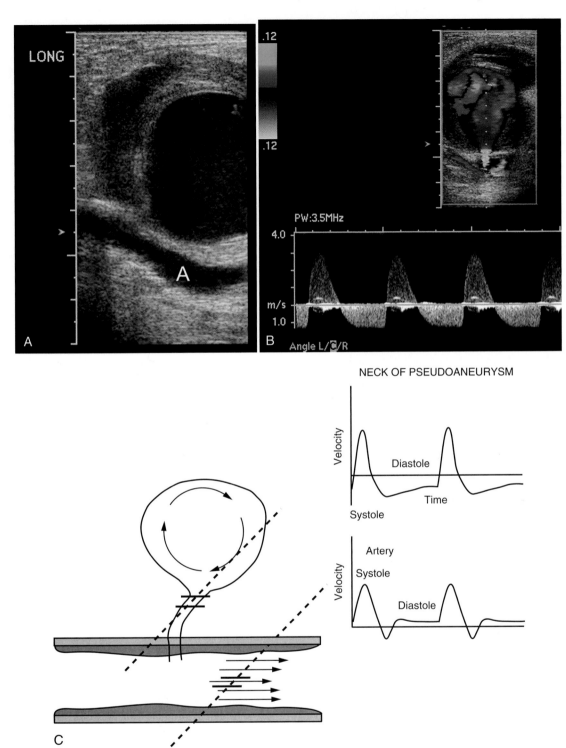

FIGURE 26-27. Femoral artery pseudoaneurysm. A, Longitudinal sonogram of the common femoral artery *(A)* shows a large perivascular fluid collection. **B,** Color Doppler sonogram shows the yin-yang pattern caused by the swirling of blood in the pseudoaneurysm cavity. Note the thin neck of communication between artery and perivascular collection. Spectral Doppler tracing shows the classic to-and-fro waveform of a pseudoaneurysm. **C,** Diagram showing blood flow as it enters the pseudoaneurysm during systole (to) when pressure is higher in the artery than in the cavity. Blood exits during diastole (fro) because the (pressure) energy that has been stored in the soft tissues surrounding the collection is now greater than diastolic pressure.

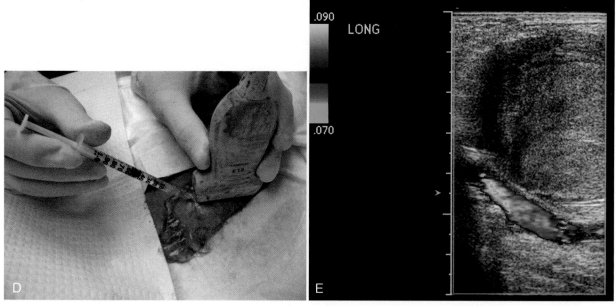

FIGURE 26-27, cont'd. D, Ultrasound-guided injection of thrombin to thrombose the pseudoaneurysm. A 25-gauge needle is attached to the 1-mL syringe containing the thrombin. **E,** Longitudinal color Doppler sonogram 2 minutes after thrombin injection shows that the lumen of the pseudoaneurysm is filled with echoes representing clot and that it has no blood flow on Doppler examination.

 26-5 and **26-6**). After ultrasound placement of a needle in the cavity of the pseudoaneurysm, up to 1000 units of thrombin is injected.[119-121] The basic protocol of using a high concentration of thrombin has been modified to use of a dilute solution of 1000 U in 10 or 20 mL of saline, with slow injection under ultrasound monitoring. The average dose of thrombin can be decreased to 192 U,[122] thereby reducing the risk of inadvertent injection in the native arteries. This technique is more efficient and has higher success rate[121,123] than compression repair.[124] Thrombin injection is also successfully applied to anti-coagulated patients.[125] Even after therapy, however, a communicating channel can persist (Fig. 26-28). Use of compression ultrasound can still be attempted, especially with smaller (<2 cm) pseudoaneurysms.[126]

Ultrasound surveillance of small pseudoaneurysms often shows spontaneous closure. Some suggest using thrombin injection even with the smaller pseudoaneurysms to reduce the cost of repeat visits.[108,127] Wide-neck pseudoaneurysms should likely be managed surgically,[128] given the risk of leakage of thrombin into the native artery and subsequent thrombosis.[129]

Another alternate therapy is the **para-aneurysm saline injection** to compress the pseudoaneurysm neck.[130] Advantages include the lack of allergic reactions, a risk with thrombin. Disadvantages include the need for large volumes of saline and accurate placement of the needle tip.

CLOSURE DEVICES

The incidence of pseudoaneurysms has apparently increased over the last decade. Kresowik et al.[131] reported

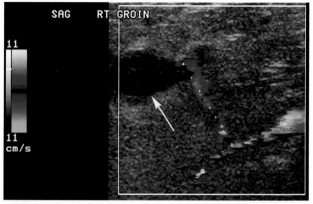

FIGURE 26-28. Persistent neck of pseudoaneurysm. Despite successful thrombosis of a pseudoaneurysm cavity *(arrow)*, the small communicating neck remains open. In most patients this will occlude spontaneously over the next few hours or days.

incidence rates almost 10 times the 0.5% rate reported in the last few decades. Explanations for this increase included use of more aggressive anticoagulation and larger-sized catheters during angioplasty and stent placement procedures. The duration needed to ensure hemostasis after femoral artery catheterization and removal of the catheter remains the most important predictor of subsequent pseudoaneurysm formation.[132]

The use of closure devices to seal the arterial entry site seems to have decreased the overall incidence of pseudoaneurysm formation.[67] When they do occur, however, pseudoaneurysms tend to be large and easily identified on ultrasound.[133] The Angio-Seal device can cause **arterial stenosis** (Fig. 26-29), or even arterial occlusion, from inadvertent displacement of the device's intra-

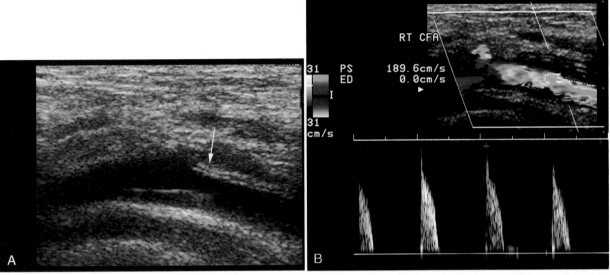

FIGURE 26-29. Arterial closure device causes stenosis of common femoral artery (CFA). A, Closure device *(arrow)* apposed to the near wall of the CFA. **B,** Partial downward displacement of this device causes a stenosis and a corresponding increase in blood flow velocity.

arterial component.[134] The key component of some closure devices is an intravascularly placed collagen "plug," which can migrate and fall into the lumen of the artery.[135] Despite this potential complication, the device can also be used in the radial artery.[136] As new closure devices become available, duplex ultrasound offers the ability to evaluate their efficacy by confirming the lack of AV fistulas and pseudoaneurysm formation.[137]

CONCLUSION

Doppler sonography of the peripheral arterial system is a cost-effective tool for the workup of various vascular pathologies. Doppler sonography is its own "gold standard" for the diagnosis of aneurysms, AV fistulas, and pseudoaneurysms. These diagnostic tasks are facilitated by the use of color Doppler blood flow imaging. Color Doppler and duplex Doppler sonography can be used to survey and study changes in flow dynamics over long segments of the peripheral arteries. The integration of this diagnostic modality as the main follow-up mechanism for patients with peripheral artery bypass operations is now well accepted. With recent concerns about contrast administration in patients with impaired renal function, Doppler sonography offers a cost-effective survey of native arterial disease by detecting lesions and helping triage patients to surgery or other therapeutic options, such as angioplasty or stent placement.

References

1. Polak JF, Karmel MI, Mannick JA, et al. Determination of the extent of lower-extremity peripheral arterial disease with color-assisted duplex sonography: comparison with angiography. AJR Am J Roentgenol 1990;155:1085-1089.

2. De Vries SO, Hunink MG, Polak JF. Summary receiver operating characteristic curves as a technique for meta-analysis of the diagnostic performance of duplex ultrasonography in peripheral arterial disease. Acad Radiol 1996;3:361-369.
3. Favaretto E, Pili C, Amato A, et al. Analysis of agreement between Duplex ultrasound scanning and arteriography in patients with lower limb artery disease. J Cardiovasc Med (Hagerstown) 2007;8:337-341.
4. Hingorani A, Ascher E, Markevich N, et al. Magnetic resonance angiography versus duplex arteriography in patients undergoing lower extremity revascularization: which is the best replacement for contrast arteriography? J Vasc Surg 2004;39:717-722.
5. Leiner T, Kessels AG, Nelemans PJ, et al. Peripheral arterial disease: comparison of color duplex ultrasound and contrast-enhanced MR angiography for diagnosis. Radiology 2005;235:699-708.
6. Visser K, Kuntz KM, Donaldson MC, et al. Pretreatment imaging workup for patients with intermittent claudication: a cost-effectiveness analysis. J Vasc Interv Radiol 2003;14:53-62.

Instrumentation
7. Barber FE, Baker DW, Nation AW, et al. Ultrasonic duplex echo-Doppler scanner. IEEE Trans Biomed Eng 1974;21:109-113.
8. Kasai C, Namekawa K, Koyano A, Omoto R. Real-time two-dimensional blood flow imaging using an autocorrelation technique. IEEE Trans Sonics Ultrasound 1985;S32:458-463.
9. Polak JF, Dobkin GR, O'Leary DH, et al. Internal carotid artery stenosis: accuracy and reproducibility of color-Doppler-assisted duplex imaging. Radiology 1989;173:793-798.

Doppler Flow Patterns
10. Ojha M, Johnston KW, Cobbold RS, Hummel RL. Potential limitations of center-line pulsed Doppler recordings: an in vitro flow visualization study. J Vasc Surg 1989;9:515-520.
11. Reneman RS, Spencer MP. Local Doppler audio spectra in normal and stenosed carotid arteries in man. Ultrasound Med Biol 1979;5:1-11.
12. Spencer MP, Reid JM. Quantitation of carotid stenosis with continuous-wave (C-W) Doppler ultrasound. Stroke 1979;10:326-330.
13. Li JC, Cai S, Jiang YX, et al. Diagnostic criteria for locating acquired arteriovenous fistulas with color Doppler sonography. J Clin Ultrasound 2002;30:336-342.
14. Middleton WD, Erickson S, Melson GL. Perivascular color artifact: pathologic significance and appearance on color Doppler ultrasound images. Radiology 1989;171:647-652.
15. Polak JF, Donaldson MC, Whittemore AD, et al. Pulsatile masses surrounding vascular prostheses: real-time ultrasound color flow imaging. Radiology 1989;170:363-366.

16. Mitchell DG. Color Doppler imaging: principles, limitations, and artifacts. Radiology 1990;177:1-10.

17. Wilkinson DL, Polak JF, Grassi CJ, et al. Pseudoaneurysm of the vertebral artery: appearance on color-flow Doppler sonography. AJR Am J Roentgenol 1988;151:1051-1052.

18. Abu-Yousef MM, Wiese JA, Shamma AR. The "to-and-fro" sign: duplex Doppler evidence of femoral artery pseudoaneurysm. AJR Am J Roentgenol 1988;150:632-634.

19. Bjork L, Leven H. Intra-arterial DSA and duplex-Doppler ultrasonography in detection of vascularized inguinal lymph node. Acta Radiol 1990;31:106-107.

20. Morton MJ, Charboneau JW, Banks PM. Inguinal lymphadenopathy simulating a false aneurysm on color-flow Doppler sonography. AJR Am J Roentgenol 1988;151:115-116.

21. Musto R, Roach MR. Flow studies in glass models of aortic aneurysms. Can J Surg 1980;23:452-455.

Peripheral Artery Disease

22. Newman AB, Siscovick DS, Manolio TA, et al. Ankle-arm index as a marker of atherosclerosis in the Cardiovascular Health Study (CHS Collaborative Research Group). Circulation 1993;88:837-845.

23. Cronenwett JL, Warner KG, Zelenock GB, et al. Intermittent claudication: current results of nonoperative management. Arch Surg 1984;119:430-436.

24. Mills JL. Infrainguinal vein graft surveillance: how and when. Semin Vasc Surg 2001;14:169-176.

25. Teo NB, Mamode N, Murtagh A, et al. Effectiveness of surveillance of infrainguinal grafts. Eur J Surg 2001;167:605-609.

26. Back MR, Novotney M, Roth SM, et al. Utility of duplex surveillance following iliac artery angioplasty and primary stenting. J Endovasc Ther 2001;8:629-637.

27. Dougherty MJ, Calligaro KD, DeLaurentis DA. The natural history of "failing" arterial bypass grafts in a duplex surveillance protocol. Ann Vasc Surg 1998;12:255-259.

28. Katsamouris AN, Giannoukas AD, Tsetis D, et al. Can ultrasound replace arteriography in the management of chronic arterial occlusive disease of the lower limb? Eur J Vasc Endovasc Surg 2001;21:155-159.

29. Koelemay MJ, Legemate DA, de Vos H, et al. Duplex scanning allows selective use of arteriography in the management of patients with severe lower leg arterial disease. J Vasc Surg 2001;34:661-667.

30. Schillinger M, Sabeti S, Dick P, et al. Sustained benefit at 2 years of primary femoropopliteal stenting compared with balloon angioplasty with optional stenting. Circulation 2007;115:2745-2749.

31. Kedora J, Hohmann S, Garrett W, et al. Randomized comparison of percutaneous Viabahn stent grafts vs prosthetic femoral-popliteal bypass in the treatment of superficial femoral arterial occlusive disease. J Vasc Surg 2007;45:10-16; discussion 16.

32. Kohler TR, Nance DR, Cramer MM, et al. Duplex scanning for diagnosis of aortoiliac and femoropopliteal disease: a prospective study. Circulation 1987;76:1074-1080.

33. Gooding GA, Effeney DJ. Ultrasound of femoral artery aneurysms. AJR Am J Roentgenol 1980;134:477-480.

34. MacGowan SW, Saif MF, O'Neill G, et al. Ultrasound examination in the diagnosis of popliteal artery aneurysms. Br J Surg 1985;72:528-529.

35. Shortell CK, DeWeese JA, Ouriel K, Green RM. Popliteal artery aneurysms: a 25-year surgical experience. J Vasc Surg 1991;14:771-776; discussion 776-779.

36. Mehta M, Champagne B, Darling 3rd RC, et al. Outcome of popliteal artery aneurysms after exclusion and bypass: significance of residual patent branches mimicking type II endoleaks. J Vasc Surg 2004;40:886-890.

37. Rajasinghe HA, Tzilinis A, Keller T, et al. Endovascular exclusion of popliteal artery aneurysms with expanded polytetrafluoroethylene stent-grafts: early results. Vasc Endovascular Surg 2006;40:460-466.

38. Antonello M, Frigatti P, Battocchio P, et al. Endovascular treatment of asymptomatic popliteal aneurysms: 8-year concurrent comparison with open repair. J Cardiovasc Surg (Torino) 2007;48:267-274.

39. Jager KA, Phillips DJ, Martin RL, et al. Noninvasive mapping of lower limb arterial lesions. Ultrasound Med Biol 1985;11:515-521.

40. Cossman DV, Ellison JE, Wagner WH, et al. Comparison of contrast arteriography to arterial mapping with color-flow duplex imaging in the lower extremities. J Vasc Surg 1989;10:522-528; discussion 528-529.

41. Fletcher JP, Kershaw LZ, Chan A, Lim J. Noninvasive imaging of the superficial femoral artery using ultrasound duplex scanning. J Cardiovasc Surg (Torino) 1990;31:364-367.

42. Mulligan SA, Matsuda T, Lanzer P, et al. Peripheral arterial occlusive disease: prospective comparison of MR angiography and color duplex ultrasound with conventional angiography. Radiology 1991;178:695-700.

43. Whelan JF, Barry MH, Moir JD. Color flow Doppler ultrasonography: comparison with peripheral arteriography for the investigation of peripheral vascular disease. J Clin Ultrasound 1992;20:369-374.

44. Moneta GL, Yeager RA, Antonovic R, et al. Accuracy of lower extremity arterial duplex mapping. J Vasc Surg 1992;15:275-283; discussion 283-284.

45. Karacagil S, Lofberg AM, Granbo A, et al. Value of duplex scanning in evaluation of crural and foot arteries in limbs with severe lower limb ischaemia: a prospective comparison with angiography. Eur J Vasc Endovasc Surg 1996;12:300-303.

46. Moneta GL, Yeager RA, Lee RW, Porter JM. Noninvasive localization of arterial occlusive disease: a comparison of segmental Doppler pressures and arterial duplex mapping. J Vasc Surg 1993;17:578-582.

47. Koelemay MJ, Legemate DA, de Vos H, et al. Can cruropedal colour duplex scanning and pulse-generated run-off replace angiography in candidates for distal bypass surgery? Eur J Vasc Endovasc Surg 1998;16:13-18.

48. Wain RA, Berdejo GL, Delvalle WN, et al. Can duplex scan arterial mapping replace contrast arteriography as the test of choice before infrainguinal revascularization? J Vasc Surg 1999;29:100-107; discussion 107-109.

49. Grassbaugh JA, Nelson PR, Rzucidlo EM, et al. Blinded comparison of preoperative duplex ultrasound scanning and contrast arteriography for planning revascularization at the level of the tibia. J Vasc Surg 2003;37:1186-1190.

50. Ascher E, Mazzariol F, Hingorani A, et al. The use of duplex ultrasound arterial mapping as an alternative to conventional arteriography for primary and secondary infrapopliteal bypasses. Am J Surg 1999;178:162-165.

51. Mazzariol F, Ascher E, Salles-Cunha SX, et al. Values and limitations of duplex ultrasonography as the sole imaging method of preoperative evaluation for popliteal and infrapopliteal bypasses. Ann Vasc Surg 1999;13:1-10.

52. Canciglia A, Mandolfino T. Infrainguinal endovascular procedures based upon the results of duplex scanning. Int Angiol 2008;27:291-295.

53. Ascher E, Markevich N, Schutzer RW, et al. Duplex arteriography prior to femoral-popliteal reconstruction in claudicants: a proposal for a new shortened protocol. Ann Vasc Surg 2004;18:544-551.

54. Elsman BH, Legemate DA, van der Heijden FH, et al. Impact of ultrasonographic duplex scanning on therapeutic decision making in lower-limb arterial disease. Br J Surg 1995;82:630-633.

55. Collier P, Wilcox G, Brooks D, et al. Improved patient selection for angioplasty utilizing color Doppler imaging. Am J Surg 1990;160:171-174.

56. Edwards JM, Coldwell DM, Goldman ML, Strandness Jr DE. The role of duplex scanning in the selection of patients for transluminal angioplasty. J Vasc Surg 1991;13:69-74.

57. Polak JF, Karmel MI, Meyerovitz MF. Accuracy of color Doppler flow mapping for evaluation of the severity of femoropopliteal arterial disease: a prospective study. J Vasc Interv Radiol 1991;2:471-476; discussion 476-479.

58. Mewissen MW, Kinney EV, Bandyk DF, et al. The role of duplex scanning versus angiography in predicting outcome after balloon angioplasty in the femoropopliteal artery. J Vasc Surg 1992;15:860-865; discussion 865-866.

59. Katzenschlager R, Ahmadi A, Minar E, et al. Femoropopliteal artery: initial and 6-month results of color duplex ultrasound-guided percutaneous transluminal angioplasty. Radiology 1996;199:331-334.

60. Sacks D, Robinson ML, Summers TA, Marinelli DL. The value of duplex sonography after peripheral artery angioplasty in predicting subacute restenosis. AJR Am J Roentgenol 1994;162:179-183.

61. Vroegindeweij D, Tielbeek AV, Buth J, et al. Directional atherectomy versus balloon angioplasty in segmental femoropopliteal artery disease: two-year follow-up with color-flow duplex scanning. J Vasc Surg 1995;21:255-268; discussion 268-269.

62. Tielbeek AV, Rietjens E, Buth J, et al. The value of duplex surveillance after endovascular intervention for femoropopliteal obstructive disease. Eur J Vasc Endovasc Surg 1996;12:145-150.

63. Damaraju S, Cuasay L, Le D, et al. Predictors of primary patency failure in Wallstent self-expanding endovascular prostheses for iliofemoral occlusive disease. Tex Heart Inst J 1997;24:173-178.

64. Spijkerboer AM, Nass PC, de Valois JC, et al. Iliac artery stenoses after percutaneous transluminal angioplasty: follow-up with duplex ultrasonography. J Vasc Surg 1996;23:691-697.

65. Ascher E, Marks NA, Hingorani AP, et al. Duplex-guided endovascular treatment for occlusive and stenotic lesions of the femoral-popliteal arterial segment: a comparative study in the first 253 cases. J Vasc Surg 2006;44:1230-1237; discussion 1237-1238.

66. Schmidt WA, Seifert A, Gromnica-Ihle E, et al. Ultrasound of proximal upper extremity arteries to increase the diagnostic yield in large-vessel giant cell arteritis. Rheumatology (Oxford) 2008;47:96-101.

67. Dangas G, Mehran R, Kokolis S, et al. Vascular complications after percutaneous coronary interventions following hemostasis with manual compression versus arteriotomy closure devices. J Am Coll Cardiol 2001;38:638-641.

68. Kochi K, Sueda T, Orihashi K, Matsuura Y. New noninvasive test alternative to Allen's test: snuff-box technique. J Thorac Cardiovasc Surg 1999;118:756-758.

69. Yokoyama N, Takeshita S, Ochiai M, et al. Direct assessment of palmar circulation before transradial coronary intervention by color Doppler ultrasonography. Am J Cardiol 2000;86:218-221.

Vascular and Perivascular Masses

70. Hedgcock MW, Eisenberg RL, Gooding GA. Complications relating to vascular prosthetic grafts. J Can Assoc Radiol 1980;31:137-142.

71. Nichols WK, Stanton M, Silver D, Keitzer WF. Anastomotic aneurysms following lower extremity revascularization. Surgery 1980;88:366-374.

72. Coughlin BF, Paushter DM. Peripheral pseudoaneurysms: evaluation with duplex ultrasound. Radiology 1988;168:339-342.

73. Helvie MA, Rubin JM, Silver TM, Kresowik TF. The distinction between femoral artery pseudoaneurysms and other causes of groin masses: value of duplex Doppler sonography. AJR Am J Roentgenol 1988;150:1177-1180.

74. Sanchez LA, Suggs WD, Veith FJ, et al. Is surveillance to detect failing polytetrafluoroethylene bypasses worthwhile? Twelve-year experience with ninety-one grafts. J Vasc Surg 1993;18:981-989; discussion 989-990.

Autologous Vein Grafts

75. Bandyk DF, Cato RF, Towne JB. A low flow velocity predicts failure of femoropopliteal and femorotibial bypass grafts. Surgery 1985;98:799-809.

76. Bandyk DF, Jorgensen RA, Towne JB. Intraoperative assessment of in situ saphenous vein arterial grafts using pulsed Doppler spectral analysis. Arch Surg 1986;121:292-299.

77. Mills JL, Harris EJ, Taylor Jr LM, et al. The importance of routine surveillance of distal bypass grafts with duplex scanning: a study of 379 reversed vein grafts. J Vasc Surg 1990;12:379-386; discussion 387-389.

78. Grigg MJ, Nicolaides AN, Wolfe JH. Detection and grading of femorodistal vein graft stenoses: duplex velocity measurements compared with angiography. J Vasc Surg 1988;8:661-666.

79. Mills JL, Wixon CL, James DC, et al. The natural history of intermediate and critical vein graft stenosis: recommendations for continued surveillance or repair. J Vasc Surg 2001;33:273-278; discussion 278-280.

80. Ranke C, Creutzig A, Alexander K. Duplex scanning of the peripheral arteries: correlation of the peak velocity ratio with angiographic diameter reduction. Ultrasound Med Biol 1992;18:433-440.

81. Buth J, Disselhoff B, Sommeling C, Stam L. Color-flow duplex criteria for grading stenosis in infrainguinal vein grafts. J Vasc Surg 1991;14:716-726; discussion 726-728.

82. Londrey GL, Hodgson KJ, Spadone DP, et al. Initial experience with color-flow duplex scanning of infrainguinal bypass grafts. J Vasc Surg 1990;12:284-290.

83. Polak JF, Donaldson MC, Dobkin GR, et al. Early detection of saphenous vein arterial bypass graft stenosis by color-assisted duplex sonography: a prospective study. AJR Am J Roentgenol 1990;154:857-861.

84. Leng GC, Whyman MR, Donnan PT, et al. Accuracy and reproducibility of duplex ultrasonography in grading femoropopliteal stenoses. J Vasc Surg 1993;17:510-517.

85. Mills JL, Bandyk DF, Gahtan V, Esses GE. The origin of infrainguinal vein graft stenosis: a prospective study based on duplex surveillance. J Vasc Surg 1995;21:16-22; discussion 22-25.

86. Ihnat DM, Mills JL, Dawson DL, et al. The correlation of early flow disturbances with the development of infrainguinal graft stenosis: a 10-year study of 341 autogenous vein grafts. J Vasc Surg 1999;30:8-15.

87. Idu MM, Blankenstein JD, de Gier P, et al. Impact of a color-flow duplex surveillance program on infrainguinal vein graft patency: a five-year experience. J Vasc Surg 1993;17:42-52; discussion 52-53.

88. Mofidi R, Kelman J, Berry O, et al. Significance of the early postoperative duplex result in infrainguinal vein bypass surveillance. Eur J Vasc Endovasc Surg 2007;34:327-332.

89. Tinder CN, Chavanpun JP, Bandyk DF, et al. Efficacy of duplex ultrasound surveillance after infrainguinal vein bypass may be enhanced by identification of characteristics predictive of graft stenosis development. J Vasc Surg 2008;48:613-618.

90. Rzucidlo EM, Walsh DB, Powell RJ, et al. Prediction of early graft failure with intraoperative completion duplex ultrasound scan. J Vasc Surg 2002;36:975-981.

91. Matsushita M, Ikezawa T, Banno H. Relationship between the diameter of the vein graft and postoperative ankle brachial pressure index following femoro-popliteal bypass. Int Angiol 2008;27:329-332.

92. Marks N, Ascher E, Hingorani AP. Treatment of failing lower extremity arterial bypasses under ultrasound guidance. Perspect Vasc Surg Endovasc Ther 2007;19:34-39.

93. Bostrom A, Karacagil S, Jonsson ML, et al. Repeat surgery without preoperative angiography in limbs with patent infrainguinal bypass grafts. Vasc Endovascular Surg 2002;36:343-350.

Dialysis Access Grafts and Fistulas

94. Weitzel WF. Preoperative hemodialysis fistula evaluation: angiography, ultrasonography and other studies, are they useful? Contrib Nephrol 2008;161:23-29.

95. Shemesh D, Goldin I, Berelowitz D, et al. Blood flow volume changes in the maturing arteriovenous access for hemodialysis. Ultrasound Med Biol 2007;33:727-733.

96. Mihmanli I, Besirli K, Kurugoglu S, et al. Cephalic vein and hemodialysis fistula: surgeon's observation versus color Doppler ultrasonographic findings. J Ultrasound Med 2001;20:217-222.

97. Singh P, Robbin ML, Lockhart ME, Allon M. Clinically immature arteriovenous hemodialysis fistulas: effect of ultrasound on salvage. Radiology 2008;246:299-305.

98. Tordoir JH, de Bruin HG, Hoeneveld H, et al. Duplex ultrasound scanning in the assessment of arteriovenous fistulas created for hemodialysis access: comparison with digital subtraction angiography. J Vasc Surg 1989;10:122-128.

99. Middleton WD, Picus DD, Marx MV, Melson GL. Color Doppler sonography of hemodialysis vascular access: comparison with angiography. AJR Am J Roentgenol 1989;152:633-639.

100. Dossabhoy NR, Ram SJ, Nassar R, et al. Stenosis surveillance of hemodialysis grafts by duplex ultrasound reduces hospitalizations and cost of care. Semin Dial 2005;18:550-557.

101. Robbin ML, Oser RF, Lee JY, et al. Randomized comparison of ultrasound surveillance and clinical monitoring on arteriovenous graft outcomes. Kidney Int 2006;69:730-735.

102. Dousset V, Grenier N, Douws C, et al. Hemodialysis grafts: color Doppler flow imaging correlated with digital subtraction angiography and functional status. Radiology 1991;181:89-94.

103. Koksoy C, Kuzu A, Erden I, et al. Predictive value of colour Doppler ultrasonography in detecting failure of vascular access grafts. Br J Surg 1995;82:50-52.

104. Villemarette P, Hower J. Evaluation of functional longevity of dialysis access grafts using color flow Doppler imaging. J Vasc Tech 1992;16:183-188.

105. Kanterman RY, Vesely TM, Pilgram TK, et al. Dialysis access grafts: anatomic location of venous stenosis and results of angioplasty. Radiology 1995;195:135-139.

Complications of Invasive Procedures

106. Fellmeth BD, Roberts AC, Bookstein JJ, et al. Postangiographic femoral artery injuries: nonsurgical repair with ultrasound-guided compression. Radiology 1991;178:671-675.

107. Zhou T, Liu ZJ, Zhou SH, et al. Treatment of postcatheterization femoral arteriovenous fistulas with simple prolonged bandaging. Chin Med J (Engl) 2007;120:952-955.

108. Kotval PS, Khoury A, Shah PM, Babu SC. Doppler sonographic demonstration of the progressive spontaneous thrombosis of pseudoaneurysms. J Ultrasound Med 1990;9:185-190.

109. Cox GS, Young JR, Gray BR, et al. Ultrasound-guided compression repair of postcatheterization pseudoaneurysms: results of treatment in one hundred cases. J Vasc Surg 1994;19:683-686.

110. Fellmeth BD, Baron SB, Brown PR, et al. Repair of postcatheterization femoral pseudoaneurysms by color flow ultrasound guided compression. Am Heart J 1992;123:547-551.

111. Dean SM, Olin JW, Piedmonte M, et al. Ultrasound-guided compression closure of postcatheterization pseudoaneurysms during concurrent anticoagulation: a review of seventy-seven patients. J Vasc Surg 1996;23:28-34, discussion 34-35.

112. DiPrete DA, Cronan JJ. Compression ultrasonography: treatment for acute femoral artery pseudoaneurysms in selected cases. J Ultrasound Med 1992;11:489-492.

113. Paulson EK, Hertzberg BS, Paine SS, Carroll BA. Femoral artery pseudoaneurysms: value of color Doppler sonography in predicting which ones will thrombose without treatment. AJR Am J Roentgenol 1992;159:1077-1081.

114. Rooker KT, Morgan CA, Haseman MK, et al. Color flow-guided repair of axillary artery pseudoaneurysm. J Ultrasound Med 1992;11:625-626.

115. Skibo L, Polak JF. Compression repair of a postcatheterization pseudoaneurysm of the brachial artery under sonographic guidance. AJR Am J Roentgenol 1993;160:383-384.

116. Kang SS, Labropoulos N, Mansour MA, Baker WH. Percutaneous ultrasound-guided thrombin injection: a new method for treating postcatheterization femoral pseudoaneurysms. J Vasc Surg 1998;27: 1032-1038.

117. Liau CS, Ho FM, Chen MF, Lee YT. Treatment of iatrogenic femoral artery pseudoaneurysm with percutaneous thrombin injection. J Vasc Surg 1997;26:18-23.

118. Walker TG, Geller SC, Brewster DC. Transcatheter occlusion of a profunda femoral artery pseudoaneurysm using thrombin. AJR Am J Roentgenol 1987;149:185-186.

119. Lennox AF, Griffin MB, Cheshire NJ, et al. Treatment of an iatrogenic femoral artery pseudoaneurysm with percutaneous duplex-guided injection of thrombin. Circulation 1999;100:e39-e41.

120. Mohler 3rd ER, Mitchell ME, Carpenter JP, et al. Therapeutic thrombin injection of pseudoaneurysms: a multicenter experience. Vasc Med 2001;6:241-244.

121. Paulson EK, Sheafor DH, Kliewer MA, et al. Treatment of iatrogenic femoral arterial pseudoaneurysms: comparison of ultrasound-guided thrombin injection with compression repair. Radiology 2000;215:403-408.

122. Reeder SB, Widlus DM, Lazinger M. Low-dose thrombin injection to treat iatrogenic femoral artery pseudoaneurysms. AJR Am J Roentgenol 2001;177:595-598.

123. Paulson EK, Nelson RC, Mayes CE, et al. Sonographically guided thrombin injection of iatrogenic femoral pseudoaneurysms: further experience of a single institution. AJR Am J Roentgenol 2001;177: 309-316.

124. Tisi PV, Callam MJ. Surgery versus non-surgical treatment for femoral pseudoaneurysms. Cochrane Database Syst Rev 2006: CD004981.

125. Brophy DP, Sheiman RG, Amatulle P, Akbari CM. Iatrogenic femoral pseudoaneurysms: thrombin injection after failed ultrasound-guided compression. Radiology 2000;214:278-282.

126. Heis HA, Bani-Hani KE, Elheis MA, et al. Postcatheterization femoral artery pseudoaneurysms: therapeutic options—a case-controlled study. Int J Surg 2008;6:214-219.

127. Stone PA, Aburahma AF, Flaherty SK. Reducing duplex examinations in patients with iatrogenic pseudoaneurysms. J Vasc Surg 2006;43:1211-1215.

128. Luedde M, Krumsdorf U, Zehelein J, et al. Treatment of iatrogenic femoral pseudoaneurysm by ultrasound-guided compression therapy and thrombin injection. Angiology 2007;58:435-439.

129. D'Ayala M, Smith R, Zanieski G, et al. Acute arterial occlusion after ultrasound-guided thrombin injection of a common femoral artery pseudoaneurysm with a wide, short neck. Ann Vasc Surg 2008;22: 473-475.

130. Finkelstein A, Bazan S, Halkin A, et al. Treatment of post-catheterization femoral artery pseudo-aneurysm with para-aneurysmal saline injection. Am J Cardiol 2008;101:1418-1422.

Closure Devices

131. Kresowik TF, Khoury MD, Miller BV, et al. A prospective study of the incidence and natural history of femoral vascular complications after percutaneous transluminal coronary angioplasty. J Vasc Surg 1991;13:328-333; discussion 333-335.

132. Katzenschlager R, Ugurluoglu A, Ahmadi A, et al. Incidence of pseudoaneurysm after diagnostic and therapeutic angiography. Radiology 1995;195:463-436.

133. Sprouse Jr LR, Botta Jr DM, Hamilton Jr IN. The management of peripheral vascular complications associated with the use of percutaneous suture-mediated closure devices. J Vasc Surg 2001;33: 688-693.

134. Kirchhof C, Schickel S, Schmidt-Lucke C, Schmidt-Lucke JA. Local vascular complications after use of the hemostatic puncture closure device Angio-Seal. Vasa 2002;31:101-106.

135. Dregelid E, Jensen G, Daryapeyma A. Complications associated with the Angio-Seal arterial puncture closing device: intra-arterial deployment and occlusion by dissected plaque. J Vasc Surg 2006; 44:1357-1359.

136. Lupattelli T, Clerissi J, Clerici G, et al. The efficacy and safety of closure of brachial access using the Angio-Seal closure device: experience with 161 interventions in diabetic patients with critical limb ischemia. J Vasc Surg 2008;47:782-788.

137. Jaff MR, Hadley G, Hermiller JB, et al. The safety and efficacy of the StarClose Vascular Closure System: the ultrasound substudy of the CLIP study. Catheter Cardiovasc Interv 2006;68:684-689.

CHAPTER 27

The Peripheral Veins

Amy Symons Ettore and Bradley D. Lewis

Chapter Outline

DIAGNOSTIC SCREENING METHODS

The clinical evaluation of the peripheral venous system is notoriously difficult and inaccurate. Accordingly, numerous imaging and nonimaging methods have been developed to aid clinicians with this diagnostic problem. These methods can be divided into three main categories.

Noninvasive, Nonimaging, Physiologic Methods

Noninvasive, nonimaging, physiologic methods rely on altered venous flow hemodynamics to infer indirectly the presence of venous disease. Examples include plethysmographic techniques and continuous wave Doppler sonography. In general, these techniques are highly operator dependent, subjective, and low in specificity and fail to define the anatomy. However, they are inexpensive and may serve useful screening functions in the hands of competent, experienced clinicians.

Invasive Imaging Methods

Conventional venography displays the anatomy of the venous system and is the historical standard of venous imaging against which all other techniques are measured. However, its high relative cost, invasive nature, and low but finite risk of contrast reaction and postveno-graphic phlebitis have led to reluctance to use it. Conventional venography also cannot provide physiologic information.

Noninvasive Imaging Methods

Real-time imaging with B-mode ultrasound, with the addition of duplex Doppler and color flow Doppler sonography, provides objective anatomic information similar to conventional venography, as well as physiologic information of venous hemodynamics. The relatively low cost, noninvasive nature, widespread availability, portability, and proven high accuracy of ultrasound have led to its primary role in the diagnosis of venous thrombosis. Sonography has also assumed a role in the evaluation of venous incompetence, preoperative vein mapping, and evaluation of the venous system for patency before the placement of venous catheters.

The peripheral venous system is amenable to evaluation by other imaging techniques as well. Computed tomography (CT) continues to evolve with the availability of multidetector helical CT. The reduced imaging times of these techniques allow vascular imaging, which is directed primarily at the arterial system (CT angiography, CTA), but which also allows exquisite depiction of the venous system (CT venography, CTV). A strategy of adding pelvic and lower extremity venous evaluation to patients undergoing multidetector CT angiography to rule out pulmonary embolism has been investigated.[1-3] The Prospective Investigation of Pulmonary Embolism

Diagnosis II (PIOPED II) multicenter study demonstrated that the sensitivity and specificity of combined pulmonary CTA and lower extremity ultrasound were equivalent to combined CTA and CTV.[3] Magnetic resonance imaging (MRI) and magnetic resonance angiography and venography (MRA and MRV) also continue to evolve and have shown promise in imaging the peripheral venous system.

With the high accuracy, portability, availability, and low cost of ultrasound, however, as well as potential radiation exposure concerns with repeated CT examinations, it is unlikely that CT or MRI will supplant ultrasound as the primary screening examination. In most centers, **sonography is the primary imaging technique for lower extremity venous evaluation;** MRI and CT serve a secondary role, usually in the search for pelvic, abdominal, or thoracic deep venous thrombosis. Conventional venography is reserved for unusual problem-solving situations.

SONOGRAPHIC TECHNIQUE

Gray-Scale Imaging

The relatively superficial location and lack of overlying bowel and skeletal structures allow high-resolution imaging of most of the peripheral veins, with few exceptions. This superficial location favors the use of higher-frequency transducers. In most patients, a 9-MHz, linear, phased array transducer optimizes gray-scale imaging of the femoropopliteal and subclavian veins. In large patients, or when the iliac veins or the inferior vena cava must be evaluated to determine the superior extent of thrombus, a 6-MHz or 4-MHz transducer may be necessary to obtain adequate depth of penetration. Higher-frequency, 9-MHz or 15-MHz transducers optimize visualization of more superficial veins, such as the great and small saphenous, brachial, and inferior calf veins. As in all areas of sonography, the highest-frequency transducer that gives adequate depth of penetration should be used to optimize spatial resolution.

Doppler Sonography

Doppler sonographic techniques include both quantitative duplex spectral analysis and qualitative color flow Doppler sonography. Both techniques have a pivotal role in identifying and objectively quantifying disease states in the peripheral veins and give sonography the ability to detect altered venous hemodynamics. This combination of anatomic and physiologic information is what makes sonography such a powerful tool in the evaluation of vascular disease. The same linear, phased array transducers are coupled with Doppler ultrasound, which typically has a lower frequency. Many phased array transducers have the ability to steer the Doppler beam at angles independent of the imaging beam. Thus, shallower Doppler angles can be used, decreasing error caused by poor Doppler angles. These considerations are even more critical in arterial evaluation. Color flow Doppler sonography is the simultaneous display of flow information in color superimposed on the gray-scale image. This qualitative information demonstrates relative blood velocity, areas of flow disturbance, and direction of blood flow. Color flow Doppler ultrasound has simplified and decreased examination times in many vascular sonographic studies. This technique permits rapid screening of long segments of the venous system and can provide critical information, especially in segments not amenable to compression, such as the subclavian veins or the leg veins in very large or obese patients. Power Doppler or Doppler Energy allows angle-independent color sonographic imaging and improves detection of very slow flow. It may have some advantages over standard color Doppler imaging in demonstrating small veins or veins with slow flow, such as calf veins.

LOWER EXTREMITY VEINS

Anatomy

The venous system of the lower extremities is divided into superficial and deep systems. In 2002, an international forum of vascular specialists recommended changing the nomenclature of the superficial veins. This newer terminology uses great (vs. greater) saphenous vein and small (vs. lesser) saphenous vein in an effort to achieve a common international standard.[4]

The **superficial system** consists of the great and small saphenous veins and their branches. The **great saphenous vein** arises from the medial aspect of the common femoral vein in the proximal thigh, inferior to the inguinal ligament but superior to the bifurcation of the common femoral vein (Fig. 27-1). The great saphenous vein then extends inferiorly to the level of the foot in the subcutaneous tissues of the medial thigh and leg. The normal great saphenous vein typically is a single vein that is 1 to 3 mm in diameter at the level of the ankle and 3 to 5 mm in diameter at the saphenofemoral junction. These measurements assume importance when this vessel is evaluated before it is harvested for use as an autologous vein graft.

The **small saphenous vein** has a variable insertion into the posterior aspect of the superior or mid popliteal vein. The small saphenous vein then travels in the subcutaneous tissues of the dorsal calf to the ankle. The small saphenous vein is normally 1 to 2 mm in diameter inferiorly and 2 to 4 mm in diameter at its junction with the popliteal vein and is also suitable for autologous graft material in many patients. Both the great and the small

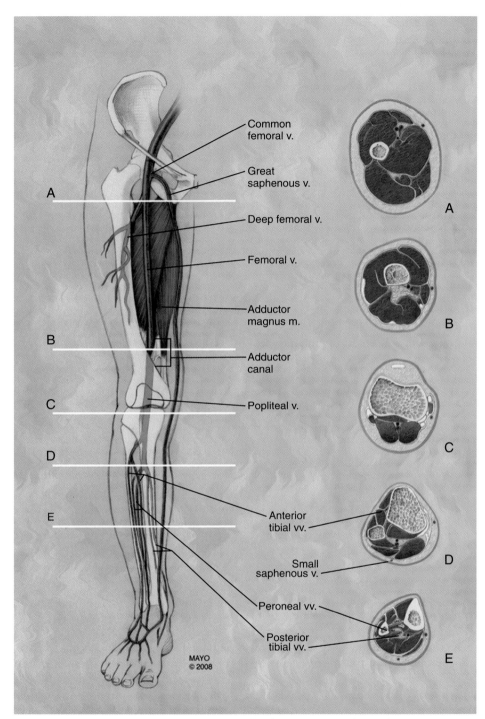

Common femoral v.

Great saphenous v.

Deep femoral v.

Femoral v.

Adductor magnus m.

Adductor canal

Popliteal v.

Anterior tibial vv.

Small saphenous v.

Peroneal vv.

Posterior tibial vv.

A

B

C

D

E

A

B

C

D

E

MAYO
© 2008

FIGURE 27-1. Anatomy of the lower extremity veins.

saphenous vein can become abnormally enlarged or varicose when superficial venous incompetence is present.

Evaluation of the lower extremity veins typically is directed at the **deep system.** The **common femoral vein** begins at the level of the inguinal ligament as the continuation of the external iliac vein and lies just medial and deep to the adjacent common femoral artery (Fig.

27-1). The common femoral vein bifurcates into the deep femoral and femoral veins in the proximal thigh 6 to 8 cm distal to the inguinal ligament and several centimeters distal to the bifurcation of the common femoral artery. The **deep (profunda) femoral vein** continues to lie medial to its respective artery as it travels deep and laterally to drain the musculature of the thigh. The deep femoral vein typically bifurcates extensively, and only the superior portion can be evaluated.

The **femoral vein** extends inferiorly in the fascial space deep to the sartorius muscle, medial to the quadriceps muscle group, and lateral to the adductor muscle group. The femoral vein remains medial to the superficial femoral artery until it passes through the adductor canal in the distal thigh. The adductor canal is formed by a separation in the tendinous insertion of the adductor magnus muscle. This canal is deep in the distal thigh and consists of dense aponeurotic and tendinous tissue. This makes visualization and compression of this segment of the inferior femoral vein difficult in large patients. The femoral vein is the continuation of the common femoral vein and is a deep vein, but its classic descriptive anatomic nomenclature "superficial" is unfortunate. Studies of family practitioners and general internists have shown a poor understanding of the anatomy of the deep venous system of the leg. One study showed that 76% of these physicians would not treat a patient with thrombosis of the femoral vein with anticoagulation because it is a "superficial" vein.[5] This suggests that radiologists should limit the use of the term *superficial femoral vein* and use the more generic term *femoral vein* instead. The **popliteal vein** is the continuation of the femoral vein as it exits the adductor canal in the popliteal space of the posterior distal thigh. At this level, the popliteal vein lies immediately superficial to the popliteal artery as it passes through the popliteal space into the upper calf. Duplication of the femoral and popliteal veins is seen in up to 20% and 35% of patients, respectively. This anatomic variant is important to keep in mind because acute deep venous thrombosis (DVT) in one branch of a paired system can be overlooked during ultrasound examination.

The first deep branches of the popliteal vein are the paired **anterior tibial veins,** which accompany the corresponding artery into the anterior compartment of the calf. These veins continue inferiorly along the anterior surface of the interosseous membrane to the dorsal aspect of the foot. Shortly after the origin of the anterior tibial veins, the tibioperoneal venous trunk bifurcates into paired peroneal and posterior tibial veins. The **peroneal veins** lie adjacent to the peroneal artery and medial to the posterior aspect of the fibula. The fibula is an important landmark for the localization of these veins. The **posterior tibial veins** accompany the artery deep in the musculature of the calf, posterior to the tibia. Visualization of the superior portion of the posterior tibial veins can be difficult in the calves of muscular or obese patients. However, these veins are easier to identify as they pass posterior to the medial malleolus and often can be evaluated in a retrograde manner.

Numerous deep veins drain the musculature of the calf. These gastrocnemial and soleal veins do not have accompanying arteries and vary in size and extent. They are a common site of acute DVT in high-risk or postop-

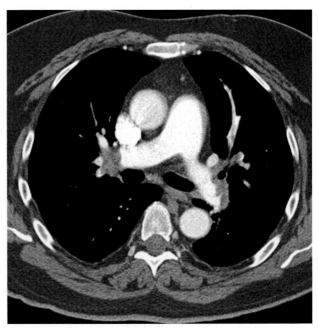

FIGURE 27-2. Acute pulmonary embolism. Contrast-enhanced 64-slice chest CT scan demonstrates acute pulmonary embolism in the pulmonary arteries bilaterally.

erative patients. Their variability often makes complete evaluation and detection of DVT suboptimal.

Deep Venous Thrombosis

The true incidence of acute DVT and its major complication, **pulmonary embolism,** is not known. In the United States the incidence of DVT and pulmonary embolism is 70 cases per 100,000 people. Each year, as many as 600,000 Americans have a pulmonary embolism (Fig. 27-2), and 100,000 die as a result.[6] Approximately 200,000 patients are hospitalized each year for the treatment of acute DVT, although the majority of patients with DVT are asymptomatic.[7,8] The difficulty in making the diagnosis results mainly from the inaccuracy of the clinical evaluation.

The signs and symptoms of acute DVT include **pain, erythema,** and **swelling**. These findings are nonspecific and can be caused by several local or systemic conditions. The presence of a palpable "cord," or thrombosed vein, most often is caused by superficial thrombophlebitis, which is not usually associated with DVT. These factors contribute to a clinical accuracy of approximately 50% for the diagnosis of acute DVT in symptomatic patients.[8-10] In fact, most hospitalized patients at high risk for developing acute venous thrombosis are asymptomatic.[8] In our vascular laboratory, only 11% of patients referred for suspected acute DVT in 2001 had positive findings on sonographic examination.

Because acute DVT is a difficult clinical diagnosis to make and may have severe complications if untreated,

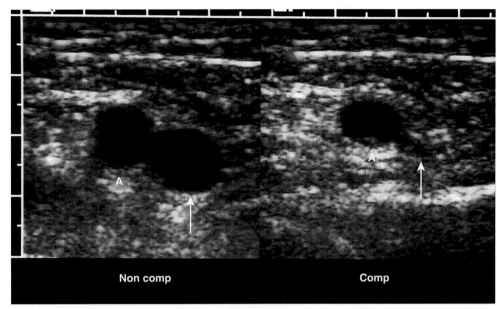

FIGURE 27-3. Normal venous compression sonography. Transverse image of the common femoral artery *(A)* and vein *(arrows)* without compression *(NON COMP)* and with compression *(COMP)* with the sonographic transducer. The normal vein collapses completely with compression.

including pulmonary embolism and postphlebitic syndrome, an accurate noninvasive method is required to establish the diagnosis. Numerous studies and extensive clinical experience have proved that sonography is an ideal technique for this purpose.

Ultrasound Examination

Evaluation of the deep venous system of the leg in patients with suspected acute DVT relies primarily on gray-scale imaging and venous compression in the transverse plane, with color flow Doppler sonography frequently added. A 9-MHz linear array transducer is suitable for most patients. With mild pressure applied to the leg by the transducer, a normal vein will collapse completely, and the vein walls will coapt (Fig. 27-3; **Video 27-1**). The degree of pressure required varies depending on the depth and location of the vein, but it is always less than that required to compress the adjacent artery.

The patient is examined in the supine position. The leg is abducted and rotated externally, with slight flexion of the knee. The standard examination begins with the superior aspect of the common femoral vein immediately distal to the inguinal ligament. The veins are visualized in the transverse plane and compressed in a stepwise fashion every 2 to 3 cm through the level of the inferior aspect of the femoral vein in the adductor canal. The proximal deep femoral vein and great saphenous vein are also visible in this plane and can be evaluated in most patients. The popliteal vein is evaluated best with the patient prone and the foot resting on a pad to maintain slight knee flexion. The left lateral decubitus position also provides adequate visualization. In these positions, transverse compression sonography can be carried out

through the popliteal trifurcation. Many modifications or additions to this standard compression ultrasound examination can be used.

Examination Modifications. The pelvic venous system is less well visualized because of its depth and overlying bowel gas. However, duplex spectral analysis of the common femoral vein while the patient performs the **Valsalva maneuver** can provide indirect evidence of patency of the pelvic veins. In normal subjects, there is constant antegrade venous flow with slight superimposed variation with each respiratory phase. During the Valsalva maneuver, a short period of flow reversal is followed by no flow because of increased intra-abdominal pressure. **With release of the Valsalva maneuver**, there is normally an abrupt increase in forward venous flow, which quickly returns to baseline (Fig. 27-4, *A*). Patients with **complete obstruction of the common or external iliac vein** will have decreased or absent flow and loss of variation with respiration. There is no change in this spectral pattern with the Valsalva maneuver (Fig. 27-4, *B*). **Sluggish venous flow** may also be appreciated with standard real-time imaging because echogenic red blood cell rouleaux become visible (**Videos 27-2 and 27-3**). The Valsalva maneuver provides indirect physiologic evidence of venous patency from the level of the common femoral vein through the inferior vena cava.

False-negative examinations may occur with this indirect portion of the examination because of nonocclusive thrombus in the iliac veins and patients with well-developed pelvic venous collaterals. Both these conditions may result in a normal response to the Valsalva maneuver. In patients with an abnormal Valsalva maneuver or a clinical suspicion of pelvic DVT, dedicated pelvic venous ultrasound can be of value. In thinner patients

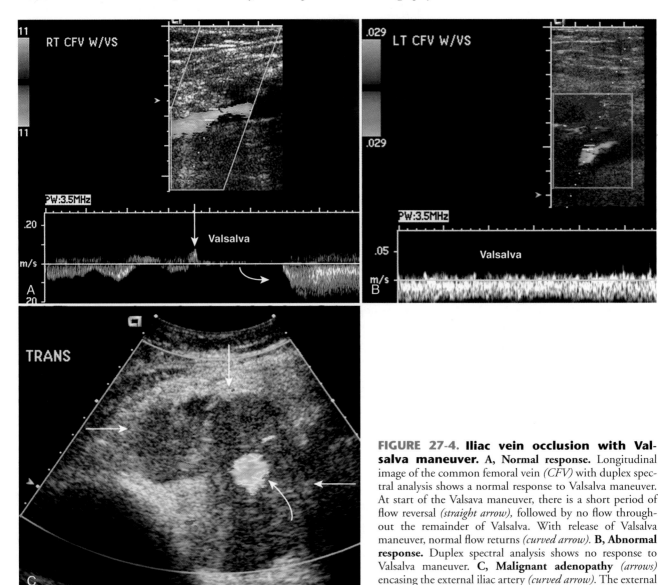

FIGURE 27-4. Iliac vein occlusion with Valsalva maneuver. A, Normal response. Longitudinal image of the common femoral vein *(CFV)* with duplex spectral analysis shows a normal response to Valsalva maneuver. At start of the Valsava maneuver, there is a short period of flow reversal *(straight arrow)*, followed by no flow throughout the remainder of Valsalva. With release of Valsalva maneuver, normal flow returns *(curved arrow)*. **B, Abnormal response.** Duplex spectral analysis shows no response to Valsalva maneuver. **C, Malignant adenopathy** *(arrows)* encasing the external iliac artery *(curved arrow)*. The external iliac vein is occluded by the adenopathy.

the iliac veins may be visualized directly. A 6-MHz or 4-MHz transducer with color flow Doppler capability may provide adequate visualization. Performing the ultrasound examination after an overnight fast decreases bowel gas and can improve visualization of the pelvic veins. If the pelvic veins are poorly seen on ultrasound and there is a high suspicion of pelvic vein DVT or extrinsic compression, contrast-enhanced CT is usually performed as the next diagnostic examination.

The addition of **color flow Doppler sonography** is a useful modification of the standard compression examination. In normal veins, color should fill the vessel lumen from wall to wall with little or no color aliasing outside the vessel lumen. **Venous flow augmentation** by squeezing the calf is often necessary to produce complete color filling. Color flow Doppler ultrasound can help in evaluating venous segments that are poorly seen because of the patient's size or the deep location of

the segment.[11] Color flow Doppler ultrasound may have some advantages over standard compression techniques in patients with chronic DVT as well.[11,12]

Evaluation of the calf veins is an additional modification of the standard examination that is aided by color flow Doppler techniques,[8-10] but the clinical value and cost-effectiveness of this evaluation are controversial. In some medical centers, the lower leg is not evaluated because it is rare for isolated calf DVT to cause significant pulmonary emboli.[13] In other medical centers, the calf is evaluated routinely in patients with localized symptoms below the knee because of the 20% incidence of clot propagation and the increased incidence of postphlebitic syndrome and significant venous insufficiency after untreated calf thrombus. Given these local practice preferences, it is possible to evaluate the tibial and peroneal veins of the calf in many patients, with a sensitivity of 92.5% and specificity of 98.7%.[12,14-16]

In 2007, the Intersocietal Commission for the Accreditation of Vascular Laboratories (ICAVL) altered its standards to require routine examination of the posterior tibial and peroneal veins during all lower extremity ultrasound examinations performed by ICAVL-accredited vascular laboratories.[17]

Patients can be positioned so they are prone, in the left lateral decubitus position, or in the sitting position. Tilting the examination table into a **reverse Trendelenburg position** or having the patient sit improves visualization by distending the calf veins and decreases the indeterminate examination rate. The **paired posterior tibial and peroneal veins** are imaged with the transducer placed over the posterior calf. Compression ultrasound in the transverse plane and color Doppler sonography with augmentation of venous flow can be used to confirm venous patency. The anterior tibial veins can be evaluated from an anterior approach. Since thrombus isolated to these veins is rare, anterior examination is not necessary if the peroneal and posterior tibial veins are well seen and normal.[12] The deep veins of the gastrocnemius and soleus muscles do not have an accompanying artery and have variable anatomy. As such, they are not routinely included in the calf vein examination at most centers. However, compression ultrasound evaluation of the muscular veins has been shown to be an accurate technique with a sensitivity and specificity similar to that of the posterior tibial and peroneal veins.[18] In centers where calf DVT is treated with anticoagulation, the **muscular calf veins** should be included as part of the ultrasound examination.

A proposed modification of the standard examination would greatly abbreviate the examination.[19,20] A limited venous compression sonographic examination of only the common femoral and popliteal veins in **symptomatic patients** would result in significant time savings, with a minimal decrease in sensitivity. It has been argued that this can be justified because of the relative rarity of isolated femoral vein or iliac vein thrombosis, because calf vein thrombosis is clinically less important, and because there will be potential cost savings from a shortened examination. Frederick et al.[21] recently reported a 4.6% incidence of isolated thrombosis of the femoral vein. It is doubtful that the cost savings of limited compression ultrasound will justify this reduced accuracy. Complete compression ultrasound from the superior aspect of the common femoral vein through the inferior aspect of the popliteal vein remains the standard of care.

Sonographic Findings

The gray-scale compression sonographic findings of acute DVT are based on direct visualization of the thrombus and lack of venous compressibility (Fig. 27-5; **Video 27-4**). Visualization of thrombus is variable, depending on the extent, age, and echogenicity of the clot. Unfortunately, some acute thrombi may be anechoic, and gray-scale imaging alone can be misleading. Therefore, the **lack of complete venous compression** is the hallmark finding of DVT. **Venous distention** by thrombus can be seen acutely in patients but is less common as the clot ages and becomes organized. Changes in vein caliber with respiration and the Valsalva maneuver are lost in patients with DVT **(Video 27-5).** This finding is present only in the proximal thigh, so it is not usually helpful below the bifurcation of the common femoral vein.

Color flow Doppler ultrasound depiction of DVT relies on identifying either a **persistent filling defect or thrombus** in the color column of the vessel lumen (Fig. 27-5) or the **absence of flow.** Color flow sonography depicts the degree of venous obstruction and any residual patent lumen. It is most helpful in deep segments of the thigh, pelvic, and calf veins.

Diagnostic Accuracy

The accuracy and clinical utility of sonographic assessment of DVT have been studied extensively. The patient population is of critical importance and should be considered in two broad groups: symptomatic and asymptomatic patients. In **symptomatic** patients, studies comparing venography with compression sonography have shown an average ultrasound sensitivity of 95% and specificity of 98%.[22] Studies of **asymptomatic**, high-risk, or postoperative patients have shown poorer results. Pooled results of six studies showed an average sensitivity of 59% and specificity of 98% in an asymptomatic population.[23] The small size, nonocclusive nature, and higher prevalence of isolated calf thrombi in this group of patients undoubtedly account for the lower sensitivity, because these are more difficult to diagnose with ultrasound than venography. Given these results, the ideal patient for sonographic evaluation has symptoms that extend above the knee.

Chronic Deep Venous Thrombosis

The ability to characterize DVT as acute or chronic is a difficult clinical and imaging problem. Serial studies of patients with acute DVT show that up to 53% have persistent abnormal findings on compression ultrasound done 6 to 24 months later.[24,25] These patients may present with postphlebitic syndrome and have symptoms that mimic those of acute DVT. Anticoagulation therapy is not indicated for these patients. Venography has been the standard imaging method for distinguishing between acute and chronic DVT. However, cost considerations and invasiveness have relegated venography to a problem-solving role in most medical centers.

As an acute thrombus ages, it undergoes fibroelastic organization, with **clot retraction, chronic occlusion, or wall thickening** of the involved segment (Fig. 27-6). These changes lead to poor visualization of the clot

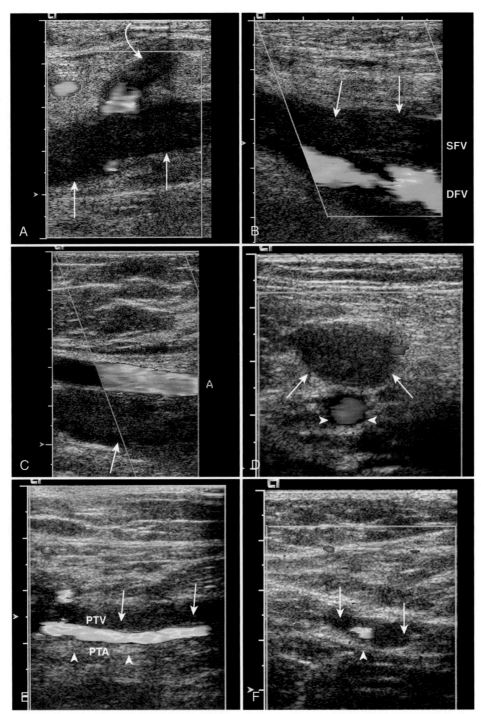

FIGURE 27-5. Acute deep venous thrombosis (DVT): spectrum of appearances. Acute hypoechoic thrombus filling and distending various deep veins of the lower extremity. **A,** Longitudinal image of acute thrombus in the common femoral vein *(straight arrows)* and great saphenous vein *(curved arrow)* at the level of the saphenofemoral junction. **B,** Longitudinal image of acute thrombus *(arrows)* in the superior aspect of the femoral vein *(SFV)*. Note patency of the superior aspect of the deep femoral vein *(DFV)*. **C,** Longitudinal image of the inferior aspect of the femoral vein showing distention by acute occlusive thrombus *(arrow)*. **D,** Transverse compression image of acute DVT in the popliteal vein *(arrows)*, which does not compress. The popliteal artery is patent *(arrowheads)*. **E,** Longitudinal, and **F,** transverse, images of acute DVT in paired posterior tibial veins *(PTV; arrows)*. The posterior tibial artery *(PTA)* is patent *(arrowheads)*.

and incomplete venous compression (**Videos 27-6** and **27-7**). Although compression sonography has a lesser role in the diagnosis of chronic DVT, color flow Doppler ultrasound often is valuable in differentiating acute from chronic DVT. Findings suggestive of chronic DVT with color flow Doppler imaging include irregular echogenic vein walls, thickening of the vein walls due to retracted thrombus, calcified retracted thrombus, decreased diameter of the venous lumina, atretic venous segments, well-developed collateral veins, associated deep venous

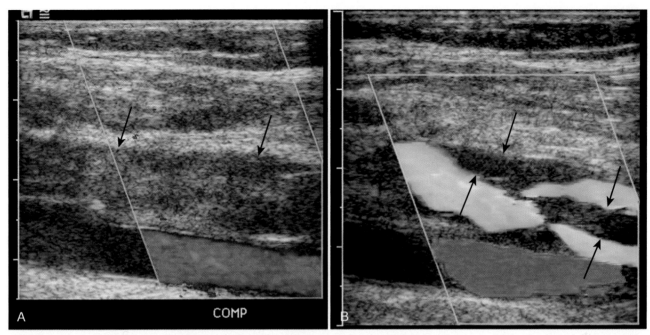

FIGURE 27-6. Evolution of acute to chronic deep venous thrombosis. A, Longitudinal color Doppler image shows acute thrombus in the popliteal vein *(arrows).* **B,** Color Doppler image after 2 months on anticoagulation therapy shows **partial recanalization** of the popliteal vein with **retracted chronic DVT** remaining *(arrows).*

insufficiency, and absence of distended veins containing hypoechoic or isoechoic thrombus (Fig. 27-7). Some centers use ultrasound to follow all patients with acute DVT until complete resolution or until changes of chronic DVT have stabilized. These patients then have baseline ultrasound studies that permit new or superimposed acute DVT to be more readily identified.

Superficial Venous Thrombosis

Superficial venous thrombosis (SVT) or superficial thrombophlebitis refers to thrombus located in the great or small saphenous vein or in superficial varicosities. SVT does not have the same clinical implications as DVT and is usually treated symptomatically with heat and aspirin. The exception is when SVT extends superiorly to within 2 cm of the deep venous system (Fig. 27-8). Generally, patients with SVT will have progression into the deep system in 11% of cases. However, almost all patients with SVT involving the superior aspect of the great saphenous vein will progress if not anticoagulated.[26] Thus, most centers anticoagulate patients with SVT involving the great or small saphenous vein if it extends to within 2 cm of the saphenofemoral or saphenopopliteal junction.

Venous Insufficiency

Pathophysiology

In many patients, deep venous insufficiency is caused by venous valvular damage following DVT. The fibroelastic organization and retraction present in the organizing thrombus secondarily involve any adjacent venous valve. This leads to deep venous insufficiency, which develops in approximately half of patients with acute DVT.[27] With venous insufficiency, there is direct transmission of the hydrostatic pressure of the standing column of fluid in the venous system to the distal leg. Clinically, this leads to leg swelling, chronic skin and pigmentation changes, woody induration, and finally, nonhealing venous stasis ulcers.

Superficial venous insufficiency leads to distended **subcutaneous varicosities** but has a much better prognosis. Perforating veins communicate from the superficial to the deep system and may also become incompetent, typically because of long-standing deep venous insufficiency.

Ultrasound Examination

The examination is performed with the patient in an upright or semi-upright position, with the body's weight supported by the contralateral leg. This positioning is necessary to create the hydrostatic pressure needed to reproduce venous insufficiency. Duplex spectral analysis is obtained at several levels of the deep and superficial venous system during provocative maneuvers. Duplex Doppler tracings in the common femoral vein and superior aspect of the great saphenous vein are obtained during Valsalva maneuver. Several spectral tracings are obtained in the deep and superficial venous systems to the level of the popliteal and saphenous veins at the knee. Reverse augmentation by squeezing the proximal thigh

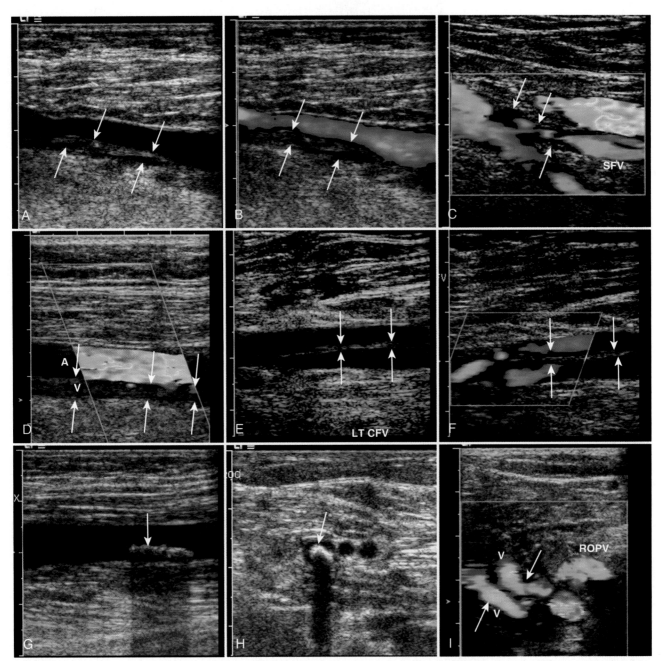

FIGURE 27-7. Chronic deep venous thrombosis. A and **B,** Longitudinal images of chronic retracted thrombus *(arrows)* along femoral vein walls. **C,** Longitudinal image of irregular wall thickening *(arrows)* of the inferior aspect of the common femoral vein and superior aspect of the femoral vein. **D,** Longitudinal image of an atretic, chronically occluded femoral vein *(arrows).* **E** and **F,** Longitudinal images of intraluminal webbing *(arrows)* in the common femoral vein. **G,** Longitudinal image of chronic calcific thrombus in the femoral vein *(arrow).* **H,** Transverse image of chronic calcific thrombus in a muscular vein of the calf *(arrow).* **I,** Transverse image of several collateral veins *(arrows)* near the popliteal vein and artery.

or standard distal venous augmentation by squeezing the calf can be used to assess for insufficiency. Distal augmentation is more reproducible and thus easier for a single examiner to perform.

Sonographic Findings

After brisk distal augmentation, the flow in normal veins is antegrade, with a very short period of flow reversal as returning blood closes the first competent venous valve (Fig. 27-9, *A*). Distal augmentation can be performed manually or with automated devices that inflate every 5 to 10 seconds. The automated devices provide more reproducible calf compression and increase the ease of the examination. **Insufficient veins** have a greater degree of reversed flow for a longer period (Fig. 27-9, *B*; **Videos 27-8** and **27-9**). Quantification schemes have been proposed by evaluating peak flow during venous reflux and

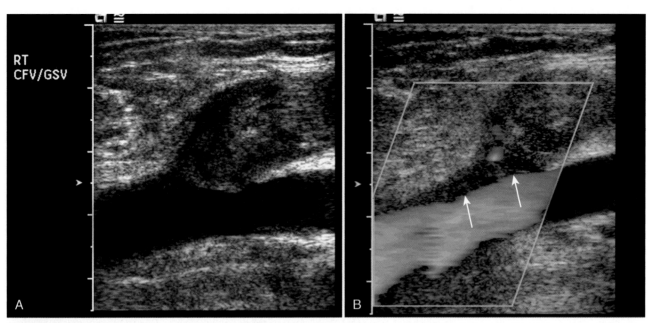

FIGURE 27-8. Superficial venous thrombosis with deep venous extension. A, Longitudinal gray-scale, and **B,** color Doppler, images of the right great saphenous vein and saphenofemoral junction. Echogenic thrombus extends from the great saphenous vein along the anterior wall of the common femoral vein *(arrows)*.

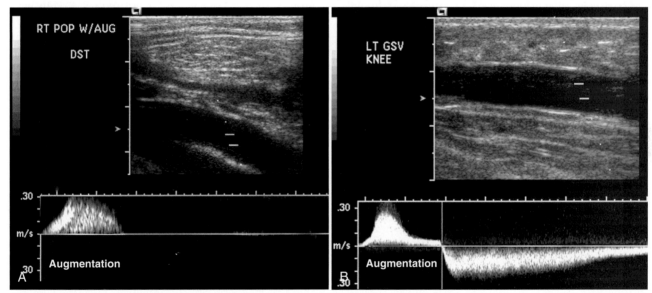

FIGURE 27-9. Venous insufficiency. A, Duplex spectral analysis of the popliteal vein shows a normal waveform with distal augmentation. Note no reversal of flow following distal augmentation. **B,** Duplex spectral analysis of the great saphenous vein shows **prolonged reflux** after distal augmentation, consistent with severe superficial venous insufficiency.

measuring the length of time that reflux occurs. These quantification schemes are somewhat subjective and need to be validated in each vascular laboratory.

Venous Mapping

Vein Harvest for Autologous Grafts

Ultrasound mapping and marking are helpful in many patients before a vein is harvested as autologous graft material for a peripheral arterial bypass graft. Any super-

ficial vein can be used, but the great saphenous vein is the most suitable for graft purposes. The examination is performed with the patient in the supine or reverse Trendelenburg position. A tourniquet or blood pressure cuff that is inflated to 50 mm Hg and placed around the proximal thigh can be used to increase venous distention and to aid in mapping. The great saphenous vein is identified and marked from the level of the saphenofemoral junction to as far inferiorly as possible. All major branch points should also be marked to aid the surgeon. A superficial vein typically needs to be larger than 3 mm

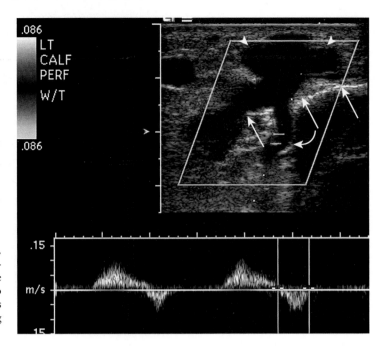

FIGURE 27-10. Incompetent perforating vein.
Gray-scale image and spectral analysis of a dilated perforating vein *(curved arrow)* passing through the fascial plane *(arrows)* between the subcutaneous fat and musculature into a superficial varicosity *(arrowheads).* Duplex spectral analysis shows reversed flow in the perforating vein indicating incompetence.

in diameter, but not varicose, to be suitable graft material. The small saphenous vein, cephalic vein, and basilic vein are secondary choices and can be used if the great saphenous vein has already been harvested or is inadequate.

Insufficient Perforating Vein Marking

Newer surgical techniques of subfascial endoscopic ligation of insufficient perforating veins are being used in some medical centers to treat chronic venous stasis changes and nonhealing venous ulcers. These techniques are aided by accurate localization and marking of insufficient venous perforators. The majority of perforating veins are located below the knee in the medial calf. In an upright patient, distended perforating veins are visible as they pass from the subcutaneous tissues through the superficial fascia into the deep muscles of the calf. These are easily visible on standard gray-scale imaging, and insufficiency can be documented with duplex spectral analysis and flow augmentation (Fig. 27-10). Competent perforating veins are much smaller in caliber and often are difficult or impossible to visualize.

UPPER EXTREMITY VEINS

Anatomy

Venous return from the arm is primarily through the superficial cephalic and basilic veins. The **cephalic vein** travels in the subcutaneous fat of the lateral aspect of the arm. The cephalic vein joins with the deep venous system at the medial aspect of the axillary vein or the lateral aspect of the subclavian vein (Fig. 27-11). The **basilic**

vein is located superficially in the medial aspect of the arm. At the level of the teres major muscle, it joins with the paired deep brachial veins. The **brachial veins** are smaller, deeper, and adjacent to the brachial artery. The level where the brachial and basilic veins join, at the teres major muscle, defines the lateral aspect of the axillary vein. The **axillary vein** is adjacent and superficial to the axillary artery as it passes from the teres major muscle to the first rib through the axilla.

As the axillary vein crosses the first rib, it becomes the lateral portion of the subclavian vein. The **subclavian vein** is inferior and superficial to the adjacent artery as it passes medially deep to the clavicle. The medial portion of the subclavian vein receives the smaller external jugular vein and the larger internal jugular vein in the base of the neck to form the brachiocephalic (innominate) vein. The **internal jugular vein** extends from the jugular foramen in the base of the skull to the confluence with the subclavian vein. The internal jugular vein travels in the carotid sheath and is superficial and lateral to the common carotid artery in the anterior neck. The left and right internal jugular veins are often unequal in size. The **brachiocephalic vein** is formed by the confluence of the subclavian and internal jugular veins. The right brachiocephalic vein travels along the superficial aspect of the superior right mediastinum. The left brachiocephalic vein is longer and passes from the left superior mediastinum to the right, just deep to the sternum. The right and left brachiocephalic veins join to form the superior vena cava.

Clinical Background

The most common indication for ultrasound evaluation of upper extremity veins is to identify venous thrombo-

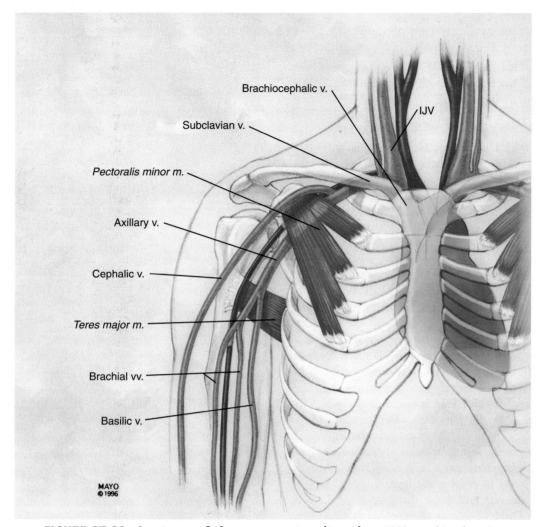

FIGURE 27-11. **Anatomy of the upper extremity veins.** *IJV,* Internal jugular vein.

sis. The cause and clinical significance of acute DVT of the upper extremity differ from those of acute DVT of the lower extremity. Most cases of arm DVT are thought to be caused by the presence of a **central venous catheter or pacemaker lead (Video 27-10).** Of patients with central venous catheters, 26% to 67% develop thrombosis, although the majority are asymptomatic.[28,29] **Radiation therapy, effort-induced thrombosis,** and **malignant obstruction** are causes of venous obstruction that are more common in the thorax and arm than in the leg. Although the cause of upper extremity DVT differs from that of the lower extremity, the pathophysiology of its evolution is similar.

The sequelae of upper extremity thrombosis are less severe than those of lower extremity thrombosis. Only 10% to 12% of patients with arm DVT develop pulmonary emboli, and the majority of these are insignificant[30-32] **(Video 27-11).** The development and manifestations of venous stasis and venous insufficiency caused by DVT in the arm are less common and less severe than in the leg. Chronic swelling, skin changes,

and nonhealing venous ulcers are rare in the arm because of two major factors. First, multiple extensive collateral venous pathways usually develop in the arm and upper thorax after an episode of thrombosis or venous obstruction. Second, the arm veins are not exposed to the high hydrostatic pressure of leg veins. Chronic occlusion related to intravenous catheter use and venous thrombosis has made obtaining suitable central venous access difficult in many hospitalized and chronically ill patients. Sonography is ideal for identifying suitable sites for venous access. In difficult cases, direct real-time ultrasonic guidance can be used for placement of venous catheters.

Venous Thrombosis

Ultrasound Examination

Evaluation of the venous system of the upper thorax and arm typically extends from the superior aspect of the brachiocephalic veins through the axillary or brachial veins. The internal jugular veins are also studied. The patient is positioned supine, with the arm to be examined slightly abducted and rotated externally. The patient's head is turned slightly to the opposite side. The highest-frequency transducer that still provides adequate depth of penetration is used. Typically, a 9-MHz linear array transducer is used for the internal jugular vein and the arm veins through the axillary vein. A 6-MHz transducer with color Doppler ultrasound capability is often necessary to visualize the subclavian vein.

Evaluation of the venous system of the upper thorax and arm presents several technical challenges different from the lower extremity. First, the overlying skeletal structures and the lung make direct visualization and examination of the inferior aspects of the brachiocephalic veins and the superior vena cava impossible. Second, the clavicle precludes compression ultrasound of the subclavian vein. Third, the typical development of large venous collateral pathways in patients with venous obstruction can be confusing or may lead to false-negative sonographic results if they are not recognized as collateral pathways. For these reasons, color flow Doppler sonography, attention to detail, and knowledge of the normal anatomic relationships are crucial.

The **internal jugular vein** is examined initially with compression sonography in the transverse plane and is followed inferiorly to its junction with the subclavian and brachiocephalic veins. An inferiorly angled, coronal, supraclavicular approach with color flow Doppler sonography is necessary to evaluate the superior portion of the brachiocephalic vein and the medial portion of the subclavian vein. Duplex Doppler sonographic analysis of the inferior internal jugular vein, superior brachiocephalic vein, and medial subclavian vein is helpful to assess transmitted cardiac pulsatility and respiratory phasicity. Due to the proximity to the heart, duplex Doppler spectral tracings in these sites will show greater transmitted pulsatility than in the leg veins. Loss of this pulsatility may be caused by a more central venous obstruction (Fig. 27-12). Comparison of these Doppler ultrasound waveforms with those from the contralateral arm is often helpful to confirm the presence or absence of venous obstruction. Response to Valsalva maneuver or a brisk inspiratory sniff can also be observed and may help evaluate venous patency. When a normal patient sniffs, the internal jugular vein or subclavian vein will decrease in diameter, and spectral analysis will show an increase in blood velocity. Patients with central brachiocephalic vein or superior vena cava obstruction lose this response (Fig. 27-13).

The **subclavian vein** is difficult to visualize completely. A coronal, supraclavicular, inferiorly angled approach is used medially, and a coronal, infraclavicular, superiorly angled approach is used laterally. The venous segment deep to the clavicle often is imaged incompletely. Because of the overlying clavicle, color flow Doppler sonography is necessary to confirm complete

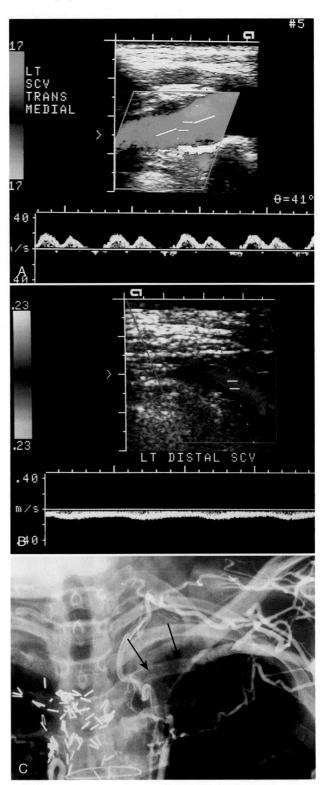

FIGURE 27-12. Comparison of normal and obstructed subclavian veins. A, Normal subclavian vein *(SCV)* with color flow Doppler sonography and spectral analysis. There is complete color filling and normal transmitted cardiac pulsations. **B, Loss of the transmitted cardiac pulsations.** Color flow Doppler and spectral analysis in another patient shows the subclavian vein is patent but has reversed flow direction. **C, Subclavian vein occlusion** *(arrows)* with numerous collateral vessels on venogram.

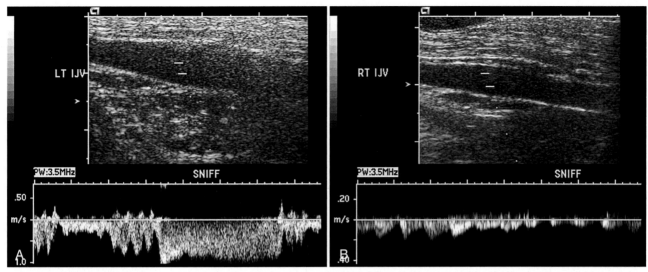

FIGURE 27-13. Normal and abnormal response to sniff test. A, Duplex spectral analysis of the internal jugular vein shows an increase in blood flow velocity with inspiratory sniff, a **normal response suggestive of central venous patency. B,** Duplex spectral analysis of the contralateral internal jugular vein shows no increase in blood flow velocity with inspiratory sniff, an **abnormal response suggestive of brachiocephalic or superior vena cava obstruction.**

venous patency. The examiner should also confirm the normal inferior superficial relationship of the vein with the adjacent artery. This will avoid the pitfall of confusing well-developed collateral vessels for a patent subclavian vein in patients with chronic venous occlusion. The axillary and upper arm veins can also be evaluated with transverse compression or color flow Doppler ultrasound. The extent of the examination into the arm depends on the clinical indication, but typically it is continued through the bifurcation of the axillary vein into the brachial veins.

Sonographic Findings

The normal and abnormal findings in the upper extremity veins mirror those seen in the lower extremity veins. Patients with venous thrombosis have incomplete collapse of the vein with compression. Thrombus or an intraluminal filling defect is visible in the color column of the vein with color flow Doppler ultrasound (Fig. 27-14). Absent or decreased cardiac pulsatility with duplex spectral analysis and abnormal response to an inspiratory sniff are also helpful. Abundant, well-developed collateral vessels are common because of long-standing venous occlusion.

Diagnostic Accuracy

The accuracy of ultrasound versus venography in patients with acute DVT of the upper extremity has not been studied as extensively as in the lower extremity. The available literature shows sensitivity ranging from 78% to 100% and specificity of 92% to 100%.[33-35] The lower accuracy in the upper extremity compared with the lower

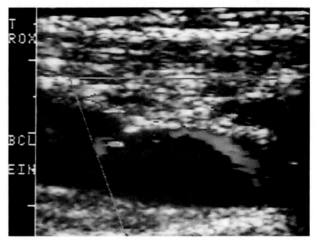

FIGURE 27-14. Acute subclavian vein thrombosis. Color flow Doppler sonography of the subclavian vein shows extensive hypoechoic thrombus with minimal peripheral flow remaining.

extremity is a result of the greater number of technical challenges facing the examiner.

References

Diagnostic Screening Methods
1. Hunsaker AR, Zou KH, Poh AC, et al. Routine pelvic and lower extremity CT venography in patients undergoing pulmonary CT angiography. AJR Am J Roentgenol 2008;190:322-326.
2. Kalva SP, Jagannathan JP, Hahn PF, Wicky ST. Venous thromboembolism: indirect CT venography during CT pulmonary angiography—should the pelvis be imaged? Radiology 2008;246:605-611.
3. Goodman LR, Stein PD, Matta F, et al. CT venography and compression sonography are diagnostically equivalent: data from PIOPED II. AJR Am J Roentgenol 2007;189:1071-1076.

Lower Extremity Veins

4. Caggiati A, Bergan JJ, Gloviczki P, et al. Nomenclature of the veins of the lower limbs: an international interdisciplinary consensus statement. J Vasc Surg 2002;36:416-422.

5. Bundens WP, Bergan JJ, Halasz NA, et al. The superficial femoral vein: a potentially lethal misnomer. JAMA 1995;274:1296-1298.

6. Anderson Jr FA, Wheeler HB, Goldberg RJ, et al. A population-based perspective of the hospital incidence and case-fatality rates of deep vein thrombosis and pulmonary embolism. The Worcester DVT Study. Arch Intern Med 1991;151:933-938.

7. Sandler DA, Martin JF. Autopsy-proven pulmonary embolism in hospital patients: are we detecting enough deep vein thrombosis? J R Soc Med 1989;82:203-205.

8. Salzman EW. Venous thrombosis made easy. N Engl J Med 1986; 314:847-848.

9. Haeger K. Problems of acute deep venous thrombosis. I. The interpretation of signs and symptoms. Angiology 1969;20:219-223.

10. Barnes RW, Wu KK, Hoak JC. Fallibility of the clinical diagnosis of venous thrombosis. JAMA 1975;234:605-607.

11. Lewis BD, James EM, Welch TJ, et al. Diagnosis of acute deep venous thrombosis of the lower extremities: prospective evaluation of color Doppler flow imaging versus venography. Radiology 1994;192:651-655.

12. Rose SC, Zwiebel WJ, Nelson BD, et al. Symptomatic lower extremity deep venous thrombosis: accuracy, limitations, and role of color duplex flow imaging in diagnosis. Radiology 1990;175:639-644.

13. Gottlieb RH, Widjaja J, Mehra S, Robinette WB. Clinically important pulmonary emboli: does calf vein ultrasound alter outcomes? Radiology 1999;211:25-29.

14. Atri M, Herba MJ, Reinhold C, et al. Accuracy of sonography in the evaluation of calf deep vein thrombosis in both postoperative surveillance and symptomatic patients. AJR Am J Roentgenol 1996;166:1361-1367.

15. Polak JF, Culter SS, O'Leary DH. Deep veins of the calf: assessment with color Doppler flow imaging. Radiology 1989;171:481-485.

16. Gottlieb RH, Widjaja J, Tian L, et al. Calf sonography for detecting deep venous thrombosis in symptomatic patients: experience and review of the literature. J Clin Ultrasound 1999;27:415-420.

17. Intersocietal Commission for the Accreditation of Vascular Laboratories. ICAVL standards for accreditation in noninvasive vascular testing. II. Vascular laboratory operations–peripheral venous testing. http://www.icavl.org/icavl/pdfs/venous2007.pdf. Accessed October 2008.

18. Krunes U, Teubner K, Knipp H, Holzapfel R. Thrombosis of the muscular calf veins–reference to a syndrome which receives little attention. Vasa 1998;27:172-175.

19. Pezzullo JA, Perkins AB, Cronan JJ. Symptomatic deep vein thrombosis: diagnosis with limited compression ultrasound. Radiology 1996;198:67-70.

20. Bernardi E, Camporese G, Buller HR, et al. Serial 2-point ultrasonography plus D-dimer vs whole-leg color-coded Doppler ultrasonography for diagnosing suspected symptomatic deep vein thrombosis: a randomized controlled trial. JAMA 2008;300:1653-1659.

21. Frederick MG, Hertzberg BS, Kliewer MA, et al. Can the ultrasound examination for lower extremity deep venous thrombosis be abbreviated? A prospective study of 755 examinations. Radiology 1996;199:45-47.

22. Cronan JJ. Venous thromboembolic disease: the role of ultrasound. Radiology 1993;186:619-630.

23. Weinmann EE, Salzman EW. Deep-vein thrombosis. N Engl J Med 1994;331:1630-1641.

24. Cronan JJ, Leen V. Recurrent deep venous thrombosis: limitations of ultrasound. Radiology 1989;170:739-742.

25. Baxter GM, Duffy P, MacKechnie S. Colour Doppler ultrasound of the post-phlebitic limb: sounding a cautionary note. Clin Radiol 1991;43:301-304.

26. Chengelis DL, Bendick PJ, Glover JL, et al. Progression of superficial venous thrombosis to deep vein thrombosis. J Vasc Surg 1996;24:745-749.

27. Van Haarst EP, Liasis N, van Ramshorst B, Moll FL. The development of valvular incompetence after deep vein thrombosis: a 7-year follow-up study with duplex scanning. Eur J Vasc Endovasc Surg 1996;12:295-299.

Upper Extremity Veins

28. Bonnet F, Loriferne JF, Texier JP, et al. Evaluation of Doppler examination for diagnosis of catheter-related deep vein thrombosis. Intensive Care Med 1989;15:238-240.

29. McDonough JJ, Altemeier WA. Subclavian venous thrombosis secondary to indwelling catheters. Surg Gynecol Obstet 1971;133:397-400.

30. Horattas MC, Wright DJ, Fenton AH, et al. Changing concepts of deep venous thrombosis of the upper extremity: report of a series and review of the literature. Surgery 1988;104:561-567.

31. Becker DM, Philbrick JT, Walker FB. Axillary and subclavian venous thrombosis: prognosis and treatment. Arch Intern Med 1991;151:1934-1943.

32. Monreal M, Lafoz E, Ruiz J, et al. Upper-extremity deep venous thrombosis and pulmonary embolism: a prospective study. Chest 1991;99:280-283.

33. Knudson GJ, Wiedmeyer DA, Erickson SJ, et al. Color Doppler sonographic imaging in the assessment of upper-extremity deep venous thrombosis. AJR Am J Roentgenol 1990;154:399-403.

34. Baxter GM, Kincaid W, Jeffrey RF, et al. Comparison of colour Doppler ultrasound with venography in the diagnosis of axillary and subclavian vein thrombosis. Br J Radiol 1991;64:777-781.

35. Morton MJ, James EM, Welch TJ, et al. Duplex and color Doppler imaging in the evaluation of upper extremity and thoracic inlet deep venous thrombosis (exhibit). AJR Am J Roentgenol 1994;162(Suppl):192.

Index

Page numbers followed by *f* indicate figures; *t*, tables; *b*,
boxes.

Fetus (Continued)
  movements of, musculoskeletal development and, 1390
  musculoskeletal system of, 1389-1423. See also Musculoskeletal system, fetal.
  neck of. See Neck, fetal.
  normal sonographic appearance of, 1043f
  orbits of, 1172-1178. See also Orbits, fetal.
  pancreas of, 1334
  presentation of, determination of, 1045-1046, 1047f
  reduction of, in multifetal pregnancy, 1160-1161, 1549
    complications of, 1549
    indications for, 1549
    technique for, 1549
  situs of, determination of, 1045-1046, 1047f
  small bowel of, 1334-1338, 1335f-1336f
  small-for-gestational age, 1466, 1473-1474
  spine of, 1245-1272. See also Spine, fetal.
  spleen of, 1334
  stomach of, 1327-1329, 1328f, 1329b, 1330f-1331f, 1330t
  surgery on, ultrasound-guided, 1551-1552, 1552f
  surveillance of, 1472-1498. See also Surveillance, fetal.
  transfusion for, 1549
  urinary tract of, 1353-1357. See also Urinary tract, fetal.
  urogenital tract of, 1353-1388
  weight of
    assessment of, in relation to gestational age, 1463-1464, 1463t, 1464f
    estimation of, 1462-1463
      versus gestational age, 1464, 1464f
      percentile of, versus gestational age, 1464, 1464f
      recommended approach to, 1463, 1463t
Fibrillar echotexture, of tendons, 907, 908f
Fibrinous peritonitis, 528f
Fibrochondrogenesis, 1407
Fibroelastosis, endocardial, fetal, 1318-1319, 1320f
  heart block and, 1438
Fibroids, uterine, 556-558, 556b, 557f-558f, 558b
  in first trimester, 1114
Fibrointimal hyperplasia, venous bypass graft stenosis from, 1011-1013
Fibrolamellar carcinoma, 129
Fibrolipomas, of filum terminale, pediatric, 1745, 1748f-1749f
Fibroma(s)
  bladder, pediatric, 1969-1970
  cardiac, fetal, 1318
  gastrointestinal, endosonographic identification of, 305
  ovarian, 591-592, 592f
  simulating anterior abdominal wall hernias, 522, 522f
Fibromatosis, ovarian edema differentiated from, 1932-1933
Fibromatosis coli, 1721-1725, 1726f
  pediatric, 2002-2003, 2003f
Fibromuscular dysplasia
  carotid flow disturbances in, 962
  of internal carotid artery, 979-981, 981f
  renal artery stenosis and, 461, 463f
Fibronectin, fetal, in prediction of spontaneous preterm birth, 1533
Fibrosarcoma(s), simulating anterior abdominal wall tumors, 522, 522f
Fibrothorax, sonographic appearance of, 1769
Fibrous pseudotumor, epididymal, 863f, 864

Fibrous sheaths, 902-903
Field of view, in obstetric sonography, 1062
Filar cyst, in newborn, 1735, 1738f
Filariasis, 339
Filling defect, persistent, in deep venous thrombosis, 1029
Filum terminale, in pediatric spine, 1735, 1737f
  fibrolipomas of, 1745, 1748f-1749f
  tight, 1745, 1749f
Finger(s)
  syndactyly of, in triploidy, 1138f
  tendons of, normal sonographic appearance of, 908-910, 913f-915f
Finite amplitude distortion, in soft tissue, 37, 38f
Finnish nephrosis, hyperechogenic kidneys in, 1366-1367
Fistula(s)
  arteriovenous. See Arteriovenous (AV) fistulas.
  bladder, 342, 343f
  cholecystoenteric, 183
  choledochoduodenal, 183
  in Crohn's disease, 278-280, 281f-282f
  dialysis, 1013-1014, 1014f
  dorsal enteric, pediatric, 1750
  in imperforate anus, 1905
  perianal, perianal inflammatory disease in, 310
  tracheoesophageal, fetal
    congenital high airway obstruction with, 1281-1282
    in VACTERL sequence, 1329
  vesicocutaneous, 342
  vesicoenteric, 342
  vesicoureteral, 342
  vesicovaginal, 342
Fistulous communications, complicating invasive peripheral artery procedures, 1014-1015, 1016f
Fitz-Hugh-Curtis syndrome, pediatric, 1942
Flash artifact, 57
Flexor digitorum profundus muscle, tendons of, normal sonographic appearance of, 907-908
Flexor digitorum superficialis muscle, tendons of, normal sonographic appearance of, 907-908
Flexor hallucis longus tendon, injection of, 941, 941f
Flexor muscles, of elbow, 907
Flexor tendons, of fingers, 913f, 915f
Fluid, in neonatal/infant brain imaging, 1559
Fluorescence in situ hybridization, for amniotic fluid analysis, 1543
Fluorescent in situ hybridization, in hydrops diagnosis, 1448
Fluoroscopic guidance, for drainage catheter placement, 626
Focal depth, in obstetric sonography, 1062
Focal nodular hyperplasia, 118-119, 119f-121f
  characterization of, with microbubble contrast agents, 112f, 113, 114t
  hepatic, pediatric, 1814
Focused abdominal sonography for trauma (FAST), 527
  in children, 1841
Folic acid, in spina bifida prevention, 1253-1255
Follicular adenomas, thyroid, pediatric, 1709-1710, 1710f
Follicular carcinoma, of thyroid, 709f, 720, 721b, 725f
  pediatric, 1710-1711

Follicular cysts, 573, 575-576
  pediatric, 1930
Fontanelle
  anterior
    compression of, in hydrocephalus, resistive index and, 1647-1648, 1648f
    neonatal/infant brain imaging through, 1559, 1560f
      coronal planes in, 1560f
        Doppler, 1637, 1639f
      Doppler, 1637, 1638f
      sagittal planes in, 1564f
  mastoid, neonatal/infant brain imaging through, 1559, 1565f, 1566-1567, 1567f
    Doppler, 1638, 1640f
  posterior, neonatal/infant brain imaging through, 1559, 1564-1566, 1565f-1566f
  posterolateral, neonatal/infant brain imaging through, Doppler, 1638, 1640f
Foot (feet)
  fetal
    deformities of, 1415-1420
    length of, measurement of, 1393, 1393f
    rocker-bottom, 1418f, 1420
    in skeletal dysplasias, 1396
  injection of, 938
    superficial peritendinous and periarticular, 939-941, 942f
  pediatric, congenital anomalies of, 2001-2002
  tendons of, normal sonographic appearance of, 909f, 916-918
Foramen magnum approach
  for Doppler imaging of neonatal/infant brain, 1638, 1640f
  for transcranial Doppler, 1655-1657, 1658f
Foramen of Bochdalek, diaphragmatic hernia through, 1285
Foramen of Magendie, neonatal/infant, in mastoid fontanelle imaging, 1566-1567
Foramen ovale, 1297, 1298f, 1305, 1305f
  in fetal circulation, 1472
  sonographic appearance of, 1305-1306, 1307f
Foraminal flap, sonographic appearance of, 1302f, 1307f
Foregut cysts, pediatric, 1713
Foregut malformations, bronchopulmonary, pediatric, 1791, 1793f
Forehead, fetal, abnormalities of, 1170f, 1172, 1172b, 1173f-1174f
Foreign body(ies)
  atelectasis from, 1783f
  in gastrointestinal tract, 304
  musculoskeletal, 2000, 2000f
  pediatric vaginitis from, 1942
Fornices
  fetal, normal sonographic appearance of, 1199
  in lobar holoprosencephaly, 1218
Fournier's gangrene, 869
  pediatric, 1955
Fracture(s)
  fetal, in skeletal dysplasias, 1392f, 1395
  pediatric
    metaphyseal, 1999-2000
    rib, 1798
Frame rate
  in obstetric sonography, 1062
  in renal artery duplex Doppler sonography, 463
Fraser syndrome, laryngeal atresia in, 1281
Fraunhofer zone, of beam, 8-9